Anesthesia and Co-Existing Disease

Anesthesia and Co-Existing Disease

FOURTH EDITION

Robert K. Stoelting, M.D.
Professor and Chair
Department of Anesthesia
Indiana University School of Medicine
Indianapolis, Indiana

Stephen F. Dierdorf, M.D.
Professor
Department of Anesthesia
Indiana University School of Medicine
Indianapolis, Indiana

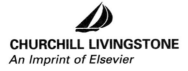

CHURCHILL LIVINGSTONE
An Imprint of Elsevier

CHURCHILL LIVINGSTONE
An Imprint of Elsevier

The Curtis Center
Independence Square West
Philadelphia, Pennsylvania 19106

Library of Congress Cataloging-in-Publication Data

Anesthesia and co-existing disease / [edited by] Robert K. Stoelting, Stephen F. Dierdorf—4th ed.

p. ; cm.

Includes bibliographical references and index.
ISBN 0–443–06604–3

1. Anesthesia—Complications.   2. Therapeutics, Surgical.   I. Stoelting, Robert K.
II. Dierdorf, Stephen F.
[DNLM: 1. Anesthesia—adverse effects.   2. Anesthetics. WO 245 A578 2002]

RD87 .A53 2002

617.9′6041—dc21   2001047235

ANESTHESIA AND CO-EXISTING DISEASE   ISBN 0–443–06604–3

Copyright © 2002, 1993, 1988, 1983 by Churchill Livingstone

Printed in the United States of America.

Last digit is the print number: 9   8   7   6   5   4   3

Preface to the Fourth Edition

This fourth edition of *Anesthesia and Co-Existing Disease* is published nearly 10 years after the third edition appeared in 1993. As with the previous three editions, the Editor's goal is to provide readers with current and concise descriptions of the pathophysiology of diseases, and the impact, if any, on the management of anesthesia. Common diseases such as diabetes mellitus, ischemic heart disease, and asthma receive detailed discussions whereas rare diseases are discussed based on unique features that these diseases might present in the perioperative period that could be of importance in the management of anesthesia. Some chapter titles have been changed from the third edition to better reflect the chapter's content. New figures and tables have been added to the fourth edition.

As with the previous three editions of this textbook, *Anesthesia and Co-Existing Disease* is the product of the Editors. We believe this provides the readers with a consistency in style and an absence of duplication of information in differing areas of the textbook. It is believed, that this fourth edition of *Anesthesia and Co-Existing Disease* can serve both as an introductory source of information and as a reference book for review. Therefore, this textbook should be equally valuable to the physician trainee and to the anesthesiologist.

The Editors again wish to recognize the invaluable secretarial help of Deanna M. Walker in the preparation of the manuscript.

Robert K. Stoelting, M.D.
Stephen F. Dierdorf, M.D.

Preface to the First Edition

Optimal management of anesthesia extends beyond an understanding of the pharmacology of drugs used during the intraoperative period and a dexterity in performance of technical procedures. Specifically, a knowledge of the pathophysiology of co-existing disease regardless of the reason for surgery and an understanding of the implications of concomitant drug therapy are mandatory for the optimal management of anesthesia in an individual patient. The goal of *Anesthesia and Co-Existing Disease* is to provide a concise description of the pathophysiology of disease states and their medical treatment that is relevant to the care of the patient in the perioperative period. Diseases or characteristics unique to the pediatric, geriatric, and pregnant patient are considered in separate chapters. There is a liberal use of illustrations and tables to reinforce written material. Discussions of disease states often include a section designated Management of Anesthesia. This section is designed to relate the impact of co-existing disease to the selection of drugs, techniques, and monitors to be employed in the perioperative period.

We feel that *Anesthesia and Co-Existing Disease* can serve both as an introductory source of information and as a reference for review. Therefore, this book should be equally valuable to the beginner or the individual with training and experience in the administration of anesthesia. Although several authors have contributed to this undertaking, a consistency in style is assured by virtue of the Editors' roles as the final "authors" so as to make the entire book read as if written by a single individual.

The Editors wish to recognize the invaluable secretarial help of Deanna Walker in preparation of manuscripts. We salute the contagious enthusiasm of Lewis Reines, President of Churchill Livingstone, in the initial formulation of the idea for this book. In addition, the superb cooperation of our copy editor, Donna Balopole, permitted us to continue to make important additions to the book as new information and references became available. As a result, we have been able to achieve our desire to provide a work which is current to within 6 months of publication. Finally, we are grateful to our colleagues and families for their understanding and support during the time the book was in preparation.

Robert K. Stoelting, M.D.
Stephen F. Dierdorf, M.D.

Contents

1

Ischemic Heart Disease

Ischemic heart disease, which reflects the presence of atherosclerosis in coronary arteries (coronary artery disease), is present in an estimated 30% of patients who undergo surgery annually in the United States.[1] The aging of the population increases the likelihood that patients undergoing surgery will have co-existing ischemic heart disease. Angina pectoris, acute myocardial infarction, and sudden death are often the first manifestations of ischemic heart disease. Cardiac dysrhythmias are probably the major cause of sudden death in patients with ischemic heart disease. The two most important risk factors for the development of atherosclerosis involving the coronary arteries are male gender and increasing age (Table 1–1). Three additional risk factors are hypercholesterolemia, systemic hypertension, and cigarette smoking. Other proposed risk factors include diabetes mellitus, obesity, a sedentary life style, and a family history of premature development of ischemic heart disease. An association between psychological traits (anxiety, hostility, stress) and ischemic heart disease has not been documented.[2]

■ ANGINA PECTORIS

The coronary artery circulation normally supplies sufficient blood flow to meet the demands of the myocardium in response to widely varying workloads. An imbalance between coronary blood flow (supply) and myocardial oxygen consumption (demand) can precipitate ischemia, which frequently manifests as angina pectoris.[3] When the imbalance becomes extreme, congestive heart failure, electrical instability and cardiac dysrhythmias, and myocardial infarction may result. Angina pectoris reflects intracardiac release of adenosine during ischemia.

Table 1–1 • Risk Factors for the Development of Ischemic Heart Disease

Male gender
Increasing age
Hypercholesterolemia
Systemic hypertension
Cigarette smoking
Diabetes mellitus
Obesity
Sedentary lifestyle
Family history (premature development of ischemic heart disease)

Stimulation of adenosine receptors slows atrioventricular nodal conduction and decreases contractility, thereby improving the balance between myocardial oxygen demand and delivery. Atherosclerosis is the most common cause of myocardial ischemia resulting in angina pectoris. Other causes of impaired coronary blood flow resulting in angina pectoris include vasoactive materials from platelets, endothelial damage, and coronary artery spasm.

Diagnosis

Angina pectoris is typically retrosternal chest discomfort, usually perceived as pain but often described as pressure or heaviness.[3] Discomfort typically radiates to the neck, left shoulder, left arm, or lower jaw and occasionally to the back, down the right arm, or down both arms. Although angina may be perceived as epigastric discomfort resembling indigestion, the pain usually does not radiate far below the level of the diaphragm. Some patients describe angina as shortness of breath, mistaking a sense of chest constriction as dyspnea. The patient's need to take a deep breath, rather than to breathe rapidly, often identifies shortness of breath as an anginal equivalent. Patients with unstable angina pectoris (new onset of progressively more severe angina pectoris) and those with non-Q wave myocardial infarctions (ST segment elevation in contrast to ST segment depression characteristic of Q wave myocardial infarctions) often are clinically indistinguishable until hours or days later when results of cardiac enzyme tests are available.[4] Angina pectoris usually lasts several minutes; a sharp pain that lasts only a few seconds or a dull ache that lasts for hours is rarely caused by myocardial ischemia. Physical exertion, emotional tension, and cold weather may also induce angina; rest and/or nitroglycerin usually relieve it promptly. Noncardiac chest pain is usually transient, exacerbated by chest wall movement, and associated with tenderness over the involved area, which is often a costochondral joint. Retrosternal sharp pain exacerbated by deep breathing, coughing, or variation in body position suggests pericarditis. Esophageal spasm can produce severe substernal pressure that may be confused with angina pectoris. Because the esophagus consists of smooth muscle, administration of nitroglycerin is likely to relieve the pain.

Electrocardiography

Standard Electocardiography

The standard electrocardiogram (ECG) may be normal in the absence of angina pectoris. Conversely, myocardial ischemia is confirmed when ST segment depression on the ECG, which is characteristic of subendocardial ischemia, coincides in time with an episode of anginal chest pain. Variant angina is diagnosed by ST segment elevation on the ECG, which is characteristic of extensive transmural ischemia. T wave changes on the ECG during angina pectoris include transient symmetrical T wave inversion. Other patients with chronically inverted T waves in association with pathologic Q waves from a prior myocardial infarction may manifest a return of the T waves to the normal upright position ("pseudonormalization") during angina pectoris.

Exercise Electrocardiography

Exercise electrocardiography is useful for establishing the patient's left ventricular function and thus the prognosis; it is less useful for establishing the diagnosis of ischemic heart disease, especially in patients who clinically manifest typical angina pectoris. Exercise testing is not always possible because of noncardiac causes (peripheral vascular disease and associated claudication, lung disease, arthritis) or the presence of conditions that interfere with interpretation of the exercise ECG (paced ventricular rhythm, preexisting ST segment depression associated with left ventricular hypertrophy or digitalis administration, preexcitation syndrome). The presence of severe aortic stenosis prohibits exercise testing.

The minimum criterion for an abnormal ST segment response is at least 1 mm of horizontal or downsloping ST segment depression or elevation occurring during or within 4 minutes after exercise. The greater the degree of ST segment depression or elevation, the greater the likelihood of more severe coronary artery disease. Likewise, the prognosis is poor if the ST segment abnormality is associated with angina pectoris, poor exercise capacity, or a decrease in systolic blood pressure during exercise.

Exercise electrocardiography is less accurate for detecting ischemic heart disease than imaging tests, but it is more cost-effective.[3]

Noninvasive Imaging Tests

Coronary artery calcification can be measured by electron-beam computed tomography. Noninvasive imaging tests for the diagnosis of ischemic heart disease are most likely to be recommended when exercise electrocardiography is not possible or it is difficult to interpret ST segment changes on the ECG. For patients who cannot exercise, intravenous infusion of dobutamine or institution of artificial cardiac pacing to provide progressively more rapid heart rates provides adequate cardiac stress. Alternatively, cardiac stress can be produced by administering a coronary vasodilator such as adenosine or dipyridamole, which dilates normal coronary arteries but evokes minimal to no change in the diameters of atherosclerotic coronary arteries. After inducing cardiac stress by these interventions, it is possible to use echocardiography to assess myocardial function or radionuclide tracer scanning to assess myocardial perfusion.

Echocardiography

Echocardiographic wall motion analysis is performed after stressing the heart by dobutamine infusion or pacing. An intravenous echocardiographic contrast dye can enhance the accuracy of stress echocardiography. The ventricular wall motion abnormalities induced by stress correspond to the site of myocardial ischemia, thereby localizing the obstructive coronary lesion. In contrast, exercise electrocardiography and associated ST segment changes indicate the presence of ischemic heart disease but do not reliably predict the location of the obstructive coronary lesion.

Nuclear Stress Imaging

Nuclear stress imaging is useful for assessing coronary perfusion. Tracers (thallium, technetium) can be detected over the myocardium (single photon emission computed tomography techniques) that correspond to coronary blood flow. A significant coronary obstructive lesion causes less flow and thus less tracer activity. Exercise increases the difference in tracer activity between normal and underperfused regions because coronary blood flow increases markedly with exercise except in regions distal to the coronary artery obstruction. The magnitude of the perfusion abnormality is the most important prognostic indicator.

Coronary Angiography

Coronary angiography provides the most information about the condition of the coronary arteries and is indicated in patients with angina pectoris despite maximal medical regimens and in those whose occupations could place others at risk (airline pilots). In many of these patients, revascularization provides the best treatment for pain relief and improved prognosis. Surgical bypass is most effective when the diseased coronary artery is of reasonable size, has a high grade proximal stenosis, and is free of significant distal plaques. The most suitable atherosclerotic lesion for coronary angioplasty is discrete, concentric, proximal, noncalcified, and less than 5 mm in length. Coronary angiography is also useful for establishing the diagnosis of nonatherosclerotic coronary artery disease such as coronary artery spasm.

Coronary artery bypass surgery is likely to improve survival among patients with multivessel disease and an ejection fraction of less than 40%. Echocardiography and left ventricular angiography are the two principal methods for measuring the ejection fraction and for assessing left ventricular contractility. The presence of hypokinetic or akinetic areas of the left ventricle connote a poor prognosis. Extensive myocardial fibrosis from prior myocardial infarctions is unlikely to be improved by surgical revascularization (coronary artery bypass graft, or CABG). Conversely, some patients with chronic ischemic heart disease have chronically impaired myocardial function that manifests improved contractility ("hibernating myocardium") following surgical revascularization.

The two most important prognostic determinants in patients with coronary artery disease are the anatomic extent of the atherosclerotic disease as revealed by coronary angiography and the state of left ventricular function (ejection fraction). Left main coronary artery disease is the most dangerous anatomic lesion and is associated with an unfavorable prognosis after medical therapy. Coronary angiography cannot predict which plaques are most likely to rupture and initiate acute coronary syndromes.[4] Plaques most likely to rupture and lead to formation of an occlusive thrombus have a thin fibrous cap and a large lipid core containing an increased number of macrophages. These features predict an increased risk of myocardial infarction independent of the degree of coronary artery stenosis determined to be present on coronary angiography. Indeed, unstable angina pectoris and myocardial infarction most often result from rupture of a plaque that produced less than 50% stenosis.[3]

Treatment

Treatment of ischemic heart disease includes lifestyle modification, pharmacologic therapy, and revascularization.[3] Treatment that prolongs life has the highest priority. In this regard, surgical revascularization (CABG) for significant left main or three-vessel coronary artery obstruction is useful. In many patients with stable angina pectoris and one- or two-vessel disease antianginal medical therapy, percutaneous transluminal coronary angioplasty (PTCA), or CABG is acceptable.

Lifestyle Modification

The process of atherosclerosis may be slowed by eliminating some risk factors; this can be done by cessation of smoking, maintenance of an ideal body weight through diet (low fat, low cholesterol) and regular aerobic exercise, and treatment of systemic hypertension. Lowering the low density lipoprotein (LDL) level by diet or drugs [3-hydroxy-3-methylglutaryl coenzyme A (HMG-CoA) reductase inhibitors] is associated with a substantial decrease in the risk of death due to cardiac events. Drug treatment is appropriate when the LDL cholesterol level exceeds 130 mg/dl with the goal of decreasing it to less than 100 mg/dl.[3] Systemic hypertension increases the risk of coronary events as a result of direct vascular injury, left ventricular hypertrophy, and increased myocardial oxygen demand. Lowering systemic blood pressure from hypertensive levels (ideally less than 140/90 mmHg) decreases the risk of myocardial infarction, congestive heart failure, and cerebrovascular accident. β-Adrenergic blockers and long-acting calcium channel blockers are especially useful for managing systemic hypertension in patients with angina pectoris. If left ventricular dysfunction accompanies systemic hypertension, an angiotensin-converting enzyme (ACE) inhibitor or an angiotensin receptor blocker is a therapeutic option.

Medical Treatment of Ischemia

Antiplatelet drugs, β-blockers, calcium channel blockers, and nitrates are utilized in the medical treatment of ischemic heart disease.

Antiplatelet Drugs

Low-dose aspirin therapy (75 to 325 mg daily) decreases the risk of cardiac events in patients with stable or unstable angina pectoris and is recommended for all patients with ischemic heart disease unless contraindicated or not tolerated.[3, 4] Clopidogrel effectively inhibits platelet aggregation and may decrease the combined risk of ischemic stroke and myocardial infarction more effectively than aspirin. Platelet glycoprotein IIb/IIIa receptor antagonists inhibit platelet adhesion, activation, and aggregation. Administration of these drugs may be particularly useful in patients in whom placement of an intracoronary stent is anticipated.[4, 5]

Antithrombin Drugs

The combination of aspirin and intravenous infusion of unfractionated heparin is recommended for treatment of unstable angina.[4] The disadvantage of unfractionated heparin is the variability in dose response due to its binding with plasma proteins other than antithrombin. Unlike unfractionated heparin, low-molecular-weight heparin provides a more predictable pharmacologic profile, long plasma half-life, and a practical means of administration (subcutaneous) without the need to monitor the activated partial thromboplastin time. The combination of warfarin [international normalized ratio (INR) 2.0 to 2.5] and aspirin may be superior to monotherapy with aspirin alone during the weeks following the initial presentation of unstable angina pectoris.

β-Blockers

β-Blockers are the initial choice of therapy for patients with symptoms of myocardial ischemia characterized as chronic stable angina pectoris. Evidence supporting the use of β-blockers in the management of patients with unstable angina pectoris is limited.[4] Chronic administration of β-blockers also decreases the risk of death and myocardial reinfarction in patients who have experienced a myocardial infarction, presumably by decreasing myocardial oxygen demand.[4, 6] This benefit occurs even in patients in whom β-blockers have traditionally been considered to be contraindicated (congestive heart failure, pulmonary disease, advanced age).[6] Drug-induced blockade of β_1-adrenergic receptors (atenolol, metoprolol, acebutolol) results in heart rate slowing and decreased myocardial contractility that is greater during activity than at rest. The result is a decrease in myocardial oxygen demand with a subsequent decrease in ischemic events during exertion. The decrease in heart rate also increases diastolic perfusion time, which may contribute to improved myocardial perfusion. β_2-Adrenergic blockade, as associated with administration of propranolol and nadolol, could increase the risk of bronchospasm in patients with reactive airway disease and increase the manifestations of peripheral vascular disease. Despite the differences between β_1- and β_2-effects, all β-blockers seem to be equally effective in the treatment of angina pectoris. β-Blockers are contraindicated in the presence of atrioventricular heart block and unstable congestive heart failure. Diabetes mellitus is not a contraindication to β-blocker therapy, although these drugs may mask the sympathetic nervous system signs of hypoglycemia. The most common side effects of β-blocker therapy are fatigue and insomnia.

Calcium Channel Blockers

Long-acting calcium channel blockers are comparable to β-blockers in terms of relieving angina pectoris and are uniquely effective for decreasing the frequency and severity of angina pectoris due to coronary artery spasm. They are not as effective as β-blockers for decreasing the incidence of myocardial reinfarction. The effectiveness of calcium channel blockers is due to their ability to decrease vascular smooth muscle contractility, resulting in increased coronary blood flow. Short-acting calcium channel blockers (verapamil, nifedipine, diltiazem) are not recommended, as they may increase sympathetic nervous system activity, with associated adverse cardiac events. Calcium channel blockers are contraindicated in patients with severe congestive heart failure. Common side effects of calcium channel blocker therapy are hypotension, peripheral edema, and headache.

Organic Nitrates

Organic nitrates decrease the frequency, duration, and severity of angina pectoris and increase the amount of exercise needed before the onset of ST segment depression on the ECG.[7] These drugs dilate coronary arteries and collateral vessels, thereby improving coronary blood flow, whereas decreased peripheral vascular resistance results in decreased left ventricular outflow impedance and myocardial oxygen consumption. The venodilating effect of nitrates decreases venous return thereby decreasing left ventricular filling pressure, volume, and myocardial oxygen consumption. Nitrates are relatively contraindicated in the presence of hypertrophic obstructive cardiomyopathy and severe aortic stenosis. Nitrates should not be used within 24 hours of administering sildenafil because this combination may induce severe hypotension. Administration of sublingual nitroglycerin tablets or spray provides prompt relief of angina pectoris. For long-term therapy, long-acting nitrate preparations (isosorbide, nitroglycerin ointment or patches) are equally effective. The most common side effect of nitrate treatment is headache, whereas hypotension may occur in hypovolemic patients. The therapeutic value of organic nitrates is compromised by the rapid development of tolerance during sustained therapy.[7] In this regard, for long-term use nitrates should be administered with one daily nitrate-free interval of at least 8 hours to prevent the development of nitrate tolerance.

Revascularization

Revascularization by CABG, PTCA (including atherectomy, laser therapy), or placement of coronary artery stents is indicated when optimal medical therapy fails to control the symptoms of ischemic heart disease, principally angina pectoris. Revascularization is also indicated for specific anatomic coronary artery obstruction (left main stenosis of more than 70%, combinations of two- or three vessel disease that includes a proximal left anterior descending artery stenosis of more than 70%), and evidence of impaired left ventricular contractility (decreased ejection fraction).[4] The use of coronary artery stents with PTCA decreases the rate of restenosis and the need for repeat PTCA.[8] PTCA is effective for relief of angina pectoris but does not decrease the risk of myocardial infarction or death to a greater extent than medical therapy.[3] Revascularization (CABG) requiring cardiopulmonary bypass may be associated with postoperative cognitive dysfunction (transient to persistent) during the postoperative period, especially in elderly patients (see Chapter 33).

■ ACUTE MYOCARDIAL INFARCTION

Mortality due to acute myocardial infarction ("acute coronary artery syndrome") remains significant but has been decreasing over the past several years, presumably reflecting the value of early therapeutic interventions (thrombolytic therapy, aspirin, heparin, decrease in known risk factors for coronary artery disease).[9] Coronary angiography has documented that nearly all myocardial infarctions are caused by thrombotic occlusion of a coronary artery. In this regard, atherosclerotic plaques rich in lipid-laden macrophages are susceptible to sudden plaque disruption and hemorrhage into the vessel wall, resulting in abrupt partial or total occlusion of the coronary artery. Although stenosis of the coronary artery (more than 70%) is typically required to produce angina pectoris, such stenoses tend to have dense fibrotic caps and are less likely to rupture than are mild to moderate coronary artery stenoses, which are generally more lipid laden.

Long-term prognosis following occurrence of an acute myocardial infarction is determined principally by the severity of left ventricular dysfunction, the presence and degree of residual ischemia, and the potential for malignant ventricular dysrhythmias. Most deaths that occur during the first year after discharge from the hospital occur within the first 3 months. Nevertheless, ventricular function can be substantially improved during the weeks following an acute myocardial infarction, particularly in patients in whom early reperfusion was achieved. Therefore measuring ventricular function 2 to 3 months after myocardial infarction is a more accurate predictor of long-term prognosis than measuring it during the early acute stages.[9]

Pathophysiology

Acute coronary artery syndrome represents a hypercoagulable state. It has been presumed that focal disruption of an atheromatous plaque triggers a coagulation response with subsequent generation of thrombin and occlusion of the coronary artery. Fibrinolytic enzymes, such as tissue plasminogen activator and urokinase plasminogen activator, are important for preventing fibrin deposition within the vascular bed of the heart. Thrombosis of a coronary artery arises when an atherosclerotic plaque ruptures and alters the local hemostatic mechanisms in the coronary circulation.

There is increasing recognition that atherosclerosis may be an inflammatory disease.[10,11] The presence of inflammatory cells in atherosclerotic plaques suggests that inflammation is important in the cascade of events leading to plaque rupture. Indeed, serum markers of inflammation, such as C-reactive proteins and fibrinogen, are increased in those at greatest risk for coronary artery disease. It is somewhat paradoxical that plaques that rupture and lead to occlusion of a coronary artery are rarely flow-restrictive. By contrast, flow-restrictive plaques that produce angina pectoris and stimulate the development of collateral circulation tend to be "mature" and less likely to rupture.

Diagnosis

Diagnosis of acute myocardial infarction requires the presence of at least two of three criteria: (1) clinical history of angina pectoris; (2) serial electrocardiographic changes indicative of myocardial infarction; and (3) rise and fall of serum cardiac enzyme markers.[9] Approximately two-thirds of patients describe a new onset of angina pectoris or a change in their anginal pattern during the 30 days preceding an acute myocardial infarction. In approximately one-fourth of patients myocardial infarction is associated with mild symptoms or none at all. On physical examination patients often appear anxious, and sinus tachycardia is common. Hypotension caused by left or right ventricular dysfunction or cardiac dysrhythmias may be present. Moist rales may represent congestive heart failure due to left ventricular dysfunction. The appearance of a cardiac murmur may reflect ischemic mitral regurgitation. Other potential causes of the patient's chest pain (pulmonary embolism, aortic dissection, spontaneous pneumothorax, pericarditis, cholecystitis) should be considered.

Electrocardiography

The ECG is valuable for confirming the diagnosis of an acute myocardial infarction and selecting the most appropriate therapy. It is recommended that patients presenting with clinical symptoms of an acute myocardial infarction undergo electrocardiography within 10 minutes of arrival at the hospital. If ST segment elevation is present on the ECG of patients with chest pain typical of angina pectoris, there is more than 90% likelihood that an acute myocardial infarction has occurred. Nevertheless, an estimated 50% of patients with acute myocardial infarctions do not manifest ST segment elevation on the ECG. ST segment depression, T wave inversion, and bundle branch block on the ECG are less specific than ST segment elevation but are supportive of the diagnosis of acute myocardial infarction, especially in the presence of angina pectoris.

Laboratory Studies

Troponin is a cardiac-specific protein and marker for acute myocardial infarction; and an increase in the circulating concentration of this enzyme occurs early after myocardial injury. Troponin is more specific than CK-MB for determining myocardial injury. Cardiac troponins (troponin T or I) increase within 4 hours after myocardial injury and remain elevated for several days. When used together, elevated troponin levels and electrocardiography are powerful predictors of adverse cardiac events in patients with anginal pain. In the absence of ST segment elevation on the ECG, the presence of relative lymphocytopenia suggests the occurrence of an acute myocardial infarction.

Imaging Studies

Echocardiography reveals regional wall motion abnormalities in most patients who experience an acute myocardial infarction. Patients with typical ECG evidence of acute myocardial infarction do not require evaluation with echocardiography. Echocardiography is most useful in patients with left bundle branch block or an abnormal ECG tracing (but without ST segment elevation) and in whom the diagnosis of acute myocardial infarction is uncertain. The time required to perform perfusion imaging with thallium limits the usefulness of radionuclide imaging for early diagnosis of acute myocardial infarction.

Treatment

Early initiation of treatment in patients experiencing an acute myocardial infarction reduces morbidity and mortality. Aspirin is administered to all patients as soon as acute myocardial infarction is diagnosed and is continued indefinitely. Pain relief, usually provided by intravenous administration of morphine, is important to decrease the stimulus to catecholamine release and associated increases in myocardial oxygen requirements.

Reperfusion Therapy

Thrombolytic therapy [streptokinase, tissue plasminogen activator (t-PA), reteplase], ideally initiated within 30 to 60 minutes of arrival to the hospital especially in patients with ST segment elevation on the ECG, restores normal antegrade blood flow in the occluded artery. The most feared complication of thrombolytic therapy is intracerebral hemorrhage, which is more likely in elderly patients and those with a history of systemic hypertension. Patients with gastrointestinal bleeding and recent surgery are also at increased risk for bleeding. There is evidence that intracoronary stenting plus platelet glycoprotein IIb/IIIa blockade with abciximab leads to a greater degree of myocardial salvage and a better clinical outcome than does fibrinolysis with t-PA.[12] Thrombolytic therapy is not recommended in patients with ECG findings other than ST segment elevation or bundle branch block.

Direct Coronary Angioplasty

Coronary angioplasty without antecedent thrombolytic therapy may be superior to thrombolytic therapy alone. In this regard, PTCA is preferable for restoring flow to an occluded coronary artery when the facility's resources permit this treatment to be achieved within 1 to 2 hours. Surgical backup may be needed, as about 5% of patients with acute myocardial infarction who undergo immediate PTCA require emergency surgery for failed angioplasty or because coronary artery anatomy precludes PTCA.

The combined use of intracoronary stents and a platelet glycoprotein IIb/IIIa inhibitor during emergent PTCA ("facilitated angioplasty") may maximize achievement of normal antegrade flow and decrease the need for subsequent revascularization procedures. Even in the absence of ST segment elevation, PTCA or CABG surgery may be indicated in patients with critical coronary artery stenosis. However, PTCA is not routinely recommended in all patients following thrombolytic therapy.

Coronary Artery Bypass Graft Surgery

Coronary artery bypass grafting can also restore blood flow in an occluded coronary artery, but reperfusion can usually be achieved more promptly with thrombolytic therapy and direct coronary angioplasty. Emergency CABG surgery is usually reserved for patients in whom immediate angiography reveals coronary anatomy that precludes PTCA, patients experiencing failed angioplasty, and those with evidence of infarction-related ventricular septal defect or mitral regurgitation.

Adjunctive Medical Therapy

Intravenous heparin therapy is commonly administered for 3 to 5 days following thrombolytic therapy. β-Blockers are associated with significantly decreased in-hospital and long-term mortality that includes myocardial reinfarction.[6] Early administration of β-blockers may decrease the size of the infarct by decreasing the heart rate, systemic blood pressure, and myocardial contractility. In the absence of contraindications, it is recommended that all patients receive intravenous β-blockers as early as possible following acute myocardial infarction regardless of whether they undergo reperfusion therapy. β-Blocker therapy is continued indefinitely. All patients with large anterior myocardial infarctions and significant left ventricular dysfunction (ejection fraction less than 40%) should be treated with angiotensin-converting enzyme (ACE) inhibitors. Treatment with an ACE inhibitor may become routine therapy for all patients who survive a myocardial infarction regardless of the ejection fraction or the presence of congestive heart failure. It does not appear that administration of nitroglycerin to patients receiving early thrombolytic therapy is of any benefit. In the absence of ventricular dysrhythmias, prophylactic administration of intravenous lidocaine or other cardiac antidysrhythmia agents is not recommended. Lidocaine may increase mortality following acute myocardial infarction because of an increase in the incidence of bradydysrhythmias and associated asystole.[9] Calcium channel antagonists should not be administered routinely following an acute myocardial infarction but, rather, reserved for patients with persistent myocardial ischemia despite optimal use of aspirin, β-blockers, nitrate therapy, and intravenous heparin. Evidence does not support routine administration of magnesium in patients receiving early reperfusion therapy, although magnesium is indicated in patients with acute myocardial infarction associated with torsade de pointes ventricular tachycardia.

Complications of Acute Myocardial Infarctions

Complications of acute myocardial infarctions reflect effects on the heart and other organ systems that are dependent on adequate tissue blood flow for optimal function.

Cardiac Dysrhythmias

Cardiac dysrhythmias, especially ventricular dysrhythmias, are a common cause of death during the early period following an acute myocardial infarction.[9]

Ventricular Fibrillation

Ventricular fibrillation occurs in 3% to 5% of patients with acute myocardial infarction, with the peak incidence during the first 4 hours after the event. Prophylactic lidocaine is no longer recommended assuming electrical defibrillation can be promptly accomplished. β-Blockers may decrease the early occurrence of ventricular fibrillation and should be administered to patients who have no contraindications. Hypokalemia is a risk factor for ventricular fibrillation. When ventricular fibrillation occurs, rapid defibrillation with 200 to 300 joules should be administered. Ventricular fibrillation is associated with high mortality when it occurs in patients with coexisting hypotension and/or congestive heart failure.

Ventricular Tachycardia

Ventricular tachycardia (three or more consecutive ventricular beats) is common with acute myocardial infarction, although short periods of nonsustained ventricular tachycardia are believed not to predispose to sustained ventricular tachycardia or ventricular fibrillation. Sustained or hemodynamically significant ventricular tachycardia is treated with prompt electrical cardioversion. Prolonged periods of asymptomatic ventricular tachycardia are initially treated with intravenous administration of lidocaine, procainamide, or amiodarone.

Atrial Fibrillation

Atrial fibrillation is the most common atrial dysrhythmia, occurring in more than 10% of patients following acute myocardial infarction.[9] Atrial fibrillation may result from an acute increase in left atrial pressure caused by left ventricular dysfunction or atrial ischemia as a result of occlusion of a coronary artery, usually the right coronary artery. The incidence of atrial fibrillation is decreased in patients receiving thrombolytic therapy. When atrial fibrillation is hemodynamically significant, cardioversion should be performed promptly. In patients in whom atrial fibrillation is well tolerated, β-blocker therapy is indicated.

Bradydysrhythmias and Heart Block

Sinus bradycardia is common following acute myocardial infarction, particularly in patients with inferior myocardial infarctions, perhaps reflecting increased parasympathetic nervous system activity or acute ischemia of the sinus node or atrioventricular node. Treatment with atropine and a temporary artificial cardiac pacemaker is needed only when hemodynamic compromise manifests as increased angina pectoris, hypotension, or congestive heart failure. Second- or third-degree atrioventricular heart block occurs in approximately 20% of patients with inferior myocardial infarctions and may require a temporary artificial cardiac pacemaker for a few hours to days following the myocardial infarction.

Pericarditis

Pericarditis is a common complication of acute myocardial infarction and may cause anterior chest pain, which may be confused with continuing or recurring myocardial ischemia. In contrast to the pain of myocardial ischemia, discomfort associated with pericarditis is accentuated by inspiration. Diffuse ST segment elevation on the ECG may be present. Pericardial effusion occurs in about one-third of patients after acute myocardial infarction. Specific treatment of pericarditis is rarely required, but corticosteroids often relieve symptoms dramatically. Dressler syndrome (postmyocardial infarction syndrome) is a delayed form of acute pericarditis that develops in about 3% of patients anywhere between the first week and many months after an acute myocardial infarction.

Mitral Regurgitation

Mild mitral regurgitation due to ischemic injury to papillary muscles and ventricular walls to which they attach is common after acute myocardial infarction. Severe mitral regurgitation caused by acute myocardial infarction is rare and typically results from partial or complete rupture of a papillary muscle. Severe mitral regurgitation is more likely to occur following an acute inferior myocardial infarction than following an acute anterior myocardial infarction. Acute severe mitral regurgitation typically results in pulmonary edema and cardiogenic shock. Prompt surgical therapy is recommended. Treatment designed to decrease left ventricular afterload, as produced by intravenous nitroprusside and an intra-aortic balloon counterpulsation pump, decreases the regurgitant volume and increases forward blood flow and cardiac output; it may be helpful as a temporizing measure.

Ventricular Septal Defect

The characteristic holosystolic murmur of ventricular septal defects following acute myocardial infarctions (more likely after an anterior than an inferior infarction) may be difficult to distinguish from that of severe mitral regurgitation. Surgical repair is necessary especially when the ventricular defect is associated with congestive heart failure. Mortality associated with surgical repair of postinfarction ventricular septal defects is about 20%.[9] As with mitral regurgitation, pharmacologically induced afterload reduction (intravenous nitroprusside) or its mechanical equivalent (intra-aortic balloon counterpulsation pump) may be beneficial.

Congestive Heart Failure and Cardiogenic Shock

Acute myocardial infarction may be complicated by some degree of left ventricular dysfunction (presence of a third heart sound) as reflected by increased left ventricular end-diastolic pressure and pulmonary congestion (decreased PaO_2).[13] The term "cardiogenic shock" is restricted to the hypotension and oliguria that persist after the relief of pain, abatement of excess parasympathetic nervous system activity, correction of hypovolemia, and treatment of cardiac dysrhythmias. In this regard, cardiogenic shock is an advanced form of acute congestive heart failure in which the cardiac output is insufficient to maintain adequate perfusion of the kidneys and other vital organs. Systolic blood pressure is often less than 60 mmHg, and there may be associated pulmonary edema and arterial hypoxemia. Pulseless electrical activity (electromechanical dissociation) may also accompany cardiogenic shock. The patient in whom cardiogenic shock develops is likely to have experienced infarction of more than 40% of the left ventricular myocardium.

The initial treatment of cardiogenic shock is to decrease the left ventricular afterload with vasodilator drugs such as nitroglycerin during invasive monitoring of systemic blood pressure and cardiac filling pressures. Dopamine and dobutamine may be administered in attempts to improve cardiac output, whereas digitalis is probably of no value in the treatment of cardiogenic shock. An attempt to restore coronary blood flow in the infarct-related artery by means of thrombolytic therapy, PTCA, or surgical revascularization may be indicated. Circulatory assist devices may be considered as a means of sustaining viable cardiac output until surgical revascularization can be performed or the feasibility of cardiac transplantation established. In this regard, left ventricular assist devices provide significantly more cardiac output than intra-aortic balloon counterpulsation. The intra-aortic balloon is programmed to the ECG so it deflates just before systole and inflates during diastole. Presystolic deflation of the balloon decreases systemic blood pressure and afterload, which decreases cardiac work and myocardial oxygen requirements. Inflation of the balloon during diastole increases diastolic blood pressure and thus improves coronary blood flow and myocardial oxygen delivery. Intravenous infusion of a combination of catecholamines and vasodilators may serve as a pharmacologic alternative to mechanical counterpulsation with the intra-aortic balloon.

Myocardial Rupture

Myocardial rupture, a catastrophic complication of an acute myocardial infarction, requires emergency surgery. Echocardiography can quickly confirm the diagnosis. Mortality exceeds 50% even under the best of conditions.

Right Ventricular Infarction

Right ventricular infarction occurs in approximately one-third of patients with acute inferior left ventricular infarction, whereas isolated right ventricular infarctions are unusual.[9, 14] The right ventricle has a more favorable oxygen supply/demand ratio than the left ventricle resulting from a smaller ventricular muscle mass as well as improved oxygen delivery due to the biphasic nature of coronary blood flow during both systole and diastole.[14] The clinical triad of hypotension, clear lung fields, and increased jugular venous pressure in a patient with an inferior myocardial infarction is virtually pathognomonic for right ventricular infarction. Echocardiography is useful for diagnosing right ventricular infarction (right ventricular dilation, right ventricular wall asynergy, abnormal interventricular septal motion), and radionuclide ventriculography is utilized for estimating the right ventricular ejection fraction. Cardiogenic shock, although uncommon, is the most serious complication of right ventricular infarction. Many of these patients develop atrial fibrillation, and third-degree atrioventricular heart block is common (as many as 50% of patients) and may imply a poor prognosis in the presence of an inferior myocardial infarction.

Recognition of right ventricular infarction is important, as pharmacologic treatment that decreases right ventricular filling (nitrates, diuretics) may be undesirable. Third-degree atrioventricular heart block should be treated rapidly with dual atrial and ventricular pacing, recognizing the value of atrioventricular synchrony for maintaining ventricular filling of the ischemic noncompliant right ventricle. Intravascular volume replacement is useful for maintaining cardiac output; administration of an inotrope (dopamine) may be necessary if hypotension persists despite fluid infusion.

Cerebrovascular Accident

Infarction of the anterior wall and apex of the left ventricle results in thrombus formation in the apex of the left ventricle, with systemic embolization and the possibility of an ischemic cerebrovascular accident in about 15% of patients.[9] Echocardiography is used to detect thrombus formation in the left ventricle. Left ventricular thrombus formation is an indication for anticoagulation with intravenous heparin followed by warfarin. Thrombolytic therapy may cause hemorrhagic stroke, most commonly during the first 24 hours following treatment. Its use is associated with a high mortality rate.

PREOPERATIVE ASSESSMENT OF PATIENTS WITH KNOWN OR SUSPECTED ISCHEMIC HEART DISEASE

The risk of perioperative death due to cardiac causes is less than 1% for patients who do not have ischemic heart disease as evidenced by the history or ECG signs of myocardial infarction, angina pectoris, or angiographically documented coronary artery disease.[1] In contrast, the risk of perioperative myocardial infarction is at least twice as great in patients with known or suspected coronary or atherosclerotic vascular disease. In patients undergoing pe-

ripheral vascular or aortic surgery, the combined risk of death due to cardiac causes approaches 29%.[15] In stable patients undergoing elective major noncardiac surgery, six independent predictors of major cardiac complications (ventricular fibrillation, third-degree atrioventricular heart block, pulmonary edema, death) have been described (Table 1–2).[16] These predictors do not include prior CABG surgery, preoperative ST-T wave changes on the ECG, current treatment with β-adrenergic antagonists, the presence of critical aortic stenosis, the presence of abnormal cardiac rhythms, and advanced age. The absence of these factors from the list of cardiac risk factors should not be viewed as evidence that they are not worrisome prognostic factors; indeed, they might be important predictors in patients undergoing emergency operations.[16] Furthermore, in the presence of a history of ischemic heart disease, congestive heart failure, and diabetes mellitus, the risk of cardiovascular complications during the following 6 months is increased even if major perioperative complications do not occur.[16]

Perioperative risk can also be estimated on the basis of the patient's exercise tolerance.[1] Patients who can perform activities such as strenuous walking or climbing a flight of stairs without cardiac symptoms or who can increase their heart rates with exercise have a lower risk of perioperative cardiac

Table 1–2 • Cardiac Risk Index for Patients Undergoing Elective Major Noncardiac Surgery

High risk surgery
  Abdominal aneurysm
  Peripheral vascular operation
  Thoracotomy
  Major abdominal operation
Ischemic heart disease
  History of myocardial infarction
  History of a positive exercise test
  Current complaints of angina pectoris
  Use of nitrate therapy
  Q waves on electrocardiogram
Congestive heart failure
  History of congestive heart failure
  History of pulmonary edema
  History of paroxysmal nocturnal dyspnea
  Physical examination showing bilateral rales or S_3 gallop
  Chest radiograph showing pulmonary vascular redistribution
Cerebrovascular disease
  History of stroke
  History of transient ischemic attack
Insulin-dependent diabetes mellitus
Preoperative serum creatinine concentration >2 mg/dl

Adapted from Lee TH, Marcantonio ER, Mangione CM, et al. Derivation and prospective validation of a simple index for prediction of cardiac risk of major noncardiac surgery. Circulation 1999;100:1043–9.

complications than patients who are unable to perform such tasks. It is necessary to recognize that the patient's peripheral vascular disease may limit exercise tolerance resulting in an underestimation of the significance of co-existing coronary artery disease.

It has been argued that the routine clinical evaluation before surgery is not sufficiently sensitive or specific for risk assessment, leading to the recommendation that specialized testing (exercise electrocardiography, echocardiography, radionuclide ventriculography, dipyridamole-thallium scintigraphy) be considered in selected patients. The higher costs associated with specialized testing may be justifiable if otherwise unavailable information that improves patient outcome is obtained; but it is unclear which, if any, subgroups of patients need or benefit from such testing.[1] The primary challenge is to distinguish patients who require little or no preoperative testing from those for whom specialized testing is beneficial.

History

An important goal of the history is to elicit from the patient the severity, progression, and functional limitations introduced by ischemic heart disease. Myocardial ischemia, left ventricular dysfunction, and cardiac dysrhythmias are usually responsible for the symptoms (angina pectoris, dyspnea, limited exercise tolerance, peripheral edema) of ischemic heart disease (see "Angina Pectoris"). Symptoms of ischemic heart disease may be absent at rest, emphasizing the importance of evaluating the patient's responses to various physical activities such as walking or climbing stairs. Limited exercise tolerance in the absence of significant lung disease is the most striking evidence of decreased cardiac reserve. If a patient can climb two to three flights of stairs without symptoms, it is likely that cardiac reserve is adequate. Dyspnea following the onset of angina pectoris suggests the presence of acute left ventricular dysfunction due to myocardial ischemia. It is important to recognize the presence of incipient congestive heart failure preoperatively, as the added stress of anesthesia, surgery, fluid replacement, and postoperative pain may result in overt congestive heart failure.

Silent Myocardial Ischemia

Silent myocardial ischemia does not evoke angina pectoris and usually occurs at a heart rate and systemic blood pressure substantially lower than that present during exercise-induced myocardial ischemia. Asymptomatic evidence of myocardial ischemia on the ECG may accompany mental stress. A history of ischemic heart disease or an abnormal ECG suggestive of a prior myocardial infarction is associated with an increased incidence of silent myocardial ischemia.[17] It is estimated that nearly 75% of ischemic episodes in patients with symptomatic ischemic heart disease are not associated with angina pectoris, and 10% to 15% of acute myocardial infarctions are silent.[17] Treatment of silent myocardial ischemia is the same as for classic angina pectoris. The mortality due to myocardial infarction in patients with silent myocardial ischemia is similar to that in patients with classic chest pain.

Prior Myocardial Infarction

A history of myocardial infarction is important information for the preoperative evaluation. It is common practice to delay elective operations for some time (up to 6 months) following an acute myocardial infarction. Retrospective studies of large groups of adult patients have suggested that the incidence of myocardial reinfarction during the perioperative period is influenced by the time elapsed since the previous myocardial infarction.[18, 19] Hemodynamic monitoring using intra-arterial and pulmonary artery catheter monitoring (alternatively, transesophageal echocardiography) and prompt pharmacologic treatment or fluid infusion to treat hemodynamic alterations from the normal range may decrease the risk of perioperative myocardial reinfarction in high risk patients.[18, 19] There is evidence that intraoperative myocardial ischemia, most often associated with tachycardia, increases the likelihood of intraoperative or postoperative myocardial infarction.[20]

Co-existing Noncardiac Diseases

The history obtained from these patients should elicit symptoms and information relevant to co-existing noncardiac diseases. For example, patients with ischemic heart disease are likely to exhibit peripheral vascular disease. A history of syncope may reflect seizure disorders or cardiac dysrhythmias. Cough is often pulmonary rather than cardiac in origin. It may be difficult to differentiate dyspnea due to cardiac dysfunction from that due to chronic lung disease, although patients with ischemic heart disease often complain of associated orthopnea and paroxysmal nocturnal dyspnea. Chronic obstructive pulmonary disease is predictable in patients with a long history of cigarette smoking. Diabetes mellitus is the most likely endocrine disease encountered in patients with ischemic heart disease.

Current Medications

Preoperative awareness of medications used for medical management of ischemic heart disease is important, as these drugs may exert potentially adverse effects during anesthesia. Medical treatment for ischemic heart disease is designed to decrease myocardial oxygen requirements and to improve coronary blood flow. These goals are most often achieved by the use of β-antagonists, nitrates, and calcium entry blockers (see "Angina Pectoris").

Effective β-blockade is suggested by a resting heart rate of 50 to 60 beats/min. Routine physical activity is expected to increase the heart rate 10% to 20%. There is no evidence that β-antagonists adversely enhance negative inotropic effects of volatile anesthetics, and the accepted practice is to continue these drugs throughout the perioperative period. Atropine, 0.4 to 0.6 mg IV, is the initial treatment when excessive negative inotropic or chronotropic effects of β-antagonists manifest during the perioperative period. Atropine is effective because its vagolytic action permits sympathetic nervous system innervation of the heart to emerge. Isoproterenol, 2 to 5 μg/min IV, adjusted to the desired heart rate is the specific pharmacologic antagonist for excessive β-antagonist activity. Depending on the magnitude of the β-blockade, a larger dose of isoproterenol may be necessary. Dobutamine is also an effective catecholamine for reversal of adverse cardiac effects due to β-antagonist therapy. High doses of dopamine, as may be required to antagonize β-blockade, could result in undesirable increases in systemic vascular resistance due to relatively unopposed α stimulation. Calcium works at areas other than β-receptors to increase myocardial contractility in the presence of drug-induced β-blockade. For this reason, conventional doses of calcium, 500 to 1000 mg IV, are effective. The postoperative period is a time when inadvertent acute withdrawal of β-antagonist therapy may occur, resulting in rebound increases in systemic blood pressure and heart rate.

Preoperative therapy with calcium entry blockers introduces the theoretical possibility of adverse interactions with anesthetic drugs.[21] For example, myocardial depression and peripheral vasodilation produced by volatile anesthetic drugs could be exaggerated by similar effects of the calcium entry blockers. Despite this theoretical risk there is no evidence that myocardial depression or cardiac conduction disturbances are accentuated in patients being treated with calcium entry blockers and subsequently receiving volatile anesthetic drugs.[22, 23] Calcium entry blockers may potentiate the effects of depolarizing and nondepolarizing muscle relaxants and exaggerate disease states associated with skeletal muscle weakness.[24] Pharmacologic antagonism of neuromuscular blockade may be impaired because of diminished presynaptic release of acetylcholine in the presence of calcium entry blockers.

Physical Examination

The physical examination in patients with ischemic heart disease is often normal. Nevertheless, signs of left ventricular failure must be sought (see Chapter 6). A carotid bruit may indicate previously unrecognized cerebrovascular disease. Orthostatic hypotension may reflect attenuated autonomic nervous system activity due to treatment with antihypertensive drugs. Peripheral edema is usually a late finding in patients with left ventricular failure and is most often due to venous insufficiency. Examination of the jugular venous pulse for abnormalities reflects right ventricular failure as does peripheral edema. Auscultation of the chest may reveal evidence of left ventricular dysfunction (S_3 gallop) and incipient pulmonary edema. Evaluation of the patient's upper airway and the anticipated technical ease of laryngoscopy for tracheal intubation and determination of peripheral venous sites is useful.

Specialized Preoperative Testing

Specialized preoperative testing includes electrocardiography, echocardiography, radionuclide ventriculography, and thallium scintigraphy.[1] Noninvasive preoperative testing should be reserved for patients in whom the results are critical for guiding therapy. In patients with coronary artery disease who show strongly positive results on noninvasive tests (marked cardiac ischemic changes at minimal exertion) a possible recommendation is coronary artery revascularization prior to noncardiac surgery.

Electrocardiography

Preoperative testing that includes tests wherein there is an increase in the patient's heart rate is appealing because perioperative increases in myocardial oxygen consumption and development of myocardial ischemia are often accompanied by tachycardia. For this reason, preoperative exercise stress testing may be considered especially in patients with known atherosclerotic disease.[1] Nevertheless, exercise tolerance appears to be more important than the response during the exercise ECG, suggesting that preoperative exercise stress testing is not routinely indicated in patients with stable coronary artery disease and acceptable exercise tolerance.[1] Because the exercise ECG produces a number of false negative and false positive results, its predictive value is limited.[25]

Preoperative ambulatory electrocardiography when performed in patients with coronary artery disease often reveals silent episodes of myocardial ischemia during the 48 hours preceding surgery and has been viewed as an independent predictor of adverse postoperative outcomes in some reports.[26,27] Overall, although ambulatory electrocardiography appears to be useful in patients with known coronary artery disease or peripheral vascular disease, its precise role in relation to other specialized diagnostic tests remains undefined.[1] Ambulatory electrocardiographic monitoring is less useful than the exercise ECG for detecting myocardial ischemia. Patients with stable coronary artery disease do not require repeated ECGs at frequent intervals.[25]

Echocardiography

Preoperative transthoracic or transesophageal echocardiography is useful for diagnosing left ventricular dysfunction due to a prior myocardial infarction and for assessing the presence of cardiac valve disease. There is no evidence, however, that resting echocardiography adds appreciably to the information provided by routine clinical and electrocardiographic data for predicting adverse outcomes.[1] Echocardiographic wall motion analysis during the infusion of dipyridamole or dobutamine (pharmacologic stress) is an accurate technique for evaluating ischemic heart disease, particularly in patients with no history of prior myocardial infarction. Nevertheless, the precise role of stress echocardiography in predicting postoperative events remains unclear.[1] Echocardiographic examination should be utilized to confirm or deny clinical findings, not as a substitute for the history and physical examination.

Radionuclide Ventriculography

Radionuclide ventriculography quantitates left and right ventricular contractile and diastolic function. This test is useful in patients with congestive heart failure or valvular heart disease who are being considered for cardiac surgery including cardiac valve replacement or cardiac transplantation. Determining the ejection fraction with radionuclide ventriculography does not appear to provide information for predicting perioperative myocardial infarction beyond that provided by the preoperative history and physical examination. An ejection fraction less than 50% may predict an increased risk of postoperative congestive heart failure in patients undergoing abdominal aortic surgery.[28]

Thallium Scintigraphy

Physical limitations, such as claudication or orthopedic disease (arthritis), may alter the patients' ability to exercise, thereby limiting the usefulness of exercise stress testing. Dipyridamole-thallium testing, which mimics the coronary vasodilator response associated with exercise, may be useful, especially in patients with peripheral vascular disease. Defects or "cold spots" on the nuclear scan denote areas of probable myocardial ischemia or infarction. Nevertheless, thallium redistribution has not been shown to correlate with an increased incidence of perioperative myocardial infarction, prolonged myocardial ischemia, or other adverse outcomes.[28] In this regard, the cost-effectiveness of thallium scintigraphy is best when this test is restricted to patients who cannot exercise and whose risk for perioperative cardiac complications cannot be estimated on the basis of clinical factors.

Computed Tomography and Magnetic Resonance Imaging

High speed computed tomography (CT) can visualize coronary artery calcification. Intravenous administration of radiographic contrast medium enhances the clarity of the images. Magnetic resonance imaging (MRI), compared with CT, provides greater image clarity and can even delineate the proximal portions of the coronary arterial circulation. CT and MRI are more expensive and less mobile than echocardiography, so echocardiography is more likely to be utilized for imaging the coronary circulation. When anatomic questions persist despite performance of echocardiography, it may be useful to examine the patient utilizing CT or MRI.

Positron Emission Tomography

Positron emission tomography is a highly sophisticated technique that demonstrates regional myocardial blood flow and metabolism.[25] It may be utilized to delineate coronary artery disease and myocardial viability.

MANAGEMENT OF ANESTHESIA IN PATIENTS WITH KNOWN OR SUSPECTED ISCHEMIC HEART DISEASE UNDERGOING NONCARDIAC SURGERY

The goal of preoperative cardiac assessment is to identify patients at increased risk for adverse perioperative cardiac events including myocardial infarction. In this regard, perioperative myocardial infarction is a complex entity, that can be precipitated by a number of pathophysiologic mechanisms, including increases in myocardial oxygen consumption, alterations in coagulation that precipitate thrombosis, and changes in vascular tone and endothelial function.[26] No single test can assess all these factors, and tests that assess only one factor do not predict events associated with other mechanisms. Furthermore, intraoperative and postoperative stress responses are important determinants of perioperative cardiac morbidity. For example, myocardial ischemia on emergence from anesthesia and surgery increases the risk of cardiac events in the hospital and following discharge from the hospital.[1] Therefore the value of a cardiac risk index based only on preoperative factors is inherently limited for predicting intraoperative or postoperative adverse cardiac events (Table 1–2).[1] Anesthesia for elective noncardiac surgery in patients with ischemic heart disease may be associated with adverse cardiac events, especially myocardial infarction.[29] Perhaps the most reliable indicator of adverse postoperative cardiac events in patients undergoing noncardiac surgery is myocardial ischemia during the first 48 hours following surgery. It is possible that the postoperative outcome can be improved by monitoring and treating patients who are known to be at increased risk of myocardial ischemia after surgery.

Preoperative Preparation and Medication

High risk patients probably benefit from optimal preoperative antiischemia and antihypertension therapy as well as pharmacological and psychological attempts to decrease anxiety, which could evoke sympathetic nervous system activation with accompanying increases in systemic blood pressure and heart rate. Increased myocardial oxygen requirements resulting from the effects of sympathetic nervous system activation may manifest as myocardial ischemia that is first recognized when these patients arrive in the operating room. In many patients these ECG changes are characterized as silent ischemia, as they are not accompanied by angina pectoris or hemodynamic abnormalities. It is not clear if these episodes of silent myocardial ischemia differ from those that occur in the same patients during their normal daily activity.[30] It is possible that "new" myocardial ischemia observed during anesthesia is simply the manifestation of silent ischemia that was present before the operation.[31]

Anxiety reduction is achieved by both psychological and pharmacologic approaches. Patients are more likely to arrive in the operating room in a relaxed state if there has been a preoperative visit during which the anesthetic sequence was explained in detail. Pharmacologic sedation can be achieved with many drugs or combinations of drugs, and the choice often reflects the personal preference and experience of the anesthesiologist. The goal of drug administration is to produce maximum sedation and amnesia without undesirable degrees of circulatory and ventilatory depression. A useful approach to preoperative medication for patients with ischemic heart disease is administration of morphine, 10 to 15 mg IM, plus scopolamine, 0.4 to 0.6 mg IM, with or without an orally administered benzodiazepine. Scopolamine is valuable because of its profound sedative and amnesic effects without producing undesirable changes in heart rate.

Drugs used for medical management of patients with ischemic heart disease are continued throughout the perioperative period, including in some instances administration of these drugs with the preoperative medication.[23] Abrupt withdrawal of a β-blocker or antihypertensive drug may result in undesirable increases in sympathetic nervous system activity. Application of nitroglycerin ointment may be considered, and patients should have ready access to sublingual nitroglycerin during the period preceding anesthesia induction. Administration of H_2-receptor antagonists to patients with ischemic heart disease does not seem to produce adverse effects, although these drugs have the theoretical ability to contribute to coronary artery vasoconstriction by virtue of leaving H_1-mediated coronary artery constricting effects relatively unopposed.

Intraoperative Management

The intraoperative anesthetic techniques utilized should permit modulation of sympathetic nervous system responses and prompt control of hemodynamic variables.[17] The basic challenge during induction and maintenance of anesthesia for patients with ischemic heart disease is to prevent myocardial ischemia. This goal is logically achieved by maintaining the balance between myocardial oxygen delivery and myocardial oxygen requirements. Intraoperative events associated with persistent tachycardia, systolic hypertension, sympathetic nervous system stimulation, arterial hypoxemia, or diastolic hypotension can adversely influence this delicate balance (Table 1–3). An increase in heart rate is more likely than systemic hypertension to produce signs of myocardial ischemia on the ECG especially when the heart rate exceeds 110 beats/min (Fig. 1–1).[32] When the heart rate is less than 110 beats/min, the

Table 1–3 • Intraoperative Events that Influence the Balance Between Myocardial Oxygen Delivery and Myocardial Oxygen Requirements

Decreased oxygen delivery
  Decreased coronary blood flow
    Tachycardia
    Diastolic hypotension
    Hypocapnia (coronary artery vasoconstriction)
    Coronary artery spasm
  Decreased oxygen content
    Anemia
    Arterial hypoxemia
    Shift of the oxyhemoglobin dissociation curve to
      the left
  Increased preload (wall tension)
Increased oxygen requirements
  Sympathetic nervous system stimulation
    Tachycardia
    Systemic hypertension
    Increased myocardial contractility
    Increased afterload

incidence of myocardial ischemia is random and silent, being unrelated to heart rate. Conceptually, a rapid heart rate increases myocardial oxygen requirements and decreases the time during diastole for coronary blood flow (and thus delivery of oxygen) to occur. Conversely, increased oxygen requirements produced by systemic hypertension tend to be offset by improved perfusion through pressure-dependent atherosclerotic coronary arteries. Iatrogenic hyperventilation of the patient's lungs, which greatly decreases the $PaCO_2$, is avoided, as hypocapnia may evoke coronary artery vasoconstriction. In the final analysis, maintenance of the balance between myocardial oxygen requirements and myocardial oxygen delivery is probably more important than the specific anesthetic technique or drugs selected to produce anesthesia (isoflurane, desflurane, sevoflurane, opioids) and skeletal muscle relaxation.[31, 33, 34] Although isoflurane may cause decreased coronary vascular resistance, predisposing to coronary artery steal syndrome, there is no evidence that this drug increases the incidence of intraoperative myocardial ischemia when administered to patients with steal-prone coronary artery anatomy.[35]

It is important to avoid persistent and excessive changes in heart rate and systemic blood pressure. A common recommendation is to strive to maintain the patient's heart rate and systemic blood pressure within 20% of the normal awake value. Nevertheless, most episodes of intraoperative myocardial ischemia seen on the ECG occur in the absence of hemodynamic changes, suggesting that it is unlikely that this form of myocardial ischemia will be predictably preventable by the anesthesiologist.[26] In this regard, as many as 45% of patients are shown to have myocardial ischemia by thallium scans during tracheal intubation.[36] These episodes of silent myocardial ischemia are probably due to regional decreases in myocardial perfusion and oxygenation, which are of doubtful significance and very likely are identical to episodes that occur in these same patients during their daily activities in the absence of angina pectoris.

Induction of Anesthesia

Induction of anesthesia in patients with ischemic heart disease can be accomplished with intravenous administration of several induction drugs. Ketamine is not a likely choice because associated increases in heart rate and systemic blood pressure could transiently increase myocardial oxygen requirements. Tracheal intubation is facilitated by administration of succinylcholine or a nondepolarizing muscle relaxant.

Myocardial ischemia may accompany sympathetic nervous system stimulation that results from direct laryngoscopy and tracheal intubation. Short-duration direct laryngoscopy (15 seconds or less) may be useful for minimizing the magnitude and duration of circulatory stimulation associated with tracheal intubation. When the duration of direct laryngoscopy is not likely to be brief or when systemic hypertension already exists, it is reasonable to consider additional drugs to minimize the pressor re-

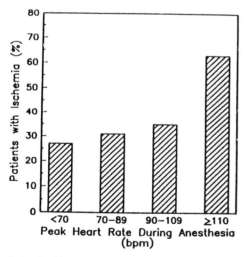

Figure 1–1 • Incidence of intraoperative myocardial ischemia is unrelated to heart rate (''silent ischemia'') until the heart rate exceeds about 110 beats/min. (From Slogoff S, Keats AS. Does chronic treatment with calcium entry blocking drugs reduce perioperative myocardial ischemia? Anesthesiology 1988;68:676–680, with permission.)

sponse produced by direct laryngoscopy and tracheal intubation. For example, laryngotracheal lidocaine, 2 mg/kg, administered just before placing the tube in the trachea, decreases the magnitude and duration of the systemic blood pressure increase evoked by direct laryngoscopy and tracheal intubation. Likewise lidocaine, 1.5 mg/kg IV, administered about 90 seconds before beginning direct laryngoscopy is efficacious in some patients. An alternative to lidocaine is nitroprusside, 1 to 2 μg/kg IV, administered 15 seconds before beginning direct laryngoscopy.[37] This dose of nitroprusside effectively attenuates the pressor but not the heart rate response to direct laryngoscopy. Continuous infusion of esmolol, 100 to 300 μg/kg/min IV, before and during direct laryngoscopy is useful for blunting the increase in heart rate evoked by tracheal intubation.[38] A small dose of fentanyl, 1 to 3 μg/kg IV (or equivalent doses of other short-acting opioids), administered before initiating direct laryngoscopy may also be useful for blunting the circulatory responses evoked by tracheal intubation. Although the rationale for these drug interventions is apparent, it must be recognized that the value and efficacy of these interventions is unknown, even in highly selected patients.

The continuous infusion of nitroglycerin, 0.25 to 1.0 μg/kg/min IV, has been used as prophylaxis against the development of coronary vasospasm in vulnerable patients. Despite the logic of this treatment, controlled studies have not consistently confirmed that this approach decreases the incidence of intraoperative myocardial ischemia.[39] The incidence of systemic hypertension, as produced by tracheal intubation is less in patients receiving a continuous infusion of nitroglycerin.[39]

Maintenance of Anesthesia

Drugs administered for maintenance of anesthesia are logically selected on the basis of the patient's presumed left ventricular function as determined by the preoperative evaluation. In patients with normal left ventricular function, tachycardia and systemic hypertension are likely to develop in response to intense stimulation, as during direct laryngoscopy or painful surgical stimulation. Controlled myocardial depression using a volatile anesthetic (isoflurane, desflurane, sevoflurane) may be useful in such patients to minimize increased sympathetic nervous system activity and subsequent increases in myocardial oxygen requirements. The volatile anesthetic may be administered alone or in combination with nitrous oxide. Equally acceptable for maintenance of anesthesia is use of a nitrous oxide–opioid technique, with addition of a volatile anesthetic to treat any undesirable increases in systemic blood pressure that may accompany painful surgical stimulation. Overall, volatile anesthetics may be beneficial in patients with ischemic heart disease by virtue of decreasing myocardial oxygen requirements, or they may be detrimental because of drug-induced decreases in systemic blood pressure and associated decreases in coronary perfusion pressure.

Patients with severely impaired left ventricular function, as associated with a prior myocardial infarction, may not tolerate anesthetic-induced myocardial depression. Short-acting opioids may be selected for these patients rather than volatile anesthetics. For severely compromised patients, a high-dose opioid (fentanyl 50 to 100 μg/kg IV or equivalent doses of other short-acting opioids) may be utilized as the sole anesthetic. The addition of nitrous oxide, benzodiazepines, or low-dose volatile anesthetic to the opioid is needed if total amnesia cannot be ensured with the opioid alone. The addition of nitrous oxide or volatile anesthetic to opioid infusions may be associated with myocardial depression, which is not present when any of these drugs is administered alone.

Regional anesthesia is an acceptable technique for patients with ischemic heart disease. Despite decreases in myocardial oxygen requirements produced by peripheral sympathetic nervous system blockade, it is important to realize that flow through coronary arteries narrowed by atherosclerosis is pressure-dependent. Therefore decreases in systemic blood pressure associated with epidural or spinal anesthesia should not be permitted to persist based on the erroneous notion that patients are protected by decreases in myocardial oxygen requirements. Prompt treatment of a decrease in systemic blood pressure that exceeds 20% of the preblock value with intravenous infusion of fluids or administration of sympathomimetic drugs such as ephedrine and/or phenylephrine is often recommended. A disadvantage of using fluid infusion to treat regional anesthesia-induced hypotension is the interval necessary for this treatment to become effective.

Choice of Muscle Relaxant

The choice of nondepolarizing muscle relaxants for administration to patients with ischemic heart disease may be influenced by the impact these drugs could have on the balance between myocardial oxygen delivery and myocardial oxygen requirements. In this regard, muscle relaxants with minimal to no effects on heart rate and systemic blood pressure (vecuronium, rocuronium, cisatracurium) are attractive choices for patients with ischemic heart disease. Histamine release and the resulting systemic blood pressure effects produced by atracurium and mivacurium are usually modest and transient, especially if the dose is administered over 30 to 45 seconds. Myocardial ischemia has been described in patients with ischemic heart disease and receiving pancuronium, presumably reflecting the usually modest increases in heart rate and systemic blood pressure produced by this drug.[40] Overall, however, pancuronium has been used without apparent adverse effects in many patients with ischemic heart disease. In fact, circulatory changes produced by pancuronium may be useful for offsetting negative inotropic and chronotropic effects of drugs used for anesthesia. This may be especially useful when the anesthesiologist considers the opioid-induced bradycardia to be excessive. The notion that coexisting β-blocker therapy prevents pancuronium-induced increases in heart rate may not be correct, as this drug most likely increases heart rate by a vagolytic, not a sympathomimetic, mechanism.

Reversal of nondepolarizing neuromuscular blockade with an anticholinesterase–anticholinergic drug combination can be safely accomplished in patients with ischemic heart disease. Glycopyrrolate, which is viewed as having minimal chronotropic effects compared with atropine, may be preferred as the anticholinergic drug if excessive increases in heart rate are a concern. Nevertheless, marked increases in heart rate rarely occur with the pharmacologic reversal of nondepolarizing muscle relaxants, and atropine seems as acceptable as glycopyrrolate for inclusion with the anticholinesterase drug.

Monitoring

Perioperative monitoring is influenced by the complexity of the operative procedure and the severity of the ischemic heart disease. An important goal when selecting monitors (ECG, pulmonary artery catheter, transesophageal echocardiography) for patients with ischemic heart disease is early detection of intraoperative myocardial ischemia (Fig. 1–2).[41] Most myocardial ischemia occurs in the absence of hemodynamic alterations; therefore one should be cautious when endorsing routine use of expensive, complex monitors to detect myocardial ischemia. Indeed, electrocardiography, pulmonary capillary wedge monitoring, and transesophageal echocardiography are acceptable methods for detecting intraoperative myocardial ischemia, but the sensitivity and specificity vary greatly.[41]

Electrocardiography

The simplest, most cost-effective method for detecting perioperative myocardial ischemia is moni-

toring the patient's ECG.[1, 41] The diagnosis of myocardial ischemia by ECG changes focuses principally on changes in the ST segment characterized as depression or elevation of at least 1 mm. T wave inversion and R wave changes are also associated with myocardial ischemia, although numerous factors (particularly electrolyte changes) can produce these changes. The depth of ST segment depression parallels the severity of myocardial ischemia. Because visual detection of ST segments changes on the ECG is unreliable, computerized analysis has been incorporated into ECG monitors.[41] This analysis of ST segment trends offers a simple, noninvasive method for detecting myocardial ischemia especially in high risk patients.

Events other than myocardial ischemia that may cause ST segment abnormalities on the ECG include cardiac dysrhythmias, cardiac conduction disturbances, digitalis therapy, electrolyte abnormalities, and hyperthermia. Nevertheless, in patients with known or suspected coronary artery disease it is reasonable for the anesthesiologist to assume that intraoperative ST segment changes represent myocardial ischemia. The occurrence of intraoperative ST segment changes in high risk patients, is linked to an increased incidence of perioperative myocardial infarction and cardiac events. Furthermore, the duration of the ST segment changes correlates positively with the incidence of perioperative myocardial infarction.

The choice of ECG leads used to monitor patients to detect significant ST segment changes recognizes that leads II and V_5 detect most of the significant ST segment changes. There is a predictable correlation between the lead of the ECG that reflects myocardial ischemia and the anatomic distribution of the diseased coronary artery (Table 1–4). For example, the V_5 lead (fifth interspace in the anterior axillary line) reflects myocardial ischemia present in that portion of the left ventricle supplied by the left anterior descending coronary artery. Lead II is more likely to reflect myocardial ischemia that occurs in the distribution of the right coronary artery. Lead II is also useful for identifying P waves and for subsequent analysis of cardiac rhythm disturbances.

Pulmonary Artery Catheter

Intraoperative myocardial ischemia may manifest as acute increases in pulmonary capillary wedge pressures owing to changes in systolic performance and ventricular compliance.[41] If myocardial ischemia is global or involves the papillary muscle, V waves are indicative of papillary muscle dysfunction and subsequent mitral regurgitation. Nonischemic causes of increased pulmonary capillary

Intraoperative Monitors for Ischemia

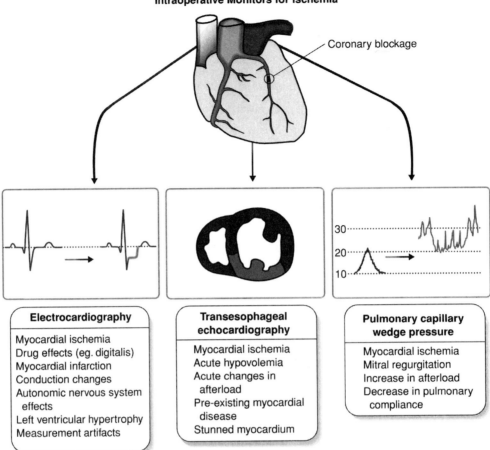

Figure 1–2 • Causes of changes characteristic of myocardial ischemia on intraoperative monitors. (From Fleisher LA. Real-time intraoperative monitoring of myocardial ischemia in noncardiac surgery. Anesthesiology 2000;92:1183–8. © 2000, Lippincott Williams & Wilkins, with permission.)

wedge pressures include acute increases in ventricular afterload, decreases in pulmonary venous compliance, and mitral regurgitation due to nonischemic mechanisms. If only small regions of myocardium become ischemic, the overall ventricular compliance and pulmonary capillary wedge pressure may remain unchanged. Furthermore, in contrast to monitoring the ECG, the pulmonary capillary wedge pressure is measured only intermittently; and the pulmonary artery end-diastolic pressure is even less sensitive than the pulmonary capillary wedge pressure for detecting a change in ventricular compliance. Rather than use the pulmonary artery catheter to monitor for intraoperative myocardial ischemia, it may be more useful to use the pulmonary capillary wedge pressure to guide treatment of myocardial

Table 1–4 • Relation of Electrocardiogram Leads to Areas of Myocardial Ischemia

ECG Lead	Coronary Artery Responsible for Ischemia	Area of Myocardium That May Be Involved
II, III, aVF	Right coronary artery	Right atrium Right ventricle Sinoatrial node Atrioventricular node
I, aVL	Circumflex coronary artery	Lateral aspects of left ventricle
V_3–V_5	Left anterior descending coronary artery	Anterolateral aspects of left ventricle

ischemia.[41] Specifically, pulmonary capillary wedge pressures can be used to guide fluid replacement. In addition to guiding volume replacement, placing a pulmonary artery catheter permits measurement of cardiac output and calculation of systemic vascular resistance, information essential for evaluating the response to vasopressors, vasodilators, and inotropic drugs.

Indications for placing a pulmonary artery catheter are influenced by the information likely to be derived versus the cost of the catheter.[42] The value of the pulmonary artery catheter for intraoperative myocardial ischemia monitoring is questionable, and it is not possible to show that use of a pulmonary artery catheter is associated with improved outcome. Nevertheless, the value and safety of pulmonary artery catheter monitoring in selected patients is widely accepted.[43] The central venous pressure and pulmonary capillary wedge pressure correlate in patients with ischemic heart disease when the ejection fraction is more than 0.5 and there is no evidence of left ventricular dysfunction.[44] Conversely, when the ejection fraction is less than 0.5, there is no longer a predictable correlation; changes in the filling pressures may even be in opposite directions.

Transesophageal Echocardiography

The development of new regional ventricular wall motion abnormalities (ventricular dysfunction), as detected by transesophageal echocardiography, is the accepted standard for the intraoperative diagnosis of myocardial ischemia.[41, 45] In patients in whom myocardial ischemia develops, regional ventricular wall motion abnormalities occur before ECG changes. In addition to myocardial ischemia, segmental wall motion abnormalities may occur in response to acute hypovolemia in patients with co-existing left ventricular dysfunction and acute increases in afterload, as accompanies acute cross-clamping of the abdominal or thoracic aorta. Limitations regarding the use of transesophageal echocardiography include its cost and the need for extensive training in its interpretation. Because the probe cannot be placed until after anesthesia induction, there is a critical period during which myocardial ischemia may develop in the absence of this monitoring. Routine monitoring of intraoperative myocardial ischemia using transesophageal echocardiography seems to have minimal additive value over analysis of ST segments on the ECG.

Intraoperative Treatment of Myocardial Ischemia

Treatment of myocardial ischemia is likely to be instituted when ST segment changes on the ECG

reach 1 mm in patients at high risk for developing myocardial ischemia. Prompt, aggressive pharmacologic treatment of changes in heart rate and/or systemic blood pressure is indicated. A persistent increase in heart rate is often treated with intravenous administration of a β-blocker such as esmolol. An excessive increase in systemic blood pressure without evidence of myocardial ischemia is often treated with nitroprusside. Nitroglycerin is a more appropriate choice when myocardial ischemia is associated with a normal to modestly elevated systemic blood pressure. In this situation nitroglycerin-induced decreases in preload facilitate improved subendocardial blood flow, but do not decrease systemic blood pressure to the point that coronary perfusion pressure is jeopardized.

Hypotension is likely to be treated with sympathomimetic drugs to restore promptly the perfusion through pressure-dependent atherosclerotic coronary arteries. A drug is often chosen that increases systemic blood pressure by increasing myocardial contractility and systemic vascular resistance. In this regard, ephedrine may be superior to a relatively pure α-adrenergic drug such as phenylephrine. Nevertheless, co-existing β-blockade may convert ephedrine to a predominantly α-agonist similar to phenylephrine. Furthermore, the dose of phenylephrine needed to constrict arteries is less than the dose needed to constrict veins, thus reducing the likelihood of drug-induced coronary artery vasoconstriction by stimulation of α-receptors in coronary arteries.

In addition to drugs, intravenous infusion of fluids to restore systemic blood pressure is useful, as myocardial oxygen requirements for volume work of the heart are less than those for pressure work. The risk of rapid infusion of fluids is increased preload, leading to decreased subendocardial perfusion and ischemia. Regardless of the treatment, it is important to realize that prompt restoration of systemic blood pressure is the goal so as to maintain pressure-dependent flow through coronary arteries narrowed by atherosclerosis.

Postoperative Period

Continuous ECG monitoring is useful for detecting postoperative myocardial ischemia, which is often asymptomatic. Postoperative myocardial ischemia predicts adverse in-hospital and long-term cardiac events.[1] Decreases in body temperature that occur intraoperatively may predispose to shivering on awakening, leading to abrupt, excessive increases in myocardial oxygen requirements. Attempts to minimize decreases in body temperature and provision of supplemental oxygen are of obvious importance. Postoperative pain may result in activation of the sympathetic nervous system, leading to increased myocardial oxygen requirements and myocardial ischemia. This emphasizes the unique importance of providing adequate postoperative pain relief to patients with ischemic heart disease. Suppression of pain is also important to facilitate deep breathing and coughing, which may decrease the likelihood of atelectasis and the development of pneumonia. In this regard, it is of interest that postoperative myocardial reinfarction often occurs 48 to 72 hours postoperatively, a period that could correspond to discontinuation of supplemental oxygen and less aggressive treatment of pain.

Adverse neurologic outcomes following CABG surgery are the result of damage to the brain, spinal cord, and peripheral nerves.[46] Central nervous system injury ranges from subtle changes in personality, behavior, and cognitive function (cognitive dysfunction is detectable in 30% to 79% of patients) to fatal brain injury.[46] It is often presumed that microemboli (air, calcium) are responsible for cerebral dysfunction following operations that require cardiopulmonary bypass. Peripheral nerve injury, especially brachial plexus stretch injuries, are not uncommon following cardiac surgery and are most likely due to stretching effects on the brachial plexus owing to the median sternotomy. Selective damage to the fibers that become the ulnar nerve may erroneously suggest compression injury to this nerve at the condylar groove following cardiac surgery.

■ HEART TRANSPLANTATION

Heart transplantation is most often utilized for patients with end-stage heart failure due to dilated cardiomyopathy or ischemic heart disease.[47] Preoperatively, the ejection fraction is often less than 0.2. Irreversible pulmonary hypertension is a contraindication to heart transplantation. In this regard, the principal indication for heart-lung transplantation is fixed pulmonary hypertension in patients with end-stage cardiac disease. Heart-lung donors are scarce, as pulmonary injury is likely in victims of fatal accidents, and tracheal intubation may predispose to pneumonia.

Management of Anesthesia

Management of anesthesia for cardiac transplantation may include ketamine and/or benzodiazepines for induction of anesthesia plus opioids to provide analgesia during surgery.[48] Alternatively, opioids may be used for induction and maintenance of anesthesia. Volatile anesthetics, especially in high doses, may produce undesirable degrees of direct myocardial depression and peripheral vasodilation. Nitrous oxide is seldom selected because of additive depressant effects in the presence of opioids and concern about enlargement of an accidental air embolus that may occur when large blood vessels are opened during the surgical procedure. Nondepolarizing neuromuscular blocking drugs with little likelihood of decreasing systemic blood pressure because of histamine release are often selected. The ability of pancuronium to increase heart rate and systemic blood pressure modestly may be desirable in these patients. Airway equipment, including the anesthetic delivery tubing, is sterile and handled using aseptic techniques. Bacterial filters may be placed on the inhalation and exhalation limbs of the anesthetic delivery tubing. Many patients undergoing heart transplantation have abnormal coagulation, reflecting passive congestion of the liver due to chronic congestive heart failure.

The operative technique consists of cardiopulmonary bypass and anastomosis of the aorta, pulmonary artery, and left and right atria. Immunosuppressive drugs (cyclosporine, azathioprine, corticosteroids) are usually initiated during the preoperative period. Intravascular catheters are placed using aseptic techniques. It is necessary to withdraw the central venous pressure catheter or pulmonary artery catheter back into the internal jugular vein when the recipient's heart is removed. The catheter is then repositioned with the donor heart in place. Placing of these catheters into the central circulation through the left internal jugular vein leaves the right internal jugular vein available as an access site to perform cardiac biopsies during the postoperative period.

After cessation of cardiopulmonary bypass, an inotropic drug such as isoproterenol may be needed briefly to maintain myocardial contractility and heart rate. Therapeutic attempts to lower pulmonary vascular resistance may be necessary and include administration of isoproterenol or vasodilating prostaglandin preparations.[49] The denervated transplanted heart initially assumes an intrinsic heart rate of about 110 beats/min, reflecting the absence of normal vagal tone. Stroke volume responds to augmented preload by the Frank-Starling mechanism, emphasizing that these patients tolerate hypovolemia poorly. The transplanted heart responds to direct-acting catecholamines (may be even more sensitive than normal hearts); drugs that act by indirect mechanisms (ephedrine) have less intense effects. The heart rate is not likely to change in response to administration of anticholinergic or anticholinesterase drugs.

Postoperative Complications

Early postoperative morbidity following heart transplant surgery is most often related to sepsis and rejection. The most common early cause of death after heart transplantation is opportunistic infection, reflecting immunosuppressive therapy. Transvenous right ventricular endomyocardial biopsies are performed to provide early warning of otherwise clinically asymptomatic allograft rejection. The onset of congestive heart failure and the development of cardiac dysrhythmias are late signs of severe transplant rejection. Chronic cyclosporine treatment is associated with drug-induced systemic hypertension that is often resistant to antihypertensive therapy.[50] Nephrotoxicity is also associated with cyclosporine therapy. Chronic corticosteroid use may result in skeletal demineralization (osteoporosis, aseptic necrosis of weight-bearing joints) and glucose intolerance.

Late complications include the development of allograft coronary artery disease and an increased incidence of cancer.[47] Diffuse obliterative coronary arteriopathy affects increasing numbers of cardiac transplant recipients over time, and its ischemic sequelae comprise the principal limitation for long-term survival. The disease is restricted to the allograft and is present in about 50% of recipients after 5 years. The accelerated appearance of coronary artery disease may reflect a chronic rejection process taking place in the endothelium of the allograft's arteries. This process is not unique to cardiac allografts and is thought to be analogous to the chronic immunologically mediated changes seen in other organ allografts (chronic rejection of the kidney, obliterative bronchiolitis in the lungs, vanishing bile duct syndrome in the liver). The clinical sequelae of this obliterative disease reflect myocardial ischemia with its attendant left ventricular dysfunction, cardiac dysrhythmias, and sudden death. The prognosis for transplant recipients with angiographically established coronary artery disease is poor, especially after an ischemic event.

Any medical regimen involving long-term immunosuppression is associated with an increased incidence of cancer, especially lymphoproliferative disease and cutaneous cancers. Malignancy is responsible for a significant portion of mortality in heart transplant patients. Most posttransplantation lymphoproliferative disease is related to infection with the Epstein-Barr virus.[47]

Anesthetic Considerations in Heart Transplant Recipients

Heart transplant patients present unique anesthesia issues related to the pharmacodynamic behavior and hemodynamic function of the transplanted and denervated heart, side effects of immunosuppression, risk of infection, possible drug interactions with complex drug therapies, and the potential for allograft rejection.[51,52] If epidural or spinal anesthesia is planned, clotting studies and platelet counts are likely to be considered. Allograft rejection results in progressive deterioration of cardiac function and is the main cause of late mortality in heart transplant patients. The presence of infection should always be ruled out preoperatively, as infection is a significant cause of morbidity and mortality following heart transplantation. Upper gastrointestinal bleeding may be present, and hepatobiliary and pancreatic dysfunction are relatively common after heart transplantation. Perioperative invasive monitoring requires fully aseptic techniques and should be selected in terms of the risk/benefit ratio. When hepatic and renal function are normal, there is no contraindication to the use of any anesthetic drug.[52]

Cardiac Innervation

The transplanted heart has no sympathetic, parasympathetic, or sensory innervation; and the loss of vagal influences results in a higher than normal resting heart rate.[52] Unpredictable reinnervation of the transplanted heart may occur. There are two P waves on the ECG after heart transplantation. The native pacemaker remains intact in individuals in whom a cuff of atrium is left to permit surgical anastomosis to the grafted heart. Because the native P wave cannot traverse the suture line, it has no influence on the chronotropic activity of the heart. Carotid sinus massage and the Valsalva maneuver have no effect on the heart rate. There is no sympathetic nervous system response to direct laryngoscopy and tracheal intubation, and the denervated heart may have a more blunted heart rate response to inadequate depths of anesthesia or analgesia. The transplanted heart is unable to increase its heart rate acutely in response to hypovolemia or hypotension but responds acutely instead with an increase in stroke volume (classic Frank–Starling mechanism).[47] The subsequent increases in cardiac output are dependent on venous return until the heart rate increases after about 5 to 6 minutes in response to circulating catecholamines. Because α- and β-adrenergic receptors remain intact, the transplanted heart eventually responds to circulating catecholamines.

Cardiac dysrhythmias may occur in heart transplant patients perhaps reflecting a lack of vagal innervation and/or increased circulating concentrations of endogenous catecholamines. At rest, the patient's heart rate reflects the intrinsic rate of depolarization at the donor sinoatrial node in the absence of any vagal tone. First-degree atrioventricular heart block is common following heart transplantation, and some patients require an external artificial cardiac pacemaker for treatment of bradydysrhythmias. A surgical transplant technique that preserves the anatomic integrity of the right atrium by using anastomoses at the level of the superior and inferior vena cava rather than at the midatrial level results in better preservation of tricuspid valve function and sinoatrial node function. Afferent denervation typically renders the patient incapable of experiencing the subjective sensation of angina pectoris in response to myocardial ischemia, although there is some evidence that limited sympathetic nervous system reinnervation of the transplanted heart does occur.[53]

Responses to Drugs

Catecholamine responses are different in the recipient's transplanted heart, as intact sympathetic nerves are required for normal uptake and metabolism of catecholamines.[52] Receptor density in the transplanted heart seems unchanged, however, and responses to direct-acting sympathomimetic drugs are intact. Epinephrine has an augmented inotropic effect in transplanted hearts. Dopamine's inotropic effects are principally due to release of norepinephrine; and in denervated hearts the resulting effects are principally dopaminergic with a less effective inotropic effect than in normal hearts, whereas isoproterenol and dobutamine have similar effects in both normal and denervated hearts. Indirect-acting sympathomimetics such as ephedrine have blunted effects on denervated hearts.

Vagolytic effects of drugs such as atropine are ineffective for increasing the heart rate, and a positive inotropic drug such as isoproterenol may be needed. Pancuronium does not increase the heart rate. Neostigmine usually has no chronotropic effect on denervated hearts.

Preoperative Evaluation

Heart transplant recipients may present with ongoing rejection manifesting as myocardial dysfunction, accelerated coronary atherosclerosis, or cardiac dysrhythmias. All preoperative drug therapy is continued; and proper functioning of an external pacemaker, if in place, is confirmed. Cyclosporine-induced systemic hypertension may require treatment, which may include calcium channel-blocking drugs or ACE inhibitors. The serum creatinine concentration may be increased as evidence of cyclosporine-induced nephrotoxicity. Anesthetic drugs excreted mainly by renal clearance mechanisms may be avoided. Adequate intravascular fluid volume is important to confirm preoperatively, as heart transplant patients are preload-dependent.

Management of Anesthesia

Experience suggests that heart transplant patients undergoing subsequent noncardiac surgery have monitoring and anesthetic requirements (inhaled and intravenous anesthetics) similar to those of nontransplant patients undergoing the same procedures.[51] Adequate intravascular fluid volume is important to maintain intraoperatively because these patients are preload-dependent and the denervated heart is unable to respond promptly with a compensatory increase in heart rate to sudden shifts in blood volume. Invasive hemodynamic monitoring is a consideration if the planned surgical procedure is associated with the potential for large intravascular fluid volume shifts. Transesophageal echocardiography may be an alternative to invasive monitoring (central venous catheter, pulmonary artery catheter) in these patients. General anesthesia is usually selected, as there is a possibility of impaired responses to hypotension after spinal or epidural anesthesia. Goals of anesthesia include avoidance of significant vasodilation and acute decreases in preload. Although volatile anesthetics may produce direct myocardial depression, they are usually well tolerated in heart transplant patients who do not present with significant degrees of heart failure.[52] Despite reports of cyclosporine-induced enhanced neuromuscular blockade, it does not appear that these patients have dose requirements for muscle relaxants that differ from those of nontransplant patients. It seems prudent to exercise appropriate aseptic techniques in these patients in view of their likely increased susceptibility to infection.

References

1. Mangano D, Goldman L. Preoperative assessment of patients with known or suspected coronary disease. N Engl J Med 1995;333:1750–7
2. O'Malley PG, Jones DL, Feuerstein IM, et al. Lack of correlation between psychological factors and subclinical coronary artery disease. N Engl J Med 2000;343:1298–304
3. Fenster PE, Sox HC, Alpert J. Ischemic heart disease: angina pectoris. Sci Am Med 2000;1–16
4. Yeghizarians Y, Braunstein JB, Askari A, et al. Unstable angina pectoris. N Engl J Med 2000;342:101–13

5. Bhatt DL, Topol EJ. Current role of platelet glycoprotein IIb/IIIa inhibitors in acute coronary syndromes. JAMA 2000; 284:1549–58

6. Gottlieb SS, McCarter RJ, Vogel RA. Effect of beta-blockade on mortality among high-risk and low-risk patients after myocardial infarction. N Engl J Med 1998;339:489–97

7. Parker JD, Parker JO. Nitrate therapy for stable angina pectoris. N Engl J Med 1998;338:520–31

8. Suwaidi JA, Berger PB, Holmes DR. Coronary artery stents. JAMA 2000;284:1828–36

9. Berger PB. Acute myocardial infarction. Sci Am Med 2000; 1–16

10. Packard CJ, O'Reilly DSJ, Caslake MJ, et al. Lipoprotein-associated phospholipase A₂ as an independent predictor of coronary heart disease. N Engl J Med 2000;343:1148–55

11. Lindahl B, Toss H, Siegbahn A, et al. Markers of myocardial damage and inflammation in relation to long-term mortality in unstable coronary artery disease. N Engl J Med 2000; 343:1139–47

12. Schomig A, Kastrati A, Dirschinger J, et al. Coronary stenting plus platelet glycoprotein IIb/IIIa blockade compared with tissue plasminogen activator in acute myocardial infarction. N Engl J Med 2000;343:385–91

13. Goldberg RJ, Gore JM, Alpert JS, et al. Cardiogenic shock after acute myocardial infarction: incidence and mortality from a community-wide perspective, 1975–1988. N Engl J Med 1991;325:1117–22

14. Kinch JW, Ryan TJ. Right ventricular infarction. N Engl J Med 1994;330:1211–7

15. Wong T, Detsky AS. Preoperative cardiac risk assessment for patients having peripheral vascular surgery. Ann Intern Med 1992;116:743–53

16. Lee TH, Marcantonio ER, Mangione CM, et al. Derivation and prospective validation of a simple index for prediction of cardiac risk of major noncardiac surgery. Circulation 1999;100:1043–9

17. Muir AD, Reeder MK, Foex P, et al. Perioperative silent myocardial ischemia: incidence and predictors in a general surgical population. Br J Anaesth 1991;67:373–7

18. Rao TLK, Jacobs EH, El-Etr AA. Reinfarction following anesthesia in patients with myocardial infarction undergoing noncardiac operations. Anesth Analg 1991;71:231–5

19. Shah KB, Kleinman BS, Sami H, et al. Reevaluation of perioperative myocardial infarction in patients with prior myocardial infarction undergoing noncardiac operations. Anesth Analg 1991;71:231–5

20. Slogoff S, Keats AS. Does perioperative myocardial ischemia lead to postoperative myocardial infarction? Anesthesiology 1985;62:107–14

21. Reves JG, Kissin I, Lell WA, et al. Calcium entry blockers: uses and implications for anesthesiologists. Anesthesiology 1982;57:504–18

22. Merin RG. Calcium channel blocking drugs and anesthetics: is the drug interaction beneficial or detrimental? Anesthesiology 1987;66:111–3

23. Henling CE, Slogoff S, Kodali SV, et al. Heart block after coronary artery bypass-effect of chronic administration of calcium-entry blockers and beta-blockers. Anesth Analg 1984;63:515–20

24. Durant NN, Kraynack BJ, Gintautas J. Neuromuscular and electrocardiographic responses to verapamil in dogs. Anesth Analg 1983;62:50–4

25. Alpert JS. Approach to the cardiac patient. Sci Am Med 2000;1–8

26. Mangano DT. Perioperative cardiac morbidity. Anesthesiology 1990;72:153–84

27. Epstein SE, Quyyumi AA, Bonow RO. Myocardial ischemia: silent or symptomatic. N Engl J Med 1988;318:1038–43

28. Baron J-F, Mundler O, Bertrand M, et al. Dipyridamole-thallium scintigraphy and gated radionuclide angiography to assess cardiac risk before abdominal aortic surgery. N Engl J Med 1994;330:663–9

29. Hollenberg M, Mangano DT, Browner WS, et al. Predictors of postoperative myocardial ischemia in patients undergoing noncardiac surgery. JAMA 1992;268:205–9

30. DeBono DP, Rose EL. Silent myocardial ischemia in preoperative patients: what does it mean, and what should be done about it? Br J Anaesth 1986;65:539–42

31. Slogoff S, Keats AS. Randomized trial of primary anesthetic agents on outcome of coronary artery bypass operations. Anesthesiology 1989;70:179–88

32. Slogoff S, Keats AS. Does chronic treatment with calcium entry blocking drugs reduce perioperative myocardial ischemia? Anesthesiology 1988;68:676–80

33. Tuman K, McCarthy R, Spies B, et al. Does choice of anesthetic agent significantly affect outcome after coronary artery surgery? Anesthesiology 1989;70:189–98

34. Leung JM, Goehner P, O'Kelly BF, et al. Isoflurane anesthesia and myocardial ischemia: comparative risk versus sufentanil anesthesia in patients undergoing coronary artery bypass graft surgery. Anesthesiology 1991;74:838–47

35. Slogoff S, Keats AS, Dear WE, et al. Steal-prone coronary anatomy and myocardial ischemia associated with four primary anesthetic agents in humans. Anesth Analg 1991; 72:22–7

36. Kleinman B, Henkin RE, Glisson SN, et al. Qualitative evaluation of coronary flow during anesthetic induction using thallium-201 perfusion scans. Anesthesiology 1986;64:157–64

37. Stoelting RK. Attenuation of blood pressure response to laryngoscopy and tracheal intubation with sodium nitroprusside. Anesth Analg 1979;58:116–9

38. Menkhaus PG, Reves JG, Kissin I, et al. Cardiovascular effects of esmolol in anesthetized humans. Anesth Analg 1985; 64:327–34

39. Gallagher JD, Moore RA, Jose AB, et al. Prophylactic nitroglycerin infusions during coronary artery bypass surgery. Anesthesiology 1986;64:785–9

40. Thomson IR, Putnins CL. Adverse effects of pancuronium during high-dose fentanyl anesthesia for coronary artery bypass grafting. Anesthesiology 1985;62:708–13

41. Fleisher LA. Real-time intraoperative monitoring of myocardial ischemia in noncardiac surgery. Anesthesiology 2000; 92:1183–8

42. Practice guidelines for pulmonary artery catheterization: a report by the American Society of Anesthesiologists Task Force on Pulmonary Artery Catheterization. Anesthesiology 1993;78:380–94

43. Murdoch SD, Cohen AT, Bellamy MC. Pulmonary artery catheterization and mortality in critically ill patients. Br J Anaesth 2000;85:611–5

44. Mangano DT. Monitoring pulmonary artery pressure in coronary artery disease. Anesthesiology 1980;53:364–70

45. Practice guidelines for perioperative transesophageal echocardiography: a report by the American Society of Anesthesiologists and the Society of Cardiovascular Anesthesiologists Task Force on Transesophageal Echocardiography. Anesthesiology 1996;84:986–1006

46. Arrowsmith JE, Grocott HP, Reves JG, et al. Central nervous system complications of cardiac surgery. Br J Anaesth 2000; 84:378–93

47. Hunt SA. Current status of cardiac transplantation. JAMA 1998;280:1692–8

48. Demas K, Wyner J, Mihm FG, et al. Anaesthesia for heart transplantation: a retrospective study and review. Br J Anaesth 1986;58:1357–64

49. Casella ES, Humphrey LS. Bronchospasm after cardiopulmonary bypass in a heart-lung- transplant recipient. Anesthesiology 1988;69:135–8

50. Scherrer U, Vissing SF, Morgan BJ, et al. Cyclosporine-induced sympathetic activation and hypertension after heart transplantation. N Engl J Med 1990;323:693–9

51. Cheng DCH. Anaesthesia for noncardiac surgery in heart-transplanted patients. Can J Anaesth 1993;40:981–6

52. Kostopanagiotou G, Smyrniotis V, Arkadopoulos N, et al. Anesthetic and perioperative management of adult transplant recipients in nontransplant surgery. Anesth Analg 1999;89:613–22

53. Stark RP, McGinn AL, Wilson RF. Chest pain in cardiac-transplant recipients: evidence of sensory reinnervation after cardiac transplantation. N Engl J Med 1991;324:1791–4

2

Valvular Heart Disease

Improvements in the prognosis of patients with valvular heart disease most likely reflect more effective noninvasive monitoring of ventricular function, improved prosthetic heart valves, advances in cardiac valve reconstruction techniques, and the development of guidelines for selecting the proper timing for surgical intervention.[1, 2] Furthermore, advances in minimally invasive surgical techniques may make cardiac valve procedures more easily tolerated by patients.

Valvular heart disease places a hemodynamic burden on the left and/or right ventricle that is initially tolerated as the cardiovascular system compensates for the overload. Hemodynamic overload eventually leads to cardiac muscle dysfunction, congestive heart failure, and sometimes sudden death. It is important to determine if the cardiac valvular disease is severe enough to cause morbidity and mortality; and if so, to determine the optimal medical therapy and the best time for surgical intervention to minimize morbidity.[1]

Management of the patient with valvular heart disease during the perioperative period requires an understanding of the hemodynamic alterations that accompany dysfunction of the cardiac valves. The most frequently encountered cardiac valve lesions produce pressure overloads (mitral stenosis, aortic stenosis) or volume overloads (mitral regurgitation, aortic regurgitation) on the left atrium or left ventricle. Drug selection during the perioperative period for patients with valvular heart disease is based on the likely effects of drug-induced changes in cardiac rhythm, heart rate, systemic blood pressure, systemic vascular resistance, and pulmonary vascular resistance relative to the pathophysiology of the heart disease.

▌PREOPERATIVE EVALUATION

Preoperative evaluation of patients with valvular heart disease includes assessment of (1) the severity of the cardiac disease; (2) the degree of impaired myocardial contractility; and (3) the presence of associated major organ system disease (pulmonary, renal, hepatic). Recognition of compensatory mechanisms for maintaining cardiac output (increased sympathetic nervous system activity, cardiac hypertrophy) and consideration of drug therapy are important. This information can be obtained from the history and physical examination and a review of laboratory data. The presence of a prosthetic heart valve introduces special considerations to the preoperative evaluation of patients, especially when noncardiac surgery is planned.

History and Physical Examination

Questions designed to define the patient's exercise tolerance are useful for evaluating cardiac reserve in the presence of valvular heart disease. In this regard it may be helpful to classify patients according to the criteria established by the New York Heart Association (Table 2–1). Congestive heart failure (CHF) is a frequent companion of chronic valvular heart disease. When myocardial contractility is impaired, patients may complain of dyspnea, orthopnea, and fatigability. A compensatory increase in sympathetic nervous system activity may manifest as anxiety, diaphoresis, and resting tachycardia. In support of the diagnosis of CHF is the presence of basilar chest rales, jugular venous distension, and a third heart sound, as determined on physical examination. Ideally, elective surgery is deferred until CHF can be treated and myocardial contractility optimized.

Disease of a cardiac valve rarely occurs without an accompanying murmur, reflecting turbulent blood flow across the valve. The character, location, intensity, and direction of radiation of a heart murmur provide a clue to the location and severity of the cardiac valve lesion (Fig. 2–1).[3] During systole the aortic and pulmonic valves are open, and the mitral and tricuspid valves are closed. Therefore a heart murmur that occurs during systole is due to stenosis of the aortic or pulmonic valves or incompetence of the mitral or tricuspid valves. During diastole the aortic and pulmonic valves are closed, and the mitral and tricuspid valves are open. Therefore a heart murmur during diastole is due to stenosis of the mitral or tricuspid valves or incompetence of the aortic or pulmonic valves.

Cardiac dysrhythmias are seen with all types of valvular heart disease. Atrial fibrillation is the most common with rheumatic mitral valve disease associated with enlargement of the left atrium. Initially, atrial fibrillation is paroxysmal, but after several years this cardiac dysrhythmia often becomes persistent.

Angina pectoris may occur in patients with valvular heart disease, even in the absence of ischemic heart disease. It reflects increased myocardial oxygen demand due to increased cardiac muscle mass that exceeds the ability of even normal coronary arteries to deliver adequate amounts of oxygen. Furthermore, valvular heart disease and ischemic heart disease frequently co-exist. Indeed, 50% of patients with aortic stenosis who are older than 50 years of age have associated ischemic heart disease. The presence of coronary artery disease in patients with mitral or aortic valve disease worsens the long-term prognosis. Mitral regurgitation due to ischemic heart disease is associated with increased mortality.[1]

Drug Therapy

Drug therapy in patients with valvular heart disease is likely to include digitalis preparations and diuret-

---

| ▬ **Table 2–1** • New York Heart Association |
| ▬ Classification of Patients with Heart Disease |

Class	Description
I	Asymptomatic
II	Symptoms with ordinary activity but comfortable at rest
III	Symptoms with minimal activity but comfortable at rest
IV	Symptoms at rest

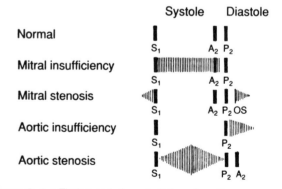

Figure 2–1 • Timing and characteristics of cardiac murmurs in relation to systole and diastole. (From Fishman MC, Hoffman AR, Klausner RD, et al. Medicine. Philadelphia, JB Lippincott, 1981, p 42, with permission.)

ics. Digitalis is most often administered to increase myocardial contractility and to slow ventricular heart rate responses in patients with atrial fibrillation. Slowing the ventricular heart rate response prolongs the duration of diastole and thus improves left ventricular filling. An adequate digitalis effect for heart rate control is indicated by ventricular heart rates slower than 80 beats/min at rest that increases no more than 15 beats/min with mild physical activity. In the absence of adequate preoperative heart rate control, activation of the sympathetic nervous system, as during tracheal intubation or in response to surgical stimulation, may adversely increase the heart rate with subsequent decreases in the diastolic filling time and stroke volume. Digitalis toxicity is suggested by prolongation of the PR intervals on the electrocardiogram (ECG), as well as by patient complaints related to gastrointestinal dysfunction. Vulnerability to the development of digitalis toxicity is increased when concomitant diuretic therapy has led to total body depletion of potassium.

Laboratory Data

The ECG often exhibits characteristic changes due to valvular heart disease. For example, broad and notched P waves suggest the presence of left atrial enlargement typical of mitral stenosis. Ventricular hypertrophy is mirrored by the presence of left or right axis deviation on the ECG. The size and shape of the heart and great vessels and vascular markings in the lungs are evaluated on chest radiographs. On posteroanterior chest radiographs, heart size should not exceed 50% of the internal width of the thoracic cage. The shadow of the left heart border from above downward represents the aorta, pulmonary artery, left atrium, and left ventricle; on the right side the shadow is due to the superior vena cava and right atrium. Enlargement of the left atrium can result in elevation of the left bronchus and an increase in the angle of the carina to more than 90 degrees. Vascular markings in the peripheral lungs fields may be sparse in the presence of severe pulmonary hypertension.

Valvular heart disease can interfere with oxygenation and ventilation, as reflected by measurements of arterial blood gases and pH. For example, chronic increases in left atrial pressure are reflected back into the pulmonary veins and eventually into the lung interstitium. These changes can produce an alteration in the relation of the ventilation-to-perfusion matching and the development of pulmonary edema leading to decreases in PaO_2.

Transvalvular pressure gradients determined at the time of cardiac catheterization provide useful information about the severity of the valvular heart disease. Mitral and aortic stenoses are considered to be present when transvalvular pressure gradients are more than 10 mmHg and 50 mmHg, respectively. These limits are valid only in the absence of CHF. For example, when CHF accompanies aortic stenosis, transvalvular pressure gradients of only 20 mmHg signify severe valvular heart disease. The magnitude of V waves on tracings of the pulmonary artery occlusion pressures can be a clinically useful measure of the severity of mitral regurgitation (Fig. 2–2).[4] In patients with mitral stenosis or mitral regurgitation, measurements of pulmonary artery pressures and right ventricular filling pressures may provide evidence of pulmonary hypertension and right ventricular failure. Coronary artery angiography may provide evidence of ischemic heart disease in patients with valvular heart disease. Indeed, mitral regurgitation secondary to papillary muscle dysfunction may reflect myocardial ischemia or a prior myocardial infarction.

Doppler echocardiography is essential for noninvasive evaluation of valvular heart disease (Table 2–2). Echocardiography is particularly useful for evaluating the significance of systolic ejection murmurs in suspected aortic stenosis and for detecting the presence of mitral stenosis. This technique permits both determination of the valve orifice area and assessment of the transvalvular pressure gradients. Doppler echocardiography with color flow mapping allows assessment of the magnitude of valvular regurgitation.

Presence of Prosthetic Heart Valves

Prosthetic heart valves may be mechanical or bioprosthetic.[5] Mechanical valves, composed primarily of metal or carbon alloys, are classified according to their structure, such as caged-ball, single tilting disk, or bileaflet tilting disk valves. Bioprostheses may be heterografts, composed of porcine or bovine tissues mounted on metal supports, or homografts, which are preserved human aortic valves.

Prosthetic valves differ from one another with regard to durability (longevity), thrombogenicity, and hemodynamic profile. Mechanical valves are highly durable, most lasting at least 20 to 30 years, whereas bioprosthetic valves often fail within 10 to 15 years and require replacement. Mechanical valves are thrombogenic and therefore require long-term anticoagulant therapy. Because bioprosthetic valves have a low thrombogenic potential, long-term anticoagulation is not required in these pa-

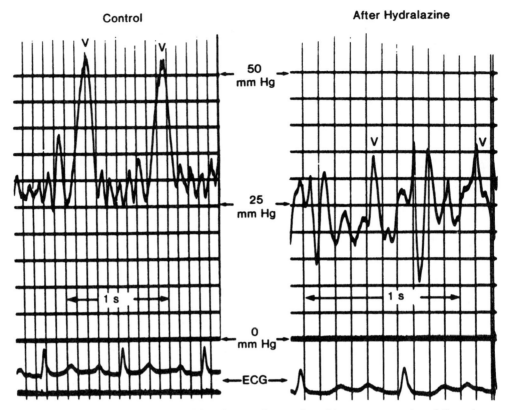

Figure 2–2 • Regurgitant blood flow into the left atrium produces a large V wave on a tracing of the pulmonary artery occlusion pressure from a patient with mitral regurgitation. Administration of a vasodilator (hydralazine) decreases resistance to forward ejection of the left ventricular stroke volume. As a result, the volume of regurgitant flow into the left atrium is less, and the magnitude of the V wave is decreased. (From Greenberg BH, Rahimtoola SH. Vasodilator therapy for valvular heart disease. JAMA 1981;246:269–72, with permission.)

tients. Mechanical valves are preferred for patients who are young or have a life expectancy of more than 10 to 15 years and for those who require long-term anticoagulation therapy for other reasons, such as atrial fibrillation. Bioprosthetic valves are preferred in patients who are elderly or who cannot take long-term anticoagulation medications.

Table 2–2 • Doppler Echocardiography and Valvular Heart Disease

Determine significance of cardiac murmurs (most often aortic stenosis)
Identify hemodynamic abnormalities associated with physical findings (most often mitral regurgitation)
Determine transvalvular pressure gradient
Determine orifice area of cardiac valve
Determine ventricular ejection fraction
Diagnose cardiac valve regurgitation
Evaluate prosthetic cardiac valve function

Assessment of Prosthetic Heart Valve Function

Prosthetic heart valve dysfunction is suggested by changes in the intensity or quality of previously audible sounds, the appearance of a new murmur, or changes in the characteristics of existing murmurs.[5] For patients in whom prosthetic valve dysfunction is suspected, cinefluoroscopy is a rapid, inexpensive technique for evaluating mechanical valve function, although it cannot visualize the leaflets of bioprosthetic valves. Transthoracic echocardiography can be used to assess sewing ring stability and leaflet motion of bioprosthetic valves, but mechanical valves may be difficult to visualize because of echo reverberations from the metal. Transesophageal echocardiography provides a higher resolution image and is utilized whenever dysfunction of prosthetic mitral valves is suspected. Magnetic resonance imaging is used if prosthetic valve regurgitation or paravalvular leakage is suspected but not adequately visualized by echocardiography. Cardiac catheterization permits measurement of transvalvular pressure gradients across bioprosthetic valves, and the effective orifice area can be calculated from this information.

Complications Associated with Prosthetic Heart Valves

The presence of prosthetic heart valves introduces the possibility of significant associated complications that may have to be considered during the preoperative evaluation of patients (Table 2–3).[5] Because of the risk of thromboembolism, patients with mechanical prosthetic heart valves require long-term anticoagulant therapy. Subclinical intravascular hemolysis, evidenced by increased serum lactic dehydrogenase concentrations, decreased serum haptoglobin concentrations, and reticulocytosis, is noted in most patients with normally functioning mechanical prosthetic heart valves. The incidence of cholecystitis is increased in patients with prosthetic heart valves, presumably reflecting chronic low-grade intravascular hemolysis. Severe hemolytic anemia is uncommon and when present usually indicates paravalvular leakage due to partial dehiscence of the valve or endocarditis. Antibiotic prophylaxis may be recommended for patients with prosthetic heart valves undergoing a dental or surgical procedure to decrease the risk of endocarditis.

Management of Anticoagulation in Patients with Prosthetic Heart Valves

Anticoagulation can be continued in patients with prosthetic heart valves who are scheduled for minor surgery such as dental extractions in which blood loss is expected to be minimal.[5] When major surgical procedures with significant blood loss are planned, it is common to discontinue warfarin 3 to 5 days preoperatively in an effort to minimize perioperative bleeding. In patients with mechanical prosthetic heart valves it is recommended that intravenous heparin be administered following discontinuation of the warfarin and up until 2 to 4 hours before surgery. Postoperatively, heparin therapy is resumed and continued until effective anticoagulation is achieved with oral therapy.

Table 2–3 • Complications Associated with Prosthetic Heart Valves

Valve thrombosis
Systemic embolization
Structural failure of bioprosthetic valves
Hemolysis
Paravalvular regurgitation
Endocarditis

Anticoagulant therapy is particularly important during pregnancy in parturients with prosthetic heart valves, as the incidence of systemic embolization is greatly increased.[3] Warfarin administration during the first trimester of pregnancy is associated with embryopathy and fetal death. For this reason, warfarin is discontinued when pregnancy is a possibility, and subcutaneous heparin is administered until delivery. Low-dose aspirin therapy is safe for the mother and child and may be used in conjunction with anticoagulant therapy in women at high risk for thromboembolism.

▌ MITRAL STENOSIS

Mitral stenosis, a sequela of rheumatic heart disease, primarily affects females.[1] Patients with mitral stenosis typically exhibit dyspnea on exertion, orthopnea, and paroxysmal nocturnal dyspnea as evidence of left ventricular dysfunction, although left ventricular contractility is usually normal in patients with mitral stenosis. When aortic and/or mitral regurgitation accompany mitral stenosis, there is likely to be evidence of left ventricular dysfunction, as reflected by increased left ventricular end-diastolic pressure.

Pathophysiology

Mitral stenosis is characterized by mechanical obstruction to left ventricular diastolic filling secondary to progressive decreases in the orifice of the mitral valve. This valvular obstruction produces increases in left atrial volumes and pressures. Left ventricular filling and stroke volume in the presence of mild mitral stenosis are usually maintained at rest by increased left atrial pressures. Stroke volume, however, may decrease during stress-induced tachycardia or when an effective atrial contraction is lost, as during atrial fibrillation.

Pulmonary venous pressure is increased in association with increased left atrial pressure. The result is transudation of fluid into the pulmonary interstitial space, decreased pulmonary compliance, and increased work of breathing, leading to progressive dyspnea on exertion. Overt pulmonary edema is likely when the pulmonary venous pressure exceeds the oncotic pressure of plasma proteins. If increases in the pressures are gradual, however, there is a concomitant increase in lymphatic drainage from the lungs; and thickening of capillary basement membranes enables patients to tolerate increased pulmonary venous pressures without the development of pulmonary edema.

Diagnosis

Echocardiography is the premier noninvasive diagnostic tool for assessing the severity of mitral stenosis and for judging the applicability of balloon mitral valvotomy. Echocardiography can be used to calculate valve area and the severity of the stenosis. Patients are likely to become symptomatic when the size of the mitral valve orifice (4 to 6 cm^2) has decreased at least 50%. When the mitral valve area is less than 1 cm^2, a mean atrial pressure of about 25 mmHg is necessary to maintain an adequate resting cardiac output. Pulmonary hypertension is likely when the left atrial pressure is chronically increased above 25 mmHg. When the transvalvular pressure gradient is higher than 10 mmHg (normal less than 5 mmHg) it is likely that the mitral stenosis is severe. When it is severe, the addition of stress such as sepsis, atrial fibrillation, pulmonary embolism, or pregnancy may precipitate acute decompensation, most often manifesting as pulmonary edema.

Clinically, mitral stenosis is recognized by the characteristic opening snap that occurs early during diastole and by a rumbling diastolic heart murmur best heard at the cardiac apex (Fig. 2–1).[5] The opening snap is caused by vibrations set in motion when the mobile but stenosed valve initially opens. Calcification of the valve may result in disappearance of the opening snap. Left atrial enlargement is often visible on chest radiographs as straightening of the left heart border, widening of the carinal angle, and displacement of a barium-filled esophagus on a lateral view. There may be evidence of pulmonary edema on chest radiographs. In the absence of atrial fibrillation, large biphasic P waves on the ECG suggest left atrial enlargement. Atrial fibrillation is present in about one-third of patients with severe mitral stenosis, occurring most often when the left atrium is greatly enlarged. Stasis of blood in the distended left atrium predisposes to the formation of thrombi, especially with the onset of atrial fibrillation. Venous thrombosis is also encouraged by the low cardiac output and decreased physical activity characteristic of these patients.

Treatment

Prophylaxis against infective endocarditis is the only medical therapy for mitral stenosis that is utilized in asymptomatic patients in normal sinus rhythm.[1] When mild symptoms of mitral stenosis develop, diuretics usually decrease the left atrial pressure and relieve symptoms. If atrial fibrillation develops, heart rate control may be achieved with digoxin, β-blockers, or calcium channel-blocking drugs. Control of the heart rate is critical, as tachycardia further impairs left ventricular filling and increases left atrial pressure. Anticoagulant therapy is required in patients with mitral stenosis and atrial fibrillation, as the risk of systemic embolization is greatly increased.

Surgical correction of mitral stenosis is indicated when symptoms increase or evidence of pulmonary hypertension develops.[1] Catheter balloon valvotomy often provides mechanical relief at this time in the progression of the disease. In the presence of heavy valvular calcification the treatment is open commissurotomy, valve reconstruction, or mitral valve replacement.

Management of Anesthesia

Management of anesthesia for noncardiac surgery in patients with mitral stenosis includes avoidance of events that may further decrease the cardiac output (Table 2–4). The development of atrial fibrillation with rapid ventricular response rates may significantly decrease cardiac output and produce pulmonary edema. Treatment consists of cardioversion starting with 25 watt/sec or, alternatively, intravenous administration of β-antagonists such as esmolol to decrease the heart rate to less than 110 beats/min. Digoxin, 0.25 to 0.50 mg IV over 10 minutes, is useful when more sustained but not immediate control of heart rate is needed. Increases in the central blood volume, as produced by excess perioperative fluid administration, head-down position, or autotransfusion via uterine contractions, can precipitate CHF, pulmonary edema, or atrial fibrillation.

In patients with severe mitral stenosis, sudden decreases in systemic vascular resistance may not be tolerated, as systemic blood pressure can be maintained only by increases in heart rate. If necessary, systemic blood pressure and systemic vascular resistance may be maintained with sympathomimetic drugs, such as ephedrine or phenylephrine.

Table 2–4 • Anesthetic Considerations in Patients with Mitral Stenosis

Avoid sinus tachycardia or rapid ventricular response rates during atrial fibrillation

Avoid marked increases in central blood volume, as associated with overtransfusion or head-down position

Avoid drug-induced decreases in systemic vascular resistance

Avoid events, such as arterial hypoxemia and hypoventilation, that may exacerbate pulmonary hypertension and evoke right ventricular failure

The advantage of ephedrine is its β-agonist effect, which serves to increase myocardial contractility; whereas any drug-induced tachycardia would be undesirable. Phenylephrine eliminates concerns regarding increases in heart rate, but increases in ventricular afterload that follow administration of this predominantly α-agonist drug can decrease the left ventricular stroke volume. Pulmonary hypertension and right ventricular failure may be precipitated by numerous factors, including hypercarbia, hypoxemia, hyperinflation of the lungs, and increases in lung water. If pulmonary hypertension and right ventricular failure develop, inotropic support with dopamine, 3 to 10 μg/kg/min IV, and pulmonary vasodilation with nitroprusside, 0.1 to 0.5 μg/kg/min IV, may be useful.

Preoperative Medication

Preoperative medication of patients with mitral stenosis is designed to decrease anxiety and any associated likelihood of adverse circulatory responses produced by tachycardia. The best drug or drug combination for decreasing anxiety is not known, but it must be appreciated that such patients can be more susceptible than normal individuals to the ventilatory depressant effects of sedative drugs. Furthermore, use of anticholinergic drugs is controversial because of concern that adverse increases in heart rate could occur. Therefore when anticholinergic drugs are included in the preoperative medication, it may be prudent to select scopolamine or glycopyrrolate, as these drugs have fewer chronotropic effects than those evoked by atropine.

Prophylactic antibiotics instituted during the preoperative period for protection against the development of infective endocarditis are usually recommended for patients with mitral stenosis scheduled for dental or surgical procedures. For patients taking digoxin to control the ventricular heart rate response during atrial fibrillation, this drug should be continued during the preoperative period. Because diuretic therapy is likely, serum potassium concentrations are often measured preoperatively. In addition, the presence of orthostatic hypotension may be evidence of diuretic-induced hypovolemia. It is acceptable to continue anticoagulant therapy for minor surgery, whereas for major surgery likely to be associated with significant blood loss the common practice is to discontinue warfarin 3 to 5 days before surgery and substitute heparin.[1]

Induction of Anesthesia

Induction of anesthesia in the presence of mitral stenosis can be achieved with available intravenous induction drugs, with the possible exception of ketamine, which may be avoided because of its propensity to increase the heart rate. Tracheal intubation is usually facilitated by administration of muscle relaxants that are unlikely to induce cardiovascular changes related to histamine release or to affect conduction of cardiac impulses through the atrioventricular node. The occurrence of ventricular dysrhythmias after administration of succinylcholine to patients with mitral stenosis and taking digoxin is not a consistent observation.

Maintenance of Anesthesia

Drugs used for maintenance of anesthesia should be associated with minimal changes in heart rate and systemic and pulmonary vascular resistance. Furthermore, the drugs should not greatly decrease myocardial contractility. These goals are most closely achieved with combinations of nitrous oxide and opioids or low concentrations of volatile anesthetic drugs. Although nitrous oxide can evoke pulmonary vascular constriction and increase pulmonary vascular resistance, it seems unlikely that the magnitude of this change would justify avoiding this drug in patients with mitral stenosis (Fig. 2–3).[6,7] When co-existing pulmonary hypertension

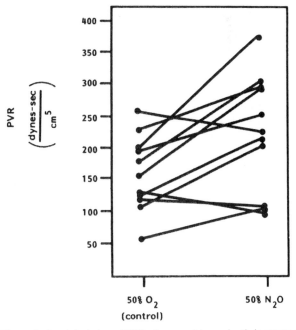

Figure 2–3 • Inhalation of 50% nitrous oxide modestly increased pulmonary vascular resistance in 8 of 11 patients with co-existing pulmonary hypertension due to mitral valve disease. (From Hilgenberg JC, McCammon RL, Stoelting RK. Pulmonary and systemic vascular responses to nitrous oxide in patients with mitral stenosis and pulmonary hypertension. Anesth Analg 1980;59:323–6, with permission.)

is severe, however, nitrous oxide may be more likely to increase pulmonary vascular resistance significantly.[8]

Muscle relaxants with minimal effects on the heart rate, systemic blood pressure, and systemic vascular resistance are useful in patients with mitral stenosis. In this regard, pancuronium is not a likely selection because of its ability to increase the speed of transmission of cardiac impulses through the atrioventricular node, which could lead to excessive increases in heart rate. Such increases seem particularly likely in the presence of atrial fibrillation, as the ventricular response to atrial impulses is determined by the degree of atrioventricular conduction. There is no reason to avoid pharmacologic reversal of nondepolarizing muscle relaxants, although the adverse effects of any drug-induced tachycardia deserves consideration. Theoretically, combining anticholinesterase drugs with glycopyrrolate, rather than atropine, would be more appropriate, as glycopyrrolate is likely to evoke fewer chronotropic effects than atropine.

Light anesthesia and surgical stimulation can lead to systemic hypertension and decreased cardiac output owing to increased systemic and pulmonary vascular resistance. When this occurs, intravenous infusions of nitroprusside may effectively decrease systemic vascular resistance.[9] Nitroprusside-induced decreases in systemic vascular resistance are also associated with increased left ventricular stroke volume, particularly when co-existing pulmonary hypertension is severe or when mitral regurgitation co-exists with mitral stenosis (Fig. 2–4).[9] Intraoperative fluid replacement is carefully titrated, as these patients are susceptible to volume overload and the development of pulmonary edema. Likewise, the head-down position is not well tolerated, as pulmonary blood volume is already increased.

Monitoring

Use of invasive monitoring depends on the complexity of the operative procedure and the magnitude of physiologic impairment by mitral stenosis. Monitoring asymptomatic patients without evidence of pulmonary congestion is probably no different from monitoring patients without valvular heart disease. Conversely, transesophageal echocardiography may be useful in patients with symptomatic mitral stenosis undergoing major operative procedures, especially those associated with significant blood loss. Continuous monitoring of intra-arterial systemic blood pressure and atrial filling pressures may also be a consideration in these patients. These monitors are helpful for confirming the adequacy of cardiac function, intravascular fluid volume, ven-

tilation, and oxygenation. An increase in right atrial pressure could reflect nitrous oxide-induced pulmonary vasoconstriction, suggesting the need to discontinue inhalation of this drug.

Postoperative Management

Postoperatively, patients with mitral stenosis are at risk of developing pulmonary edema and right heart failure. Pain, hypoventilation with respiratory acidosis, and arterial hypoxemia may be the events responsible for increasing heart rate or pulmonary vascular resistance. This emphasizes the usefulness of continuing cardiac monitoring during the postoperative period. Decreased pulmonary compliance and increased oxygen cost of breathing often accompany mitral stenosis. These changes may necessitate mechanical support of ventilation during the postoperative period, particularly after major thoracic or abdominal surgery. Relief of postoperative pain with neuraxial techniques is an important consideration in selected patients.

■ MITRAL REGURGITATION

Mitral regurgitation is usually due to rheumatic fever and is almost always associated with mitral stenosis. Isolated mitral regurgitation in the absence of mitral stenosis is often acute, as in the presence of an acute myocardial infarction or rupture of a chordae tendineae secondary to infective endocarditis. Another cause of mitral regurgitation is dilation of the mitral valve annulus due to left ventricular hypertrophy.

Pathophysiology

Left atrial volume overload is the principal pathophysiologic change produced by mitral regurgitation. Indeed, the basic hemodynamic derangement in mitral regurgitation is a decrease in forward left ventricular stroke volume, as part of the stroke volume is regurgitated through the incompetent mitral valve back into the left atrium. Patients with regurgitant fractions of more than 0.6 are considered to have severe mitral regurgitation. The fraction of left ventricular stroke volume that enters the left atrium depends on the (1) size of the mitral valve orifice; (2) heart rate, which determines the duration of the ventricular ejection; and (3) pressure gradients across the mitral valve. Such gradients depend on compliance of the left ventricle and on the impedance of left ventricular ejection into the aorta. Phar-

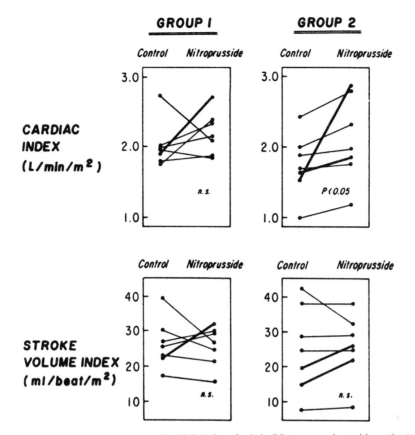

Figure 2–4 • Cardiovascular effects of nitroprusside (0.2–4.0 µg/kg/min IV) were evaluated in patients with pure mitral stenosis (group 1) and in patients with mixed mitral stenosis and mitral regurgitation (group 2) with (*heavy lines*) or without (*fine lines*) severe co-existing pulmonary hypertension. Nitroprusside-induced decreases in systemic vascular resistance were not detrimental in either group; patients with severe co-existing pulmonary hypertension had the most favorable response. (From Stone JG, Hoar PF, Faltas AN, et al. Nitroprusside and mitral stenosis. Anesth Analg 1980;59:662–5, with permission.)

macologic interventions that increase or decrease systemic vascular resistance also have an important impact on the regurgitant fraction of the stroke volume.

Patients with isolated mitral regurgitation are less dependent on properly timed left atrial contractions for left ventricular filling than are patients with mitral or aortic stenosis. Indeed, conversion from atrial fibrillation (present in about one-third of patients with mitral regurgitation) to normal sinus rhythm produces minimal changes in cardiac output. Patients with rheumatic fever-induced mitral regurgitation are most likely to exhibit marked left atrial enlargement and associated atrial fibrillation. Myocardial ischemia is unlikely in the presence of mitral regurgitation because the increased ventricular wall tension is quickly dissipated as the stroke volume is rapidly ejected into the aorta and left atrium. Furthermore, when mitral regurgitation develops gradually, the compliant left atrium is able to accom-

modate increased regurgitant volumes without increases in left atrial pressure. Severe mitral regurgitation may be exhibited as left atrial and ventricular hypertrophy on the ECG and chest radiograph.

The frequent combination of mitral regurgitation and mitral stenosis results in increased volume and pressure work by the heart. In this situation increased flow rates across the stenotic valve secondary to regurgitation markedly increase left atrial pressure. Atrial fibrillation, pulmonary edema, and pulmonary hypertension develop earlier in these patients than in those with isolated mitral regurgitation.

Diagnosis

Mitral regurgitation is recognized by the presence of a holosystolic apical murmur (Fig. 2–1).[5] Chronic mitral regurgitation is compensated for by the development of eccentric cardiac hypertrophy and cardiac enlargement detectable on physical examination. Echocardiography confirms enlargement of the left ventricular chamber, and color flow examination of the mitral valve establishes the pattern of disturbed flow caused by regurgitation across the mitral valve.[3] Echocardiography provides only a semiquantitative estimate of the severity of mitral regurgitation. The presence of V waves on recordings of the pulmonary artery occlusion pressures reflects regurgitant flow through the mitral valve (Fig. 2–2).[4] The size of the V waves correlates with the magnitude of the regurgitant flow.

Treatment

Unlike stenotic cardiac valve lesions, regurgitant cardiac valve lesions may progress insidiously, causing left ventricular damage before symptoms have developed.[1] In this regard, surgical treatment of mitral regurgitation is recommended when ejection fractions are less than 0.6. Mitral valve repair is preferred, as the operative mortality is less and outcome better than in patients undergoing mitral valve replacement. This reflects the important role of the mitral valve apparatus in sustaining left ventricular function. For this reason, even when the mitral valve is replaced, attempts are made to conserve the subvalvular apparatus and continuity of the papillary muscles. Absence of these structures causes distortion of the left ventricular contractile geometry (papillary muscles can no longer contribute to shortening of the left ventricular axis, resulting in premature circumferential shortening of cardiac muscle) and impairment of left ventricular ejection during systole. After mitral valve replacement, the dilated left ventricle is suddenly exposed to increased resistance to ventricular ejection as the low-resistance left atrial "pop off" has been removed.[1] Most patients can compensate for this change, but in patients with marked prior deterioration of left ventricular function the loss of ejection into the highly compliant left atrium may contribute to the development of CHF. Although vasodilators have been useful for medical management of acute mitral regurgitation, there is no apparent benefit to long-term use of these drugs.

Management of Anesthesia

Management of anesthesia for noncardiac surgery in patients with mitral regurgitation includes avoidance of events that may further decrease cardiac output (Table 2–5). Maintenance of normal to slightly increased heart rates is recommended, as forward left ventricular stroke volume is likely to be heart rate-dependent. In this regard, sudden bradycardia may result in abrupt left ventricular volume overload. Likewise, sudden increases in systemic vascular resistance can cause acute decompensation of the left ventricle. Patients with left ventricular failure due to this mechanism may benefit from drug-induced afterload reduction with nitroprusside combined with a cardiac inotrope such as dopamine to increase myocardial contractility. Because left ventricular dysfunction usually accompanies mitral regurgitation, even minimal drug-induced myocardial depression is undesirable. Overall, anesthesia management is designed to avoid a decrease in heart rate or increase in systemic vascular resistance that would potentially decrease the forward left ventricular stroke volume. Conversely, cardiac output can be improved by modest increases in heart rate and decreases in systemic vascular resistance.

Prophylactic antibiotics instituted during the preoperative period for protection against the development of infective endocarditis are usually recommended for patients with mitral regurgitation who are scheduled for dental or surgical procedures. General anesthesia is the usual choice for patients with mitral regurgitation undergoing a surgical procedure. Although a decrease in systemic vascular resistance is theoretically beneficial, the uncontrolled nature of this response with regional anesthesia detracts from the use of epidural or spinal anesthesia.

Induction of Anesthesia

Induction of anesthesia in the presence of mitral regurgitation can be achieved with available intravenous induction drugs, keeping in mind the importance of avoiding excessive and abrupt changes in systemic vascular resistance or a decrease in the heart rate. Bradycardia that may accompany administration of succinylcholine is undesirable.

Table 2–5 • Anesthetic Considerations in Patients with Mitral Regurgitation

Avoid sudden decreases in heart rate
Avoid sudden increases in systemic vascular resistance
Minimize drug-induced myocardial depression
Monitor the magnitude of regurgitant flow with echocardiography and/or a pulmonary artery catheter (size of the V wave)

Maintenance of Anesthesia

In the absence of severe left ventricular dysfunction, maintenance of anesthesia is often provided by nitrous oxide plus volatile anesthetics. Volatile anesthetics can be administered to attenuate the undesirable increases in systemic blood pressure and systemic vascular resistance that can accompany surgical stimulation. Although a specific volatile anesthetic has not been demonstrated to be superior, the usual increase in heart rate and decrease in systemic vascular resistance plus the minimal negative depressant effects on myocardial contractility associated with administration of isoflurane, desflurane, and sevoflurane should be acceptable. When myocardial function is severely compromised, as in the presence of acute mitral regurgitation due to papillary muscle dysfunction or rupture of a chordae tendineae, use of an opioid anesthetic, which minimizes the likelihood of drug-induced myocardial depression, may be considered. Selection of muscle relaxants may be influenced by the likely circulatory effects associated with certain of these drugs. In this regard, pancuronium, which generally produces a modest increase in heart rate, would potentially contribute to maintenance of the forward left ventricular stroke volume.

Ventilation of the lungs is often controlled and adjusted to maintain near-normal $PaCO_2$. The pattern of ventilation should provide sufficient time between breaths for venous return to occur. Maintenance of intravascular fluid volume with prompt replacement of blood loss is important for maintaining cardiac filling volumes and ejection of optimal forward left ventricular stroke volumes.

Monitoring

Minor operations performed on patients with asymptomatic mitral regurgitation probably do not require invasive monitoring. In the presence of severe mitral regurgitation, the use of invasive monitoring is helpful for detecting the onset of an undesirable degree of myocardial depression and for facilitating intravenous fluid replacement. Transesophageal echocardiography is useful for monitoring mitral valve function, myocardial contractility, and the adequacy of the intravascular fluid volume. Alternatively, a pulmonary artery catheter may be useful, especially if peripheral vasodilating drugs are administered in attempts to increase the forward left ventricular stroke volume. Measuring cardiac output by thermodilution confirms the response to a decrease in systemic vascular resistance produced by drugs such as nitroprusside. It should be appreciated that regurgitation of blood into the left atrium produces V waves on tracings of pulmonary artery occlusion pressures. Changes in V wave amplitude can assist in estimating the magnitude of mitral regurgitation (Fig. 2–2).[4] Pulmonary artery occlusion pressure is a poor measure of the left atrial volume or left ventricular end-diastolic volume. With acute mitral regurgitation, however, the left atrium is less compliant; and changes in pulmonary artery occlusion pressures are more likely to correlate with changes in the left atrial and left ventricular end-diastolic pressures.

■ MITRAL VALVE PROLAPSE

Mitral valve prolapse is defined as billowing of the posterior mitral leaflet into the left atrium during systole; it is associated with the auscultatory finding of a midsystolic click and a late systolic murmur (click-murmur syndrome). The syndrome of mitral valve prolapse has been portrayed as the most common form of valvular heart disease (prevalence is 5% to 10% of the U.S. population and is even higher among young women).[10–12] Nevertheless, using more specific and standardized echocardiographic criteria, the true incidence of mitral valve prolapse is low (2.4% of the population), and unexplained cerebral events cannot be demonstrated to occur at a more frequent incidence than in control patients.[10–12] Though it is a predominantly benign condition, devastating complications have been ascribed to mitral valve prolapse, including cerebral embolic events, infective endocarditis, severe mitral regurgitation requiring surgical replacement, and sudden death. Only patients with abnormal mitral valve morphology appear to be at risk for complications. Indeed, there is a subgroup of patients with mitral valve prolapse in whom infective endocarditis or severe mitral regurgitation may develop that requires mitral valve surgery. The risk of sudden death in patients with hemodynamically insignificant mitral valve prolapse is not increased. Conversely, patients with markedly myxomatous mitral valves and a history of syncope are considered to be at increased risk for sudden death.

Diagnosis

The definitive diagnosis of mitral valve prolapse is based on echocardiographic findings.[10–13] Patients with redundant and thickened leaflets on echocardiography are considered to have a primary (anatomic) form of mitral valve prolapse. This form of mitral valve prolapse generally occurs in patients with connective tissue diseases (Marfan syndrome, von Willebrand syndrome, muscular dystrophy, cardiomyopathy) or in elderly men. Patients with mild bowing and normal-appearing leaflets are thought to have a normal variant (functional) of mitral valve function, and their risk of adverse events is probably no different than that of the general population. Patients with primary mitral valve prolapse require prophylaxis against infective endocarditis, whereas prophylaxis is probably not necessary for patients with normal-variant mitral valve prolapse and no murmur.

Cardiac dysrhythmias commonly associated with mitral valve prolapse are nonspecific and include both supraventricular (sinus tachycardia, atrial fibrillation, atrial flutter, junctional tachycardia) and ventricular (premature ventricular contractions, nonsustained or sustained ventricular tachycardia) dysrhythmias. In addition to cardiac dysrhythmias, conduction abnormalities are not uncommon in patients with mitral valve prolapse. For example, the ECG often shows T wave abnormalities as evidence of repolarization abnormalities.

Management of Anesthesia

Management of anesthesia for noncardiac surgery in patients with mitral valve prolapse includes the principles outlined for patients with mitral regurgitation (Table 2–5). An important concept is recognition that increased left ventricular emptying in these patients can accentuate mitral valve prolapse leading to acute mitral regurgitation. Perioperative events that can increase left ventricular emptying include (1) increased sympathetic nervous system activity, (2) decreased systemic vascular resistance, and (3) assumption of the upright (sitting) posture. Symptoms of mitral valve prolapse often occur in the setting of decreased left ventricular filling, which may be produced by hypovolemia. Conversely, vasoconstriction that occurs in response to surgical stimulation in the presence of minimal depressant effects of anesthetic drugs could decrease left ventricular emptying and increase left ventricular volume, thus decreasing the probability of mitral valve prolapse.[13] However, increased sympathetic nervous system activity and catecholamine release associated with this vasoconstriction also increase myocardial contractility, which could worsen mitral valve prolapse and aggravate cardiac dysrhythmias. Overall, anesthetic management is significantly influenced by the patient's degree of mitral regurgitation.[13]

Preoperative Evaluation

Preoperative evaluation should focus on distinguishing patients with purely functional disease from those with significant mitral regurgitation.[13] Functional mitral valve prolapse is most often present in women younger than 45 years of age. These patients may be receiving β-blockers to control tachycardia, and the drugs should be continued throughout the perioperative period. The presence of mitral valve prolapse uncomplicated by other symptoms is probably not sufficient reason to request a preoperative ECG or chest radiograph. Although the ECG frequently shows premature ventricular contractions and repolarization abnormalities, there is no evidence that these findings predict intraoperative events. Despite multiple case reports suggesting an association between mitral valve prolapse and intraoperative cardiac dysrhythmias, there is no clear cause-and-effect relation. Nevertheless, optimization of preoperative electrolytes seems prudent to minimize the risk of intraoperative cardiac dysrhythmias. In the absence of other symptoms, finding an isolated cardiac systolic click murmur probably does not warrant a preoperative consultation with a cardiologist.

Patients with an anatomic variant of mitral valve prolapse are likely to be older men who often manifest symptoms of mild to moderate CHF, including exercise intolerance, orthopnea, and dyspnea on exertion.[13] These patients may be receiving numerous drugs including diuretics, digoxin, and angiotensin-converting enzyme (ACE) inhibitors. Physical examination often reveals a midsystolic to holosystolic murmur and possibly an S_3 gallop with signs of pulmonary congestion and echocardiographic evidence of mitral regurgitation.

Premedication of patients with functional or anatomic mitral valve prolapse should produce anxiolysis without causing tachycardia, which could decrease ventricular volume and possibly accentuate mitral valve prolapse and mitral regurgitation. The use of atropine as a preoperative medication is influenced by the realization that an increased heart rate may be undesirable.

Antibiotic prophylaxis for protection against infective endocarditis is likely to be recommended in patients with systolic murmurs. Patients with a history of functional mitral valve prolapse or a midsystolic cardiac click-murmur without echocardiographic evidence of mitral valve prolapse are at low risk for infective endocarditis and do not benefit from prophylactic antibiotic therapy.[10, 13] The risk of fatal anaphylactic reactions to antibiotics may be greater than the risk of infective endocarditis in patients with isolated and asymptomatic functional mitral valve prolapse. Antibiotic prophylaxis is not necessary for tracheal intubation or fiberoptic bronchoscopy but is probably indicated if nasotracheal intubation is planned.

Selection of Anesthesia Technique

Most patients with mitral valve prolapse have normal left ventricular function. Consequently, volatile anesthetics should be well tolerated by these patients. Furthermore, any volatile anesthetic-induced myocardial depression could be useful for offsetting concomitant vasodilating effects of these drugs, which could decrease left ventricular volume and increase mitral regurgitation. There is no clinical evidence that contraindicates the use of regional anesthesia in patients with mitral valve prolapse, although the associated decrease in systemic vascular resistance is theoretically undesirable.[13] The impact of an anesthetic-induced decrease in systemic vascular resistance on the left ventricular volume can be offset by repletion of intravascular fluid volume with crystalloid solutions prior to institution of the regional anesthetic.

Induction of Anesthesia

Most patients with mitral valve prolapse have been treated with diuretics preoperatively, resulting in intravascular fluid volume deficits that may be unmasked by the vasodilating effects of drugs administered for anesthesia induction. Therefore these patients may benefit from preoperative fluid administration given to optimize the intravascular fluid volume prior to induction of anesthesia. At the same time it is important to keep in mind the risk of pulmonary congestion and left ventricular overdistension due to overzealous intravenous fluid administration.[13]

During induction of anesthesia with available drugs one must consider the need to avoid sudden and prolonged decreases in systemic vascular resistance. The myocardial depressant and peripheral vasodilating effects of barbiturates and propofol can be undesirable in patients with hemodynamically significant mitral valve prolapse. Etomidate causes minimal myocardial depression and alterations in sympathetic nervous system activity, suggesting that this drug may be an attractive choice for induction of anesthesia in the presence of symptomatic mitral valve prolapse.[13] The use of ketamine is not encouraged based on its ability to stimulate the sympathetic nervous system with associated increases in systemic vascular resistance, which could accentuate mitral regurgitation.

Maintenance of Anesthesia

Maintenance of anesthesia is designed to minimize sympathetic nervous system activation secondary to painful intraoperative stimulation. Volatile anesthetics, combined with nitrous oxide and/or opioids, may be useful for attenuating sympathetic nervous system activity, keeping in mind the importance of titrating drug doses to minimize the likelihood of undesirable decreases in systemic vascular resistance.

Patients with hemodynamically significant mitral valve prolapse may not tolerate the dose-dependent cardiac depressant effects of volatile anesthetics. Low concentrations (about 0.5 MAC) of isoflurane, desflurane, and sevoflurane may decrease the regurgitant fraction through the mitral valve, but these effects are not readily predictable. An alternative to volatile anesthetics in the presence of severe hemodynamic dysfunction related to mitral valve prolapse is the use of opioids combined with modest doses of volatile anesthetics. In the presence of mitral regurgitation and increased pulmonary vascular resistance, administration of nitrous oxide may cause a further increase in pulmonary artery pressures. Potent vasodilators such as nitroprusside, nitroglycerin, and hydralazine may be carefully titrated to maximize forward left ventricular stroke volume. In the presence of adequate hydration, vasodilators have the added benefit of decreasing left ventricular end-diastolic volume and pressure. There are no clinical data to support the use of one muscle relaxant over another in the presence of isolated mitral valve prolapse, although drug-induced hemodynamic alterations (vagolysis, histamine release) deserve consideration when selecting specific drugs.[13]

Unexpected ventricular cardiac dysrhythmias may occur during anesthesia especially during operations performed in the head-up or sitting positions, presumably reflecting increased left ventricular emptying and accentuation of mitral valve prolapse. Lidocaine and β-antagonists such as esmolol are useful for treating cardiac dysrhythmias. Digoxin is not an appropriate choice in the presence of mitral valve prolapse for treating perioperative cardiac dysrhythmias and may contribute to the development of malignant ventricular dysrhythmias.[13] Ventricular fibrillation has been described during induction of anesthesia in a child with previously undiagnosed mitral valve prolapse.[14]

Prompt replacement of blood loss and generous intravenous fluid maintenance replacement can likely blunt any adverse effects caused by positive-pressure ventilation of the lungs. Furthermore, a high intravascular fluid volume helps maintain forward left ventricular stroke volume should acute increases in the magnitude of mitral regurgitation occur intraoperatively. If vasopressors are needed, an α-agonist such as phenylephrine is acceptable. Production of controlled hypotension with vasodilator drugs is an unlikely choice, as the associated decrease in systemic vascular resistance could enhance mitral valve prolapse.

Monitoring

The ECG is monitored for prompt detection of cardiac dysrhythmias that may occur in patients with mitral valve prolapse. Transesophageal echocardiography is utilized to monitor and assess the degree of mitral regurgitation.[13] A pulmonary artery catheter may be placed to complement information from echocardiography and to permit measurement of cardiac output and calculation of systemic vascular resistance. Pulmonary artery catheter measurements may be correlated with echocardiography to establish trends that may be followed postoperatively when the pulmonary artery catheter remains after removing the echocardiography probe. In the absence of hemodynamically significant mitral valve prolapse, monitoring pulmonary artery pressures is probably not necessary.

■ AORTIC STENOSIS

Aortic stenosis is usually an idiopathic disease resulting from degeneration and calcification of the aortic leaflets.[1] Stenosis is more likely to occur in persons born with bicuspid aortic valves than in those with normal tricuspid aortic valves. Evidence of aortic stenosis is more likely to develop earlier (30 to 40 years old) in life in individuals with bicuspid aortic valves than in those with tricuspid aortic valves (60 to 80 years old). Aortic stenosis is associated with the same risk factors (systemic hypertension, hypercholesterolemia) as those for ischemic heart disease. The incidence of sudden death is increased in patients with aortic stenosis especially after the onset of symptoms.

Pathophysiology

Obstruction to ejection of blood into the aorta due to decreases in the area of the aortic valve orifice necessitates increases in left ventricular pressures to maintain forward stroke volume. Critical aortic stenosis capable of causing symptoms and sudden death is characterized by transvalvular pressure gradients higher than 50 mmHg and an aortic valve orifice area less than 0.8 cm^2 (normal 2.5 to 3.5 cm^2). Furthermore, aortic stenosis is almost always associated with some degree of aortic regurgitation. Angina pectoris may occur in patients with aortic stenosis despite the absence of coronary artery atherosclerosis. It reflects increased myocardial oxygen requirements owing to the increased amounts of ventricular muscle associated with concentric myocardial hypertrophy as well as increased myocardial oxygen requirements due to the increased afterload. Furthermore, myocardial oxygen delivery is decreased owing to compression of subendocardial coronary blood vessels by the increased left ventricular systolic pressure. The origin of syncope in patients with aortic stenosis is controversial but may reflect exercise-induced decreases in systemic vascular resistance that remains uncompensated because cardiac output is restricted by the stenotic valve. CHF is due to diastolic dysfunction (increased left ventricular wall thickness) and/or systolic dysfunction (increased afterload, decreased myocardial contractility).

Diagnosis

The classic clinical symptoms of aortic stenosis are angina pectoris, dyspnea on exertion, and syncope often associated with exertion. Auscultation reveals a characteristic systolic ejection murmur radiating into the neck that is best heard in the aortic area (second right intercostal space) (Fig. 2–1).[5] Because many patients with aortic stenosis are asymptomatic, it is important to listen for this heart murmur in those scheduled for surgery. Chest radiographs may show a prominent ascending aorta due to poststenotic dilation, whereas the ECG demonstrates evidence of left ventricular hypertrophy.

Echocardiography with Doppler examination of the aortic valve provides a more accurate assessment of the severity of aortic stenosis than does clinical evaluation.[1] Thickening and calcification of the aortic valve combined with decreased mobility of the valve leaflets is evident on echocardiography. Assessment of transvalvular pressure gradients and the area of the aortic valve is provided by echocardiography. Echocardiography is also useful for determining the extent of left ventricular hypertrophy and for estimating left ventricular ejection. Cardiac catheterization and coronary angiography may be necessary when the severity of aortic stenosis cannot be determined by echocardiography.

Treatment

Except for antibiotic prophylaxis against infective endocarditis, there is no effective medical therapy for aortic stenosis.[1] In asymptomatic patients with aortic stenosis, it appears to be relatively safe to continue medical management and to delay surgery until symptoms develop.[15] The presence of moderate or severe valvular calcification may identify patients with a poor prognosis, and these patients may be considered for aortic valve replacement before symptoms develop. Indeed, the only effective treatment is relief of the mechanical obstruction to left ventricular ejection by surgical replacement of the diseased aortic valve. Mortality approaches 75% within 3 years after aortic stenosis becomes symptomatic unless the valve is surgically replaced.[1] Although most patients with aortic stenosis are elderly, the prognosis with surgery even in this age group is acceptable. Balloon aortic valvotomy for adult acquired aortic stenosis is useful only for palliation of the disease in patients who are not candidates for aortic valve replacement because of other medical conditions.

Aortic valve replacement usually relieves the symptoms of aortic stenosis dramatically, and the ejection fraction increases. Nevertheless, there is a subgroup of patients in whom the ejection fraction remains low and symptoms persist after aortic valve replacement. There are differences in the ventricular geometry of men and women, characterized as thicker ventricular walls and higher ejection fractions in women. Preoperative recognition of these differences may be important because postoperative management of low cardiac output requires volume expansion rather than the use of inotropic drugs.[1]

Management of Anesthesia

Management of anesthesia for noncardiac surgery in patients with aortic stenosis includes avoidance of events that may further decrease the cardiac output (Table 2–6). There is no evidence that elective noncardiac surgery is associated with increased morbidity and mortality in these patients.[16] General anesthesia is often selected in preference to epidural or spinal anesthesia because peripheral sympathetic nervous system blockade produced by regional anesthesia can lead to undesirable decreases in systemic vascular resistance.

Preservation of normal sinus rhythm is desirable, as the left ventricle is dependent on properly timed

---

Table 2–6 • Anesthetic Considerations in Patients with Aortic Stenosis

Maintain normal sinus rhythm
Avoid bradycardia
Avoid sudden increases or decreases in systemic vascular resistance
Optimize intravascular fluid volume to maintain venous return and left ventricular filling

---

atrial contractions to ensure an optimal left ventricular end-diastolic volume. Indeed, loss of normal atrial contractions, as during junctional rhythm or atrial fibrillation, may produce significant decreases in stroke volume and systemic blood pressure. The heart rate is important as it determines the time available for filling the ventricles and ejection of the forward left ventricular stroke volume. For example, marked, sustained increases in heart rate can decrease the time for left ventricular filling and ejection, leading to undesirable decreases in stroke volume. Likewise, sudden decreases in heart rate can lead to acute overdistension of the left ventricle. In view of the obstruction to left ventricular ejection, it is important to recognize that decreased systemic vascular resistance may be associated with large decreases in systemic blood pressure and subsequent decreases in coronary blood flow. Conversely, increased systemic vascular resistance and systemic blood pressure can lead to a decreased stroke volume. It is important to have available a direct-current defibrillator when anesthesia is administered to patients with aortic stenosis. External cardiac massage is unlikely to be effective should cardiac arrest occur, as it is difficult to create an adequate stroke volume across a stenotic aortic valve using mechanical compression of the patient's sternum.

Preoperative Medication

Prophylactic antibiotics are instituted during the preoperative period for protection against the development of infective endocarditis in patients with aortic stenosis who are scheduled for dental or surgical procedures. Preoperative medication is tailored to minimize the likelihood of decreases in systemic vascular resistance.

Induction of Anesthesia

Induction of anesthesia in the presence of aortic stenosis can be achieved with available intravenous induction drugs. Tracheal intubation is facilitated by administration of muscle relaxants. Bradycardia that may be associated with the administration of succinylcholine is undesirable. Interventions to prevent this rare response (increased heart rate is the more common response) may be considered, including prior administration of anticholinergic drugs.

Maintenance of Anesthesia

Maintenance of anesthesia is most often accomplished with a combination of nitrous oxide and volatile anesthetics or opioids. A disadvantage of volatile drugs (especially halothane) is depression of sinoatrial node automaticity, which may lead to junctional rhythm and loss of properly timed atrial contractions. Furthermore, when left ventricular function is severely impaired by aortic stenosis, it is useful to avoid any additional depression of myocardial contractility with volatile anesthetics. Decreased systemic vascular resistance produced by high concentrations of isoflurane, desflurane, or sevoflurane would be undesirable; in contrast, clinical experience has shown that low concentrations of these drugs are unlikely to be associated with undesirable responses. Maintenance of anesthesia with nitrous oxide plus opioids or with opioids alone in high doses (fentanyl 50 to 100 μg/kg IV or equivalent doses of other potent opioids) has been recommended for patients with marked left ventricular dysfunction attributable to aortic stenosis. Nondepolarizing neuromuscular blocking drugs with minimal effects on the circulation are useful, although modest increases in systemic blood pressure and heart rate as typically produced by pancuronium are acceptable. Intravascular fluid volume is maintained by prompt replacement of blood loss and liberal administration (5 ml/kg/hr) of intravenous fluids.

The onset of junctional rhythm or bradycardia during anesthesia and surgery usually requires prompt treatment with intravenous atropine. Persistent tachycardia can be treated with β-antagonists such as esmolol, keeping in mind that these patients may be dependent on endogenous β-adrenergic activity to maintain left ventricular stroke volume especially in the presence of increased systemic vascular resistance that occurs in response to surgical stimulation. Supraventricular tachycardia should be promptly terminated with electrical cardioversion. Lidocaine is kept available, as these patients have a propensity to develop ventricular cardiac dysrhythmias.

Monitoring

Intraoperative monitoring of patients with aortic stenosis may utilize an ECG lead that reliably reflects myocardial ischemia. The magnitude of the surgery and the severity of the aortic stenosis influence the decision to utilize an intra-arterial catheter, transesophageal echocardiography, or a pulmonary artery catheter. These monitors help determine whether intraoperative hypotension is due to hypovolemia or CHF. It should be remembered that pulmonary artery occlusion pressures may overestimate left ventricular end-diastolic pressures because of the decreased compliance of the left ventricle that accompanies chronic aortic stenosis.

Regional Anesthesia

Spinal or epidural anesthesia and the associated sympathetic nervous system blockade has been considered undesirable in patients with aortic stenosis. The concern is that anesthetic-induced peripheral sympathetic nervous system blockade could rapidly decrease systemic vascular resistance, with decreased venous return to the heart and decreased coronary artery perfusion pressures. In patients with aortic stenosis, concentric ventricular hypertrophy renders the myocardium susceptible to myocardial ischemia even in the absence of coronary artery disease. Large decreases in systemic vascular resistance could initiate a cycle of hypotension-induced myocardial ischemia, subsequent ventricular dysfunction, and worsening hypotension.[17] If a regional anesthetic is selected, it may be useful to consider the more likely gradual onset of peripheral sympathetic nervous system blockade after epidural anesthesia, in contrast to spinal anesthesia. Alternatively, continuous spinal anesthesia has been described for elderly patients with severe aortic stenosis undergoing surgical repair of hip fractures.[18]

▮ AORTIC REGURGITATION

Aortic regurgitation results from disease of the aortic leaflets or of the aortic root that distorts the leaflets, preventing their coaptation.[1] Common causes of leaflet abnormalities that result in aortic regurgitation are infective endocarditis and rheumatic fever. Aortic root causes of aortic regurgitation include idiopathic root dilation associated with systemic hypertension and aging, thoracic aortic dissection, collagen vascular diseases, and Marfan syndrome. Acute aortic regurgitation is usually due to infective endocarditis, which complicates surgical replacement of the diseased valve.

Pathophysiology

The basic hemodynamic derangement in patients with aortic regurgitation is a decrease in forward left ventricular stroke volume because of regurgitation of part of the ejected stroke volume from the aorta back into the left ventricle. The magnitude of the regurgitant volume depends on (1) the time available for the regurgitant flow to occur, which is determined by the heart rate; and (2) the pressure gradient across the aortic valve, which is dependent on the systemic vascular resistance. The magnitude of aortic regurgitation is decreased by tachycardia and peripheral vasodilation. With chronic aortic regurgitation, left ventricular hypertrophy results in a large total stroke volume that is entirely ejected into the aorta, imposing increased afterload on the left ventricle. Indeed, afterload can be as high with aortic regurgitation as it is with aortic stenosis.[1] Increased myocardial oxygen requirements secondary to left ventricular hypertrophy plus a characteristic decrease in aortic diastolic pressure, which decreases coronary blood flow, may manifest as angina pectoris due to subendocardial ischemia in the absence of ischemic heart disease.

The left ventricle usually tolerates chronic increases in left ventricular volume overload. When left ventricular failure does occur, however, left ventricular end-diastolic volume increases precipitously, and evidence of pulmonary edema is likely. Indeed, a helpful indicator of left ventricular function in the presence of aortic regurgitation is the echocardiographic determination of end-systolic volume and ejection fraction, both of which remain normal until left ventricular function becomes impaired.

Compared with patients who have chronic aortic regurgitation, patients with acute aortic regurgitation experience sudden increases in ventricular volume before left ventricular hypertrophy can occur. This limits the effectiveness of compensatory mechanisms, such as increased heart rate and myocardial contractility, with the end result often being decreased cardiac output and hypotension.

Diagnosis

Aortic regurgitation is recognized by its characteristic diastolic blowing murmur best heard along the left sternal border plus peripheral signs of a hyperdynamic circulation that include a widened pulse pressure, decreased diastolic blood pressure, and bounding peripheral pulses (Fig. 2–1).[5] In addition to the typical murmur of aortic regurgitation, a diastolic rumble (Austin Flint murmur) may also be heard over the cardiac apex. Echocardiography with Doppler examination of the aortic valve and aortography during cardiac catheterization is useful for confirming the clinical impression gained from the physical examination and for quantitating the severity of the aortic regurgitation. In the presence of chronic aortic regurgitation, there is likely to be evidence of left ventricular enlargement on the chest radiograph and ECG. In contrast to aortic stenosis, sudden death related to aortic regurgitation is rare.

As with mitral regurgitation, symptoms of aortic regurgitation may not appear until left ventricular dysfunction is advanced. Symptoms at this stage usually reflect left ventricular failure (dyspnea, or-

thopnea, fatigue) and angina pectoris in the absence of coronary artery disease. Increased stroke volume associated with aortic regurgitation may result in systolic hypertension and increased afterload on the left ventricle, which is as great as that created by aortic stenosis.

Treatment

Surgical replacement of the diseased aortic valve is recommended before the onset of permanent left ventricular damage, even in asymptomatic patients. After aortic valve replacement, left ventricular afterload is decreased and the ejection fraction improves. A general rule is that surgical treatment of aortic regurgitation is indicated before the ejection fraction decreases to less than 0.55 or the end-systolic dimension exceeds 55 mm.[1] Alternatives to aortic valve replacement include a pulmonary autograft (Ross procedure) and aortic valve reconstruction.

Medical therapy of aortic regurgitation is based on decreasing the left ventricular afterload with drug-induced vasodilation. In this regard, intravenous infusions of nitroprusside may be useful for improving the forward left ventricular stroke volume when acute aortic regurgitation results in left ventricular volume overload and decreased cardiac output. The use of nifedipine in asymptomatic patients with aortic regurgitation and normal left ventricular function can delay the need for surgery for several months.[1]

Management of Anesthesia

Management of anesthesia for noncardiac surgery in patients with aortic regurgitation is designed to maintain the forward left ventricular stroke volume (Table 2–7). In this regard it is useful to maintain the patient's heart rate above 80 beats/min, as bradycardia, by increasing the duration of ventricular diastole, leads to acute left ventricular volume overload. Abrupt increases in systemic vascular re-

Table 2–7 • Anesthetic Considerations in Patients with Aortic Regurgitation

Avoid sudden decreases in heart rate
Avoid sudden increases in systemic vascular resistance
Minimize drug-induced myocardial depression

sistance can precipitate left ventricular failure, requiring treatment with peripheral vasodilators such as nitroprusside. Aortic regurgitation usually produces left ventricular impairment, and anesthetic-induced depression of myocardial contractility may be undesirable. Left ventricular failure may be treated with afterload reduction provided by nitroprusside and cardiac inotropes such as dopamine to increase myocardial contractility. Overall, modest increases in heart rate and modest decreases in systemic vascular resistance are reasonable goals for management of anesthesia. Still, it should be recognized that these patients may be exquisitely sensitive to peripheral vasodilation.

Prophylactic antibiotics instituted during the preoperative period for protection against the development of infective endocarditis are usually recommended for patients with aortic regurgitation who are scheduled for dental or surgical procedures. General anesthesia is the usual choice for patients with aortic regurgitation. Although decreased systemic vascular resistance is theoretically beneficial, the uncontrolled nature of this response with regional anesthesia detracts from the use of epidural or spinal anesthesia.

Induction of Anesthesia

Induction of anesthesia in the presence of aortic regurgitation can be achieved with available intravenous induction drugs. Ketamine may be advantageous by virtue of its ability to accelerate the heart rate, but the accompanying increase in resistance to ejection of the forward left ventricular stroke volume due to increased systemic vascular resistance could be undesirable. Nevertheless, when intravascular fluid volume is judged to be decreased, the use of ketamine for induction of anesthesia is an acceptable choice. Bradycardia that may be associated with administration of succinylcholine is undesirable, and interventions to prevent this rare occurrence (increased heart rate is the more common response) may be considered, including prior administration of anticholinergic drugs.

Maintenance of Anesthesia

In the absence of severe left ventricular dysfunction, maintenance of anesthesia is often provided with nitrous oxide plus volatile anesthetics and/or opioids. Although a specific volatile anesthetic has not been demonstrated to be superior, the usual increased heart rate and decreased systemic vascular resistance with little evidence of direct myocardial depression characteristic of isoflurane, desflurane, and sevoflurane make these drugs acceptable

choices. When left ventricular function is severely compromised, use of an opioid (fentanyl 50 to 100 μg/kg IV or an equivalent short-acting opioid) as the sole drug for maintenance of anesthesia may be the best way to provide adequate amnesia without producing additional cardiac depression. It is important to consider the possibility of exaggerated myocardial depression, which may occur when nitrous oxide or a benzodiazepine is added to an opioid.[19,20] Muscle relaxant selection is influenced by the likely circulatory effects produced by these drugs. Drugs with minimal to no effects on systemic blood pressure and heart rate may be most attractive, although modest increases in heart rate associated with administration of pancuronium could contribute to the maintenance of forward left ventricular stroke volume.

Ventilation of the lungs is often mechanically controlled and adjusted to maintain the $PaCO_2$ near normal. This pattern of ventilation should provide sufficient time between breaths for venous return to occur. Maintenance of intravascular fluid volume with prompt replacement of blood loss is important for maintaining cardiac filling and ejection of an optimal forward left ventricular stroke volume. Preoperative fluid loading and intravenous infusions of nitroprusside may be useful for maintaining cardiac output during surgery (Fig. 2–5).[21] Bradycardia and junctional rhythm may require prompt treatment with intravenous atropine.

Monitoring

Minor operations performed in patients with asymptomatic aortic regurgitation probably do not require invasive monitoring. In view of the possibility of myocardial ischemia, it is useful to monitor an ECG lead likely to detect this change. In the presence of severe aortic regurgitation, monitoring with transesophageal echocardiography and/or a pulmonary artery catheter is helpful for early recognition of undesirable degrees of myocardial depression and for facilitating intravenous fluid replacement. The response to administration of peripheral vasodilating drugs can be followed by measuring cardiac output and calculating the systemic vascular resistance made possible by data obtained from a pulmonary artery catheter.

■ TRICUSPID REGURGITATION

Tricuspid regurgitation is usually functional, reflecting dilation of the right ventricle due to pulmonary hypertension. Indeed, tricuspid regurgitation often accompanies pulmonary hypertension and

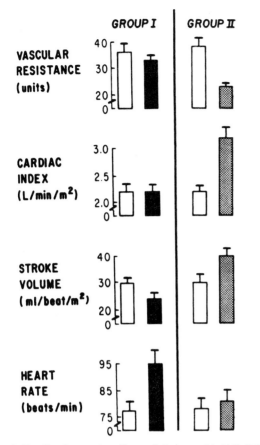

GROUP I   GROUP II

VASCULAR
RESISTANCE
(units)

CARDIAC
INDEX
(L/min/m²)

STROKE
VOLUME
(ml/beat/m²)

HEART
RATE
(beats/min)

Figure 2–5 • Cardiovascular effects of nitroprusside (1.3–3.7 µg/ kg/min IV) (*dark bars*) compared with the control (*clear bars*) were determined in patients with mitral and/or aortic regurgitation with (group II) or without (group I) preoperative fluid loading. The combination of afterload reduction and preload augmentation (group II) produced more desirable circulatory responses than afterload reduction alone (group I). Preoperative fluid loading was with approximately 2 L of lactated Ringer's solution. (From Stone JG, Hoar PF, Calabro JR, et al. Afterload reduction and preload augmentation of patients with cardiac failure and valvular regurgitation. Anesth Analg 1980;59:737–42, with permission.)

right ventricular volume overload due to left ventricular failure produced by aortic or mitral valve disease. A significant incidence of tricuspid regurgitation secondary to infective endocarditis is also associated with intravenous drug abuse. Tricuspid regurgitation is invariably associated with tricuspid stenosis when valve dysfunction is the result of prior rheumatic fever.

Pathophysiology

The basic hemodynamic consequence of tricuspid regurgitation is right atrial volume overload, which

is well tolerated. The high compliance of the right atrium and vena cavae result in minimal increases in right atrial pressures, even in the presence of large regurgitant volumes. Even surgical removal of the tricuspid valve, as in patients with infective endocarditis, is usually well tolerated. Although pure tricuspid regurgitation is relatively benign, the addition of right ventricular pressure overload as produced by left ventricular failure or pulmonary hypertension often leads to right ventricular failure. This causes an increased magnitude of regurgitation through an incompetent tricuspid valve, further decreasing the left ventricular stroke volume owing to decreased pulmonary blood flow. The combination of right ventricular failure and left ventricular underloading can cause right atrial pressures to exceed left atrial pressures, potentially leading to a right-to-left intracardiac shunt through an incompletely closed foramen ovale. Annuloplasty, rather than tricuspid valve replacement, is often the preferred surgical treatment of tricuspid regurgitation.

Management of Anesthesia

Management of anesthesia in patients with tricuspid regurgitation is similar whether the regurgitation is isolated or associated with aortic or mitral valve disease. Intravascular fluid volume and central venous pressures are maintained in high normal ranges to facilitate adequate right ventricular stroke volume and left ventricular filling. High intrathoracic pressure due to positive-pressure ventilation of the lungs or drug-induced venodilation decreases venous return and eventually compromises the left ventricular stroke volume. Likewise, events known to increase pulmonary vascular resistance, such as arterial hypoxemia and hypercarbia, should be avoided.

A specific anesthetic drug combination or technique cannot be recommended for anesthesia management in patients with tricuspid regurgitation. Nevertheless, a volatile anesthetic that could produce pulmonary vasodilation is a consideration, and ketamine is useful by virtue of its ability to maintain venous return. Nitrous oxide is a weak pulmonary vasoconstrictor when combined with opioids and could increase the magnitude of tricuspid regurgitation by this mechanism. If nitrous oxide is administered, it may be helpful to monitor the central venous pressure and consider the possible role of nitrous oxide should unexpected increases in right atrial pressures occur. Intraoperative monitors include measurement of right atrial filling pressures to guide intravenous fluid replacement and to detect adverse effects of the anesthetic drugs or technique on the amount of tricuspid regurgitation. Intravenous infusion of air through the tubing used to deliver intravenous fluids must be guarded against in view of the possibility of a right-to-left intracardiac shunt through an incompletely closed foramen ovale.

References

1. Carabello BA, Crawford FA. Valvular heart disease. N Engl J Med 1997;337:32–41
2. Griffin BP. Valvular heart disease. Sci Am Med 2000;1–14
3. Fishman MC, Hoffman AR, Klausner RD, et al. Medicine. Philadelphia, JB Lippincott, 1981, p 42
4. Greenberg BH, Rahimtoola SH. Vasodilator therapy for valvular heart disease. JAMA 1981;246:269–72
5. Vongpatanasin W, Hillis LD, Lange RA. Prosthetic heart valves. N Engl J Med 1996;335:407–16
6. Hilgenberg JC, McCammon RL, Stoelting RK. Pulmonary and systemic vascular responses to nitrous oxide in patients with mitral stenosis and pulmonary hypertension. Anesth Analg 1980;59:323–6
7. Konstadt SN, Reich DL, Thys DM. Nitrous oxide does not exacerbate pulmonary hypertension or ventricular dysfunction in patients with mitral valvular disease. Can J Anaesth 1990;37:13–7
8. Schulte-Sasse U, Hess W, Tarnow J. Pulmonary vascular responses to nitrous oxide in patients with normal and high pulmonary vascular resistance. Anesthesiology 1982;57:9–13
9. Stone JG, Hoar PF, Faltas AN, et al. Nitroprusside and mitral stenosis. Anesth Analg 1980;59:662–5
10. Nishimura RA, McGoon MD. Perspectives on mitral-valve prolapse. N Engl J Med 1999;341:48–50
11. Freed LA, Levy D, Levine RA, et al. Prevalence and clinical outcome of mitral-valve prolapse. N Engl J Med 1999;341:1–7
12. Gilon D, Buonanno FS, Joffe MM, et al. Lack of evidence of an association between mitral-valve prolapse and stroke in young patients. N Engl J Med 1999;341:8–13
13. Hanson EW, Neerhut RK, Lynch C. Mitral valve prolapse. Anesthesiology 1996;85:178–95
14. Moritz HA, Parnass SM, Mitchell JS. Ventricular fibrillation during anesthetic induction in a child with undiagnosed mitral valve prolapse. Anesth Analg 1997;85:59–61
15. Rosenhek R, Binder T, Porenta G, et al. Predictors of outcome in severe, asymptomatic aortic stenosis. N Engl J Med 2000;343;611–7
16. O'Keefe JH, Shub C, Rettke SR. Risk of noncardiac surgical procedures in patients with aortic stenosis. Mayo Clin Proc 1989;64:400–5
17. Loubser P, Suh K, Cohen S. Adverse effects of spinal anesthesia in a patient with idiopathic hypertrophic subaortic stenosis. Anesth Analg 1984;60;228–30
18. Collard CD, Eappen S, Lynch EP, et al. Continuous spinal anesthesia with invasive hemodynamic monitoring for surgical repair of the hip in two patients with severe aortic stenosis. Anesth Analg 1995;81:195–8
19. Stoelting RK, Gibbs PS. Hemodynamic effects of morphine and morphine-nitrous oxide in valvular heart disease and coronary artery disease. Anesthesiology 1973;38:45–52
20. Tomicheck RC, Rosow CE, Philbin DM, et al. Diazepam-fentanyl interaction: hemodynamic and hormonal effects in coronary artery surgery. Anesth Analg 1983;62:881–4
21. Stone JG, Hoar PF, Calabro JR, et al. Afterload reduction and preload augmentation improve the anesthetic management of patients with cardiac failure and valvular regurgitation. Anesth Analg 1980;59:737–42

3

Congenital Heart Disease

Congenital anomalies of the heart and cardiovascular system occur in 7 to 10 per 1000 live births (0.7% to 1.0%).[1] Congenital heart disease is the most common form of congenital disease and accounts for approximately 30% of the total incidence of all congenital diseases. With the decline in rheumatic heart disease, congenital heart disease has become the principal cause of heart disease with 10% to 15% of afflicted children having associated congenital anomalies of the skeletal, genitourinary, or gastrointestinal systems. Nine congenital heart lesions comprise more than 80% of congenital heart disease, with a wide range of more unusual and complex lesions comprising the remainder (Table 3–1).[1] The population of adults with congenital heart disease, surgically corrected or uncorrected, is estimated to exceed 1 million persons in the United States.[2] As a result, it is not uncommon for adult patients with congenital heart disease to present for noncardiac surgery.[3]

Transthoracic and transesophageal echocardiography have facilitated early, accurate diagnosis of congenital heart disease. Fetal cardiac ultrasonography has permitted early diagnosis of congenital heart defects, allowing subsequent perinatal management in specialized tertiary care centers. Imaging modalities, such as cardiac magnetic resonance imaging and three-dimensional echocardiography, have increased the understanding of complex cardiac malformations and allowed visualization of blood flow and vascular structures.[4] Cardiac catheterization and selective angiocardiography are the most definitive diagnostic procedures available for use in patients with congenital heart disease.

Advances in molecular biology have provided new understanding of the genetic basis of congenital heart disease.[4] Chromosomal abnormalities are as-

Table 3–1 • Classification and Incidence of Congenital Heart Disease

Disease	Incidence (%)
Acyanotic defects	
Ventricular septal defect	35
Atrial septal defect	9
Patent ductus arteriosus	8
Pulmonary stenosis	8
Aortic stenosis	6
Coarctation of the aorta	6
Atrioventricular septal defect	3
Cyanotic defects	
Tetralogy of Fallot	5
Transposition of the great vessels	4

Table 3–3 • Common Problems Associated with Congenital Heart Disease

Infective endocarditis
Cardiac dysrhythmias
Complete heart block
Hypertension (systemic or pulmonary)
Erythrocytosis
Thromboembolism
Coagulopathy
Brain abscess
Increased plasma uric acid concentration
Sudden death

sociated with an estimated 10% of congenital cardiovascular lesions. Two-thirds of these lesions occur in patients with trisomy 21; the other one-third are found in patients with karyotypic abnormalities, such as trisomy 13 and trisomy 18, and in patients with Turner syndrome. The remaining 90% of congenital cardiovascular lesions are postulated to be multifactorial in origin as a result of interactions of several genes with or without external factors (rubella, ethanol abuse, lithium, maternal diabetes mellitus). A widely used acronym, CATCH-22 (cardiac defects, abnormal facies, thymic hypoplasia, cleft palate, hypocalcemia) depicts a congenital heart disease syndrome attributed to defects in chromosome 22. An increased incidence of congenital heart disease in the offspring of affected adult patients suggests a role for single-gene defects in isolated congenital heart disease.

Signs and symptoms of congenital heart disease in infants and children often include dyspnea, slow physical development, and the presence of a cardiac murmur (Table 3–2). The diagnosis of congenital heart disease is apparent during the first week of life in about 50% of afflicted neonates and before 5 years of age in virtually all remaining patients. Echocardiography is the initial diagnostic step if congenital heart disease is suspected. Certain complications are likely to accompany the presence of congenital heart disease (Table 3–3). For example, infective endocarditis is a risk associated with most congenital cardiac anomalies. Cardiac dysrhythmias are not usually a prominent feature of congenital heart disease. Sudden death occasionally occurs in patients who undergo surgical correction of congenital heart disease, presumably reflecting myocardial scarring or damage to the cardiac conduction system.

ACYANOTIC CONGENITAL HEART DISEASE

Acyanotic congenital heart disease is characterized by a left-to-right intracardiac shunt (Table 3–4). The ultimate result of this intracardiac shunt, regardless of its location, is increased pulmonary blood flow with pulmonary hypertension, right ventricular hypertrophy, and eventually congestive heart failure. The younger the patient at the time of operation, the greater is the likelihood that pulmonary vascular resistance will normalize. In older patients, if pulmonary vascular resistance is one-third or less of the systemic vascular resistance, progressive pulmo-

Table 3–2 • Signs and Symptoms of Congenital Heart Disease

Infants
  Tachypnea
  Failure to gain weight
  Heart rate > 200 beats/min
  Heart murmur
  Congestive heart failure
  Cyanosis
Children
  Dyspnea
  Slow physical development
  Decreased exercise tolerance
  Heart murmur
  Congestive heart failure
  Cyanosis
  Clubbing of digits
  Squatting
  Hypertension

Table 3–4 • Congenital Heart Defects Resulting in a Left-to-Right Intracardiac Shunt or Its Equivalent

Secundum atrial septal defect
Primum atrial septal defect (endocardial cushion defect)
Ventricular septal defect
Aorticopulmonary fenestration

nary vascular disease after corrective surgery is unlikely. The onset and severity of clinical symptoms vary with the site and magnitude of the vascular shunt.

Atrial Septal Defect

Atrial septal defect (ASD) accounts for about one-third of the congenital heart disease detected in adults, with the frequency in females two to three times that in males.[2] Anatomically, an ASD may take the form of ostium secundum in the region of the fossa ovalis (often located near the center of the interatrial septum and varying from a single opening to a fenestrated septum), ostium primum (endocardial cushion defect characterized by a large opening in the interatrial septum), or sinus venosus located in the upper atrial septum (Fig. 3–1). Secundum ASDs account for 75% of all ASDs. Additional cardiac abnormalities may occur with each type of defect and include mitral valve prolapse (ostium secundum) and mitral regurgitation due to a cleft in the anterior mitral valve leaflet (ostium primum). Most ASDs occur as a result of spontaneous genetic mutations.

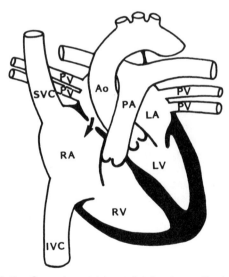

Figure 3–1 • Secundum atrial septal defect located in the center of the interatrial septum. Blood flow along a pressure gradient from the left atrium (LA) to the right atrium (RA). The resulting left-to-right intracardiac shunt is associated with increased blood flow through the pulmonary artery (PA). A decrease in systemic vascular resistance or an increase in pulmonary vascular resistance decreases the pressure gradient across the defect, leading to a decrease in the magnitude of the shunt. Ao, aorta; IVC, inferior vena cava; RV, right ventricle; PV, pulmonary vein; LV, left ventricle; SVC, superior vena cava.

The physiologic consequences of ASDs are the same regardless of the anatomic location and reflect the shunting of blood from one atrium to the other; the direction and magnitude of the shunt are determined by the size of the defect and the relative compliance of the ventricles. A small defect (less than 0.5 cm in diameter) is associated with a small shunt and no hemodynamic sequelae. When the diameter of the ASD approaches 2 cm it is likely that left atrial blood is being shunted to the right atrium (the right ventricle is more compliant than the left ventricle) resulting in increased pulmonary blood flow. A systolic ejection murmur audible in the second left intercostal space may be mistaken for an innocent flow murmur. The electrocardiogram (ECG) may reflect right axis deviation and incomplete right bundle branch block. Atrial fibrillation and supraventricular tachycardia may accompany an ASD that remains uncorrected into adulthood. The chest radiograph is likely to reveal prominent pulmonary arteries. Transesophageal echocardiography and Doppler color flow echocardiography are useful for detecting and determining the location of ASDs.

Signs and Symptoms

Because they initially produce no symptoms or striking findings on physical examination, ASDs may remain undetected for years. A small defect with minimal right-to-left shunting (ratio of pulmonary flow to systemic flow is less than 1.5) usually causes no symptoms and therefore does not require closure. When pulmonary blood flow is 1.5 times the systemic blood flow, the ASD should be surgically closed to prevent right ventricular dysfunction and irreversible pulmonary hypertension. Symptoms due to large ASDs include dyspnea on exertion, supraventricular dysrhythmias, right heart failure, paradoxical embolism, and recurrent pulmonary infections. Prophylaxis against infective endocarditis is not recommended for patients with an ASD unless a concomitant valvular abnormality (mitral valve prolapse or mitral valve cleft) is present.

Management of Anesthesia

An ASD associated with a left-to-right intracardiac shunt has only minor implications for the management of anesthesia. For example, so long as the systemic blood flow remains normal, the pharmacokinetics of inhaled drugs are not significantly altered despite the increased pulmonary blood flow.[5] Conversely, increased pulmonary blood flow could dilute drugs injected intravenously. It is unlikely, however, that this potential dilution will alter the clinical response to these drugs, as the pulmonary circulation time is brief. Another effect of increased pulmonary blood flow is that positive-pressure ventilation of the lungs is well tolerated.

Any change in systemic vascular resistance during the perioperative period could have important implications for the patient with an ASD. For example, drugs or events that produce prolonged increases in systemic vascular resistance should be avoided, as this change favors an increase in the magnitude of the left-to-right shunt at the atrial level. This is particularly true with a primum ASD defect associated with mitral regurgitation. Conversely, decreases in systemic vascular resistance, as produced by volatile anesthetics or increases in pulmonary vascular resistance due to positive-pressure ventilation of the lungs, tend to decrease the magnitude of the left-to-right shunt.

Another consideration for management of anesthesia in the presence of ASDs is the need to provide prophylactic antibiotics to protect against infective endocarditis when a cardiac valvular abnormality is present. In addition, meticulously avoiding the entrance of air into the circulation, as can occur through tubing used to deliver intravenous solutions, is imperative. Transient supraventricular dysrhythmias and atrioventricular conduction defects are common during the early postoperative period after surgical repair of an ASD.

Ventricular Septal Defect

Ventricular septal defect (VSD) is the most common congenital cardiac abnormality in infants and children (Fig. 3–2). A large number of VSDs close spontaneously by the time a child reaches 2 years of age. Anatomically, about 70% of these defects are located in the membranous portion of the intraventricular septum, 20% in the muscular portion of the septum, 5% just below the aortic valve causing aortic regurgitation, and 5% near the junction of the mitral and tricuspid valve (atrioventricular canal defect).[2] Echocardiography with Doppler flow confirms the presence and location of the VSD, and color-flow mapping provides information about the magnitude and direction of the intracardiac shunt. Cardiac catheterization and angiography confirm the presence and location of the VSD and determine the magnitude of the intracardiac shunting and the pulmonary vascular resistance.

Signs and Symptoms

The physiologic significance of a VSD depends on the size of the defect and the relative resistance in the

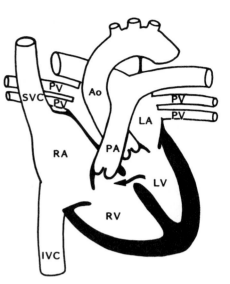

Figure 3–2 • Ventricular septal defect located just below the muscular ridge that separates the body of the right ventricle (RV) from the pulmonary artery (PA) outflow tract. Blood flow is along a pressure gradient from the left ventricle (LV) to the RV. The resulting left-to-right intracardiac shunt is associated with pulmonary blood flow that exceeds the stroke volume of the LV. A decrease in systemic vascular resistance decreases the pressure gradient across the defect and reduces the magnitude of the shunt.

systemic and pulmonary circulations. If the defect is small, there is minimal functional disturbance as pulmonary blood flow is only modestly increased. If the defect is large, the ventricular systolic pressures equalize; and the magnitude of systemic and pulmonary blood flow is determined by the relative vascular resistances of these two circulations. Initially, systemic vascular resistance exceeds pulmonary vascular resistance, and left-to-right intracardiac shunting predominates. Over time the pulmonary vascular resistance increases, and the magnitude of the left-to right intracardiac shunting declines; eventually the shunt may become right-to-left with the development of arterial hypoxemia (cyanosis).

The murmur of a moderate to large VSD is holosystolic and is loudest at the lower left sternal border. The ECG and chest radiograph remain normal in the presence of a small VSD. When the VSD is large there is evidence of left atrial and ventricular enlargement on the ECG. If pulmonary hypertension develops, the QRS axis shifts to the right, and right atrial and ventricular enlargement are noted on the ECG.

The natural history of a VSD depends on the size of the defect and the pulmonary vascular resistance.[2] Adults with small defects and normal pulmonary arterial pressures are generally asymptomatic, and pulmonary hypertension is unlikely to develop.

These patients are at risk of developing infective endocarditis but do not require surgical correction of the VSD. In the absence of surgical correction a large VSD eventually leads to left ventricular failure or pulmonary hypertension with right ventricular failure. Surgical closure of the defect is recommended in these patients, if the magnitude of the pulmonary hypertension is not prohibitive. Once the pulmonary/systemic vascular resistance ratio exceeds 0.7, the risk of surgical closure is prohibitive.[2]

Management of Anesthesia

Antibiotic prophylaxis to protect against infective endocarditis is indicated when noncardiac surgery is planned in patients with VSDs. The pharmacokinetics of inhaled and injected drugs are not significantly altered by a VSD. As with an ASD, acute and persistent increases in systemic vascular resistance or decreases in pulmonary vascular resistance are undesirable, as these changes can accentuate the magnitude of the left-to-right intracardiac shunt at the ventricular level. In this regard, volatile anesthetics (which decreases systemic vascular resistance) and positive-pressure ventilation of the patient's lungs (which increases pulmonary vascular resistance) are well tolerated. However, there may be increased delivery of depressant drugs to the heart if coronary blood flow is increased to supply the hypertrophied ventricles. Conceivably, increasing the inspired concentrations of volatile anesthetics to achieve rapid induction of anesthesia, as is often done in normal children, could result in excessive depression of the heart before central nervous system depression is achieved.

Right ventricular infundibular hypertrophy may be present in patients with VSDs. Normally, this is a beneficial change, as it increases the resistance to right ventricular ejection, leading to a decrease in the magnitude of the left-to-right intracardiac shunt. Nevertheless, perioperative events that exaggerate this obstruction to right ventricular outflow, such as increased myocardial contractility or hypovolemia, must be minimized. Therefore these patients are often anesthetized with volatile anesthetics. In addition, intravascular fluid volume should be maintained by prompt replacement of lost blood.

Anesthesia for placement of a pulmonary artery band is often achieved with drugs that provide minimal cardiac depression. Muscle relaxants are used to prevent patient movement. If bradycardia or systemic hypotension develops during surgery, it may be necessary to remove the pulmonary artery band promptly. Continuous monitoring of the systemic

blood pressure with an intra-arterial catheter is helpful. Administration of positive end-expiratory pressure may be useful in the presence of congestive heart failure but should be discontinued when the pulmonary artery band is in place. The high mortality rate associated with pulmonary artery banding has led to attempted complete surgical correction at an early age using cardiopulmonary bypass. Third-degree atrioventricular heart block may follow surgical closure if the cardiac conduction system is near the VSD. Premature ventricular beats may reflect the electrical instability of the ventricle due to surgical ventriculotomy. The risk of ventricular tachycardia, however, is low if postoperative ventricular filling pressures are normal.

Patent Ductus Arteriosus

Patent ductus arteriosus (PDA) is present when the ductus arteriosus (which arises just distal to the left subclavian artery and connects the descending aorta to the left pulmonary artery) fails to close spontaneously shortly after birth (Fig. 3–3). In the fetus the ductus arteriosus permits pulmonary arterial blood to bypass the deflated lungs and enter the descending aorta for oxygenation in the placenta. In full-term newborns the ductus arteriosus closes within 24 to 48 hours after delivery, but in preterm newborns the ductus arteriosus frequently fails to close.

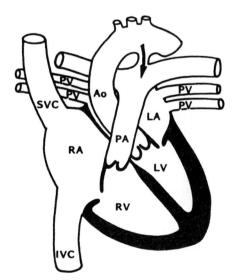

Figure 3–3 • Patent ductus arteriosus connecting the arch of the aorta (Ao) with the pulmonary artery (PA). Blood flow is from the high pressure Ao into the PA. The resulting aorta-to-pulmonary artery shunt (left-to-right shunt) leads to increased pulmonary blood flow. A decrease in systemic vascular resistance or an increase in pulmonary vascular resistance decreases the magnitude of the shunt through the ductus arteriosus.

When the ductus arteriosus fails to close spontaneously after birth the result is continuous flow of blood from the aorta to the pulmonary artery. The pulmonary/systemic blood flow ratio depends on the pressure gradient from the aorta to the pulmonary artery, the pulmonary/systemic vascular resistance ratio, and the diameter and length of the ductus arteriosus. The PDA can usually be visualized on echocardiography, with Doppler studies confirming the continuous flow into the pulmonary circulation. Cardiac catheterization and angiography make it possible to quantify the magnitude of the shunting and the pulmonary vascular resistance and to visualize the PDA.

Signs and Symptoms

Most patients with a PDA are asymptomatic and have only modest left-to-right shunts. This cardiac defect is often detected during a routine physical examination, at which time a characteristic continuous systolic and diastolic murmur is heard. If the left-to-right shunt is large, there may be evidence of left ventricular hypertrophy on the ECG and chest radiograph. If pulmonary hypertension develops, right ventricular hypertrophy is apparent. The presence of a PDA increases the risk of infective endocarditis. Surgical ligation of a PDA is associated with low mortality and is unlikely to require cardiopulmonary bypass. Without surgical closure, most patients remain asymptomatic until adolescence, when pulmonary hypertension and congestive heart failure may occur. Once severe pulmonary hypertension develops, surgical or percutaneous closure is contraindicated.

Treatment

It is estimated that 70% of preterm infants delivered before 28 weeks' gestation require medical or surgical closure of a PDA. Surgical ligation of a PDA can be performed in neonatal intensive care units with low morbidity and mortality rates. Nevertheless, risks of surgical closure are significant and include intracranial hemorrhage, infections, and recurrent laryngeal nerve paralysis especially in infants born at less than 28 weeks' gestation. Inhibition of prostaglandin synthesis with nonselective cyclooxygenase inhibitors (COX-1, COX-2) appears to be an effective alternative to surgery for closure of a PDA in neonates. Indomethacin, a nonselective cyclooxygenase inhibitor utilized for this purpose, has replaced surgery as the preferred therapy for PDA.[6] Adverse side effects of indomethacin include decreased mesenteric, renal, and cerebral blood flow. Ibuprofen is a nonselective cyclooxygenase inhibitor that can be used effectively to treat PDA, and it has less effect on organ blood flow than indomethacin.[7]

Management of Anesthesia

Antibiotic prophylaxis for protection against infective endocarditis is recommended for patients with PDAs who are scheduled for noncardiac surgery. When surgical closure of the PDA is planned through a left thoractomy, appropriate preparations must be taken in anticipation of the possibility of large blood loss should control of the PDA be lost during attempted ligation. Anesthesia with volatile anesthetics is useful, as these drugs tend to lower systemic blood pressure, lessening the danger of the PDA escaping from the vascular clamp or tearing as it is being divided. Furthermore, the decreased systemic vascular resistance produced by volatile anesthetics may improve systemic blood flow by decreasing the magnitude of the left-to-right shunt. Likewise, positive-pressure ventilation of the patient's lungs is well tolerated, as increased airway pressure increases pulmonary vascular resistance, thereby decreasing the pressure gradient across the PDA. Conversely, increases in systemic vascular resistance or decreases in pulmonary vascular resistance should be avoided, as these changes would increase the magnitude of the left-to-right shunt. Continuous monitoring of systemic blood pressure by a catheter placed in a peripheral artery is helpful during the operation.

Ligation of the PDA is often associated with significant systemic hypertension during the postoperative period. This hypertension can be managed with continuous infusion of vasodilator drugs such as nitroprusside. Long-acting antihypertensive drugs can be gradually substituted for nitroprusside if systemic hypertension persists.

Aorticopulmonary Fenestration

Aorticopulmonary fenestration is characterized by a communication between the left side of the ascending aorta and the right wall of the main pulmonary artery, just anterior to the origin of the right pulmonary artery. This communication is due to failure of the aorticopulmonary septum to fuse and completely separate the aorta from the pulmonary artery. Clinical and hemodynamic manifestations of an aorticopulmonary communication are similar to those associated with a large PDA. The diagnosis is facilitated by echocardiography and angiocardiography. Treatment is surgical and requires the use of cardiopulmonary bypass. Management of anesthesia entails the same principles as described for patients with PDAs.

Aortic Stenosis

Bicuspid aortic valves occur in 2% to 3% of the U.S. population, and an estimated 20% of these patients have other cardiovascular abnormalities, such as PDA or coarctation of the aorta (see Chapter 2).[2] The deformed bicuspid aortic valve is not stenotic at birth; but with time, thickening and calcification of the leaflets (usually not apparent before 15 years of age) occurs with resulting immobility. Transthoracic echocardiography with Doppler flow studies permits accurate assessment of the severity of the aortic stenosis and of left ventricular function. Cardiac catheterization is performed to determine the presence of concomitant coronary artery disease.

Aortic stenosis is associated with a systolic murmur that is audible over the aortic area (second right intercostal space) and often radiates into the neck. Most patients with congenital aortic stenosis are asymptomatic until adulthood. Infants with severe aortic stenosis, however, may present with congestive heart failure. Findings in patients with supravalvular aortic stenosis may include characteristic appearances in which the facial bones are prominent, the forehead is rounded, and the upper lip is pursed. Strabismus, inguinal hernia, dental abnormalities, and moderate mental retardation are commonly present. The ECG in the presence of congenital aortic stenosis typically reveals left ventricular hypertrophy. Depression of the ST segment on the ECG is likely during exercise, particularly if the pressure gradient across the aortic valve is more than 50 mmHg. Chest radiographs show left ventricular hypertrophy with or without poststenotic dilation of the aorta. Angina pectoris in the absence of coronary artery disease reflects the inability of coronary blood flow to meet increased myocardial oxygen requirements of the hypertrophied left ventricle. Syncope can occur when the pressure gradient across the aortic valve exceeds 50 mmHg. In the presence of aortic stenosis, the myocardium must generate an intraventricular pressure that is two to three times normal, whereas pressure in the aorta remains within a physiologic range. The resulting concentric myocardial hypertrophy leads to increased myocardial oxygen requirements. Furthermore, the high velocity of blood flow through the stenotic area predisposes to the development of infective endocarditis and is associated with poststenotic dilation of the aorta. In adults with symptomatic aortic stenosis (syncope, angina pectoris, congestive heart failure) the indicated treatment is surgical valve replacement (see Chapter 2).

Pulmonic Stenosis

Pulmonic stenosis producing obstruction to right ventricular outflow is valvular in 90% of patients; in the remainder it is supravalvular or subvalvular.[2] Supravalvular pulmonic stenosis often co-exists with other congenital cardiac abnormalities (ASD, VSD, PDA, tetralogy of Fallot). It is a common feature of Williams syndrome, which is characterized by infantile hypercalcemia and mental retardation. Subvalvular pulmonic stenosis usually occurs in association with a VSD. Valvular pulmonic stenosis is typically an isolated abnormality, but it may occur in association with a VSD. Severe pulmonic stenosis is characterized by transvalvular pressure gradients of more than 80 mmHg or right ventricular systolic pressures of more than 100 mmHg. Echocardiography and Doppler flow studies can determine the site of the obstruction and the severity of the stenosis. Treatment of pulmonic stenosis is with percutaneous balloon valvuloplasty.

Signs and Symptoms

In asymptomatic patients the presence of pulmonic stenosis is identified by the presence of a loud systolic ejection murmur, best heard at the second left intercostal space. The intensity and duration of the cardiac murmur parallel the severity of the pulmonic stenosis. Dyspnea may occur on exertion, and eventually right ventricular failure with peripheral edema and ascites develops. If the foramen ovale is patent, right-to-left intracardiac shunting of blood may occur, causing cyanosis and clubbing.

Management of Anesthesia

Management of anesthesia is designed to avoid increases in right ventricular oxygen requirements. Therefore excessive increases in heart rate and myocardial contractility are undesirable. The impact of changes in pulmonary vascular resistance are minimized by the presence of fixed obstruction of the pulmonic valve. As a result, increases in pulmonary vascular resistance due to positive-pressure ventilation of the lungs are unlikely to produce significant increases in right ventricular afterload and oxygen requirements. These patients are extremely difficult to resuscitate if cardiac arrest occurs because external cardiac compression is not highly effective in forcing blood across a stenotic pulmonic valve. Therefore decreases in systemic blood pressure should be promptly treated with sympathomimetic drugs. Likewise, cardiac dysrhythmias or increases in heart rate that become hemodynamically significant should be rapidly corrected, using such drugs as lidocaine, propranolol, or esmolol. An electrical defibrillator should be available when anesthesia is administered to patients with pulmonic stenosis.

Spinal and epidural anesthesia, as for parturients in labor, may be avoided because of the potential cardiovascular side effects associated with pulmonic stenosis. Nevertheless, continuous spinal analgesia utilizing an opioid has been described as an alternative for labor analgesia in a patient with severe pulmonic stenosis.[8]

Coarctation of the Aorta

Coarctation of the aorta typically consists of a discrete, diaphragm-like ridge extending into the aortic lumen just distal to the left subclavian artery at the site of the aortic ductal attachment (ligamentum arteriosum). This anatomic manifestation is known as postductal coarctation of the aorta and is most likely to manifest in young adults. Less commonly the coarctation is immediately proximal to the left subclavian artery (preductal); this situation is most likely to present in infants. Coarctation of the aorta is more common in males and may occur in conjunction with a bicuspid aortic valve, PDA, mitral stenosis or regurgitation, aneurysms of the circle of Willis, and gonadal dysgenesis (Turner syndrome).[2]

Signs and Symptoms

Most adults with coarctation of the aorta are asymptomatic, and the problem is diagnosed during a routine physical examination when systemic hypertension is detected in the arms in association with diminished or absent femoral arterial pulses. Characteristically, systolic blood pressure is higher in the arms than in the legs, but the diastolic pressure is similar, resulting in widened pulse pressure in the arms. The femoral arterial pulses are weak and delayed. Systemic hypertension presumably reflects ejection of the left ventricular stroke volume into the fixed resistance created by the narrowed aorta. A harsh systolic ejection murmur is present along the left sternal border and in the back, particularly over the area of the coarctation. In the presence of preductal coarctation of the aorta, there is no difference in the systemic blood pressures in the arms and legs. Extensive collateral arterial circulation to the distal body through the internal thoracic, intercostal, scapular, and subclavian arteries is likely in the presence of coarctation of the aorta. In this regard a systolic murmur may be heard in the back, reflecting this collateral blood flow.

The ECG shows signs of left ventricular hypertrophy. On the chest radiograph increased collateral flow through the intercostal arteries causes symmetrical notching of the posterior third of the third through eighth ribs.[2] Notching is not seen in the anterior ribs, as the anterior intercostal arteries are not located in costal grooves. The coarctation may be visible as an indentation of the aorta with prestenotic or poststenotic dilation of the aorta, producing the "reversed E," or "3," sign. The coarctation may be visualized with echocardiography, and Doppler examination makes it possible to estimate the transcoarctation pressure gradient. Computed tomography, magnetic resonance imaging, and contrast aortography provide precise anatomic information regarding the location and length of the coarctation and the degree of collateral circulation.

When clinical symptoms of a previously unrecognized coarctation of the aorta manifest, they are usually characterized as headache, dizziness, epistaxis, and palpitations. Occasionally diminished blood flow to the legs causes claudication. Women with coarctation of the aorta are at increased risk for aortic dissection during pregnancy. Complications of coarctation of the aorta include systemic hypertension, left ventricular failure, aortic dissection, premature ischemic heart disease presumably related to chronic hypertension, infective endocarditis, and cerebral vascular accidents due to rupture of intracerebral aneurysms. Patients with known coarctation of the aorta should be given prophylactic antibiotics prior to dental or surgical procedures.

Treatment

Surgical resection of the coarctation of the aorta should be considered for patients with a transcoarctation pressure gradient of more than 30 mmHg. Although balloon dilation is a therapeutic alternative, the procedure is associated with a higher incidence of subsequent aortic aneurysm and recurrent coarctation than surgical resection.

Management of Anesthesia

Management of anesthesia for surgical resection of coarctation of the aorta must consider: (1) the adequacy of perfusion to the lower portion of the body during cross-clamping of the aorta; (2) the propensity for systemic hypertension during cross-clamping of the aorta; and (3) the risk of neurologic sequelae due to ischemia of the spinal cord (see Chapter 10). Blood flow to the anterior spinal artery is augmented by radicular branches of the intercostal arteries and may be compromised during cross-clamping of the aorta for surgical resection of coarctation of the aorta. Paraplegia after surgical resection of coarctation of the aorta is a rare complication. Continuous monitoring of systemic blood pressure above and below the coarctation is achieved by placing a catheter in the right radial artery and a femoral artery. By monitoring these pressures simultaneously it is possible to evaluate the adequacy of the collateral circulation during periods of aortic cross-clamping. Mean arterial pressures in the lower extremities should be at least 40 mmHg to ensure adequate blood flow to the kidneys and spinal cord. If the systemic blood pressure cannot be maintained above this level it may be necessary to use partial circulatory bypass. Somatosensory evoked potentials are useful for monitoring spinal cord function and the adequacy of its blood flow during cross-clamping of the aorta. Nevertheless, case reports of paraplegia despite normal somatosensory evoked potentials suggest that monitoring posterior (sensory) cord function does not ensure adequate blood flow to the anterior (motor) portion of the spinal cord (see Chapter 10). Excessive increases in systolic blood pressure during cross-clamping of the aorta may adversely increase the work of the heart and make surgical repair more difficult. In this situation, the use of volatile anesthetics is helpful for maintaining normal systemic blood pressures. If systemic hypertension persists, continuous intravenous infusions of nitroprusside should be considered. The disadvantages of lowering the systemic blood pressure to normal levels are excessively decreased perfusion pressure in the lower part of the body and inadequate blood flow to the kidneys and spinal cord.

Postoperative Management

Immediate postoperative complications include paradoxical hypertension, possible sequelae of a bicuspid aortic valve (infective endocarditis and aortic regurgitation), and paraplegia. Baroreceptor reflexes, activation of the renin-angiotensin-aldosterone system, and excessive release of catecholamines have been implicated as possible causes of immediate postoperative systemic hypertension. Regardless of the etiology, intravenous administration of nitroprusside with or without esmolol effectively controls the systemic blood pressure during the early postoperative period. Longer-acting antihypertensive drugs may be needed if hypertension persists. Paraplegia manifesting during the immediate postoperative period is assumed to reflect ischemic damage to the spinal cord during the aortic cross-clamping required for surgical resection of the

coarctation. Abdominal pain may occur during the postoperative period and is presumably due to sudden increases in blood flow to the gastrointestinal tract, leading to increased vasoactivity.

The incidence of persistent or recurrent systemic hypertension and the survival rate are influenced by the patient's age at the time of surgery. Most of the patients who undergo surgery during childhood are normotensive 5 years later, whereas those who undergo surgery after 40 years of age often manifest persistent systemic hypertension.[2]

▌ CYANOTIC CONGENITAL HEART DISEASE

Cyanotic congenital heart disease is characterized by a right-to-left intracardiac shunt with associated decreases in pulmonary blood flow and the development of arterial hypoxemia (Table 3–5).[2] The magnitude of shunting determines the severity of arterial hypoxemia. Erythrocytosis secondary to chronic arterial hypoxemia results in a risk of thromboembolism, especially when the hematocrit exceeds 70%. Patients with secondary erythrocytosis may exhibit coagulation defects most likely owing to deficiencies of vitamin K-dependent clotting factors in the liver and defective platelet aggregation. Development of a brain abscess is a major risk in patients with cyanotic congenital heart disease. The onset of a brain abscess often mimics a stroke. Survival in the presence of a right-to-left intracardiac shunt requires a communication between the systemic and pulmonary circulations. Tetralogy of Fallot is the prototype of these defects. Most children with cyanotic congenital heart disease do not survive to adulthood without surgical intervention. Principles for the management of anesthesia are the same for all the cyanotic congenital cardiac defects.

Tetralogy of Fallot

Tetralogy of Fallot, the most common cyanotic congenital heart defect, is characterized by a large single VSD, an aorta that overrides the right and left ventri-

Table 3–5 • Congenital Heart Defects Resulting in a Right-to-Left Intracardiac Shunt

Tetralogy of Fallot
Eisenmenger syndrome
Ebstein's anomaly (malformation of the tricuspid valve)
Tricuspid atresia
Foramen ovale

cles, obstruction to right ventricular outflow (sub-valvular, valvular, supravalvular, pulmonary arterial branches), and right ventricular hypertrophy (Fig. 3–4).[9] Several abnormalities may occur in association with tetralogy of Fallot, including right aortic arch, ASD ("pentalogy of Fallot"), and coronary arterial anomalies. Right ventricular hypertrophy occurs because the VSD permits continuous exposure of the right ventricle to the high pressures present in the left ventricle. Right-to-left intracardiac shunting occurs because of increased resistance to flow in the right ventricular outflow tract, the severity of which determines the magnitude of the shunt. Because the resistance to flow across the right ventricular outflow tract is relatively fixed, changes in systemic vascular resistance (drug-induced) may affect the magnitude of the shunt. Decreases in systemic vascular resistance increase right-to-left intracardiac shunting and accentuate arterial hypoxemia, whereas increases in systemic vascular resistance (squatting) decrease left-to-right intracardiac shunting with resultant increases in pulmonary blood flow.

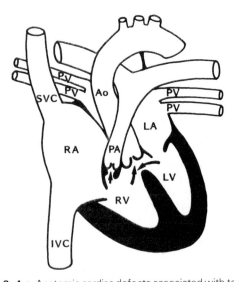

Figure 3–4 • Anatomic cardiac defects associated with tetralogy of Fallot. Defects include (1) ventricular septal defect, (2) aorta (Ao) overriding the pulmonary artery (PA) outflow tract, (3) obstruction to blood flow through a narrowed PA or stenotic pulmonic valve, and (4) right ventricular hypertrophy. Obstruction to PA outflow results in a pressure gradient that favors blood flow across the ventricular septal defect from the right ventricle (RV) to the left ventricle (LV). The resulting right-to-left intracardiac shunt combined with obstruction to ejection of the stroke volume from the RV leads to marked decreases in pulmonary blood flow and the development of arterial hypoxemia. Any event that increases pulmonary vascular resistance or decreases systemic vascular resistance increases the magnitude of the shunt and accentuates arterial hypoxemia.

Diagnosis

Echocardiography is used to establish the diagnosis and assess the presence of associated abnormalities, the level and severity of the obstruction to right ventricular outflow, the size of the main pulmonary artery and its branches, and the number and location of the VSDs.[9] Right-to-left shunting through the VSD is visualized by color Doppler imaging, and the severity of the right ventricular outflow tract obstruction can be determined by spectral Doppler measurement. Cardiac catheterization further confirms the diagnosis and permits confirmation of anatomic and hemodynamic data, including the location and magnitude of the right-to-left shunt, the level and severity of the right ventricular outflow obstruction, the anatomic features of the right ventricular outflow obstruction, the anatomic features of the right ventricular outflow tract and the main pulmonary artery and its branches, and the origin and course of the coronary arteries.[9] Magnetic resonance imaging can also provide much of this information.

Signs and Symptoms

Most patients with tetralogy of Fallot have cyanosis from birth or beginning during the first year of life. The most common auscultatory finding is an ejection murmur heard along the left sternal border resulting from blood flow across the stenotic pulmonic valve. Congestive heart failure rarely develops because the large VSD permits equilibration of intraventricular pressures and cardiac workload. Chest radiographs show evidence of decreased lung vascularity, and the heart is "boot shaped" with an upturned right ventricular apex and a concave main pulmonary arterial segment. The ECG is characterized by changes of right axis deviation and right ventricular hypertrophy. Arterial oxygen desaturation is present even when breathing 100% oxygen (PaO_2 usually less than 50 mmHg). Compensatory erythropoiesis is proportional to the magnitude of the arterial hypoxemia. The $PaCO_2$ and arterial pH (pHa) are usually normal. Squatting is a common feature of children with tetralogy of Fallot. It is speculated that squatting increases the systemic vascular resistance by kinking the large arteries in the inguinal area. The resulting increase in systemic vascular resistance tends to decrease the magnitude of the right-to-left intracardiac shunt, which leads to increased pulmonary blood flow and subsequent improvement in arterial oxygenation.

Hypercyanotic Attacks

Hypercyanotic attacks are characterized by sudden spells of arterial hypoxemia associated with worsening cyanosis, tachypnea, and in some instances loss of consciousness, seizures, cerebrovascular accidents, and even death.[9] These attacks can occur without obvious provocation but are often associated with crying or exercise. Their mechanism is not known, but the most likely explanation is a sudden decrease in pulmonary blood flow due to spasm of the infundibular cardiac muscle or decreased systemic vascular resistance.

Treatment of hypercyanotic attacks is influenced by the cause of the pulmonary outflow obstruction.[10] When symptoms reflect a dynamic infundibular obstruction (spasm), appropriate treatment is administration of β-adrenergic antagonists such as esmolol or propranolol. Indeed, chronic oral propranolol therapy is indicated in patients who have recurrent hypercyanotic attacks caused by spasm of the outflow tract muscle. If the cause is decreased systemic vascular resistance, treatment is intravenous administration of fluids and/or phenylephrine. Sympathomimetic drugs that display β-agonist properties are not selected, as they may accentuate the spasm of the infundibular cardiac muscle. Recurrent hypercyanotic attacks indicate the need for surgical correction of the abnormalities associated with tetralogy of Fallot.

These attacks do not occur in adolescents or adults. Adults with tetralogy of Fallot manifest dyspnea and limited exercise tolerance. They may also have complications of chronic cyanosis including erythrocytosis, hyperviscosity, abnormalities of hemostasis, cerebral abscess or stroke, and infective endocarditis.

Cerebrovascular Accident

Cerebrovascular accidents are common in children with severe tetralogy of Fallot. Cerebrovascular thrombosis or severe arterial hypoxemia may be the explanation for these adverse responses. Dehydration and polycythemia may contribute to thrombosis. Hemoglobin concentrations exceeding 20 g/dl are common in these patients.

Cerebral Abscess

A cerebral abscess is suggested by the abrupt onset of headache, fever, and lethargy followed by persistent emesis and the appearance of seizure activity. The most likely cause is arterial seeding into areas of prior cerebral infarction.

Infective Endocarditis

Infective endocarditis is a constant danger in patients with tetralogy of Fallot and is associated with a high mortality rate. Antibiotics should be administered to protect against this serious possibility whenever dental or surgical procedures are planned in these patients.

Treatment

Treatment of tetralogy of Fallot is complete surgical correction (closure of the VSD with a Dacron patch and relief of right ventricular outflow obstruction by placing a synthetic graft) when patients are extremely young.[9] Without surgery, mortality exceeds 50% by 3 years of age. Pulmonic regurgitation due to an incompetent pulmonic valve usually results from surgical correction of the cardiac defects characteristic of tetralogy of Fallot but poses no major hazard unless the distal pulmonary arteries are hypoplastic, in which case volume overload of the right ventricle secondary to regurgitant blood flow may result. A major complication of complete surgical repair is difficulty achieving surgical hemostasis. Platelet dysfunction and hypofibrinogenemia are common in these patients and may contribute to postoperative bleeding problems. Right-to-left intracardiac shunting often develops through the foramen ovale during the postoperative period. Shunting through the foramen ovale acts as a safety valve if the right ventricle is unable to function at the same efficiency as the left ventricle.

In the past, infants underwent one of three palliative procedures to increase pulmonary blood flow. All three palliative procedures involved anastomosis of a systemic artery to a pulmonary artery in an effort to increase pulmonary blood flow and improve arterial oxygenation. These palliative procedures were the Waterston procedure (side-to-side anastomosis of the ascending aorta and the right pulmonary artery), the Potts operation (side-to-side anastomosis of the descending aorta to the left pulmonary artery), and the Blalock-Taussig operation (end-to-side anastomosis of the subclavian artery to the pulmonary artery). Often, however, these procedures were associated with long-term complications such as pulmonary hypertension, left ventricular volume overload, and distortion of the pulmonary arterial branches.

Management of Anesthesia

Management of anesthesia for patients with tetralogy of Fallot requires a thorough understanding of those events and drugs that can alter the magnitude of the right-to-left intracardiac shunt. For example, when shunt magnitude is acutely increased, there are associated decreases in pulmonary blood flow and PaO_2. Furthermore, the magnitude of the right-to-left shunt may alter the pharmacokinetics of both inhaled and injected drugs.

The magnitude of a right-to-left intracardiac shunt can be increased by (1) decreased systemic vascular resistance, (2) increased pulmonary vascular resistance, and (3) increased myocardial contractility, which accentuates infundibular obstruction to ejection of blood by the right ventricle. In many respects, resistance to ejection of blood into the pulmonary artery outflow tract is relatively fixed, and hence the magnitude of the shunt is inversely proportional to the systemic vascular resistance. Pharmacologically induced responses that decrease systemic vascular resistance (volatile anesthetics, histamine release, ganglionic blockade, α-adrenergic blockade) increase the magnitude of the right-to-left shunt and accentuate arterial hypoxemia. Pulmonary blood flow can be decreased by increases in pulmonary vascular resistance that accompany such intraoperative ventilatory maneuvers as intermittent positive airway pressure or positive end-expiratory pressure. Furthermore, the loss of negative intrapleural pressure on opening the chest increases pulmonary vascular resistance and the magnitude of the shunt. Nevertheless, the advantages of controlled ventilation of the lungs during operations usually offset this potential hazard. Indeed, arterial oxygenation does not predictably deteriorate in patients with tetralogy of Fallot, either with the institution of positive pressure ventilation of the lungs or after opening of the chest.

Preoperative Preparation

Preoperatively, it is important to avoid dehydration by maintaining oral feedings in extremely young patients or by providing intravenous fluids before the patient's arrival in the operating room. Crying associated with intramuscular administration of drugs used for preoperative medication can lead to hypercyanotic attacks.[10] For this reason, it may be prudent to avoid administering drugs by this route until patients are in highly supervised environments and the ability to treat hypercyanotic attacks is optimal (see "Hypercyanotic Attacks"). β-Adrenergic antagonists should be continued until the induction of anesthesia in patients receiving these drugs for prophylaxis against hypercyanotic attacks.

Induction of Anesthesia

Induction of anesthesia in patients with tetralogy of Fallot is often accomplished with ketamine (3 to 4 mg/kg IM or 1 to 2 mg/kg IV). The onset of anesthesia after ketamine injection may be associated with improved arterial oxygenation, presumably reflecting increased pulmonary blood flow due to ketamine-induced increases in systemic vascular resistance, which can lead to a decrease in the magnitude of the right-to-left intracardiac shunt. Ketamine has also been alleged to increase pulmonary vascular resistance, which would be undesirable in patients with a right-to-left shunt. The efficacious response to ketamine of patients with tetralogy of Fallot, however, suggests that this concern is not clinically significant. Tracheal intubation is facilitated by administration of muscle relaxants. It should be remembered that the onset of action of drugs administered intravenously may be more rapid in the presence of right-to-left shunts, as the dilutional effect in the lungs is decreased. For this reason it may be prudent to decrease the rate of intravenous injection of depressant drugs in these patients.

Induction of anesthesia with a volatile anesthetic, such as sevoflurane (alternatively halothane) is acceptable but must be accomplished with caution and careful monitoring of systemic oxygenation.[11] Although decreased pulmonary blood flow speeds the achievement of anesthetic concentrations, the hazard of decreased systemic blood pressure plus decreased systemic vascular resistance is great. Indeed, hypercyanotic attacks can occur during administration of low concentrations of volatile anesthetics.

Maintenance of Anesthesia

Maintenance of anesthesia is often achieved with nitrous oxide combined with ketamine. The advantage of this combination is preservation of the systemic vascular resistance. Nitrous oxide may also increase pulmonary vascular resistance, but this potentially adverse effect is more than offset by its beneficial effects on systemic vascular resistance (no change or modest increase). The principal disadvantage of using nitrous oxide is the associated decrease in the inspired oxygen concentration. Theoretically, increased inspired oxygen concentrations could decrease pulmonary vascular resistance, leading to increased pulmonary blood flow and improved PaO_2. Therefore it seems prudent to limit the inspired concentration of nitrous oxide to 50%. The use of an opioid or benzodiazepine may also be considered during maintenance of anesthesia, but the dose and rate of administration must be adjusted to minimize decreased systemic blood pressure and systemic vascular resistance.

Intraoperative skeletal muscle paralysis may be provided with pancuronium in view of its ability to maintain systemic blood pressure and systemic vascular resistance. An increase in heart rate associated with pancuronium is helpful for maintaining left ventricular cardiac output. Alternative nondepolarizing neuromuscular blocking drugs are often selected with consideration given to the ability of some of these drugs, when administered rapidly in high doses, to evoke the release of histamine with associated decreases in systemic vascular resistance and systemic blood pressure.

Ventilation of the patient's lungs should be controlled, but it must be appreciated that excessive positive airway pressure may adversely increase the resistance to blood flow through the lungs. Intravascular fluid volume must be maintained with intravenous fluid administration, as acute hypovolemia tends to increase the magnitude of the right-to-left intracardiac shunt. In view of the predictable erythrocytosis, it is probably not necessary to consider blood replacement until about 20% of the patient's blood volume has been lost. It is crucial that meticulous care be taken to avoid infusion of air through the tubing used to deliver intravenous solutions, as it could lead to systemic air embolization. α-Adrenergic agonist drugs such as phenylephrine must be available to treat undesirable decreases in systemic blood pressure caused by decreased systemic vascular resistance.

Patient Characteristics Following Surgical Repair of Tetralogy of Fallot

Although patients with surgically repaired tetralogy of Fallot are usually asymptomatic, their survival is often shortened because of sudden death, presumably due to cardiac causes.[9] Ventricular cardiac dysrhythmias are common in patients following surgical correction of tetralogy of Fallot. Patients with surgically repaired tetralogy of Fallot often develop atrial fibrillation or flutter. Right bundle branch block is frequent, whereas third-degree atrioventricular heart block is uncommon. Pulmonic regurgitation may develop as a consequence of surgical repair of the right ventricular outflow tract, eventually leading to right ventricular hypertrophy and dysfunction. An aneurysm may form at the site where the right ventricular outflow tract was repaired.

Eisenmenger Syndrome

Patients in whom a left-to-right intracardiac shunt is reversed, as a result of increased pulmonary vascular resistance, to a level that equals or exceeds the systemic vascular resistance are said to have Eisenmenger syndrome. It is presumed that exposure of the pulmonary vasculature to increased blood flow and pressure, as may accompany a VSD or ASD, results in pulmonary obstructive disease. As obliteration of the pulmonary vascular bed progresses, the pulmonary vascular resistance, increases until it equals or exceeds systemic vascular resistance and the intracardiac shunt is reversed. Shunt reversal occurs in about 50% of patients with an untreated VSD and about 10% of patients with an untreated ASD. The murmur associated with these cardiac defects disappears when Eisenmenger syndrome develops.

Signs and Symptoms

Cyanosis and decreased exercise tolerance occur as right-to-left intracardiac shunting develops.[9] Palpitations are common and are most often due to the onset of atrial fibrillation or atrial flutter. Arterial hypoxemia stimulates erythrocytosis, leading to increased blood viscosity and associated visual disturbances, headache, dizziness, and paresthesias. Hemoptysis may occur as a result of pulmonary infarction or rupture of dilated pulmonary arteries, arterioles, or aorticopulmonary collateral vessels. Abnormal coagulation and thrombosis often accompany arterial hypoxemia and erythrocytosis. The possibility of a cerebral vascular accident or brain abscess is increased. Syncope most likely reflects inadequate cardiac output. Sudden death is a risk in patients with Eisenmenger syndrome. The ECG shows right ventricular hypertrophy.

Treatment

No treatment has proved effective in producing sustained decreases in pulmonary vascular resistance, although intravenous epoprostenol may be beneficial.[9] Phlebotomy with isovolemic replacement should be undertaken in patients with moderate or severe symptoms of hyperviscosity. Pregnancy is discouraged in women with Eisenmenger syndrome. Lung transplantation with repair of the cardiac defect or combined heart-lung transplantation is an option for selected patients with this syndrome. The presence of irreversibly increased pulmonary vascular resistance contraindicates surgical correction of the congenital heart defect that was responsible for the original left-to-right intracardiac shunt.

Management of Anesthesia

Management of anesthesia for patients with Eisenmenger syndrome undergoing noncardiac surgery is based on maintenance of preoperative levels of systemic vascular resistance and recognizing that increases in right-to-left intracardiac shunting are likely if sudden vasodilation occurs. Continuous intravenous infusions of norepinephrine have been reported to maintain systemic vascular resistance during the perioperative period.[12] Minimization of blood loss with the development of hypovolemia and the prevention of iatrogenic paradoxical embolization are important considerations. It may be useful to perform prophylactic phlebotomy with isovolumic replacement in patients with hematocrits above 65%.[9] Preoperative administration of antiplatelet drugs is not encouraged, as intraoperative blood loss may be associated with the impaired coagulation that accompanies chronic arterial hypoxemia and erythrocytosis. Opioids have been administered safely for preoperative and postoperative analgesia.

Laparoscopic procedures may pose an increased risk to these patients, as insufflation of the peritoneal cavity with carbon dioxide may cause increases in the $PaCO_2$, resulting in acidosis, hypotension, and cardiac dysrhythmias.[12] Efforts to maintain normocapnia may be accompanied by increases in airway pressures and pulmonary vascular resistance, especially as the intra-abdominal pressure increases. These events may be further exaggerated by placing the patient in the head-down position. Early tracheal extubation in these patients is preferable because of the deleterious effects of positive pressure ventilation.

Despite the potential for undesirable decreases in systemic blood pressure and systemic vascular resistance, the successful management of anesthesia using epidural anesthesia has been described in patients undergoing tubal ligation and cesarean section.[13, 14] If epidural anesthesia is selected, it seems prudent not to add epinephrine to the local anesthetic solution injected into the epidural space. This recommendation is based on the observation that peripheral β-agonist effects produced by the epinephrine absorbed from the epidural space into the systemic circulation could exaggerate decreases in systemic blood pressure and systemic vascular resistance associated with epidural anesthesia.

Ebstein's Anomaly

Ebstein's anomaly is an abnormality of the tricuspid valve in which the valve leaflets are malformed or displaced downward into the right ventricle.[9] As a result, the right ventricle has a small distal effective portion and an atrialized proximal portion. The tricuspid valve is usually regurgitant but may also be stenotic. Most patients with Ebstein's anomaly have an interatrial communication (ASD, patent foramen ovale) through which there may be right-to-left shunting of blood.

Signs and Symptoms

The severity of the hemodynamic derangements in patients with Ebstein's anomaly depends on the degree of displacement and the functional status of the tricuspid valve leaflets.[9] As a result, the clinical presentation of Ebstein's anomaly varies from congestive heart failure in neonates to the absence of symptoms in adults in whom the anomaly is discovered incidentally. Neonates often manifest cyanosis and congestive heart failure that worsens after the ductus arteriosus closes, thereby decreasing pulmonary blood flow. Older children with Ebstein's anomaly may be diagnosed because of an incidental murmur, whereas adolescents and adults are likely to present with supraventricular dysrhythmias that lead to congestive heart failure, worsening cyanosis, and occasionally syncope. Patients with Ebstein's anomaly and an interatrial communication are at risk of paradoxical embolization, brain abscess, congestive heart failure, and sudden death.

The severity of cyanosis depends on the magnitude of the right-to-left shunt. A systolic murmur caused by tricuspid regurgitation is usually present at the left lower sternal border. Hepatomegaly resulting from passive hepatic congestion due to increased right atrial pressures may be present. The ECG is characterized by tall and broad P waves (resembling right bundle branch block), and first-degree atrioventricular heart block is common. Paroxysmal supraventricular and ventricular tachydysrhythmias may occur; and as many as 20% of patients with Ebstein's anomaly have ventricular preexcitation by way of accessory electrical pathways between the atrium and ventricle (Wolff-Parkinson-White syndrome) (see Chapter 4).[15] In patients with severe disease (marked right-to-left shunting and minimal functional right ventricle) marked cardiomegaly is present that is largely due to right atrial enlargement.

Echocardiography is used to assess right atrial dilation, distortion of the tricuspid valve leaflets, and the severity of the tricuspid regurgitation or stenosis. The presence and magnitude of interatrial shunting can be determined by color Doppler imaging studies. Enlargement of the right atrium may be so massive that the apical portions of the lungs are compressed, resulting in restrictive pulmonary disease.

The hazards of pregnancy in parturients with Ebstein's anomaly include deterioration in right ventricular function due to increased blood volume and cardiac output, increased right-to-left shunting and arterial hypoxemia if an ASD is present, and cardiac dysrhythmias. Pregnancy-induced hypertension may result in the development of congestive heart failure in these women.

Treatment

Treatment of Ebstein's anomaly is based on the prevention of associated complications including antibiotic prophylaxis against infective endocarditis and administration of diuretics and digoxin for management of congestive heart failure. Patients with supraventricular dysrhythmias are treated pharmacologically or with catheter ablation if an accessory pathway is present. In severely ill patients with Ebstein's anomaly, an arterial shunt from the systemic circulation to the pulmonary circulation is created to increase pulmonary blood flow and thus decrease cyanosis. Further surgery to create a univentricular heart (Fontan procedure) may also be considered in neonates (see "Tricuspid Atresia"). Repair or replacement of the tricuspid valve in conjunction with closure of the interatrial communication is recommended for older patients who have severe symptoms despite medical therapy. Complications of surgery to correct Ebstein's anomaly include third-degree atrioventricular heart block, persistence of supraventricular dysrhythmias, residual tricuspid regurgitation after valve repair, and prosthetic valve dysfunction when the tricuspid valve is replaced.[9]

Management of Anesthesia

Hazards during anesthesia in patients with Ebstein's anomaly include accentuation of arterial hypoxemia due to increases in the magnitude of the right-to-left intracardiac shunt and the development of supraventricular tachydysrhythmias.[16] Increased right atrial pressures may indicate the presence of right ventricular failure. In the presence of a probe-patent foramen ovale (present in about 30% of patients), an increase in right atrial pressure above the pressure in the left atrium can lead to a right-to-left intracardiac shunt through the foramen ovale. Unexplained arterial hypoxemia or paradoxical air embolism during the perioperative period may be due to shunting of blood or air through a previously closed foramen ovale. The delayed onset of pharmacologic effects after intravenous administration of drugs during anesthesia most likely reflects pooling and dilution in an enlarged right atrium. Epidural analgesia has been utilized safely for labor and delivery.[15]

Tricuspid Atresia

Tricuspid atresia is characterized by arterial hypoxemia, a small right ventricle, a large left ventricle, and marked decreases in pulmonary blood flow. Poorly oxygenated blood from the right atrium passes through an ASD into the left atrium, mixes with oxygenated blood, and then enters the left ventricle, from which it is ejected into the systemic circulation. Pulmonary blood flow is via a VSD, PDA, or bronchial vessels.

Treatment

A Fontan procedure (anastomosis of the right atrial appendage to the right pulmonary artery to bypass the right ventricle and provide a direct atriopulmonary communication) is used to treat tricuspid atresia. This operation is also used to treat pulmonary artery atresia.

Management of Anesthesia

Management of anesthesia for patients undergoing Fontan procedures has been successfully achieved with opioids or volatile anesthetics.[17] Immediately after cardiopulmonary bypass and continuing into the early postoperative period, it is important to maintain increased right atrial pressures (16 to 20 mmHg) to facilitate pulmonary blood flow. An increase in pulmonary vascular resistance due to acidosis, hypothermia, peak airway pressures above 15 cmH$_2$O, or reactions to the tracheal tube may cause right-sided heart failure. Early tracheal extubation and spontaneous ventilation are desirable. Positive inotropic drugs (dopamine) with or without vasodilators (nitroprusside) are often required to optimize cardiac output and maintain low pulmonary vascular resistance. Pleural effusions, ascites, and edema of the lower extremities are not uncommon postoperatively and usually resolve within a few weeks. Right atrial pressure equal to the pulmonary artery pressure remains elevated after this operation, averaging 15 mmHg.

Although absence of a contractile right ventricle is compatible with long-term survival, the adaptability of the circulatory system is restricted. This decreased capacity of a single ventricle to respond to an increased workload may have a significant impact on the management of these patients for another operation. In this regard, subsequent management of anesthesia in patients who have undergone Fontan procedures is facilitated by monitoring the central venous pressure (which equals the pulmonary artery pressure in these patients) to assess the intravascular fluid volume and to detect sudden impairment of left ventricular function and increased pulmonary vascular resistance.[17] The value of monitoring the central venous pressure reflects the absence of a contractile right ventricle and the impaired ability of a single ventricle to adapt to acute increases in afterload that may necessitate prompt administration of positive inotropic drugs. Insertion of a thermodilution pulmonary artery catheter in patients after a Fontan repair may be technically difficult secondary to the unusual anatomy. No information is available regarding the accuracy of thermodilution cardiac output measurements in such patients.

Transposition of the Great Arteries

Transposition of the great arteries results from failure of the truncus arteriosus to spiral, resulting in the aorta arising from the anterior portion of the right ventricle and the pulmonary artery arising from the left ventricle (Fig. 3–5). There is complete separation of the pulmonary and systemic circulations such that systemic venous blood traverses the right atrium, right ventricle, aorta, and systemic circulation; and pulmonary venous blood traverses the left atrium, left ventricle, pulmonary artery, and lungs.[9] Survival is possible only if there is communication between the two circulations in the form of a VSD, ASD, or PDA.

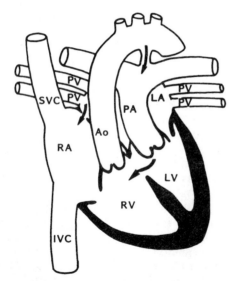

Figure 3–5 • Transposition of the great arteries. The right ventricle (RV) and left ventricle (LV) are not connected in series. Instead, the two ventricles function as parallel and independent circulations, with the aorta (Ao) arising from the RV and the pulmonary artery (PA) arising from the LV. Survival is not possible unless mixing of blood between the two circulations occurs through an atrial septal defect, ventricular septal defect, or patent ductus.

Signs and Symptoms

Persistent cyanosis and tachypnea at birth may be the first clues to the presence of transposition of the great arteries. Congestive heart failure is often present, reflecting left ventricular failure due to volume overload created by the left-to-right intracardiac shunt necessary for survival. The ECG is likely to demonstrate right axis deviation and right ventricular hypertrophy, as the right ventricle is the systemic ventricle. Classically, the cardiac silhouette on the chest radiograph is described as being "egg-shaped with a narrow stalk."[9]

Treatment

The immediate management of transposition of the great arteries involves creating intracardiac mixing or increasing the degree of mixing. This goal is accomplished with infusions of prostaglandin E to maintain patency of the ductus arteriosus and/or creating an ASD (Rashkind procedure).[9] Administration of oxygen may decrease pulmonary vascular resistance and increase pulmonary blood flow. Diuretics and digoxin are administered to treat congestive heart failure.

Two surgical switch procedures have been used to treat complete transition of the great arteries. The initial surgical procedure, known as the "atrial switch" operation (Mustard or Senning operation), involved resection of the atrial septum and its replacement with a baffle to direct the systemic venous blood into the left ventricle and pulmonary venous blood across the tricuspid valve into the right ventricle. This operation has been replaced by the "arterial switch" operation in which the pulmonary artery and ascending aorta are transected above the semilunar valves and coronary arteries are then switched, so the aorta is connected to the left ventricle and the pulmonary artery is connected to the right ventricle.[9]

Management of Anesthesia

Management of anesthesia in the presence of transposition of the great arteries must take into account separation of the pulmonary and systemic circulations. Drugs administered intravenously are distributed with minimal dilution to organs such as the heart and brain. Therefore doses and rates of injection of intravenously administered drugs may have to be decreased. Conversely, the onset of anesthesia produced by inhaled drugs is delayed, as only small amounts of the inhaled drug reach the systemic circulation. In the final analysis, induction and maintenance of anesthesia are often accomplished with ketamine combined with muscle relaxants to facilitate tracheal intubation. Ketamine can be supplemented with opioids or benzodiazepines for maintenance of anesthesia. Nitrous oxide has limited application in these patients, as it is important to administer high inspired oxygen concentrations. The potential cardiac depressant effects of volatile anesthetics detract from the use of these drugs. Selection of muscle relaxants is influenced by the desire to avoid histamine-induced changes in systemic blood pressure. The ability of pancuronium to increase the heart rate and systemic blood pressure modestly may be useful.

Dehydration must be avoided during the perioperative period. These patients may have hematocrits in excess of 70%, which may contribute to the high incidence of cerebral venous thrombosis. This finding suggests that oral fluids should not be withheld from these patients for prolonged periods. If fluids cannot be ingested orally, an intravenous infusion should be initiated during the preoperative period. Atrial dysrhythmias and conduction disturbances may occur postoperatively.

Mixing of Blood Between the Pulmonary and Systemic Circulations

Rare congenital heart defects that result in mixing of blood from the pulmonary and systemic circulations manifest as cyanosis and arterial hypoxemia of varying severity depending on the magnitude of the pulmonary blood flow. As a result of the mixing of blood from both circulations, pulmonary arterial blood has higher oxygen saturation than that of systemic venous blood, and systemic arterial blood has lower oxygen saturation than that of pulmonary venous blood.

Truncus Arteriosus

Truncus arteriosus refers to the congenital cardiac defect in which a single arterial trunk serves as the origin of the aorta and pulmonary artery (Fig. 3–6). This single arterial trunk overrides both ventricles, which are connected through a VSD. Mortality is high, with the median age of survival at about 5 to 6 weeks.

Signs and Symptoms

Presenting signs and symptoms of truncus arteriosus include cyanosis and arterial hypoxemia, failure to thrive, and congestive heart failure early in life. Peripheral pulses may be accentuated owing to the rapid diastolic runoff of blood into the pulmonary

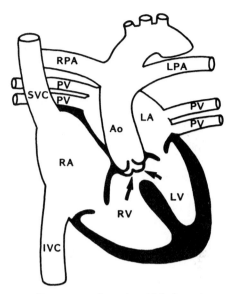

Figure 3–6 • Truncus arteriosus in which the pulmonary artery (RPA, right pulmonary artery; LPA, left pulmonary artery) and aorta (Ao) arise from a single trunk that overrides the left ventricle (LV) and right ventricle (RV). This trunk receives blood from both ventricles by virtue of a ventricular septal defect.

circulation. Auscultation of the chest and evaluation of the ECG do not give predictable information and are not diagnostic. Chest radiography reveals cardiomegaly and increased vascularity of the lung fields. The diagnosis is confirmed by angiocardiography performed during cardiac catheterization.

Treatment

Surgical treatment of truncus arteriosus includes banding of the right and left pulmonary arteries if pulmonary blood flow is excessive. In addition, an associated VSD can be closed so only left ventricular output enters the truncus arteriosus. When this is done, a Dacron conduit with a valve is also placed between the right ventricle and pulmonary artery.

Management of Anesthesia

Management of anesthesia in the presence of truncus arteriosus is influenced by the magnitude of the pulmonary blood flow. When pulmonary blood flow in increased, the use of positive end-expiratory pressure is beneficial and may serve to decrease the symptoms of congestive heart failure. Increased pulmonary blood flow may be associated with evidence of myocardial ischemia on the ECG. When myocardial ischemia that occurs intraoperatively does not respond to (1) intravenous administration of phenylephrine or fluids or (2) the use of positive end-expiratory pressure, consideration may be given to temporary banding of the pulmonary artery to increase systemic and coronary blood flow.[18] Patients with decreased pulmonary blood flow and arterial hypoxemia should be managed as described for tetralogy of Fallot.

Partial Anomalous Pulmonary Venous Return

Partial anomalous pulmonary venous return is characterized by the presence of left or right pulmonary veins that empty into the right side of the circulation rather than the left atrium. In about one-half of cases, the aberrant pulmonary veins drain into the superior vena cava. In the remaining cases, pulmonary veins enter the right atrium, inferior vena cava, azygos vein, or coronary sinus. Partial anomalous pulmonary venous return may be more common than appreciated, suggested by the presence of this anomaly in about 0.5% of routine autopsies.

The onset and severity of symptoms produced by this abnormality depend on the amount of pulmonary blood flow routed through the right side of the heart. Fatigue and exertional dyspnea are the most frequent initial manifestations, usually appearing during early adulthood. Cyanosis and congestive heart failure are likely if more than 50% of the pulmonary venous flow enters the right side of the circulation.

Angiography is the most useful technique for confirming the diagnosis of partial anomalous pulmonary venous return. Cardiac catheterization usually demonstrates normal intracardiac pressures and increased oxygen saturations of blood in the right side of the heart. Treatment is by surgical repair.

Total Anomalous Pulmonary Venous Return

Total anomalous pulmonary venous return is characterized by drainage of all four pulmonary veins into the systemic venous system. The most common presentation of this defect, accounting for about one-half of cases, is drainage of the four pulmonary veins into the left innominate vein in association with a left-sided superior vena cava. Oxygenated blood reaches the left atrium by way of an ASD. PDA is present in about one-third of patients.

Signs and Symptoms

Total anomalous pulmonary venous return presents clinically as congestive heart failure in 50% of patients by 1 month of age and in 90% by 1 year. It is definitively diagnosed by angiocardiography. Mortality is about 80% by 1 year of age unless it is surgically corrected using cardiopulmonary bypass.

Management of Anesthesia

Management of anesthesia in the presence of total anomalous pulmonary venous return may include positive end-expiratory pressure applied to the airways in an attempt to decrease excessive pulmonary blood flow. Patients who present with pulmonary edema should undergo positive-pressure ventilation through a tube placed in the trachea before cardiac catheterization. Operative manipulation of the right atrium, which is tolerated by normal patients, may result in obstruction to flow into the right atrium in these patients, manifesting as sudden decreases in systemic blood pressure and the onset of bradycardia. Intravenous transfusions may be hazardous, as any increase in right atrial pressure is transmitted directly to the pulmonary veins, leading to the possibility of pulmonary edema.

Hypoplastic Left Heart Syndrome

Hypoplastic left heart syndrome is characterized by left ventricular hypoplasia, mitral valve hypoplasia, aortic valve atresia, and hypoplasia of the ascending aorta.[19] Extracardiac congenital anomalies do not usually accompany this syndrome. There is complete mixing of pulmonary venous and systemic venous blood in a single ventricle, which is connected in parallel to both the pulmonary and systemic circulations. Systemic blood flow is dependent on a PDA. In addition to ductal patency, infant survival depends on a balance between systemic vascular resistance and pulmonary vascular resistance, as both circulations are supplied from a single ventricle in a parallel fashion. An abrupt decrease in pulmonary vascular resistance after delivery results in increased pulmonary blood flow at the expense of systemic blood flow (pulmonary steal phenomenon). When this occurs, coronary and systemic blood flow are inadequate, leading to metabolic acidosis, high-output cardiac failure, and ventricular fibrillation, despite increasingly high PaO_2 values (Fig. 3–7).[19] Alternatively, any postnatal event that leads to increased pulmonary vascular resistance can decrease the pulmonary blood flow so severely that arterial hypoxemia worsens, leading to progressive metabolic acidosis and circulatory collapse (Fig. 3–7).[19] Because rapid changes in pulmonary vascular resistance occur during the postnatal period, the necessary fine balance between pulmonary vascular resistance and systemic vascular resistance is unstable and difficult to maintain.

Treatment

Treatment of hypoplastic left heart syndrome is surgical, beginning with a palliative procedure that

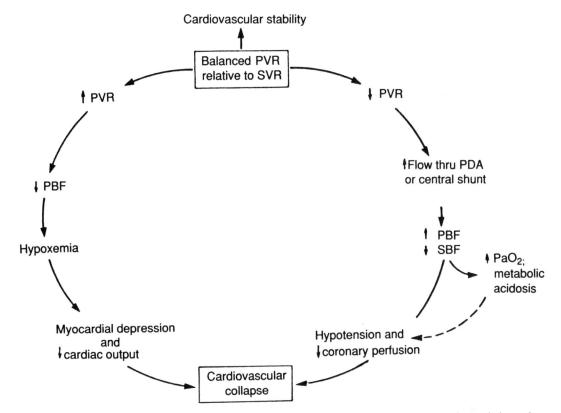

Figure 3–7 • Cardiovascular stability in the presence of hypoplastic left heart syndrome requires a balance between pulmonary vascular resistance (PVR) relative to systemic vascular resistance (SVR). An abrupt decrease in PVR after delivery can result in excessive pulmonary blood flow (PBF) relative to systemic blood flow (SBF) with cardiovascular collapse despite the absence of arterial hypoxemia. Conversely, postnatal changes that increase PVR can lead to cardiovascular collapse in the presence of arterial hypoxemia. (From Hansen DD, Hickey PR. Anesthesia for hypoplastic left heart syndrome: use of high-dose fentanyl in 30 neonates. Anesth Analg 1986;65:127–32, with permission.)

eliminates the need for continued patency of the ductus arteriosus. Preoperatively, continuous intravenous infusions of prostaglandins may be useful for preventing physiologic closure of the ductus arteriosus. In addition, administration of cardiac inotropes and sodium bicarbonate may be necessary.

The palliative procedure consists of reconstructing the ascending aorta using the proximal pulmonary artery (Fig. 3–8).[19] A systemic-to-pulmonary shunt to provide pulmonary blood flow is placed between the reconstructed aorta and the distal pulmonary artery. Typically, infants are placed on cardiopulmonary bypass to permit production of whole-body hypothermia; reconstruction of the aorta is then accomplished during 40 to 60 minutes of circulatory arrest. The central shunt is placed after reinstitution of cardiopulmonary bypass and during rewarming. The completed palliative procedure leaves the single right ventricle connected in parallel to the systemic circulation and pulmonary circulation. The stage is set, however, for later correction

with a Fontan procedure when pulmonary vascular resistance has decreased to adult levels (see "Tricuspid Atresia"). The Fontan procedure plus elimination of the systemic-to-pulmonary shunt separates the two circulations and facilitates development of normal arterial oxygen saturation.

Management of Anesthesia

An umbilical artery and intravenous catheter are usually placed before the arrival of these infants in the operating room. After instituting monitoring, induction of anesthesia is often accomplished with fentanyl (50 to 75 μg/kg IV) administered simultaneously with pancuronium.[19] There is also a suggestion that deep anesthesia with opioids continued for 24 hours postoperatively is effective in attenuating the hormonal and metabolic responses to stress in these critically ill neonates leading to decreased morbidity and mortality, compared with neonates receiving lighter anesthesia.[20] Nevertheless, it seems

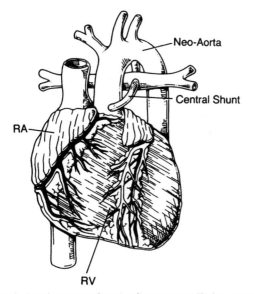

Figure 3–8 • Anatomy after the first-stage palliative procedure for hypoplastic left heart syndrome during the neonatal period. The ascending aorta has been reconstructed from the proximal pulmonary artery to form a neo-aorta. (From Hansen DD, Hickey PR. Anesthesia for hypoplastic left heart syndrome: use of high-dose fentanyl in 30 neonates. Anesth Analg 1986;65:127–32, with permission.)

unjustified to conclude from the limited number of patients studied that deep anesthesia is always safer than light anesthesia in such critically ill patients.[21]

These infants are vulnerable to the development of ventricular fibrillation due to inadequate coronary blood flow before the palliative procedure. The danger of ventricular fibrillation and borderline cardiac status argues against the use of volatile anesthetics in these infants. The infant's lungs are ventilated and a tracheal tube is placed. A crystalloid solution (10 to 15 ml/kg IV) is often infused before cardiopulmonary bypass is instituted. After induction of anesthesia and tracheal intubation, ventilation of the patient's lungs is adjusted on the basis of arterial blood gas measurements. A high PaO_2 implies excessive pulmonary blood flow at the expense of the systemic circulation. Indeed, if the initial PaO_2 is more than 100 mmHg, maneuvers to increase pulmonary vascular resistance and decrease pulmonary blood flow are instituted. For example, a decrease in the volume of ventilation leads to increases in $PaCO_2$ and decreases in pHa, resulting in increased pulmonary vascular resistance and decreased pulmonary blood flow. If the PaO_2 remains unacceptably high, institution of positive end-expiratory pressure leads to increased lung volumes and further increases in pulmonary vascular resistance. In extreme cases,

temporary occlusion of one pulmonary artery serves to decrease the PaO_2.

Dopamine or isoproterenol is administered when necessary for inotropic support at the conclusion of cardiopulmonary bypass. The selection of specific inotropic drugs is influenced by pulmonary vascular resistance. The most frequent problem after cardiopulmonary bypass is too little pulmonary blood flow with associated arterial hypoxemia (PaO_2 less than 20 mmHg).[19] Attempts to improve the PaO_2 include hyperventilation of the lungs to produce a low $PaCO_2$ (20 to 25 mmHg) and to increase the pHa plus infusion of isoproterenol to decrease pulmonary vascular resistance. A PaO_2 higher than 50 mmHg after cardiopulmonary bypass may indicate inadequate systemic blood flow and the likely occurrence of progressive metabolic acidosis unless steps are taken to decrease pulmonary blood flow.

MECHANICAL OBSTRUCTION OF THE TRACHEA

The trachea can be obstructed by circulatory anomalies that produce a vascular ring or by dilation of the pulmonary artery secondary to absence of the pulmonic valve. These lesions must be considered when evaluating a child with unexplained stridor or other evidence of upper airway obstruction. The possibility of an undiagnosed vascular ring should be considered in the differential diagnosis of airway obstruction that follows placement of a nasogastric tube or an esophageal stethoscope.

Double Aortic Arch

Double aortic arch results in a vascular ring that can produce pressure on the trachea and esophagus. Compression resulting from this pressure can be manifested as inspiratory stridor, difficulty mobilizing secretions, and dysphagia. Patients with this cardiac defect usually prefer to lie with the neck extended, as flexion of the neck often accentuates compression of the trachea.

Surgical transection of the smaller aortic arch is the treatment of choice for symptomatic patients. During surgery the tracheal tube should be placed beyond the area of tracheal compression if this can be safely accomplished without producing endobronchial intubation. It must be appreciated that esophageal stethoscopes or nasogastric tubes can cause occlusion of the trachea if the tracheal tube remains above the level of vascular compression. Clinical improvement after surgical transection is often prompt. Tracheomalacia due to prolonged compression of the trachea, however, can jeopardize the patency of the trachea.

Aberrant Left Pulmonary Artery

Tracheal or bronchial obstruction can occur when the left pulmonary artery is absent and the arterial supply to the left lung is derived from a branch of the right pulmonary artery passing between the trachea and esophagus. This anatomic arrangement has been referred to as vascular sling, as a complete ring is not present. The sling can cause obstruction of the right mainstem bronchus, the distal trachea, or rarely the left mainstem bronchus.

Clinical manifestations of an aberrant left pulmonary artery include stridor, wheezing, and occasionally arterial hypoxemia. In contrast to a true vascular ring, esophageal obstructions are rare; and the stridor produced by this defect is usually present during exhalation rather than inspiration. Chest radiographs may demonstrate an abnormal separation between the esophagus and the trachea. Hyperinflation or atelectasis of either lung may be present. Angiography is the most accurate approach for confirming the diagnosis.

Surgical division of the aberrant left pulmonary artery at its origin and redirection of its course anterior to the trachea, with anastomosis to the main pulmonary artery, is the treatment of choice. During the first months of life, surgical correction with deep hypothermia without cardiopulmonary bypass may be considered. Theoretically, continuous positive airway pressure or positive end-expiratory pressure should relieve the airway obstruction and associated stridor in these cases.

Absent Pulmonic Valve

Absence of the pulmonic valve results in dilation of the pulmonary artery, which can result in compression of the trachea and left mainstem bronchus. This lesion may occur as an isolated defect or in conjunction with tetralogy of Fallot. Symptoms include signs of tracheal obstruction and occasionally the development of arterial hypoxemia and congestive heart failure. Any increase in pulmonary vascular resistance, as may occur with arterial hypoxemia or hypercarbia, accentuates airway obstruction. Tracheal intubation and maintenance of 4 to 6 mmHg of continuous positive airway pressure can be used to keep the trachea distended, reducing the magnitude of airway obstruction. Definitive treatment

consists of inserting a tubular graft with an artificial pulmonic valve.

References

1. Findlow D, Doyle E. Congenital heart disease in adults. Br J Anaesth 1997;78:24–30
2. Brickner ME, Hillis LD, Lange RA. Congenital heart disease in adults. N Engl J Med 2000;342:256–63
3. Baum VC, Perloff JK. Anesthetic implications of adults with congenital heart disease. Anesth Analg 1993;76:1342–58
4. Mullen MP. Adult congenital heart disease. Sci Am Med 2000;1–10
5. Eger EI II. Effect of ventilation/perfusion abnormalities. In: Eger EI II (ed) Anesthetic Uptake and Action, Baltimore, Williams & Wilkins, 1974, pp 146–59
6. Clyman RI. Ibuprofen and patent ductus arteriosus. N Engl J Med 2000;343:728–30
7. Van Overmeire B, Smets K, Lecoutere D, et al. A comparison of ibuprofen and indomethacin for closure of patent ductus arteriosus. N Engl J Med 2000;343:674–81
8. Ransom DM, Leicht CH. Continuous spinal analgesia with sufentanil for labor and delivery in a parturient with severe pulmonary stenosis. Anesth Analg 1995;80:418–21
9. Brickner ME, Hillis LD, Lange RA. Congenital heart disease in adults. N Engl J Med 2000;342:334–42
10. Greeley WJ, Stanley TE, Ungerleider RM, et al. Intraoperative hypoxemic spells in tetralogy of Fallot, an echocardiographic analysis of diagnosis and treatment. Anesth Analg 1989;68:815–9
11. Greeley WJ, Bushman BA, Davis DP, et al. Comparative effects of halothane and ketamine on systemic arterial oxygen saturation in children with cyanotic heart disease. Anesthesiology 1986;65:666–8
12. Sammut MS, Paes ML. Anaesthesia for laparoscopic cholecystectomy in a patient with Eisenmenger's syndrome. Br J Anaesth 1997;79:810–2
13. Spinnato JA, Kraynack BJ, Cooper MW. Eisenmenger's syndrome in pregnancy: epidural anesthesia for elective cesarean section. N Engl J Med 1981;304:1215–6
14. Weiss BM, Zemp L, Seifert B, et al. Outcome of pulmonary vascular disease in pregnancy: a systematic overview from 1978 through 1996. J Am Coll Cardiol 1998;31:1650–9
15. Groves ER, Groves JB. Epidural analgesia for labour in a patient with Ebstein's anomaly. Can J Anaesth 1995;42:77–9
16. Elsten JL, Kim YD, Hanowell ST, et al. Prolonged induction with exaggerated chamber enlargement in Ebstein's anomaly. Anesth Analg 1981;60:909–10
17. Hosking MP, Beynen F. Repair of coarctation of the aorta in a child after a modified Fontan's operation: anesthetic implications and management. Anesthesiology 1989;71:312–5
18. Wong RS, Baum VC, Sangivan S. Truncus arteriosus: recognition and therapy of intraoperative cardiac ischemia. Anesthesiology 1991;74:378–80
19. Hansen DD, Hickey PR. Anesthesia for hypoplastic left heart syndrome: use of high-dose fentanyl in 30 neonates. Anesth Analg 1986;65:127–32
20. Anand KJS, Hickey PR. Halothane-morphine compared with high-dose sufentanil for anesthesia and postoperative analgesia in neonatal cardiac surgery. N Engl J Med 1992;326:1–9
21. Larson CP. Anesthesia in neonatal cardiac surgery. N Engl J Med 1992;327:124

4

Abnormalities of Cardiac Conduction and Cardiac Rhythm

The incidence of intraoperative cardiac dysrhythmias depends on the definition (any cardiac dysrhythmia versus only potentially dangerous cardiac dysrhythmias), continuous surveillance versus casual observation, patient characteristics, and the nature of the surgery.[1, 2] For example, the incidence of cardiac dysrhythmias in patients undergoing cardiothoracic surgery with continuous monitoring of the electrocardiogram (ECG) exceeds 90%. In most of these patients the observed cardiac dysrhythmias did not require treatment. Factors that determine how a patient tolerates a cardiac dysrhythmia include the heart rate, duration of the dysrhythmia, and the presence and severity of any underlying cardiac disease. The importance of cardiac dysrhythmias relates to the effects of the specific cardiac rhythm disturbance on the cardiac output and the possible interactions of antidysrhythmic drugs with drugs administered to produce anesthesia and skeletal muscle relaxation.

MECHANISMS OF CARDIAC DYSRHYTHMIAS

Cardiac dysrhythmias that occur during the perioperative period can usually be explained on the basis of abnormalities of cardiac impulse conduction (reentry) or impulse formation (automatic or ectopic).

Reentry Pathways

Reentry accounts for most premature beats and tachydysrhythmias. Conditions necessary for reentry include two pathways over which cardiac impulses are conducted at different velocities (Fig. 4–1).[3] One pathway conducts the cardiac impulse

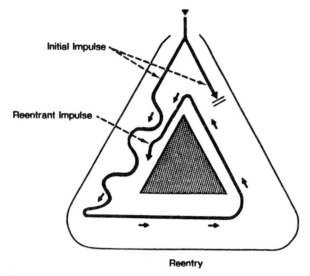

Figure 4–1 • Essential requirement for initiation of reentry excitation is a unilateral block that prevents uniform anterograde propagation of the initial cardiac impulse. Under appropriate conditions this same cardiac impulse can traverse the area of blockade in a retrograde direction and become a reentrant cardiac impulse. (From Akhtar M. Management of ventricular tachyarrhythmias. JAMA 1982;247:671–4. Copyrighted 1982 American Medical Association, with permission.)

forward (antegrade), whereas the other pathway conducts the reentering cardiac impulse backward (retrograde). In the retrograde pathway antegrade conduction is usually blocked or delayed, but retrograde conduction remains intact. Pharmacologic or physiologic events may alter the crucial balance between conduction velocities and refractory periods of dual pathways, resulting in initiation or termination of reentry cardiac dysrhythmias (Table 4–1).

Automaticity

Automatic cardiac dysrhythmias are due to enhanced automaticity of a focus in the heart capable of undergoing spontaneous depolarization (repetitive firing) analogous to that of the sinus node. Automaticity refers to the slope of phase 4 depolarization of the cardiac action potential (Fig. 4–2). Increasing the slope of phase 4 depolarization or decreasing the resting membrane potential leads to enhanced automaticity manifesting as an accelerated heart rate and ventricular irritability (Table 4–2). Conversely, a decrease in the slope of phase 4 depolarization slows the heart rate (Table 4–2). Examples of automatic cardiac dysrhythmias are bradydysrhythmias and disturbances of atrioventricular or intraventricular conduction.

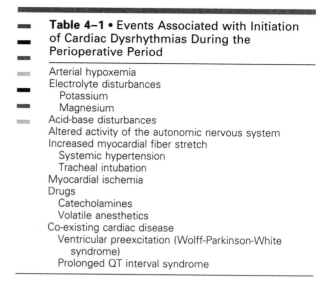

Table 4–1 • Events Associated with Initiation of Cardiac Dysrhythmias During the Perioperative Period

Arterial hypoxemia
Electrolyte disturbances
  Potassium
  Magnesium
Acid-base disturbances
Altered activity of the autonomic nervous system
Increased myocardial fiber stretch
  Systemic hypertension
  Tracheal intubation
Myocardial ischemia
Drugs
  Catecholamines
  Volatile anesthetics
Co-existing cardiac disease
  Ventricular preexcitation (Wolff-Parkinson-White syndrome)
  Prolonged QT interval syndrome

■ DIAGNOSIS OF CARDIAC DYSRHYTHMIAS

Electrocardiography

The ECG is essential for diagnosing cardiac conduction and rhythm disturbances. The normal ECG consists of three waveforms, designated the P wave (atrial depolarization), QRS complex (ventricular depolarization), and T wave (ventricular repolarization) (Fig. 4–2). The PR interval is the time necessary for the cardiac impulse to pass through the atrioventricular (AV) node. Transmission of the cardiac impulse is through a specialized conduction system present in the atria and ventricles (Fig. 4–3). The following questions should be asked when interpreting the ECG.[2]

1. What is the heart rate?
2. Are P waves present? What is the relation of the P waves to the QRS complex?
3. What is the duration of the PR interval?
4. What is the duration of the QRS complex?
5. Is the ventricular rhythm regular?
6. Are there early cardiac beats or abnormal pauses after the QRS complex?

It is important to confirm the presence of a P wave for each QRS complex. Lead II of the ECG reflects P waves most predictably and is the lead most often selected for analysis of cardiac dysrhythmias during the preoperative period. Inverted P waves are present when an abnormal pathway exists for conduc-

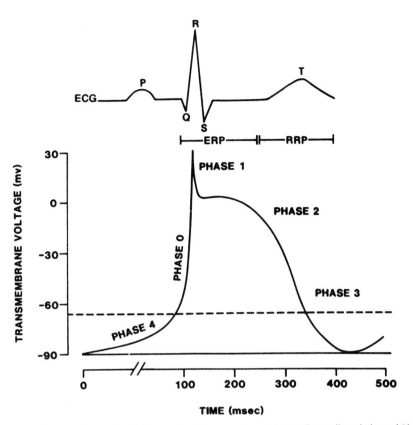

Figure 4–2 • Transmembrane action potential generated by an automatic cardiac cell and the relation of this action potential to events depicted on the electrocardiogram (ECG). Phase 4 undergoes spontaneous depolarization from the resting membrane potential (−90 mV) until the threshold potential (*broken line*) is reached. Depolarization (phase 0) occurs when the threshold potential is reached and corresponds to the QRS complex on the ECG. Phases 1 through 3 represent repolarization, with phase 3 corresponding to the T wave on the ECG. The effective refractory period (ERP) is the time during which cardiac impulses cannot be conducted, regardless of the intensity of the stimulus. During the relative refractory period (RRP), a stronger than normal stimulus can initiate an action potential. The action potential from a contractile cardiac cell differs from an automatic cardiac cell in that phase 4 does not undergo spontaneous depolarization.

Table 4–2 • Events that Alter the Slope of Phase 4 Depolarization

Increase slope
  Arterial hypoxemia
  Hypercarbia
  Acute hypokalemia
  Hyperthermia
  Catecholamines
  Sympathomimetic drugs
  Systemic hypertension
Decrease slope
  Vagal stimulation
  Positive airway pressure
  Acute hyperkalemia
  Hypothermia

tion of the cardiac impulse or when atrial (ectopic) sites other than the sinoatrial (SA) node exist. The PR interval is 0.12 to 0.20 second when the heart rate is normal. This interval is prolonged when there is increased delay of conduction of the cardiac impulse through the AV node and is shortened in the presence of a junctional rhythm. The QRS complex is normally 0.05 to 0.10 second in duration. Abnormal intraventricular conduction of the cardiac impulse is suggested by a QRS complex that exceeds 0.12 second. A pathologic Q wave is present when its duration exceeds 0.04 second. The ST segment is normally isoelectric but can be elevated up to 1 mm in standard and precordial leads in the absence of any cardiac abnormality. The ST segment, however, is never normally depressed. The T wave is in the same direction as the QRS complex and should not exceed 5 mm in amplitude in standard leads or 10 mm in precordial leads. The QT interval must be

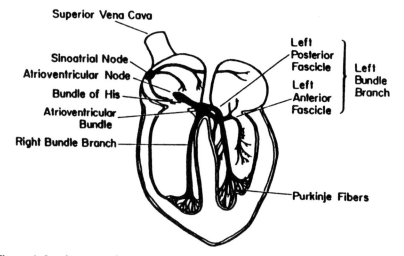

Figure 4–3 • Anatomy of the conduction system for transmission of cardiac impulses.

corrected for heart rate but normally is less than one-half the preceding RR interval.

Ambulatory Electrocardiographic Monitoring

Ambulatory electrocardiographic monitoring (Holter monitoring) is most useful for (1) documenting the occurrence of life-threatening cardiac dysrhythmias, (2) assessing the efficacy of antidysrhythmic drug therapy, and (3) detecting the occurrence of silent (asymptomatic ischemia). Transtelephone (telemetry) transmission of the ECG may be used to delineate the nature of a cardiac dysrhythmia that occurs infrequently. Semiautomated analysis of several hours of recordings facilitates rapid interpretation.

TREATMENT OF CARDIAC DYSRHYTHMIAS

It is useful to consider and correct events responsible for evoking cardiac dysrhythmias before initiating antidysrhythmic drug therapy or placing an artificial cardiac pacemaker (Table 4–1). In this regard, establishing physiologic values for PaO_2, $PaCO_2$, pH, and plasma concentrations of potassium and magnesium, and normalization of autonomic nervous system activity is important. It is not commonly appreciated that alkalosis is even more likely than acidosis to produce ventricular dysrhythmias. Bradycardia can result in ventricular dysrhythmias by causing temporal dispersion of refractory periods among Purkinje fibers.

Antidysrhythmia Drugs

Antidysrhythmia drugs are administered when correction of identifiable precipitating events is not sufficient to suppress cardiac dysrhythmias (Table 4–3). These drugs act by altering electrophysiologic characteristics of the myocardial cells. For example, most antidysrhythmia drugs suppress automaticity in cardiac pacemaker cells by decreasing the slope of phase 4 depolarization. Prolongation of the effective refractory period (quinidine, procainamide, propranolol) serves to eliminate reentry circuits by converting unidirectional blockade to total bidirectional blockade. Conversely, facilitation of cardiac impulse conduction (phenytoin, lidocaine) serves to eliminate unidirectional blockade, thereby preventing cardiac dysrhythmias due to a reentry pathway. Antidysrhythmia drugs may also produce characteristic changes (increased PR interval, prolonged QRS duration) on the ECG. The effectiveness of a specific antidysrhythmic drug is determined by the underlying cardiac conduction or rhythm disturbance (Table 4–3).

Most ventricular cardiac dysrhythmias that require pharmacologic treatment during the perioperative period are responsive to lidocaine. Lidocaine decreases the automaticity of ectopic cardiac pacemakers and increases the threshold for ventricular fibrillation. Supraventricular tachydysrhythmias are not suppressed by lidocaine. Treatment of ventricular premature beats is with a loading dose of lidocaine, 1 to 2 mg/kg IV, followed by a continuous intravenous infusion of 1 to 4 mg/min to maintain a therapeutic plasma concentration of 2 to 5 μg/ml. In the presence of decreases in hepatic blood flow, as associated with general anesthesia, it may be nec-

Table 4–3 • Cardiac Antidysrhythmia Drugs

Drug	Indication	Side Effects
Lidocaine	Ventricular premature beats Ventricular tachydysrhythmias Recurrent ventricular fibrillation	Accumulation with decreased hepatic blood flow Central nervous system toxicity Direct myocardial depression Peripheral vasodilation
Adenosine	Supraventricular tachycardia including that associated with accessory tracts	Peripheral vasodilation (flushing) Dyspnea Angina pectoris Bronchospasm (theoretical) Denervation hypersensitivity in heart transplant patients
Verapamil	Supraventricular tachycardia Atrial fibrillation Atrial flutter	Direct myocardial depression Hypotension Bradycardia Enhanced cardiac impulse transmission through accessory pathways
Digoxin	Atrial tachydysrhythmias Atrial fibrillation Atrial flutter	Toxicity especially in the presence of renal dysfunction and/or hypokalemia Enhance cardiac impulse transmission through accessory pathways
Propranolol	Atrial fibrillation Atrial flutter Supraventricular tachycardia Ventricular tachydysrhythmias Digitalis-induced ventricular dysrhythmias	Sinus bradycardia Direct myocardial depression Bronchoconstriction Lethargy
Procainamide	Ventricular tachydysrhythmias Ventricular premature beats Atrial fibrillation due to accessory pathways	Direct myocardial depression Hypotension Peripheral vasodilation Paradoxical ventricular tachycardia Lupus erythematosus-like syndrome Accumulation with renal dysfunction Potentiation of nondepolarizing neuromuscular blocking drugs
Amiodarone	Supraventricular tachydysrhythmias Ventricular tachydysrhythmias Prevent recurrence of atrial fibrillation Improve response to defibrillation	Prolonged elimination half-time Bradycardia Hypotension Pulmonary fibrosis Postoperative ventilatory failure Skeletal muscle weakness Peripheral neuropathies Hepatitis Cyanotic discoloration of the face Corneal deposits Thyroid dysfunction
Bretylium	Recurrent ventricular fibrillation Recurrent ventricular dysrhythmias	Initial hypertension Peripheral vasodilation Hypotension Accumulation with renal dysfunction Aggravates digitalis toxicity

essary to decrease the lidocaine dose. In usual therapeutic doses, lidocaine does not alter the PR, QRS, or QT intervals on the ECG and has minimal negative inotropic effects. An excessive plasma concentration of lidocaine may decrease conduction of the cardiac impulse through the AV node and His-Purkinje system and evoke seizures followed by coma. Large doses of lidocaine (5 mg/kg IV) administered to animals may increase the intensity and duration of neuromuscular blockade produced by nondepolarizing muscle relaxants.[4]

Electrical Cardioversion

Cardiac dysrhythmias most responsive to electrical cardioversion are atrial flutter, atrial fibrillation, and ventricular tachycardia, although any ectopic tachydysrhythmia that is unresponsive to antidysrhythmia drug therapy can often be successfully terminated with cardioversion. The only exception is the group of digitalis-induced cardiac dysrhythmias; which are refractory to cardioversion; cardioversion can also trigger more serious ventricular dysrhythmias. Cardioversion carries the risk of systemic embolization in patients with atrial fibrillation, which accounts for the recommendation that elective cardioversion be preceded by anticoagulation if the dysrhythmia has been present for more than 48 hours.

Elective cardioversion is performed with intravenous sedation (propofol, etomidate, methohexital), and resuscitation equipment should be immediately available. Drugs such as atropine and lidocaine (ventricular ectopy is common after treatment) and equipment for emergency artificial cardiac pacing should be available in case underlying SA node dysfunction manifests after successful cardioversion. The electrical discharge is delivered by means of two chest electrodes (one placed anteriorly and one posteriorly), beginning at 50 to 100 joules and increasing in increments of 50 to 100 joules as necessary. High energy levels may be needed in the patient with a thickened thorax, a problem often seen in association with pulmonary emphysema. Even with repeated shocks there does not appear to be a significant risk of inflicting damage to the myocardium. Because of the short duration of the electrical current required (2 to 3 ms), it is possible to program the device delivering the current (cardioverter) to be discharged by the R wave of the ECG. Thus the current is delivered during the QRS complex, and the discharge does not occur during the relative refractory period of the cardiac action potential (R on T phenomenon), when an electrical stimulus might evoke ventricular tachycardia or ventricular fibrillation.

Radiofrequency Catheter Ablation

Radiofrequency catheter ablation utilizes an electrode catheter to produce small, well demarcated areas of thermal injury that destroys areas of myocardial tissue or an anatomically specific segment of the cardiac conduction system that is critical to the initiation or maintenance of cardiac dysrhythmias. Cardiac dysrhythmias that have a focal origin or involve a narrow anatomically defined isthmus of the cardiac conduction system are more likely to be amenable to ablation therapy than are cardiac dysrhythmias with multiple foci. Cardiac dysrhythmias amenable to radiofrequency catheter ablation include reentrant supraventricular cardiac dysrhythmias (AV nodal reentrant tachycardia, AV reciprocating tachycardia as is often present in Wolff-Parkinson-White syndrome) and certain ventricular dysrhythmias (idiopathic ventricular tachycardia).

The multipolar electrode catheter is inserted percutaneously under local anesthesia into a femoral, subclavian, internal jugular, or brachial vein and positioned in the heart under fluoroscopic guidance. Conscious sedation is administered to the patient, with the procedure likely to be performed on an outpatient basis.

Artificial Cardiac Pacemakers

It is estimated that 1 million people in the United States have permanent artificial cardiac pacemakers.[5] Indications for placing artificial cardiac pacemakers include sinus node dysfunction ("sick sinus syndrome"), AV heart block, bifascicular or trifascicular heart block, neurogenic syncope, and cardiomyopathy. Temporary artificial cardiac pacing is often required when transient heart block follows cardiopulmonary bypass. A pulmonary artery catheter with a pacing electrode may be selected if simultaneous pressure monitoring and pacing capabilities are required. The physiologic basis for the effectiveness of an artificial cardiac pacemaker is that the myocardium contracts when stimulated.

An artificial cardiac pacemaker can be inserted intravenously (endocardial lead) or by the subcostal approach (epicardial or myocardial lead). Transvenous insertion sites include the internal jugular, external jugular, femoral, and antecubital veins. Electrical impulses are formed in the pulse generator and transmitted to the endocardial or myocardial surface of the heart resulting in a mechanically induced contraction.

Programmable Pacemakers

Artificial cardiac pacemaker systems consist of a lithium-iodine battery that generates electrical impulses (pulse generator) and pacing electrode leads (Table 4–4).[5] Electrical impulses originating in the pulse generator are transmitted through the specialized leads to excite endocardial cells and produce a propagating wave of depolarization in the myocardium. Electronic circuitry can modulate the frequency and amount of current flow and, in addition, sense spontaneous electrical activity in the heart through the leads. Commonly programmable features of external cardiac pacemakers include pacing mode, output, sensitivity, rate, refractory period, and rate adaptation.[5]

Pacing Modes

A four letter generic code is used to describe the various pacing modalities of artificial cardiac pacemakers (Tables 4–5, 4–6).[5] The first letter denotes the cardiac chamber being paced; the second letter denotes the cardiac chamber or chambers where sensing occurs; and the third letter indicates the type

Table 4–4 • Definition of Terms Used to Describe Artificial Cardiac Pacemakers

Term	Definition
Pulse generator	Consists of the energy source (battery) and electrical circuits necessary for pacing and sensory functions
Implanted or external	Anatomic placement of the pulse generator relative to the skin
Lead	Insulated wire connecting the pulse generator to the electrode
Electrode	Exposed metal end of electrode in contact with endocardium or epicardium (myocardium)
Endocardial pacing	Right atrium or right ventricle stimulated following transvenous insertion of the lead
Epicardial pacing	Right atrium or right ventricle stimulated following insertion of the electrode into the myocardium under direct vision
Unipolar pacing	Describes placement of the negative (stimulating) electrode in the atrium or ventricle and the positive (ground) electrode distant from the heart (metallic portion of the pulse generator in subcutaneous tissue)
Bipolar pacing	Describes placement of the negative and positive electrode in the cardiac chamber being paced
Stimulation threshold	Minimal amount of current (amperes) or voltage (volts) necessary to cause contraction of the cardiac chamber being stimulated
Resistance	Measure of the combined resistance of the electrode–lead–myocardial interface as calculated using Ohm's law with values for current and voltage thresholds; normal 350–1000 ohms
R wave sensitivity	Minimal voltage of intrinsic R wave necessary to activate the sensing circuit of the pulse generator and thus inhibit or trigger the pacing circuit (an R wave sensitivity of about 3 mV on an external pulse generator maintains ventricle-inhibited pacing)
Hysteresis	Difference between intrinsic heart rate at which pacing begins (about 60 beats/min) and the pacing rate (72 beats/min)

of response the pacemaker makes to a sensed signal. In most dual-chamber pacing modes, the atrial pacemaker output is inhibited when an atrial signal is sensed; and if no intrinsic ventricular activity is sensed by the end of a programmable AV interval, ventricular output is activated; if intrinsic ventricular activity is sensed, however, the ventricular output is inhibited.[5] The fourth letter, originally developed to describe programmable functions, is now used to designate the presence of rate-adaptive abilities, wherein the paced rates vary with metabolic demands, as might occur during exercise.[5] A fifth letter may also be used to indicate the presence of antitachycardia pacing capabilities, although most such capabilities are now incorporated into automatic implantable defibrillators.

DDD Pacing

Dual-chamber DDD pacemakers provide the important benefits of maintaining AV synchrony and min-

imizing the incidence of the pacemaker syndrome. Atrial events, both sensed and paced, initiate or trigger the AV interval so AV synchrony is maintained over a wide range of sinus rhythm heart rates. The DDD pacing mode permits the artificial pacemaker to respond to increases in the sinus node discharge rate, as during exercise. Hemodynamic improvements with AV synchrony pacing reflect more efficient left ventricular filling with up to 20% augmentation of left ventricular stroke volume. Maintenance of AV synchrony in patients with sick sinus syndrome may be associated with a decreased incidence of atrial fibrillation and thromboembolic events.

Pacemaker Syndrome

Pacing with DDD pacemakers has decreased the incidence of the pacemaker syndrome, which manifests as a constellation of symptoms associated with ventricular pacing, including syncope, weakness,

Table 4–5 • Generic Code for Identifying and Describing Pacemaker Function

First Letter	Second Letter	Third Letter	Fourth Letter
Cardiac chamber paced	Cardiac chamber in which electrical activity is sensed	Response of generator to sensed R wave and P wave	Programmable functions of the generator
V—ventricle	V—ventricle	T—triggering	P—programmable (rate and/or output only)
A—atrium	A—atrium	I—inhibited	M—multiprogrammable
D—dual (atrium and ventricle)	D—dual	D—dual	C—communicating
	O—none (asynchronous)	O—none (asynchronous)	O—none (fixed function)

Table 4–6 • Artificial Cardiac Pulse Generators

Description	Letter number*			
	I	II	III	IV
Single-chamber pacing modes				
Asynchronous (fixed rate) atrial pacing	A	O	O	
Asynchronous (fixed rate) ventricular pacing	V	O	O	
Noncompetitive (demand) atrial pacing; electrical output inhibited by intrinsic atrial depolarization (P wave)	A	A	I	
Noncompetitive (demand) ventricular pacing; electrical output inhibited by intrinsic ventricular depolarization (R wave)	V	V	I	
Triggered atrial pacing; electrical output triggered by intrinsic atrial depolarization (P wave)	A	A	T	
Triggered ventricular pacing; electrical output triggered by intrinsic ventricular depolarization (R wave)	V	V	T	
Dual-chamber pacing modes				
Paces and senses in atrium and ventricle	D	D	D	
Senses in both the atrium and ventricle, but the only response to a sensed event is inhibition	D	D	I	
Rate-adaptive pacemakers				
Single-chamber	A	A	I	R
Single-chamber	V	V	I	R
Dual-chamber	D	D	I	R
Dual-chamber	D	D	D	R

* See Table 4–5 for definitions of letter numbers.

orthopnea, paroxysmal nocturnal dyspnea, and pulmonary edema. The pathophysiologic features of the pacemaker syndrome may reflect decreases in cardiac output and hypotension, which result from the loss of atrial contributions to left ventricular filling. Furthermore, increases in atrial pressures result from contraction of the atrium against closed mitral and tricuspid valves, which occurs when the ventricle is paced (VVI mode). Activation of baroreceptors from inappropriate atrial stretch can lead to reflex peripheral vasodilation. Symptoms of the pacemaker syndrome are usually eliminated by any pacing mode that allows restoration of AV synchrony.

DDI Pacing

In the DDI pacing mode, there is sensing in both the atrium and ventricle, but the only response to a sensed event is inhibition (inhibited pacing of the atrium and ventricle). The pacemaker does not deliver an atrial stimulus if it senses atrial activity. The AV-interval timer starts only after a paced atrial event. DDI pacing is useful when there are frequent atrial tachydysrhythmias that might be inappropriately tracked by a DDD pacemaker, resulting in rapid paced ventricular rates.

Rate-Adaptive Pacemakers (AAIR, VVIR, DDIR, DDDR)

A rate-adaptive pacemaker is considered for patients who do not have an appropriate chronotropic response to increases in metabolic demand (exercise). AV synchrony contributes more to cardiac output at rest and at low levels of exercise, whereas rate adaptation is more important at higher levels of exercise. Sensors are designed so the pulse generator can mimic the responses of normal heart rates to increases in metabolic demands. Sensors most often respond to changes in motion or minute ventilation.

Choice of Pacing Mode

The choice of pacing mode depends on the primary indication for the artificial pacemaker.[5] If the patient has SA node disease and no evidence of disease of the AV node or His bundle, an atrial pacemaker (AAI) can be placed, as the rate of progression to second- or third-degree AV heart block is less than 1% per year. In the presence of accompanying disease of the AV node or His bundle, or the need for drug treatment to slow AV node conduction (β-adrenergic blockers, calcium channel blockers) a dual-chamber (DDD) system is appropriate. Patients with sinus node disease, AV node disease, or fascicular disease whose heart rates do not respond to increases in metabolic demands should be considered for placement of rate-adaptive pacing systems. Individuals experiencing intermittent episodes of symptomatic bradycardia due to SA node or AV node disease may benefit from placement of a single chamber ventricular (VVI) pacemaker. Neurocardiogenic syncope due to carotid sinus hypersensitivity or vasovagal syncope is treated with a dual-chamber pacemaker. Dual chamber pacing systems that allow control of the AV rate are utilized for managing patients with hypertrophic cardiomyopathies.

Artificial Pacemaker Failure

Early pacemaker failures are usually due to electrode displacement or breakage, whereas failures that occur more than 6 months after implantation are most often due to premature battery depletion or a faulty pulse generator. The development of lithium batteries with a projected longevity of 8 to 20 years has greatly decreased the need to replace pacemakers for battery failure. Because dual-chamber pacemakers require a greater output of energy than single-chamber units, they have shorter life spans. Although VVI pacemakers can be expected to function for 10 to 15 years, most dual-chamber pacemakers have projected life spans of 7 to 10 years.

Cardiac dysrhythmias may be evoked by artificial cardiac pacemakers, especially dual-chamber devices. Improved shielding of artificial cardiac pacemakers has largely eliminated earlier problems related to external electrical fields (microwaves, electrocautery, magnetic resonance imaging) manifesting as inhibition of ventricular-inhibited pacemakers. Many artificial cardiac pacemakers are now designed such that external electrical fields change the pacemaker rhythm to an asynchronous mode rather than shut off the unit. Many functions of an artificial cardiac pacemaker can be adjusted using a magnetically activated potentiometer held externally in proximity to the pulse generator. A demand pacemaker may be overridden by the intrinsic heart rate if this heart rate is more rapid, or the pacemaker can be momentarily converted to an asynchronous mode by placing a magnet externally over the pulse generator. An acute myocardial infarction near the site of electrode placement may interfere with the electrode–tissue interface and result in artificial cardiac pacemaker failure.

Noninvasive Transcutaneous Cardiac Pacing

An alternative to emergency transvenous artificial cardiac pacemaker placement is noninvasive transcutaneous cardiac pacing.[6] Judicious placement of cutaneous chest and back electrodes over areas of minimal skeletal muscle mass and delivery of low-density constant-current impulses permits effective cardiac stimulation with little or no skeletal muscle or cutaneous activation. Hemodynamic responses to noninvasive transcutaneous cardiac pacing are similar to those produced by right ventricular cardiac pacing. Noninvasive transcutaneous cardiac pacing is an option in clinical situations (bradydysrhythmias, cardiac arrest owing to asystole) that require emergency pacing. Noninvasive transcutaneous cardiac pacing may be of value when applied early during witnessed bradyasystolic arrest, whereas transvenous pacing does not improve the outcome after cardiac arrest.[6] This form of cardiac pacing may be useful for elective overdrive suppression of hemodynamically unstable tachydysrhythmias. It may also become useful for prophylaxis in patients with artificial cardiac pacemakers or those with left bundle branch block who are undergoing central hemodynamic monitoring.

Transvenous Implantable Cardioverter-Defibrillator

The transvenous implantable cardioverter-defibrillator (ICD) detects ventricular tachycardia or fibrillation and terminates the dysrhythmia by overdrive pacing or delivery of a synchronized high energy shock. The ICD system consists of a subcutaneously implanted generator, rate-sensing leads, and electrodes to deliver high-energy shocks via wire mesh patch electrodes applied directly to the epicardial surface of the heart. For patients with a history of ventricular fibrillation, the ICD is programmed to deliver high-energy shocks when it detects tachycardia. Patients with a history of monomorphic ventricular tachycardia may benefit from overdrive pacing. The ICD is costly and invasive, which limits its widespread use.

Surgery in Patients with Artificial Cardiac Pacemakers

The presence of artificial cardiac pacemakers in patients scheduled for surgery unrelated to the pacemaker introduces special considerations to the preoperative evaluation and subsequent management of anesthesia.

Preoperative Evaluation

Preoperative evaluation of the patient with an artificial cardiac pacemaker in place includes determining the reason for placing the pacemaker and assessment of its present function (Table 4–5). A preoperative history of vertigo or syncope may reflect dysfunction of the artificial cardiac pacemaker. The rate of discharge of an atrial or ventricular asynchronous cardiac pacemaker (usually 70 to 72 beats/ min) is a useful indicator of pulse generator function. A 10% decrease in heart rate from the initial fixed discharge rate may reflect battery failure. An irregular heart rate may reflect competition of the pulse generator with the patient's intrinsic heart rate or failure of the pulse generator to sense R waves. The ECG is evaluated to confirm one-to-one capture, as evidenced by a pacemaker spike for every palpated peripheral pulse. The ECG is not a diagnostic aid in patients in whom the intrinsic heart rate is greater than the preset pacemaker rate. In such cases proper functioning of a ventricular synchronous or sequential artificial cardiac pacemaker can be confirmed by demonstrating the appearance of captured beats on the ECG when the pacemaker is converted to the asynchronous mode by placing an external converter magnet over the pulse generator. Attempting to slow the heart rate by massaging the carotid sinus is not recommended, as dislodgement of an arteriosclerotic plaque is a risk, whereas the Valsalva maneuver may not lower the intrinsic heart rate sufficiently to confirm the functioning of the artificial cardiac pacemaker. A chest radiograph is useful for confirming and evaluating the intactness of the pacemaker's electrodes.

Management of Anesthesia

Management of anesthesia in patients with artificial cardiac pacemakers includes (1) monitoring to confirm continued functioning of the pulse generator and (2) ensuring the ready availability of equipment and drugs to maintain an acceptable intrinsic heart rate should the artificial cardiac pacemaker unexpectedly fail (Table 4–7). If electrocautery interferes with the ECG, placing a finger on a peripheral pulse or auscultation through an esophageal stethoscope confirms continued cardiac activity. Insertion of a pulmonary artery catheter does not disturb epicardial electrodes but might become entangled in, or dislodge, a recently placed transvenous (endocardial) electrode. Dislodgement of endocardial electrodes, however, has not been observed when these electrodes have been in place for more than 4 weeks.[5]

Table 4–7 • Management of Anesthesia in Patients with an Artificial Cardiac Pacemaker

Continuous monitoring of the electrocardiogram
Continuous monitoring of a peripheral pulse
Electrical defibrillator present
External convert magnet available
Drugs prepared (atropine, isoproterenol)

The choice of drugs to produce anesthesia is not altered by the presence of a properly functioning artificial cardiac pacemaker. An artificial cardiac pacemaker that is functioning normally preoperatively should continue to function intraoperatively without incident.

Improved shielding of artificial cardiac pacemakers has largely eliminated the problem of electromagnetic interference from electrocautery in which the electrical artifact was sensed as an intrinsic myocardial potential (R wave) by the pacemaker, resulting in inhibition of the pulse generator. Nevertheless, the possibility of this external suppression is a consideration and is the reason for the recommendation that drugs (atropine, isoproterenol) be promptly available should the artificial cardiac pacemaker unexpectedly fail.[7] An external converter magnet may be used to convert the pacemaker to an asynchronous mode. Despite improved shielding of artificial cardiac pacemakers, it is still a reasonable recommendation to place the ground plate for the electrocautery as far as possible from the pulse generator to minimize detection of the current by the pulse generator. Furthermore, it is useful to keep the electrocautery current as low as possible and to apply electrocautery in short bursts, especially when the current is being applied in close proximity to the pulse generator.[8] Paradoxically, the use of a repetitive electrical stimulus delivered by a peripheral nerve stimulator (twitch mode at a frequency of 2 Hz) placed ipsilateral to the artificial cardiac pacemaker generator, has been used intraoperatively for deliberate suppression of a malfunctioning ventricular-inhibited pacemaker.[9]

Ventricular fibrillation in a patient with a permanent artificial cardiac pacemaker is managed in a conventional manner, with the exception that the defibrillator paddles should not be placed directly over the pulse generator. An acute increase in stimulation threshold may follow external defibrillation, causing a loss of capture and the need for prompt insertion of a transvenous artificial cardiac pacemaker or use of noninvasive transcutaneous cardiac pacing.[10] Presumably, electrical defibrillation results in endocardial burns and fibrosis at the electrode–endocardium interface, resulting in an increased stimulation threshold and emphasizing the need to administer the lowest effective dose of electrical energy.

There is no evidence that anesthetic drugs or events likely to be associated with the perioperative period alter the stimulation threshold of artificial cardiac pacemakers (Table 4–8). Nevertheless, it seems prudent to avoid events (hyperventilation of the patient's lungs, drug-induced diuresis) that acutely increase or decrease plasma potassium concentrations.

Table 4–8 • Factors that Could Alter Stimulation Threshold of Artificial Cardiac Pacemakers

Hyperkalemia (succinylcholine)
Hypokalemia (hyperventilation)
Arterial hypoxemia
Myocardial ischemia/infarction
Catecholamines

Conceivably, succinylcholine could increase the stimulation threshold by virtue of an acute increase in the plasma potassium concentration or could inhibit a normally functioning artificial cardiac pacemaker by causing contraction of skeletal muscle groups (myopotential inhibition) interpreted as intrinsic R waves by the pulse generator. For example, unipolar pulse generators of an artificial cardiac pacemaker system may be inhibited by skeletal muscle myopotentials (fasciculations) produced by succinylcholine.[10] For this reason it has been recommended that when succinylcholine is to be administered to patients with unipolar demand pacemakers the pacemaker be switched to an asynchronous mode using a precordial magnet,[10] although use of such a magnet may increase the risk of cardiac dysrhythmias secondary to the R on T phenomenon and may allow unintentional reprogramming of certain pacemakers. It is unclear whether attenuation of succinylcholine-induced skeletal muscle fasciculations by prior administration of nonparalyzing doses of nondepolarizing muscle relaxants decreases the risk of myopotential inhibition of the pulse generator. Clinical experience suggests that succinylcholine is usually a safe drug in the patient with an artificial cardiac pacemaker; and if myopotential inhibition does occur, it is generally transient and asymptomatic. A rare occurrence is transvenous pacemaker failure associated with positive-pressure ventilation of the lungs, which may reflect an abrupt volume change in the heart and cardiac septal deviation causing loss of electrode contact with the endocardial surface of the myocardium.[11]

Anesthesia for Artificial Cardiac Pacemaker Insertion

A functioning artificial cardiac pacemaker should be in place or noninvasive transcutaneous cardiac pacing available before induction of anesthesia for permanent artificial cardiac pacemaker placement, as there is a risk that third-degree AV heart block may deteriorate to cardiac arrest. Drugs such as isoproterenol and atropine should be available for prompt administration should decreases in heart rate become a consideration before functioning of the artificial cardiac pacemaker is established. The patient's arm should not be placed in hyperextension when the brachial vein has been used for insertion of the transvenous pacemaker. The presence of a transvenous pacemaker creates a situation in which there is a direct connection between an external electrical source and the endocardium, predisposing patients to the risk of ventricular fibrillation due to microshock levels of electrical currents.

DISTURBANCES OF CARDIAC IMPULSE CONDUCTION

Disturbances of cardiac impulse conduction are classified according to the site of the conduction block relative to the AV node (Table 4–9). Heart block that occurs above the AV node is usually benign and transient, whereas heart block that develops below the AV node tends to be progressive and permanent.

First-Degree Atrioventricular Heart Block

First-degree AV heart block is arbitrarily defined as a PR interval on the ECG that is more than 0.2 second at a heart rate of 70 beats/min. This prolonged PR interval reflects a delay in passage of cardiac impulses through the AV node. Commonly, a prolonged PR interval is the result of degeneration of the cardiac conduction system that accompanies aging. Other causes are use of digitalis, ischemia of the AV node as may occur with diaphragmatic myocardial infarction, and enhanced parasympathetic nervous system activity. Aortic regurgitation

Table 4–9 • Classification of Heart Block

First-degree AV heart block
Second-degree AV heart block
Mobitz type 1 (Wenckebach)
Mobitz type 2
Unifascicular heart block
Left anterior hemiblock
Left posterior hemiblock
Right bundle branch block
Left bundle branch block
Bifascicular heart block
Right bundle branch block plus left anterior hemiblock
Right bundle branch block plus left posterior hemiblock
Third-degree (trifascicular, complete) heart block
Nodal
Infranodal

AV, atrioventricular.

is commonly accompanied by first-degree heart block, which is usually asymptomatic. Intravenous administration of atropine effectively speeds conduction of cardiac impulses through the AV node.

Second-Degree Atrioventricular Heart Block

Second-degree AV heart block is categorized as Mobitz type 1 block (Wenckebach) or Mobitz type 2 block. Mobitz type 1 block is caused by delayed conduction of cardiac impulses through the AV node. There is progressive prolongation of the PR interval until a beat is entirely blocked (dropped beat), followed by a repeat of this sequence. By contrast, Mobitz type 2 block reflects disease of the His-Purkinje conduction system (infranodal block), characterized by sudden interruption of the conduction of a cardiac impulse without prior prolongation of the PR interval on the ECG. Mobitz type 2 block has a more serious prognosis than type 1 block, as it frequently progresses to third-degree AV heart block. Treatment of Mobitz type 2 block may include placing of an artificial cardiac pacemaker.

Unifascicular Heart Block

Block of conduction of cardiac impulses over the left anterior or posterior fascicle of the left bundle branch is characterized as unifascicular heart block, or hemiblock. Block of the left anterior fascicle of the left bundle branch is designated left anterior hemiblock. Left posterior hemiblock is uncommon, as the posterior fascicle of the left bundle branch is larger and better perfused than the anterior fascicle. Although hemiblock is a form of intraventricular heart block, the duration of the QRS complex is normal or only minimally prolonged.

Right Bundle Branch Block

Right bundle branch block (RBBB) is due to block of conduction of the cardiac impulse over the right bundle branch, which is present in about 1% of hospitalized adult patients. RBBB is recognized on the ECG by QRS complexes that exceed 0.1 second in duration and by broad RSR complexes in leads V_1 and V_3. RBBB does not always imply cardiac disease and is often of no clinical significance. Incomplete RBBB (QRS complex duration 0.09 to 0.10 second) is frequently present in patients with increased right ventricular pressures, as produced by chronic pulmonary disease or an atrial septal defect.

Left Bundle Branch Block

Left bundle branch block (LBBB) is recognized on the ECG as a QRS complex more than 0.12 second in duration and by wide notched R waves in all leads. Incomplete LBBB is present when the duration of the QRS complex on the ECG is 0.10 to 0.12 second in duration. LBBB, in contrast to RBBB, is often associated with ischemic heart disease; or it may reflect left ventricular hypertrophy accompanying chronic systemic hypertension or cardiac valve disease. The appearance of LBBB has been observed during anesthesia (especially when the heart rate exceeds 115 beats/min or in the presence of systemic hypertension) and may signal an acute myocardial infarction.[12] It is difficult to diagnose a myocardial infarction on the ECG in the presence of LBBB. The wide QRS complexes characteristic of LBBB can be mistaken for ventricular tachycardia.

The presence of LBBB may have special implications for insertion of a pulmonary artery catheter.[13] For example, RBBB occurs during insertion of a pulmonary artery catheter in about 5% of patients with ischemic heart disease. Theoretically, third-degree AV heart block could occur if there is catheter-induced RBBB in a patient with co-existing LBBB. Nevertheless, clinical experience has not confirmed an increased incidence of third-degree AV heart block in such patients during insertion of a pulmonary artery catheter.

Bifascicular Heart Block

Bifascicular heart block is present when RBBB is associated with block of one of the fascicles of the left bundle branch. RBBB plus left anterior hemiblock (anterior fascicle of the left bundle) is the most frequent combination, present on about 1% of all the ECGs recorded from adults. Each year about 1% to 2% of these patients progress to third-degree AV heart block. The combination of RBBB and left posterior hemiblock (posterior fascicle of the left bundle branch) is infrequent; but in contrast to left anterior hemiblock, it often progresses to third-degree AV heart block. Insertion of an artificial cardiac pacemaker, however, is recommended only when symptomatic bradydysrhythmias occur.

A theoretical concern in patients with bifascicular heart block is that perioperative events (changes in systemic blood pressure, arterial oxygenation, plasma electrolyte concentrations) might compromise the conduction of cardiac impulses in the one remaining intact fascicle, leading to the sudden onset of third-degree AV heart block.[14] There is no evidence, however, that surgery performed with general or regional anesthesia predisposes patients with co-exisitng bifascicular heart block to the development of third-degree AV heart block.[15] For this reason, prophylactic placement of an artificial cardiac pacemaker is not recommended before anesthesia for elective surgery. This recommendation is based on the clinical course of patients with co-existing bifascicular heart block who had normal preoperative PR intervals on the ECG and who denied a history of unexplained syncope that might suggest the prior occurrence of transient third-degree AV heart block. Conceivably, a temporary transvenous artificial cardiac pacemaker can be placed before a major surgical procedure when the preoperative ECG shows a prolonged PR interval or when there is a history of unexplained syncope. Nevertheless, even symptomatic patients with bifascicular heart block have undergone uneventful surgery without prior placement of an artificial cardiac pacemaker.[14, 15]

Third-Degree Atrioventricular Heart Block

Third-degree AV heart block ("complete heart block") is characterized by the complete absence of conduction of cardiac impulses from the atria to the ventricles. Continued activity of the ventricles is due to stimulation from an ectopic cardiac pacemaker distal to the site of the conduction block. When the conduction block is near the AV node, the heart rate is 45 to 55 beats/min, and the QRS complex on the ECG appears normal. When the conduction block is below the AV node (infranodal), the heart rate is 30 to 40 beats/min, and the QRS complex on the ECG is wide. The onset of third-degree AV heart block may be signaled by an episode of vertigo and syncope. Syncope associated with a seizure is designated an Adams-Stokes attack. Congestive heart failure may occur when the stroke volume is unable to offset the decreased cardiac output produced by the bradycardia accompanying third-degree AV heart block. The most common cause of third-degree AV heart block in adults is primary fibrous degeneration of the cardiac conduction system associated with aging (Lenegre's disease) (Table 4–10). Degenerative changes in tissues adjacent to the mitral valve annulus can also interrupt the cardiac conduction system (Lev's disease). Congenital third-degree AV heart block is almost always at the level of the AV node.

Treatment of third-degree AV heart block consists of placing a permanent artificial cardiac pacemaker. Prior placement of a transvenous pacemaker or availability of noninvasive transcutaneous cardiac pacing is common before induction of anesthesia for

Table 4–10 • Causes of Third-Degree Atrioventricular Heart Block

Primary fibrotic degeneration of the cardiac conduction system (Lenegre's disease, Lev's disease)
Ischemic heart disease (myocardial infarction)
Cardiomyopathy
Myocarditis
Ankylosing spondylitis
Iatrogenic after cardiac surgery
Congenital
Increased parasympathetic nervous system activity
Drugs (digoxin, β-adrenergic antagonists)
Electrolyte disturbances (hyperkalemia)

inserting a permanent artificial cardiac pacemaker. Isoproterenol, 1 to 4 μg/min IV, may be useful along with atropine, to maintain an acceptable heart rate (chemical pacemaker) until the permanent artificial cardiac pacemaker is functional. Antidysrhythmia drugs may suppress ectopic ventricular pacemakers; and for this reason probably should not be administered to patients with third-degree AV heart block in the absence of an artificial cardiac pacemaker.

DISTURBANCES OF CARDIAC RHYTHM

Cardiac dysrhythmias that arise in the atria or AV node are classified as supraventricular dysrhythmias. Cardiac dysrhythmias that arise below the AV node are classified as ventricular dysrhythmias.

Sinus Tachycardia

Sinus tachycardia is defined as a heart rate of more than 120 beats/min. It is due to acceleration of the normal discharge rate of the SA node. An increased heart rate during the preoperative period may reflect anxiety, pain, sepsis, hypovolemia, fever, or congestive heart failure. Light anesthesia relative to the surgical stimulus may produce tachycardia. Intraoperatively, causes of tachycardia other than light anesthesia include arterial hypoxemia, hypoglycemia, hyperthyroidism, and malignant hyperthermia. Treatment of sinus tachycardia depends on the cause of the increased heart rate. When sinus tachycardia results in myocardial ischemia, intravenous administration of a β-adrenergic antagonist such as esmolol may be considered.

Inappropriate sinus tachycardia is an infrequent cardiac dysrhythmia that may be persistent or episodic. It is often precipitated by arising from a reclining or sitting position (postural orthostatic tachycardia). The tachycardia is frequently accompanied by symptoms of dizziness and syncope. β-Adrenergic antagonists and calcium channel blockers may be used to alleviate inappropriate sinus tachycardia.

Sinus Bradycardia

Sinus bradycardia is defined as a heart rate of less than 60 beats/min. It is due to deceleration of the normal discharge rate of the SA node. It may be a normal finding in physically active patients with high degrees of parasympathetic nervous system activity (athletic heart syndrome). Unexpected cardiac arrest has been described in a well trained athlete during spinal anesthesia, perhaps reflecting parasympathetic nervous system predominance enhanced by anesthesia-induced blockade of the cardioaccelerator nerves.[16] An acute diaphragmatic myocardial infarction and the presence of severe pain represent conditions in which discharge of the SA node can be normally slow. Severe nocturnal bradycardia should arouse suspicion of obstructive sleep apnea.

Among the volatile anesthetic drugs, halothane is most likely to decrease the heart rate by decreasing the automaticity of the SA node.[17] Other factors that slow the heart rate by depressing SA node automaticity, rather than by vagal stimulation, include β-adrenergic antagonist drugs, hypothermia, hypothyroidism, and icterus. In the presence of carotid sinus hypersensitivity, prolonged asystole can follow even minimal pressure on the carotid sinus. Reflex bradycardia may occur with traction on the ocular muscles (oculocardiac reflex) and with traction on the abdominal mesentery (celiac plexus stimulation); it can also occur during laryngoscopy, laparoscopy, and electroconvulsive therapy.[17] Drugs associated with reflex bradycardia are opioids and succinylcholine. Intravenous administration of atropine is the treatment of choice when heart rate slowing becomes hemodynamically significant.

Spinal and Epidural Anesthesia

Bradycardia and asystole are rare but recognized complications of spinal anesthesia.[18–22] Intraoperative bradycardia can be a warning sign of impending cardiovascular collapse.[20] A prospective study of 40,640 cases of spinal anesthesia found an incidence of cardiac arrest of 6.4 per 10,000 patients.[19] Closed claims analysis of complications during spinal anesthesia were often associated with bradycardia preceding cardiac arrest. Although reported less often, bradycardia and asystole have also been described in patients receiving epidural anesthesia.[23]

Pathophysiology

The underlying mechanism or mechanisms responsible for bradycardia and asystole during spinal and epidural anesthesia are not known.[22, 23] Proposed theories include reflex-induced bradycardia resulting from decreased venous return or unopposed parasympathetic nervous system activity resulting from spinal or epidural-induced thoracic sympathectomy. Neuraxial blockade may lead to decreased venous return to the heart, which may activate vagal reflexes (baroreceptors, stretch receptors in the sinus node, paradoxical Bezold-Jarisch response) that cause bradycardia. In addition to these myocardial reflexes, blockade of cardiac accelerators originating from the thoracic sympathetic ganglia (T1–4) may alter the balance of autonomic nervous system input to the heart, resulting in the emergence of relatively unopposed parasympathetic influences on the SA node and AV node. Nevertheless, there is evidence that even a T4 sensory level does not produce total sympathetic blockade, which challenges the concept of spinal or epidural anesthesia-induced thoracic sympathectomy as the most likely explanation for bradycardia and asystole. Secondary factors, including opioid administration, sedation, hypercarbia, concurrent medical illnesses, and chronic drug therapy may contribute to the development of bradycardia. For example, co-existing first-degree AV heart block may predispose to bradycardia and progression to second-degree (Mobitz type 2) or third-degree AV heart block during spinal anesthesia.[21, 22]

Although the mechanism of lumbar neuraxial anesthesia-induced bradycardia or asystole is debatable, the final pathway is most likely an absolute or relative increase in parasympathetic nervous system activity. In this regard, nausea, a parasympathetic event, may be the first symptom associated with the subsequent onset of bradycardia.

Clinical Manifestations

Bradycardia, asystole, or both may develop suddenly (seconds or minutes) from a prior normal or even increased heart rate.[23] In other patients heart rate slowing is progressive. In most patients pulse oximetry confirms acceptable oxygen saturations prior to the onset of bradycardia, suggesting a primary cardiac mechanism. Hypovolemia may predispose to acute bradycardia during neuraxial blockade. Inflation of a lower limb tourniquet may result in a decrease in preload, thereby providing conditions favorable for the development of bradydysrhythmias. Bradycardia during neuraxial blockade occurs over wide age ranges and American

Society of Anesthesiologists (ASA) physical status classifications, and with or without sedation. It seems that bradycardia can occur at any time during neuraxial blockade, but most often it is seen about 60 minutes after institution of the anesthetic. The sensory level of anesthesia is not necessarily a predictor of bradycardia. Indeed, the risk of bradycardia and asystole may persist into the postoperative period even after the sensory and motor blockades have diminished.[22, 23]

Treatment

Prompt pharmacologic treatment (atropine, ephedrine, epinephrine) supported by precordial pacing thumps is the recommended treatment for bradydysrhythmias associated with spinal or epidural anesthesia.[23, 24] Bradycardia may occur despite prophylactic therapy with atropine and/or intravenous fluids. Continuous monitoring of the ECG and oxygen saturation is essential, as is vigilance on the part of the anesthesiologist with the recognition that this complication may occur suddenly and without warning.

Sinus Node Dysfunction

Dysfunction of the SA node (also referred to as sick sinus syndrome) is a common cause of bradycardia. The prevalence of sinus-node dysfunction is estimated to be as high as 1 in 600 patients over the age of 65 years; the syndrome accounts for about 50% of all artificial cardiac pacemaker insertions.[25] Episodes of supraventricular tachycardia may punctuate periods of bradycardia. In an afflicted patient the SA node seems to be depressed and more vulnerable to other exogenous influences, such as vagal stimulation and certain drugs. Many patients are asymptomatic, although syncope and palpitations are often described. Bradycardia may contribute to the development of congestive heart failure, whereas tachycardia can precipitate angina pectoris in patients with ischemic heart disease.

The combination of supraventricular tachycardia and sinus bradycardia in patients with SA node dysfunction is problematic, as suppression of SA node automaticity may result in syncope when the tachycardia terminates. Therapy to control the ventricular rate during tachycardia by blocking AV conduction with β-adrenergic antagonists, calcium channel blockers, or digoxin may not be possible in the absence of an artificial cardiac pacemaker because drug-induced depression of SA node function is not desirable. In this regard, placing an artificial cardiac pacemaker and pacing are indicated when drugs required for control of the ventricular

response rate could cause bradycardia during periods of normal sinus rhythm. Atrium-based pacing is preferred in patients with SA node dysfunction because it decreases the incidence of atrial fibrillation and thromboembolism. Long-term anticoagulation may be recommended in view of the increased incidence of systemic embolism in the presence of this syndrome.

Syncope

Syncope (transient loss of consciousness with concurrent loss of postural tone followed by spontaneous recovery) is most often due to vasovagal reactions (bradydysrhythmias). Other causes of syncope are tachydysrhythmias, heart block, obstruction to left ventricular outflow, and orthostatic hypotension. Syncope must be differentiated from seizures and other states of altered consciousness, such as vertigo and narcolepsy. It is estimated that syncope accounts for 1% to 6% of hospital admissions and 3% of emergency room visits.

Atrial Premature and Junctional Premature Beats

Atrial premature and junctional premature beats arise from an ectopic cardiac pacemaker in the atria or near the AV node. These premature beats are recognized on the ECG by the presence of early, abnormally shaped P waves. The duration of the corresponding QRS complex is normal because activation of the ventricles occurs via a normal conduction pathway. When aberrant conduction of cardiac impulses occurs, however, the configuration of the QRS complex is widened and may mimic a ventricular premature beat. A distinguishing feature is that atrial premature beats, unlike ventricular premature beats, are generally not followed by compensatory pauses. Atrial premature beats can occur in patients with or without heart disease. It is usually insignificant, except when it precedes the onset of a tachydysrhythmia. Acceleration of the heart rate, as produced by the intravenous administration of atropine, usually abolishes atrial premature beats.

Supraventricular Tachycardia

Supraventricular tachycardia is any tachydysrhythmia that requires atrial or AV junctional tissue for its initiation and maintenance.[26] The term "paroxysmal atrial tachycardia," used to describe supraventricular tachycardia that begins and ends abruptly, is no longer recommended, as it is likely that many of these dysrhythmias arise in the AV junction and not the atrial muscle. AV nodal reentrant tachycardia (AVNRT) is the most common type of supraventricular tachycardia (average heart rate 160 to 180 beats/min) and occurs three times more often in women than in men. Atrial fibrillation and atrial flutter are considered supraventricular tachycardias, but their electrophysiology and treatment are distinctly different from other forms of supraventricular tachycardia.[26]

Mechanisms

Supraventricular tachycardia is often due to a reentry circuit in which there is anterograde conduction over the slow AV nodal pathway and retrograde conduction over the fast conduction pathway. Other mechanisms for supraventricular tachycardia are enhanced automaticity of latent pacemaker cells at sites other than the SA node and enhanced impulse initiation caused by membrane currents that may be due to premature stimulation. AVNRT accounts for more than 50% of patients who develop supraventricular tachycardia.

Treatment

Because AVNRT is usually hemodynamically stable, urgent treatment is not required. Initial treatment is often with vagal maneuvers including carotid sinus massage, performance of a Valsalva maneuver, or stimulation of the posterior pharynx. The carotid sinus is located below the site of maximum pulsation of the carotid artery in the patient's neck, usually immediately lateral to the thyroid cartilage. In the absence of carotid bruits detectable by auscultation, firm external pressure is applied over the carotid sinus for 10 to 20 seconds during constant monitoring of the ECG. Application of pressure over the right carotid sinus is more likely to be successful than compression applied over the left carotid sinus. If vagal maneuvers are not effective, pharmacologic treatment is directed toward blocking AV nodal conduction.

Adenosine

Adenosine, an α_1-adrenergic agonist with a rapid onset and brief duration of action, is the drug of choice for pharmacologic termination of AVNRT. Adenosine is administered intravenously with its effects becoming apparent within 15 to 30 seconds. Most SA node reentry and AVNRT episodes are terminated by a single dose of adenosine (6 mg IV). If the initial 6 mg dose is not effective, two subsequent doses of 12 mg each may be administered about 2 minutes apart. Adenosine often causes flushing and in some patients is associated with angina pectoris and dyspnea. In patients with asthma, bronchospasm triggered by intravenous administration of adenosine remains a theoretical but clinically undocumented complication.[26] Heart transplant patients may manifest a denervation hypersensitivity to adenosine. Multifocal atrial tachycardia, atrial flutter, and atrial fibrillation are not likely to respond to adenosine.

Calcium Channel-Blocking Drugs

Intravenous administration of calcium channel-blocking drugs, including verapamil and diltiazem, is also useful for terminating supraventricular tachycardia. Verapamil, 75 to 150 μg/kg IV over about 2 minutes, has a longer duration of action than adenosine, which may be an advantage for preventing the return of tachycardia but a disadvantage if it causes hypotension. Calcium channel-blocking drugs are preferable for treating patients with atrial tachycardia, as this dysrhythmia rarely responds to adenosine. Intravenous digoxin (because of its delayed onset of action) and intravenous β-adrenergic antagonists (because of their negative inotropic and possible bronchoconstrictive effects) offer no real advantages over adenosine or calcium channel-blocking drugs. Electrical cardioversion may be used when drug therapy is not promptly effective and the tachycardia is associated with hypotension and/or angina pectoris.

Long-term medical therapy of patients who experience repeated episodes of supraventricular tachycardia includes verapamil, digoxin, or propranolol. Radiofrequency catheter ablation has also been used to treat patients with AVNRT.

Atrial Flutter

Atrial flutter is a paroxysmal disturbance that usually lasts only a few minutes to hours before spontaneously converting to normal sinus rhythm or atrial fibrillation.[2] On the ECG atrial flutter is characterized by an absolutely regular atrial rate at 250 to 320 beats/min with varying degrees of AV block, often 2:1. The baseline of the ECG reveals flutter waves (F waves), resulting in a sawtooth pattern. Atrial flutter occurs most often in patients with chronic pulmonary disease, dilated cardiomyopathy, ethanol intoxication, thyrotoxicosis, and following cardiothoracic surgery (see "Postoperative Atrial Tachydysrhythmias").

Drugs do not reliably slow the ventricular response rate or convert atrial flutter to normal sinus rhythm. Digoxin is not recommended for acute ventricular rate reduction, whereas calcium channel-blocking drugs or β-adrenergic antagonists alone or in combination with digoxin may be effective. In the presence of hemodynamically significant atrial flutter the treatment of choice is elective cardioversion. If cardioversion fails to restore normal sinus rhythm or converts atrial flutter to atrial fibrillation, higher energy levels may be used or the patient may be allowed to remain in atrial fibrillation.

Atrial Fibrillation

Atrial fibrillation is the most common sustained cardiac dysrhythmia, present in about 0.4% of the U.S. population. The incidence of atrial fibrillation increases with age, being present in 1% of individuals 60 years of age, increasing to 5% for those 70 to 75 years of age, and exceeding 10% in those older than 80 years of age.[27] Transthoracic echocardiography is useful for evaluating atrial size, ventricular function, and cardiac valve function. The most common underlying cardiovascular diseases associated with atrial fibrillation are systemic hypertension and ischemic heart disease. Valvular heart disease, congestive heart failure, and diabetes mellitus are independent risk factors for atrial fibrillation. Atrial fibrillation is a common postoperative cardiac dysrhythmia, particularly in elderly patients undergoing cardiothoracic surgery.[28]

Mechanism

Atrial fibrillation occurs as a result of intra-atrial reentry pathways and is sustained by the propagation of multiple reentrant circuits with continuously changing, wandering pathways determined by local atrial refractoriness and excitability.[27] The dysrhythmia is characterized on the ECG as totally chaotic atrial activity at a frequency that often exceeds 400 beats/min. The rapid, disordered atrial activation results in loss of coordinated atrial contractions, with irregular electrical inputs to the AV node and His-Purkinje system leading to sporadic ventricular contractions. P waves are absent on the ECG, and the ventricular response rate is highly variable, sometimes exceeding 140 beats/min in the absence of treatment.

Clinical Manifestations

Although atrial fibrillation may present as an asymptomatic finding on the physical examination or ECG, more commonly the loss of AV synchrony and the rapid heart rates associated with this cardiac dysrhythmia result in significant symptoms.[21] Symptoms may range from palpitations to angina pectoris, congestive heart failure, pulmonary edema, and systemic hypotension. Atrial fibrillation is often associated with fatigue and generalized weakness. The most clinically important consequences of atrial fibrillation are thromboembolic events (stroke) and the development of atrial and/or ventricular cardiomyopathy. Formation of thrombi in the atria is due to stasis of blood in these cardiac chambers associated with loss of coordinated atrial contractions. The absence of synchronized atrial contractions combined with rapid ventricular response rates can decrease cardiac output to the point that congestive heart failure occurs.

Treatment

Treatment of atrial fibrillation is intended to restore and sustain normal sinus rhythm.

Electrical Cardioversion

Electrical cardioversion is the most effective method for converting atrial fibrillation to normal sinus rhythm. The goals of cardioversion are to relieve symptoms of congestive heart failure, improve cardiac function by restoring atrial contractility, and reduce the risk of thromboembolism. Before undergoing elective direct-current cardioversion patients are fasted for solid foods for at least 6 hours, electrolyte imbalances are corrected, and toxic drug levels are excluded as causes of the cardiac dysrhythmia. Digoxin may be withheld on the morning of scheduled cardioversion. Anesthesia for elective cardioversion is with short-acting intravenous drugs (propofol, etomidate); and monitoring includes pulse oximetry and continuous recording of the ECG. The electrical current is delivered such that the shock is synchronized to the QRS complex on the ECG to minimize the risk of inducing ventricular fibrillation. Supplemental administration of oxygen is commonly utilized.

Drug Therapy

The ventricular heart rate is typically controlled with drugs that slow AV nodal conduction. In this regard, digoxin is a frequent selection, as it exerts a vagotonic effect on the AV node. β-Adrenergic antagonists and calcium channel-blocking drugs are also utilized to control the ventricular heart rate; but unlike digoxin, these drugs may exert negative inotropic effects. Amiodarone may be the most effective drug for preventing the recurrence of atrial fibrillation.[29]

Anticoagulation

Individuals with valvular heart diseases and atrial fibrillation are at increased risk for stroke and are routinely treated with anticoagulants.[30] Oral warfarin therapy is most often utilized, although aspirin therapy may be sufficient for individuals considered to be at low risk for thromboembolic complications.

Postoperative Atrial Tachydysrhythmias

Atrial tachydysrhythmias are common during the early postoperative period (first 2 to 4 days), especially in elderly patients following cardiothoracic surgery.[28] It is estimated that more than one-third of patients who are older than 70 years of age experience postoperative atrial tachydysrhythmias. Patients with cardiac valve disease or a history of postoperative atrial tachydysrhythmias are at increased risk for developing this dysrhythmia following a subsequent operation.

Thromboembolic complications including stroke are particularly likely in patients who develop atrial fibrillation. Based on echocardiography the potential for thromboembolic complications develops early after the onset of atrial fibrillation, which is why prompt anticoagulant therapy with heparin is recommended for treating postoperative atrial fibrillation. In addition to prompt anticoagulation, a drug that produces AV nodal inhibition is administered. Unless contraindicated, a β-adrenergic antagonist is given to control the ventricular response rate. A calcium channel-blocking drug such as diltiazem is selected if a β-adrenergic antagonist is contraindicated. Digoxin may be selected for patients in whom left ventricular dysfunction accompanies atrial fibrillation. If there is no spontaneous reversion to normal sinus rhythm within 24 hours, elective electrical cardioversion is a consideration.[28]

Junctional Rhythm

Junctional (nodal) rhythm is due to the activity of an ectopic cardiac pacemaker in the tissues surrounding the AV node. The cardiac impulse initiated by this pacemaker travels to the ventricles in a normal manner but is also conducted retrograde into the atria. Depending on the site of the junctional pacemaker, the P wave precedes the QRS complex, but the PR interval is less than 0.1 second follows the QRS complex, or is obscured by it. A junctional rhythm leading to decreased cardiac output and systemic blood pressure is not infrequent during general anesthesia, especially when halothane is be-

ing administered. Intravenous administration of atropine is the initial treatment for hemodynamically significant junctional rhythms.

Wandering Atrial Pacemaker

The wandering atrial pacemaker reflects the presence of multiple atrial ectopic pacemakers. The ECG shows P waves with different configurations, and the PR intervals vary with each QRS complex. Treatment is necessary only when the loss of coordinated atrial contractions leads to decreased systemic blood pressure; when this occurs, intravenous atropine is usually effective.

Ventricular Ectopy (Ventricular Premature Beats)

Ventricular premature beats arise from single (unifocal) or multiple (multifocal) ectopic cardiac pacemaker sites located below the AV node. Characteristic findings on the ECG serve to identify ventricular premature beats (Table 4–11). A vulnerable period exists during diastole, corresponding to the relative refractory period of the cardiac action potential (roughly the middle third of the T wave) (R on T phenomenon), during which time ventricular premature beats may initiate repetitive ventricular responses, including ventricular tachycardia or ventricular fibrillation (Fig. 4–2).

Prognosis

The prognostic significance of ventricular ectopy depends on the presence and severity of left ventricular dysfunction. In the absence of structural heart disease, asymptomatic ventricular ectopy is benign, with no demonstrable risk of sudden death, even in the presence of ventricular tachycardia.[31] Nevertheless, ventricular ectopy in the form of ventricular premature beats most often reflects a cardiac abnor-

---

Table 4–11 • Characteristic Appearance of Ventricular Premature Beats on the Electrocardiogram

Premature occurrence
Absence of a P wave preceding the QRS complex
Wide and often bizarre-appearing QRS complex
ST segment in a direction opposite the QRS complex
Inverted T wave
Compensatory pause after the premature beat

mality (Table 4–12). For example, ventricular premature beats occur in as many as 95% of patients with an acute myocardial infarction. In patients with chronic myocardial ischemia, the presence of ventricular premature beats is directly correlated with the severity of ischemic heart disease and left ventricular dysfunction. The most common conditions in which ventricular premature beats predispose to life-threatening ventricular dysrhythmias are myocardial ischemia, valvular heart disease causing pressure or volume overload on the ventricles, cardiomyopathies, prolonged QT intervals on the ECG, and the presence of electrolyte abnormalities, especially hypokalemia. The presence of frequent ventricular premature beats 7 to 10 days after an acute myocardial infarction is associated with a markedly increased risk of life-threatening cardiac dysrhythmias. Typically, benign ventricular premature beats tend to disappear with exercise, whereas an increased frequency with exercise is often considered to reflect underlying cardiac disease.

Because the significance of ventricular ectopy depends on the presence of left ventricular dysfunction, echocardiography is a useful diagnostic test. It provides information regarding regional wall motion abnormalities, cardiac valvular lesions, and left ventricular ejection fraction.

Treatment

Ventricular premature beats should be treated when they are frequent (more than 6 beats/min), are multifocal, occur in salvos of three or more, or take place during the vulnerable period on the T wave (R on T phenomenon), as these characteristics are associated with an increased incidence of ventricular tachycardia and fibrillation. The first step in the treatment of ventricular premature beats is to eliminate the underlying cause, such as arterial hypo-

xemia or other events associated with excessive sympathetic nervous system activity. If ventricular premature beats persist despite correction of the underlying cause or are hemodynamically significant, the initial drug of choice is lidocaine, 1 to 2 mg/kg IV. This initial dose may be followed with a continuous infusion, 1 to 4 mg/min IV, to maintain a therapeutic blood level and continued suppression of the ectopic ventricular pacemaker. Lidocaine does not effectively suppress ventricular premature beats due to mechanical irritation of the heart, as might be produced by an intracardiac catheter.

Ventricular Tachycardia

Ventricular tachycardia is present when three or more consecutive ventricular premature beats occur at a calculated heart rate of more than 120 beats/min. The QRS complexes on the ECG are widened, reflecting aberrant intraventricular conduction of cardiac impulses, and there are no discernible P waves. Without the aid of His bundle electrocardiography it may be difficult to distinguish supraventricular tachycardia with aberrant conduction from reentrant ventricular tachycardia. Ventricular tachycardia is common after an acute myocardial infarction and in the presence of inflammatory or infectious diseases of the heart. Digitalis toxicity may manifest as ventricular tachycardia. Torsade de pointes, an unusual form of ventricular tachycardia, is initiated by a ventricular premature beat in the setting of abnormal ventricular repolarization characterized by prolongation of the QT interval on the ECG (see "Congenital Long QT Syndrome").

Treatment of hemodynamically significant ventricular tachycardia consists of prompt electrical cardioversion. If ventricular tachycardia is well tolerated hemodynamically, it is acceptable to administer lidocaine, 1 to 2 mg/kg IV, as a rapid injection followed by a continuous infusion of 1 to 4 mg/min IV to maintain an effective plasma concentration. Procainamide, 100 mg every 2 minutes IV up to a maximum dose of 2 g, may effectively convert ventricular tachycardia to a supraventricular rhythm. When lidocaine and procainamide are ineffective, bretylium, 5 mg/kg IV, may be considered.

Ventricular Fibrillation

Ventricular fibrillation is the most common cause of sudden cardiac death, with most of the victims having underlying ischemic heart disease.[2] Ventricular tachycardia often precedes the onset of ventricular fibrillation. Ventricular fibrillation is charac-

---

Table 4–12 • Conditions Associated with the Development of Ventricular Premature Beats

Normal heart
Arterial hypoxemia
Myocardial ischemia
Myocardial infarction
Myocarditis
Sympathetic nervous system activation
Hypokalemia
Hypomagnesemia
Digitalis toxicity
Caffeine
Cocaine
Alcohol
Mechanical irritation (central venous or pulmonary artery catheter)

terized on the ECG by chaotic asynchronous contraction of the ventricles with no visible QRS complexes. There is no associated stroke volume, emphasizing the need for prompt institution of cardiopulmonary resuscitation.

Electrical defibrillation is the only effective treatment for converting ventricular fibrillation to a rhythm capable of generating spontaneous cardiac output. This electrical treatment should be instituted as soon as possible, as cardiac output, coronary blood flow, and cerebral blood flow are extremely low despite properly performed external cardiac compression. For example, cerebral blood flow and coronary blood flow may be less than 10% of normal during external cardiac compression.[32] Evidence suggests that external cardiac compression alone is as effective as external cardiac compression combined with mouth-to-mouth ventilation during the period before electrical defibrillation can be applied.[33] When ventricular fibrillation is refractory to electrical treatment, administration of amiodarone, lidocaine, or bretylium may improve the response to electrical defibrillation. Recurrent ventricular tachycardia or fibrillation that can result in the sudden death of a cardiac arrest survivor may be treated by placing a transvenous ICD (see "Transvenous Implantable Cardioverter-Defibrillator").

VENTRICULAR PREEXCITATION SYNDROMES

The normal conduction system of the heart limits antegrade propagation of electrical impulses traveling from the atria to the ventricles to a single conduction pathway through the AV node and His-Purkinje system.[34] This single connecting pathway between the atria and the ventricles results in a delay in activation of the ventricles sufficient to optimize mechanical function without creating the opportunity for reentrant tachycardia.

The presence of alternate ("accessory") pathways that function as electrically active muscular bridges that bypass the normal AV nodal conduction of cardiac impulses creates the potential for reentrant tachycardia. It is estimated that accessory AV pathways for conduction of cardiac impulses between the atria and ventricles are present in 0.1% to 0.3% of the U.S. population. Accessory pathways are congenital and most likely reflect remnants of fetal AV muscular connections left in place by incomplete development of the annulus fibrosis. The most prominent manifestation of ventricular preexcitation by cardiac impulses traveling via accessory AV pathways is the Wolff-Parkinson-White (WPW) syndrome (Fig. 4–4). The accessory pathways of the WPW syndrome usually have conduction properties similar to those of the myocardium and unlike the AV node. Thus after conducting an electrical impulse through the atria, this same SA node impulse can travel down both the AV node and the accessory pathway to activate the ventricles, with ventricular activation occurring earlier at sites near the accessory pathway than at sites activated normally by the His-Purkinje system.

Clinical Manifestations

Symptomatic tachydysrhythmias associated with the WPW syndrome typically begin during early adulthood; and pregnancy is associated with the initial manifestation of the syndrome in some women.[35] The first manifestation of WPW syndrome may appear during the perioperative period.[36] In some patients the first manifestation of WPW syn-

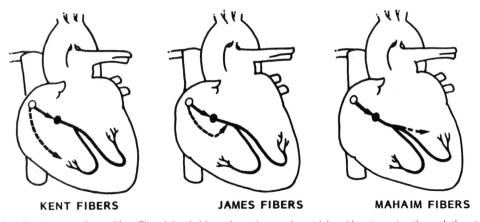

KENT FIBERS   **JAMES FIBERS**   **MAHAIM FIBERS**

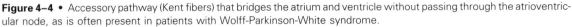

Figure 4–4 • Accessory pathway (Kent fibers) that bridges the atrium and ventricle without passing through the atrioventricular node, as is often present in patients with Wolff-Parkinson-White syndrome.

drome is sudden death presumably due to ventricular fibrillation. The estimated incidence of sudden death in patients with WPW syndrome is 0.15% per patient-year.[35]

Paroxysmal palpitations with or without dizziness, syncope, dyspnea, or angina pectoris are common in the presence of the tachydysrhythmia associated with the WPW syndrome. The diuresis that often occurs about 30 to 60 minutes after the onset of the tachycardia may be related to the production of atrial natriuretic factor during the tachycardia.

Electrocardiographic Findings

Ventricular preexcitation causes an earlier than normal deflection on the ECG, designated a delta wave. Delta waves can mimic the Q waves of a myocardial infarction.[37] AV reciprocating tachycardia (AVRT) is the most common tachydysrhythmia in patients with WPW syndrome. It is classified as orthodromic or antidromic. The orthodromic form of AVRT is more common and is characterized as narrow QRS complex tachycardia, reflecting conduction of cardiac impulses from the atrium through the normal AV node–His Purkinje system and return of impulses from the ventricle to the atrium using the accessory pathway. This tachydysrhythmia is generally initiated by an atrial or ventricular premature beat that is blocked in one of the AV conduction pathways. The less common antidromic form of AVRT is characterized as wide complex QRS tachycardia, reflecting conduction of cardiac impulses from the atrium to the ventricle through the accessory pathway to activate the ventricles eccentrically, resulting in a wide QRS complex. Impulses then travel retrograde from the ventricles to the atria via the AV node–His Purkinje system. Antidromic AVRT may be difficult to distinguish from ventricular tachycardia on the ECG. Atrial fibrillation and atrial flutter are less common but potentially more serious tachydysrhythmias in patients with WPW syndrome because they can result in rapid ventricular response rates and, in rare instances, ventricular fibrillation.

Treatment

Acute treatment of tachydysrhythmias in patients with WPW syndrome depends on the characteristics of the dysrhythmia presentation (Table 4–13).[34] Long-term management of tachydysrhythmias in patients with WPW syndrome may include antidysrhythmia drugs or radiofrequency catheter ablation of the accessory pathways.[27, 35]

Table 4–13 • Management of Cardiac Dysrhythmias in Patients with Wolff-Parkinson-White Syndrome

Orthodromic AV reciprocating tachycardia (narrow complex)
    Vagal maneuvers (carotid sinus massage, Valsalva maneuver, stimulation of the posterior pharynx)
    Adenosine
    Verapamil
Antidromic AV reciprocating tachycardia (wide complex)
    Procainamide (systolic blood pressure > 90 mmHg)
    Electrical cardioversion (systolic blood pressure < 90 mmHg)
Atrial fibrillation
    Procainamide
    Electrical cardioversion if hemodynamic instability

AV, atrioventricular.

Orthodromic AVRT

Treatment of orthodromic AVRT (narrow complex) should begin with vagal maneuvers (carotid sinus massage, Valsalva maneuver, stimulation of the posterior pharynx), which often terminate this tachydysrhythmia. When vagal maneuvers are not promptly successful, adenosine, 6 to 12 mg IV, is indicated. If this drug is not successful, verapamil can be administered.

Antidromic AVRT

Treatment of antidromic AVRT (wide complex) is intended to block conduction of the cardiac impulses along the accessory pathway. In this regard, adenosine slows AV node conduction and would not be expected to be effective in the treatment of wide complex AVRT. The brief duration of adenosine, however, means that its administration in the presence of this tachydysrhythmia is unlikely to cause difficulty. Conversely, verapamil should not be administered to patients with wide complex AVRT because its hypotensive effect plus an inability to block cardiac impulse conduction along accessory pathways may worsen the existing hemodynamics and even predispose to the development of ventricular fibrillation. Digoxin is not recommended, as it, like verapamil, does not slow conduction via the accessory pathways.

In the presence of antidromic AVRT and a systolic blood pressure higher than 90 mmHg, intravenous administration of procainamide, 10 mg/kg IV infused at a rate not to exceed 50 mg/min, is indicated. Procainamide depresses conduction of cardiac impulses via the accessory pathways and thus may slow the ventricular response rate and terminate the wide complex tachydysrhythmia.

Electrical cardioversion is indicated should systolic blood pressure decrease to less than 90 mmHg during intravenous infusion of procainamide. Likewise, electrical cardioversion is indicated if drug therapy does not slow the ventricular response rate.

Atrial Fibrillation

Atrial fibrillation associated with anterograde conduction via accessory pathways and the risk of ventricular fibrillation is treated with intravenous administration of procainamide. Verapamil and digoxin are not recommended, as these drugs block conduction of cardiac impulses through the AV node and may accelerate conduction through accessory pathways. Electrical cardioversion is utilized in the presence of hemodynamic instability caused by atrial fibrillation.

Management of Anesthesia

Patients with known WPW syndrome presenting for elective or emergency surgery should continue to receive the antidysrhythmia drugs that are being administered to maintain normal sinus rhythm.[22, 38] The goal during management of anesthesia is to avoid any event (increased sympathetic nervous system activity due to anxiety or hypovolemia) or drug (digoxin, verapamil) that could enhance anterograde conduction of cardiac impulses through accessory pathways. Logic suggests avoidance of drugs in the preoperative medication that are known to have the potential to increase the heart rate. Although atropine has been used as a preoperative medication in patients with WPW syndrome without adverse responses, scopolamine or glycopyrrolate are equally acceptable choices if administration of anticholinergic drugs is deemed appropriate. Reduction of anxiety with preoperative medication is desirable but no specific drug has proven superior. Likewise, sedation is an important consideration for decreasing anxiety when a regional anesthetic technique is selected. Drugs known to be effective in the management of tachydysrhythmias associated with the WPW syndrome must be immediately available, as must be the ability to perform electrical cardioversion promptly should the tachydysrhythmia become hemodynamically significant (Table 4–13).

Induction of Anesthesia

Induction of anesthesia can be achieved with a variety of drugs (propofol, etomidate, thiopental, opioids) administered intravenously.[39, 40] Ketamine would be an unlikely option based on its known ability to increase sympathetic nervous system activity. Droperidol increases the refractory period of accessory pathways, but the large doses (200 to 600 μg/kg IV) required renders its use here clinically impractical.[41] Thiopental has been alleged to increase aberrant conduction of cardiac impulses, but this has not been substantiated by clinical use of this drug. Propofol has been associated with normalization of the ECG (disappearance of the delta wave on the ECG as evidence of ventricular preexcitation due to conduction of cardiac impulses over accessory pathways) during induction of anesthesia in a patient with known WPW syndrome.[40] Nevertheless, there is evidence that propofol has no effect on the refractory period of accessory pathways, making it an appropriate drug to use for anesthesia during radiofrequency catheter ablation procedures.

Tracheal intubation is often facilitated with neuromuscular blocking drugs that lack the ability to increase sympathetic nervous system activity directly or reflexly due to hypotension caused by histamine-induced peripheral vasodilation. It seems logical to establish an adequate depth of anesthesia with volatile anesthetics or injected drugs prior to initiating direct laryngoscopy for tracheal intubation.

Maintenance of Anesthesia

Maintenance of general anesthesia should be designed to minimize the likelihood of increased sympathetic nervous system activity, as may accompany direct laryngoscopy for tracheal intubation or abrupt changes in the intensity of painful surgical stimulation. Volatile anesthetics in appropriate concentrations decrease sympathetic nervous system activity and seem to be a logical choice for maintenance of anesthesia. In this regard, it is useful to consider the potential for abrupt large increases in the delivered concentrations of desflurane to produce transient increases in sympathetic nervous system activity.[42] Although rarely used, there is evidence that enflurane uniquely increases the refractory period of accessory pathways and thus may be a useful drug in patients with WPW syndrome.[43] Nitrous oxide is often combined with the volatile anesthetic being administered to patients with WPW syndrome.

Muscle relaxants used during maintenance of anesthesia should not be associated with the potential to increase sympathetic nervous system activity or to increase the heart rate. In this regard, pancuronium is an unlikely choice for patients with known WPW syndrome. Short-acting muscle relaxants that may not require pharmacologic antagonism with an anticholinesterase-anticholinergic drug mixture are theoretically useful. Nevertheless, the decision to antagonize nondepolarizing muscle relaxants pharmacologically must be individualized, as clinical experience is too limited to offer a recommendation.

Monitoring

The degree of invasive monitoring during anesthesia is influenced by the complexity of the surgery and the presence of concomitant cardiac disease. An intra-arterial catheter is often useful, whereas monitoring left ventricular function with transesophageal echocardiography or a pulmonary artery catheter is usually not necessary for noncardiac surgery. Indeed, placement of a central venous catheter or pulmonary artery catheter could theoretically predispose to the development of tachydysrhythmias. Nevertheless, a pulmonary artery catheter with the ability to deliver artificial cardiac pacing may be useful in selected patients.

CONGENITAL LONG QT SYNDROME

The congenital long QT syndrome (Romano Ward syndrome) is an autosomal dominant disorder that usually presents as syncope during childhood or adolescence. It is due to recurrent bouts of rapid polymorphic ventricular tachycardia known as torsade de pointes.[44] In the absence of ECG confirmation of a cardiac dysrhythmia, syncope may be confused with a seizure disorder. Syncope may be triggered by sympathetic nervous system stimulation, as produced by exercise or fright. Association of this syndrome with deafness (Jervell and Lange-Nielsen syndrome) is rare. Sudden death is a risk, especially as part of the sudden infant death syndrome (SIDS).[45] Indeed, 50% of infants who die of SIDS have prolonged QT intervals corrected for heart rate (QTc). The presence of a QTc longer than 440 ms during the first week of life increases the risk of SIDS by 41%. Spontaneous mutations in the long QT syndrome genes may manifest as SIDS.[46] The hallmark of the long QT syndrome is prolongation of the QTc interval (exceeding 460 to 480 ms) on the ECG. Females have a longer QTc and a higher incidence of torsade de pointes tachycardia than males and more frequently develop torsade de points after administration of drugs that modify potassium or sodium currents (conductance) to lengthen cardiac repolarization. About one-third of patients have a resting heart rate of less than 60 beats/min. The relation between sympathetic nervous system activation and cardiac dysrhythmias led to the hypothesis that long QT syndrome was caused by an abnormality in cardiac sympathetic innervation. More recent evidence describes mutation defects in four genes encoding sodium and potassium ion channels mediating myocardial depolarization.[31]

Acquired long QT interval syndrome may be due to drugs (droperidol, quinidine, tricyclic antidepressants) or metabolic disorders; or it may accompany subarachnoid hemorrhage. Right (but not left) radical neck dissection may result in an increase in the QT interval on the ECG with associated cardiac dysrhythmias during the postoperative period (Fig. 4–5).[47]

Treatment

The prognosis of those with untreated long QT syndrome is poor, with sudden death a particular risk in the presence of congenital deafness, history of syncope, female gender, and documentation of prior ventricular tachycardia.[31] Suppression of sympathetic nervous system activity with a β-adrenergic antagonist or left thoracic sympathectomy via a supraclavicular approach is the recommended treatment. Temporary treatment is a left stellate ganglion block intended to abolish the sympathetic nervous system imbalance that exists between the left and right cardiac nerves.[47] A successful stellate ganglion block is indicated by shortening of the QT interval on the ECG. The effect of a left stellate ganglion

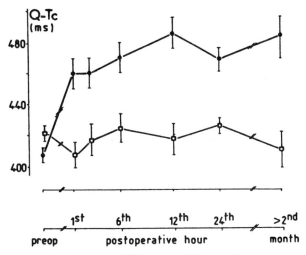

Figure 4–5 • Corrected QT intervals (QTc) in milliseconds were prolonged on the electrocardiogram in patients following a right radical neck dissection (*solid symbols*) but not after a left radical neck dissection (*clear symbols*). Mean ± SE. (From Otenni JC, Pottecher T, Bronner G, et al. Prolongation of the Q-T interval and sudden cardiac arrest following right radical neck dissection. Anesthesiology 1983;59:358–61, with permission.)

block is only transient; therefore it is used only to control acute cardiac dysrhythmias, assess whether surgical sympathectomy might be successful, and as preoperative preparation of patients unresponsive to medical therapy who require emergency surgery.

Management of Anesthesia

A preoperative ECG to rule out congenital long QT syndrome is useful in the presence of a family history of sudden death or in the presence of congenital deafness and a history of unexplained syncope. In patients presenting with a prolonged QTc interval, the choice of anesthetic drugs deserves special consideration. For example, isoflurane and sevoflurane, but not halothane, have been shown to prolong the QTc interval in otherwise healthy children and adults (especially females) as well as patients with a preexisting prolonged QTc.[44, 48, 49] Ventricular tachycardia torsade de pointes during sevoflurane anesthesia has been described.[50] Overall, the clinical experience is too limited to clearly select one volatile drug to the exclusion of another, but the potential effect of a drug on the QT interval deserves prospective consideration in patients presenting with long QT interval syndrome.

Events known to prolong the QT interval on the ECG are avoided, such as abrupt increases in sympathetic nervous system activity associated with preoperative anxiety or noxious stimulation intraoperatively and acute hypokalemia due to iatrogenic hyperventilation of the patient's lungs. In this regard, it seems logical to provide pharmacologic preoperative medication to decrease anxiety. Inclusion of anticholinergic drugs in the preoperative medication, however, is questionable in view of the possible alteration in the balance of sympathetic and parasympathetic nervous system activity that can accompany administration of such drugs. Consideration may be given to establishing β-blockade or performing a prophylactic left stellate ganglion block prior to induction of anesthesia in patients believed to be at risk.

Induction of anesthesia has been safely accomplished with available intravenous induction drugs, although propofol is an attractive selection based on its reported ability to shorten the QT interval.[44] Ketamine would be an unlikely choice because of its sympathetic nervous system stimulating effects. Tracheal intubation is attempted only after establishing a depth of anesthesia deemed sufficient to blunt the effect of noxious stimulation. Prior administration of opioids and/or volatile anesthetics may facilitate this goal. Tracheal extubation may be performed when the patient is still anesthetized to minimize sympathetic nervous system stimulation associated with this event.

The choice of muscle relaxants is guided by the desire to avoid drugs that could stimulate the sympathetic nervous system or evoke the release of histamine. Nevertheless, succinylcholine and pancuronium have been administered to patients with this syndrome without incident. Pharmacologic reversal of nondepolarizing neuromuscular blockade does not seem to have an adverse effect on the QT interval in these patients.

An electrical defibrillator should be promptly available, as the likelihood of perioperative ventricular fibrillation is increased. A β-adrenergic antagonist (esmolol) is useful for treating acute ventricular dysrhythmias that develop intraoperatively. Lidocaine and procainamide are not recommended, as these drugs prolong the QT interval on the ECG of normal patients. Nevertheless, lidocaine has been described as effectively reversing intraoperative ventricular tachycardia in a patient with long QT syndrome.[51] The ability of phenytoin to shorten the QT interval on the ECG is the rationale for administering this drug orally during the postoperative period.

References

1. Atlee J, Bosnjak Z. Mechanisms for cardiac dysrhythmias during anesthesia. Anesthesiology 1990;72:347–74
2. Atlee JL. Perioperative cardiac dysrhythmias: diagnosis and management. Anesthesiology 1997;86:1397–424
3. Akhtar M. Management of ventricular tachyarrhythmias. JAMA 1982;247:671–4
4. Harrah MD, Way WL, Katzung BG. The potentiation of neuromuscular blocking agents by quinidine. Anesthesiology 1970;33:406–10
5. Kusumoto FM, Goldschlager N. Cardiac pacing. N Engl J Med 1996;334:89–98
6. Kelly JS, Royster RL. Noninvasive transcutaneous cardiac pacing. Anesth Analg 1989;69:229–38
7. Mangar D, Atlas GM, Kane PG. Electrocautery-induced pacemaker malfunction during surgery. Can J Anaesth 1991;38:616–8
8. Domino KB, Smith TC. Electrocautery-induced reprogramming of a pacemaker using a precordial magnet. Anesth Analg 1983;62:609–12
9. Ducey JP, Fincher CW, Baysinger CL. Therapeutic suppression of a permanent ventricular pacemaker using a peripheral nerve stimulator. Anesthesiology 1991;75:533–6
10. Finer SR. Pacemaker failure on induction of anaesthesia. Br J Anaesth 1991;66:509–12
11. Thiagarajah S, Azar I, Agres M, et al. Pacemaker malfunction associated with positive-pressure ventilation. Anesthesiology 1983;58:565–6
12. Edelman JD, Hurlbert BJ. Intermittent left bundle branch block during anesthesia. Anesth Analg 1981;59:628–30
13. Thomson IR, Dalton BC, Lappas DG, et al. Right bundle-branch block and complete heart block caused by the Swan Ganz catheter. Anesthesiology 1979;51:359–62

14. Rooney S-M, Goldiner PL, Muss E. Relationship of right bundle-branch block and marked left axis deviation to complete heart block during general anesthesia. Anesthesiology 1976;44:64–6
15. Coriat P, Harari A, Ducardonet A, et al. Risk of advanced heart block during extradural anaesthesia in patients with right bundle branch block and left anterior hemiblock. Br J Anaesth 1981;53:545–8
16. Kreutz JM, Mazuzan JE. Sudden asystole in a marathon runner: the athletic heart syndrome and its anesthetic implications. Anesthesiology 1990;73:1266–8
17. Doyle DJ, Mark PWS. Reflex bradycardia during surgery. Can J Anaesth 1990;37:219–22
18. Caplan RA, Ward RJ, Posner K, et al. Unexpected cardiac arrest during spinal anesthesia: a closed claims analysis of predisposing factors. Anesthesiology 1988;68:5–11
19. Auroy Y, Narchi P, Messiah A, et al. Serious complications related to regional anesthesia: results of a prospective survey in France. Anesthesiology 1997;87:479–86
20. Youngs PJ, Littleford J. Arrhythmias during spinal anesthesia. Can J Anaesth 2000;47:385–90
21. Shen C-L, Hung Y-C, Chen P-J, et al. Mobitz type II block during spinal anesthesia. Anesthesiology 1999;90:1477–8
22. Jordi E-M, Marsch SCU, Strebel S. Third degree heart block and asystole associated with spinal anesthesia. Anesthesiology 1998;89:257–60
23. Liguori GA, Sharrock NE. Asystole and severe bradycardia during epidural anesthesia in orthopedic patients. Anesthesiology 1997;86:250–7
24. Gibbons JJ, Ditto FF. Sudden asystole after spinal anesthesia treated with the "pacing thump." Anesthesiology 1991;75:705
25. Mangrum JM, DiMarco JP. The evaluation and management of bradycardia. N Engl J Med 2000;342:703–9
26. Ganz LI, Friedman PL. Supraventricular tachycardia. N Engl J Med 1995;332:162–73
27. Falk RH. Atrial fibrillation. N Engl J Med 2001;344:1067–78
28. Ommen SR, Odell JA, Stanton MS. Atrial arrhythmias after cardiothoracic surgery. N Engl J Med 1997;336:1429–34
29. Roy D, Talajic M, Dorian P, et al. Amiodarone to prevent recurrence of atrial fibrillation. N Engl J Med 2000;342:913–20
30. Stern S, Altkorn D, Levinson W. Anticoagulation for chronic atrial fibrillation. JAMA 2000;283:2901–3
31. Langberg JJ, DeLurgio DB. Ventricular arrhythmias. Sci Am Med 1999;1–12
32. White BC, Wiegenstein JG, Winegar CD. Brain ischemic anoxia. Mechanisms of injury. JAMA 1984;251:1586–90
33. Hallstrom A, Cobb L, Johnson E, et al. Cardiopulmonary resuscitation by chest compression alone or with mouth-to-mouth ventilation. N Engl J Med 2000;342:1546–53
34. Tchou PJ, Trohman RG. Supraventricular tachycardia. Sci Am Med 1999;1–7
35. Calkins H. Catheter ablation for cardiac arrhythmias. Sci Am Med 1999;1–6
36. Lubarsky D, Kaufman B, Turndorf H. Anesthesia unmasking benign Wolff-Parkinson-White syndrome. Anesth Analg 1989;68:172–4
37. Lustik SJ, Wojtczak J, Chhibber AK. Wolff-Parkinson-White syndrome simulating inferior myocardial infarction in a cocaine abuser for urgent dilation and evacuation of the uterus. Anesth Analg 1999;89:609–12
38. Irish CL, Mukin JM, Guiraudon GM. Anaesthetic management for surgical cryoablation of accessory conduction pathways: a review and report of 181 cases. Can J Anaesth 1988;35:634–40
39. Gomez-Arnau J, Marques-Montes J, Avello F. Fentanyl and droperidol effects on the refractoriness of the accessory pathway in the Wolff-Parkinson-White syndrome. Anesthesiology 1983;58:307–13
40. Seki S, Ichimiya T, Tsuchida H, et al. A case of normalization of Wolff-Parkinson-White syndrome conduction during propofol anesthesia. Anesthesiology 1999;90:1779–81
41. Sharpe MD, Dobkowski WB, Murkin JM, et al. Propofol has no direct effect on sinoatrial node function or on normal atrioventricular and accessory pathway conduction in Wolff-Parkinson-White syndrome during alfentanil/midazolam anesthesia. Anesthesiology 1995;82:888–95
42. Weiskopf RB, Moore MA, Eger EI, et al. Rapid increase in desflurane concentration is associated with greater transient cardiovascular stimulation than with rapid increases in isoflurane concentration in humans. Anesthesiology 1994;80:1035–45
43. Sharpe MD, Dobkowski WB, Murkin JM, et al. The electrophysiologic effects of volatile anesthetics and sufentanil on the normal atrioventricular conduction system and accessory pathways in Wolff-Parkinson-White syndrome. Anesthesiology 1994;80:63–70
44. Kleinsasser A, Kuenszberg E, Loeckinger A, et al. Sevoflurane, but not propofol, significantly prolongs the Q-T interval. Anesth Analg 2000;90:25–7
45. Schwartz PJ, Stramba-Badiale M, Segantini A, et al. Prolongation of the QT interval and the sudden infant death syndrome. N Engl J Med 1998;338:1709–14
46. Schwartz PJ, Priori SG, Dumaine R, et al. A molecular link between the sudden infant death syndrome and the long-QT syndrome. N Engl J Med 2000;343:263–6
47. Otteni JC, Pottecher T, Bronner G, et al. Prolongation of the Q-T interval and sudden cardiac arrest following right radical neck dissection. Anesthesiology 1983;59:358–61
48. Michaloudis D, Fradidakis O, Lefaki T, et al. Anaesthesia and the QT interval in humans: the effects of isoflurane and halothane. Anaesthesia 1996;51:219–24
49. Gallagher JD, Weindling SN, Anderson G, et al. Effects of sevoflurane in a patient with congenital long QT syndrome. Anesthesiology 1998;89:1569–73
50. Abe K, Takada K, Yoshiya I. Intraoperative torsade de points ventricular tachycardia and ventricular fibrillation during sevoflurane anesthesia. Anesth Analg 1998;86:701–2
51. Adu-Gyanfi Y, Said A, Chowdhary UM, et al. Anaesthetic-induced ventricular tachyarrhythmia in Jervell and Lange-Nielsen syndrome. Can J Anaesth 1991;38:358–61

5

Systemic Hypertension

An adult (18 years of age or older) is considered to manifest systemic hypertension (be "hypertensive") when the systolic/diastolic blood pressures are 140/90 mmHg or more on at least two occasions measured at least 1 to 2 weeks apart (Table 5–1).[1] Based on this definition, systemic hypertension is the most common circulatory derangement in the United States, affecting approximately 24% of adults. The incidence of systemic hypertension increases progressively with age, and the risk of systemic hypertension is higher in the African-American population (Fig. 5–1).[2] Systemic hypertension is a significant risk factor for the development of ischemic heart disease and is a major cause of congestive heart failure, cerebral vascular accident (stroke), arterial aneurysm, and end-stage renal disease (Fig. 5–2). It is estimated that fewer than one-third of patients with systemic hypertension in the United States are aware of their condition and are adequately treated.[3]

▌ PATHOPHYSIOLOGY

Systemic hypertension is characterized as essential hypertension when a cause for the increased blood pressure cannot be identified. It is called secondary hypertension when a known etiology is present.

Essential Hypertension

Essential hypertension, which accounts for more than 95% of all cases of hypertension, is characterized by a familial incidence and inherited biochemical abnormalities. Pathophysiologic factors implicated in the genesis of essential hypertension include increased sympathetic nervous system ac-

Table 5–1 • Classification of Systemic Blood Pressure for Adults*

Category	Systolic blood pressure (mmHg)	Diastolic blood pressure (mmHg)
Optimal	<120	<80
Normal	<130	<85
High normal	130–139	85–89
Systemic hypertension		
Stage 1 (mild)	140–159	90–99
Stage 2 (moderate)	160–179	100–109
Stage 3 (severe)	≥180	≥110

* Adults are defined as individuals 18 years of age and older.
Adapted from The sixth report of the Joint National Committee on Prevention, Detection, Evaluation and Treatment of High Blood Pressure (JNC VI). Arch Intern Med 1997;157:2413–20.

tivity as may accompany the response to psychosocial stress, overproduction of sodium-retaining hormones and vasoconstrictors, high sodium intake, inadequate dietary intake of potassium and calcium, increased renin secretion, deficiencies of vasodilators such as prostaglandins and nitric oxide, and the presence of medical diseases such as diabetes mellitus and obesity. A final common pathway to genetically related essential hypertension is salt and water retention. An estimated 40% of persons with essential hypertension also manifest hypercholesterolemia (serum cholesterol levels higher than 240 mg/dl). Hypertension, insulin resistance, dyslipidemia, and obesity often occur concomitantly. Alcohol and tobacco use are associated with essential hypertension. Sleep-disordered breathing (obstructive sleep apnea), which is present in a substantial proportion of the adult population, causes temporary increases in systemic blood pressure in association with arterial hypoxemia, arousal, and activation of the sympathetic nervous system. There is evidence that sleep-disordered breathing leads to sustained systemic hypertension independent of known confounding factors such as obesity.[4] Indeed, an estimated 30% of hypertensive patients manifest sleep-disordered breathing.

A history of ischemic heart disease, angina pectoris, left ventricular hypertrophy, congestive heart failure, cerebrovascular disease, stroke, peripheral vascular disease, or renal insufficiency suggests end-organ disease due to chronic, poorly controlled essential hypertension. The laboratory evaluation is intended to document target organ damage and includes blood urea nitrogen and serum creatinine assays to quantify renal function. Hypokalemia in the presence of essential hypertension suggests primary aldosteronism. Fasting blood glucose concentrations are evaluated, as 50% of hypertensive patients manifest glucose intolerance. An electrocardiogram (ECG) is useful for detecting evidence of ischemic heart disease or left ventricular hypertrophy associated with essential hypertension.

Secondary Hypertension

Secondary hypertension has a demonstrable etiology but accounts for fewer than 5% of all cases of systemic hypertension. In this regard, renovascular hypertension due to renal artery stenosis is the most common cause of secondary hypertension (Table 5–2). The likelihood of renal artery stenosis as a cause of systemic hypertension is increased when the diastolic blood pressure exceeds 125 mmHg. The presence of an upper abdominal bruit strongly suggests the presence of renal artery stenosis. Magnetic resonance imaging angiography can confirm the clinical diagnosis. The natural history of renal artery stenosis is progressive arterial occlusion with loss of renal function.

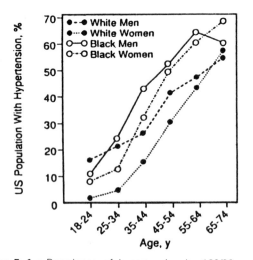

Figure 5–1 • Prevalence of hypertension (> 160/90 mmHg) among the adult population in the United States. (From Tjoa HI, Kaplan NM. Treatment of hypertension in the elderly. JAMA 1990;264:1015–18, with permission.)

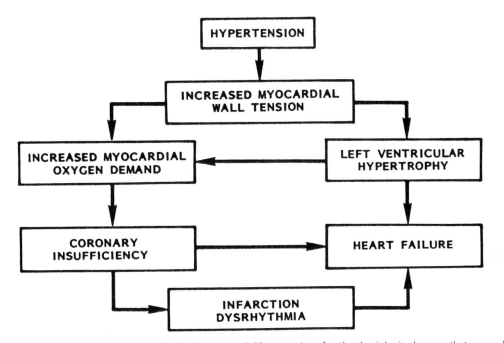

Figure 5–2 • Chronic increases in systemic blood pressure initiate a series of pathophysiologic changes that may culminate in congestive heart failure.

Primary aldosteronism produces secondary hypertension associated with hypokalemia. The presence of an adrenal adenoma or hyperplastic adrenal gland as the source of increased aldosterone secretion is confirmed by abdominal computed tomography or magnetic resonance imaging. Pheochromocytoma is a rare cause of secondary hypertension.

TREATMENT OF ESSENTIAL HYPERTENSION

Decreasing systemic blood pressure by lifestyle modification and pharmacologic means is intended to decrease cardiovascular morbidity and mortality. The standard goal of pharmacologic therapy is to decrease the systemic blood pressure to less than 140/90 mmHg. Treatment resulting in normalization of systemic blood pressure has been particularly successful for decreasing the incidence of cerebrovascular accidents. Likewise, decreasing systemic blood pressure by pharmacologic means decreases the morbidity and mortality associated with ischemic heart disease. Drug treatment of systemic hypertension has beneficial effects in that it slows or prevents progression to more severe systemic hypertension and the development of congestive heart failure and renal failure. The benefits of antihypertensive drug therapy appear to be greater in elderly patients than in young patients.

Patient Selection

Patients with concomitant risk factors (hypercholesterolemia, diabetes mellitus, tobacco abuse, family history, age older than 60 years) and evidence of target organ damage (angina pectoris, prior myocardial infarction, left ventricular hypertrophy, cerebrovascular disease, nephropathy, retinopathy, peripheral vascular disease) are most likely to benefit from immediate initiation of pharmacologic therapy. Patients who do not manifest clinical evidence of cardiovascular disease or target organ damage may benefit from a trial of lifestyle modification and subsequent reevaluation before initiation of pharmacologic therapy.

Lifestyle Modification

Lifestyle modifications of proven value for lowering systemic blood pressure include weight reduction or prevention of weight gain, moderation of alcohol intake, increased physical activity, maintenance of recommended levels of dietary calcium and potassium, and moderation of dietary sodium. Cessation of tobacco use is critical, as smoking is an independent risk factor for cardiovascular disease.

Weight loss is closely related to decreased systemic blood pressure and may be the most efficacious of all nonpharmacologic interventions in the

Table 5–2 • Causes of Secondary Hypertension

Systolic and diastolic hypertension
  Renal
    Renal vascular disease
    Renal parenchymal disease
    Renal transplantation
    Renin-secreting tumors
  Endocrine
    Primary aldosteronism
    Pheochromocytoma
    Cushing syndrome
    Acromegaly
    Hyperparathyroidism
  Pregnancy-induced hypertension (eclampsia)
  Sleep-disordered breathing (obstructive sleep apnea)
  Coarctation of the aorta
  Postoperative hypertension
  Neurologic disorders
    Increased intracranial pressure
    Spinal cord injury
    Guillain-Barré syndrome
    Dysautonomia
  Drugs
    Glucocorticoids
    Mineralocorticoids
    Cyclosporine
    Sympathomimetics
    Tyramine and monoamine oxidase inhibitors
    Nasal decongestants
  Chronic essential hypertension
  Sudden withdrawal from antihypertensive drug
    therapy (central acting and β-adrenergic
    antagonists)
Isolated systolic hypertension
  Aging with associated aortic rigidity
  Increased cardiac output
    Thyrotoxicosis
    Anemia
    Aortic regurgitation
  Decreased peripheral vascular resistance
    Arteriovenous shunts
    Paget's disease of bone

treatment of systemic hypertension. Weight loss also enhances the efficacy of antihypertensive drugs. Alcohol consumption is associated with increased blood pressure, and excessive use of alcohol may cause resistance to antihypertensive therapy. However, moderate alcohol ingestion has been shown to decrease overall cardiovascular risks in the general population.[5] At least 30 minutes of moderate intensity physical activity, such as brisk walking or bicycling (preferably once a day), can lower systemic blood pressure in normotensive and hypertensive individuals.

There is an inverse relation between dietary potassium and calcium intake and systemic blood pressure in the general population. The antihypertensive efficacy of dietary salt restriction is questionable, although small but consistent decreases in systemic blood pressure have been reported.[6] It is possible that the role of sodium restriction in lowering blood pressure is most beneficial in only a subset of patients with low renin activity (the elderly and African-Americans). Sodium restriction can minimize diuretic-induced hypokalemia and may enhance the ease of blood pressure control with diuretic therapy. Additional benefits of salt restriction include protection from osteoporosis and fractures by decreasing urinary calcium excretion and favorable effects on left ventricular hypertrophy. Salt substitutes in which sodium is replaced with potassium are useful for hypertensive patients who do not have renal dysfunction.

Pharmacologic Therapy

Initiation of drug therapy always includes lifestyle modifications. After drug therapy is initiated, patients are seen every 1 to 4 weeks to titrate the antihypertensive drug dosage and then every 3 to 4 months once the desired blood pressure is achieved. Long-acting drugs are preferred initially because patient compliance and consistency of blood pressure control are superior with once-a-day dosing. When monotherapy is unsuccessful, a second drug, usually of a different class, is added. A large variety of antihypertensive drugs are available, and many of these drugs present unique and potentially significant side effects (Table 5–3).[7]

The choice of antihypertensive therapy may be influenced by the presence of cardiovascular risk factors and evidence of target organ damage. In the absence of these conditions (representing a small proportion of hypertensive patients) the selection of diuretics or β-adrenergic antagonist drugs for initial monotherapy is often recommended. For patients with co-existing diabetes mellitus or a history of congestive heart failure (systolic dysfunction) there may be compelling indications for selecting angiotensin-converting enzyme (ACE) inhibitor drugs for the initial therapy of systemic hypertension. In patients with a history of prior myocardial infarctions, selection of β-antagonist drugs lacking intrinsic sympathomimetic activity may be preferred. In elderly patients with isolated systolic hypertension and the associated risks of prostatic hypertrophy and osteoporosis, selection of diuretics or calcium channel-blocking drugs may be preferred.

TREATMENT OF SECONDARY HYPERTENSION

Treatment of secondary hypertension is often surgical. Pharmacologic therapy is reserved for patients in whom surgical therapy is not possible.

Table 5–3 • Antihypertensive Drugs, Associated Side Effects, and Special Considerations

Drugs	Side effects	Special considerations
Diuretics		
Thiazides	Hypokalemia	May enhance digitalis toxicity
	Hyperuricemia	May precipitate acute gout
	Glucose intolerance	May be ineffective in renal failure
	Hypercholesterolemia	May decrease lithium clearance
	Hypertriglyceridemia	
	Sexual dysfunction	
	Alkalosis	
Loop diuretics	Same as for thiazides	Effective in renal failure
		May precipitate gout or enhance digitalis toxicity
		Hyponatremia especially in elderly patients
Potassium-sparing drugs	Hyperkalemia	
Amiloride	Sexual dysfunction	
Spironolactone	Gynecomastia	
Adrenergic antagonists		
β-Adrenergic antagonists	Bradycardia	Do not use in patients with asthma or COPD
	Bronchospasm	Do not use in patients with CHF, sick sinus syndrome, or heart block
	Congestive heart failure	Use cautiously in patients with diabetes mellitus and peripheral vascular disease
	Hypertriglyceridemia	
	Mask hypoglycemia	
	Sedation	Abrupt discontinuation may result in rebound sympathetic nervous system stimulation
	Sexual dysfunction	
Centrally acting drugs		
Methyldopa	Drowsiness	Rebound hypertension may occur when abruptly discontinued
	Dry mouth	May cause liver damage
	Fatigue	May cause hemolytic anemia (Coombs' test)
		Decreases anesthetic requirements
Reserpine	Fatigue	Do not use in patients with a history of mental depression
	Nasal congestion	
	Sexual dysfunction	Decreases anesthetic requirements
Clonidine	Sedation	Decreases anesthetic requirements
	Bradycardia	Abrupt discontinuation may result in rebound hypertension
	Xerostomia	
		May be an analgesic alone or in combination with neuraxial opioids
α_1-Adrenergic antagonists		
Prazosin	First-dose syncope	Use cautiously in elderly patients
	Orthostatic hypotension	Unlikely to elicit reflex tachycardia
	Fluid retention	Hypotension during neuraxial blockade may be exaggerated as compensatory vasoconstriction is blocked
Combined α- and β-adrenergic antagonists		
Labetalol	Bronchospasm	Use cautiously in patients with asthma or COPD
	Orthostatic hypotension	
	Fatigue	Use cautiously in patients with CHF, sick sinus syndrome, or heart block
Vasodilators	Tachycardia	May precipitate angina pectoris in patients with ischemic heart disease
Hydralazine	Headache	
	Fluid retention	
	Sodium retention	
	Positive antinuclear antibody	Lupus syndrome may occur
Minoxidil	Hypertrichosis	May cause or aggravate pleural effusion
Angiotensin-converting enzyme inhibitors		
Benazepril	Cough	May be associated with hemodynamic instability and hypotension during general anesthesia especially if large fluid shifts are associated with the surgical procedure
Captopril	Rhinorrhea	
Enalapril	Angioedema	
Lisinopril	Rash	
Moexipril	Hyperkalemia	May cause neutropenia in patients with autoimmune collagen diseases
	Proteinuria	May cause reversible acute renal failure in patients with renal artery stenosis
	Loss of taste	May cause fetal toxicity
		NSAIDs may antagonize antihypertensive effects

Table continued on following page

Table 5–3 • Antihypertensive Drugs, Associated Side Effects, and Special Considerations *Continued*

Drugs	Side effects	Special considerations
Angiotensin II receptor antagonists		
Irbesartan	Dizziness	May be associated with hypotension following the induction of anesthesia
Losartan		
Valsartan		May cause reversible acute renal failure in patients with renal artery stenosis
		May cause fetal toxicity
Calcium channel-blocking drugs	CHF	
	Hypotension	
	Heart block	
	Syncope	
	Hepatic dysfunction	
Verapamil	Bradycardia	Use cautiously in patients with CHF or heart block

CHF, congestive heart failure; COPD, chronic obstructive pulmonary disease; NSAIDs, nonsteroidal antiinflammatory drugs.
Adapted from Oparil S, Calhoun DA. High blood pressure. Sci Am Med 2000;1–16.

Surgical Therapy

Surgical therapy is reserved for identifiable causes of secondary hypertension, and includes revascularization via angioplasty, surgery for a stenotic renal artery, or adrenalectomy for a unilateral adrenal adenoma or pheochromocytoma. Renal artery stents are useful for maintaining renal artery patency.

Pharmacologic Therapy

For patients in whom renal artery revascularization is not possible, blood pressure control may be attempted with ACE inhibitors alone or in combination with diuretics. Renal function and serum potassium concentrations must be carefully monitored when ACE inhibitor therapy is initiated in these patients. Bilateral primary aldosteronism in women is treated with an aldosterone antagonist such as spironolactone, whereas amiloride is used in men because spironolactone sometimes causes gynecomastia.

HYPERTENSIVE CRISIS

Definition

Hypertensive crisis is arbitrarily defined as acute diastolic blood pressure increases above 130 mmHg.[8] The need for emergency treatment of a hypertensive crisis is determined more by the rate of increase in blood pressure than the absolute blood pressure. For example, patients with chronic systemic hypertension can tolerate higher systemic blood pressures than previously normotensive individuals. Encephalopathy rarely develops in patients with chronic systemic hypertension until the diastolic blood pressure exceeds 150 mmHg, whereas parturients with pregnancy-induced hypertension may develop signs of encephalopathy with diastolic blood pressures lower than 100 mmHg.

Pharmacologic Therapy

Patients with evidence of acute or ongoing target-organ damage (encephalopathy, congestive heart failure, renal insufficiency as reflected by oliguria and proteinuria) require prompt pharmacologic interventions to lower the systemic blood pressure, generally by means of intravenous therapy in a high intensity monitoring environment. The goal when treating most hypertensive emergencies is to decrease the diastolic blood pressure promptly but gradually. A precipitous decrease in the systemic blood pressure to normotensive levels is not recommended, as it may provoke target organ ischemia or infarction. Typically, the desired decrease in mean arterial pressure is less than 20% during the first 2 hours of treatment. Subsequent additional decreases in systemic blood pressure are achieved gradually over the next 24 to 48 hours.

For most types of hypertensive crisis (encephalopathy, congestive heart failure, subarachnoid hemorrhage, renal insufficiency, postoperative), nitroprusside, 0.5 to 10.0 μg/kg/min IV, is the drug of choice for treatment. The immediate onset of action of nitroprusside and its short duration of action allow effective minute-by-minute titration. Placing an intra-arterial catheter to monitor systemic blood pressure continuously may be recommended during treatment with nitroprusside. Hydralazine may increase intracranial pressure and so is not likely to be selected for treatment of hypertensive emergencies associated with encephalopathy. Nitroglycerin is an appropriate choice to treat a hypertensive crisis in the presence of myocardial ischemia or cocaine overdose. Use of labetalol or β-adrenergic antagonists to treat a hypertensive crisis due to cocaine overdose may not be optimal, as β-adrenergic blockade may accentuate cocaine-induced coronary artery vasospasm. Lowering the systemic blood pressure in the presence of a dissecting thoracic aneurysm may be achieved with a combination of nitroprusside and β-adrenergic antagonists.

MANAGEMENT OF ANESTHESIA IN PATIENTS WITH ESSENTIAL HYPERTENSION

Perioperative management of patients with essential hypertension who are scheduled for elective or emergency surgery is similar (Table 5–4). Despite earlier suggestions that antihypertensive drugs should be discontinued preoperatively, it is now accepted that drugs that effectively control systemic blood pressure in treated individuals should be continued throughout the perioperative period to ensure optimum medical control of systemic blood pressure. Emergency surgery in patients with

Table 5–4 • Management of Anesthesia for Hypertensive Patients

Preoperative evaluation
  Determine adequacy of systemic blood pressure control
  Review pharmacology of drugs being administered to control systemic blood pressure (orthostatic hypotension, bradycardia, sedation, anesthetic requirements)
  Evaluate for evidence of end-organ damage
    Angina pectoris
    Left ventricular hypertrophy
    Congestive heart failure
    Cerebrovascular disease
    Stroke
    Peripheral vascular disease
    Renal insufficiency
Induction of anesthesia
  Anticipate exaggerated systemic blood pressure changes
  Limit duration of direct laryngoscopy
Maintenance of anesthesia
  Administer a volatile anesthetic to blunt hypertensive responses
  Monitor for myocardial ischemia
Postoperative management
  Anticipate periods of systemic hypertension
  Maintain monitoring of end-organ function

poorly or uncontrolled systemic hypertension introduces the question of the safe level for maintenance of the systemic blood pressure during the perioperative period. In this situation, an acceptable approach is to permit the systemic blood pressure to decrease to about 140/90 mmHg, assuming that this blood pressure is not associated with evidence of target organ ischemia (brain, heart, kidneys).

Preoperative Evaluation

Preoperative evaluation of patients with essential hypertension should determine the adequacy of systemic blood pressure control. Antihypertensive drug therapy that has rendered patients normotensive preoperatively should be continued throughout the perioperative period. It seems reasonable to support the concept that hypertensive patients should be rendered normotensive before undergoing elective surgery. This notion is based on the observation that the incidence of hypotension and evidence of myocardial ischemia on the ECG during the maintenance of anesthesia is increased in patients who remain hypertensive prior to the induction of anesthesia.[9, 10] Furthermore, decreases in systemic blood pressure during anesthesia are likely to be greater in hypertensive than in normotensive patients.[11] However, increases in systemic blood pressure during the intraoperative period are more likely to occur in patients with a history of essential hypertension regardless of the degree of preoperative blood pressure control (Table 5–5).[11]

Despite the desire to render patients normotensive before elective surgery, there is no evidence that the incidence of postoperative complications is increased when hypertensive patients (diastolic blood pressure as high as 110 mmHg) undergo elective operations (Table 5–5).[11] Nevertheless, coexisting systemic hypertension may increase the incidence of postoperative myocardial reinfarction in patients with a history of prior myocardial infarction as well as the incidence of neurologic complications in patients undergoing carotid endarterectomy surgery.[12, 13]

It is not uncommon for the systemic blood pressure on admission to the hospital to be increased ("white coat syndrome"), reflecting patient anxiety during the preoperative period. Subsequent systemic blood pressures are often lower. The subset of patients who manifest anxiety-related increases in systemic blood pressure related to hospital admission are also likely to display exaggerated pressor responses to direct laryngoscopy for tracheal intubation and are more likely than other patients to expe-

Table 5–5 • Risk of General Anesthesia and Elective Surgery in Hypertensive Patients

Preoperative systemic blood pressure status	Incidence of perioperative hypertensive episodes (%)	Incidence of postoperative cardiac complications (%)
Normotensive	8*	11
Treated and rendered normotensive	27	24
Treated but remains hypertensive	25	7
Untreated and hypertensive	20	12

* $P < 0.05$ compared with other groups in the same column.
Data from Goldman L, Caldera DL. Risk of general anesthesia and elective operation in the hypertensive patient. Anesthesiology 1979;50:285–92.

rience perioperative myocardial ischemia or to require vasodilator therapy intraoperatively.[14]

Evidence of End-Organ Damage

The presence of associated end-organ damage (angina pectoris, left ventricular hypertrophy, congestive heart failure, cerebrovascular disease, stroke, peripheral vascular disease, renal insufficiency) is evaluated preoperatively by the ECG and renal function tests. Patients with essential hypertension are always suspect for incipient congestive heart failure and are presumed to have ischemic heart disease until proven otherwise. Symptoms of cerebrovascular disease may be reflected by dizziness or syncope with changes in head position, as may be necessary for direct laryngoscopy during tracheal intubation and subsequent positioning for surgery. Essential hypertension is associated with shifts to the right of the curve for autoregulation of cerebral blood flow. This shift suggests that, in most cases, cerebral blood flow is more dependent on perfusion pressure than in normotensive adults. Evidence of peripheral vascular disease may influence placement of an intra-arterial catheter for intraoperative monitoring of systemic blood pressure. Renal insufficiency secondary to chronic systemic hypertension places patients at increased risk and signals a widespread hypertensive disease process.

Antihypertensive Drug Therapy

There is no evidence that antihypertensive drug therapy adversely alters the course or conduct of anesthesia. Nevertheless, it is useful to review the pharmacology and potential side effects of antihypertensive drugs being used to treat essential hypertension prior to the induction of anesthesia (Table 5–4).[15] In this regard, many drugs used to treat essential hypertension interfere with autonomic nervous system function. Preoperatively, this may manifest as orthostatic hypotension. During anesthesia exaggerated decreases in systemic blood pressure, as are associated with blood loss, positive airway pressure, or sudden changes in body position, could reflect impaired compensatory peripheral vascular vasoconstriction due to inhibitory effects of antihypertensive drugs on the sympathetic nervous system. Despite the possible presence of drug-induced impairment of sympathetic nervous system activity, there is extensive clinical experience supporting the conclusion that administration of vasopressors, such as ephedrine, results in predictable and appropriate systemic blood pressure responses in these patients.[16] A compelling reason to continue antihypertensive drug therapy throughout the perioperative period is the risk of rebound hypertension should these drugs (especially β-adrenergic antagonists and clonidine) be abruptly discontinued during the immediate preoperative period. Antihypertensive drugs that act independently of the autonomic nervous system (ACE inhibitors) do not seem to be associated with rebound hypertension should treatment be abruptly discontinued.

Bradycardia may be a manifestation of selective impairment of sympathetic nervous system activity. There is no evidence, however, that heart rate responses to surgical stimulation or surgical blood loss are absent in patients treated with antihypertensive drugs. Likewise, clinical experience does not support the theoretical possibility that exaggerated decreases in heart rate could occur when drugs that normally increase parasympathetic nervous system activity, such as an anticholinesterase drug, are administered during anesthesia. Decreased anesthetic requirements seem to parallel the sedative effects produced by certain antihypertensive drugs. This is particularly prominent with clonidine. Hypokalemia (less than 3.5 mEq/L) despite potassium supplementation is a common preoperative finding in patients being treated with diuretics. Nevertheless, this drug-induced hypokalemia has not been documented to increase the incidence of cardiac dysrhythmias in either awake or anesthetized patients.[17] Hyperkalemia is a consideration in patients being treated with ACE inhibitors who are also receiving potassium supplementation or experiencing renal dysfunction.

ACE Inhibitors

Despite acceptance of the concept that antihypertensive drug therapy should be continued throughout the perioperative period, there is a risk that hemodynamic instability and hypotension may occur during anesthesia in patients receiving ACE inhibitors.[18–20] Anesthetic-induced hypotension is mainly due to decreased sympathetic nervous system vasoconstrictive responses. In this regard, surgical procedures involving major body fluid shifts have been associated with hypotension in patients being treated with ACE inhibitors. Exaggerated hypotension attributed to continued ACE inhibitor therapy has been responsive to crystalloid fluid infusions, administration of sympathomimetic drugs such as ephedrine and/or phenylephrine. In patients with hypotension resistant to sympathomimetics, a vasopressin agonist such as terlipressin may be effective.[19] Titrating and decreasing the doses of anesthetic drugs often prevents the appearance or limits the magnitude of hypotension attributed to ACE inhibitors. Equally important is maintenance of intravascular fluid volume during surgery in patients treated chronically with ACE inhibitors.[19]

An alternative to continuing treatment with ACE inhibitors in patients considered to be at high risk for intraoperative hypovolemia and subsequent hypotension is to discontinue the drugs 24 to 48 hours preoperatively.[19, 20] The disadvantage of this approach is the potential loss of control of systemic blood pressure and the detrimental effects on some regional tissue circulation, especially that of the heart and kidneys.

Angiotensin II Antagonists

Angiotensin II antagonists (AIIA) are effective in the treatment of systemic hypertension by virtue of inhibiting angiotensin II from binding to its receptor, resulting in increased angiotensin II and normal plasma bradykinin concentrations. As with ACE inhibitors, blockade of the renin-angiotensin system increases the potential hypotensive effects of induction of anesthesia. Hypotension requiring vasoconstrictor treatment occurs more often after the induction of anesthesia in patients being chronically treated with AIIA than in those in whom treatment had been discontinued on the day before surgery.[21] For this reason it may be recommended that AIIA be discontinued on the day before surgery.[21]

Induction of Anesthesia

Induction of anesthesia with rapidly acting intravenous drugs is acceptable, recognizing that an exaggerated decrease in systemic blood pressure may occur, particularly if systemic hypertension is present preoperatively. This most likely reflects drug-induced peripheral vasodilation in the presence of a decreased intravascular fluid volume, as is likely in the presence of diastolic hypertension. Ketamine is not a likely choice for induction of anesthesia in hypertensive patients, as its circulatory stimulant effects could theoretically exaggerate existing systemic hypertension. It is possible that systemic blood pressure decreases during induction of anesthesia are more noticeable in patients receiving ACE inhibitors preoperatively for control of their essential hypertension.[18]

Direct laryngoscopy and tracheal intubation may result in exaggerated increases in systemic blood pressure in patients with essential hypertension, even if these patients have been treated with antihypertensive drugs and are rendered normotensive preoperatively.[9] Evidence of myocardial ischemia on the ECG of patients with ischemic heart disease is most likely to occur in association with the increased systemic blood pressure and heart rate that accompany direct laryngoscopy and tracheal intubation.[10] This increased incidence of myocardial ischemia is consistent with increased diastolic intracavitary pressures in the left ventricle that compress subendocardial arteries, as well as increased myocardial oxygen requirements attributable to tachycardia. It is possible that drugs administered for intravenous induction of anesthesia cannot adequately or predictably suppress circulatory responses evoked by tracheal intubation. For this reason it may be prudent, in selected patients judged to be at increased risk for the development of myocardial ischemia, to increase the concentrations of inhaled volatile anesthetics or to inject a potent opioid prior to initiating direct laryngoscopy. Intravenous opioid administration should be timed so the peak effects of the opioids are predictably matched with the stimulus of the laryngoscopy and tracheal intubation. In this regard, alfentanil and remifentanil have more rapid effect–site equilibration times (time from intravenous injection to peak effect at the target organ) than do fentanyl and sufentanil (Fig. 5–3).[22] Therefore the administration of alfentanil (15 to 30 μg/kg IV) or remifentanil (1 μg/kg IV) can be timed to coincide with injection of the intravenous induction drugs, whereas it seems more appropriate to inject fentanyl (50 to 150 μg/kg IV) or sufentanil (10 to 30 μg/kg IV) about 3 minutes before the anticipated

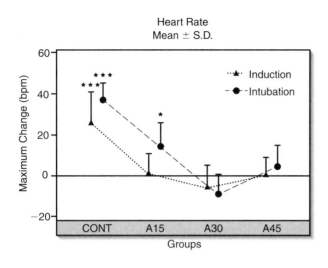

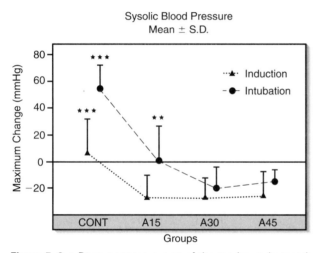

Figure 5–3 • Dose-response curves of the maximum (percent) changes in heart rate and systolic blood pressure in response to induction of anesthesia and tracheal intubation. (A15, alfentanil 15 μg/kg IV; A30, alfentanil 30 μg/kg IV; A45, alfentanil 45 μg/kg IV; Cont, control). Heart rate and systemic blood pressure responses to tracheal intubation were blunted in these patients with prior administration of alfentanil 15 to 30 μg/kg IV. (From Miller DR, Martineau RJ, O'Brien H, et al. Effect of alfentanil on the hemodynamic and catecholamine response to tracheal intubation. Anesth Analg 1993;76:1040–6. © 1993, Lippincott Williams & Wilkins, with permission.)

induction of anesthesia. There are data suggesting that sympathetic nervous system responses to painful stimulation are not blocked until volatile anesthetic concentrations equivalent to about 1.5 MAC are achieved.[23] During the short period available during a typical anesthetic induction it is unlikely that 1.5 MAC of a volatile anesthetic can be reliably achieved, although poorly soluble anesthetics such

as desflurane and sevoflurane are more likely to be compatible with this goal than the more soluble isoflurane.

In addition to anesthetic depth, the duration of direct laryngoscopy is important for limiting the pressor responses to this painful stimulus. Direct laryngoscopy that does not exceed 15 seconds in duration is helpful for minimizing systemic blood pressure increases evoked by direct laryngoscopy and tracheal intubation.[24] In addition, topical administration of laryngotracheal lidocaine, 2 mg/kg, immediately before placing the tracheal tube may attenuate additional pressor responses produced by tracheal intubation.[25] Alternatively, lidocaine 1.5 mg/kg IV, administered about 1 minute before the induction of anesthesia may be useful for attenuating pressor responses. When the duration of direct laryngoscopy is likely to exceed 15 seconds, it may be useful to inject nitroprusside, 1 to 2 μg/kg IV, just before beginning direct laryngoscopy in an attempt to attenuate the systemic blood pressure response produced by tracheal intubation.[26] Esmolol, 100 to 200 mg IV, about 15 seconds before the induction of anesthesia is an alternative to nitroprusside and has the advantage, like alfentanil, of attenuating both the heart rate and systemic blood pressure responses to tracheal intubation (Fig. 5–3).[22,27] Regardless of the drugs administered before initiating direct laryngoscopy, it should be appreciated that excessive depressant drug effects during attempts to blunt a usually benign and transient hemodynamic response can produce hypotension that is more undesirable than the transient stimulatory effects produced by direct laryngoscopy and tracheal intubation.

Maintenance of Anesthesia

The goal during maintenance of anesthesia is to adjust the depth of anesthesia to minimize wide fluctuations in systemic blood pressure. In this regard, a technique that includes a volatile anesthetic is useful for permitting rapid adjustment of the depth of anesthesia in response to changes in systemic blood pressure. Indeed, management of intraoperative blood pressure lability with the anesthetic technique may be more important than preoperative control of systemic hypertension.[11]

Regional anesthesia is an acceptable option for hypertensive patients, recognizing that a need for high sensory levels of anesthesia and associated sympathetic nervous system denervation could unmask unsuspected hypovolemia. It is important to recognize that chronic systemic hypertension is often associated with hypovolemia and ischemic heart disease, which means that decreases in systemic blood pressure are more likely to result in myocardial ischemia.

Intraoperative Hypertension

The most likely intraoperative change in systemic blood pressure is systemic hypertension produced by painful stimulation. Indeed, the incidence of perioperative hypertensive episodes is increased in patients diagnosed as having essential hypertension, even in those previously rendered normotensive with drug therapy (Table 5–5).[11] Volatile anesthetics are useful for attenuating the activity of the sympathetic nervous system, which is responsible for pressor responses. Isoflurane, desflurane, and sevoflurane produce dose-dependent decreases in systemic blood pressure, reflecting decreases in systemic vascular resistance and to a lesser extent direct myocardial depression and decreased cardiac output. There is no evidence that one volatile anesthetic drug is preferable to another, although the poor blood solubility of desflurane and sevoflurane compared with isoflurane may permit more rapid changes in alveolar concentrations and hence the depth of anesthesia with these less soluble drugs.

A nitrous oxide–opioid technique is also acceptable for maintaining anesthesia. If this approach is selected, however, it is likely that volatile anesthetics will be needed at various times to control undesirable increases in systemic blood pressure, as may occur during periods of abruptly increased surgical stimulation. Continuous intravenous infusions of nitroprusside are alternatives to the use of volatile anesthetics for maintaining normotension during the intraoperative period. Labetalol may also be administered to blunt the systemic blood pressure and heart rate responses evoked by painful stimulation. There is no evidence that a specific muscle relaxant is the best selection for patients with essential hypertension. Although pancuronium can modestly increase systemic blood pressure, there is no evidence that this pressor response is exaggerated by the presence of essential hypertension.

Intraoperative Hypotension

Hypotension that occurs during maintenance of anesthesia may be treated by decreasing the delivered concentrations of volatile anesthetics and by increasing the infusion rates of crystalloid or colloid solutions. Sympathomimetic drugs such as ephedrine or phenylephrine may be necessary to restore vital organ perfusion pressures until the underlying cause of hypotension can be corrected. Despite the predictable suppressant effect of many antihypertensive drugs on the autonomic nervous system,

extensive clinical experience has confirmed that the response to sympathomimetic drugs is both appropriate and predictable. Intraoperative hypotension in patients being treated with ACE inhibitors has been described as being responsive to administration of intravenous fluids and/or sympathomimetic drugs. Another cause of an abrupt decrease in systemic blood pressure is the sudden onset of junctional cardiac rhythm. In this regard, avoidance of marked decreases in $PaCO_2$ and delivery of high concentrations of volatile anesthetics minimize the likelihood of this cardiac rhythm. Persistent junctional rhythm associated with decreases in systemic blood pressure may be treated with intravenous administration of atropine.

Monitoring

The selection of monitors for patients with essential hypertension is influenced by the complexity of the surgery. The ECG is particularly useful for recognizing the occurrence of myocardial ischemia during painful stimulation, such as that caused by direct laryngoscopy and tracheal intubation. Invasive monitoring using an intra-arterial catheter and pulmonary artery catheter may be useful if extensive surgery is planned and there is evidence of left ventricular dysfunction. Transesophageal echocardiography is also a useful method for monitoring left ventricular function and the adequacy of intravascular fluid volume replacement.

Postoperative Management

Hypertension during the early postoperative period (often in the postanesthesia care unit) is a likely response in patients with a preoperative diagnosis of essential hypertension. The mechanism is not known but likely reflects exaggerated sympathetic nervous system activity with or without relative hypervolemia related to intraoperative fluid replacement. The development of postoperative systemic hypertension warrants prompt assessment and treatment to decrease the risk of myocardial ischemia, cardiac dysrhythmias, congestive heart failure, stroke, and bleeding. If hypertension persists despite adequate treatment of postoperative pain, it may be necessary to administer vasodilator drugs such as hydralazine, 2.5 to 10.0 mg IV every 10 to 20 minutes, or nitroprusside. If nitroprusside is selected, the dose is titrated (0.5 to 10.0 $\mu g/kg/min$ IV) to produce the desired systolic blood pressure with the aid of continuous intra-arterial blood pressure monitoring. Alternatively, labetalol 0.1 to 0.5 mg/kg every 10 minutes, may be useful for controlling acute postoperative systemic hypertension.[28]

References

1. The sixth report of the Joint National Committee on Prevention, Detection, Evaluation, and Treatment of High Blood Pressure (JNC VI). Arch Intern Med 1997:2413–20
2. Tjoa HI, Kaplan NM. Treatment of hypertension in the elderly. JAMA 1990;264:1015–8
3. Burt VL, Culter JA, Higgins M, et al. Trends in the prevalence, awareness, treatment, and control of hypertension in the adult US population: data from the health examinations surveys, 1960–1991. Hypertension 1995;26:60–9
4. Peppard PE, Young T, Palta M, et al. Prospective study of the association between sleep-disordered breathing and hypertension. N Engl J Med 2000;342:1378–84
5. Rimm ED, Giovannucci EL, Willett WC, et al. Prospective study of alcohol consumption and risk of coronary disease in men. Lancet 1991;338:464–70
6. Midgley JP, Matthew AG, Greenwood CMT, et al. Effect of reduced dietary sodium on blood pressure: a meta-analysis of randomized controlled trials. JAMA 1996;275:1590–6
7. Oparil S, Calhoun DA. High blood pressure. Sci Am Med 2000;1–16
8. Gifford RW. Management of hypertensive crises. JAMA 1991;266:829–35
9. Prys-Roberts C. Anaesthesia and hypertension. Br J Anaesth 1984;56:711–24
10. Stone JG, Foex P, Sear JW, et al. Risk of myocardial ischaemia during anaesthesia in treated and untreated hypertensive patients. Br J Anaesth 1988;61:675–9
11. Goldman L, Caldera DL. Risks of general anesthesia and elective operation in the hypertensive patient. Anesthesiology 1979;50:285–92
12. Steen PA, Tinker JH, Tarhan S. Myocardial reinfarction after anesthesia and surgery: an update: incidence, mortality and predisposing factors. JAMA 1978;239:2566–70
13. Asiddas CB, Donegan JHY, Whitesell RC, et al. Factors associated with perioperative complications during carotid endarterectomy. Anesth Analg 1982;61:631–7
14. Bedford RF, Feinstein B. Hospital admission blood pressure: a predictor for hypertension following endotracheal intubation. Anesth Analg 1980;59:367–70
15. Husserl FE, Messerli FH. Adverse effects of antihypertensive drugs. Drug 1981;22:188–210
16. Katz RL, Weintraub HD, Papper EM. Anesthesia, surgery, and rauwolfia. Anesthesiology 1964;25:142–7
17. Vitez TS, Soper LE, Wong KC, et al. Chronic hypokalemia and intraoperative dysrhythmia. Anesthesiology 1985;63:130–3
18. Coriat P, Richer C, Douraki T, et al. Influence of chronic angiotensin-converting enzyme inhibition on anesthetic induction. Anesthesiology 1994;81:299–307
19. Colson P, Ryckwaert F, Coriat P. Renin angiotensin system antagonists and anesthesia. Anesth Analg 1999;89:1143–55
20. Licker M, Schweizer A, Hohn L, et al. Cardiovascular responses to anesthetic induction in patients chronically treated with angiotensin-converting enzyme inhibitors. Can J Anesth 2000;47:433–40
21. Bertrand M, Godet G, Meersschaert K, et al. Should the angiotensin II antagonists be discontinued before surgery? Anesth Analg 2001;92:26–30
22. Miller DR, Martineau RJ, O'Brien H, et al. Effect of alfentanil on the hemodynamic and catecholamine response to tracheal intubation. Anesth Analg 1993;76:1040–6
23. Roizen MF, Horrigan RW, Frazer BM. Anesthetic doses blocking adrenergic (stress) and cardiovascular responses to incision MAC BAR. Anesthesiology 1981;54:390–8
24. Stoelting RK. Blood pressure and heart rate changes during short duration laryngoscopy for tracheal intubation: influence of viscous or intravenous lidocaine. Anesth Analg 1978;57:197–9
25. Stoelting RK. Circulatory changes during direct laryngoscopy and tracheal intubation: influence of duration of laryngoscopy with or without prior lidocaine. Anesthesiology 1977;47:381–3
26. Stoelting RK. Attenuation of blood pressure response to laryngoscopy and tracheal intubation with sodium nitroprusside. Anesth Analg 1979;58:116–9
27. Sheppard S, Eagle CJ, Sturnin L. A bolus dose of esmolol attenuates tachycardia and hypertension after tracheal intubation. Can J Anaesth 1990;37:202–5
28. Leslie JB, Kalayjian RW, Sirgo MA, et al. Intravenous labetalol for treatment of postoperative hypertension. Anesthesiology 1987;67:413–6

6

Congestive Heart Failure

Chronic heart failure (congestive heart failure, CHF) is a major health problem in the United States, affecting about 1% of adults. Despite advances in therapy mortality remains high.[1,2] There are new and better drugs for treatment of CHF, but there is evidence from large trials that progression of heart failure is common; and the mortality rate continues to approach 40% during the first 4 years following the diagnosis of CHF.[3] CHF is a complex of symptoms (fatigue, dyspnea, congestion) related to the inadequate perfusion of tissues during exertion and often to the retention of fluid. The principal cause of CHF is impairment of the heart's ability to fill or empty the left ventricle.[2] In this regard CHF is most often due to: (1) cardiac valve abnormalities; (2) impaired myocardial contractility secondary to ischemic heart disease or cardiomyopathy; (3) systemic hypertension; or (4) pulmonary hypertension (cor pulmonale). The most common cause of right ventricular failure is left ventricular failure. Guidelines for the treatment of CHF stress the importance of documenting the presence of the signs and symptoms of expanded left ventricular volume (imaging of the left ventricle for size and function), early intervention with angiotensin-converting enzyme (ACE) inhibitors, and diagnosing correctable myocardial ischemia and cardiac valve dysfunction.[2,4]

Management of CHF cannot be confined to the treatment of symptoms. The processes that contribute to the left ventricular dysfunction (progressive dilation and remodeling of the left ventricle) may progress independently from the development of symptoms (Fig. 6–1).[2] Treatment to prevent or delay the progression of left ventricular dysfunction may be quite different from treatment intended to relieve symptoms and improve the patient's quality of life.

105

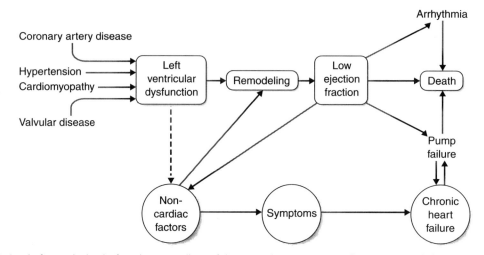

Figure 6–1 • Left ventricular dysfunction, regardless of the cause (coronary artery disease, systemic hypertension, cardiomyopathy, valvular heart disease), results in progressive remodeling of the ventricular chamber leading to dilation and a low ejection fraction. Cardiac dysrhythmias, progressive cardiac failure, and premature death are likely. Noncardiac factors (neurohormonal stimulation, vasoconstriction, renal sodium retention) may be stimulated by left ventricular dysfunction and ultimately contribute to remodeling of the left ventricle and symptoms (dyspnea, fatigue, edema) considered characteristic of the clinical syndrome of congestive heart failure. (From Cohn JN. The management of chronic heart failure. N Engl J Med 1996;335:490–8. Copyright 1996 Massachusetts Medical Society, with permission.)

Indeed, the short-term relief of symptoms attributed to CHF may have little relation to the progression of cardiac dysfunction over time.

The symptoms of CHF are only weakly related to the severity of left ventricular dysfunction, although the magnitude of the dysfunction is closely linked to mortality. A normal-size heart on the chest radiograph and an absence of edema or pulmonary rales do not exclude the diagnosis of CHF. Structural changes in the myocardium and vasculature contribute to progression of left ventricular dysfunction. It is likely that these structural changes, if allowed to progress, adversely affect the prognosis of patients with a history of myocardial infarction.

MANIFESTATIONS OF LEFT VENTRICULAR DYSFUNCTION

Decreased ventricular systolic wall motion reflects systolic dysfunction, whereas ventricular diastolic dysfunction is characterized by increased end-diastolic pressures in a chamber of normal size.[2]

Systolic Heart Failure

Ischemic heart disease usually results in localized defects in ventricular systolic contraction, whereas cardiomyopathy results in global ventricular dysfunction. Systemic hypertension and cardiac valve disease may produce chronic pressure or volume overloads that alter the structure and function of the left ventricle. Ventricular dysrhythmias are common in patients with left ventricular dysfunction.

A decreased ejection fraction, a hallmark of chronic left ventricular systolic dysfunction, is closely related to the increase in the volume of the left ventricle (Fig. 6–1).[2] Measuring the left ventricular ejection fraction via echocardiography, radionuclide imaging, or ventriculography provides the quantification necessary to document the severity of ventricular systolic dysfunction. An ejection fraction less than 0.45, with or without symptoms of CHF, is often viewed as evidence of left ventricular dysfunction. Chest radiographs are not sensitive methods for assessing the size or function of the left ventricle, whereas the electrocardiogram (ECG) of patients with substantial left ventricular dysfunction is almost always abnormal.[2] Decreased diastolic compliance, which manifests as impaired filling of the left ventricle during diastole, may be part of any type of left ventricular dysfunction.

Diastolic Heart Failure

Symptomatic CHF in patients with normal or near-normal left ventricular systolic function is most likely due to diastolic dysfunction.[5] The prevalence of diastolic heart failure is age-dependent, increasing from less than 15% among patients younger than

45 years of age to 35% among those older than 65 years of age.[6] With diastolic heart failure, the left ventricle has decreased compliance and cannot adequately fill at normal diastolic pressures. Factors that predispose to decreased diastolic distensibility include myocardial edema, fibrosis, hypertrophy, aging, and pressure overload (essential hypertension).[2] Ischemic heart disease, long-standing essential hypertension, and progressive aortic stenosis are the most common causes of diastolic CHF. In contrast to systolic heart failure, diastolic heart failure affects women more than men.

Diagnosis

Clinical signs and symptoms do not reliably differentiate systolic dysfunction from diastolic dysfunction. The absence of cardiomegaly on chest radiography is a useful clue, but demonstration of normal ejection fractions is usually necessary to establish the correct diagnosis. Signs of systemic or pulmonary venous congestion in patients with a left ventricular chamber of normal size are considered evidence that diastolic ventricular dysfunction is the predominant mechanism of CHF.

Treatment

Treatment of patients with diastolic CHF is empirical. Current treatment includes avoidance of excessive sodium intake, cautious use of diuretics (to relieve pulmonary congestion without excessive decreases in preload), restoration and maintenance of normal sinus rhythm at a heart rate that optimizes ventricular filling, and correction of precipitating factors, such as acute myocardial ischemia and systemic hypertension.[5, 7] No drugs have been documented to improve diastolic distensibility selectively. Long-acting nitrates and diuretics alleviate symptoms of diastolic CHF by lowering the preload, but they do not alter the natural history of the disease.

The best treatment for diastolic CHF is prevention. In the presence of hypertensive pulmonary edema, early detection and optimal control of systemic hypertension are the key preventive steps. In this regard it is estimated that fewer than one-third of patients with systemic hypertension in the United States are aware of their condition and are adequately treated.[8]

HEMODYNAMIC PARAMETERS OF VENTRICULAR FUNCTION

The hemodynamic parameters of ventricular function likely to be altered by CHF are the cardiac output, ejection fraction, and ventricular end-diastolic pressure.

Cardiac Output

Cardiac output is the product of stroke volume and heart rate. Stroke volume is determined by myocardial contractility, synchronous contraction of all portions of the ventricle, afterload, and most importantly venous return. In the presence of left ventricular dysfunction the resting cardiac output may be normal but unable to increase in response to exercise, whereas more severe CHF is associated with decreased cardiac output (less than 2.5 L/min/m²). When cardiac output cannot increase, any enhanced extraction of oxygen by peripheral tissues lowers the oxygen content of venous blood, leading to an increased arterial-venous oxygen content difference.

A heart with properly functioning valves can adequately accept venous return (preload) and eject it against systemic vascular resistance (afterload). The heart can be overloaded by an increase in the volume of blood it must eject forward (aortic or mitral regurgitation) or by an increase in the resistance against which it must eject blood (systemic hypertension, aortic stenosis). Adaptive mechanisms that allow the heart to maintain its cardiac output with changes that may predispose to CHF include the (1) Frank-Starling relation, (2) inotropic state, (3) afterload, (4) heart rate, and (5) myocardial hypertrophy and dilation. In addition, alterations in sympathetic nervous system activity and humoral-mediated responses occur in the presence of CHF.

Frank-Starling Relation

The Frank-Starling relation describes the increases in stroke volume that accompany progressive increases in the left or right ventricular end-diastolic volumes, which are closely related to end-diastolic pressures (Fig. 6–2). Stroke volume is increased because the tension developed by contracting muscle is greater when the resting length of that muscle is increased. The magnitude of the stroke volume increase produced by the increased resting tension of ventricular muscle fibers depends on myocardial contractility. For example, when myocardial contractility is decreased, as in the presence of CHF, a lower stroke volume is achieved relative to any given left ventricular end-diastolic filling pressure (Fig. 6–1). Constriction of a venous capacitance vessel shifts blood centrally, which helps maintain cardiac output by the Frank-Starling relation.

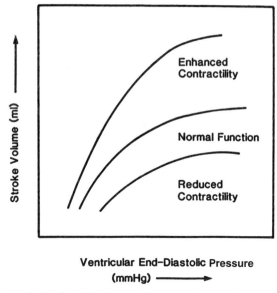

Figure 6–2 • Frank-Starling relation states that stroke volume is directly related to the ventricular end-diastolic pressure.

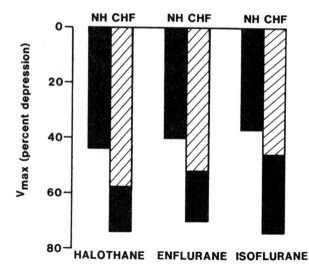

Figure 6–3 • Effect of equipotent concentrations (1 MAC) of volatile anesthetics on maximal velocity of shortening (V_{max}) of isolated papillary muscles taken from adult cats with normal hearts (NH) or experimentally induced congestive heart failure (CHF) were studied. The presence of CHF had an additive depressant effect on V_{max} in the presence of volatile anesthetics. (From Kemmotsu O, Hashimoto Y, Shimosato S. The effects of halothane, enflurane, and isoflurane on performance of isolated papillary muscles from failing hearts. Anesthesiology 1974;40:252–60, with permission.)

Inotropic State

The inotropic state describes myocardial contractility as reflected by the velocity of contraction developed by cardiac muscle. The maximum velocity of contraction is referred to as V_{max}. When the inotropic state of the heart is increased, as in the presence of catecholamines, V_{max} is increased. Conversely, V_{max} is decreased when myocardial contractility is impaired, as in CHF. Volatile anesthetics have been shown to decrease V_{max}, and this effect is additive to the decrease produced by CHF alone (Fig. 6–3).[9] In clinical practice the rate of increase in intraventricular pressure (dp/dt) simulates V_{max} and is used as an approximation of the inotropic state of the heart.

Congestive heart failure is associated with depletion of catecholamines in the heart, with subsequent decreases in myocardial contractility. In contrast to depletion of myocardial catecholamines, the plasma concentrations and urinary excretion of catecholamines are invariably increased in patients in CHF. Furthermore, there are decreases in the density of β-adrenergic receptors in the cardiac muscle of failing hearts and decreased inotropic responses to β-agonist stimulation.

Afterload

Afterload is the tension the ventricular muscle must develop to open the aortic or pulmonic valve. The afterload presented to the left ventricle is increased in the presence of systemic hypertension. The for-

ward left ventricular stroke volume in patients with CHF can be increased by administering peripheral vasodilating drugs.

Heart Rate

In the normal heart the ventricular filling time parallels the heart rate, such that changes in heart rate are associated with the opposite change in stroke volume, and cardiac output is unlikely to change. Conversely, in the presence of CHF and low cardiac output the stroke volume is relatively fixed, with any increase in cardiac output being dependent on heart rate increases. Increases in myocardial contractility that accompany increases in heart rate are known as the rate-treppe phenomenon. Tachycardia is an expected finding in the presence of CHF, reflecting activation of the sympathetic nervous system.

Myocardial Hypertrophy and Dilation

Myocardial hypertrophy represents compensatory mechanisms that develop in response to chronic pressure overloads (mitral stenosis, aortic stenosis, systemic hypertension, pulmonary hypertension), whereas cardiac dilation occurs in response to volume overloads (mitral regurgitation, aortic regurgitation). Myocardial hypertrophy helps overcome pressure overloads on the heart but has limitations because hypertrophied cardiac muscle functions at a lower inotropic state than does normal cardiac muscle. Cardiac dilation leads to compensatory increases in cardiac output by the Frank-Starling relation. Increased cardiac wall tension produced by the enlarged ventricular radius is also associated with increased myocardial oxygen requirements and decreased cardiac efficiency.

Sympathetic Nervous System Activity

Arteriolar and venous constriction occur in the presence of CHF. Arteriolar constriction serves to maintain systemic blood pressure despite decreased cardiac output, whereas increased venous tone shifts blood from peripheral sites to the central circulation, thereby enhancing venous return and maintaining cardiac output by the Frank-Starling relation. Furthermore, arteriolar constriction causes redistribution of blood from the kidneys, splanchnic organs, skeletal muscles, and skin to maintain coronary and cerebral blood flow despite overall decreases in cardiac output. Decreased renal blood flow (as low as 25% of normal) evokes increased renal tubular absorption of sodium and water, resulting in increased blood volume and enhanced cardiac output by the Frank-Starling relation. These compensatory peripheral responses, although effective in compensating for hypovolemic states such as acute blood loss, can contribute to a vicious circle in the presence of CHF. For example, fluid retention, increased venous return, and increased afterload impose more work on the failing myocardium and can further decrease cardiac output. Interruption of this vicious circle is the rationale for treating CHF with peripheral vasodilators and ACE inhibitors (see ''Pharmacologic Therapy'').

Humoral-Mediated Responses

Atrial natriuretic factor is stored in atrial muscle and released in response to increases in atrial pressures, as produced by tachycardia or hypervolemia. This hormone increases the glomerular filtration rate, leading to natriuresis and diuresis. In addition, it suppresses aldosterone secretion and the release of antidiuretic hormone.

Ejection Fraction

Normally, the left ventricle ejects 56% to 78% of its volume during systole, resulting in an ejection fraction (stroke volume/end-diastolic volume ratio) of 0.56 to 0.78. The ejection fraction as measured by angiographic techniques, radioisotope imaging, or echocardiography is diminished by decreased myocardial contractility, increased afterload, or asynchrony of left ventricular contraction.

End-Diastolic Pressure

End-diastolic pressure that parallels end-diastolic volume is increased in the presence of CHF. It can also be increased in the presence of a poorly compliant (stiff) ventricle, even in the absence of an increase in ventricular volume (see ''Frank-Starling Relation''). Left ventricular end-diastolic pressure is normally less than 12 mmHg, whereas right ventricular end-diastolic pressure is normally less than 5 mmHg. In the absence of mitral valve disease, mean left atrial pressures parallel left ventricular end-diastolic pressures. Likewise, in the absence of increased pulmonary vascular resistance or mitral valve disease, pulmonary artery end-diastolic pressures reflect the left ventricular end-diastolic pressures. Manifestations of left atrial enlargement on the ECG (P wave lasts longer than 0.1 second and has an M-shaped configuration on lead II) correlates with increases in left atrial pressure.

DIAGNOSIS OF CONGESTIVE HEART FAILURE

The diagnosis of CHF is based on the history, physical examination, and interpretation of laboratory and diagnostic tests. Symptoms of CHF are principally those of systemic and venous congestion due to increased cardiac ventricular filling pressures.[2] In addition, patient fatigue and organ system dysfunction are most likely related to inadequate cardiac output in response to stress. The hallmark of decreased cardiac reserve and low cardiac output is fatigue at rest or with minimal exertion. Associated decreases in cerebral blood flow may produce confusion, and decreases in renal blood flow may lead to prerenal azotemia characterized by a disproportionate increase in blood urea nitrogen concentration relative to the serum creatinine concentration.

The most prominent physical sign in patients experiencing left ventricular failure is moist rales in the lungs, often associated with tachypnea. These extraneous sounds may be confined to lung bases in patients with a mild degree of left ventricular failure, or they may be generalized in those with acute pulmonary edema. Compensatory increases in sympathetic nervous system activity manifest as resting tachycardia and peripheral vasoconstriction, which helps maintain systemic blood pressure and blood flow to the heart and brain despite decreased cardiac output. Unexplained resting tachycardia during the preoperative period suggests CHF, particularly if the patient is elderly or is known to have co-existing heart disease. A third heart sound (S_3 gallop or ventricular diastolic gallop) indicates significant left ventricular dysfunction and may be the first sign of CHF. This heart sound is due to blood entering and distending a relatively noncompliant left ventricle.

Vascular and neuroendocrine responses are responsible for abnormalities of regional blood flow, renal retention of sodium, and pulmonary congestion that leads to symptoms recognized clinically as evidence of CHF. Activation of the renin-angiotensin system and the sympathetic nervous system may also contribute to progressive structural changes in the peripheral vasculature and heart (remodeling of the left ventricle).

Signs and Symptoms

The pathophysiologic hallmarks of CHF are (1) decreased cardiac output, (2) increased ventricular end-diastolic pressures, (3) peripheral vasoconstriction, and (4) metabolic acidosis. Conceptually, left ventricular failure results in signs and symptoms of pulmonary edema, whereas right ventricular failure results in systemic venous hypertension and associated peripheral edema.

Dyspnea

Dyspnea, which reflects increased work of breathing owing to stiffness of the lungs produced by interstitial pulmonary edema, is one of the earliest subjective symptoms of left ventricular failure. Initially, this symptom occurs only with exertion. It can be quantitated by asking the patient how many flights of stairs can be climbed or the distance that can be walked at a normal pace before dyspnea occurs. Patients experiencing angina pectoris may interpret substernal discomfort as breathlessness.

Orthopnea

Orthopnea reflects the inability of a failing left ventricle to handle increased venous return associated with the recumbent position. A dry, nonproductive cough that develops with assumption of the supine position and is relieved by sitting up is the equivalent of orthopnea owing to pulmonary congestion. The orthopneic cough differs from the productive

morning cough characteristic of patients with chronic bronchitis.

Paroxysmal Nocturnal Dyspnea

Paroxysmal nocturnal dyspnea is shortness of breath that awakens the patient from sleep. This symptom must be differentiated from anxiety-provoked hyperventilation or wheezing owing to accumulation of secretions in patients with chronic bronchitis. Wheezing caused by pulmonary congestion (cardiac asthma) is typically accompanied by radiographic evidence of pulmonary congestion, which distinguishes this response from that due to sputum accumulation in the airways.

Acute Pulmonary Edema

Acute pulmonary edema reflecting movement of fluid into the alveoli is the ultimate manifestation of left ventricular failure. Systemic blood pressure is often increased. Other signs of sympathetic nervous system stimulation such as tachycardia and vasoconstriction are often present. Bubbling rales are diffusely present with or without wheezes. Pulmonary artery occlusion pressures are likely to be higher than 30 mmHg in the presence of acute pulmonary edema. When left atrial pressures remain normal, pulmonary edema is characterized as noncardiogenic, reflecting direct damage to the alveolar epithelium, pulmonary capillary walls, or both. The ratio of the colloid osmotic pressure of the edema fluid relative to that of the plasma differentiates pulmonary edema due to left ventricular failure (ratio is less than 0.6) from that due to noncardiogenic causes (ratio approaches 1.0, reflecting a high protein content).

The initial treatment of acute pulmonary edema includes placing the patient in a head-up position, delivering humidified oxygen by face mask, and administering morphine (5 to 10 mg IV) to decrease venous return to the heart. A rapid-acting diuretic such as furosemide (10 to 40 mg IV) is administered; early in therapy digoxin is used only to control atrial tachydysrhythmias. Dopamine is probably the preferred inotrope because it maintains systemic vascular resistance and enhances renal blood flow. In patients who have high systemic vascular resistance, however, dobutamine, which has relatively little effect on systemic vascular resistance, may be selected. The determination of arterial blood gases and pH is useful, and monitoring systemic and pulmonary arterial pressures may be indicated.

Chest Radiography

The earliest radiographic sign of left ventricular failure and associated pulmonary venous hypertension is evidence of distension of the pulmonary veins in the upper lobes of the lungs. Perivascular edema appears as a hilar and perihilar haze. The hilus appears large, with ill-defined margins. Septal edema on a chest radiograph is described as Kerley's lines, reflecting edematous interlobular septae in the upper lung fields (Kerley A lines), lower lung fields (Kerley B lines), or basilar regions of the lungs producing a honeycomb pattern (Kerley C lines). Subpleural edema indicates extension of interstitial pulmonary edema to the periphery of the lungs. Alveolar edema typically produces homogeneous densities in the lung fields, resembling a butterfly pattern when the distribution is central, bilateral, and symmetrical. Pleural effusions and pericardial effusions may accompany CHF, particularly if it is biventricular. Radiographic changes of pulmonary edema may lag behind acute increases of left atrial pressures by up to 12 hours. Likewise, radiographic patterns of pulmonary congestion may persist for 1 to 4 days after normalization of cardiac filling pressures.

Systemic Venous Congestion

The hallmark of right ventricular failure is systemic venous congestion, classically evidenced by jugular venous distension. For example, distension of the external jugular veins above the clavicles of patients in the sitting position suggests right ventricular failure. In the presence of normal right ventricular function, the increased venous return produced by inspiration and associated negative intrathoracic pressure is easily propelled into the pulmonary circulation. By contrast, in the presence of right ventricular failure, any increase in venous return causes a further increase, rather than a normal decrease, in jugular venous pressure. This distension of neck veins with inspiration is known as Kussmaul's sign. A similar response may be seen in patients with constrictive pericarditis or cardiac tamponade.

Organomegaly

The liver is typically the first organ to become engorged with blood in the presence of right ventricular failure. If the engorgement is rapid, right upper quadrant pain and tenderness may occur, reflecting distension of the liver against its capsule. When moderate liver congestion is present the results of liver function tests may be mildly elevated, and when liver engorgement is severe the prothrombin time may be prolonged. Ascites is a late manifestation of right ventricular failure and is most likely to occur in patients with CHF owing to constrictive pericarditis or tricuspid stenosis.

Peripheral Edema

Peripheral edema, which is usually dependent and often characterized as pitting, is an early sign of right ventricular failure. It reflects a combination of venous congestion and sodium and water retention. Ankle edema caused by local venous or lymphatic obstruction, cirrhosis of the liver, or hypoalbuminemia is differentiated from similar edema attributable to right ventricular failure by the absence of jugular venous distension with inspiration.

THERAPEUTIC GOALS IN THE MANAGEMENT OF CONGESTIVE HEART FAILURE

Short-term therapeutic goals in patients with CHF are to relieve symptoms of circulatory congestion, increase tissue perfusion, and improve the quality of life.[2] Long-term therapeutic goals are to prolong life by slowing or reversing the progressive left ventricular dysfunction (ventricular remodeling) that results in a dilated ventricular chamber and the low ejection fraction that is characteristic of CHF. At present, there are no reliable measures of the effectiveness of therapy for achieving this goal.

Pharmacologic Therapy

Drugs utilized to relieve symptoms of CHF include ACE inhibitors, diuretics, peripheral vasodilators, and digitalis preparations.[2] ACE inhibitors alleviate symptoms and prolong survival in patients with CHF. Antidysrhythmia drugs are not currently recommended to suppress ventricular dysrhythmias except in the event of ventricular fibrillation. In this regard, implanted defibrillators may be a more effective therapeutic intervention. Although thromboembolism is a potential risk in patients with CHF, routine prophylactic anticoagulation is not indicated, as the incidence of thromboembolic events is low.[10] Conversely, patients with CHF who are considered to be at particularly high risk for thromboembolism (history of thromboembolism, atrial fibrillation) are likely candidates for anticoagulant therapy. First-generation calcium-blocking drugs with significant negative inotropic effects (verapamil, diltiazem, nifedipine) and nonsteroidal anti-inflammatory drugs are not likely to be recommended for patients with evidence of CHF.

ACE Inhibitors

ACE inhibitors (enalapril, captopril, ramipril) are often administered as part of the long-term therapeutic management of CHF. Enalapril may be administered to patients with low ejection fractions even in the absence of symptoms of CHF. Symptomatic relief and improved exercise tolerance may require the highest tolerated conventional dose of an ACE inhibitor. An advantage of ACE inhibitors given to relieve symptoms of CHF is conservation of potassium by decreasing aldosterone secretion. Side effects of ACE inhibitors include hypotension (usually moderate and asymptomatic), azotemia (serum creatinine concentrations greater than 2.5 mg/dl), and development of a nonproductive cough. The combination of hydralazine and isosorbide dinitrate is useful for improving exercise tolerance and survival in patients with CHF who cannot tolerate or who do not respond to ACE inhibitors.

Diuretics

Diuretics can relieve circulatory congestion and the accompanying pulmonary and peripheral edema.[2] Drug-induced decreases in atrial and ventricular diastolic pressures may subsequently decrease diastolic stress on the ventricular wall, thereby preventing the persistent cardiac distension that interferes with subendocardial perfusion and negatively affects myocardial metabolism and function. Potassium supplementation may be needed in patients treated chronically with diuretics. Alternatively, potassium-sparing diuretics may minimize potassium loss, although these drugs are not potent natriuretic diuretics. Excessive doses of diuretics may cause hypovolemia, prerenal azotemia, and an undesirably low cardiac output. In the absence of symptoms of circulatory congestion, diuretics may induce neurohormonal activation, which could have deleterious effects.

Vasodilators

Vasodilators that relax arterial and venous vascular smooth muscle result in decreased resistance to left ventricular ejection and increased venous capacitance.[2] In patients with dilated left ventricles, administration of vasodilators results in increased stroke volume and decreased ventricular filling pressures. Intravenous infusion of nitroprusside and to a lesser extent nitroglycerin produce these pharmacologic effects. Such effects can be sustained by daily administration of hydralazine and isosorbide dinitrate or ACE inhibitors. It is not known if vasodilators administered to patients with adequate left ventricular function (remodeling of the left ventricle not yet present) results in improved survival. In the presence of symptoms of CHF due to diastolic dysfunc-

tion, administration of vasodilators that increase venous capacitance may be most effective.

Digitalis

Digitalis enhances inotropy of cardiac muscle and at the same time decreases activation of the sympathetic nervous system and the renin-angiotensin system. The latter effects are related to the ability of digitalis to restore the inhibitory effects of cardiac baroreceptors on the sympathetic nervous system outflow from the central nervous system. The therapeutic efficacy of digoxin in patients with CHF and normal sinus rhythm is controversial.[2] The suggestion that digoxin has an adverse effect on survival has not been substantiated. Digoxin has not been shown to benefit patients with asymptomatic left ventricular dysfunction. When digoxin is administered to patients with normal sinus rhythm, the dose should be adjusted to avoid the risk of toxic effects. In this regard, measurement of serum digoxin concentrations is not usually necessary to ensure maintenance of nontoxic serum concentrations. Digoxin is excreted primarily by the kidneys, and its clearance (normally about one-third of the daily dose) is closely related to creatinine clearance. In this regard, daily doses of digoxin should be adjusted to replace the drug eliminated by the kidneys. Sensitivity to digoxin can be increased during the perioperative period if there are associated decreases in renal function.

Prophylactic Administration of Digitalis

Prophylactic administration of digoxin to patients scheduled for elective operations without evidence of CHF is controversial. The disadvantage of such prophylaxis is administration of a drug with a small therapeutic-to-toxic dose difference to patients with no clinical indications for the drug. Furthermore, differentiation of anesthetic-induced cardiac dysrhythmias from those due to digitalis toxicity may be difficult.[11] Indeed, such events as increased sympathetic nervous system activity, decreased serum potassium concentrations, and decreased renal function are likely to occur intraoperatively, thereby enhancing the chances of increased pharmacologic effects from circulating digitalis. Despite these theoretical disadvantages, there is evidence that patients with limited cardiac reserves may benefit from prophylactic administration of digoxin. For example, preoperative administration of digoxin (0.75 mg PO in divided doses the day before surgery and 0.25 mg before induction of anesthesia) decreases the incidence of atrial fibrillation in elderly patients undergoing thoracic or abdominal surgery.[12] Prophylactic digoxin also decreases evidence of impaired cardiac function in patients with ischemic heart disease who are recovering from anesthesia (Fig. 6–4).[13] Therefore it is reasonable to conclude that the beneficial effects of prophylactic digoxin administered to selected patients outweigh the potential risk of digitalis toxicity. Certainly, there are no data to support discontinuing digoxin preoperatively, especially if the drug is being administered for heart rate control.

Digitalis Toxicity

Digitalis toxicity is always a hazard in patients being treated with this drug. Factors that predispose to digitalis toxicity are hypokalemia, hypercalcemia, hypomagnesemia, and arterial hypoxemia. During the preoperative period, digitalis toxicity should be suspected in patients who complain of anorexia or nausea, especially if hypokalemia is also present.

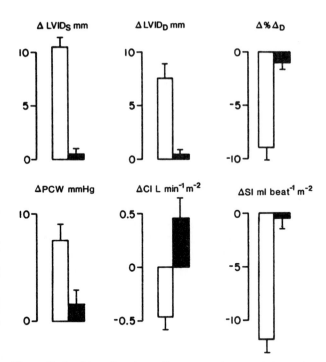

Figure 6–4 • M-mode echocardiograms and systemic hemodynamics were measured in patients with ischemic heart disease and receiving digoxin (10 μg/kg IV) 48, 24, and 3 hours before surgery (*solid bars*) or not receiving digoxin (*clear bars*). Values represent differences in preoperative and postoperative measurements. CI, cardiac index; LVID, left ventricular dimensions during systole (S) or diastole (D); PCW, pulmonary capillary wedge; SI, stroke index. (Redrawn from Pinaud MLF, Blanloeil YAG, Souron RJ. Preoperative prophylactic digitalization of patients with coronary artery disease—a randomized echocardiographic and hemodynamic study. Anesth Analg 1983;62:865–9, with permission.)

Cardiac Manifestations of Digitalis Toxicity. Cardiac dysrhythmias are the first evidence of digitalis toxicity in about one-third of patients. Although no specific cardiac dysrhythmia is pathognomonic for digitalis toxicity, ventricular premature beats (particularly bigeminy) and various forms of atrioventricular heart block are common. Depression of ST segments and T waves on the ECG are nonspecific changes that do not necessarily indicate digitalis toxicity. Ventricular fibrillation is the most frequent cause of death due to digitalis toxicity.

Treatment of Digitalis-Induced Cardiac Dysrhythmias. Treatment of digitalis toxicity includes the correction of predisposing events (especially hypokalemia), administration of drugs (lidocaine, phenytoin, atropine) to treat cardiac dysrhythmias, and insertion of a temporary transvenous pacemaker if complete heart block is present.

Plasma Digitalis Concentration. The wide range of overlap between therapeutic and toxic plasma concentrations of digoxin (therapeutic plasma concentrations 1.0 to 1.5 ng/ml) has cast doubt on the usefulness of the plasma digoxin concentration as the sole indicator of digitalis toxicity. Nevertheless, serum digoxin concentrations above 3 ng/ml usually reflect a toxic level of the drug.

Surgery in the Presence of Digitalis Toxicity. Proceeding with anesthesia and surgery in the presence of suspected or confirmed digitalis toxicity depends entirely on the urgency of the surgery. Certainly, elective operations should be delayed until digitalis toxicity subsides. When the surgical disease is life-threatening, it is necessary to proceed with the operative procedure despite digitalis toxicity. In this situation, events or drugs, such as ketamine, that stimulate the sympathetic nervous system should be avoided. Halothane, and by inference other volatile anesthetics, has been shown to antagonize the cardiac effects of digitalis in animals.[14] This finding suggests that a volatile anesthetic is a reasonable choice in the presence of digitalis toxicity. Hyperventilation of the lungs, which can acutely lower serum potassium concentrations, must be avoided. Drugs to treat digitalis-induced cardiac dysrhythmias must be readily available (see "Treatment of Digitalis-Induced Cardiac Dysrhythmias"). Calcium decreases binding of digitalis to cardiac tissues and thus directly antagonizes the cardiotoxic effects of digitalis preparations. Conversely, potassium intensifies digitalis-induced heart block and depresses the automaticity of ectopic pacemakers in the ventricles, leading to complete heart block. This emphasizes the importance of measuring the serum potassium concentration before administering supplemental potassium. If renal function is normal and heart block is not present, it is acceptable to administer potassium (0.025 to 0.050 mEq/kg IV) to suppress life-threatening cardiac dysrhythmias associated with digitalis toxicity.

Lidocaine (0.5 to 1.0 mg/kg IV) is useful as the initial treatment of digitalis-induced ventricular irritability not accompanied by hypokalemia. Therapeutic serum concentrations of lidocaine suppress ectopic ventricular cardiac pacemakers without affecting myocardial contractility or prolonging conduction of cardiac impulses through the atrioventricular node. Lidocaine is not highly effective in the management of digitalis-induced supraventricular dysrhythmias. For treatment of these cardiac dysrhythmias the drug of choice is phenytoin, 20 mg/min IV, until cardiac dysrhythmias disappear or a total dose of 1000 mg is reached. Atropine can be administered to increase the heart rate by offsetting excessive parasympathetic nervous system activity produced by a toxic plasma concentration of digitalis. Propranolol effectively suppresses the increased cardiac automaticity produced by digitalis toxicity, but its tendency to slow conduction of cardiac impulses through the atrioventricular node limits its usefulness when conduction block is present. When the heart rate remains slow despite appropriate drug therapy, it may be necessary to insert a temporary transvenous cardiac pacemaker.

Life-threatening digitalis toxicity can be treated by administering antibodies (Fab fragments) to the drug, thereby decreasing the plasma concentration of digitalis available to attach to cardiac cell membranes. External electrical cardioversion must be used with caution in the treatment of digitalis-induced supraventricular dysrhythmias, as even more severe cardiac dysrhythmias, including ventricular fibrillation, have occurred after this treatment in the presence of digitalis toxicity.

Nonpharmacologic Management

Sodium restriction effectively decreases the patient's requirements for diuretics. Regular exercise prevents deconditioning and enhances the quality of life. It is unknown if regular exercise alters the progressive remodeling of the left ventricle associated with chronic CHF. Recurrent episodes of CHF due to left ventricular ischemia may be treated with angioplasty or bypass surgery. Increasingly severe symptoms in the presence of correctable cardiac valve lesions may be alleviated surgically. Heart transplantation can be dramatically effective, but the limited supply of donors renders this treatment unrealistic in most patients.

Ventricular assist devices (extracorporeal membrane oxygenation, implantable pulsatile devices) are mechanical pumps that take over function of the damaged ventricle and facilitate restoration of normal hemodynamics and end-organ blood flow.[5] These devices are most useful in patients who require ventricular assistance to allow the heart to rest and recover its function (unload the left ventricle, decrease myocardial work, improve subendocardial perfusion) and those who require mechanical support while awaiting heart transplantation. Bleeding, right-sided heart failure, venous air embolism, thromboembolism, infections, and progressive multisystem organ failure are the most common causes of morbidity and mortality associated with the use of left ventricular assist devices.[5]

New Management Approaches

The steady progression of CHF and high mortality despite conventional pharmacologic therapy has led to interest in the possible efficacy of other drug therapies.[2] For example, β-adrenergic antagonists such as metoprolol, despite their potentially adverse effect on left ventricular function, have a favorable effect on the course and prognosis of some patients experiencing CHF. Second-generation β-adrenergic antagonists that also have vasodilating effects may delay the progression of CHF and protect against sudden death. Calcium-blocking drugs such as felodipine and amlodipine with greater vasodilating effects than first-generation calcium-blocking drugs may augment vasodilation induced by ACE inhibitors. It is possible that drugs that inhibit the sympathetic nervous system or the renin-angiotensin system may be efficacious in the management of CHF.

SURGERY IN THE PRESENCE OF CONGESTIVE HEART FAILURE

Elective operations are not recommended for patients with evidence of CHF. In fact, the presence of CHF has been described as the single most important factor for predicting postoperative cardiac morbidity.[15] If surgery cannot be delayed, drugs and techniques chosen to provide anesthesia are often selected with the goal of optimizing cardiac output. Dehydration or fluid overload during the perioperative period may contribute to the development of CHF.

General Anesthesia

Ketamine is useful for induction of anesthesia in the presence of CHF. Volatile anesthetics must be administered cautiously in view of the dose-dependent cardiac depressant effects associated with these drugs. Cardiac depression produced by the combined effects of volatile anesthetics and CHF is greater than that present in the absence of CHF (Fig. 6–3).[9] Opioids, benzodiazepines, and possibly etomidate are acceptable considerations, as they produce little or no direct myocardial depression. It must be remembered, however, that addition of nitrous oxide to opioids or the combination of benzodiazepines and opioids is associated with significant depression of cardiac output and systemic blood pressure.[16, 17] Propofol causes greater decreases in systemic blood pressure than thiopental, but this is more likely due to peripheral vasodilation than direct myocardial depression.

In the presence of severe CHF, the use of opioids as the only drug for maintenance of anesthesia may be justified. Positive-pressure ventilation of the lungs may be beneficial by decreasing pulmonary congestion and improving arterial oxygenation. Monitoring is adjusted to the complexity of the operation. Invasive monitoring of arterial pressure and cardiac filling pressures (pulmonary artery catheter, transesophageal echocardiography) is justified when a major operation is necessary in the presence of CHF. Support of cardiac output with drugs such as dopamine or dobutamine may be necessary during the perioperative period.

Drug interactions in patients treated with digitalis should be anticipated. For example, succinylcholine or other drugs that can abruptly increase parasympathetic nervous system activity could theoretically have additive effects with digitalis. Nevertheless, clinical experience does not support the occurrence of an increased incidence of cardiac dysrhythmias in patients treated with digitalis and receiving succinylcholine.[18] Sympathomimetics with β-agonist effects and pancuronium may increase the likelihood of cardiac dysrhythmias in patients treated with digitalis. Calcium may accentuate the effects of previously therapeutic serum concentrations of digitalis. Hyperventilation of the lungs, which acutely lowers the serum potassium concentration, must be avoided in patients treated with digitalis.

Regional Anesthesia

Regional anesthesia is acceptable for peripheral operations in the presence of CHF. In fact, modest decreases in systemic vascular resistance secondary to peripheral sympathetic nervous system blockade may permit increased cardiac output. Nevertheless, decreased systemic vascular resistance produced by epidural or spinal anesthesia is not predictable or easy to control. Therefore regional anesthesia should probably not be selected over general anesthesia if the only reason is the belief that regional anesthesia improves cardiac output.

References

1. Givertz MM. Underlying causes and survival in patients with heart failure. N Engl J Med 2000;342:1120–2
2. Cohn JN. The management of chronic heart failure. N Engl J Med 1996;335:490–8
3. SOLVD Investigators. Effect of enalapril on survival in patients with reduced left ventricular ejection fractions and congestive heart failure. N Engl J Med 1991;325:293–302
4. Guidelines for the evaluation and management of heart failure: report of the American College of Cardiology / American Heart Association Task Force on Practice Guidelines (Committee on Evaluation and Management of Heart Failure). Circulation 1995;92:2764–84
5. Goldstein DJ, Oz MC, Rose EA. Implantable left ventricular assist devices. N Engl J Med 1998;339:1522–33
6. Dec GW, Hutter AM. Congestive heart failure. Sci Am Med 1998;1–17
7. Vasan RFS, Benjamin EJ. Diastolic heart failure: no time to relax. N Engl J Med 2001;344:56–9
8. Burt VL, Culter JA, Higgins M, et al. Trends in the prevalence, awareness, treatment, and control of hypertension in the adult US population: data from the health examination surveys, 1960–91. Hypertension 1995;26:60–9
9. Kemmotsu O, Hashimoto Y, Shimosato S. The effects of halothane, enflurane and isoflurane on contractile performance of isolated papillary muscles from failing hearts. Anesthesiology 1974;40:252–60
10. Tchou PJ, Kadri N, Anderson J, et al. Automatic implantable cardioverter defibrillators and survival of patients with left ventricular dysfunction and malignant ventricular arrhythmias. Ann Intern Med 1988;109:529–34
11. Chung DC. Anaesthetic problems associated with the treatment of cardiovascular disease. I. Digitalis toxicity. Can Anaesth Soc J 1981;28:6–16
12. Chee TP, Prakash NS, Desser KB, et al. Postoperative supraventricular arrhythmias and the role of prophylactic digoxin in cardiac surgery. Am Heart J 1982;104:974–7
13. Pinaud MLJ, Blanloeil YAG, Souron RJ. Preoperative prophylactic digitalization of patients with coronary artery disease: a randomized echocardiographic and hemodynamic study. Anesth Analg 1983;62:865–9
14. Morrow DH, Townley NT. Anesthesia and digitalis toxicity: an experimental study. Anesth Analg 1964;43:510–9
15. Goldman L, Caldera DL, Nussbaum SR, et al. Multifactorial index of cardiac risk in noncardiac surgical procedures. N Engl J Med 1977;297:845–50
16. Stoelting RK, Gibbs PS. Hemodynamic effects of morphine and morphine-nitrous oxide in valvular heart disease and coronary artery disease. Anesthesiology 1973;38:45–52
17. Tomicheck RC, Rosow CE, Philbin DM, et al. Diazepam-fentanyl interaction: hemodynamic and hormonal effects in coronary artery surgery. Anesth Analg 1983;62:881–4
18. Bartolone RS, Rao TLK. Dysrhythmias following muscle relaxant administration in patients receiving digitalis. Anesthesiology 1983;58:567–9

7

Cardiomyopathies

Cardiomyopathies comprise a diverse group of disorders characterized by myocardial dysfunction unrelated to the usual causes of heart disease, notably coronary artery disease, cardiac valve dysfunction, and essential hypertension. Common to all cardiomyopathies is progressive, life-threatening congestive heart failure. The etiology of cardiomyopathies includes many diverse factors (Table 7–1). Familial analyses have demonstrated that cardiomyopathy may have a genetic basis in children and adults.[1] Cardiomyopathies are classified on a morphologic and hemodynamic basis as (1) dilated, (2) restrictive, (3) hypertrophic, and (4) obliterative (Table 7–2). Features of more than one type of cardiomyopathy may be present in any individual.

◼ IDIOPATHIC DILATED CARDIOMYOPATHY

Idiopathic dilated cardiomyopathy is a primary myocardial disease of unknown cause characterized by left ventricular or biventricular dilation, impaired myocardial contractility, decreased cardiac output, and increased ventricular filling pressures (Table 7–2).[2] Convincing associations have been reported between idiopathic dilated cardiomyopathy and essential hypertension, the use of β-adrenergic agonists, and moderate alcohol consumption. Familial and genetic factors may be important in the etiology of idiopathic dilated cardiomyopathy, as 20% of patients with this cardiomyopathy have a first-degree relative with a decreased ejection fraction and cardiomegaly. African-Americans have an increased risk of developing idiopathic dilated cardiomyopathy. A viral etiology in some patients is suggested by the frequent occurrence of a febrile illness preceding the onset of cardiac dysfunction. Idio-

Table 7–1 • Etiology of Cardiomyopathies

Idiopathic
Ischemic
Infectious
    Viral (human immunodeficiency virus)
    Bacterial
Toxic
    Alcohol
    Daunorubicin
    Doxorubicin
    Cocaine
Systemic
    Muscular dystrophy
    Myotonic dystrophy
    Collagen vascular diseases
    Sarcoidosis
    Pheochromocytoma
    Acromegaly
    Thyrotoxicosis
    Myxedema
Infiltrative
    Amyloidosis
    Hemochromatosis
    Primary or metastatic tumors
Nutritional
Familial (genetic)

pathic dilated cardiomyopathy may occur in peripartum patients, most often manifesting 1 to 6 weeks after delivery. The clinical course is unpredictable, although most deaths occur within 3 years of the diagnosis owing to progressive congestive heart failure. Ventricular cardiac dysrhythmias and sudden death are common in patients with idiopathic dilated cardiomyopathy.

Clinical Presentation

Most patients are first seen between the ages of 20 and 50 years, although idiopathic dilated cardiomyopathy may also affect children and the elderly. The most common initial manifestation is congestive heart failure. Chest pain on exertion that may be indistinguishable from angina pectoris occurs as an initial symptom in some patients. Hemodynamic abnormalities that predict a poor prognosis include an ejection fraction of less than 0.25, left ventricular end-diastolic dilatation and a hypokinetic left ventricle on echocardiography, pulmonary capillary wedge pressures higher than 20 mmHg, a cardiac index less than 2.5 L/min/m^2, systemic hypotension, pulmonary hypertension, and increased central venous pressure. Ventricular dilation may be so marked that functional mitral or tricuspid regurgitation occurs. The electrocardiogram (ECG) is likely to show evidence of left ventricular hypertrophy, ST and T wave abnormalities, and bundle branch block. Cardiac dysrhythmias are common and include ventricular premature beats and atrial fibrillation. Chest radiographs may show evidence of cardiac enlargement involving all four cardiac chambers, with ventricular dilatation being the most distinguishing morphologic feature of idiopathic dilated cardiomyopathy. Systemic embolization is common, reflecting formation of mural thrombi in dilated and hypokinetic cardiac chambers.

Treatment

General supportive measures include adequate rest, weight control, abstinence from tobacco use, moder-

Table 7–2 • Classification of Cardiomyopathies on Morphologic and Hemodynamic Basis

Parameter	Classification, by Type of Cardiomyopathy			
	Dilated	Restrictive	Hypertrophic	Obliterative
Morphology	Biventricular dilation	Decreased ventricular compliance	Hypertrophy of left ventricle and usually interventricular septum	Thickened endocardium or mural thrombi
Ventricular volume	Marked increase	Normal to modest increase	Normal to modest decrease	Modest decrease
Ejection fraction	Marked decrease	Normal to modest decrease	Marked increase	Normal to modest decrease
Ventricular compliance	Normal to modest decrease	Marked decrease	Marked decrease	Marked decrease
Ventricular filling pressure	Marked increase	Marked increase	Normal to modest increase	Modest increase
Stroke volume	Marked decrease	Normal to modest decrease	Normal to modest increase	Normal to modest decrease

ation of alcohol consumption, and decreased physical activity during periods of cardiac decompensation.[2] Vasodilator therapy is considered the standard initial treatment for patients with symptomatic left ventricular dysfunction due to idiopathic dilated cardiomyopathy. Clinical trials have confirmed the efficacy of certain vasodilators, particularly the angiotensin-converting enzyme (ACE) inhibitor enalapril, and smooth muscle-relaxing drugs such as hydralazine and isosorbide dinitrate.

Patients with idiopathic dilated cardiomyopathy are at risk for systemic or pulmonary embolization because blood stasis in the hypocontractile ventricle leads to activation of coagulation processes. The risk is greatest in patients with severe left ventricular dysfunction, atrial fibrillation, a history of thromboembolism, or echocardiographic evidence of thrombus. For this reason anticoagulation with warfarin may be instituted in patients with idiopathic dilated cardiomyopathy and symptomatic congestive heart failure. Long-term anticoagulation is often adjusted to prolong the prothrombin time to an international normalized ratio of 2.0 to 3.0.

Although asymptomatic, nonsustained ventricular tachycardia is common in patients with idiopathic dilated cardiomyopathy, suppression of this cardiac dysrhythmia with drug therapy does not improve survival. Indeed, antidysrhythmia therapy for suppression of asymptomatic ventricular cardiac dysrhythmias may introduce the risk of life-threatening cardiac dysrhythmias. Placing an automatic cardioverter-defibrillator can decrease the risk of sudden death in patients with congestive heart failure who have survived a prior cardiac arrest and in whom pharmacologic therapy has failed.

Digitalis effectively controls the symptoms of congestive heart failure in patients with idiopathic dilated cardiomyopathy and normal sinus rhythm. Unlike digitalis, oral inotropic drugs (amrinone, milrinone, enoxamine) do not predictably improve exercise tolerance when administered alone or in combination with digitalis.

Idiopathic dilated cardiomyopathy remains the principal indication for heart transplantation in adults and children.[2] Patients most likely to benefit from heart transplantation are formerly vigorous persons under the age of 60 years with intractable symptoms of congestive heart failure despite optimal medical therapy. Transplantation is usually deferred in patients with moderate symptoms or in those with idiopathic dilated cardiomyopathy of less than 6 months' duration, as substantial improvement in ventricular performance may occur spontaneously.

Management of Anesthesia

Goals during the management of anesthesia in patients with idiopathic dilated cardiomyopathy include (1) avoidance of drug-induced myocardial depression, (2) maintenance of normovolemia, and (3) prevention of increased ventricular afterload. Excessive cardiovascular depression in response to induction of anesthesia in patients with a history of alcohol abuse may reflect unsuspected idiopathic dilated cardiomyopathy.[3] Conversely, when the expected sedative responses fail to occur after intravenous injection, it may reflect a slow circulation time. These patients are vulnerable to drug overdoses if additional drugs are administered on the erroneous assumption that an inadequate dose was injected. During maintenance of anesthesia, the dose-dependent direct myocardial depression produced by volatile anesthetics must be considered, although the vasodilating properties of certain volatile anesthetics are theoretically desirable. Opioids are associated with benign effects on cardiac contractility but when used alone may not produce unconsciousness. Administration of opioids with nitrous oxide or benzodiazepines may result in unexpected depression of myocardial contractility. Surgical stimulation that produces undesirable increases in heart rate may be treated with β-antagonists such as esmolol, keeping in mind the potential for these drugs to cause cardiac depression. Skeletal muscle paralysis is provided by nondepolarizing muscle relaxants that lack significant cardiovascular effects. Intravenous infusion of crystalloid solutions or blood should be guided by cardiac filling pressures to decrease the likelihood of volume overload. By permitting determination of cardiac output and cardiac filling pressures, a pulmonary artery catheter facilitates early recognition of the need for inotropic support or administration of peripheral vasodilating drugs. Prominent A waves on venous pressure tracings reflect decreased ventricular compliance, whereas prominent V waves reflect functional incompetence of the tricuspid or mitral valves owing to cardiac dilation. Intraoperative hypotension is logically treated with vasopressors such as ephedrine, which provide some degree of β-stimulation. Conversely, predominant α-stimulation, as produced by phenylephrine, could theoretically evoke adverse increases in left ventricular afterload, owing to increased systemic vascular resistance.

Regional anesthesia may be an alternative to general anesthesia in selected patients with idiopathic dilated cardiomyopathy.[4] For example, epidural anesthesia produces changes in preload and afterload that mimic pharmacologic goals in the treatment of idiopathic dilated cardiomyopathy. Clinical experience is limited, however, and caution is indicated to avoid an abrupt onset of blockade of sympathetic nervous system innervation.

■ RESTRICTIVE CARDIOMYOPATHY

Restrictive cardiomyopathy is the least common of the cardiomyopathies, with cardiac amyloidosis and idiopathic disease being the most common etiologies in the United States. The diagnosis of restrictive cardiomyopathy should be considered in patients presenting with congestive heart failure but no evidence of cardiomegaly or systolic dysfunction. The condition usually results from increased stiffness of the myocardium, which causes pressures within the ventricles to increase precipitously with only small increases in volume.[5] There is impaired ventricular filling, but systolic function usually remains normal. Because restrictive cardiomyopathy affects both ventricles, it may cause symptoms and signs of right and/or left ventricular failure.

Clinical Presentation

The clinical presentation in patients with restrictive cardiomyopathy may resemble constrictive pericarditis (Table 7–2) (see Chapter 9). A clinical history suggestive of pericarditis makes the diagnosis of constrictive pericarditis more likely. In contrast to the eventual equalization of cardiac filling pressures that characterize constrictive pericarditis, restrictive cardiomyopathy tends to cause more impairment of left than right ventricular filling (left ventricular end-diastolic pressures are often higher than right ventricular end-diastolic pressures). As a result, left heart filling pressures are typically higher than those recorded on the right side of the heart. In advanced cases all the signs of congestive heart failure are present except cardiomegaly. Peripheral edema and ascites are present in advanced cases. Idiopathic restrictive cardiomyopathy often presents with thromboembolic complications. Cardiac conduction disturbances are particularly common with amyloidosis and sarcoidosis. Atrial fibrillation is common in patients with idiopathic restrictive cardiomyopathy and cardiac amyloidosis. Angina pectoris does not occur except in those with amyloidosis, where it may be the presenting symptom. In elderly patients restrictive cardiomyopathy remains a diagnosis of exclusion and it must be differentiated from age-related changes in diastolic compliance.[5]

Treatment

Symptomatic treatment of restrictive cardiomyopathy includes administration of diuretics to treat venous congestion in the pulmonary and systemic circulations. Excessive effects of diuretics may decrease ventricular filling pressures, leading to decreased cardiac output, hypoperfusion, and hypotension. Digoxin is used with caution, as it is potentially dysrhythmogenic, especially in patients with amyloidosis. The development of atrial fibrillation with removal of the atrial contribution to ventricular filling may worsen existing diastolic dysfunction, and rapid ventricular responses may further compromise cardiac output. Maintenance of normal sinus rhythm is important, and medications such as amiodarone may be needed for this purpose.[5] If cardioversion is utilized to treat atrial fibrillation, particularly in the presence of amyloidosis, the abnormal sinus node may fail as an effective pacemaker. When cardiac conduction system disease is severe, implantation of an artificial external pacemaker may be considered. With cardiac sarcoidosis, malignant ventricular dysrhythmias are common and may necessitate treatment with an implantable defibrillator. Because stroke volume tends to be fixed in the presence of restrictive cardiomyopathy, the onset of bradycardia may precipitate acute congestive heart failure. Anticoagulation with warfarin is likely in view of the risk of embolic complications, especially in patients with atrial fibrillation and low cardiac output. Cardiac transplantation may be a consideration in patients with refractory symptoms due to idiopathic restrictive cardiomyopathy. Conversely, cardiac transplantation is not usually considered a viable option in patients with restrictive cardiomyopathy due to systemic disorders (amyloidosis, sarcoidosis), as the disease may recur in the transplanted heart.

Management of Anesthesia

Management of anesthesia for patients with restrictive cardiomyopathy utilizes the same principles described for patients with cardiac tamponade (see Chapter 9). Because stroke volume is relatively fixed, it is important to sustain a normal sinus rhythm and avoid abrupt decreases in the heart rate. Maintenance of venous return and intravascular fluid volume is essential for maintaining cardiac output. The presence of anticoagulation may influence the decision to select regional anesthesia.

■ HYPERTROPHIC CARDIOMYOPATHY

Hypertrophic cardiomyopathy is a complex cardiac disease with unique pathophysiologic characteristics and a great diversity of morphologic, functional, and clinical features.[6] The disease affects patients of all ages, and the prevalence in the general population may approach 1 in 500. As such, hypertrophic cardiomyopathy can be viewed as a common genetic malformation of the heart. The disease may be caused by a mutation in one of four genes that encode proteins in the cardiac sarcomere. There are numerous other mutations as well that may occur in the genes of the sarcomere such that the precise molecular defect responsible for hypertrophic cardiomyopathy often differs in unrelated patients.

Clinical Presentation

The clinical course varies widely, with most patients remaining asymptomatic throughout life; some have symptoms of severe congestive heart failure, however, and others die suddenly presumably due to ventricular tachydysrhythmias, often in the absence of previous symptoms (see "Sudden Death"). The principal symptoms of hypertrophic cardiomyopathy are angina pectoris, syncope (may represent aborted sudden death), tachydysrhythmias, and congestive heart failure. Angina pectoris relieved by assumption of the recumbent position is suggestive of hypertrophic cardiomyopathy, presumably reflecting an increase in left ventricular size that accompanies this position change, which decreases left ventricular outflow obstruction.

Massive cardiac hypertrophy (maximal wall thickness of 35 mm or more) in adults is characteristic of hypertrophic cardiomyopathy. Echocardiography reveals a large variation in the location and extent of the cardiac hypertrophy. In its severest form, there is hypertrophy of the left ventricular chamber, which becomes elongated and slit-like (Table 7–2). Even in the presence of severe left ventricular outflow obstruction, ejection fractions are usually more than 0.8, reflecting the hypercontractile condition of the heart. Marked left ventricular hypertrophy makes these patients particularly vulnerable to myocardial ischemia, especially when endocardial blood flow is decreased because of excessive pressures in the left ventricle. Mitral regurgitation reflects interference with movement of the septal leaflet of the mitral valve by the hypertrophied interventricular septum. Alternatively, septal hypertrophy may result in left ventricular outflow obstruction that is constant or intermittent (dynamic). The degree of left ventricular outflow obstruction is influenced by (1) myocardial contractility, (2) preload, and (3) afterload (Table 7–2).

Cardiac murmurs may reflect the presence of left ventricular outflow obstruction or mitral regurgitation in patients with hypertrophic cardiomyopathy. Indeed, hypertrophic cardiomyopathy may be confused with aortic or mitral valve disease. Characteristic of these murmurs is their marked variation with different maneuvers. For example, the Valsalva maneuver decreases the left ventricular chamber size, which then increases left ventricular outflow obstruction. In addition, because left ventricular systolic pressures increase, the murmur of mitral regurgitation intensifies as well. Nitroglycerin and standing (versus recumbency) likewise increases the loudness of the murmur. Hypertrophic cardiomyopathy should be considered in otherwise asymptomatic patients in whom a systolic murmur develops during long-standing systemic hypertension.

Chest radiographs and the ECG typically depict left ventricular hypertrophy. In asymptomatic patients, marked unexplained left ventricular hypertrophy may be the only sign of the disease. Because of massive hypertrophy of the interventricular septum, abnormal Q waves resembling those seen with myocardial infarction may be present on the ECG. The diagnosis of hypertrophic cardiomyopathy should be considered in young patients whose ECGs suggest a prior myocardial infarction, although as many as 15% of patients with hypertrophic cardiomyopathy show no evidence of left ventricular hypertrophy on the ECG. Systemic embolization is a common complication of atrial fibrillation in patients with hypertrophic cardiomyopathy.

Echocardiography is useful for demonstrating asymmetrical hypertrophy of the interventricular septum and for estimating pressure gradients across the left ventricular outflow tract. When the septal thickness/left ventricular free wall thickness ratio exceeds 1.3 : 1.0, a diagnosis of hypertrophic cardiomyopathy should be considered.

Cardiac catheterization may demonstrate evidence of mitral regurgitation or the presence of increased left ventricular end-diastolic pressures as a consequence of decreased left ventricular compliance. Decreased left ventricular compliance produces increases in the height of A waves on the venous pressure tracing that may exceed 30 mmHg. If left ventricular outflow obstruction is present, there are demonstrable pressure gradients between the left ventricle and aorta. Provocative measures such as Valsalva maneuvers may be required to evoke evidence of left ventricular outflow obstruction during echocardiography or cardiac catheterization, emphasizing the dynamic nature of this obstruction. Left ventricular angiography characteristically shows a small hyperdynamic chamber.

Sudden Death

Sudden death is a recognized complication of hypertrophic cardiomyopathy. In this regard, the magnitude of hypertrophic cardiomyopathy is directly related to the risk of sudden death and is a strong, independent predictor of the prognosis.[7] Young individuals with massive hypertrophy and even those with few or no symptoms deserve consideration for an intervention to prevent sudden death. Most patients with mild hypertrophy are at low risk for sudden death. Sudden death due to fatal cardiac dysrhythmias is especially likely to occur in patients between the ages of 10 and 30 years. For this reason, there is general agreement that known afflicted patients should not participate in competitive sports because of the risk of sudden death.

Treatment

The diverse clinical and genetic features of hypertrophic cardiomyopathy make it impossible to define precise guidelines for management (Fig. 7–1).[6] Despite the difficulty of establishing a prognosis in patients with hypertrophic cardiomyopathy, it is

recognized that some of these patients are at high risk for sudden death and must be treated aggressively. Pharmacologic therapy to improve diastolic filling and possibly decrease myocardial ischemia is the primary means of relieving the symptoms of hypertrophic cardiomyopathy. This is the only therapeutic option for patients without left ventricular outflow obstruction, who comprise most of the patients with hypertrophic cardiomyopathy. Invasive interventions to remove the outflow gradient surgically are considered in only about 5% of patients who have both marked outflow obstruction and severe symptoms unresponsive to medical therapy.[6]

Medical Therapy

β-Adrenergic blocking drugs and verapamil have been used extensively to treat hypertrophic cardiomyopathy.[6] The beneficial effects of β-blockers on dyspnea, angina pectoris, and exercise tolerance are likely due to the decreased heart rate with conse-

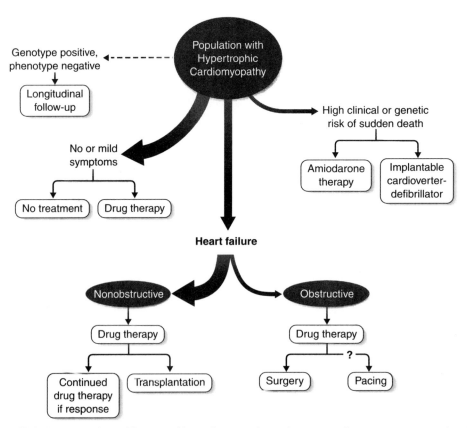

Figure 7–1 • Clinical presentations of hypertrophic cardiomyopathy and corresponding treatment strategies. Size of the *arrows* indicates the approximate proportion of patients in each subgroup. *Dashed arrow* indicates uncertainties as to the size of this subgroup. (From Spirito P, Seidman CE, McKenna WJ, et al. The management of hypertrophic cardiomyopathy. N Engl J Med 1997;336:775–85. Copyright 1997 Massachusetts Medical Society, with permission.)

quent prolongation of diastole and increased passive ventricular filling. β-Blockers may also lessen myocardial oxygen requirements and decrease the outflow gradient during exercise and increased sympathetic nervous system activity. Verapamil has beneficial effects on symptoms of hypertrophic cardiomyopathy because it improves ventricular filling and likely decreases myocardial ischemia. Patients who develop congestive heart failure despite treatment with β-blockers or verapamil may improve with the addition of diuretics. However, because many of these patients have diastolic dysfunction and require relatively high filling pressures to achieve adequate ventricular filling, it is necessary to administer diuretics with caution. There is no evidence that a β-blocker or verapamil protects patients with hypertrophic cardiomyopathy from sudden death. For patients with hypertrophic cardiomyopathy who are considered to be at high risk for sudden death from ventricular tachydysrhythmias, the available therapeutic options (amiodarone, implantable cardioverter-defibrillator) are the same as for patients with coronary artery disease or idiopathic dilated cardiomyopathy.[6]

Atrial fibrillation is an important cardiac dysrhythmia because it often develops in patients with hypertrophic cardiomyopathy and is associated with an increased risk of thromboembolism, congestive heart failure, and sudden death.[6] Paroxysmal episodes of atrial fibrillation may cause rapid clinical deterioration by decreasing diastolic filling and cardiac output, usually as a consequence of the rapid ventricular rate. In contrast, chronic atrial fibrillation is often well tolerated if the heart rate is adequately controlled. Amiodarone is considered the most effective antidysrhythmia drug for the prevention of recurrences of atrial fibrillation. β-Blockers and verapamil can usually control the heart rate in patients with chronic atrial fibrillation. Anticoagulant therapy is indicated in those with recurrent or chronic atrial fibrillation.

Surgical Therapy

The small subgroup of patients with hypertrophic cardiomyopathy who have both large outflow gradients (50 mmHg or more) and severe symptoms of congestive heart failure despite medical therapy are candidates for surgery.[6] Surgical reduction of the outflow gradient is usually achieved by removing a small amount of cardiac muscle from the ventricular septum (myotomy-myectomy). Replacement of the mitral valve has been used as an alternative to myotomy-myectomy. Surgery abolishes or greatly decreases left ventricular outflow gradients in most patients. Intraoperative echocardiography is useful for determining the extent of surgical resection and for defining mitral valve structure. Marked decreases in the intraventricular systolic and end-diastolic pressures are the most tangible consequence of surgery, which may favorably influence left ventricular filling and myocardial oxygen requirements.[6]

Nonsurgical Techniques to Relieve Left Ventricular Outflow Obstruction

Dual chamber pacing may be associated with a decrease in the outflow gradients and symptomatic improvement in patients with hypertrophic cardiomyopathy who are unresponsive to medical therapy. Not all reports, however, suggest favorable responses to this nonsurgical intervention.[8]

Management of Anesthesia

Management of anesthesia in patients with hypertrophic cardiomyopathy is directed toward minimizing left ventricular outflow obstruction. In this regard, any drug or event that decreases myocardial contractility or that increases preload or afterload decreases the left ventricular outflow obstruction (Table 7–3). For example, dose-dependent cardiac depression produced by volatile anesthetics and

Table 7–3 • Factors Influencing Left Ventricular Outflow Obstruction in Patients with Hypertrophic Cardiomyopathy

Events that increase outflow obstruction
  Increased myocardial contractility
    β-Adrenergic stimulation (catecholamines)
    Digitalis
    Tachycardia
  Decreased preload
    Hypovolemia
    Vasodilators (nitroglycerin, nitroprusside)
    Tachycardia
    Positive-pressure ventilation
  Decreased afterload
    Hypotension
    Vasodilators
    Hypovolemia
Events that decrease outflow obstruction
  Decreased myocardial contractility
    β-Adrenergic blockade (esmolol)
    Volatile anesthetics (halothane)
    Calcium entry blockers
  Increased preload
    Hypervolemia
    Bradycardia
  Increased afterload
    α-Adrenergic stimulation (phenylephrine)
    Hypervolemia

expansion of the intravascular fluid volume distends the left ventricle and increases stoke volume. Conversely, intraoperative events associated with increased myocardial contractility are not desirable, as these events may increase left ventricular outflow obstruction (Table 7–3). Overall, the risk associated with general anesthesia seems acceptable in patients with hypertrophic cardiomyopathy.[9] However, anesthesia and surgery in patients with previously unrecognized hypertrophic cardiomyopathy may manifest intraoperatively as unexpected hypotension and sudden increases in the intensity of a systolic murmur, typically in association with acute hemorrhage or drug-induced vasodilation.[10, 11] The incidence of ischemic heart disease is increased in these patients, which may subsequently increase the risk of anesthesia and surgery.[9]

Preoperative Medication

Ideally, preoperative medication decreases anxiety and the associated activation of the sympathetic nervous system. Administration of anticholinergic drugs such as atropine is questionable, as tachycardia could increase left ventricular outflow obstruction. Conversely, scopolamine produces desirable sedation when used in conjunction with other central nervous system depressant drugs. Changes in heart rate are unlikely after administration of scopolamine. Expansion of intravascular fluid volume during the preoperative period is useful for maintaining intraoperative stroke volume and minimizing the adverse effects of positive-pressure ventilation of the patient's lungs.

Induction of Anesthesia

Induction of anesthesia with intravenous drugs is acceptable, remembering the importance of avoiding sudden drug-induced decreases in systemic vascular resistance. Modest degrees of direct myocardial depression are acceptable. In this regard, ketamine is not a likely choice, as increased myocardial contractility could increase left ventricular outflow obstruction and decrease stroke volume. The duration of direct laryngoscopy should be brief to minimize activation of the sympathetic nervous system. Administration of volatile anesthetics or β-antagonists before initiating direct laryngoscopy is a consideration when attempting to blunt the sympathetic nervous system responses likely to be evoked by direct laryngoscopy and tracheal intubation.

Maintenance of Anesthesia

Maintenance of anesthesia is designed to produce mild depression of myocardial contractility and, at the same time, preserve intravascular fluid volume and systemic vascular resistance. Nitrous oxide combined with volatile anesthetics that predictably decrease myocardial contractility, such as halothane, is acceptable. Theoretically, other volatile anesthetics are less ideal choices than halothane, as these drugs tend to produce more peripheral vasodilation than halothane and thus decrease the calculated systemic vascular resistance. Nevertheless, there is no evidence that volatile anesthetics other than halothane are predictably detrimental when administered to patients with hypertrophic cardiomyopathy. Opioids are not a likely choice for maintenance of anesthesia, as they do not produce myocardial depression and can decrease systemic vascular resistance. The combination of opioids with nitrous oxide, however, may be associated with direct myocardial depression and modest increases in systemic vascular resistance.[12] Hemodynamic changes (hypotension, increased venous capacitance, decreased venous return) that may accompany high levels of sensory anesthesia as produced by spinal or epidural anesthesia could contribute to increases in left ventricular outflow obstruction.[13]

Nondepolarizing muscle relaxants that have minimal to no effects on the systemic circulation are logical choices for the production of skeletal muscle relaxation if needed to facilitate surgical exposure. An increased heart rate, as may accompany administration of pancuronium, is not desirable. Likewise, drug-induced histamine release and the subsequent hypotension that may occur in response to rapid intravenous injection of large doses of atracurium and possibly mivacurium are to be avoided.

Invasive monitoring of the systemic blood pressure and cardiac filling pressures is helpful. Transesophageal echocardiography and Doppler color flow imaging provide useful information, particularly with respect to intraoperative left ventricular and mitral valve function as well as intravascular fluid volume.[14] When intraoperative hypotension occurs in response to decreased preload or afterload, drugs with predominantly α-adrenergic activity, such as phenylephrine, 50 to 100 μg IV, are useful for normalizing systemic blood pressure. Drugs with β-adrenergic agonist activity, such as ephedrine, dopamine, or dobutamine, are not recommended for treating hypotension, as drug-induced increases in myocardial contractility and heart rate can increase left ventricular outflow obstruction.[11] Prompt replacement of blood loss and titration of intravenous fluid administration guided by clinical criteria, which may include measurement of cardiac filling pressures and monitoring via transesophageal echocardiography, is important for maintaining the systemic blood pressure. Increasing the delivered concentrations of volatile anesthetics is useful for treating persistent systemic hypertension. Vasodilators such as nitroprusside or nitroglycerin are not used to lower systemic blood pressure in these patients, as decreased systemic vascular resistance could accentuate left ventricular outflow obstruction (Table 7–3).

Maintenance of normal sinus rhythm in patients with hypertrophic cardiomyopathy is important, as ventricular filling is dependent on left atrial contractions. A change from sinus rhythm to junctional rhythm is treated by decreasing the delivered concentration of volatile anesthetic. If this cardiac dysrhythmia persists, intravenous administration of atropine may be helpful. β-Antagonists such as propranolol and esmolol are indicated to slow persistently increased heart rates. Controlled hypotension, as may be considered for certain intracranial and spinal operations, presents conflicting therapeutic goals for the management of patients with hypertrophic cardiomyopathy.[15]

Parturients

Pregnancy and delivery are usually well tolerated in patients with hypertrophic cardiomyopathy despite pregnancy-induced decreases in systemic vascular resistance and the risk of impaired venous return owing to uterine compression of the inferior vena cava.[16] Parturients with hypertrophic cardiomyopathy may present major anesthetic challenges at term, as events such as catecholamine release and "bearing down" (Valsalva maneuver) may increase left ventricular outflow obstruction. Many clinicians believe that regional anesthesia should be avoided in these patients because of the vasodilation associated with sympathetic nervous system blockade, which may lead to critical decreases in preload and afterload; instead, they recommend general anesthesia with a volatile anesthetic, such as halothane, in the event that cesarean section is needed. Nevertheless, epidural anesthesia has been successfully administered to these patients with emphasis on central venous pressure monitoring and maintaining euvolemia or slight hypervolemia.[16] Should hypotension unresponsive to fluid administration occur following institution of regional anesthesia, phenylephrine may be preferred to increase the afterload because of its brief duration of action. Ropivacaine has been proposed as a useful local anesthetic to produce regional anesthesia based on its lower cardiotoxicity compared with bupivacaine and slower onset (less effect on hemodynamic effects) than that of lidocaine. Oxytocin must be administered carefully because of its vasodilating properties (and compensatory tachycardia) and the abrupt inflow of large amounts of blood into the central circulation as a consequence of uterine contractions, which can adversely affect cardiac performance.[16]

Pulmonary edema has been observed in parturients with hypertrophic cardiomyopathy after delivery, emphasizing the delicate fluid requirements of these patients.[17] Treatment of pulmonary edema associated with regional anesthesia in the presence of hypertrophic cardiomyopathy may include a fluid bolus to increase venous return and esmolol to slow the heart rate, decrease myocardial contractility, and allow a prolonged diastolic filling time to decrease the left ventricular outflow obstruction.[18] Diuretics, digoxin, nitrates, or inotropes to treat pulmonary edema in this situation could worsen the edema by provoking further left ventricular outflow obstruction.

▌ OBLITERATIVE CARDIOMYOPATHY

Obliterative cardiomyopathy is considered by some to be a variant of restrictive cardiomyopathy, characterized by marked decreases in ventricular compliance (Table 7–2). This cardiomyopathy may occur in association with hypereosinophilia syndromes that are accompanied by the eosinophilic infiltration of multiple organs. Cardiac dysrhythmias, cardiac conduction disturbances, systemic embolization, and tricuspid and mitral regurgitation are common. Medical therapy may include corticosteroids.

▌ PERIPARTUM CARDIOMYOPATHY

Peripartum cardiomyopathy is a rare congestive cardiomyopathy of unknown cause that occurs during the peripartum period (defined as 1 month before full-term delivery to 5 months after delivery) in women with no history of heart disease (Table 7–4).[19] The estimated incidence of this cardiomyopathy is 1 : 3000 to 1 : 4000 live births. Risk factors for peripartum cardiomyopathy include multiparity, advanced maternal age, multifetal pregnancy, gesta-

Table 7–4 • Defining Characteristics of Peripartum Cardiomyopathy

Onset of left ventricular dysfunction during the last month of pregnancy or within 5 months of delivery
Absence of an identifiable cause
Absence of known heart disease prior to the last month of pregnancy
Left ventricular dysfunction demonstrated by echocardiography

tional hypertension, and being African-American. Possible causes of this disease include viral myocarditis, abnormal immune responses to pregnancy, and maladaptive responses to the hemodynamic stresses of pregnancy.

Diagnosis

The diagnosis of peripartum cardiomyopathy is based on the onset of unexplained left ventricular dysfunction and echocardiographic documentation of new left ventricular systolic dysfunction during the limited period surrounding parturition. The diagnosis presents a challenge, as many parturients in the final month of pregnancy experience dyspnea, fatigue, and peripheral edema. There are no specific criteria for differentiating subtle symptoms of congestive heart failure from normal late pregnancy, so it is important to maintain a high index of suspicion. Clinical conditions that may mimic congestive heart failure, such as amniotic and pulmonary emboli, should be excluded when considering the diagnosis.

Treatment

The goal of treatment is to alleviate symptoms of congestive heart failure. In this regard, diuretics, vasodilators, and digoxin are likely to be selected. ACE inhibitors are teratogenic during pregnancy but are useful for treating affected parturients following delivery. Alternatives to this class of drugs during pregnancy are hydralazine and nitrites. Thromboembolic complications are not uncommon, and the use of anticoagulants is often recommended. Heart transplantation may be considered.

Prognosis

The prognosis appears to depend on normalization of the left ventricular size and function within 6 months after delivery. The mortality rate ranges from 25% to 50%, and most deaths occur within 3 months after delivery as a result of progression of congestive heart failure or sudden death associated with cardiac dysrhythmias or thromboembolic events.

Management of Anesthesia

The management of anesthesia in parturients with peripartum cardiomyopathy requires assessment of cardiac status and careful planning of the analgesia and/or anesthesia required for delivery. Continuous intravenous infusions of remifentanil with or without propofol may be useful for providing cardiovascular stability in parturients who require cesarean section.[20] Regional anesthesia might provide desirable decreases in afterload, but associated effects on hemodynamic status may be less predictable.

References

1. Kelly DP, Strauss AW. Inherited cardiomyopathies. N Engl J Med 1994;330:913–9
2. Dec GW, Fuster V. Idiopathic dilated cardiomyopathy. N Engl J Med 1994;331:1564–75
3. Hanson CW. Asymptomatic cardiomyopathy presenting as cardiac arrest in the day surgical unit. Anesthesiology 1989;71:982–4
4. Amaranath L, Eskandiari S, Lockrem J, et al. Epidural analgesia for total hip replacement in a patient with dilated cardiomyopathy. Can Anaesth Soc J 1986;33:84–8
5. Kushwaha SS, Fallon JT, Fuster V. Restrictive cardiomyopathy. N Engl J Med 1997;336:267–76
6. Spirito P, Seidman CE, McKenna WJ, et al. The management of hypertrophic cardiomyopathy. N Engl J Med 1997;336:775–85
7. Spirito P, Bellone P, Harris KM, et al. Magnitude of left ventricular hypertrophy and risk of sudden death in hypertrophic cardiomyopathy. N Engl J Med 2000;342:1778–85
8. Nishimura RA, Trusty JM, Hayes DL, et al. Dual-chamber pacing for hypertrophic obstructive cardiomyopathy: a randomized, double-blind, crossover study. J Am Coll Cardiol 1997;29:435–41
9. Thompson RC, Liberthson RR, Lowenstein E. Perioperative anesthetic risk of noncardiac surgery in hypertrophic obstructive cardiomyopathy. N Engl J Med 1989;320:755–61
10. Lanier W, Prough DS. Intraoperative diagnosis of hypertrophic obstructive cardiomyopathy. Anesthesiology 1984;60:61–3
11. Pearson J, Reves JG. Unusual cause of hypotension after coronary artery bypass grafting: idiopathic hypertrophic subaortic stenosis. Anesthesiology 1984;60:592–4
12. Stoelting RK, Gibbs PS. Hemodynamic effects of morphine and morphine-nitrous oxide in valvular heart disease and coronary artery disease. Anesthesiology 1973;38:45–52
13. Loubser P, Suh K, Cohen S. Adverse effects of spinal anesthesia in a patient with idiopathic hypertrophic subaortic stenosis. Anesthesiology 1984;60:228–30
14. Stanley TH, Rankin JS. Idiopathic hypertrophic subaortic stenosis and ischemia mitral regurgitation: the value of intraoperative transesophageal echocardiography and Doppler color flow imaging in guiding operative therapy. Anesthesiology 1990;72:1083–5
15. Freilich JD, Jacobs BR. Anesthetic management of cerebral aneurysm resection in a patient with idiopathic hypertrophic subaortic stenosis. Anesth Analg 1990;71:558–60
16. Autore C, Brauneis S, Apponi F, et al. Epidural anesthesia for cesarean section in patients with hypertrophic cardiomyopathy: a report of three cases. Anesthesiology 1999;90:1205–7
17. Tester MY, Hudson R, Naugler-Colville MA, et al. Pulmonary oedema in two parturients with hypertrophic obstructive cardiomyopathy (HOCM). Can J Anaesth 1990;37:469–73
18. Wulfson HD, LaPorta RF. Pulmonary oedema after lithotripsy in a patient with hypertrophic subaortic stenosis. Can J Anaesth 1993;40:465–7
19. Pearson GD, Veille J-C, Rahimtoola S, et al. Peripartum cardiomyopathy. JAMA 2000;283:1183–8
20. McCarroll CP, Paxton LD, Elliott P, et al. Use of remifentanil in a patient with peripartum cardiomyopathy requiring caesarean section. Br J Anaesth 2001;86:135–8

8

Cor Pulmonale and Pulmonary Hypertension

■ COR PULMONALE

Cor pulmonale is right ventricular enlargement that develops secondary to pulmonary hypertension.[1-4] It is the third most common cardiac disorder in persons older than 50 years of age, after ischemic heart disease and hypertensive heart disease. Men are afflicted five times more often than women. It is estimated that 10% to 30% of patients admitted to the hospital with congestive heart failure (CHF) exhibit cor pulmonale.

Chronic obstructive pulmonary disease (COPD) with associated loss of pulmonary capillaries and arterial hypoxemia leading to pulmonary vascular vasoconstriction is the most likely cause of cor pulmonale. If the pulmonary vascular vasoconstriction is sustained, it produces hypertrophy of vascular smooth muscle and irreversibly increases the pulmonary vascular resistance. Alveolar hypoxia, when generalized, is the most potent known stimulus for pulmonary vasoconstriction. When alveolar hypoxia is localized, the associated pulmonary vasoconstriction (hypoxic pulmonary vasoconstriction) acts to divert blood flow to better oxygenated alveoli, thereby optimizing ventilation-to-perfusion relations and arterial oxygenation. Systemic acidosis also promotes pulmonary vasoconstriction and acts synergistically with arterial hypoxemia.

The prognosis for patients with cor pulmonale is determined by the pulmonary disease responsible for initiating the increase in pulmonary vascular resistance. In patients with COPD in whom arterial oxygenation can be maintained at near-normal levels, the prognosis for longevity is favorable. Prognosis is poor for patients in whom cor pulmonale is the result of gradual destruction of pulmonary vessels by intrinsic pulmonary vascular disease or pulmonary fibrosis. These anatomic changes produce irreversible alterations in the pulmonary vasculature, resulting in fixed increases of pulmonary vascular resistance.

Signs and Symptoms

Clinical manifestations of cor pulmonale are often nonspecific and tend to be obscured by co-existing COPD. As right ventricular function becomes more impaired, dyspnea increases and effort-related syncope may occur. Right heart catheterization demonstrates increased mean pulmonary artery pressures (higher than 20 mmHg) and normal pulmonary artery occlusion pressures. Pulmonary hypertension is considered moderate when the mean pulmonary artery pressure exceeds 35 mmHg. Accentuation of the pulmonic component of the second heart sound and a diastolic murmur due to incompetence of the pulmonic valve connote severe pulmonary artery hypertension. The A wave of the right atrial pressure tracing becomes prominent, reflecting enhanced right atrial contraction in response to decreased right ventricular compliance. Doppler ultrasonography usually demonstrates some evidence of tricuspid regurgitation, even in the absence of an audible murmur. Overt right ventricular failure is evidenced by increased jugular venous pressure, hepatosplenomegaly, and peripheral dependent edema. Patients with COPD are often cigarette smokers and are therefore likely to have ischemic heart disease, which may result in left ventricular dysfunction along with right ventricular failure.

The rate at which right ventricular dysfunction develops depends on the magnitude of pressure increases in the pulmonary circulation and on the rapidity with which this increase occurs. For example, pulmonary embolism may produce right ventricular failure with mean pulmonary artery pressures as low as 30 mmHg. By contrast, when pulmonary hypertension develops gradually, as with COPD, and the right ventricle has time to compensate, CHF rarely occurs until the mean pulmonary artery pressure exceeds 50 mmHg.[5] In patients with COPD, acute right ventricular failure may develop during pulmonary infections. This CHF may reverse spontaneously with successful treatment of pulmonary infections, presumably reflecting a concomitant decrease in pulmonary vascular resistance.

Chest Radiography

Right ventricular hypertrophy is reflected by decreases in the retrosternal space seen on the lateral projection of chest radiographs. Prominence of the main pulmonary artery and decreased pulmonary vascular markings are suggestive of pulmonary hypertension. In patients with COPD, dramatic changes in heart size characteristically occur between episodes of acute pulmonary dysfunction and recovery.

Electrocardiography

The electrocardiogram (ECG) in the presence of cor pulmonale may show signs of right atrial and ventricular hypertrophy. Right atrial hypertrophy is suggested by peaked P waves in leads II, III, and aVF. Right axis deviation and a partial or complete right bundle branch block are often seen on the ECG when right ventricular hypertrophy is present.

Treatment

Treatment of cor pulmonale is intended to decrease the workload of the right ventricle by decreasing pulmonary vascular resistance (Table 8–1). This goal is best achieved by returning the PaO_2, $PaCO_2$, and arterial pH to normal, assuming that the pulmonary artery and arteriolar vasoconstriction is reversible. This assumption is likely to be valid in the presence of COPD, particularly during exacerbations caused by acute pulmonary infection. By contrast, pulmonary vascular resistance is unlikely to be responsive to treatment when anatomic occlusive lesions are responsible for pulmonary artery hypertension.

Supplemental administration of oxygen to maintain the PaO_2 higher than 60 mmHg [pulse oximetry (SpO_2) above 90%] decreases the mortality due to cor pulmonale and improves cognitive function and quality of life.[1] Uncontrolled oxygen administration entails some risk, especially if hypoxic stimulation is necessary to maintain alveolar ventilation. Almitrine is a carotid body stimulant that improves ventilation-to-perfusion matching without altering minute ventilation.[1]

Long-term anticoagulation with warfarin-type drugs or the administration of antiplatelet drugs is often recommended as prophylaxis against thrombus formation, which may result in pulmonary em-

---

Table 8–1 • Treatment of Cor Pulmonale

Supplemental oxygen
Diuretics
Digitalis
Vasodilators
Anticoagulants
Antibiotics
Heart-lung transplantation

boli. Indeed, low cardiac output and a sedentary lifestyle are consistent with an increased incidence of thrombus formation in patients with cor pulmonale. A small pulmonary embolism that would likely have little effect on normal individuals could have catastrophic consequences in patients with pulmonary hypertension.

Diuretics and digitalis may be administered for treatment of CHF that does not respond to correction of arterial blood gases. Diuretics must be administered with care, as drug-induced metabolic alkalosis may aggravate ventilatory insufficiency by depressing the effectiveness of carbon dioxide as a stimulus to breathing. Moreover, diuresis may increase blood viscosity by further increasing the hematocrit. Digitalis must be used cautiously, as the risk of drug toxicity is increased in the presence of arterial hypoxemia, acidosis, and electrolyte imbalance, which are common in patients with cor pulmonale. Despite the initial enthusiasm for administration of calcium channel-blocking drugs as vasodilator therapy, only about one-third of patients respond.[5] If vasodilation occurs primarily in the systemic circulation without an adequate increase in cardiac output, systemic hypotension results. Prompt treatment with antibiotics minimizes an additional increase in pulmonary vascular resistance associated with pulmonary infections. Invading organisms are most often strains of *Haemophilus* or pneumococci, which are usually sensitive to ampicillin or, alternatively, to cephalosporins. When cor pulmonale is progressive despite maximum medical therapy, transplantation of one or two lungs or a heart-lung transplant can provide dramatic relief of cardiorespiratory failure.[1]

Management of Anesthesia

It is recommended that elective operations in patients with cor pulmonale be postponed until the reversible components of co-existing COPD are treated. Preoperative preparation is directed toward (1) eliminating and controlling acute and chronic pulmonary infections, (2) reversing bronchospasm, (3) improving secretion clearance, (4) expanding collapsed of poorly ventilated alveoli, (5) hydration, and (6) correcting any electrolyte imbalance. Arterial blood gases and pH are often determined to provide guidelines for management of patients, both intraoperatively and postoperatively.

Preoperative Medication

Preoperative medication should not include drugs that are likely to depress ventilation excessively. Although opioids are the most potent in this regard, any medication that produces sedation can result in depressed ventilation. Often a preoperative interview allays the patient's apprehension, eliminating the need for pharmacologic premedication. The depressant effects of anticholinergic drugs on mucociliary activity and the possible impairment of secretion clearance may outweigh the advantages of including these drugs in the preoperative medication. If a specific case requires anticholinergic drugs, an alternative is to administer them intravenously, just before induction of anesthesia.

Induction of Anesthesia

Induction of anesthesia is usually accomplished with the intravenous injection of rapidly acting induction drugs, taking care to avoid abrupt decreases in systemic vascular resistance in the presence of a fixed increase in pulmonary vascular resistance. Adequate depth of anesthesia should be present before tracheal intubation, as this stimulus in lightly anesthetized patients can elicit reflex bronchospasm. Furthermore, increases in systemic and pulmonary vascular resistance may accompany tracheal intubation, especially when the concentration of anesthetic drugs is low.[6]

Maintenance of Anesthesia

Maintenance of anesthesia is usually with volatile anesthetics combined with adjuvant drugs. It is likely that volatile anesthetics are as effective as bronchodilators. Large doses of opioids are avoided, as they could contribute to prolonged depression of ventilation during the postoperative period. Nitrous oxide may produce pulmonary artery vasoconstriction and further increases in pulmonary vascular resistance.[7, 8] For this reason it may be prudent to monitor right atrial pressures to provide an early warning that nitrous oxide is causing increased and undesirable degrees of pulmonary hypertension. Conversely, there are also data demonstrating that administration of nitrous oxide does not exacerbate pulmonary hypertension.[9] The choice of nondepolarizing muscle relaxants is not critical, although histamine release with administration of certain of these drugs might have adverse effects on airway and pulmonary vascular resistance.

Intermittent positive-pressure breathing is most often selected for intraoperative management of ventilation in patients with cor pulmonale. Although positive pressure applied to the airways and alveoli can increase pulmonary vascular resistance, this potentially adverse effect is usually more than offset by improved arterial oxygenation. Improved arterial oxygenation during positive-pressure ventilation of the patient's lungs presumably reflects better ventilation-to-perfusion distribution. An excessive decrease in the $PaCO_2$ during controlled ventilation of the lungs should be avoided, as metabolic alkalosis could produce hypokalemia. This is particularly important in patients being treated with digitalis, as acute decreases in serum potassium concentrations can predispose to digitalis toxicity. Humidification of the inhaled gases helps maintain hydration and liquefaction of secretions.

Regional anesthetic techniques are appropriate considerations for superficial surgery or operations on the extremities of patients with cor pulmonale. Operations that would require high sensory levels of anesthesia are not optimally performed with regional anesthesia in patients with pulmonary hypertension, as any decrease in systemic vascular resistance in the presence of fixed increases in pulmonary vascular resistance could produce undesirable degrees of systemic hypotension.

Monitoring

Intraoperative monitoring of patients with cor pulmonale is influenced by the invasiveness of the operation. An intra-arterial catheter permits frequent determination of arterial blood gases and pH and subsequent adjustments in inspired concentrations of oxygen. Continuous monitoring of SpO_2 and end-tidal CO_2 concentrations decreases the need for frequent analysis of arterial blood gases and pH. A right atrial catheter provides useful information regarding right ventricular function and the safety of intravenous infusions of fluids. Abrupt increases in right atrial pressures during the intraoperative period signal right ventricular dysfunction, which mandates a search for the cause of the sudden increases in pulmonary vascular resistance, as can be produced by unrecognized arterial hypoxemia, hypoventilation, or drugs such as nitrous oxide. Furthermore, maintenance of adequate right heart filling pressures is necessary to ensure optimal right ventricular stroke volume. When left ventricular dysfunction accompanies cor pulmonale and the magnitude of the surgery includes the likelihood of large fluid volume replacement, it may be helpful to place a pulmonary artery catheter, which facilitates regulation of intravascular fluid volume and cardiac output with volume infusions or inotropic drugs.

▌ PRIMARY PULMONARY HYPERTENSION

Primary pulmonary hypertension is characterized by sustained increases of pulmonary artery pressures without a demonstrable cause.[2-4] The diagnostic criteria include mean pulmonary artery pressures higher than 25 mmHg at rest or more than 30 mmHg with exercise and the exclusion of left-sided cardiac valvular disease, myocardial disease, congenital heart disease, and any clinically important respiratory, connective tissue, or chronic thromboembolic disease. Pulmonary vascular disease with features similar to primary pulmonary hypertension can occur in patients with portal hypertension, acquired immunodeficiency syndrome, or a history of cocaine abuse and in those who take appetite suppressant drugs (serotonin uptake inhibitor drugs and amphetamines).

Estimates of the incidence of primary pulmonary hypertension range from one to two cases per million people in the general population. Elements responsible for pulmonary hypertension in these patients include (1) pulmonary vascular vasoconstriction, (2) vascular wall remodeling, and (3) thrombosis in situ. The hemodynamic stresses of pregnancy are poorly tolerated by women with primary pulmonary hypertension; and sudden deterioration, particularly during the immediate postpartum period, can be fatal. Oral contraceptives are not recommended for birth control, as their use may exacerbate pulmonary hypertension. The median period of survival after diagnosis is 2.5 years, and most patients succumb to progressive right-sided heart failure. Sudden death accounts for about 7% of deaths.[4]

Classification

A treatment-based classification of pulmonary hypertension divides the disease into five distinct categories (Table 8–2).[3] These heterogeneous diseases have similar characteristic pathologic changes, including in situ thrombosis, smooth muscle hypertrophy, and intimal proliferation. Right heart catheterization is essential to confirm the diagnosis of pulmonary hypertension, determine the prognosis, and assign therapy.

Diagnosis

The major obstacles to establishing a clinical diagnosis of pulmonary hypertension during the early course of the disease are the nonspecific nature of the symptoms and the subtlety of the signs of less advanced disease.[4] Dyspnea is the most common reason for seeking medical attention, and fatigability is a common early symptom. Angina pectoris and syncope, particularly with exertion, are indicative

Table 8–2 • Diagnostic Classification of
Pulmonary Hypertension

Pulmonary hypertension associated with diseases of the
   respiratory system or arterial hypoxemia
     Chronic obstructive pulmonary disease
     Interstitial pulmonary fibrosis
     Cystic fibrosis
     Chronic alveolar hypoxemia (altitude)
Pulmonary venous hypertension
     Mitral valve disease
     Chronic left ventricular dysfunction
     Pulmonary veno-occlusive disease
Pulmonary hypertension due to chronic thrombotic and/
   or embolic disease
     Thromboembolic obstruction of proximal pulmonary
      arteries
     Obstruction of distal pulmonary arteries
Pulmonary arterial hypertension
     Primary pulmonary hypertension (sporadic, familial)
     Pulmonary arterial hypertension related to collagen
      vascular diseases (scleroderma, lupus
      erythematosus, rheumatoid arthritis)
     Pulmonary arterial hypertension related to congenital
      systemic-to-pulmonary shunts (Eisenmenger
      syndrome, AIDS, drugs, toxins)
Pulmonary hypertension due to disorders directly
   affecting the pulmonary vasculature
     Inflammatory
     Pulmonary capillary hemangiomatosis

AIDS, acquired immunodeficiency syndrome.
Adapted from Gaine S. Pulmonary hypertension. JAMA 2000;
284:3160–8.

of more severe limitations in cardiac output. Approximately 10% of patients, usually women, report symptoms of Raynaud's phenomenon. There is a correlation between the distance walked during a 6 minute walk test and the severity of pulmonary hypertension. This noninvasive test may be useful for monitoring the response to therapy.

Echocardiography can rule out congenital, valvular, and myocardial disease and may provide a means for estimating pulmonary artery systolic pressures. The results of ventilation-perfusion scanning are normal or reveal a patchy distribution of tracer, particularly with pulmonary veno-occlusive disease. Pulmonary arteriography is useful when perfusion lung scans are inconclusive.

Arterial hypoxemia is almost always present, reflecting (1) ventilation-to-perfusion imbalance due to increased perfusion of poorly ventilated alveoli, (2) mixed venous hypoxemia due to depression of the cardiac output, and (3) shunting of blood through a patent foramen ovale. Pulmonary hemodynamics are markedly deranged with increases in pulmonary artery pressures to levels three or more times normal, increased right atrial pressures, and decreased cardiac output. Pulmonary artery occlusion pressures are usually normal owing to the pat-

ency of the larger pulmonary veins and the patchy nature of the disease process in the veins.

Treatment

Primary pulmonary hypertension is a progressive disease for which there is no cure.[4] Right heart catheterization and a vasodilator trial are undertaken to determine the approach to therapy (Fig. 8–1).[3] Patients who exhibit favorable acute responses are treated long term with calcium channel-blocker therapy. The most widely used drugs for long-term therapy are the calcium channel blockers nifedipine and diltiazem, which produce sustained improvements in an estimated 30% of patients. Nonresponders are considered for continuous intravenous epoprostenol (prostacyclin) therapy as a bridge to transplantation or as definitive long-term therapy.

The rationale for vasodilator therapy is based on the observation that vasoconstriction is a prominent feature of the disease. Continuous intravenous administration of epoprostenol alleviates symptoms and improves survival in patients with advanced primary pulmonary hypertension, and it has potential benefit in patients with other forms of pulmonary arterial hypertension. Intravenously administered epoprostenol serves as a test for pulmonary vascular responsiveness with a 20% decrease in pulmonary vascular resistance defined as a positive response.[10, 11] Epoprostenol must be administered by continuous intravenous infusion, as it has a short half-life in the circulation and is inactivated by the acidic pH present in the stomach. The drug is delivered with a portable infusion pump attached to a permanent indwelling central venous catheter. Aerosolized epoprostenol may be an alternative route of administration. Side effects that may accompany epoprostenol administration include bleeding due to platelet inhibition, a significant decrease in systemic vascular resistance with associated hypotension and arterial hypoxemia, and complications associated with the drug delivery system.[12] Iloprost, a prostacyclin analogue, is a potent pulmonary vasodilator when administered as an aerosol for treatment of pulmonary hypertension.[13]

The action of nitric oxide is most specific to the pulmonary vascular bed. Indeed, inhaled nitric oxide decreases the extent to which extracorporeal membrane oxygenation is needed in neonates with hypoxemic respiratory failure and pulmonary hypertension.[14] Nitric oxide treatment may be complicated by platelet inhibition, methemoglobinemia, formation of toxic nitrate metabolites, and the technical requirements for its application.

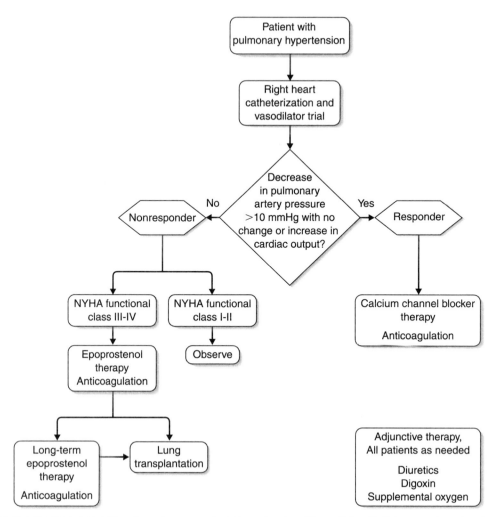

Figure 8–1 • Treatment algorithm for pulmonary arterial hypertension. (From Gaine S. Pulmonary hypertension. JAMA 2000;284:3160–8. Copyrighted 2000, American Medical Association, with permission.)

Anticoagulation may be recommended based on the increased risk of thrombosis and thromboembolism in the presence of sluggish pulmonary blood flow, dilation of the right heart, venous stasis, and the limitations in physical activity imposed by the disease. Diuretics are useful for decreasing preload in patients with right heart failure, particularly when hepatic congestion and ascites are present. Patients with arterial hypoxemia may experience symptomatic improvement with supplemental oxygen. Lung transplantation and combined heart-lung transplantation have been performed in some patients with end-stage primary pulmonary hypertension in whom maximal medical therapy fails.

Management of Anesthesia

Management of anesthesia for patients with primary pulmonary hypertension should follow the same principles as described for patients with cor pulmonale. Management of cesarean delivery utilizing epidural anesthesia has been described in a parturient with primary pulmonary hypertension.[15] General anesthesia and mechanical ventilation has been associated with circulatory failure following induction of anesthesia.[16]

References

1. Palevsky HI, Fishman AP. Chronic cor pulmonale: etiology and management. JAMA 1991;263:2347–53
2. Staton GW, Ingram RH. Pulmonary hypertension, cor pulmonale, and primary pulmonary hypertension. Sci Am Med 2000;1–9
3. Gaine S. Pulmonary hypertension. JAMA 2000;284:3160–8
4. Rubin LJ. Primary pulmonary hypertension. N Engl J Med 1997;336:111–7
5. Robotham JL. Cardiovascular disturbance in chronic respiratory insufficiency. Am J Cardiol 1981;47:941–9

6. Sorensen MB, Jacobsen E. Pulmonary hemodynamics during induction of anesthesia. Anesthesiology 1977;46:246–51

7. Hilgenberg JC, McCammon RL, Stoelting RK. Pulmonary and systemic vascular responses to nitrous oxide in patients with mitral stenosis and pulmonary hypertension. Anesth Analg 1980;59:323–6

8. Schulte-Sasse U, Hess W, Tarnow J. Pulmonary vascular responses to nitrous oxide in patients with normal and a high pulmonary vascular resistance. Anesthesiology 1982; 57:9–13

9. Konstadt SN, Reich DL, Thys DM. Nitrous oxide does not exacerbate pulmonary hypertension or ventricular dysfunction in patients with mitral valvular disease. Can J Anaesth 1990;37:613–7

10. McLaughlin VV, Genthner DE, Panella MM, et al. Reduction in pulmonary vascular resistance with long-term epoprostenol (prostacyclin) therapy in primary pulmonary hypertension. N Engl J Med 1988;338:273–7

11. Fishman AP. Pulmonary hypertension: beyond vasodilator therapy. N Engl J Med 1998;338:321–2

12. Schroeder RA, Wood GL, Plotkin JS, et al. Intraoperative use of inhaled PGI_2 for acute pulmonary hypertension and right ventricular failure. Anesth Analg 2000;91:291–5

13. Hoeper MM, Schwarze M, Ehlerding S, et al. Long-term treatment of primary pulmonary hypertension with aerosolized iloprost, a prostacyclin analogue. N Engl J Med 2000; 342:1866–70

14. Clark RH, Kueser TJ, Walker MW, et al. Low-dose nitric oxide therapy for persistent pulmonary hypertension of the newborn. N Engl J Med 2000;342:469–74

15. Weiss BM, Maggiorini M, Jenni R, et al. Pregnant patient with primary pulmonary hypertension: inhaled pulmonary vasodilators and epidural anesthesia for cesarean delivery. Anesthesiology 2000;92:1191–4

16. Hohn L, Schweizer A, Morel DR, et al. Circulatory failure after anesthesia induction in a patient with severe primary pulmonary hypertension. Anesthesiology 1999;91:1943–5

9

Pericardial Diseases

Pericardial diseases have diverse causes that may result in responses that are clinically and pathologically similar.[1] The three clinicopathologic responses to pericardial injury are characterized as acute pericarditis, pericardial effusion, and constrictive pericarditis. Cardiac tamponade is a possibility whenever pericardial fluid accumulates under pressure. Management of anesthesia in patients with pericardial diseases is facilitated by an understanding of alterations in cardiovascular function produced by specific pericardial diseases.[2]

■ ACUTE PERICARDITIS

Viral infections are often presumed to be the cause of acute pericarditis that occurs as a primary illness (Table 9–1).[1] Because most cases of acute pericarditis follow a transient and uncomplicated clinical course, the syndrome is often termed "acute benign pericarditis." Acute benign pericarditis unaccompanied by cardiac tamponade or substantial pericardial effusion rarely progresses to constrictive pericarditis. Dressler syndrome is a delayed form of acute pericarditis that may follow an acute myocardial infarction.

Diagnosis

The clinical diagnosis of acute pericarditis is based on the presence of chest pain, pericardial friction rub, and changes on the electrocardiogram (ECG).[1] Chest pain associated with acute pericarditis typically has an acute onset and is described as severe pain over the anterior chest. This pain typically worsens with inspiration, which helps distinguish it from pain due to myocardial ischemia. Low grade

135

Table 9–1 • Causes of Acute Pericarditis with or without Pericardial Effusion

Infectious etiology
  Viral
  Bacterial
  Fungal
  Tuberculosis (often associated with acquired
      immunodeficiency syndrome)
Postmyocardial infarction (Dressler syndrome)
Posttraumatic (cardiac surgery, pacemaker lead,
    pressure monitoring catheters)
Metastatic disease
Drug-induced (minoxidil, procainamide)
Mediastinal radiation
Systemic diseases
  Rheumatoid arthritis
  Systemic lupus erythematosus
  Scleroderma

fever and sinus tachycardia are often present. Auscultation of the chest often reveals friction rubs ("to and fro") especially when the symptoms are acute. Inflammation of the superficial myocardium is the most likely explanation for diffuse ST segment elevation on the ECG. The diffuse distribution, or absence, of reciprocal ST segment depression distinguishes these changes produced by acute pericarditis from ECG changes typical of myocardial infarction. Depression of the PR segment on the ECG reflects superficial injury of the atrial myocardium and may be the earliest sign of acute pericarditis on the ECG. Acute pericarditis in the absence of an associated pericardial effusion does not alter cardiac function.

Treatment

Symptomatic relief of the pain due to acute pericarditis is often provided by oral analgesics such as codeine. Salicylates or nonsteroidal antiinflammatory drugs (NSAIDs) may be useful for decreasing pericardial inflammation. Corticosteroids such as prednisone usually relieve symptoms of acute pericarditis, but this therapy is reserved for patients who do not respond to conventional therapy, as symptoms are likely to recur when the corticosteroids are discontinued.

Relapsing Pericarditis

Acute pericarditis due to any cause may follow a recurrent or chronic relapsing course.[1] In many patients the symptoms of relapsing pericarditis are subjective (weakness, fatigue, headache) and are as-

sociated with chest discomfort. Treatment includes colchicine, methylprednisolone, or immunosuppression produced by prednisone or azathioprine.

Pericarditis After Cardiac Surgery

The postcardiotomy syndrome presents primarily as acute pericarditis.[1] The cause of this syndrome is presumed to be infective or autoimmune. A similar response may follow blunt or penetrating trauma, hemopericardium, or epicardial pacemaker implantation.

PERICARDIAL EFFUSION AND CARDIAC TAMPONADE

Pericardial fluid may accumulate in the pericardial cavity with virtually any form of pericardial disease.[1] The fluid may be a transudate or exudate and is often serosanguineous when the pericardial disease reflects cancer or tuberculosis or is related to dialysis or radiation. Hemopericardium occurs in the presence of coagulopathy, trauma, myocardial rupture due to an acute myocardial infarction, and aortic dissection. Acute pericarditis with pericardial effusion often occurs in patients with end-stage renal disease who are on dialysis. Pericardial effusions develop frequently in patients with Hodgkin's disease or other lymphomas. Neoplastic pericardial effusions are common causes of cardiac tamponade in nonsurgical patients.

Signs and Symptoms

The physiologic effects of pericardial effusions depend on whether the fluid is under increased pressure. If pericardial effusions develop gradually, the pericardium stretches sufficiently to accommodate volumes that may exceed 2000 ml. Conversely, if pericardial effusions develop abruptly, volumes as small as 200 ml may result in increased intrapericardial pressures and the development of cardiac tamponade. As pericardial pressures increase, the right atrial and central venous pressures rise in parallel such that central venous pressure readings are accurate reflections of intrapericardial pressures.

Cardiac Tamponade

Cardiac tamponade manifests as a spectrum of hemodynamic abnormalities of varying severity rather than as an all-or-none phenomenon.[1] Many of the initial manifestations of cardiac tamponade mimic those of pulmonary embolism.

Depending on the severity of the cardiac tamponade, systemic blood pressure may be decreased or maintained in the normal range for that patient. Central venous pressure is almost always increased, except for rare instances of low-pressure cardiac tamponade, which may occur in the presence of hypovolemia. In this regard, monitoring right atrial pressures may be useful for determining whether cardiac tamponade is present. Activation of the sympathetic nervous system occurs during attempts to maintain cardiac output and systemic blood pressure by virtue of tachycardia and peripheral vasoconstriction. Cardiac output is maintained so long as pressure in the central veins exceeds the right ventricular end-diastolic pressure. A persistent, progressive increase in intrapericardial fluid pressure eventually results in equalization of right and left atrial pressures and right ventricular end-diastolic pressures at about 20 mmHg as measured with a pulmonary artery catheter. The exception may be accumulation of blood and clots over the right ventricle, as may follow cardiac surgery, where the right atrial pressure is increased but the pulmonary artery occlusion pressure remains normal.

Paradoxical pulse (decrease in systolic blood pressure of more than 10 mmHg during inspiration) is present in patients with cardiac tamponade (Fig. 9–1). This hemodynamic change associated with inspiration reflects selective impairment of diastolic filling of the left ventricle. Ultimately, accumulation of fluid increases the intrapericardial pressure, leading to impaired diastolic filling of the heart, decreased stroke volume, and hypotension.

Cardiac tamponade may be the cause of low cardiac output syndrome during the early postoperative period after cardiac surgery. Cardiac tamponade may occur as a complication of various invasive procedures in the cardiac catheterization laboratory and intensive care unit. Perforation of the heart and subsequent cardiac tamponade may result from central venous catheters that have been placed in the right atrium rather than the superior vena cava.[3]

Loculated Pericardial Effusions

Loculated pericardial effusions may selectively compress one or more chambers of the heart, producing localized cardiac tamponade. This response is most often seen following cardiac surgery, when blood accumulates behind the sternum and selectively compresses the left ventricle and left atrium. Similar responses may be present following anterior chest wall trauma. Transesophageal echocardiography is superior to transthoracic echocardiography for demonstrating localized pericardial effusions.

Diagnosis

Echocardiography is the most accurate and practical method for diagnosing pericardial effusions and cardiac tamponade. Echocardiography detects pericardial effusions as small as 20 ml and reveals characteristic changes with effusions larger than 100 ml.[1] Computed tomography is also useful for detecting both pericardial effusions and pericardial thickening. Magnetic resonance imaging provides information similar to that gained with computed tomography. The ECG often shows nonspecific low voltage in the presence of large pericardial effusions. Electrical alternans may occur, especially when the pericardial effusion is large, and is most often caused by metastatic lesions. Pericardiocentesis may be useful for diagnosing metastatic disease or infection.

The diagnosis of cardiac tamponade is based on combinations of clinical findings and a high index of suspicion, as no single change is pathognomonic (Table 9–2).[1] Echocardiography, although definitive for diagnosing pericardial effusion, is not always confirmatory of cardiac tamponade. The presence of early diastolic inward wall motion of the right atrial or right ventricular wall ("collapse"), reflecting the similarity of intracavitary and intrapericardial pressures, is helpful for confirming the presence of cardiac tamponade.

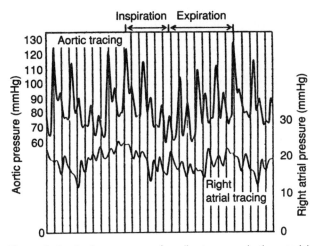

Figure 9–1 • In the presence of cardiac tamponade the arterial blood pressure decreases more than 10 mmHg during inspiration as a reflection of a concomitant decrease in left ventricular stroke volume. This contrasts with the opposite response observed during inspiration in the absence of cardiac tamponade, accounting for its designation as a paradoxical pulse (pulsus paradoxus).

Table 9–2 • Signs and Symptoms of Cardiac Tamponade

Increased central venous pressure
Activation of the sympathetic nervous system
Equalization of atrial filling pressures and pulmonary artery end-diastolic pressures
Decreased voltage and electrical alternans on the electrocardiogram
Paradoxical pulse
Hypotension

Treatment

Mild cardiac tamponade can be managed conservatively in some patients, but removal of fluid is required for definitive treatment and should be performed in most instances when the central venous pressure is increased.[1] Pericardial fluid may be removed by pericardiocentesis or by surgical techniques that include subxiphoid pericardiostomy, thoracoscopic pericardiostomy, or thoractomy. Removal of small amounts of pericardial fluid often results in dramatic decreases in intrapericardial pressures. Acute cardiac tamponade may be due to hemopericardium caused by aortic dissection, penetrating cardiac trauma, or acute myocardial infarction; when it occurs following cardiac surgery, it requires immediate surgery.

Temporizing measures designed to maintain stroke volume until definitive surgical treatment of cardiac tamponade can be instituted include expanding the intravascular fluid volume, administering catecholamines to increase myocardial contractility, and correcting metabolic acidosis.[2] Expansion of intravascular fluid volume can be achieved by intravenous infusion of colloid or crystalloid solutions (500 ml over 5 to 10 minutes). Volume infusions that increase right atrial pressures to 25 to 30 mmHg may be necessary to offset the effects of increased intrapericardial pressures on venous return. Despite the time-honored acceptance of intravascular fluid volume expansion for emergency treatment of cardiac tamponade, improvement in hemodynamic function may be limited, and pericardiocentesis should not be delayed.[4]

Continuous intravenous infusion of isoproterenol or other catecholamines may be an effective temporizing measure for increasing myocardial contractility and the heart rate, although the beneficial effects of these drugs seen in animals with experimentally induced cardiac tamponade have not been reproduced in patients.[5] Atropine may be necessary to treat the bradycardia that results from vagal reflexes evoked by increased intrapericardial pressures. High doses of dopamine, which increase systemic

vascular resistance, could be undesirable. Vasodilator drugs, such as nitroprusside or hydralazine, could theoretically improve cardiac output, but their use should be considered only when the intravascular fluid volume has been replenished. As with intravascular fluid volume replacement, pericardiocentesis should never be delayed in preference to drug therapy.

Correction of metabolic acidosis is essential. Metabolic acidosis owing to low cardiac output in the presence of cardiac tamponade is treated with intravenous administration of sodium bicarbonate, 0.5 to 1.0 mEq/kg. Correction of metabolic acidosis is important, as increased hydrogen ion concentrations can depress myocardial contractility and attenuate the positive inotropic effects of catecholamines.

Management of Anesthesia

Institution of general anesthesia and positive-pressure ventilation of the patient's lungs in the presence of cardiac tamponade that is hemodynamically significant can result in life-threatening hypotension. Reasons for hypotension include anesthetic-induced peripheral vasodilation, direct myocardial depression, and decreased venous return. In this regard, pericardiocentesis performed with local anesthesia is often preferred for initial management of patients who are hypotensive owing to low cardiac output produced by cardiac tamponade.[6] Ketamine, administered intravenously, can provide sedation in selected patients.[2]

After the hemodynamic status has been improved by percutaneous pericardiocentesis, it may be considered acceptable to induce general anesthesia and institute positive-pressure ventilation of the patient's lungs to permit surgical exploration and more definitive treatment of cardiac tamponade. Induction and maintenance of anesthesia with ketamine or a benzodiazepine plus nitrous oxide are acceptable. The circulatory effects of pancuronium make it useful for producing skeletal muscle relaxation in these patients. Monitors often include intra-arterial and central venous pressure catheters.

When it is not possible to relieve the intrapericardial pressure that is causing cardiac tamponade before the induction of anesthesia, the goal must be to maintain cardiac output. Anesthetic-induced decreases in myocardial contractility, systemic vascular resistance, and heart rate are avoided. Increased intrathoracic pressure caused by straining or coughing during induction of anesthesia or by controlled ventilation of the lungs may further decrease venous return in the presence of increased intrapericardial pressures (Fig. 9–2).[7] For these reasons it may be prudent to avoid vigorous positive-pressure

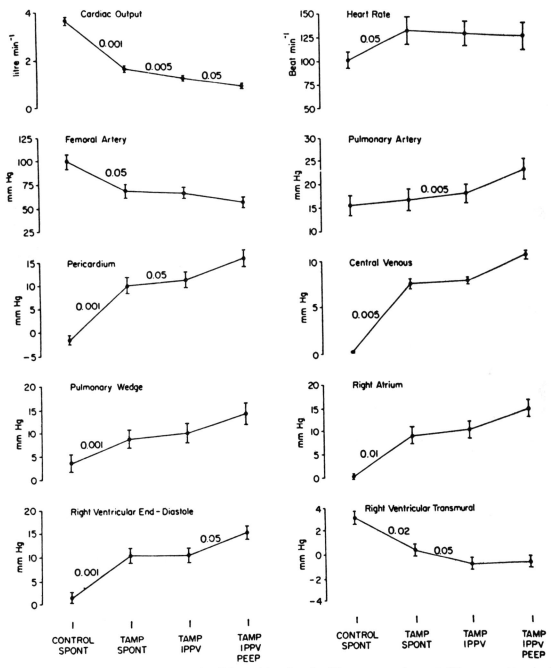

Figure 9–2 • Cardiac output and pleural, pericardial, arterial, and cardiac filling pressures (mean ± SE) measured in animals during different modes of ventilation in the presence of acute cardiac tamponade. IPPV, intermittent positive-pressure ventilation; PEEP, positive end-expiratory pressure; SPONT, spontaneous breathing; TAMP, cardiac tamponade. (From Moller CT, Schoonbee CB, Rosendorff C. Haemodynamics of cardiac tamponade during various modes of ventilation. Br J Anaesth 1979;51:409–15, with permission.)

ventilation of the patient's lungs until the chest is opened and drainage of the pericardial fluid is imminent. Ketamine is useful for induction and maintenance of anesthesia, as it increases myocardial contractility, systemic vascular resistance, and the heart rate. Induction of anesthesia with benzodiazepines, followed by maintenance of anesthesia with nitrous oxide plus fentanyl and pancuronium for skeletal muscle relaxation, has also been utilized successfully in these patients.[8] Continuous monitoring of the systemic blood pressure and central venous pressure should be initiated before induction of anesthesia. Maintenance of increased central venous pressures with generous administration of intravenous fluids is indicated to maintain venous return. Continuous intravenous infusion of a catecholamine, such as isoproterenol, dopamine, or dobutamine, may be useful for maintaining cardiac output until the cardiac tamponade can be relieved by surgical drainage. In addition, personnel and equipment should be available to perform emergency pericardiocentesis in case circulatory collapse occurs after induction of anesthesia.

■ CONSTRICTIVE PERICARDITIS

Constrictive pericarditis is most often idiopathic or due to previous cardiac surgery or radiotherapy. Tuberculosis may also cause constrictive pericarditis. Chronic constrictive pericarditis is characterized by fibrous scarring and adhesions that obliterate the pericardial cavity, resembling a "rigid shell" around the heart.[1] Calcification may develop in long-standing cases. Subacute constrictive pericarditis is more common than chronic calcific pericarditis, and the resulting constriction is fibroelastic.

Signs and Symptoms

Increased venous pressure in patients who do not have other symptoms of heart disease suggests the presence of constrictive pericarditis. As the pericardial pressures increase, the right atrial and central venous pressures rise in parallel, such that central venous pressure readings are accurate reflections of the intrapericardial pressure. Although constrictive pericarditis involves both sides of the heart, the dominant manifestations are those of right ventricular failure with venous congestion, hepatosplenomegaly, and ascites. Increased and eventual equalization of right atrial pressures, pulmonary artery end-diastolic pressures, and pulmonary artery occlusion pressures may occur in the presence of both constrictive pericarditis and cardiac tamponade.

Atrial dysrhythmias (atrial fibrillation or flutter) are common in patients with chronic constrictive pericarditis, presumably reflecting involvement of the sinoatrial node by the disease process.

Constrictive pericarditis is similar to cardiac tamponade in that both conditions impede diastolic filling of the heart and result in increased central venous pressure and ultimately decreased cardiac output.[1] Diagnostic signs, however, are different for the two conditions. Paradoxical pulse is a regular feature of cardiac tamponade but is insignificant or absent in the presence of constrictive pericarditis. Kussmaul's sign (increased venous pressure with inspiration) occurs in some patients with constrictive pericarditis but is not present in patients with cardiac tamponade. An early diastolic sound ("pericardial knock") is often heard in patients with constrictive pericarditis but does not occur in the presence of cardiac tamponade.

Diagnosis

Constrictive pericarditis is difficult to diagnose and is often erroneously attributed to liver disease or idiopathic pericardial effusions.[1] The clinical diagnosis of constrictive pericarditis depends on confirmation of increased central venous pressure in patients who may not have other obvious signs or symptoms of heart disease. Heart size and lung fields usually appear normal on chest radiography, and the ECG shows only minor, nonspecific abnormalities. Echocardiography is nondiagnostic in many instances, although the appearance of abnormal septal motion and pericardial thickening suggest the presence of constrictive pericarditis. Transesophageal echocardiography and chest computed tomography are superior to transthoracic echocardiography for demonstrating pericardial thickening. Pulsed-wave Doppler studies show exaggerated respiratory variation in the mitral and tricuspid diastolic flow velocities in most cases of constrictive pericarditis and cardiac tamponade. Cardiac catheterization shows characteristic abnormalities, including increased central venous pressures, nondilated and normally contracting right and left ventricles, and near-equilibration of right- and left-sided cardiac filling pressures. Many features considered characteristic of constrictive pericarditis may also be present in patients with cardiac amyloidosis and idiopathic restrictive cardiomyopathy (Table 9–3).[1]

Treatment

Constrictive pericarditis occasionally resolves spontaneously when it develops as a complication of

Table 9–3 • Clinical Features that Differentiate Constrictive Pericarditis from Cardiac Amyloidosis and Idiopathic Restrictive Cardiomyopathy

Clinical Feature	Constrictive Pericarditis	Cardiac Amyloidosis	Idiopathic Restrictive Cardiomyopathy
Early diastolic sound (S_3 or "pericardial knock")	Frequent	Occasional	Occasional
Late diastolic sound (S_4)	Rare	Frequent	Frequent
Atrial enlargement	Mild or absent	Marked	Marked
Atrioventricular or intraventricular conduction defect	Rare	Frequent	Frequent
QRS voltage	Normal or low	Low	Normal or high
Mitral or tricuspid regurgitation	Rare	Frequent	Frequent
Paradoxical pulse	Frequent but usually mild	Rare	Rare
Exaggerated variation in mitral and tricuspid flow velocity with respiration	Usual	Rare	Rare

Data from Hancock EW. Diseases of the pericardium, cardiac tumors, and cardiac trauma. Sci Am Med 1999;1–10.

acute pericarditis. In nearly all patients, however, treatment of constrictive pericarditis is surgical stripping and removal of both layers of the adherent constricting pericardium which may result in massive bleeding from the epicardial surfaces of the heart. Cardiopulmonary bypass may be used to facilitate the surgical procedure, especially if hemorrhage is difficult to control. Unlike cardiac tamponade, in which hemodynamic improvement occurs promptly, surgical removal of constricting pericardium is not immediately followed by decreases in right atrial pressures or an increase in cardiac output. Typically, right atrial pressures return to normal within 3 months after surgery. The absence of immediate hemodynamic improvement may reflect disuse atrophy due to prolonged constriction of myocardial muscle fibers or persistent constrictive effects from sclerotic epicardium, which is not removed with the parietal pericardium. Inadequate long-term relief following surgical removal of the constricting pericardium may reflect associated myocardial disease, particularly in patients with radiation-induced pericardial disease.

Management of Anesthesia

In the absence of hypotension caused by increased intrapericardial pressure, anesthetic drugs and techniques that do not excessively depress myocardial contractility, decrease systemic blood pressure, slow the heart rate, or interfere with venous return are most likely to be selected. Combinations of opioids, benzodiazepines, and nitrous oxide with or without low doses of volatile anesthetics are acceptable for maintaining anesthesia. Muscle relaxants with mini-

mal circulatory effects are useful choices, although modest increases in heart rate, as associated with administration of pancuronium, are acceptable. Preoperative optimization of intravascular fluid volume is important in these patients. When hemodynamic compromise due to increased intrapericardial pressure is present, treatment and management of anesthesia are as described for cardiac tamponade (see "Cardiac Tamponade").

Invasive monitoring of arterial and venous pressures is helpful, as removal of adherent pericardium may be tedious and is often associated with decreased systemic blood pressure and cardiac output. Cardiac dysrhythmias are common during surgical removal of adherent pericardium, presumably reflecting direct mechanical stimulation of the heart. In this regard, cardiac antidysrhythmia drugs and an electrical defibrillator should be promptly available. Venous access and appropriate intravenous fluids and blood products are necessary to treat the occasional massive blood loss associated with pericardiectomy.

Postoperative ventilatory insufficiency may necessitate continued mechanical ventilation of the lungs. Cardiac dysrhythmias and low cardiac output may require treatment during the postoperative period. An infrequent complication of subtotal pericardiectomy is pneumopericardium.

References

1. Hancock EW. Diseases of the pericardium, cardiac tumors, and cardiac trauma. Sci Am Med 1999;1–10

2. Lake CL. Anesthesia and pericardial disease. Anesth Analg 1983;62:431–43
3. Collier PE, Goodman GB. Cardiac tamponade caused by central venous catheter perforation of the heart: a preventable complication. J Am Coll Surg 1995;181:459–61
4. Kerber RE, Gascho JA, Litchfield R, et al. Hemodynamic effects of volume expansion and nitroprusside compared with pericardiocentesis in patients with acute cardiac tamponade. N Engl J Med 1982;307:929–31
5. Martins JB, Manuel JB, Marcus ML, et al. Comparative effects of catecholamines in cardiac tamponade: experimental and clinical studies. Am J Cardiol 1980;46:59–66
6. Stanley TH, Weidauer HE. Anesthesia for the patient with cardiac tamponade. Anesth Analg 1973;52:110–4
7. Moller CT, Schoonbee CG, Rosendorff C. Haemodynamics of cardiac tamponade during various modes of ventilation. Br J Anaesth 1979;51:409–15
8. Konchigere HN, Levitsky S. Anesthetic considerations for pericardiectomy in uremic pericardial effusion. Anesth Analg 1976;55:378–82

10

Aneurysms of the Thoracic and Abdominal Aorta

Diseases of the aorta are most often aneurysmal; occlusive diseases are more likely to occur in peripheral arteries. Aneurysms of the aorta may involve the ascending or descending portions of the thoracic aorta or the portion of the aorta below the diaphragm. The initiating event of the aortic dissection is a tear in the intima of the vessel wall. Blood surges through the tear into a false lumen separating the intima from the adventitia for various distances.[1] The origin of the side branches arising from this portion of the aorta may be compromised and the aortic valve rendered incompetent. Blood in the false lumen can reenter the true lumen anywhere along the course of the aortic dissection. Alternatively, rupture of the aorta occurs most frequently in the pericardial space and left pleural cavity.

■ ANEURYSMS OF THE THORACIC AORTA

Dissection of the aorta can originate anywhere along the length of the aorta, but the most common point of origin is the ascending thoracic aorta within a few centimeters of the aortic valve. The second most common location is the descending thoracic aorta just distal to the origin of the left subclavian artery in the region of insertion of the ligamentum arteriosus. Aneurysm is the most common condition of the thoracic aorta requiring surgical treatment.[1]

Classification

Two classifications are widely used for aortic dissection (Fig. 10–1).[1] The DeBakey classification includes types I through III. In type I the intimal tear usually originates in the proximal ascending aorta, and the

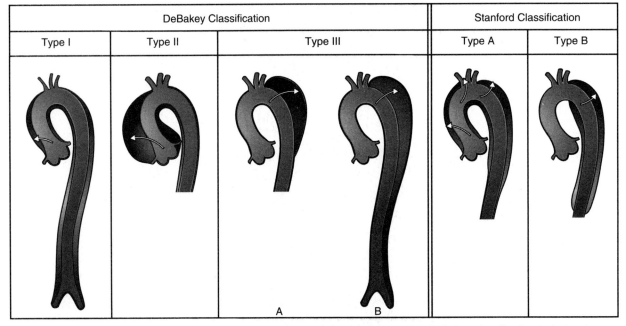

DeBakey Classification			Stanford Classification	
Type I	Type II	Type III	Type A	Type B

Figure 10–1 • The two most widely used classifications of aortic dissection. The DeBakey classification includes three types: type I, the intimal tear usually originates in the proximal ascending aorta and the dissection involves the ascending aorta; type II, the dissection is confined to the ascending aorta; type III, the dissection may be confined to the descending thoracic aorta (type IIIa) or may extend into the abdominal aorta and iliac arteries (type IIIb). The dissection may extend proximally to involve the arch and the ascending aorta. The Stanford classification has two types: type A, all cases in which the ascending aorta is involved by the dissection, with or without involvement of the arch or the descending aorta; type B, cases in which the descending thoracic aorta is involved, with or without proximal (retrograde) or distal (anterograde) extension. (From Kouchoukos NT, Dougenis D. Surgery of the thoracic aorta. N Engl J Med 1997;336:1876–88. Copyright 1997 Massachusetts Medical Society, with permission.)

dissection involves the ascending aorta, arch, and variable lengths of the descending and abdominal aorta. In type II the dissection is confined to the ascending aorta. In type III the dissection may be confined to the descending thoracic aorta (type IIIa) or may extend into the abdominal aorta and iliac arteries (type IIIb). The dissection may also extend proximally to involve the arch and the ascending aorta. The Stanford classification describes thoracic aneurysms as type A or B. Type A includes all cases in which the ascending aorta is involved by the dissection, with or without involvement of the arch or the descending aorta. Type B includes all cases in which the descending thoracic aorta is involved, with or without proximal (retrograde) or distal (anterograde) extension. Mortality is greatly increased when thoracic aortic dissection remains untreated by surgery for more than 14 days.

Etiology

Systemic hypertension is the single most important risk factor for thoracic aortic dissection. Other fac-

tors predisposing to thoracic aortic dissection include cystic medial degeneration of the aorta, Marfan syndrome, a bicuspid aortic valve, aortic coarctation, pregnancy, disorders of connective tissues (Ehlers-Danlos syndrome), manipulation of and operations on the thoracic aorta, and blunt trauma. Deceleration injuries, as may result from automobile accidents, are important causes of blunt trauma related thoracic aortic aneurysms, with the dissection most often involving the distal descending thoracic aorta at its point of fixation to the thorax by the ligamentum arteriosus just distal to the origin of the left subclavian artery. Blunt trauma to the thoracic aorta or heart must be considered in any patient with severe chest injury (see "Myocardial Contusion"). The chest trauma may seem so trivial that associated injury to the thoracic aorta is not suspected. Aortic dissection predominates in men, but there is also an association with pregnancy. For example, about one-half of all aortic dissections in women younger than 40 years of age occur during pregnancy, usually during the third trimester.[2] Iatrogenic aortic dissection may occur as a complication of cardiopulmonary bypass at the site of aortic cannulation. Aortic dissection may also arise where the aorta has been cross-clamped or incised, as for aortic valve replacement or proximal anastomosis of a venous bypass graft.

Signs and Symptoms

Many patients with thoracic aortic aneurysms are asymptomatic at the time of presentation, and the aneurysms are detected during testing for other disorders.[1,3] Symptoms due to thoracic aneurysms typically reflect impingement of the aneurysm on adjacent structures. Hoarseness results from stretching of the left recurrent laryngeal nerve; stridor is due to compression of the trachea; dysphagia is due to impingement on the lumen of the esophagus; dyspnea results from compression of the lungs; and plethora and edema result from compression of the superior vena cava. Patients with aneurysms of the thoracic aorta associated with dilation of the aortic valve annulus may present with signs of aortic regurgitation and congestive heart failure.

The acute onset of sharp pain in the anterior part of the chest, in the neck, or between the shoulders is the typical presenting symptom of thoracic aortic dissection. The pain often migrates as the dissection advances along the aorta. Patients with aortic dissection often appear as if they are in shock (vasoconstricted), yet the systemic blood pressure may be elevated, especially in those with distal dissection. Other symptoms and signs in patients with acute thoracic aorta dissections reflect occlusion of branches of the aorta, which may manifest as diminution or absence of peripheral pulses. Neurologic complications of aortic dissection include stroke caused by occlusion of the carotid arteries, ischemic peripheral neuropathy associated with obvious ischemia of the arms or legs, and paraparesis or paraplegia owing to impairment of the blood supply to the spinal cord. Myocardial infarction may reflect occlusion of coronary arteries by proximal aortic dissection. Gastrointestinal ischemia is possible. Renal artery obstruction manifests as increases in serum creatinine concentrations. Retrograde dissection into the sinus of Valsalva with rupture into the pericardial space leading to cardiac tamponade is a major cause of death. Approximately 90% of patients with acute dissection of the ascending aorta who are not treated surgically die within 3 months.

Diagnosis

Findings on the chest radiograph (widening of the mediastinum) may be diagnostic of a thoracic aortic aneurysm. Nevertheless, enlargement of the ascending aorta may be confined to the retrosternal area, so the aortic silhouette appears normal. Computed tomography is a commonly used noninvasive technique to diagnose thoracic aortic disease. The principal disadvantage of computed tomography is the need to inject contrast medium for precise delineation of the aortic disease. The use of contrast medium may be contraindicated in patients with allergies to contrast agents or with renal insufficiency. Magnetic resonance imaging has the advantage of not requiring the use of contrast medium.[1]

Transesophageal echocardiography with color Doppler imaging is used to diagnose thoracic aortic disease and for the care of these patients during the perioperative period. Aortography is usually required for patients undergoing elective operations on the thoracic aorta. The major disadvantages of aortography are the risk of allergic reactions after injection of contrast medium and the risk of renal failure in patients with impaired renal function.

Preoperative Evaluation

Because myocardial infarction, respiratory failure, renal failure, and stroke are the principal causes of morbidity and mortality after operations on the thoracic aorta, preoperative assessment of the function of these organ systems is recommended.[1] Assessment for the presence of myocardial ischemia (electrocardiogram) and valvular dysfunction is important. In some patients preoperative angioplasty or coronary artery bypass grafting during surgery on the thoracic aorta is indicated.

A history of cigarette smoking and the presence of chronic obstructive pulmonary disease (COPD) are important indicators of respiratory failure after thoracic aorta surgery. Spirometric tests and arterial blood gas analysis may be useful predictors of postoperative respiratory failure in these patients. If reversible airway obstruction is present, antibiotics and bronchodilators are considerations. Cessation of smoking is also advisable.

The presence of preoperative renal dysfunction is the most important predictor of acute renal failure after operations on the thoracic aorta. Adequate preoperative hydration and avoidance of hypotension, low cardiac output, and hypovolemia during the perioperative period are important for decreasing the incidence of postoperative renal failure. Duplex imaging of the carotid arteries and angiography of the brachiocephalic and intracranial arteries may be performed preoperatively in patients with a history of stroke or transient ischemic attacks. Patients with more than 80% to 90% stenosis of one or both common or internal carotid arteries may be considered for carotid endarterectomy before elective operations on the thoracic aorta.

Indications for Surgery

A number of important technical advances have decreased the risks of operations on the thoracic aorta.[1] These advances include the use of adjuncts such as distal aortic perfusion, profound hypothermia and circulatory arrest, monitoring evoked potentials in the brain and spinal cord, and cerebrospinal fluid drainage. Postoperative complications associated with thoracic aneurysm resection are increased in patients with co-existing pulmonary insufficiency or coronary artery disease.

Ascending Aorta

All patients with acute dissections involving the ascending aorta should be considered candidates for surgery. The most commonly performed procedure is replacement of the ascending aorta and aortic valve with a composite graft containing a Dacron graft and a mechanical valve prosthesis.

Aortic Arch

In patients with acute aortic arch dissections, resection of the aortic arch (segment of the thoracic aorta that extends from the proximal origin of the innominate artery to the distal origin of the left subclavian artery) is indicated. Operations on the aortic arch usually require hypothermic cardiopulmonary bypass and a period of circulatory arrest. With current techniques, a period of circulatory arrest up to 30 to 40 minutes at body temperatures of 15°C to 18°C are tolerated by most patients.[4] Focal and diffuse neurologic deficits are the major complications associated with resection of aneurysms of the aortic arch, occurring in 3% to 18% of patients.

Descending Thoracic Aorta

For patients with degenerative or chronic aneurysms, elective resection is advisable if the aneurysms exceed 5 to 6 cm in diameter or if symptoms are present. Most patients with type B (DeBakey type III) acute descending thoracic aorta dissections can be treated initially with medical therapy, which consists of (1) monitoring the systemic blood pressure (most often continuous intra-arterial monitoring) and urinary output and (2) administering drugs to control the systemic blood pressure (nitroprusside) and the force of left ventricular contraction

(β-adrenergic antagonists). Surgery is indicated for patients with signs of impending rupture (persisting pain, hypotension, left-sided hemothorax) and those with ischemia of the legs or abdominal viscera, renal failure, paraparesis, or paraplegia. Endovascular placement of intraluminal stent grafts to treat patients with aneurysms of the descending thoracic aorta may be particularly useful in elderly individuals or those with co-existing medical conditions (systemic hypertension, COPD, renal insufficiency) that would significantly increase the risk of conventional operative treatments.

Unique Risks of Surgery

Surgical resection of thoracic aortic aneurysms, and to a lesser extent abdominal aortic aneurysms, is associated with a risk of spinal cord ischemia (anterior spinal artery syndrome) with resulting paraparesis or paraplegia. Likewise, cross-clamping and unclamping the aorta introduces the potential for adverse hemodynamic responses, especially during resection of thoracic aortic aneurysms, as the cross-clamp must be placed near the heart.

Anterior Spinal Artery Syndrome

An uncommon but devastating complication of cross-clamping the thoracic aorta for thoracic aneurysm resection surgery is ischemic damage to the anterior spinal cord (Fig. 10–2).[5] The frequency of spinal cord injury ranges from 0.2% after elective repair of infrarenal abdominal aortic aneurysms to as high as 40% in the setting of acute dissections or ruptures involving the descending thoracic aorta.[5, 6] Anterior spinal artery syndrome may also follow retroperitoneal surgery (nephrectomy, pancreatic resection) when the artery of Adamkiewicz originates from the lumbar portion of the aorta. Manifestations of the anterior spinal artery syndrome include flaccid paralysis of the lower extremities. Bowel and bladder dysfunction are common, but sensation and proprioception are usually spared.

Risk Factors

The risk of paraplegia during thoracic aortic surgery is determined by the interaction of four independent processes: (1) decreases in spinal blood flow; (2) rate of neuronal metabolism; (3) postischemia reperfusion; and (4) postreperfusion blood flow. Because the main mechanism of paraplegia associated with cross-clamping the descending thoracic aorta lies in spinal cord ischemia and reperfusion, the duration

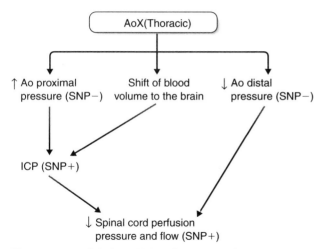

Figure 10–2 • Spinal cord blood flow and perfusion pressures during thoracic aortic occlusion, with or without sodium nitroprusside (SNP) infusion. The changes (*arrows*) represent the response to aortic cross-clamping per se. Ao, aortic; AoX, aortic cross-clamping; ICP, intracranial pressure; SNP+, SNP aggravates the effect of cross-clamping; SNP−, SNP counteracts the effect of cross-clamping; ↑ and ↓, increase and decrease, respectively. (From Gelman S. The pathophysiology of aortic cross-clamping and unclamping. Anesthesiology 1995;82:1026–60. © 1995, Lippincott Williams & Wilkins, with permission.)

of cross-clamping is influential. In this regard, a brief period of thoracic aortic cross-clamping (less than 30 minutes) or the use of partial circulatory assistance or a shunt may decrease the likelihood of this complication following resection of a descending thoracic aortic aneurysm.[5, 7] In addition, a combination of other factors including intercostal reimplantation whenever possible, cerebrospinal fluid drainage, maintenance of proximal systemic hypertension during cross-clamping, reduction of spinal cord metabolism by moderate hypothermia, barbiturates and avoidance of hyperglycemia, and the use of mannitol, steroids, and calcium channel antagonists may further reduce the risk of postoperative spinal cord dysfunction in patients undergoing thoracoabdominal aortic aneurysm resection.[5]

Spinal Cord Blood Supply

The anatomy of the blood supply of the spinal cord is the reason cross-clamping of the thoracic aorta may introduce the risk of spinal cord ischemia. The spinal cord is supplied by one anterior spinal artery and two posterior spinal arteries. The anterior spinal artery relies on reinforcement of its blood supply by six to eight medullary arteries, the most important and largest of which is the artery of Adamkiewicz. Multiple levels of the spinal cord do not receive feeding medullary branches, thus leaving

watershed areas that are particularly susceptible to ischemic injury. The tenuous collateral anastomosis of the anterior spinal artery in the midthoracic region places segments of the spinal cord in jeopardy during aortic occlusion or hypotension. Damage may result from surgical dissection of the artery of Adamkiewicz (because the origin is unknown) or exclusion of the origin of the artery by cross clamps (usually applied between T5 and L1). Cross-clamping the proximal descending thoracic aorta interrupts the blood supply to the area of the spinal cord supplied by the aortic segment distal to the clamp.[8] If the artery of Adamkiewicz arises from the portion of the aorta that is cross-clamped, the pressure in the anterior spinal artery may be much less than the pressure in the distal aorta.

Hemodynamic Responses to Aortic Cross-Clamping

Aortic cross-clamping and unclamping are associated with severe homeostatic disturbances in virtually all organ systems in the body, as reflected by expected decreases in blood flow distal to the aortic clamp and substantial increases in blood flow above the occlusion (Fig. 10–3).[5] Hemodynamic responses to cross-clamping the aorta consist of increased systemic blood pressure and increased systemic vascu-

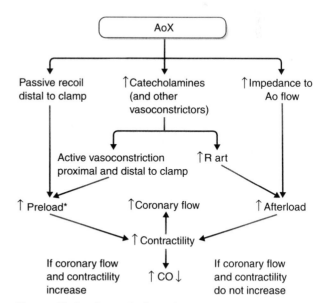

Figure 10–3 • Systemic hemodynamic responses to aortic cross-clamping. Preload does not necessarily increase. If during infrarenal aortic cross-clamping the blood volume shifts into the splanchnic vasculature, preload does not increase. Ao, aortic; AoX, aortic cross-clamping; R art, arterial resistance; ↑ and ↓, increase and decrease, respectively. (From Gelman S. The pathophysiology of aortic cross-clamping and unclamping. Anesthesiology 1995;82:1026–60. © 1995, Lippincott Williams & Wilkins, with permission.)

lar resistance with no significant changes in heart rate. In most but not all instances cardiac output decreases. Systemic hypertension is the most dramatic, consistent component of the hemodynamic responses to aortic cross-clamping and is attributed to increased impedance to aortic outflow (increased systemic vascular resistance and afterload). In addition, there is blood volume redistribution caused by collapse and constriction of the venous vasculature distal to the aortic cross-clamp and a subsequent increase in preload (Fig. 10–4).[5] Evidence of blood volume redistribution is the increase in filling pressures (central venous pressure, pulmonary capillary occlusion pressure, left ventricular end-diastolic pressure) that often accompanies cross-clamping the

thoracic aorta. Substantial differences in hemodynamic responses observed after aortic cross-clamping at different levels (supraceliac versus infraceliac aortic cross-clamping) may result in part from different patterns of blood volume redistribution. Preload may not increase if the aorta is clamped distal to the celiac artery, in which case the blood volume from the distal venous vasculature may be redistributed into the splanchnic vasculature without associated increases in preload. Increases in afterload and preload require an increase in myocardial contractility, which results in autoregulatory increases in coronary blood flow. If coronary blood flow and myocardial contractility are not increased, decompensation is likely to follow. Indeed, echocar-

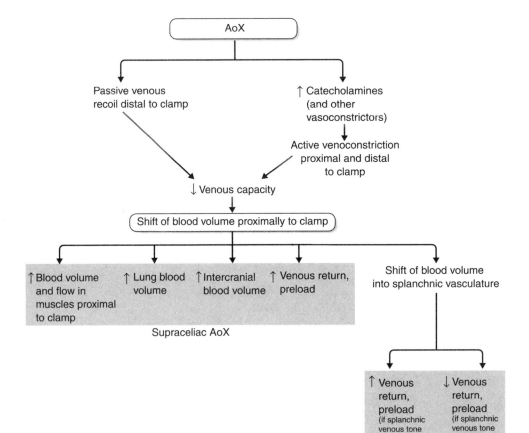

Figure 10–4 • Blood volume redistribution during aortic cross-clamping. This scheme depicts the reason for the decrease in venous capacity, which results in blood volume redistribution from the vasculature distal to the aortic occlusion to the vasculature proximal to the occlusion. If the aorta is occluded above the splanchnic system, the blood volume travels to the heart, increasing preload and blood volume in all organs and tissues proximal to the clamp. However, if the aorta is occluded below the splanchnic system, blood volume may shift into the splanchnic system or into the vasculature of other tissues proximal to the clamp. The distribution of this blood volume between the splanchnic and nonsplanchnic vasculature determines changes in preload. AoX, aortic cross-clamping; ↑ and ↓, increase and decrease, respectively. (From Gelman S. The pathophysiology of aortic cross-clamping and unclamping. Anesthesiology 1995;82:1026–60. © 1995, Lippincott Williams & Wilkins, with permission.)

diography often indicates abnormal wall motion of the left ventricle, suggesting the presence of myocardial ischemia.

The level of aortic cross-clamping is important to the degree and pattern of hemodynamic changes. Changes in mean arterial pressure, filling pressures, end-diastolic and end-systolic left ventricular areas, ejection fraction, and wall motion abnormalities as assessed by transesophageal echocardiography are minimal during infrarenal aortic cross-clamping but dramatic during supraceliac aortic cross-clamping.[5] Furthermore, systemic vascular resistance increases and cardiac output decreases with increasing duration of aortic cross-clamping. Hemodynamic responses to aortic cross-clamping seem to be blunted in patients with aortic occlusive disease.

Pulmonary damage associated with aortic cross-clamping and unclamping is reflected by increases in pulmonary vascular resistance (particularly with unclamping of the aorta), increases in capillary membrane permeability, and development of pulmonary edema. The mechanisms involved may include pulmonary hypervolemia and the effects of various mediators, mainly prostaglandins, oxygen free radicals, the renin-angiotensin system, and the complement cascade.

Cross-clamping the thoracic aorta markedly decreases perfusion pressures to organs below the clamp, although collateral vessels may deliver some blood to distal structures. For example, cross-clamping the thoracic aorta just distal to the left subclavian artery is associated with severe decreases (85% to 94%) in spinal cord blood flow and renal blood flow, glomerular filtration rate, and urinary output.[5] Infrarenal aortic cross-clamping is associated with large increases in renal vascular resistance and up to 30% decreases in renal blood flow. Renal dysfunction results from renal hypoperfusion and involves activation of the renin-angiotensin system, the sympathetic nervous system, and other mediators. Renal failure following aortic surgery almost always results from acute tubular necrosis. Ischemia-reperfusion insults to the kidneys play a central role in the pathogenesis of this renal failure.

Cross-clamping the thoracic aorta is associated not only with decreases in distal aortic-anterior spinal artery pressures but also with increases in cerebrospinal fluid pressure and decreases in the compliance of the spinal fluid space. Presumably, intracranial hypertension during aortic cross-clamping is due to systemic hypertension above the clamp, producing redistribution of the blood volume (intracranial hypervolemia) and engorgement of the intracranial compartment. In this regard, cerebrospinal fluid drainage may increase spinal cord

blood flow, diminish reperfusion hypervolemia, and decrease the incidence of neurologic complications.[5]

Aortic cross-clamping is associated with the formation and release of hormonal factors (activation of the sympathetic nervous system and increased concentrations of epinephrine and norepinephrine, renin-angiotensin system) and other mediators (prostaglandins, oxygen free radicals, complement cascade). These mediators may aggravate or blunt the harmful effects of aortic cross-clamping and unclamping. Overall, injury to the spinal cord, lungs, kidneys, and abdominal viscera is principally due to ischemia and subsequent reperfusion of organs distal to the aortic cross-clamp (local effects) or to release of mediators from ischemic and reperfused tissues (distant effects).[5]

Pharmacologic interventions intended to offset the hemodynamic effects of aortic cross-clamping, especially the thoracic aorta, are often related to the effects of the administered drug on arterial and/or venous capacitance, emphasizing the importance of blood volume redistribution evoked by aortic cross-clamping. For example, vasodilators such as nitroprusside and nitroglycerin often reduce aortic cross-clamping-induced decreases in cardiac output. The most plausible explanation for this effect is drug-induced decreases in systemic vascular resistance and afterload and increased venous capacitance with subsequent increases in the ejection fraction and cardiac output. Volatile anesthetics decrease the ability of the myocardium to increase its contractility in response to aortic cross-clamping.

It is important to recognize that perfusion pressures distal to the aortic cross-clamp are decreased and are directly dependent on the proximal systemic pressures above the aortic cross-clamp.[5] Blood flow through the tissues (kidneys, liver, spinal cord) distal to the aortic occlusion, which occurs through existing collateral vessels, is pressure-dependent and decreases dramatically during aortic cross-clamping. Therefore blood flow distal to the aortic occlusion depends on perfusion pressures and not cardiac output or volume load. Drugs such as nitroprusside decrease both proximal and distal aortic pressures. Vasoconstrictors may constrict vasculature above the aortic clamp more than below the clamp because the nonischemic tissues are likely to respond better to vasopressors than the ischemic and acidotic tissues.

Clinically, drugs and volume replacement must be adjusted to maintain distal perfusion pressures even if it results in increased systemic blood pressures proximal to the clamp. Strategies for myocardial preservation during and after aortic cross-clamping include decreasing afterload and normalizing preload, coronary blood flow, and contractility. Modalities such as temporary shunts, reimplantation of arteries supplying distal tissues (spinal cord), and hypothermia may influence the choice of drugs and endpoints of treatment.

Hemodynamic Responses to Aortic Unclamping

Unclamping the thoracic aorta is associated with substantial (70% to 80%) decreases in systemic vascular resistance and systemic blood pressure (Fig. 10–5).[5] Cardiac output may increase, decrease, or remain unchanged. Left ventricular end-diastolic pressures decrease, and myocardial blood flow increases. Reactive hyperemia is one of the important components of the response to aortic unclamping. Gradual release of the aortic clamp is recommended to allow time for volume replacement and to slow the washout of the vasoactive and cardiodepressant mediators from ischemic tissues.

The principal explanations for unclamping hypotension include (1) central hypovolemia caused by the pooling of blood into reperfused tissues distal to the aortic occlusion; (2) hypoxia-mediated vasodilation with subsequent increases in vascular (venous) capacity in the extremities below the occlusion; and (3) accumulation of vasoactive and myocardium-depressant metabolites.[5] Vasodilation and hypotension may be further aggravated by transient increases in carbon dioxide release from tissues and increases in oxygen consumption following unclamping. Correction of metabolic acidosis does not significantly influence the degree of hypotension during unclamping of the aorta, which may reflect failure of sodium bicarbonate to correct acidosis in the tissues and walls of the blood vessels. It is even conceivable that oxygen free radical-induced increases in microvascular permeability and subsequent loss of intravascular fluid volume are responsible in part for the hypovolemia and hypotension observed during unclamping of the aorta.

Management of Anesthesia

Management of anesthesia in patients undergoing thoracic aneurysm resection requires special considerations for monitoring the systemic blood pressure, neurologic function, and intravascular fluid volume, as well as pharmacologic interventions to control systemic hypertension during the period of aortic cross-clamping. Proper monitoring is more important than the drugs selected for anesthesia in patients undergoing resection of a thoracic aortic aneurysm.

Monitoring Systemic Blood Pressure

Surgical repair of a thoracic aortic aneurysm (or coarctation of the aorta) requires aortic cross-clamping just distal to the left subclavian artery or between the left subclavian and left common carotid arteries. For these reasons monitoring the systemic blood pressure must be via an artery in the right upper extremity, as occlusion of the aorta proximal to the left subclavian artery would prevent recording the blood pressure in the left upper extremity. Loss of arterial blood pressure tracings from an artery in the right upper extremity during cross-clamping of the thoracic aorta occurs if the innominate artery is occluded. Monitoring the systemic blood pressure above (right radial artery) and below (femoral artery) the aneurysm is useful. This approach permits assessment of cerebral perfusion pressures as well as perfusion pressures to the kidneys during aortic cross-clamping.

Blood flow through the tissues below the aortic cross-clamp is dependent on perfusion pressures rather than on preload and cardiac output. There-

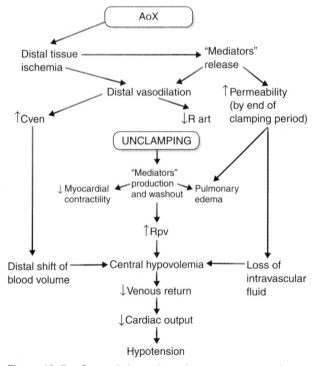

Figure 10–5 • Systemic hemodynamic responses to aortic unclamping. AoX, aortic cross-clamping; Cven, venous capacitance; R art, arterial resistance; Rpv, pulmonary vascular resistance; ↑ and ↓, increase and decrease, respectively. (From Gelman S. The pathophysiology of aortic cross-clamping and unclamping. Anesthesiology 1995;82:1026–60. © 1995, Lippincott Williams & Wilkins, with permission.)

fore during cross-clamping of the thoracic aorta, proximal and distal aortic pressures should be maintained as high as the heart can withstand unless other modalities (temporary shunts, hypothermia, or reimplantation of arteries supplying tissues distal to aortic cross-clamping) are implemented.[5] Drugs such as sympathomimetics and vasodilators may be needed to adjust perfusion pressures above and below the level of the aortic cross-clamp. Esmolol has been used to provide systemic blood pressure control comparable to that seen with nitroprusside but without the likelihood of the reflex tachycardia and decreased PaO_2 that may accompany administration of vasodilators.[9] A common recommendation is to maintain the mean arterial pressure near 100 mmHg in the upper part of the body and above 50 mmHg in the portion of the body distal to the aortic cross-clamp. The use of vasodilators to treat systemic blood pressure elevations above the level of the aortic cross-clamp must be balanced against the likely undesirable decreases in perfusion pressures below the clamp. Indeed, nitroprusside may decrease spinal cord perfusion pressures by decreasing the distal aortic pressures below the aortic cross-clamp and by increasing cerebral spinal fluid pressure secondary to cerebral vasodilation (Fig. 10–2).[5] For this reason it may be prudent to limit the use of drugs that decrease proximal aortic pressures and at the same time cause cerebral vasodilation. Use of a temporary external heparinized shunt to bypass the occluded thoracic aorta (proximal aorta to femoral artery) may be considered when attempting to maintain distal circulation to the kidneys and spinal cord. Alternatively, left heart bypass may be performed, but the need for systemic heparinization is a possible disadvantage.

Monitoring Neurologic Function

Monitoring somatosensory evoked potentials (SEPs) or electroencephalography are methods for evaluating central nervous system (CNS) viability during the period of aortic cross-clamping. Intraoperative monitoring of SEPs has not proven reliable for detecting spinal cord ischemia and avoidance of postoperative neurologic damage.[10, 11] This is not surprising as SEP monitoring principally reflects dorsal column (sensory tracts) function, such that ischemic changes of anterior cord function (motor tracts) are not detected. For this reason, monitoring SEPs has limited value for thoracic aortic aneurysm resection. Monitoring motor evoked potentials would reflect anterior spinal cord function but is not practical as it would prohibit use of neuromuscular blocking drugs.

Monitoring Cardiac Function

During operations on the thoracic aorta, transesophageal echocardiography is invaluable for assessing the presence of atherosclerosis in the thoracic aorta, the competence of cardiac valves, ventricular function, adequacy of myocardial oxygenation, and volume replacement. A pulmonary artery catheter is commonly placed in these patients and the data so obtained complement the information derived from transesophageal echocardiography.

Monitoring Intravascular Fluid Volume

Pulmonary protection during and after the period of aortic cross-clamping consists of careful titration of fluid volume replacement and the use of diuretics such as mannitol. In the future, specific antagonists of hormonal and humoral factors that are formed and released from ischemic tissues during and after the period of aortic cross-clamping may become available.[5] Optimization of systemic hemodynamics, including circulating blood volume, represents the most effective measure for protecting the kidneys from the ischemic effects produced by aortic cross-clamping. Diuretics are often administered to maintain urine output during the period of aortic cross-clamping, but there is no clinical proof that this intervention is protective.[5]

Induction and Maintenance of Anesthesia

Induction of anesthesia and tracheal intubation must minimize undesirable increases in systemic blood pressure, which could exacerbate the aortic dissection. Selective endobronchial intubation permitting collapse of the left lung facilitates surgical exposure during resection of the thoracic aneurysm. A disadvantage of one-lung ventilation is production of an iatrogenic shunt that can lead to arterial hypoxemia despite maximum delivered concentrations of oxygen. The magnitude of this iatrogenic intrapulmonary shunt can be decreased by minimizing pulmonary blood flow through the collapsed lung. The selective application of continuous positive airway pressure (2.5 to 10 cmH_2O) to the nondependent unventilated lung may improve arterial oxygenation as well. If this does not improve arterial oxygenation, it may be beneficial to apply selective positive end-expiratory pressure (2.5 to 10 cmH_2O) to the dependent ventilated lung. General anesthesia, including volatile anesthetics and opioids, is frequently chosen for maintenance of anesthesia, as it takes advantage of the cerebral metabolic suppression produced by these drugs. The choice of neuromuscular blocking drugs may be influenced by the dependence of some of these drugs on renal clearance mechanisms.

Postoperative Management

Posterolateral thoractomy is among the most painful of surgical incisions because major muscles are transected and ribs are removed.[12] Additionally, chest tube insertion sites are often extremely painful. Amelioration of pain is essential for patient comfort and to facilitate coughing and maneuvers designed to prevent atelectasis. Pain relief is commonly provided by intrathecal or epidural placement (intermittent or continuous infusion) of opioids or local anesthetics and the institution of patient-controlled analgesia. Inclusion of local anesthetics in the solutions placed in the epidural space may produce sensory and motor anesthesia, which delays recognition of the postoperative anterior spinal artery syndrome. Moreover, when the neurologic deficit is recognized, the epidural may be erroneously implicated as a cause of postoperative paraplegia. If epidural analgesia is utilized during the immediate postoperative period, opioids may be preferred over local anesthetics to prevent masking an anterior spinal artery syndrome.[13] Drainage of cerebrospinal fluid has been reported to be effective for treating a patient developing delayed-onset paraparesis (13 hours following thoracic aneurysm resection).[14]

Patients recovering from thoracic aortic aneurysm resection are at risk for developing cardiac, ventilatory, and renal failure during the immediate postoperative period. Cerebrovascular accidents may be produced by air or thrombotic emboli that occur during surgical resection of the diseased aorta. Patients with co-existing cerebrovascular disease are probably more vulnerable to the development of CNS complications. The possibility of postoperative CNS dysfunction including paraparesis or paralysis emphasizes the importance of documenting any preoperative abnormalities. Spinal cord injury may manifest during the immediate postoperative period as paraparesis or flaccid paralysis. Delayed appearance of paraplegia during the postoperative period (12 hours to 21 days) has been associated with postoperative myocardial infarction and/or hypotension, in patients with severe atherosclerotic disease and in whom marginally adequate collateral circulation is present (artery of Adamkiewicz resected during earlier surgery).[8]

Systemic hypertension is not uncommon and may jeopardize the vascular integrity of the surgical repair and/or predispose to myocardial ischemia. The role of pain in the etiology of systemic hypertension must be considered. Institution of antihypertensive therapy with drugs such as nitroglycerin, nitroprusside, hydralazine, or labetalol may be appropriate. Some patients benefit from administration of β-antagonists to attenuate manifestations of a hyperdynamic circulation.

■ MYOCARDIAL CONTUSION

Deceleration injuries caused by sudden impact of the anterior chest wall against the automobile steering wheel may cause acute dissection of the descending thoracic aorta, and they are the most common cause of myocardial contusion. Sudden deceleration from speeds as low as 33 km/hr may injure the heart without displaying any obvious external signs of trauma on the patient's anterior chest. Because of its immediate substernal location, the right ventricle is more likely than the left ventricle to be injured.

Signs and Symptoms

Chest pain resembling angina pectoris but unrelieved by nitroglycerin may be present. The presence of chest pain and changes on the electrocardiogram (ECG) resembling myocardial infarction, especially in young patients, should prompt questions about recent chest trauma that might have seemed trivial at the time of its occurrence. The most important complications of myocardial contusion are cardiac dysrhythmias.

Blunt trauma may injure any of the cardiac valves, leading to valvular regurgitation. The most severe valvular injuries are those in which the chordae tendineae or papillary muscles of the mitral or tricuspid valve rupture or in which an aortic cusp ruptures. Pulmonary contusion may also result from blunt thoracic trauma manifesting as a diffuse nonsegmental airspace consolidation on the chest radiograph. Hemorrhage into the tracheobronchial tree may accompany pulmonary contusion.

Diagnosis

Cardiac contusion is best recognized clinically by transthoracic or transesophageal echocardiography, which shows localized areas of impaired wall motion. Wall motion abnormalities usually resolve within a few days. Serum concentrations of creatine kinase (CK) and its MB fraction (CK-MB) increase but are difficult to interpret because of the release of CK from injured skeletal muscles. In this regard, the CK-MB/total CK ratio is more useful than are the absolute levels, and the serum concentrations of cardiac troponin I are even more specific.

Treatment

Treatment of myocardial contusion is directed toward the symptoms and anticipation of possible complications. Continuous monitoring of the ECG is necessary to detect life-threatening cardiac dysrhythmias. Diffuse nonspecific ST-T segment abnormalities on the ECG are common in injured patients even in the absence of echocardiographic wall motion abnormalities. Localized changes, especially ST segment elevation, are more specific for myocardial contusion. Patients with Q wave infarct patterns and irreversible wall motion defects are likely to have a coronary artery occlusion secondary to trauma.

ANEURYSMS OF THE ABDOMINAL AORTA

Abdominal aortic aneurysms have historically been viewed as atherosclerotic, but there is little evidence to support this perception.[15] In fact, atherosclerosis may represent a secondary, nonspecific response to vessel wall injury.

Diagnosis

Clinically, abdominal aneurysms can usually be detected as pulsating masses in the absence of any other symptoms. Abdominal ultrasonography detects aneurysms with a sensitivity that approaches 100%. Computed tomography is highly sensitive for identifying abdominal aortic aneurysms and may be more accurate than ultrasonography for estimating the size of the aneurysm. In contrast to computed tomography, magnetic resonance imaging may be superior for accurate aneurysm measurement and views of the relevant vascular anatomy without exposing the patient to ionizing radiation or the need to inject contrast medium.

Treatment

Considering the low mortality associated with elective resection of abdominal aortic aneurysms, surgery is usually recommended for all aneurysms larger than 5 cm in diameter.[15] This recommendation is influenced by clinical studies suggesting that 25% to 41% of aneurysms larger than 5 cm in diameter

rupture spontaneously within 5 years. Smaller aneurysms are less likely to rupture, but removal of any clinically detectable abdominal aortic aneurysm may be justified in patients considered at low operative risk.[16] An alternative to surgery may be endovascular placement of a stent via an arteriotomy in the leg.

Preoperative Evaluation

Co-existing diseases, particularly coronary artery disease, are important to identify preoperatively in an attempt to minimize postoperative complications. Indeed, postoperative myocardial infarction is responsible for most of the postoperative deaths following elective resection of abdominal aortic aneurysms. Preoperative evaluation of cardiac function may include monitored exercise testing, echocardiography, radionuclide angiography, and dipyridamole-thallium scanning. Other adverse postoperative cardiac events are cardiac dysrhythmias and congestive heart failure. Co-existing conditions that may influence the decision to proceed with elective resection of an abdominal aortic aneurysm are COPD (vital capacity and forced expiratory volume in 1 second less than 50% of normal) and marginal renal function (serum creatinine concentrations higher than 3 mg/dl).

Rupture of an Abdominal Aortic Aneurysm

Although the diagnosis of a ruptured abdominal aortic aneurysm may be obvious, the classic triad (hypotension, back pain, a pulsatile abdominal mass) is present in only about one-half of patients.[15] Renal colic, diverticulitis, and gastrointestinal hemorrhage may be confused with ruptured abdominal aortic aneurysms.

Most abdominal aortic aneurysms rupture into the left retroperitoneum. Although the patient may be in hypovolemic shock, exsanguination is not the rule because of clotting and the tamponade effect of the retroperitoneum. So long as patients are conscious and have adequate peripheral perfusion, euvolemic resuscitation should be deferred until the aortic rupture is surgically controlled in the operating room.[15] Euvolemic resuscitation and increasing the systemic blood pressure without surgical control of bleeding from the ruptured aneurysm may lead to loss of retroperitoneal tamponade, resulting in further bleeding, hypotension, and death. In patients who are unstable with a suspected ruptured abdominal aortic aneurysm, immediate operation and control of the proximal portion of the aorta without confirmatory testing (ultrasonography, computed tomography) or optimizing the patient's preoperative condition (volume resuscitation) is mandatory.

Management of Anesthesia

Management of anesthesia for resection of abdominal aortic aneurysms must consider the high incidence of associated ischemic heart disease, systemic hypertension, COPD, diabetes mellitus, and renal dysfunction in these usually elderly patients. In view of the many complications associated with surgical resection of abdominal aortic aneurysms, it is important to monitor the intravascular fluid volume and cardiac, pulmonary, and renal function during the perioperative period. Systemic blood pressure is monitored continuously by an intra-arterial catheter, keeping in mind that perfusion of tissues distal to the aortic clamp is pressure-dependent. Pulmonary artery catheterization is indicated in most patients, as it is not always possible to predict whether central venous pressures will parallel left heart filling pressures. This is particularly true in patients with a history of previous myocardial infarction or angina pectoris or in those who exhibit signs of congestive heart failure. Echocardiography is an important monitor for evaluating cardiac responses to aortic cross-clamping and unclamping, providing an assessment of left ventricular filling volume and regional and global myocardial contractility and oxygenation. Urine output is monitored continuously. Warming of fluids and blood helps maintain body temperature.

No single anesthetic drug or technique is ideal for all patients undergoing elective surgical resection of an abdominal aortic aneurysm. Combinations of volatile drugs and opioids are commonly used with or without nitrous oxide.[17] Continuous epidural anesthesia combined with general anesthesia provides the advantages of decreased depressant drug requirements, attenuation of increased systemic vascular resistance with aortic cross-clamping, and significant alleviation of postoperative pain. Nevertheless, there is no evidence that this combination technique decreases postoperative cardiac or pulmonary morbidity compared with similar high risk patients undergoing the same abdominal aortic surgery with general anesthesia.[18] There remains, however, the possibility that postoperative epidural analgesia may favorably influence the postoperative course. Anticoagulation during abdominal aortic surgery introduces the controversy regarding placement of an epidural catheter and the remote risk of epidural hematoma formation.

Patients undergoing abdominal aortic surgery usually experience major functional extracellular fluid and blood loss. A combination of balanced salt and colloid solutions guided by appropriate monitoring of cardiac and renal function facilitates maintenance of an adequate intravascular fluid volume, cardiac output, and urine formation. Balanced salt solutions, with or without colloid solutions, should be infused during aortic cross-clamping. In this way, pulmonary artery occlusion pressures are maintained 3 to 5 mmHg above preclamp values, thereby minimizing declamping hypotension and decreased cardiac output. If urinary output is decreased (less than 50 ml/hr) despite adequate fluid and blood replacement, diuretic therapy with mannitol or furosemide may be considered. Low-dose dopamine (approximately 3 μg/kg/min IV) may also be administered to improve renal function, although the efficacy of low dose dopamine in preserving renal function during abdominal aortic aneurysm surgery is unproven.[19]

Infrarenal aortic cross-clamping and unclamping is an integral component of abdominal aortic surgery. The anticipated consequences of sudden abdominal aortic cross-clamping include increased systemic vascular resistance (afterload) and decreased venous return (see "Hemodynamic Responses to Aortic Cross-Clamping"). Nevertheless, myocardial performance and circulatory variables usually remain within acceptable ranges after the aorta is occluded at an infrarenal level, even in patients with co-existing cardiac dysfunction. Deepening of anesthesia or administration of vasodilators at the time of infrarenal aortic occlusion is necessary in some patients to maintain myocardial performance at acceptable levels.

Despite the negligible cardiovascular effects of infrarenal cross-clamping, hypotension still may occur when the cross-clamp is removed (see "Hemodynamic Responses to Aortic Unclamping"). Severe hypotension is unlikely, but transient decreases in systolic blood pressure of about 40 mmHg are not uncommon. Prevention of declamping hypotension and maintenance of a stable cardiac output are often achieved by volume loading to create pulmonary capillary occlusion pressures before cross-clamp removal that are higher than the preoperative pulmonary capillary occlusion pressures. Likewise, gradual removal of the aortic cross-clamp may minimize decreases in systemic blood pressure by allowing pooled venous blood to return to the central circulation. The role of washout of acid metabolites from ischemic extremities when the clamp is released has been questioned, as sodium bicarbonate pretreatment does not reliably blunt declamping hypotension. If hypotension persists more than about 4 minutes after removing the cross-clamp, the presence of unrecognized bleeding or inadequate volume replacement must be considered. Echocardiography at this time may be helpful for determining the adequacy of volume replacement and cardiac output.

Postoperative Management

Patients recovering from an abdominal aortic aneurysm resection are at risk for the development of cardiac, ventilatory, and renal failure during the immediate postoperative period. Assessment of graft patency and lower extremity blood flow is important. Provision of adequate analgesia, such as with neuraxial opioids with or without local anesthetics or patient-controlled analgesia, should be given priority. Pain relief is important for permitting early tracheal extubation.

Systemic hypertension is a potentially serious complication during the postoperative period that seems more likely in patients with preoperative hypertension. Overzealous intraoperative hydration and/or postoperative hypothermia with compensatory vasoconstriction may contribute to postoperative hypertension. Treatment of postoperative systemic hypertension consists of excluding contributing causes and prompt institution of antihypertensive therapy with drugs such as nitroglycerin, nitroprusside, labetalol, or hydralazine. Preoperative administration of clonidine may attenuate hyperdynamic responses during the postoperative period.

References

1. Kouchoukos NT, Dougenis D. Surgery of the thoracic aorta. N Engl J Med 1997;336:1876–88
2. Williams GM, Gott VL, Brawley RK, et al. Aortic disease associated with pregnancy. J Vasc Surg 1988;8:470–5
3. Hagan PG, Nienaber CA, Isselbacher EM, et al. The international registry of acute aortic dissection (IRAD): new insights into an old disease. JAMA 2000;283:987–1003
4. Ergin MA, Griepp EB, Lansman SL, et al. Hypothermic circulatory arrest and other methods of cerebral protection during operations on the thoracic aorta. J Card Surg 1994;9:525–37
5. Gelman S. The pathophysiology of aortic cross-clamping and unclamping. Anesthesiology 1995;82:1026–60
6. Gharagozloo F, Larson J, Dausmann MJ, et al. Spinal cord protection during surgical procedures on the descending thoracic and thoracoabdominal aorta: review of current techniques. Chest 1996;109:799–809
7. Liversay JL, Cooley DA, Ventemiglia RA, et al. Surgical experience in descending thoracic aneurysmectomy with and without adjuncts to avoid ischemia. Ann Thorac Surg 1995;39:37–46
8. Fitzgibbon DR, Glosten B, Wright I, et al. Paraplegia, epidural analgesia, and thoracic aneurysmectomy. Anesthesiology 1995;83:1355–9
9. Fenner SG, Mahoney A, Cashman JN. Repair of traumatic transection of the thoracic aorta: esmolol for intraoperative control of arterial pressure. Br J Anesth 1991;67:483–7
10. Crawford ES, Mizrahi EM, Hess OR, et al. The impact of distal aortic perfusion and somatosensory evoked potential monitoring on prevention of paraplegia after aortic aneurysm operation. J Thorac Cardiovasc Surg 1988;95:357–67
11. Loughman BA, Hal GM. Spinal cord monitoring 1989. Br J Anaesth 1989;63:589–94
12. Weissman C. Pulmonary function after cardiac and thoracic surgery. Anesth Analg 1999;88:1272–9
13. Linz SM, Charbonnet C, Mikhail MS, et al. Spinal artery syndrome masked by postoperative epidural analgesia. Can J Anaesth 1997;44:1178–81
14. Khong B, Yang H, Doobay B, et al. Reversal of paraparesis after thoracic aneurysm repair by cerebrospinal fluid drainage. Can J Anaesth 2000;47:992–5
15. Ernst CB. Abdominal aortic aneurysm. N Engl J Med 1993;328:1167–77
16. Crawford ES, Hess OR. Abdominal aortic aneurysm. N Engl J Med 1989;321:1040–1
17. Cunningham AJ. Anaesthesia for abdominal aortic surgery: a review. Part II. Can J Anaesth 1989;36:568–77
18. Baron J-F, Bertrand M, Barre E, et al. Combined epidural and general anesthesia versus general anesthesia for abdominal aortic surgery. Anesthesiology 1981;55:618–20
19. Thadhani R, Pascual M, Bonventre JV. Acute renal failure. N Engl J Med 1996;334:1448–60

11

Peripheral Vascular Disease

Peripheral arterial disease results in compromised blood flow to the extremities, especially the legs. Chronic impairment of blood flow to the extremities is most often due to atherosclerosis, whereas embolism is most likely to be responsible for acute arterial occlusions (Table 11–1). Vasculitis may also be responsible for compromised blood flow to the extremities.

■ PERIPHERAL ATHEROSCLEROSIS

Peripheral atherosclerosis (arteriosclerosis obliterans) in the extremities resembles atherosclerosis seen in the aorta, coronary arteries, and extracranial cerebral arteries. The prevalence of peripheral atherosclerosis increases with age, exceeding 70% in individuals older than 75 years of age.[1] In many instances patients do not walk sufficient distances to elicit clinical symptoms. Among patients who present with symptoms (claudication) of peripheral atherosclerosis, 80% have femoropopliteal stenoses, 40% have tibioperoneal artery stenoses, and 30% have lesions in the aorta or iliac arteries. Long-term survival is decreased in patients with peripheral atherosclerosis, with most patients dying from myocardial infarction or stroke.[2]

Risk Factors

Risk factors associated with the development of peripheral atherosclerosis are similar to those that cause ischemic heart disease: diabetes mellitus, essential hypertension, tobacco abuse, dyslipidemia, hyperhomocysteinemia, and a family history of premature atherosclerosis. The risk of developing claudication is doubled in those who smoke tobacco

157

Table 11-1 • Peripheral Vascular Disease

Chronic peripheral arterial occlusive disease
  (atherosclerosis)
    Distal abdominal aorta or iliac arteries
    Femoral arteries
    Subclavian steal syndrome
Acute peripheral arterial occlusive disease (embolism)
Systemic vasculitis
    Takayasu's arteritis (pulseless disease)
    Thromboangiitis obliterans (Buerger's disease)
    Wegener's granulomatosis
    Temporal arteritis
    Polyarteritis nodosa
Other vascular syndromes
    Schönlein-Henoch purpura
    Raynaud's phenomenon
    Moyamoya disease
    Kawasaki disease
    Coronary-subclavian steal syndrome
    Klippel-Trénaunay syndrome
    Behçet's disease

compared with nonsmokers. Furthermore, continued cigarette smoking enhances the risk of progression from stable claudication to severe limb ischemia and amputation.

Signs and Symptoms

Intermittent claudication and rest pain are the principal symptoms of peripheral atherosclerosis.[3] Intermittent claudication occurs when the metabolic requirements of exercising skeletal muscles (walking) exceeds oxygen delivery, which is compromised by stenotic vascular lesions that prevent increased blood flow during exercise. Rest pain occurs when the arterial blood supply does not meet even the minimal nutritional requirements of the skin of the affected extremity. Even minor trauma to an ischemic foot may produce an unhealing skin lesion.

Decreased or absent arterial pulses is the most reliable physical finding associated with peripheral arterial disease. Bruits auscultated in the abdomen, pelvis, and inguinal areas and decreased palpable femoral, popliteal, posterior tibial, and dorsalis pedis pulses may indicate anatomic sites of arterial stenosis. Signs of chronic leg ischemia include subcutaneous atrophy, hair loss, coolness, pallor, cyanosis, and dependent rubor.

Diagnostic Tests

Doppler ultrasonography and the resulting pulse volume waveform is used to identify arterial vessels with stenotic lesions. In the presence of severe ischemia, the arterial waveform may be entirely absent. In addition, segmental systolic blood pressure measurements [the posterior tibial (ankle)/brachial artery systolic blood pressure ratio should be more than 0.95 at rest] provide a quantitative means to assess the presence and severity of peripheral arterial stenosis. The ratio is less than 0.9 during claudication, lower than 0.4 with rest pain, and less than 0.25 with ischemic ulceration or impending gangrene. Duplex ultrasonographic scanning is a direct, noninvasive test that identifies areas of plaque formation and calcification as well as blood flow abnormalities caused by arterial stenoses. Transcutaneous oximetry is used to assess the severity of skin ischemia in patients with peripheral arterial disease. Normally, the transcutaneous oxygen tension of the resting foot is about 60 mmHg; and it may be less than 40 mmHg in patients with skin ischemia.[3] Results from noninvasive tests and clinical evaluation are usually sufficient for the diagnosis of peripheral arterial disease. Magnetic resonance imaging and contrast angiography are utilized when the diagnosis is in doubt or as a prelude to endovascular intervention or surgical reconstruction.

Treatment

Medical therapy of peripheral arterial disease includes establishment of exercise programs and identification and treatment of risk factors for atherosclerosis. Supervised exercise training programs improve the walking capacity of patients with peripheral arterial disease presumably by improving the efficiency of skeletal muscle metabolic function, as improved blood flow to the extremity cannot be demonstrated. Patients who stop smoking have a more favorable prognosis than those who continue to smoke. Aggressive lipid-lowering therapy slows the progression of peripheral atherosclerosis, although it is not known if progression of symptoms from claudication to critical limb ischemia are altered. Likewise, it is not known if aggressive treatment of diabetes mellitus alters progression of atherosclerosis. Antihypertensive drug therapy with β-adrenergic antagonists that evoke reflex peripheral cutaneous vasoconstriction are not utilized in patients with critical limb ischemia. Nevertheless, β-adrenergic antagonists do not adversely affect claudication. Overall, vasodilator drugs have not alleviated the symptoms of claudication or decreased the complication of critical limb ischemia.

Revascularization procedures are indicated in patients with disabling claudication, ischemic rest pain, or impending limb loss.[3] Revascularization can be achieved by endovascular interventions or surgical reconstruction. Percutaneous transluminal angioplasty (PTA) of iliac arteries has a high initial success rate, which may be further improved by stent placement. Femoral and popliteal artery PTA has a lower success rate than iliac artery PTA.

The operative procedures used for vascular reconstruction depend on the location and severity of peripheral arterial stenoses. Aortobifemoral bypass with a bifurcated Dacron prosthetic graft is the standard surgical procedure used to treat aortoiliac disease. Intra-abdominal aortoiliac reconstructive surgery may not be feasible in patients with severe co-morbid conditions. In these patients axillobifemoral bypass can circumvent the abdominal aorta and achieve revascularization of both legs. Femorofemoral bypass can be performed in patients with unilateral iliac artery obstruction. Infrainguinal bypass procedures utilizing saphenous vein bypass grafts or synthetic grafts include femoropopliteal and tibioperoneal reconstruction. Lumbar sympathectomy is rarely used to treat critical limb ischemia, as it is presumed that ischemic vessels are already maximally vasodilated. Amputation is utilized for patients with advanced limb ischemia in whom revascularization procedures are not possible or have failed.

The operative risk with reconstructive peripheral vascular surgery, as for abdominal aortic aneurysm resection, is primarily related to the presence of associated atherosclerotic vascular disease, particularly ischemic heart disease and cerebrovascular disease.[4] It is presumed that the increased incidence of perioperative myocardial infarction and cardiac death is due to the high prevalence of coronary artery disease in patients with peripheral vascular disease. Mortality following revascularization surgery is usually secondary to myocardial infarction in patients who manifest preoperative evidence of ischemic heart disease, congestive heart failure, or a preoperative history of coronary artery bypass grafting (CABG). In patients with advanced ischemic heart disease and claudication, treatment of the ischemic heart disease (angioplasty, CABG) may be considered before performing revascularization surgery.

Management of Anesthesia

Management of anesthesia for surgical revascularization of the lower extremities incorporates many of the same principles described for management of patients with an abdominal aneurysm (see Chapter 10).[5] For example, the principal risk during reconstructive peripheral vascular surgery is associated atherosclerosis, particularly ischemic heart disease. CABG operations are usually performed before peripheral vascular surgery in patients who have both angina pectoris and claudication. Because patients with claudication are often unable to perform treadmill exercise tests, thallium perfusion scanning during intravenous dipyridamole infusions is a useful method for detecting ischemic heart disease. Ambulatory electrocardiographic monitoring to detect evidence of myocardial ischemia, which is often asymptomatic (silent), is an alternative method for evaluating ischemic heart disease.

There is often reluctance to select epidural or spinal anesthesia for patients undergoing surgical revascularization procedures of the legs, despite some perceived advantages (increased graft blood flow, less increase in systemic vascular resistance with aortic cross-clamping, postoperative pain relief, less activation of the coagulation system) when this technique is used alone or in combination with general anesthesia. The popularity of general anesthesia is in part due to the controversy surrounding regional anesthesia, especially placing lumbar epidural catheters, in the presence of drug-induced anticoagulation (see Chapter 25). Nevertheless, placing epidural catheters before the institution of heparin anticoagulation in patients undergoing revascularization of the lower extremity is not associated with an increased incidence of untoward neurologic events.[6] Furthermore, provision of epidural analgesia after this type of surgery attenuates postoperative stress-induced hypercoagulability and may beneficially influence the outcome in high risk patients who have undergone major peripheral vascular surgery.[7]

Infrarenal aortic cross-clamping in the presence of peripheral vascular occlusive disease but adequate collateral circulation, as verified on the preoperative arteriogram, is associated with fewer hemodynamic derangements than occur in patients undergoing resection of abdominal aortic aneurysms. Likewise, minimal hemodynamic changes associated with declamping the abdominal aorta may reflect, in part, the beneficial role of the collateral circulation in preventing marked increases in lactate during the aortic cross-clamp period. In view of the decreased likelihood of major hemodynamic alterations associated with aortic cross-clamping, it may be acceptable to use a central venous pressure catheter in lieu of a pulmonary artery catheter, especially in the absence of symptomatic left ventricular dysfunction or ischemic heart disease. Monitoring left ventricular function and intravascular fluid volume may also be facilitated by use of transesophageal echocardiography.

Heparin is commonly administered before application of the aortic cross-clamp, presumably to decrease the risk of thromboembolic complications. It is now recognized, however, that distal emboli, especially to the kidneys, most likely reflect dislodgement of atheroembolic debris from the diseased aorta. Thus in the absence of major distal occlusive disease, care when manipulating and clamping the aorta to minimize the likely dislodgement of potentially embolic debris may be more important than administration of heparin. Spinal cord damage associated with surgical revascularization of the legs is unlikely, and special monitoring for this complication is not necessary.

Postoperative Management

Postoperative management includes provision of analgesia, such as with neuraxial opioids, and treatment of fluid and electrolyte derangements. Dexmedetomidine, an α_2-agonist, attenuates increases in heart rate and plasma norepinephrine concentrations during emergence from anesthesia in vascular surgery patients.[8] Dexmedetomidine also has analgesic and sedative properties without producing cardiac or ventilatory depression.[9]

Subclavian Steal Syndrome

Occlusion of the subclavian or innominate artery proximal to the origin of the vertebral artery by atherosclerotic lesions may result in reversal of flow through the ipsilateral vertebral artery into the distal subclavian artery (Fig. 11–1).[10, 11] Reversal of flow diverts blood flow from the brain to supply the arm (subclavian steal syndrome). Symptoms of central nervous system ischemia (syncope, vertigo, ataxia, hemiplegia) and/or arm ischemia are usually present. Exercise of the ipsilateral arm accentuates these hemodynamic changes and may evoke neurologic

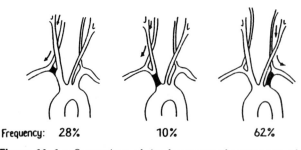

Frequency: 28%   10%   62%

Figure 11–1 • Comparison of the frequency of occurrence of left, right, and bilateral subclavian steal syndrome. (From Heidrich H, Bayer O. Symptomatology of the subclavian steal syndrome. Angiology 1969;20:406–13, with permission.)

symptoms. There is often an absent or diminished pulse in the ipsilateral arm, and the systolic blood pressure is likely to be at least 20 mmHg lower in that arm.[12] Physical examination may demonstrate a bruit over the subclavian artery. Stenosis of the left subclavian artery is responsible for this syndrome in about 70% of patients. Subclavian endarterectomy may be curative.

■ ACUTE ARTERIAL OCCLUSION

Acute arterial occlusion differs from the gradual development of occlusion caused by atherosclerosis and most often reflects systemic emboli that originate from the heart. For example, systemic emboli may arise from a mural thrombus in the left ventricle secondary to an old or recent myocardial infarction or to a dilated hypocontractile ventricle, as in the presence of idiopathic dilated cardiomyopathy. Another cardiac source of systemic emboli is valvular heart disease (particularly in those with rheumatic mitral valve disease), a prosthetic heart valve, infective endocarditis, or left atrial myxoma. Atrial fibrillation is an important factor in systemic embolism associated with valvular heart disease, and it may increase the risk of embolism even in the absence of valvular heart disease. Noncardiac causes of acute arterial occlusion include atheroemboli that originate from atheromatous lesions in the abdominal aorta or iliac or femoral artery. Aortic dissection and trauma may acutely occlude arteries by disrupting the integrity of the vessel lumen.

Signs and Symptoms

Acute arterial occlusion may result in severe extremity ischemia with associated sudden onset of intense pain, paresthesia, and motor weakness distal to the site of the arterial occlusion. There is loss of palpable peripheral pulses, cool skin, and sharply demarcated skin color changes (pallor or cyanosis) distal to the arterial occlusion. Large embolic fragments often lodge at arterial bifurcations such as the distal abdominal aorta or the femoral artery bifurcation, causing a syndrome of sudden severe pain, numbness, and pallor of the extremity.

Diagnosis

Noninvasive tests can provide additional evidence of peripheral arterial occlusion and may reveal the severity of the ischemia, but definitive treatment should not be delayed. Arteriography is used to define the site of acute arterial occlusion and the appropriateness of revascularization surgery.

Treatment

Surgical embolectomy is used to treat acute systemic embolism to a large peripheral artery. Embolectomy is rarely feasible for atheromatous embolism, but the primary lesion may be resectable, especially if it is distal to the renal artery. Once the diagnosis is confirmed, anticoagulation with heparin is initiated to prevent propagation of the thrombus. Intra-arterial thrombolysis with urokinase or recombinant human tissue plasminogen activator may restore vascular patency in acutely occluded arteries and synthetic bypass grafts. The clinical outcome is highly dependent on the severity of the associated heart disease. Amputation is necessary in some patients.

Management of Anesthesia

Management of anesthesia for surgical treatment of acute arterial occlusion due to acute systemic embolism is as described for treatment of chronic peripheral arterial disease.

■ SYSTEMIC VASCULITIS

Peripheral vascular disease may manifest as systemic vasculitis in which inflammation of the blood vessel walls presents in nonspecific ways, suggesting connective tissue disease, sepsis, or malignancy (Table 11–2).[13] The diagnosis of vasospastic disorders due to systemic vasculitis may be facilitated by biopsy of an involved organ and detection of autoantibodies directed against cytoplasmic (extranuclear) components of neutrophils. An immune mechanism generated in response to one or more factors is the most likely cause of systemic vasculitis.

Table 11–2 • Signs and Symptoms of Systemic Vasculitis

Fever
Fatigue
Weight loss
Neuropathy
Increased erythrocyte sedimentation rate
Anemia
Hypoalbuminemia

Takayasu's Arteritis

Takayasu's arteritis is a rare, idiopathic, chronic, progressive occlusive vasculitis that causes narrowing, thrombosis, or aneurysms of systemic and pulmonary arteries. Inflammatory changes are seen preferentially in large vessels such as the aorta and its branches: hence its alternative names of pulseless disease, occlusive thromboaortopathy, or aortic arch syndrome. The disease occurs most often in Oriental women. Takayasu's arteritis is definitively diagnosed on the basis of contrast angiography.

Signs and Symptoms

Clinical symptoms of Takayasu's arteritis occur as a consequence of progressive obliteration of the lumens of the aorta and its main branches (Table 11–3). Decreased perfusion to the brain owing to involvement of the carotid arteries by occlusive inflammatory and thrombotic processes may manifest as vertigo, visual disturbances, seizures, and cerebrovascular accidents with hemiparesis or hemiplegia. Bruits are often audible over stenosed carotid or subclavian vessels. Hyperextension of the patient's head may decrease carotid blood flow by placing tension on the arteries. Indeed, patients often hold their heads in flexed ("drooping") positions to prevent syncope.

Vasculitis of the pulmonary arteries occurs in about 50% of patients and may manifest as pulmonary hypertension. Ventilation-to-perfusion abnormalities owing to occlusion of small pulmonary arteries by the inflammatory process may contribute

Table 11–3 • Signs and Symptoms of Takayasu's Arteritis

Central nervous system
  Vertigo
  Visual disturbance
  Syncope
  Seizures
  Cerebral ischemia or infarction
Cardiovascular system
  Multiple occlusions of peripheral arteries
  Ischemic heart disease
  Cardiac valve dysfunction
  Cardiac conduction defects
Lungs
  Pulmonary hypertension
  Ventilation-perfusion mismatch
Kidneys
  Renal artery stenosis
Musculoskeletal system
  Ankylosing spondylitis
  Rheumatoid arthritis

to unexpected decreases in the PaO_2. Myocardial ischemia may reflect inflammation of the coronary arteries, and the cardiac valves and cardiac conduction system may be involved. Renal artery stenosis can lead to decreased renal function and to initiation of events producing renal hypertension. Ankylosing spondylitis and rheumatoid arthritis may accompany this syndrome.

Treatment

Takayasu's arteritis is treated with corticosteroids. Inhibitors of platelet aggregation or oral anticoagulants may be instituted in selected patients. Hypertension may be treated with calcium entry blockers or angiotensin-converting enzyme (ACE) inhibitors. Life-threatening or incapacitating arterial occlusions are sometimes amenable to surgical interventions.

Management of Anesthesia

Takayasu's arteritis may be encountered in patients presenting for obstetric anesthesia, incidental surgery, or such corrective vascular procedures as carotid endarterectomy. Formulation of a plan for the management of anesthesia must take into account the drugs used to treat this syndrome as well as multiple organ system involvement by vasculitis.[14] For example, chronic corticosteroid therapy may result in suppression of adrenocortical function, indicating the need for supplemental exogenous corticosteroids during the perioperative period. During the preoperative evaluation it is useful to establish the effect of changes in head position on cerebral function. In this regard, hyperextension of the patient's head during direct laryngoscopy and tracheal intubation could compromise blood flow though the carotid arteries that are diseased as a result of the vascular inflammatory process associated with this disease.

Choice of Anesthesia

Regional anesthesia may be a controversial choice in the presence of Takayasu's arteritis, especially if patients are anticoagulated. Associated musculoskeletal changes can make performance of lumbar epidural or spinal anesthesia difficult. Hypotension produced by regional anesthesia could jeopardize perfusion pressures to vital organs, especially the brain. However, regional anesthesia in awake and responsive patients is a useful method for monitoring cerebral function when disease-induced cerebrovascular disease is prominent. Both epidural and spinal anesthesia have been successfully utilized for performance of cesarean section in the presence of Takayasu's arteritis.[15–17]

General anesthesia has the advantage over regional anesthesia in that sympathectomy and subsequent decreases in systemic blood pressure can be avoided. Selection of short-acting anesthetic drugs that allow prompt awakening and evaluation of the patient's mental status seem logical.

Regardless of the techniques or drugs selected to produce anesthesia, the priority must be to maintain adequate arterial perfusion pressures during the intraoperative period. Therefore, anesthetic-induced decreased systemic blood pressure caused by decreased cardiac output or systemic vascular resistance must be recognized promptly and treated by reducing the concentration of anesthetic drugs or expanding the intravascular fluid volume. Administration of sympathomimetic drugs to maintain perfusion pressures may be helpful until the underlying cause of the decreased systemic blood pressure can be corrected. Avoidance of excessive hyperventilation of the lungs and selection of volatile anesthetics, perceived to favor maintenance of cerebral blood flow, are reasonable goals, especially in patients in whom the disease process involves the carotid arteries.[14]

Monitoring

Systemic blood pressure may be difficult to measure noninvasively in the upper extremities. Indeed, systemic blood pressure is predictably decreased in the upper extremities because of narrowing of the arterial lumens. There is a theoretical but undocumented concern regarding cannulation of arteries that may be involved by the inflammatory process characteristic of this disease. Nevertheless, a catheter placed in the radial artery is useful for confirming the presence of adequate perfusion pressures during major operations. Monitoring systemic blood pressure via a catheter placed in the femoral artery is an option, but it should be recognized that systolic blood pressure in the legs is higher than that present in the central aorta. Extreme arterial blood pressure differentials exist in some patients with Takayasu's arteritis that could affect regional blood flow. Monitoring systemic blood pressure in both the upper and lower extremities is a consideration in these patients.[18]

Constant monitoring of the electrocardiogram (ECG) and urine output may provide insight as to the adequacy of coronary blood flow and renal blood flow. Placing a pulmonary artery catheter or a transesophageal echocardiography probe is acceptable if the magnitude of the surgery so dictates.[14] In patients with known compromise of carotid blood flow, intraoperative monitoring of the electroencephalogram may be useful for detecting cerebral ischemia.

Thromboangiitis Obliterans (Buerger's Disease)

Thromboangiitis obliterans is an inflammatory vasculitis leading to occlusion of small and middle-size arteries and veins in the extremities. The disease is most prevalent in men (Asia, Eastern Europe, Israel), and the onset is typically before 45 years of age. The most important predisposing factor is tobacco use. The diagnosis of thromboangiitis obliterans can be confirmed only by biopsy of active vascular lesions.

Signs and Symptoms

Involvement of extremity arteries causes forearm, calf, or foot claudication. Severe ischemia of the hand and foot causes rest pain, ulcerations, and skin necrosis. Raynaud's phenomenon is commonly associated with thromboangiitis obliterans, and cold is recognized to exacerbate the disease process. Digital artery obstruction is evidence of Raynaud's phenomenon. Periods of vasospasm may alternate with periods of quiescence. Migratory superficial vein thrombosis develops in about 40% of patients.

Treatment

The most effective treatment for patients with thromboangiitis obliterans is smoking cessation. Surgical revascularization is usually not an option because of involvement of small distal vessels. There is no proven effective pharmacologic therapy (vasodilators, corticosteroids), and the efficacy of platelet inhibitors, anticoagulants, and thrombolytic therapy is not established.

Management of Anesthesia

Management of anesthesia in the presence of thromboangiitis obliterans requires avoidance of the events that might damage the already ischemic extremities. Positioning during surgery includes padding pressure points on the extremities. It seems prudent to increase the ambient temperature of the operating rooms and to warm and humidify the inspired gases to maintain body temperature. Noninvasive monitoring of systemic blood pressure is preferred, as theoretically placing a catheter in a diseased artery is a concern. The presence of pulmonary disease and elevated carboxyhemoglobin concentrations are considerations, as many of these patients are cigarette smokers.

The possible interaction of anesthetic drugs with peripheral vasodilators used to treat thromboangiitis obliterans and the potential need for supplemental corticosteroids are preoperative considerations. In the final analysis, regional or general anesthesia can be administered to these patients. If regional anesthetic techniques are selected, it may be prudent to omit epinephrine from the local anesthetic solutions to avoid any possibility of accentuating coexisting vasospasm.

Wegener's Granulomatosis

Wegener's granulomatosis is characterized by pathophysiologic changes due to the formation of necrotizing granulomas in inflamed vessels, such as those present in the central nervous system, airways and lungs, cardiovascular system, and kidneys (Table 11–4). Patients may present with sinusitis, pneumonia, or renal failure. The laryngeal mucosa may be replaced by granulation tissue, resulting in narrowing of the glottic opening. Vasculitis may result in occlusion of pulmonary vessels. There may be random interstitial distribution of pulmonary granulomas with surrounding infection and hemorrhage. Progressive renal failure is the most frequent cause of death in patients with Wegener's granulomatosis. Tests for antineutrophil cytoplasmic antibodies have a high degree of specificity for Wegener's granulomatosis, suggesting a role for immunologic dysfunction and hypersensitivity to un-

Table 11–4 • Signs and Symptoms of Wegener's Granulomatosis

Central nervous system
   Cerebral arterial aneurysms
   Peripheral neuropathy
Respiratory tract and lungs
   Sinusitis
   Laryngeal stenosis
   Epiglottic destruction
   Ventilation-perfusion mismatch
   Pneumonia
   Hemoptysis
   Bronchial destruction
Cardiovascular system
   Cardiac valve destruction
   Disturbances of cardiac impulse conduction
   Myocardial ischemia
   Infarction of the tips of digits
Kidneys
   Hematuria
   Azotemia
   Renal failure

identified antigens in the etiology of the vasculitis. Treatment of Wegener's granulomatosis with cyclophosphamide produces dramatic remissions in nearly all patients.

Management of anesthesia in patients with Wegener's granulomatosis requires an appreciation of the widespread organ system involvement associated with this disease.[19] The potential depressant effects of cyclophosphamide on the immune system and the association of hemolytic anemia and leukopenia with administration of this drug should be considered. Cyclophosphamide may cause decreased plasma cholinesterase activity, but prolonged skeletal muscle paralysis after administration of succinylcholine has not been described.[20]

Avoidance of trauma during direct laryngoscopy is important, as bleeding from granulomas and dislodgement of friable ulcerated tissues can occur. A smaller than expected endotracheal tube may be required if the glottic opening is narrowed by granulomatous changes. Suctioning the airway may be required to remove necrotic debris. The likely presence of pulmonary disease emphasizes the need for supplemental oxygen during the perioperative period. Arteritis that is likely to involve peripheral vessels may limit placement of an indwelling arterial catheter to monitor systemic blood pressure or the frequency with which arterial punctures can be performed to analyze arterial blood gases and pH.

A careful neurologic examination is helpful before the decision is made to recommend regional anesthesia to patients with Wegener's granulomatosis. The choice and doses of neuromuscular blocking drugs may be influenced by the magnitude of renal dysfunction produced by this disease. Implications for the use of succinylcholine in the presence of skeletal muscle atrophy owing to neuritis is a consideration. Conceivably, volatile anesthetics could be associated with exaggerated myocardial depression when the disease process involves the myocardium and cardiac valves. Monitoring the ECG is helpful for detecting cardiac conduction disturbances. Ultimately, rational administration of anesthesia to patients with Wegener's granulomatosis is based on the magnitude and type of organ system dysfunction produced by the disease.

Temporal Arteritis

Temporal arteritis is inflammation of the arteries of the head and neck, manifesting most often as headache, scalp tenderness, or jaw claudication. This diagnosis is suspected in any patient older than 50 years of age complaining of a unilateral headache. Superficial branches of the temporal arteries are often tender and enlarged. Arteritis of branches of the ophthalmic artery may lead to ischemic optic neuritis and sudden unilateral blindness. Indeed, prompt initiation of treatment with corticosteroids is indicated in patients with visual symptoms to prevent blindness. Evidence of arteritis on a biopsy of the temporal artery is present in about 90% of patients.

Polyarteritis Nodosa

Polyarteritis nodosa is a vasculitis that most often occurs in women between 20 and 60 years of age and commonly in association with hepatitis B antigenemia and allergic reactions to drugs. Small and medium-size arteries are involved with inflammatory changes, resulting in glomerulitis, myocardial ischemia, peripheral neuropathies, and seizures. Hypertension is common, presumably reflecting renal disease. Renal failure is the most common cause of death. A polyarteritis-like vasculitis may accompany acquired immunodeficiency syndrome.

The diagnosis of polyarteritis nodosa depends on histologic evidence of vasculitis on biopsy and arteriography demonstrating characteristic aneurysms. The treatment is empirical and usually includes corticosteroids and cyclophosphamide, removal of offending drugs, and treatment of underlying diseases such as cancer. The potential adverse effects of cyclophosphamide in patients treated with this drug are a consideration (see "Wegener's Granulomatosis").

Management of anesthesia in patients with polyarteritis nodosa should take into consideration the likelihood of renal or cardiac disease and the implication of co-exisitng systemic hypertension. Supplemental corticosteroids are appropriate in patients who have been receiving these drugs preoperatively for treatment of their underlying disease.

Schönlein-Henoch Purpura

Schönlein-Henoch purpura principally affects arterioles and capillaries in the skin, kidneys, gastrointestinal tract, and large joints of children. The disease is usually benign. Corticosteroids may be administered to patients with renal dysfunction.

Kawasaki Disease

Kawasaki disease (mucocutaneous lymph node syndrome) occurs primarily in children, manifesting as fever, conjunctivitis, inflammation of the mucous membranes, swollen erythematous hands and feet, truncal rashes, and cervical lymphadenopathy.[21] Vasculitis appears early in the disease. Subsequently the walls of coronary arteries and other medium-size muscular arteries may show evidence of focal segmental destruction, with coronary artery aneurysms or ectasia developing in 15% to 25% of affected children. Complications of this syndrome have included pericarditis, myocarditis, angina pectoris, myocardial infarction, and cerebral hemorrhage. This syndrome may be caused by a retrovirus, although there is no evidence of person-to-person transmission. Treatment is with gamma globulin and aspirin.

Management of anesthesia in these children should consider the possibility of intraoperative myocardial ischemia.[21] Peripheral nerve block to provide interruption of sympathetic nervous system activity to inflamed peripheral arteries may be a consideration when the viability of the digits is threatened.[22] Epidural anesthesia for cesarean section has been successfully utilized in patients with Kawasaki disease.[23]

RAYNAUD'S PHENOMENON

Raynaud's phenomenon is episodic vasospastic ischemia of the digits that affects women more often than men.[3] There is characteristic digital blanching, cyanosis, and rubor after cold exposure and rewarming. The digital discoloration is confined primarily to the fingers or toes. Blanching represents the ischemic phase of the phenomenon, which is caused by digital vasospasm. Cyanosis results when deoxygenated blood is present in the capillaries and veins. Rubor manifests with rewarming and a hyperemic phase as the digital vasospasm wanes. Burning and throbbing pain typically follow the ischemic episode. Often Raynaud's phenomenon is characterized by slow progression, which may consist of stationary periods lasting years.

Classification

Raynaud's phenomenon is categorized as primary (also called Raynaud's disease) and secondary when it is associated with other diseases, most often scleroderma, systemic lupus erythematosus, and other related immunologic disorders (Table 11–5). Raynaud's disease occurs most frequently as a mild condition in as many as 30% of young adult women, and it is usually bilateral. Conversely, secondary Raynaud's phenomenon tends to be unilateral. Secondary Raynaud's phenomenon is the first symptom to occur in most patients who develop scleroderma, although the systemic disease may not appear until many years later.

Table 11–5 • Secondary Causes of Raynaud's Phenomenon

Connective tissue diseases
   Scleroderma
   Systemic lupus erythematosus
   Rheumatoid arthritis
   Dermatomyositis
Peripheral arterial occlusive disease
   Atherosclerosis
   Thromboangiitis obliterans
   Thromboembolism
   Thoracic outlet syndrome
Neurologic syndromes
   Carpal tunnel syndrome
   Reflex sympathetic dystrophy
   Cerebral vascular accident
   Intervertebral disk herniation
Trauma
   Cold thermal injury (frostbite)
   Percussive injury (vibrating tools)
Drugs
   β-Adrenergic antagonists
   Tricyclic antidepressants
   Antimetabolites
   Ergot alkaloids
   Amphetamines

Etiology

Mechanisms postulated to cause Raynaud's phenomenon include increased sympathetic nervous system activity, heightened digital vascular reactivity to vasoconstrictive stimuli, circulating vasoactive hormones, and decreased intravascular pressures.[3] A role for increased sympathetic nervous system activity is questionable, as sympathectomy does not predictably produce beneficial effects. Patients with Raynaud's disease have increased numbers of α_2-adrenergic receptors in the digital arteries. Many patients with Raynaud's phenomenon have low systemic blood pressure. Decreased digital vascular pressures caused by proximal arterial occlusive disease or by digital vascular obstruction could increase the likelihood of digital vasospasm when vasoconstrictive stimuli occur.

Diagnosis

Noninvasive vascular tests utilized to evaluate patients with Raynaud's disease include digital pulse volume recordings and measurement of digital systolic blood pressures and digital blood flows. Measurements of the erythrocyte sedimentation rate and titers of antinuclear antibody, rheumatoid factor, cryoglobulins, and cold agglutins are useful for excluding specific secondary causes of Raynaud's phenomenon (Table 11–5). Angiography is not necessary to diagnose Raynaud's phenomenon but may be useful when digital ischemia is due to atherosclerosis or thrombosis and revascularization is a consideration.

Raynaud's phenomenon is the initial complaint in most patients with CREST syndrome (calcinosis, Raynaud's phenomenon, esophageal dysmotility, sclerodactyly, telangiectasia). Antinuclear antibodies are present in most patients with scleroderma. Raynaud's phenomenon should be distinguished from acrocyanosis, which is characterized by persistent bluish discoloration of the hands or feet that intensifies during cold exposure. Acrocyanosis affects men and women, and the prognosis is good, with loss of digital tissue being unlikely.

Treatment

Primary and secondary Raynaud's phenomenon can often be managed conservatively by protecting the hands and feet from exposure to cold. In addition to the hands and feet, the trunk and head should be kept warm to reduce the risk of reflex vasoconstriction. Pharmacologic intervention is indicated in patients who do not respond satisfactorily to conservative measures. Calcium channel-blocking drugs such as nifedipine and sympathetic nervous system antagonists such as prazosin can be used to treat Raynaud's phenomenon. In rare instances, surgical sympathectomy may be considered for treatment of persistent, severe digital ischemia. Transection of the sympathetic nervous system supply to the hand (transection of preganglionic fibers in the sympathetic chain at T2–3) does not consistently produce favorable responses. Stellate ganglion block has been observed to improve blood flow and increase the temperature in the ipsilateral hand, whereas digits on the contralateral side showed decreased pulse amplitude and temperature.[24]

Management of Anesthesia

There are no specific recommendations as to the choice of drugs to produce general anesthesia in patients with Raynaud's phenomenon. Maintaining body temperature and increasing the ambient temperature of the operating room seem logical. The systemic blood pressure is most often monitored via noninvasive techniques in view of the theoretical

risk of placing a catheter in a peripheral artery supplying a potentially ischemic extremity. In some instances the risk/benefit ratio of radial arterial cannulation in patients with Raynaud's phenomenon may be viewed as acceptable based on the presumption that the risk of ischemia complications caused by radial artery cannulation in these patients is probably low.[25] Conversely, if it is known that patients have CREST syndrome, cannulation of a larger artery (such as the femoral artery) should be considered if direct arterial monitoring of the systemic blood pressure is indicated.[25]

Regional anesthesia is acceptable for peripheral operations in patients with Raynaud's phenomenon. Indeed, regional anesthetic techniques that interrupt sympathetic nervous system innervation to an extremity are often selected for diagnostic purposes. If a regional anesthetic technique is selected, it may be prudent not to include epinephrine in the anesthetic solutions, as the catecholamine could provoke undesirable vasoconstriction.

■ MOYAMOYA DISEASE

Moyamoya disease is a rare progressive cerebrovascular occlusive disease of the internal carotid arteries and the anterior and middle cerebral arteries that affects children and young adults.[26–28] Pathophysiologically, affected patients are analogous to patients with bilateral internal carotid artery stenosis. The characteristic symptoms of the disease are transient ischemic attacks causing hemiparesis or weakness of the limbs associated with hyperventilation when crying or exercising. Adults with this disease are most likely to develop interventricular hemorrhage or subarachnoid hemorrhage, reflecting the increased incidence of cerebral aneurysms in these patients. Intracranial hemorrhage can be confused with pregnancy-induced hypertension because transient hypertension and proteinuria can complicate this event.[29] Diagnosis of intracranial hemorrhage is with noncontrast computed tomography.

Treatment

Several surgical procedures designed to augment collateral cerebral blood flow have been described to treat these patients.[26] Examples of surgical procedures include superficial temporal artery-middle cerebral artery anastomosis and encephalo-duro-arterio-synangiosis (EDAS), which is designed to promote formation of collateral blood flow to the brain's surface.[30] Medical management includes the use of antiplatelet (aspirin) and cerebral vasodilating (verapamil) drugs.

Management of Anesthesia

Management of anesthesia in patients with Moyamoya disease is influenced by the need to preserve cerebral blood flow relative to cerebral metabolic oxygen consumption ($CMRO_2$).[26, 29, 30] Factors that increase $CMRO_2$, such as painful stimuli (direct laryngoscopy, tracheal intubation, surgical incision), should be minimized by delivery of adequate concentrations of anesthetic drugs. Cerebral blood flow is optimized by maintaining normocarbia, avoiding systemic hypotension, and promptly replacing intravascular fluid losses to maintain normovolemia.[26] Volatile anesthetics would be a logical choice based on the theoretical value of drug-induced cerebral vasodilation. The presence of neurologic changes may limit the use of succinylcholine. Intraoperative monitoring of the electroencephalogram may be a consideration for detecting cerebral ischemia, although its use during performance of EDAS is limited because the surgical site over the cortex is at risk for ischemia and precludes the use of surface electrodes.[26] Increased intraoperative bleeding may reflect the effects of therapy with antiplatelet drugs. Cardiac rhythm disturbances have been reported in these patients during anesthesia and surgery. Patients with a history of seizures should be maintained on anticonvulsant medications.

Seizures and temporary hemiparesis have been described after administration of spinal anesthesia to a patient with Moyamoya disease.[31] It is possible that circulatory changes induced by spinal anesthesia altered the cerebral blood flow sufficiently to produce focal cerebral ischemia in the presence of co-existing cerebrovascular disease.

CORONARY-SUBCLAVIAN STEAL SYNDROME

A rare complication of using the internal mammary artery for coronary revascularization is the coronary-subclavian steal syndrome. This syndrome occurs when the development of a proximal incomplete stenosis in the left subclavian artery produces reversal of blood flow through the patent internal mammary artery graft (Fig. 11–2).[12] The steal syndrome is characterized by angina pectoris, signs of central nervous system ischemia, and a decrease in systolic blood pressure of at least 20 mmHg in the ipsilateral arm. Bilateral upper extremity brachial artery blood pressure measurements may be useful for the preop-

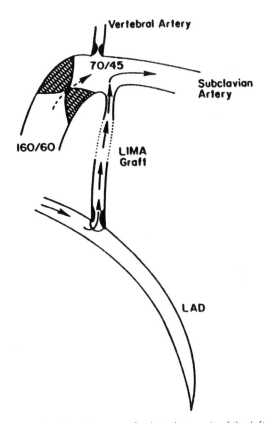

Figure 11–2 • Development of subtotal stenosis of the left subclavian artery may produce reversal of flow through a patent internal mammary graft (LIMA), thereby diverting flow (coronary-subclavian steal syndrome) destined for the left anterior descending coronary artery (LAD). (From Martin JL, Rock P. Coronary-subclavian steal syndrome: anesthetic implications and management in the perioperative period. Anesthesiology 1988;68:933–6, with permission.)

erative evaluation of patients with internal mammary artery-to-coronary artery bypass grafts. Angina pectoris associated with coronary-subclavian steal syndrome requires surgical bypass grafting. Management of anesthesia in these patients includes application of the same principles recommended for patients with ischemic heart disease due to atherosclerosis.

KLIPPEL-TRÉNAUNAY SYNDROME

Klippel-Trénaunay syndrome is characterized by port-wine hemangiomas (neck, trunk, extremities) associated with spinal cord arteriovenous malformations. Spinal cord lesions may bleed spontaneously after straining or coughing. Spinal or epidural anesthesia seems an unlikely choice in these patients.[32]

BEHÇET'S DISEASE

Behçet's disease is a chronic relapsing inflammatory disorder of unknown etiology that manifests as oral aphthous ulcers, painful genital ulcers, and uveitis.[33] Repeated attacks of uveitis can cause blindness. Involvement of the gastrointestinal tract, central nervous system, and large vessels is common. The bowel symptoms of Behçet's disease must be distinguished from those of Crohn's disease and ulcerative colitis. Neurologic symptoms may resemble multiple sclerosis. Erythema nodosum is common in female patients and usually occurs on the front of the legs. Monarthritis or polyarthritis develops in about half of patients. The joints most frequently affected are the knees, followed by the wrists, ankles, and elbows. In Japan the incidence is about 1 per 1000, whereas the prevalence in the United States is less than 1 per 15,000.

High-dose corticosteroids and immunosuppressants (cyclosporine) are utilized for management of gastrointestinal symptoms, central nervous system involvement, and large-vessel lesions. Topical mydriatic drugs and corticosteroids are utilized for attacks of acute uveitis. Topical corticosteroids are useful for oral and genital lesions. Colchicine has beneficial effects on mucocutaneous symptoms, presumably by inhibiting neutrophil function.

References

1. Criqui MH, Fronek A, Barrett-Connor E, et al. The prevalence of peripheral arterial disease in a defined population. Circulation 1985;76:510–9
2. Criqui MH, Langer RD, Fronek A, et al. Mortality over a period of 10 years in patients with peripheral arterial disease. N Engl J Med 1992;326:381–8
3. Creager MA. Peripheral arterial disease. Sci Am Med 1998;1–7
4. Sprung J, Abdelmalak B, Gottlieb A, et al. Analysis of risk factors for myocardial infarction and cardiac mortality after major vascular surgery. Anesthesiology 2000;93:129–40
5. Martin JL, Rock P. Coronary-subclavian steal syndrome: anesthetic implications and management in the perioperative period. Anesthesiology 1988;68:933–6
6. Conn DL. Update on systemic necrotizing vasculitis. Mayo Clin Proc 1989;64:535–46
7. Cunningham AJ. Anaesthesia for abdominal aortic surgery: a review. Can J Anaesth 1989;36:426–44; 568–77
8. Talke P, Chen R, Thomas B, et al. The hemodynamic and adrenergic effects of perioperative dexmedetomidine infusion after vascular surgery. Anesth Analg 2000;90:834–9
9. Hall JE, Uhrich TD, Barney JA, et al. Sedative, amnestic, and analgesic properties of small-dose dexmedetomidine infusion. Anesth Analg 2000;90:699–705
10. Baron HC, LaRaja RD, Rossi G, et al. Continuous epidural analgesia in the heparinized vascular surgical patient: a retrospective review of 912 patients. J Vasc Surg 1987;6:144–6
11. Tuman KJ, McCarthy RJ, March RJ, et al. Effects of epidural anesthesia and analgesia on coagulation and outcome after major vascular surgery. Anesth Analg 1991;73:696–704
12. Heidrich H, Bayer O. Symptomatology of the subclavian steal syndrome. Angiology 1969;20:406–13
13. Killen DA, Fostert JH, Gobbel WG, et al. The subclavian steal syndrome. J Thorac Cardiovasc Surg 1966;60:539–60
14. Warner MA, Hughes DR, Messick JM. Anesthetic management of a patient with pulseless disease. Anesth Analg 1983;62:532–5
15. Hampl KF, Schneider K, Skarvan J, et al. Spinal anaesthesia in a patient with Takayasu's disease. Br J Anaesth 1994;72:129–32
16. Clark AG, Al-Qatari M. Anaesthesia for caesarean section in Takayasu's disease. Can J Anaesth 1998;45:377–9
17. Henderson K, Fludder P. Epidural anaesthesia for caesarean section in a patient with severe Takayasu's disease. Br J Anaesth 1999;83:956–9
18. Meikle A, Milne B. Extreme arterial blood pressure differentials in a patient with Takayasu's arteritis. Can J Anaesth 1997;44:868–71
19. Lake CL. Anesthesia and Wegener's granulomatosis: case report and review of the literature. Anesth Analg 1978;57:353–9
20. Dillman JF. Safe use of succinylcholine during repeated anesthetics in a patient treated with cyclophosphamide. Anesth Analg 1987;66:351–3
21. McNiece WL, Krishna G. Kawasaki disease: a disease with anesthetic complications. Anesthesiology 1983;58:269–71
22. Edwards WT, Burney RG. Use of repeated nerve blocks in management of an infant with Kawasaki's disease. Anesth Analg 1988;67:1008–10
23. Alam S, Sakura S, Kosaka Y. Anaesthetic management for caesarean section in a patient with Kawasaki disease. Can J Anaesth 1995;42:1024–6
24. Omote K, Kawamatga M, Namiki A. Adverse effects of stellate ganglion block on Raynaud's phenomenon associated with progressive systemic sclerosis. Anesth Analg 1993;77:1057–60
25. Rose SH. Ischemic complications of radial artery cannulation: an association with calcinosis, Raynaud's phenomenon, esophageal dysmotility, sclerodactyly, and telangiectasia variant of scleroderma. Anesthesiology 1993;78:587–9
26. Soriano S, Sethna NF, Scott RM. Anesthetic management of children with Moyamoya syndrome. Anesth Analg 1993;77:1066–70
27. Wang N, Kuluz J, Barron M, et al. Cardiopulmonary bypass in a patient with Moyamoya disease. Anesth Analg 1997;84:1160–3
28. Sakamotoa T, Kawaguchi M, Kurehara K, et al. Risk factors for neurologic deterioration after revascularization surgery in patients with Moyamoya disease. Anesth Analg 1997;85:1060–5
29. Williams DL, Martin IL, Gully RM. Intracerebral hemorrhage and Moyamoya disease in pregnancy. Can J Anesth 2000;47:996–1000
30. Kurehara K, Ohnishi H, Touho H, et al. Cortical blood flow response to hypercapnia during anaesthesia in Moyamoya disease. Can J Anaesth 1993;40:709–13
31. Yasukawa M, Yasukawa K, Akawaga S, et al. Convulsions and temporary hemiparesis following spinal anesthesia in a child with Moyamoya disease. Anesthesiology 1988;69:1023–4
32. DeLeon-Casasola OA, Lema MJ. Epidural anesthesia in patients with Klippel-Trénaunay syndrome. Anesth Analg 1992;74:470
33. Sakane T, Taken OM, Suzuki N, et al. Behçet's disease. N Engl J Med 1999;341:1284–91

Deep-Vein Thrombosis and Pulmonary Embolism

Deep-vein thrombosis (usually involving a leg vein) and associated pulmonary embolism represent the spectrum of a single disease that is a leading cause of postoperative morbidity and mortality.[1-3] Formation of a clot inside a blood vessel is designated a *thrombus,* to distinguish it from normal extravascular clotting of blood. An *embolus* is a fragment of the thrombus that breaks off and travels in the blood until it lodges at a site of vascular narrowing. For this reason, an embolus originating in a vein commonly lodges in the pulmonary vasculature, whereas an embolus originating in an artery usually occludes a more distal, smaller artery (see Chapter 11).

Factors that predispose to thromboembolism are multiple but often include events likely to be associated with anesthesia and surgery (Table 12–1). For example, venous stasis, as is associated with postoperative immobility or pregnancy, results in failure to dilute or promptly clear activated clotting factors, thereby predisposing to thrombus formation. Any condition that causes a roughened endothelial vessel wall, such as infections, trauma, or drug-induced irritation, predisposes to thrombus formation. In addition to venous embolism, pulmonary embolism can also result from fat, air, amniotic fluid, or on rare occasions a tumor.

▌ DEEP-VEIN THROMBOSIS

Deep-vein thrombosis is detectable in a substantial number of patients older than 50 years of age who have undergone prostatectomy or hip surgery. Most of these venous thromboses are subclinical and resolve completely when mobility is restored, although some produce damage to venous valves with resulting chronic venous insufficiency. A few

Table 12–1 • Factors Predisposing
to Thromboembolism

Venous stasis
  Recent surgery (includes outpatient surgery)
  Trauma
  Lack of ambulation
  Pregnancy
  Low cardiac output (congestive heart failure,
    myocardial infarction)
  Stroke
Abnormality of the venous wall
  Varicose veins
  Drug-induced irritation
Hypercoagulable state
  Surgery
  Estrogen therapy (oral contraceptives)
  Cancer (malignant cells contain a cysteine proteinase
    that activates factor X)
  Deficiencies of endogenous anticoagulants
    (antithrombin III, protein C, protein S)
  Stress response associated with surgery
  Inflammatory bowel disease
History of previous thromboembolism
Morbid obesity
Advanced age

travel to the lungs and produce pulmonary embolism. Venous stasis, endothelial damage, and hypercoagulability, as may accompany anesthesia and surgery, predispose to venous thrombosis. Venous thrombi formed below the knees or in the arms rarely give rise to significant pulmonary emboli, whereas thrombi that extend into the iliofemoral venous system can produce life-threatening pulmonary embolism. Likewise, thrombi formed in the right atrium of patients with atrial fibrillation are common sources of pulmonary embolism.

Diagnosis

Superficial thrombophlebitis, such as may follow intravenous infusions or drug injections, are rarely associated with pulmonary embolism. Indeed, the intense inflammation that accompanies superficial thrombophlebitis leads to rapid total occlusion of the vein, making subsequent embolism unlikely. Typically the vein can be palpated as a cord-like structure surrounded by an area of erythema, warmth, and edema. The presence of fever suggests bacterial infection. Treatment of superficial vein thrombosis is usually conservative, consisting of elevating the affected site, applying heat locally and administering antibiotics for suspected bacterial infections.

Isolated calf thrombi are often asymptomatic, and the diagnosis of deep-vein thrombosis by clinical signs is unreliable. Compression ultrasonography of the femoral and popliteal veins and calf trifurcation is highly sensitive for detecting proximal vein thrombosis (popliteal or femoral vein) but less sensitive for detecting calf vein thrombosis (Fig. 12–1).[2] This method is preferred for evaluating patients with suspected deep-vein thrombosis because it is less invasive than venography and more accurate than impedance plethysmography. If the findings on initial ultrasonography are abnormal, venous thrombosis can be diagnosed with a predictive accuracy of more than 90%. If the findings are normal, anticoagulant therapy can be withheld.

Most postoperative venous thrombi arise in the lower legs, especially in soleal sinuses or in large veins draining the gastrocnemius muscles; but in at least 20% of patients who have undergone surgical procedures and in 40% to 50% of patients with skeletal muscle trauma, thrombi can originate in more proximal veins.[2] Left untreated, deep-vein thrombosis extends into larger and more proximal veins in 20% to 30% of patients, and such extension may be responsible for subsequent fatal pulmonary emboli.

Thrombophilia refers to a tendency to experience recurrent venous thromboembolism.[2] Laboratory abnormalities associated with initial and recurrent venous thromboembolism include congenital deficiencies of antithrombin III, protein C, protein S, or plasminogen; congenital resistance to activated protein C; and increased levels of anti-phospholipid antibodies. A family history of unexplained venous thrombosis may be present. The presence of cancer, recent bed rest or surgery, and immobilization of the legs or feet increase the likelihood of venous thrombosis.

Treatment

Anticoagulation is the first-line treatment for all patients with the diagnosis of deep-vein thrombosis and those with proximal-vein involvement.[1, 2] Therapy is initially with heparin (unfractionated or low-molecular-weight heparin), as this drug produces an immediate anticoagulant effect. Heparin is administered as continuous intravenous infusions or subcutaneous injections. So long as the activated partial thromboplastin time is maintained in the prescribed therapeutic range (1.5 to 2.5 times the control value), the two routes of administration are equally effective. Heparin has a narrow therapeutic window, and the responsiveness of patients varies greatly. Advantages of low-molecular-weight heparin over unfractionated heparin include a longer half-life, a more predictable dose response, and less risk of adverse bleeding events.

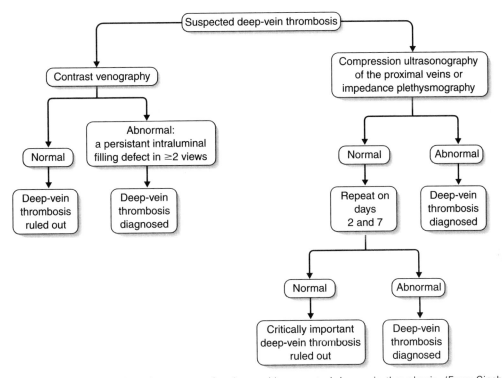

Figure 12–1 • Steps in diagnosis and treatment of patients with suspected deep-vein thrombosis. (From Ginsberg JS. Management of venous thromboembolism. N Engl J Med 1996;335:1816–28. Copyright 1996 Massachusetts Medical Society, with permission.)

An oral vitamin K antagonist (warfarin) is initiated within 24 hours of heparin therapy. Warfarin treatment is usually adjusted based on the one-stage prothrombin time, which is expressed with reference to an international standard [international normalized ratio (INR)]. Often an INR value between 2.0 and 3.0 is recommended for treating venous thromboembolic disease. Heparin is discontinued when it has been administered for at least 4 days and the INR ratio has been higher than 2.0 for two consecutive days. Oral anticoagulants may be continued for 3 months or longer.

Restoration of Venous Patency

In selected cases of deep-vein thrombosis it is possible to restore venous patency by surgical thrombectomy. This may be uniquely indicated for patients in whom the viability of a limb is threatened by an acute iliofemoral thrombosis. Inferior vena cava filters may be placed in patients who experience recurrent pulmonary embolism despite adequate anticoagulant therapy or in whom anticoagulant therapy is contraindicated. Thrombolytic treatment with plasminogen activators followed by anticoagulation may be used for early restoration of patency of a thrombosed vein.

Complications of Anticoagulation

Approximately 5% of patients treated with intravenous or subcutaneous unfractionated heparin develop major bleeding.[2] Excessive prolongation of the activated partial plasma thromboplastin time increases the risk of bleeding complications. Fewer episodes of bleeding seem to occur with the use of low-molecular-weight heparin. Approximately 3% of patients receiving unfractionated heparin develop immune-mediated thrombocytopenia (platelet counts less than 100,000 cells/mm^3), which may be complicated by extension of the co-existing venous thromboembolism or new arterial thrombosis.[2] Treatment of heparin-induced thrombocytopenia is empirical and includes discontinuation of the heparin (Fig. 12–2).[2] Long-term unfractionated heparin therapy (1 month or longer) as utilized during pregnancy (heparin does not cross the placenta) may cause osteoporosis.

Prevention of Venous Thromboembolism

Clinical Risk Factors

The presence of clinical risk factors identifies patients with the most to gain from prophylactic mea-

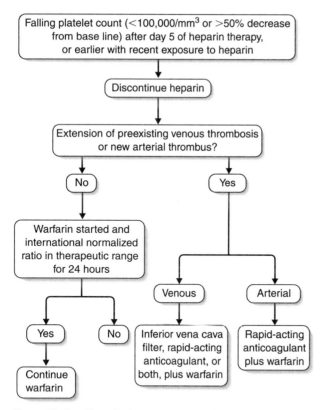

Figure 12–2 • Steps in the management of patients with venous thromboembolism and heparin-induced thrombocytopenia. (From Ginsberg JS. Management of venous thromboembolism. N Engl J Med 1996;335:1816–28. Copyright 1996 Massachusetts Medical Society, with permission.)

sures and those who should receive antithrombotic prophylaxis during periods of increased susceptibility, such as postoperatively or postpartum (Table 12–2).[1] Patients at low risk require only minimal prophylactic measures, such as early ambulation after surgery and the use of elastic stockings, which augment propulsion of blood from the ankles to the knees. The risk may be much higher in older patients (40-plus years of age) who are undergoing operations that last longer than 1 hour. The incidence of deep-vein thrombosis may exceed 60% after orthopedic procedures on the lower extremities, especially if there is a prolonged convalescence period involving bed rest. The presence of malignant disease increases the risk of thrombotic complications.

Small subcutaneous doses of heparin (minidose heparin given in doses of 5000 units two or three times daily) prevent deep-vein thrombosis in patients at moderate risk following abdominal and orthopedic surgery. The contribution of venous stasis to the pathogenesis of deep-vein thrombosis can be largely negated by contraction or compression of the calf muscles, which prevents pooling of blood in the veins of the lower extremities. Graduated-compression stockings provide adequate prophylaxis in patients at low risk for deep-vein thrombosis, and intermittent external pneumatic compression of the legs and thighs with inflatable cuffs is more protective in patients at moderate risk for deep-vein thrombosis (Table 12–2).[1]

Regional Anesthesia

The incidence of postoperative deep-vein thrombosis and pulmonary embolism in patients who have undergone total hip replacement or knee replacement is decreased by more than 50% in patients receiving epidural or spinal anesthesia compared with those undergoing the same surgery but with general anesthesia.[4–6] Nevertheless, deep-vein thrombosis still occurs, and the long-term outcome is not affected by the choice of anesthesia.[7]

Presumably, the beneficial effects of regional anesthesia compared with general anesthesia are due to vasodilation, which maximizes venous blood flow and the ability to provide optimal postoperative analgesia with associated early ambulation. Furthermore, patients receiving regional anesthesia are often given fluid loads that could decrease viscosity of blood and offset venous stasis. Local anesthetics may even exert beneficial effects by inhibiting platelet aggregation.[4] By contrast, general anesthesia may contribute to an increased incidence of deep-vein thrombosis by virtue of decreased leg blood flow, estimated to be as much as 50%. Theoretically, controlled ventilation of the lungs would further impede venous return from the legs, but the incidence of deep-vein thrombosis is not influenced by the method of ventilation.[8]

Postthrombotic Syndrome

Postthrombotic syndrome occurs as a long-term complication of proximal-vein thrombosis. It manifests as chronic leg pain associated with edema that often worsens at the end of the day. Some patients also have stasis pigmentation, induration, and skin ulceration. This syndrome is caused by venous hypertension, which usually results from valvular destruction and leads to increased ambulatory pressures in the deep calf veins. The incidence and severity of the manifestations of the postthrombotic syndrome are decreased by early, continuous treatment with compression stockings.

▌ PULMONARY EMBOLISM

Diagnosis and treatment of pulmonary embolism requires an interdisciplinary approach, combining

Table 12–2 • Risk and Predisposing Factors for the Development of Deep-Vein Thrombosis after Surgery or Trauma

Event	Low Risk	Moderate Risk	High Risk
General surgery	< 40 Years old Operation < 60 minutes	> 40 Years old Operation > 60 minutes	> 40 Years old Operation > 60 minutes Prior deep-vein thrombosis Prior pulmonary embolus Extensive trauma Major fractures
Orthopedic surgery Trauma			Knee or hip replacement Extensive soft tissue injury Major fractures Multiple trauma sites
Medical conditions	Pregnancy	Postpartum period Myocardial infarction Congestive heart failure	Stroke
Incidence of deep-vein thrombosis without prophylaxis	2%	10%–40%	40%–80%
Symptomatic pulmonary embolism	0.2%	1%–8%	5%–10%
Fatal pulmonary embolism	0.002%	0.1%–0.4%	1%–5%
Recommended steps to minimize deep-vein thrombosis	Graduated-compression stockings Early ambulation	External pneumatic compression Minidose heparin Intravenous dextran	External pneumatic compression Minidose heparin Intravenous dextran Warfarin Intracaval filters

Adapted from Weinmann EE, Salzman EW. Deep-vein thrombosis. N Engl J Med 1994;331: 1630–42.

medical, surgical, and radiologic specialties.[3] Pulmonary embolism and deep-vein thrombosis should be considered part of the same pathologic process. Despite substantial advances, the mortality and recurrence rates of pulmonary embolism remain high. Surgery predisposes patients to pulmonary embolism even as late as 1 month postoperatively.

Diagnosis

Accurate detection of pulmonary embolism remains difficult, and the differential diagnosis is extensive (Table 12–3).[3] Pulmonary embolism can accompany as well as mimic other cardiopulmonary illnesses. Clinical manifestations of pulmonary embolism are nonspecific, and the diagnosis is often difficult to establish on clinical grounds alone (Table 12–4). The most consistent manifestations of pulmonary embolism are an acute onset of dyspnea, which most likely reflects sudden increases in alveolar deadspace, and decreases in pulmonary compliance. Reflex bronchoconstriction augments airway resistance, and lung edema decreases pulmonary compliance. Pleuritic or substernal chest pain that may be indistinguishable from angina pectoris, cough, or hemoptysis often suggests a small embolism near the pleura. Breathing is likely to be rapid and shallow. Findings of right ventricular dysfunction include bulging neck veins, increased central venous pressure, right ventricular hypokinesis, and an accentuated pulmonic component of the second heart sound. Transthoracic echocardiography is particularly useful in critically ill patients suspected of having pulmonary embolism and can help identify right ventricular pressure overload as well as myocardial infarction, dissection of the aorta, or pericardial tamponade, which may mimic pulmonary embolism. Arterial blood gases may remain normal, whereas arterial hypoxemia and hypocapnia (stimulation of airway irritant receptors causes hyperventilation) are not specific for pulmonary embolism. In the presence of a patent foramen ovale or atrial septal defect, paradoxical embolism may occur, as may right-to-left shunting of blood with severe arterial hypoxemia. Changes in the electrocardiogram (ECG) are unlikely in the absence of a pulmonary embolism sufficient to cause acute cor pulmonale (peaked P waves, atrial fibrillation, right bundle branch block). The ECG is used mainly to help distinguish between massive pulmonary embolism and myocardial infarction.

Manifestations of pulmonary embolism during anesthesia are nonspecific and often transient.[9] Changes suggestive of pulmonary embolism during anesthesia include unexplained arterial hypoxemia,

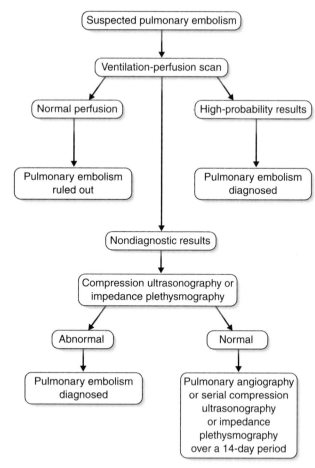

Figure 12–3 • Steps in the diagnosis of patients with clinically suspected pulmonary embolism. (From Ginsberg JS. Management of venous thromboembolism. N Engl J Med 1996; 334;1816–28. Copyright 1996 Massachusetts Medical Society, with permission.)

hypotension, tachycardia, and bronchospasm. The ECG and central venous pressure may reflect an abrupt onset of pulmonary hypertension and right ventricular dysfunction. Monitoring end-tidal carbon dioxide concentrations demonstrates increased

Table 12–3 • Differential Diagnosis of Pulmonary Embolism

Pneumonia
Asthma
Exacerbation of chronic obstructive pulmonary disease
Pulmonary edema
Thoracic aorta dissection
Pericardial tamponade
Myocardial infarction
Pneumothorax
Anxiety

Table 12–4 • Signs and Symptoms of Pulmonary Embolism

Sign/Symptom	Incidence (%)
Acute dyspnea	80–85
Tachypnea (> 20 breaths/min)	75–85
Pleuritic chest pain	65–70
Nonproductive cough	50–60
Accentuation of pulmonic valve second sound	50–60
Rales	50–60
Tachycardia (> 100 beats/min)	45–65
Fever (38°–39°C)	40–50
Hemoptysis	30

alveolar-to-arterial differences in carbon dioxide owing to ventilation of unperfused alveoli. Transesophageal echocardiography demonstrating acute dilation of the right atrium, right ventricle, and pulmonary artery may aid in the diagnosis of an intraoperative pulmonary embolus.[10] Right ventricular hypokinesis often predicts a poor clinical prognosis.

Perfusion lung scanning remains the most useful screening test to rule out clinically important acute pulmonary embolism. Venous ultrasonography is highly accurate, but normal results do not rule out pulmonary embolism if the level of clinical suspicion is moderately high. An alternative to lung scans or conventional pulmonary arteriography is computed tomography of the chest with contrast medium.

Treatment

Heparin constitutes the cornerstone of managing pulmonary embolism with an intravenous bolus of unfractionated heparin (5000 to 10,000 units) followed by continuous intravenous infusions being initiated during the diagnostic workup in patients considered to have a high clinical likelihood of pulmonary embolism.[3] Warfarin can be safely initiated once a therapeutic activated partial thromboplastin time has been achieved. The goal is an INR of 3.0, as concomitant administration of unfractionated heparin usually prolongs the INR by an additional 0.5, yielding an effective INR due to warfarin alone of 2.5. The optimal duration of anticoagulation after pulmonary embolism remains uncertain. Nevertheless, a treatment period of 6 months prevents far more recurrences than a treatment period of 6 weeks.[3]

Hypotension caused by low cardiac output may require treatment with inotropes such as isoproterenol, dopamine, or dobutamine. Isoproterenol is an attractive selection, as it is more likely than other catecholamines to decrease pulmonary vascular resistance. Nevertheless, the value of pulmonary vasodilators for managing pulmonary embolism has not been established. Tracheal intubation and institution of controlled ventilation of the patient's lungs with positive end-expiratory pressure may be necessary. Analgesics to treat pain associated with pulmonary embolism are important but must be prescribed keeping in mind the underlying instability of the cardiovascular system. Pulmonary artery embolectomy using cardiopulmonary bypass is reserved for patients with massive pulmonary embolism documented by pulmonary arteriography who are unresponsive to medical therapy.

Management of Anesthesia

Management of anesthesia for the surgical treatment of life-threatening pulmonary embolism is designed to support vital organ function and to minimize anesthetic-induced myocardial depression. Most patients arrive in the operating room with a tracheal tube in place and with ventilation of the lungs being controlled with increased inspired concentrations of oxygen. Monitoring arterial and cardiac filling pressures is recommended. It is useful to monitor right atrial filling pressures and to adjust the rate of intravenous fluid administration in an effort to optimize the right ventricular stroke volume in the presence of marked increases in afterload. It may be necessary to support cardiac output with continuous infusions of catecholamines during the operative procedure. In this regard, isoproterenol increases myocardial contractility and may decrease pulmonary vascular resistance. The disadvantage of isoproterenol is a decrease in diastolic blood pressure, which may jeopardize coronary blood flow. Dopamine and dobutamine are acceptable alternatives to isoproterenol, but neither of these catecholamines is likely to decrease pulmonary vascular resistance. In fact, large doses of dopamine may increase pulmonary vascular resistance.

Induction and maintenance of anesthesia should avoid accentuation of co-existing arterial hypoxemia, systemic hypotension, and pulmonary hypertension. Among the intravenous induction drugs, the potential adverse effects of ketamine on pulmonary vascular resistance must be considered. Anesthesia can be maintained with any drug or combination of drugs that does not produce excessive myocardial depression. Nitrous oxide is not a likely selection, considering the need to administer high concentrations of oxygen and the potential for this drug to increase pulmonary vascular resistance. Selection of nondepolarizing neuromuscular blocking drugs should consider the possible undesirable effects of drug-induced histamine release.

Removal of embolic fragments from the distal pulmonary artery may be facilitated by the application of positive-pressure ventilation of the patient's lungs when the surgeon applies suction through the arteriotomy placed in the pulmonary trunk. Although the cardiopulmonary status of these patients is perilous before surgery, significant hemodynamic improvement usually occurs postoperatively.

▌ FAT EMBOLISM

The syndrome of fat embolism to the lungs typically appears 12 to 72 hours (lucid interval) after long-bone fractures, especially of the femur or tibia.[11] Fat embolism syndrome has also been observed in association with acute pancreatitis, cardiopulmonary bypass, parenteral infusion of lipids, and liposuction.[12] The triad of arterial hypoxemia, mental confusion, and petechiae especially over the anterior neck, shoulders, and chest (caused by embolic fat) in young adults with closed tibia or femur fractures should arouse suspicion of fat embolism. Associated pulmonary dysfunction may be limited to arterial hypoxemia (always present), or it may be fulminant, progressing from tachypnea to alveolar capillary leak and adult respiratory distress syndrome. Central nervous system dysfunction ranges from confusion to seizures and coma.[13] Petechiae, especially over the neck, shoulders, and chest, occur in at least 50% of patients with clinical evidence of fat embolism. Coagulopathy and thrombocytopenia are probably related to other complications of severe trauma, including disseminated intravascular coagulation. Increased serum lipase concentrations or the presence of lipiduria is suggestive of fat embolism but may also occur after trauma in the absence of this problem. Temperature increases up to 42°C and tachycardia are often present. Magnetic resonance imaging is necessary to show the characteristic cerebral lesions during the acute stage of fat embolism syndrome.

The source of fat producing the fat embolism is undocumented but may represent disruption of the adipose architecture of bone marrow. Treatment of fat embolism syndrome includes management of acute respiratory distress syndrome and immobilization of long-bone fractures. Prophylactic administration of corticosteroids for patients at risk may be useful, but the efficacy of corticosteroids for the established syndrome has not been documented. Conceptually, corticosteroids may decrease the incidence of fat embolism syndrome by limiting the endothelial damage caused by free fatty acids.

References

1. Weinmann EE, Salzman EW. Deep-vein thrombosis. N Engl J Med 1994;331:1630–42
2. Ginsberg JS. Management of venous thromboembolism. N Engl J Med 1996;335:1816–28
3. Goldhaber SZ. Pulmonary embolism. N Engl J Med 1998; 339:93–104
4. McKenzie PJ, Wishart HY, Gray I, et al. Effects of anaesthetic technique on deep-vein thrombosis: a comparison of subarachnoid and general anaesthesia. Br J Anaesth 1985;57:853–7
5. Modig J, Maripuu E, Sahlstedt B. Thromboembolism following total hip replacement: a prospective investigation of 94 patients with emphasis on efficacy of lumbar epidural anesthesia in prophylaxis. Reg Anesth 1986;11:72–9
6. Jorgensen LN, Rasmussen LS, Neilsen PT, et al. Antithrombotic efficacy of continuous extradural analgesia after knee replacement. Br J Anaesth 1991;66:8–12
7. Davis FM, Woolner DF, Frampton C, et al. Prospective multicenter trial of mortality following general or spinal anaesthesia for hip fracture surgery in the elderly. Br J Anaesth 1987;59:1080–8
8. Coleman SA, Boyce WJ, Cosh PH, et al. Outcome after general anaesthesia for repair of fractured neck of the femur: a randomized trial of spontaneous v. controlled ventilation. Br J Anaesth 1988;60:43–7
9. Divekan VM, Kamdar BM, Pansare SN. Pulmonary embolism during anaesthesia: case report. Can Anaesth Soc J 1981;28:277–9
10. Langeron O, Goarin J-P, Pansard J-L, et al. Massive intraoperative pulmonary embolism: diagnosis with transesophageal two-dimensional echocardiography. Anesth Analg 1992;74: 148–50
11. Fabian TC. Unraveling the fat embolism syndrome. N Engl J Med 1993;339:961–3
12. Fourme T, Vieillard-Brown A, Loubieres Y, et al. Early fat embolism after liposuction. Anesthesiology 1998;89:782–4
13. Byrick RJ, Korley RE, McKee MD, et al. Prolonged coma after unreamed locked nailing of femoral shaft fracture. Anesthesiology 2001;94:163–5

13

Chronic Obstructive Pulmonary Disease

Chronic obstructive pulmonary disease (COPD) is characterized by the progressive development of airflow limitation that is not fully reversible.[1] The term *COPD* encompasses chronic obstructive bronchitis (with obstruction of small airways) and emphysema (with enlargement of air spaces and destruction of lung parenchyma, loss of lung elasticity, and closure of small airways). *Chronic bronchitis*, by contrast, is defined by the presence of a productive cough of more than 3 months duration for more than two successive years. The cough is due to hypersecretion of mucus and is not necessarily accompanied by airflow limitation. Most patients with COPD have all three pathologic conditions (chronic obstructive bronchitis, emphysema, mucous plugging), but the relative extent of emphysema and obstructive bronchitis in individual patients often varies. It is estimated that 16 million Americans suffer from chronic bronchitis and/or pulmonary emphysema. Chronic bronchitis and emphysema usually occur together as the consequence of cigarette smoking (usually of at least 10 years duration). Chronic bronchitis and emphysema are distinguished from asthma in that the abnormalities causing chronic bronchitis and emphysema are usually irreversible.

CHRONIC BRONCHITIS AND PULMONARY EMPHYSEMA

Chronic bronchitis, which follows prolonged exposure of the airways to nonspecific irritants, is characterized by hypersecretion of mucus and inflammatory changes in the bronchi. Hypersecretion of mucus and inflammation usually cause daily cough and sputum production, which helps identify this disease clinically. In contrast to chronic bronchitis, acute bronchitis is a self-limited condition of the bronchi most often caused by viral infections in association with an upper respiratory tract illness. The clinical features of chronic bronchitis can resemble or contrast with findings present in patients with pulmonary emphysema (Table 13–1). The prognosis of chronic bronchitis is poor, with death often occurring within 5 years after the first episode of acute respiratory failure.

Pulmonary emphysema is characterized by a destructive process involving the lung parenchyma that results in loss of elastic recoil of the lungs (Table 13–1). As a result, airway collapse occurs during exhalation, leading to increased airway resistance. Obstruction to expiratory airflow can also lead to the formation of bullae with compression of adjacent lung tissue. Dyspnea is severe, reflecting increased work of breathing due to loss of elastic recoil of the lungs.

Epidemiology

Cigarette smoking is the major predisposing factor for the development of COPD. The risk of death from chronic bronchitis or emphysema is 30 times higher for heavy smokers (more than 25 cigarettes daily). The forced expiratory volume in 1 second (FEV_1) can be used to assess the prevalence of COPD. Most smokers have slightly decreased expiratory flow rates, and about 10% exhibit chronic airflow obstruction (FEV_1 less than 65%). Virtually all cigarette smokers older than 60 years of age exhibit some evidence of emphysema.

The dominant feature of the natural history of COPD is progressive airflow obstruction, as reflected by decreases in FEV_1. Respiratory infections do not influence the overall course of the disease. It seems likely that lung damage is irreversible by the time chronic airflow obstruction is present in patients with chronic bronchitis and emphysema,

and the FEV_1 has decreased below the normal range. Smoking cessation at this point serves only to slow the rate of further loss of lung function. Passive exposure to cigarette smoke may cause coughing but has not been shown to lead to the development of COPD. A major unknown in the etiology of COPD is why clinically significant airway obstruction develops in only 10% to 15% of smokers.

An imbalance between protease and antiprotease results in unopposed degradation of pulmonary interstitial elastin fibers by the enzyme elastase and the early development of emphysema. The genetic absence of α_1-antitrypsin activity is present in about 0.1% of the population; emphysema develops in about 80% of these individuals.[2] Wide variability exists in the tendency toward the development of emphysema in patients with this deficiency, but those who smoke cigarettes become disabled 15 to 20 years earlier than those who do not smoke. Liver disease, most often cirrhosis, occurs in 5% to 10% of adults with α_1-antitrypsin deficiency. Heterozygotes for α_1-antitrypsin whose enzyme activity is equal to or more than 40% of normal probably are protected against the development of emphysema. Most cigarette smokers have normal plasma concentrations of α_1-antitrypsin, but chronic inhalation of cigarette smoke can increase elastase activity in the lungs. Furthermore, oxidants in cigarette smoke can inactivate α_1-antitrypsin.

Clinical Features and Diagnosis

Chronic productive cough and progressive exercise limitation due to dyspnea are the hallmarks of persistent expiratory airflow obstruction characteristic of COPD (Table 13–1). Although these symptoms are nonspecific, a diagnosis of COPD is likely in patients who are also chronic cigarette smokers. Patients with predominant chronic bronchitis present with a chronic productive cough, whereas patients with predominant emphysema complain of dys-

Table 13–1 • Comparative Features of Chronic Obstructive Pulmonary Disease

Feature	Chronic Bronchitis	Pulmonary Emphysema
Mechanism of airway obstruction	Decreased airway lumen due to mucus and inflammation	Loss of elastic recoil
Dyspnea	Moderate	Severe
Forced exhaled volume in 1 second	Decreased	Decreased
PaO_2	Marked decrease ("blue bloater")	Modest decrease ("pink puffer")
$PaCO_2$	Increased	Normal to decreased
Diffusing capacity	Normal	Decreased
Hematocrit	Increased	Normal
Cor pulmonale	Marked	Mild
Prognosis	Poor	Good

pnea. When the FEV_1 is less than 40% of normal, patients with emphysema probably experience dyspnea during activities of daily living.[1] Orthopnea is often present in patients with advanced COPD especially if increased airway secretions accompany the airflow obstruction. The orthopnea of COPD may be difficult to differentiate from that due to congestive heart failure. Transient periods of sputum discoloration commonly occur in association with respiratory tract infections. Wheezing is common in the presence of mucus accumulation in the airways and may mimic asthma. The combination of chronic bronchitis and reversible bronchospasm is referred to as asthmatic bronchitis.

Physical Examination

Physical findings vary with the severity of COPD, and during the early stages of the disease the physical examination may be normal. As expiratory airflow obstruction increases in severity, tachypnea and a prolonged expiratory phase are likely. Breath sounds are likely to be decreased, and expiratory wheezes are common especially if patients are supine.

Pulmonary Function Tests

Pulmonary function tests in dyspneic patients reveal decreases in the FEV_1/forced vital capacity (FVC) ratio and even greater decreases in the forced expiratory flow between 25% and 75% of vital capacity (FEF_{25-75}). Measurement of lung volumes reveals an increased residual volume (RV) and normal to increased functional residual capacity (FRC) and total lung capacity (TLC) (Fig. 13–1). Slowing of expiratory airflow and gas trapping behind prematurely closed airways is responsible for the increases in the RV. The advantage of increased RV and FRC in patients with COPD is an enlarged airway diameter and increased elastic recoil for exhalation. The cost to patients is the greater work of breathing at the higher lung volumes.

Chest Radiography

Radiographic abnormalities may be minimal even in the presence of advanced COPD. Hyperlucency of the lungs owing to arterial vascular deficiency in the lung periphery and hyperinflation (flattening of the diaphragm with loss of the normal domed appearance and a vertically oriented cardiac silhouette) suggest the diagnosis of emphysema. If bullae are also present, the diagnosis of emphysema is virtually certain, except only a small percentage of patients who are affected with emphysema have bul-

lae. Chronic bronchitis is rarely recognized on chest radiographs. Computed tomography of the chest can be useful for diagnosing emphysema.

Arterial Blood Gases

Arterial blood gases in the presence of advanced COPD are commonly used to categorize patients with COPD as "pink puffers" (PaO_2 usually higher than 65 mmHg and $PaCO_2$ normal to slightly decreased) or "blue bloaters" (PaO_2 usually lower than 65 mmHg and $PaCO_2$ chronically increased to more than 45 mmHg). Individuals characterized as pink puffers are typically of thin body habitus, are free of signs of right heart failure, and are usually found to have severe emphysema. Blue bloaters typically exhibit cough and sputum production, frequent respiratory tract infections, and recurrent episodes of cor pulmonale. These patients may have pathologic changes consistent with emphysema but more often meet the criteria for chronic bronchitis. The common denominator in all these patients is chronic cigarette smoking.

The consequences of the two arterial blood gas patterns on the cardiovascular system are different in patients with COPD. Patients with COPD who are characterized as "blue bloaters" develop pulmonary hypertension (arterial hypoxemia and respiratory acidosis evoke pulmonary vascular vasoconstriction) and secondary erythrocytosis due to chronic arterial hypoxemia. In response to chronic pulmonary hypertension, cor pulmonale generally develops and right ventricular hypertrophy (right axis deviation on the electrocardiogram) is present. Right ventricular failure results in systemic venous hypertension with associated jugular venous distension, peripheral edema, passive hepatic congestion, and occasionally ascites. Pleural effusions are present only if left ventricular failure also occurs.

Patients with COPD who are characterized as "pink puffers" experience emphysematous lung destruction leading to loss of pulmonary capillaries as a result of destroyed alveolar walls. The subsequent loss of the pulmonary capillary vascular bed manifests as decreased diffusing capacity, although the PaO_2 is typically only mildly depressed such that pulmonary vasoconstriction is minimal and secondary erythrocytosis does not occur. Cor pulmonale develops only rarely in these patients.

Treatment

Treatment of COPD is designed to relieve existing symptoms and slow the progressive decrease in

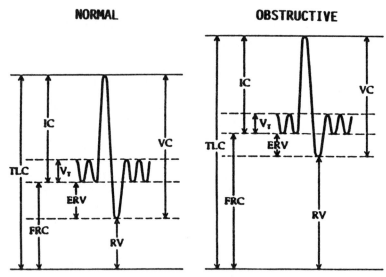

NORMAL

OBSTRUCTIVE

Figure 13–1 • Lung volumes in chronic obstructive pulmonary disease compared with normal values. In the presence of obstructive lung disease the VC is normal to decreased, the RV and FRC are increased, the TLC is normal to increased, and the RV/TLC ratio is increased. ERV, expiratory reserve volume; FRC, functional residual capacity; IC, inspiratory capacity; RV, residual volume; TLC, total lung capacity; VC, vital capacity; V_T, tidal volume.

pulmonary function that accompanies the natural course of this disease.

Cessation of Smoking and Supplemental Oxygen Administration

Cessation of smoking and chronic administration of oxygen in the presence of arterial hypoxemia are the only two therapeutic interventions that may favorably alter the natural progression of COPD.[1, 3] Smoking cessation generally causes the symptoms of chronic bronchitis to diminish or entirely disappear, and it eliminates the accelerated loss of lung function observed in those who continue to smoke. Chronic oxygen administration ("home oxygen therapy") is usually recommended if the PaO_2 is less than 55 mmHg, the hematocrit is more than 55%, or there is evidence of cor pulmonale. The goal of supplemental oxygen administration is to achieve a PaO_2 between 60 and 80 mmHg. This goal can usually be accomplished by delivering oxygen through a nasal cannula at 2 L/min. Ultimately the flow rate for oxygen is titrated to the individual patient's needs according to arterial blood gas measurements. Relief of arterial hypoxemia with supplemental oxygen administration is more effective than any known drug therapy in decreasing pulmonary vascular resistance and preventing excessive erythrocytosis with associated increases in blood viscosity.

Drug Therapy

Bronchodilators are the mainstay of current drug therapy for COPD.[1] Bronchodilators cause only a small (less than 10%) increase in FEV_1 in patients with COPD, but these drugs may alleviate symptoms by decreasing hyperinflation and thus dyspnea, and they may improve exercise tolerance, despite the fact that there is little improvement in spirometric measurements. An additional benefit of long-acting β_2-agonists in COPD patients may be a decrease in infective exacerbations, as these drugs decrease the adhesion of bacteria such as *Haemophilus influenzae* to airway epithelial cells. COPD appears to be more effectively treated by anticholinergic drugs than by β_2-agonists, in contrast to asthma, for which β_2-agonists are more effective. Inhaled corticosteroids are widely prescribed for COPD. Intermittent broad-spectrum antibiotic (ampicillin, cephalosporin, erythromycin) administration is indicated for acute episodes of worsening clinical symptoms marked by increased dyspnea, excessive sputum production, or sputum purulence. Annual vaccinations against influenza and possibly pneumococcus may be beneficial. Exacerbations of COPD may also be due to viral infections of the upper respiratory tract or may be noninfective, so antibiotic treatment is not always warranted.[1] Drug-induced diuresis may be considered for patients with cor pulmonale and right ventricular failure (peripheral edema). Diuretic-induced chloride depletion may result in hypochloremic metabolic alkalosis that depresses the ventilatory drive and may aggravate chronic carbon dioxide retention. Physical training programs can increase exercise capacity of patients with COPD despite the absence of detectable effects on the FEV_1. Prompt deconditioning occurs when the exercise program is abandoned.

Noninvasive Ventilation

Noninvasive positive-pressure ventilation with a nasal mask eliminates the need for tracheal intubation and decreases the need for mechanical ventilation during acute exacerbations of COPD.[1] Uncontrolled studies have shown that noninvasive positive-pressure ventilation used at home may improve oxygenation and decrease hospital admissions in patients with severe COPD and hypercapnia.

Lung Volume Reduction Surgery

Lung volume reduction surgery may be considered in selected patients with emphysema characterized by regions of overdistended and poorly functioning emphysematous regions.[1, 4] Surgical removal of these overdistended areas allows more normal areas of the lung to expand with resultant improvement in the FEV_1 and possibly an improvement in arterial oxygenation such that supplemental oxygen is no longer required.

Management of anesthesia for lung volume reduction surgery includes use of a double-lumen endobronchial tube to permit separation of the lungs, avoidance of nitrous oxide (which could diffuse into emphysematous bullae), and avoidance of excessive positive airway pressures (inspiratory pressures ideally less than 20 cmH_2O).[4] Positive end-expiratory pressure would not be an acceptable technique for mechanical ventilation of the lungs during lung volume reduction surgery. Monitoring central venous pressures to guide fluid management is not likely to be reliable because of gas trapping and the pulmonary tamponade effect due to large emphysematous bullae.

Preoperative Pulmonary Evaluation and Risk of Postoperative Pulmonary Complications

Preoperative pulmonary evaluation of patients with COPD is based on the recognition that postoperative pulmonary complications are predictable risks of surgery in these patients.[5] Despite the emphasis on postoperative cardiac complications, it is important to recognize that postoperative pulmonary complications are as common as cardiac complications. Important pulmonary complications (those that contribute to increased morbidity and mortality in contrast to fever or productive cough) include pneumonia, atelectasis, bronchospasm, and acute respiratory failure requiring mechanical ventilation.

Patient-Related Risk Factors

Potential patient-related risk factors for the development of postoperative pulmonary complications are smoking, the presence of existing pulmonary disease (COPD, asthma), advanced age, and poor general health.[5, 6] Despite a common assumption that obesity increases the risk of pulmonary complications, most reports in the literature have failed to confirm such an association.

Smoking

The incidence of postoperative pulmonary complications is increased in those who smoke cigarettes.[7-9] Therefore cessation of cigarette smoking during the perioperative period is prudent, although sufficient time for reversible changes to occur is not always possible.

Chronic Obstructive Pulmonary Disease

Patients with COPD are at increased risk for the development of postoperative pulmonary complications.[5] Aggressive preoperative treatment is indicated for patients with COPD who have evidence of airflow obstruction on physical examination and who do not have optimal exercise capacity. Elective surgery is deferred in the presence of acute exacerbations of COPD. Combinations of bronchodilators, antibiotics, smoking cessation, corticosteroids, and physical therapy reduce the risk of postoperative pulmonary complications in these patients.

Patients with symptomatic COPD are treated with inhaled ipratropium; inhaled β-agonists are added as needed to control the symptoms, as the combination of these two drugs produces additive effects. Although not all patients with COPD respond to corticosteroid therapy, a 2 week preoperative course of systemic corticosteroids may be considered for those who continue to have symptoms despite aggressive bronchodilator therapy. Preoperative antibiotics are reserved for patients in whom the presence of infection is suggested by changes in the character or amount of sputum. The indiscriminant use of preoperative antibiotics does not decrease the risk of postoperative pneumonia in patients undergoing operations outside the thorax.[5] The risk of postoperative pulmonary complications in patients with viral upper respiratory infections is not known, although it seems reasonable to defer elective surgery.

Procedure-Related Risk Factors

Procedure-related risk factors for the development of postoperative pulmonary complications include the site of the surgical procedure and the effects of anesthetic drugs and surgical trauma on respiratory muscle function.[5, 6]

Operative Site

The operative site is the most important predictor of the development of postoperative pulmonary complications.[5] The risk of postoperative pulmonary complications increases as the incision approaches the diaphragm and the duration of surgery exceeds 3 hours. Upper abdominal and thoracic surgery create the greatest risk for postoperative pulmonary complications, ranging from 10% to 40%. The risk is lower for laparoscopic cholecystectomy than for open cholecystectomy. Postoperative pulmonary complications are less likely following operations outside the thorax or abdomen.

Respiratory Muscle Function

Many postoperative pulmonary complications, such as atelectasis and pneumonia, seem to be related to disruption of the normal activity (coordination) of the respiratory muscles (intercostal muscles, upper abdominal muscles, diaphragm), which begins with the induction of anesthesia and may continue into the postoperative period.[6] In addition to residual effects of anesthetic drugs and neuromuscular blocking drugs, surgical trauma can also disrupt normal coordination of respiratory muscle action, leading to persistent decreases in the FRC and vital capacity (VC), with atelectasis that can last several days after surgery. The effects of surgical trauma are most pronounced following thoracic or upper abdominal surgery. The clinical impression is that atelectasis leads to pneumonia, although this progression has not been conclusively documented.

Preoperative Clinical Evaluation

The history and physical examination of patients with COPD provide a more accurate assessment of the likelihood of postoperative pulmonary complications than do pulmonary function tests and measurement of arterial blood gases.[5, 6] A history of exercise intolerance, chronic cough, or unexplained dyspnea is important to elicit during the preoperative evaluation. Evidence of decreased breath sounds, wheezing, and prolonged expiratory phases on the physical examination may predict an increased risk of postoperative pulmonary complications.

Preoperative Pulmonary Function Testing

The value of routine preoperative pulmonary function testing (spirometry) remains controversial.[5, 10] Although the results of pulmonary function testing and arterial blood gases have proved useful for predicting pulmonary function following lung resection, they do not predict the likelihood of postoperative pulmonary complications.[6] Indeed, clinical findings (smoking, diffuse wheezing, productive cough) are generally more predictive of pulmonary complications than spirometric results. Even patients at high risk as defined by spirometry (FEV_1 less than 70% of predicted, FEV_1/FVC ratio less than 65%) or arterial blood gases ($PaCO_2$ higher than 45 mmHg) can undergo surgery (including lung resection) with an acceptable risk of postoperative pulmonary complications.[5, 11] Thus pulmonary function tests should be viewed as a management tool to optimize preoperative pulmonary function but not as a means to assess risk.[6] The results of preoperative pulmonary function testing should not be used to deny surgery to patients.[5]

Preoperative spirometry may be reserved for patients scheduled to undergo thoracic or upper abdominal surgery and who have symptoms of cough, dyspnea, or exercise intolerance. Spirometry may be helpful in patients with COPD or asthma if, after clinical assessment, it is uncertain whether the degree of airflow obstruction has been optimally reduced.

Risk Reduction Strategies

Risk reduction strategies to decrease the incidence of postoperative pulmonary complications include preoperative, intraoperative, and postoperative interventions (Table 13–2).[5] Prophylaxis against the development of postoperative pulmonary complications in patients with COPD is based on restoring decreased lung volumes and facilitating production of an effective cough to remove secretions from the airways. Identification of the FRC as the most important lung volume during the postoperative period provides a specific goal of therapy.

Table 13–2 • Risk-Reduction Strategies to Decrease the Incidence of Postoperative Pulmonary Complications

Preoperative
Encourage cessation of smoking for at least 8 weeks
Treat evidence of expiratory airflow obstruction
Treat respiratory infection with antibiotics
Initiate patient education regarding lung volume expansion maneuvers

Intraoperative
Use minimally invasive surgery (laparoscopic) techniques when possible
Consider use of regional anesthesia (?)
Avoid use of long-acting neuromuscular blocking drugs (?)
Avoid surgical procedures likely to require more than 3 hours

Postoperative
Institute lung volume expansion maneuvers (voluntary deep breathing, incentive spirometry, continuous positive airway pressure)
Maximize analgesia (neuraxial opioids, intercostal nerve blocks, patient-controlled analgesia)

Adapted from: Smetana GW. Preoperative pulmonary evaluation. N Engl J Med 1999;340:937–44.

Lung Expansion Maneuvers

Lung expansion maneuvers (deep breathing exercises, incentive spirometry, chest physical therapy, positive-pressure breathing techniques) are of proven benefit for preventing postoperative pulmonary complications in high risk patients.[5, 6] These techniques decrease the risk of atelectasis by increasing lung volumes. All regimens seem to be equally efficacious in decreasing the frequency of postoperative pulmonary complications (about twofold compared with no therapy).[6, 12] Incentive spirometry is simple and inexpensive, and it provides objective goals for, and monitoring of, patient performance. Patients are given inspired volumes as goals to achieve and maintain so as to provide sustained inflation, which is important for expanding collapsed alveoli. The major disadvantage of incentive spirometry is the need for patient cooperation to accomplish the treatment. Preoperative education in lung expansion maneuvers decreases the incidence of pulmonary complications to a greater degree than if education begins after surgery. There is little evidence, however, that instituting lung expansion maneuvers preoperatively is of any value other than teaching patients the use of the technique.

Intermittent positive-pressure breathing also effectively decreases the incidence of postoperative pulmonary complications, but its cost has resulted in decreased usage. Continuous positive airway pressure is usually reserved for the prevention of postoperative pulmonary complications in patients who are not able to perform deep-breathing exercises or incentive spirometry. Nasal positive airway pressure minimizes the expected decrease in lung volumes after surgery and may decrease the incidence of postoperative pulmonary complications including atelectasis and acute respiratory failure. Nevertheless, less costly lung expansion maneuvers are available, and positive nasal airway pressure is not recommended routinely for primary prevention of postoperative pulmonary complications.

Pain Control

Relief of postoperative pain with neuraxial opioids permits tracheal extubation in patients who would otherwise require systemic opioids and sedatives to permit mechanical ventilation of the lungs and tolerance of the tracheal tube. Sympathetic nervous system blockade and loss of proprioception as produced by a local anesthetic placed in the epidural space does not accompany neuraxial opioids. Therefore early ambulation is possible in patients treated with neuraxial opioids. Ambulation serves to increase the FRC and improve arterial oxygenation, presumably by improving ventilation-to-perfusion matching. Neuraxial opioids administered after intrathoracic and upper abdominal surgery help restore the FEV_1 toward preoperative values.[13] Breakthrough pain may require treatment with opioids administered intravenously. In this regard, patient-controlled analgesia serves as a useful adjunct to neuraxial opioids. Sedation may accompany neuraxial opioid administration, and delayed depression of ventilation 6 to 12 hours after epidural opioid placement is a rare problem. Presumably, opioids are absorbed into the subarachnoid space, ultimately diffusing into the area of the fourth cerebral ventricle, where they can depress the medullary ventilatory center. This delayed depression of ventilation is more likely to occur in (1) elderly patients, (2) patients considered naive to opioids, (3) patients receiving systemic opioids as well, and (4) patients in whom poorly lipid-soluble opioids (morphine) are used.

The quality of postoperative neuraxial analgesia (epidural or spinal) is superior to that provided by parenteral administration of opioids. Nevertheless, it is not possible to document that neuraxial analgesia decreases the incidence of clinically significant postoperative pulmonary complications or is superior to parenteral opioids.[6] Rather, maneuvers to encourage deep breathing that are of proven benefit should be the focus of preventive efforts.[6] Hypotension is more common among patients receiving epidural analgesia, but it has not been confirmed to be a cause of morbidity. Postoperative neuraxial analgesia is recommended after high risk thoracic, abdominal, and major vascular surgery. Use of postoperative intercostal nerve blocks may be an option if neuraxial analgesia is ineffective or technically difficult.

Mechanical Ventilation

Continued tracheal intubation and mechanical ventilation of the patient's lungs during the immediate postoperative period may be necessary in patients with severe COPD undergoing major abdominal or intrathoracic surgery.[14] For example, it is likely that patients with preoperative FEV_1/FVC ratios less than 0.5 must continue mechanical support of ventilation during the early postoperative period after upper abdominal or intrathoracic surgery. The presence of preoperative $PaCO_2$ of more than 50 mmHg is likely to be associated with the need for postoperative mechanical ventilation. It should be appreciated that the measured $PaCO_2$ during the preoperative period may be erroneously low if the arterial puncture to obtain the blood sample for measurement was painful and produced hyperventilation. Increased plasma concentrations of bicarbonate in the presence of low or normal $PaCO_2$ suggests that acute hyperventilation is masking chronic carbon dioxide retention. When the $PaCO_2$ has been chronically increased, it is important not to correct the hypercarbia too quickly because sudden decreases in $PaCO_2$ can result in alkalemia, as the kidneys cannot instantly excrete the excess bicarbonate. This alkalemia can be associated with cardiac dysrhythmias and central nervous system stimulation culminating in seizures.

When continued mechanical ventilation of the lungs is necessary during the postoperative period, inspired concentrations of oxygen and ventilator settings should be adjusted to maintain the PaO_2 at 60 to 100 mmHg and the $PaCO_2$ in ranges that maintain the pHa at 7.35 to 7.45. Until these values can be confirmed during the postoperative period, it is customary to administer at least 50% oxygen, using tidal volumes of 10 to 15 ml/kg and breathing rates of 6 to 10 breaths/min. Institution of positive end-expiratory pressure may be a consideration if the PaO_2 cannot be maintained above 60 mmHg breathing 50% oxygen. It must be remembered that positive end-expiratory pressure may be associated with increased air trapping in patients with COPD. The decision to discontinue mechanical support of ventilation and to perform tracheal extubation is based on the patient's clinical status and the indices of pulmonary function (see Chapter 16).

Chest Physiotherapy

A combination of chest physiotherapy and postural drainage plus deep breathing exercises taught during the preoperative period may decrease the incidence of postoperative pulmonary complications. Presumably, vibrations produced on the chest wall by physiotherapy result in dislodgement of mucus plugs from peripheral airways. Appropriate positioning facilitates elimination of loosened mucus from the airways.

Management of Anesthesia

Management of anesthesia for patients with COPD undergoing elective surgery includes efforts during the preoperative period to optimize pulmonary function, intraoperative management designed to minimize residual depressant effects of anesthetic drugs on breathing, and postoperative interventions to decrease surgical pain that could contribute to impaired oxygenation and ventilation.

Preoperative Preparation

Preoperative preparation of patients with COPD includes efforts to stop smoking, treatment of reversible processes such as bronchospasm (inhaled β-agonists), and eradication of bacterial infections. Preoperative pulmonary function tests are useful tools for assessing lung function and responses to therapy, but these tests do not provide predictive information as to the likelihood of postoperative pulmonary complications.[6] The presence of expiratory airflow obstruction, demonstrated on preoperative pulmonary function tests, has been shown to predict the occurrence of bronchospasm in cigarette smokers undergoing abdominal surgery but not to predict the need for prolonged postoperative tracheal intubation.[15]

Logic supports a strong recommendation to patients to cease cigarette smoking before undergoing elective surgery, as the risk of postoperative pulmonary complications is predictably increased.[6] Although the optimal period of abstinence before elective surgery is not known, it is clear that even brief periods of abstinence improve the oxygen-carrying capacity of the patient's arterial blood. For example, the adverse effects of carbon monoxide on oxygen-carrying capacity and of nicotine on the cardiovascular system are short-lived. The elimination half-time of carbon monoxide is about 4 to 6 hours, such that smoke-free intervals of 12 to 18 hours should result in substantial decreases in carboxyhemoglobin levels. Indeed, within 12 hours after cessation of smoking the PaO_2 at which hemoglobin is 50% saturated with oxygen (P_{50}) increases from 22.9 to 26.4 mmHg and the plasma levels of carboxyhemoglobin decrease from 6.5% to 1.1%.[8] Increased plasma concentrations of carboxyhemoglobin can cause the pulse oximeter to overestimate the SpO_2. It seems unlikely, however, that the relatively low plasma carboxyhemoglobin concentrations associated with cigarette smoking can produce significant overestimations. Carbon monoxide may also have negative inotropic effects. Sympathomimetic effects of nicotine on the heart are transient, lasting only 20 to 30 minutes. Despite the favorable effects on plasma carboxyhemoglobin concentrations, short-term abstinence from cigarettes has not been proven to decrease the incidence of postoperative pulmonary complications.

Cigarette smoking causes mucus hypersecretion, impairment of mucociliary transport activity, and narrowing of the small airways. In contrast to favorable effects of short-term abstinence from smoking on carboxyhemoglobin concentrations, improved ciliary and small airway function and decreased sputum production occur slowly over periods of weeks after cigarette smoking is stopped. Indeed, the incidence of postoperative pulmonary complications after coronary artery surgery decreases only when abstinence from cigarette smoking is longer than 8 weeks (Fig. 13–2).[9]

Cigarette smoking may interfere with normal immune responses and could interfere with the ability of smokers to respond to pulmonary infection following anesthesia and surgery.[16] Return of normal immune function may require at least 6 weeks of abstinence from smoking. Some components of cigarette smoke stimulate hepatic enzymes, which could alter postoperative analgesic requirements. As with immune responses, it likely takes 6 to 8 weeks for hepatic enzyme activity to return to normal following cessation of smoking.

Selection of Anesthetic Technique

The preoperative presence of COPD does not dictate the use of specific drugs or techniques for the management of anesthesia. Regional anesthesia is most suited for operations that do not invade the peritoneum and for surgical procedures performed on the extremities.[17] Lower abdominal surgery can be performed using regional techniques, but general anesthesia is equally acceptable. General anesthesia is the usual choice for upper abdominal and intrathoracic operations. The choice of anesthetic techniques or specific anesthetic drugs does not seem to alter the incidence of postoperative pulmonary complications.[14] Studies in patients with COPD that suggest a higher incidence of postoperative acute respiratory failure in patients who receive general anesthesia might reflect the fact that the operative site dictated selection of general anesthesia rather than regional anesthesia. Whether there is a relation between the duration of anesthesia and the incidence of postoperative pulmonary complications is controversial, although some suggest that operations lasting longer than 3 hours are more likely to be associated with postoperative pulmonary complications.[5, 14]

More important than the techniques or drugs selected for anesthesia is the realization that these patients are susceptible to the development of acute respiratory failure during the postoperative period. Therefore continued tracheal intubation and me-

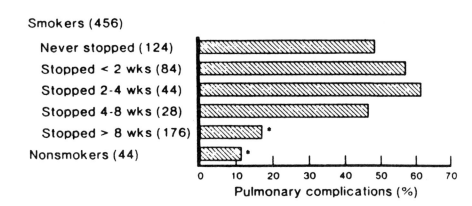

Figure 13–2 • Preoperative duration of smoking cessation and pulmonary complication rates after coronary artery bypass graft surgery. The incidence of postoperative complications in this patient population was decreased only when abstinence from cigarette smoking was longer than 8 weeks. (From Warner MA, Divertie MB, Tinker JH. Preoperative cessation of smoking and pulmonary complications in coronary artery bypass graft patients. Anesthesiology 1984;60:380–3, with permission.)

chanical ventilation of the patient's lungs may be necessary, particularly after upper abdominal or intrathoracic surgery. Alternatively, postoperative analgesia with neuraxial opioids that permit pain-free breathing during the postoperative period may permit early tracheal extubation and decrease systemic analgesic requirements with their associated depressant effects on ventilation and consciousness.

Regional Anesthesia

The risk of pulmonary complications is often viewed as being less following surgery performed with epidural or spinal anesthesia than with general anesthesia, although the literature is not consistent.[5] Regional anesthesia, such as axillary block, carries a lower risk of pulmonary complications than either spinal or general anesthesia. Nevertheless, regional anesthesia remains a useful selection in patients with COPD only when large doses of sedative drugs are not needed. For example, it must be appreciated that such patients may be extremely sensitive to the ventilatory depressant effects of sedative drugs used for systemic medication. If patient anxiety is substantial, however, small doses of a benzodiazepine, such as midazolam, in increments of 1 to 2 mg IV, can be administered with minimal likelihood of producing undesirable degrees of ventilatory depression. Elderly patients may be uniquely susceptible to depression of ventilation after receiving drugs intended to allay anxiety. Regional anesthetic techniques that produce sensory anesthesia above T6 are not recommended, as this level can lead to decreases in expiratory reserve volumes. The most important adverse effects produced by this decrease are gas flows that are inadequate to produce an effective cough, leading to reduced clearance of secretions from the airways.

General Anesthesia

General anesthesia in patients with COPD is often provided with volatile anesthetics using humidification of the inspired gases and mechanical ventilation of the lungs. Volatile anesthetics are useful because of the patient's ability to eliminate these drugs (especially desflurane and sevoflurane) rapidly through the lungs and thereby minimize residual ventilatory depression during the early postoperative period. Furthermore, volatile anesthetics may produce beneficial effects secondary to drug-induced bronchodilation.

Nitrous oxide is frequently administered in combination with a volatile anesthetic. When using nitrous oxide, one should consider the potential passage of this gas into pulmonary bullae associated with pulmonary emphysema. Conceivably, nitrous oxide could lead to enlargement and rupture of bullae resulting in development of a tension pneumothorax during anesthesia.[18] Another potential disadvantage of nitrous oxide is the limitation on the inspired concentrations of oxygen introduced by use of this anesthetic. In this regard, it is important to remember that inhaled anesthetics may attenuate regional hypoxic pulmonary vasoconstriction, leading to increased degrees of right-to-left intrapulmonary shunting. It is conceivable that increased inspired concentrations of oxygen might be necessary to offset the potential adverse consequences of this anesthetic-induced change. Nevertheless, not all studies confirm anesthetic-induced inhibition of regional hypoxic pulmonary vasoconstriction.

Opioids, although acceptable, may be less useful than inhaled anesthetics for maintenance of anesthesia in patients with COPD. For example, opioids can be associated with prolonged depression of ventilation, reflecting their slow rate of inactivation by the liver and/or elimination by the kidneys. Even the duration of depression of ventilation produced by such drugs as thiopental and midazolam may be prolonged in patients with COPD compared with that in normal individuals.[19] A higher risk of pulmonary complications has been observed in patients receiving long-acting neuromuscular blocking drugs compared with those receiving shorter-acting neuromuscular blocking drugs.[20] Presumably the longer-acting drugs are associated with postoperative hypoventilation. High inspired concentrations of nitrous oxide may be required to ensure amnesia when opioids are used for maintenance of anesthesia. In this regard, administration of adequate inspired concentrations of oxygen may be compromised by the need to administer high concentrations of nitrous oxide.

Humidification of inspired gases during anesthesia is important to prevent drying of secretions in the airways. It should be remembered that placing a tracheal tube results in bypass of nearly the entire airway humidification system. Furthermore, high flows of dry anesthetic gases intensify the need for humidification of inhaled gases. Systemic dehydration due to inadequate fluid administration during the perioperative period can result in excessive drying of secretions in the airways despite humidification of inhaled gases.

Controlled ventilation of the lungs is useful for optimizing arterial oxygenation in patients with COPD who are undergoing operations requiring general anesthesia.[21] Large tidal volumes (10 to 15 mg/kg) combined with slow inspiratory flow rates minimize the likelihood of turbulent airflow through airways and maintain optimal ventilation-to-perfusion matching. Slow breathing rates (6 to 10 breaths/min) allow sufficient time for venous return to the heart and are less likely to be associated with undesirable degrees of hyperventilation, as reflected by the $PaCO_2$. Furthermore, slow breathing rates provide sufficient time for complete exhalation to occur, which is particularly important if air trapping is to be minimized in patients with COPD. The hazard of pulmonary barotrauma in the presence of pulmonary bullae should be appreciated, particularly if high positive airway pressures are required to provide adequate ventilation of the patient's lungs. Overall, the intraoperative use of large tidal volumes and slow breathing rates are often as efficacious as positive end-expiratory pressure (PEEP) with respect to arterial oxygenation, without the detrimental cardiovascular effects produced by sustained positive airway pressure. The detrimental effects of PEEP on expiratory airflow would further detract from instituting this ventilation technique in patients with COPD.

If spontaneous breathing is permitted during anesthesia in patients with COPD, it should be appreciated that depression of ventilation produced by volatile anesthetics may be greater in patients with COPD than in individuals with normal lungs.[21] Regardless of the ventilation method selected during surgery, objective adjustments in the mode of ventilation or in settings of the mechanical ventilator are made on the basis of (1) measurements of arterial blood gases and pH, (2) continuous monitoring of the SpO_2 by pulse oximetry, and (3) continuous monitoring of the exhaled carbon dioxide concentrations by capnography.

Postoperative Care

Postoperative care of patients with COPD is intended to minimize the incidence and severity of pulmonary complications, recognizing that these patients are at increased risk for the development of acute respiratory failure (see ''Risk Reduction Strategies'') (Table 13–2). Lung volume expansion techniques and provision of postoperative analgesia, often with neuraxial opioids, are the most important interventions for preventing postoperative pulmonary complications.

The likelihood of postoperative pulmonary complications is greatest following upper abdominal and intrathoracic surgery.[5, 6] Vital capacity is decreased about 40% from the preoperative value on the day of upper abdominal surgery and does not return to near preoperative levels for 10 to 14 days.[14] In contrast to vital capacity, the FRC does not decrease until about 16 hours after upper abdominal surgery, suggesting that altered breathing patterns (altered respiratory muscle coordination) during the postoperative period are responsible for this delayed change.[10] Complete relief of postoperative pain does not restore vital capacity or FRC, further suggesting that trauma from the surgical procedure itself, in addition to altered breathing patterns, contributes to decreased lung volumes after surgery.[6]

Residual effects of anesthetic drugs may contribute to decreased PaO_2 and increased $PaCO_2$ during the immediate postoperative period. For example, anesthetics may impair regional hypoxic pulmonary vasoconstriction and blunt the ventilatory responses to carbon dioxide and to hypoxemia.[22] Decreases in the PaO_2 that persist beyond the early postoperative period most likely reflect mechanical abnormalities of the lungs, as reflected by decreases in the FRC or lack of coordination between the muscles of respiration.[6, 14] Upper abdominal surgery has the greatest effect on FRC and is followed by the largest postoperative decrease in PaO_2. Arterial oxygenation associated with decreases in the FRC may not return to preoperative levels until 10 to 14 days after surgery. With respect to abdominal operations, there is no evidence that the type of abdominal incision (transverse versus vertical) alters the incidence of postoperative pulmonary complications. The incidence of postoperative pulmonary complications, however, is dramatically less after laparoscopic cholecystectomy than after open cholecystectomy.[5]

LESS COMMON CAUSES OF EXPIRATORY AIRFLOW OBSTRUCTION

Expiratory airflow obstructions that occur less commonly than chronic bronchitis and pulmonary emphysema are bronchiectasis, cystic fibrosis, bronchiolitis obliterans, and tracheal stenosis.

Bronchiectasis

Bronchiectasis is a chronic suppurative disease of the airways that if sufficiently widespread may cause expiratory airflow obstruction similar to that seen with COPD.[1] Despite the availability of antibiotics, bronchiectasis is an important cause of chronic productive cough with purulent sputum and accounts for a significant number of patients who develop massive hemoptysis reflecting the presence of highly vascularized granulation tissues.

Pathophysiology

Bronchiectasis is characterized by a localized, irreversible dilation of a bronchus caused by destructive inflammatory processes involving the bronchial walls. Bacterial or myobacterial infections are presumed to be responsible for most cases of bronchiectasis. A typical history is that of a childhood bacterial respiratory infection complicating a viral pneumonia followed by recurrent "chest colds."[1] The most important consequence of bronchiectatic destruction of airways (continued infection from destructive organisms, most often *Pseudomonas aeruginosa*) is an increased susceptibility to recurrent or persistent bacterial infections, reflecting impaired ciliary activity and pooling of mucus in dilated airways. Once bacterial superinfection is established it is nearly impossible to eradicate, and daily expectoration of purulent sputum persists.

Diagnosis

The history of a chronic cough productive of purulent sputum is highly suggestive of bronchiectasis. Clubbing of the digits occurs in most patients with significant bronchiectasis and is a valuable diagnostic clue, as this change is not characteristic of COPD. Pulmonary function changes are unpredictable, ranging from no change to alterations characteristic of COPD or restrictive lung disease. Computed tomography provides excellent images of bronchiectatic airways and can be used to confirm the presence and extent of the disease.

Treatment

Treatment of bronchiectasis is with oral administration of antibiotics and postural drainage. Periodic culture of the sputum may guide antibiotic selection, although *Pseudomonas* is the most common organism. Significant hemoptysis can also be controlled with appropriate antibiotic therapy. Massive hemoptysis (more than 200 ml over a 24-hour period) may be treated by surgical resection of the involved lung or by selective bronchial arterial embolization under radiographic control. Postural drainage is useful for expectoration of secretions that pool distal to the diseased airways, which are likely to collapse during coughing and forced exhalation. Chest physical therapy with chest percussion and vibration is used to aid bronchopulmonary drainage. Surgical resection has played a declining role in the management of bronchiectasis during the modern antibiotic era.[1] In rare instances in which severe symptoms persist or recurrent complications occur, surgery is indicated to remove the diseased portions of the lung that are distal to the obstructive bronchial lesion.

Management of Anesthesia

Prior to elective surgery, the pulmonary status of patients with bronchiectasis is optimized by appropriate antibiotic therapy and postural drainage. Airway management may include use of a double-lumen endobronchial tube to prevent spillage of purulent sputum into normal areas of the lungs. Instrumentation of the nares may not be prudent in view of the high incidence of chronic sinusitis in these patients.

Cystic Fibrosis

Cystic fibrosis is the most common life-shortening autosomal recessive disorder. It affects an estimated 30,000 persons in the United States.[23, 24]

Pathophysiology

The cause of cystic fibrosis is a mutation in a single gene on chromosome 7 that encodes the cystic fibrosis transmembrane conductance regulator. The result of the mutation on chromosome 7 is defective chloride ion transport in epithelial cells in the lungs, pancreas, liver, gastrointestinal tract, and reproductive organs. Decreased chloride transport is accompanied by decreased transport of sodium and water, resulting in dehydrated, viscous secretions that are associated with luminal obstruction as well as destruction and scarring of various exocrine glands. As a result, pancreatic insufficiency, meconium ileus at birth, diabetes mellitus, obstructive hepatobiliary tract disease (cirrhosis and portal hypertension), and azospermia are often present. Nevertheless, the primary causes of morbidity and mortality in patients with cystic fibrosis are bronchiectasis and COPD.

Diagnosis

The presence of a sweat chloride concentration higher than 80 mEq/L plus the characteristic clinical manifestations (cough, chronic purulent sputum production, exertional dyspnea) or a family history of the disease confirm the diagnosis of cystic fibrosis.[24] Although it can add important evidence, genotyping alone cannot establish or rule out the diagnosis of cystic fibrosis, as commercially available probes are not available for all the mutations that affect the transmembrane conductance regulator. Chronic pansinusitis is almost universal with cystic fibrosis such that the presence of normal sinuses on radiographic examination is strong evidence that cystic fibrosis is not present. Malabsorption plus a response to pancreatic enzyme treatment is evidence of exocrine insufficiency associated with cystic fibrosis. Obstructive azospermia confirmed by testicular biopsy is strong evidence of cystic fibrosis. Bronchoalveolar lavage typically shows a high percentage of neutrophils (airway inflammation) in patients with cystic fibrosis. COPD is present in virtually all adult patients with cystic fibrosis and follows a relentlessly progressive course.

Treatment

Treatment of cystic fibrosis is similar to that for bronchiectasis and is directed toward alleviation of symptoms (mobilization and clearance of lower airway secretions and treatment of pulmonary infections) and correction of organ dysfunction (pancreatic enzyme replacement).[23]

Clearance of Airway Secretions

The abnormal viscoelastic properties of purulent sputum in patients with cystic fibrosis leads to its retention, resulting in airway obstruction.[23] The principal nonpharmacologic approach to enhancing clearance of pulmonary secretions is chest physical therapy with postural drainage. High-frequency chest compressions with an inflatable vest may provide an alternative method to physical therapy that is less time-consuming and does not require trained personnel.

Bronchodilator Therapy

Bronchial reactivity to histamine and other provocative stimuli is greater in patients with cystic fibrosis than in normal subjects. Bronchodilator therapy is considered if patients have an increase of 10% or more in the FEV_1 in response to an inhaled bronchodilator β-agonist or anticholinergic drug.

Reduction in Viscoelasticity of Sputum

The abnormal viscosity of airway secretions in patients with cystic fibrosis is primarily due to the presence of polymorphonuclear neutrophils and their degradation products. A purified recombinant human deoxyribonuclease that can digest extracellular degradation products decreases the viscoelasticity of sputum.

Antibiotic Therapy

Patients with cystic fibrosis have periodic exacerbations of pulmonary infections that are identified primarily on the basis of increases in pulmonary symp-toms and airway secretions (Table 13–3).[23] The choice of antibiotic therapy is based on identification and susceptibility testing of bacteria isolated from the sputum. In patients in whom oropharyngeal cultures yield no pathogens, bronchoscopy to remove lower-airway secretions may be indicated if there is no response to empirical antibiotic therapy. The most common antibiotic regimen consists of an aminoglycoside and a β-lactam antibiotic active against *Pseudomonas aeruginosa*. Many patients with cystic fibrosis are given long-term antibiotic therapy in hopes of decreasing the frequency of exacerbations of pulmonary infections and slowing the progression of pulmonary obstruction.

Management of Anesthesia

Management of anesthesia in patients with cystic fibrosis invokes the same principles as outlined for patients with COPD and bronchiectasis. Elective surgical procedures should be delayed until optimal pulmonary function can be ensured by controlling bronchial infections and facilitating removal of secretions from the airways. Vitamin K treatment may be necessary if hepatic function is poor or if absorption of fat-soluble vitamins from the gastrointestinal tract is impaired. Preoperative medication is probably unnecessary, as sedation may lead to undesirable ventilatory depression, and anticholinergic drugs may further increase the viscosity of secretions. Maintenance of anesthesia with volatile anesthetics permits the use of high inspired concentrations of oxygen and can decrease airway resistance

---

Table 13–3 • Symptoms and Signs Associated with Exacerbation of Pulmonary Infection in Patients with Cystic Fibrosis

Symptoms
Increased frequency and duration of cough
Increased sputum production
Changes in appearance of sputum
Increased dyspnea
Further decreases in exercise tolerance
Decreased appetite
Feeling of increased congestion in the chest
Signs
Increased breathing rate
Use of accessory muscles for breathing
Intercostal retractions
Change in chest auscultatory findings
Further decline in pulmonary function measurements
  consistent with obstructive lung disease
Fever and leukocytosis
Weight loss
New infiltrate on chest radiographs

Adapted from Ramsey BW. Management of pulmonary disease in patients with cystic fibrosis. N Engl J Med 1996;335:179–88.

by decreasing the tone of bronchial smooth muscles. Furthermore, volatile anesthetics are helpful for decreasing the responsiveness of hyperreactive airways characteristic of cystic fibrosis. Humidification of inspired gases is important for maintaining secretions in a less viscous state. Frequent suctioning of the patient's trachea is often necessary during the operative period.

Primary Ciliary Dyskinesia

Primary ciliary dyskinesia is characterized by congenital impairment of ciliary activity in respiratory tract epithelial cells and sperm tails (spermatozoa are alive but immobile). As a result of impaired ciliary activity in the respiratory tract, chronic sinusitis, secretory otitis media, and productive cough (failure of ciliary activity to transport mucus toward the glottic opening) are present from birth or early childhood. In addition to male infertility, fertility is decreased in females with this syndrome as oviducts have ciliated epithelium. Bronchiectasis develops in most patients. The triad of chronic sinusitis, bronchiectasis, and situs inversus is known as Kartagener syndrome.[25] It is speculated that the normal asymmetrical positioning of body organs is dependent on normal ciliary function of the embryonic epithelium. In the absence of normal ciliary function, placement of organs to the left or the right is random; moreover, as expected, about one-half of patients with congenitally nonfunctioning cilia manifest situs inversus. Isolated dextrocardia is almost always associated with congenital heart disease.

Preoperative preparation is directed at treating active pulmonary infections and determining the presence of any significant organ inversion.[26, 27] Drugs that depress ventilation or ciliary activity may be avoided in the preoperative medication regimen. In the presence of dextrocardia it is necessary to reverse the electrocardiogram leads to permit accurate interpretation. Inversion of the great vessels is a reason to select the left internal jugular vein for cannulation, thereby avoiding the thoracic duct and ensuring more direct access to the right atrium. Uterine displacement in parturients is logically to the right in these patients. Should use of a double-lumen endobronchial tube be considered, as in the presence of bronchiectasis, it is useful to appreciate the altered anatomy introduced by pulmonary inversion. For example, a left-sided tube is inserted, with the bronchial tube on the right. In view of the high incidence of sinusitis, the use of nasopharyngeal airways is a questionable selection.

Bronchiolitis Obliterans

Bronchiolitis is generally considered a disease of childhood and is most often the result of infections with respiratory syncytial virus. Bronchiolitis obliterans is a rare cause of COPD in adults. The process may accompany viral pneumonia, collagen vascular disease (especially rheumatoid arthritis), and inhalation of nitrogen dioxide ("silo filler's disease"), or it may be a sequela of graft-versus-host disease after bone marrow transplantation.[28] Nitrogen dioxide may accumulate above fresh silage and cause dyspnea, a nonproductive cough, and cardiogenic pulmonary edema. Treatment of bronchiolitis obliterans is usually ineffective, although corticosteroids may be administered in attempts to suppress inflammatory reactions involving the bronchioles. Symptomatic improvement may accompany the use of bronchodilators.

Tracheal Stenosis

Tracheal stenosis is an extreme example of COPD that typically develops after mechanical ventilation of the lungs that included prolonged translaryngeal tracheal intubation or tracheostomy. Tracheal mucosal ischemia that may progress to destruction of cartilaginous rings and subsequent circumferential constricting scar formation is minimized by the use of high residual volume cuffs on tracheal tubes in an effort to avoid excessive pressure on the underlying mucosa. Infections and systemic hypotension may contribute to events that culminate in tracheal stenosis.

Diagnosis

Tracheal stenosis becomes symptomatic when the lumen of the adult trachea is decreased to less than 5 mm. Symptoms may not develop until several weeks after tracheal extubation. Dyspnea is prominent even at rest, as these patients must use accessory muscles of breathing during all phases of the breathing cycle. Ineffective cough is present, and stridor may be audible. Patients with tracheal stenoses breathe slowly because of an inability to increase the tidal volume despite additional muscular efforts. Peak flow rates are decreased during exhalation. Flow-volume loops are likely to display flattened exhaled and inhaled portions (see Fig. 14–2). Tomograms of the trachea demonstrate tracheal narrowing in these patients.

Management of Anesthesia

Tracheal dilation is useful in some patients, but surgical resection of the stenotic tracheal segment with primary anastomosis is often required.[29] Anesthesia for tracheal resection may be complicated by total airway obstruction during surgical mobilization of the trachea. Initially, a translaryngeal tube is placed in the trachea. After surgical exposure, the distal normal trachea is opened and a sterile cuffed tube inserted and attached to the anesthetic breathing system. Maintenance of anesthesia with volatile anesthetics is useful for ensuring maximum inspired concentrations of oxygen. High-frequency ventilation is useful in selected patients. The addition of helium (50% to 75%) to the inspired gases decreases the density of these gases and may improve flow through the area of tracheal narrowing.

References

1. Barnes PJ. Chronic obstructive pulmonary disease. N Engl J Med 2000;343:269–80
2. Wulfsberg EA, Hoffmann DE, Cohen MM. Alpha-1 antitrypsin deficiency: impact of genetic discovery on medicine and society. JAMA 1994;271:217–22
3. Tarpy SP, Celli B. Long-term oxygen therapy. N Engl J Med 1995;333:710–4
4. Conacher ID. Anaesthesia for the surgery of emphysema. Br J Anaesth 1997;79:530–8
5. Smetana GW. Preoperative pulmonary evaluation. N Engl J Med 1999;340:937–44
6. Warner DO. Preventing postoperative pulmonary complications: the role of the anesthesiologist. Anesthesiology 2000;92:1467–72
7. Pearce AC, Jones RM. Smoking and anesthesia: preoperative abstinence and perioperative morbidity. Anesthesiology 1984;61:576–84
8. Kambam JR, Chen LH, Hyman SA. Effect of short-term smoking halt on carboxyhemoglobin levels and P_{50} values. Anesth Analg 1986;65:1186–8
9. Warner MA, Divertie MB, Tinker JH. Preoperative cessation of smoking and pulmonary complications in coronary artery bypass patients. Anesthesiology 1984;60:380–3
10. Crapo RO. Pulmonary-function testing. N Engl J Med 1994;331:25–30
11. Kearney DJ, Lee TH, Reilly JJ, et al. Assessment of operative risk in patients undergoing lung resection: importance of predicted pulmonary function. Chest 1994;105:753–9
12. Brooks-Brunn JA. Postoperative atelectasis and pneumonia. Heart Lung 1995;24:94–115
13. Shulman M, Sandler AN, Bradley JW, et al. Postthoracotomy pain and pulmonary function following epidural and systemic morphine. Anesthesiology 1984;61:569–75
14. Craig DB. Postoperative recovery of pulmonary function. Anesth Analg 1981;60:46–52
15. Warner DO, Warner MA, Offord KP, et al. Airway obstruction and perioperative complications in smokers undergoing abdominal surgery. Anesthesiology 1999;90:372–9
16. Kotani N, Hashimoto H, Sessler DI, et al. Smoking decreases alveolar macrophage function during anesthesia and surgery. Anesthesiology 2000;92:1268–77
17. Ravin MB. Comparison of spinal and general anesthesia for lower abdominal surgery in patients with chronic obstructive pulmonary disease. Anesthesiology 1971;35:319–22
18. Gold MI, Joseph SI. Bilateral tension pneumothorax following induction of anesthesia in two patients with chronic obstructive airway disease. Anesthesiology 1973;38:93–6
19. Gross JB, Zebrowski ME, Carel WD, et al. Time course of ventilatory depression after thiopental and midazolam in normal subjects and in patients with chronic obstructive pulmonary disease. Anesthesiology 1983;58:540–4
20. Berg H, Viby-Mogensen J, Roed J, et al. Residual neuromuscular block is a risk factor for postoperative pulmonary complications: a prospective, randomized, and blinded study of postoperative pulmonary complications after atracurium, vecuronium, and pancuronium. Acta Anaesthesiol Scand 1997;41:1095–1103
21. Pietak S, Weenig CS, Hickey RF, et al. Anesthetic effects on ventilation in patients with chronic obstructive pulmonary disease. Anesthesiology 1975;42:160–6
22. Knill RL, Clement JL. Variable effects of anaesthetics on the ventilatory response to hypoxemia in man. Can Anaesth Soc J 1982;29:93–9
23. Ramsey BW. Management of pulmonary disease in patients with cystic fibrosis. N Engl J Med 1996;335:179–88
24. Stern RC. The diagnosis of cystic fibrosis. N Engl J Med 1997;336:487–91
25. Woodring JH, Royer JM, McDonagh D. Kartagener's syndrome. JAMA 1982;247:2814–16
26. Ho AM-H, Friedland MJ. Kartagener's syndrome: anesthetic considerations. Anesthesiology 1992;77:386–8
27. Reidy J, Sischy S, Barrow V. Anaesthesia for Kartagener's syndrome. Br J Anaesth 2000;85:919–21
28. Ralph DD, Springmeyer SC, Sullivan KM, et al. Rapidly progressive airflow obstruction in marrow transplant recipients: possible association between obliterative bronchiolitis and chronic graft-versus-host disease. Am Rev Respir Dis 1984;129:641–6
29. Boyan CP, Privitera PA. Resection of stenotic trachea: a case presentation. Anesth Analg 1976;55:191–4

14

Asthma

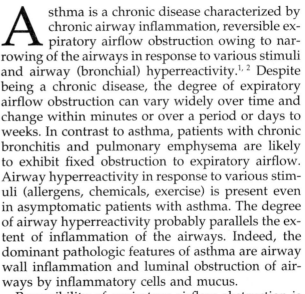

Asthma is a chronic disease characterized by chronic airway inflammation, reversible expiratory airflow obstruction owing to narrowing of the airways in response to various stimuli and airway (bronchial) hyperreactivity.[1, 2] Despite being a chronic disease, the degree of expiratory airflow obstruction can vary widely over time and change within minutes or over a period or days to weeks. In contrast to asthma, patients with chronic bronchitis and pulmonary emphysema are likely to exhibit fixed obstruction to expiratory airflow. Airway hyperreactivity in response to various stimuli (allergens, chemicals, exercise) is present even in asymptomatic patients with asthma. The degree of airway hyperreactivity probably parallels the extent of inflammation of the airways. Indeed, the dominant pathologic features of asthma are airway wall inflammation and luminal obstruction of airways by inflammatory cells and mucus.

Reversibility of expiratory airflow obstruction is characteristic of asthma, although irreversible airflow obstruction develops in some patients with asthma. Airway hyperreactivity is characteristic but not unique as patients with chronic obstructive pulmonary disease (COPD) also demonstrate increased airway responsiveness. Cigarette smokers or former cigarette smokers with chronic bronchitis who demonstrate episodic wheezing and dyspnea mimicking asthma may be diagnosed as having asthmatic bronchitis. These ambiguous situations reflect the deficiencies in the definition of a disease for which there is no pathognomonic feature or definitive diagnostic test. Nevertheless, more than a 15% increase in expiratory airflow in response to bronchodilator therapy is supportive evidence when asthma is suspected on clinical grounds.

The incidence of asthma in persons 5 to 34 years of age is nearly 5% (at least 10 million Americans, making it one of the most common chronic diseases in the United States) with the greatest incidence of new cases of asthma occurring in individuals less than 5 years of age.[3] Approximately 50% of newly diagnosed cases of asthma in persons older than 40 years of age occur in cigarette smokers with a prior diagnosis of chronic bronchitis or emphysema. In these individuals the more correct diagnosis is asthmatic bronchitis. Nevertheless, adult-onset asthma may occur in this age group in the absence of cigarette smoking. Acute exacerbations of asthma can be fatal and in some patients reflect cardiac toxicity of drugs used to treat asthma.[4]

■ PATHOGENESIS

Possible explanations for the features of asthma (airway inflammation, reversible expiratory airflow obstruction, bronchial hyperreactivity) are allergen-induced immunologic responses and abnormal autonomic nervous system regulation of airway function.

Allergen-Induced Immunologic Model

In atopic persons, repeated antigen exposure leads to synthesis and secretion of specific immunoglobulin E (IgE) antibodies. Antigens can cross-link adjacent IgE molecules, leading to the explosive release of vasoactive, bronchoactive, and chemoactive mediators (histamine, interleukins, tumor necrosis factor, leukotrienes, prostaglandins, platelet-activating factor) from mast cell granules. These chemical mediators have potentially important roles in airway inflammation, contraction, and hyperreactivity. Eosinophils infiltrate the airways during the hours following allergen exposure and may contribute to further release of mediators.

Abnormal Autonomic Nervous System Regulation of Airway Function

An alternative explanation for the features characteristic of asthma is abnormal autonomic nervous system regulation of neural function. This hypothesis is supported by increased expiratory airflow obstruction in patients with asthma being treated with a nonselective β-antagonist (propranolol), suggesting the presence of an imbalance between excitatory (bronchoconstrictor) and inhibitory (bronchodilator) neural input. It is likely that chemical mediators released from mast cells interact with the autonomic nervous system. For example, some chemical mediators can stimulate airway irritant receptors to trigger reflex bronchoconstriction, while other mediators sensitize bronchial smooth muscle to the effects of acetylcholine. In addition, stimulation of muscarinic receptors facilitates mediator release from mast cells, providing another positive feedback loop for sustained inflammation and bronchoconstriction.

■ CLINICAL MANIFESTATIONS

During periods of normal to near-normal pulmonary function, patients are likely to have no physical findings referable to their asthma. As expiratory airflow obstruction increases, a number of signs and symptoms may manifest and offer clues to the severity of the asthmatic attack. In this regard, the classic manifestations of asthma are wheezing, cough, and dyspnea.

Wheezing, the most common finding during an acute asthma attack, is the term used to describe the expiratory sound produced by turbulent gas flow through narrowed airways. As obstruction becomes more severe, wheezing becomes more prominent and is audible during earlier phases of exhalation. Forced exhalation may demonstrate wheezing that was not audible during quiet breathing. The degree of airway obstruction may change abruptly; the absence of wheezing in severe cases may reflect a parallel absence of airflow sufficient to create expiratory sounds. In contrast to the random monophasic wheezes of asthma, the presence of single monophasic wheezes that occur repetitively with consistent timing suggests focal airway obstruction, such as a bronchus narrowed by an aspirated foreign body or a neoplasm.

The characteristic cough of asthma ranges from nonproductive to the production of copious amounts of sputum that is typically mucoid and often highly tenacious. Eosinophils and their debris may cause yellow discoloration of sputum, even when infection is absent. Occasionally, cough is the only manifestation of asthma.

Dyspnea tends to vary greatly over time, depending on the severity of the expiratory airflow obstruction. In severe cases of airway obstruction the presence of "air hunger" may be the predominant symptom, and patients often insist on sitting up to ease their breathing. Chest discomfort or tightness (sensation of not being able to inhale fully) is a frequent accompaniment of dyspnea in patients with asthma and may mimic angina pectoris.

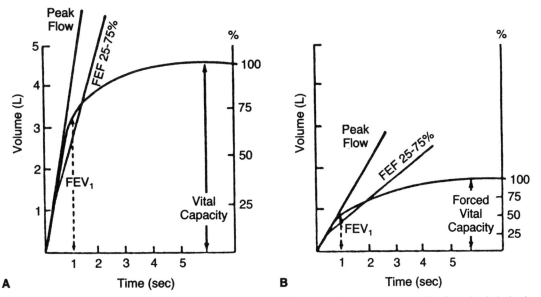

Figure 14–1 • Spirographic changes of (*A*) a normal subject and (*B*) a patient in bronchospasm. The forced exhaled volume in 1 second (FEV$_1$) is typically less than 80% of the vital capacity in the presence of obstructive airway disease. Peak flow and maximum mid-expiratory flow rate (FEF$_{25-75}$) are also decreased in these patients (*B*). (From Kingston HGG, Hirshman CA. Perioperative management of the patient with asthma. Anesth Analg 1984;63:844–55, with permission.)

The forced exhaled volume in 1 second (FEV$_1$) and the maximum mid-expiratory flow rate are direct reflections of the severity of expiratory airflow obstruction (Fig. 14–1, Table 14–1).[5] These measurements provide objective data that can be used to assess the severity and monitor the course of an exacerbation of asthma. The typical patient with asthma who presents at the hospital for treatment of an asthmatic attack has an FEV$_1$ that is less than 35% of normal and a maximum mid-expiratory flow rate that is 20% of normal or lower. Flow-volume loops show characteristic downward scooping of the expiratory limb of the loop (Fig. 14–2).[5] Flow-volume loops in which the inhaled and exhaled portion of the loop are flat helps distinguish wheezing caused by upper airway obstruction (foreign body,

tracheal stenosis, mediastinal tumor) from asthma. During moderate to severe asthma attacks, the functional residual capacity may increase as much as 1 to 2 L, whereas total lung capacity usually remains within the normal range. Diffusing capacity of the lungs for carbon monoxide is not decreased in patients with asthma. Residual abnormalities as detected by pulmonary function tests may persist for several days after an acute asthmatic attack despite the absence of symptoms.

Mild asthma is usually accompanied by normal PaO$_2$ and PaCO$_2$. Tachypnea and hyperventilation observed during an acute asthmatic attack therefore do not reflect arterial hypoxemia but, rather, neural reflexes in the lungs. Indeed, hypocarbia and respiratory alkalosis are the most common arterial blood

Table 14–1 • Severity of Expiratory Airflow Obstruction

Severity	FEV$_1$* (% predicted)	FEF$_{25-75}$* (% predicted)	PaO$_2$† (mmHg)	PaCO$_2$† (mmHg)
Mild (asymptomatic)	65–80	60–75	> 60	< 40
Moderate	50–64	45–59	> 60	< 45
Marked	35–49	30–44	< 60	> 50
Severe (status asthmaticus)	< 35	< 30	< 60	> 50

FEV$_1$ forced exhaled volume in 1 second; FEF$_{25-75}$, forced exhaled flow at 25% to 75% of forced vital capacity.
* See Figure 14–1 for definitions.
† Values are estimates.
Data from Kingston HGG, Hirshman CA. Perioperative management of the patient with asthma. Anesth Analg 1984;63:844–55.

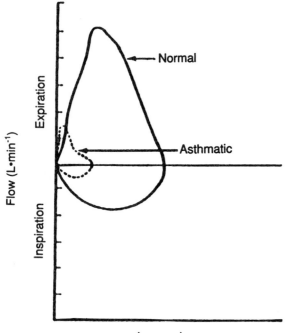

Figure 14-2 • Flow–volume curve of a normal person and an asthmatic individual. (From Kingston HGG, Hirshman CA. Perioperative management of the patient with asthma. Anesth Analg 1984;63:844–55, with permission.)

gas findings in the presence of asthma. As the severity of expiratory airflow obstruction increases, the associated ventilation-to-perfusion mismatching may result in PaO_2 less than 60 mmHg while breathing room air. The $PaCO_2$ is likely to increase when the FEV_1 is less than 25% of the predicted value. Fatigue of the skeletal muscles necessary for breathing may contribute to the development of hypercarbia.

Chest radiographs may demonstrate hyperinflation of the lungs but are more useful for ruling out pneumonia or congestive heart failure, which may be confused with asthma. The electrocardiogram may show evidence of acute right heart failure and ventricular irritability during acute asthmatic attacks.

DIAGNOSIS

No single laboratory test can confirm the diagnosis of asthma. Nevertheless, a test for bronchodilator responsiveness can provide supportive evidence when asthma is suspected on clinical grounds. In patients with baseline expiratory airflow obstruction, increases (more than 15%) in airflow after inhalation of a bronchodilator suggests asthma. Unfortunately, false-positive and false-negative responses to a bronchodilator occur in patients with asthma. Because asthma is episodic, its diagnosis may be suspected, even if pulmonary function is normal.

The differential diagnosis of asthma may include viral tracheobronchitis, restrictive pulmonary diseases (sarcoidosis), rheumatoid arthritis and associated bronchiolitis, and extrinsic compression (thoracic aneurysm, mediastinal neoplasm) or intrinsic compression (epiglottitis, croup) causing upper airway obstruction. Upper airway obstruction produces characteristic flow-volume loops, and tracheal tomograms using computed tomography may be helpful. A history of recent trauma, surgery, or tracheal intubation may be present in patients with upper airway obstruction mimicking asthma. Congestive heart failure and pulmonary embolism may cause dyspnea and wheezing. Wheezing in association with pulmonary edema has been characterized as "cardiac asthma." Improvement after inhaled bronchodilator administration does not exclude cardiac asthma as a cause of wheezing.

ETIOLOGIC FORMS OF ASTHMA

Asthma is not a single disease. Rather, it comprises a group of disorders with various etiologies.

Allergen-Induced-Immunologic Asthma

Allergen-induced (IgE-mediated) asthma is the most common form of reversible expiratory airflow obstruction. Patients with allergen-induced asthma commonly have other atopic manifestations, such as allergic rhinitis and allergic dermatitis. A genetic predisposition is suggested by the common presence of a family history of asthma. Peripheral blood eosinophilia and increased plasma concentrations of IgE support the diagnosis of atopic disease. Presumably, inhalation of antigens evokes the release of chemical mediators from mast cells, leading to bronchoconstriction, edema of the bronchial mucosa, and secretion of viscous mucus.

Exercise-Induced Asthma

Exercise-induced asthma describes patients with increased airway reactivity in whom vigorous physical activity triggers acute airway narrowing and expiratory airflow obstruction.[6] A more accurate description of this response would be exercise-induced bronchospasm. To emphasize the underlying pathogenesis, the term "thermally induced asthma" has been proposed to emphasize the association with fluxes in heat and water that develop in the tracheobronchial tree during warming and humidification of large volumes of air.[6] Exercise-induced asthma is seen most often in children and young adults because of their high levels of physical activity.

Nocturnal Asthma

Nocturnal exacerbations of asthma may reflect sleep-related changes in airway tone, circadian variations in circulating catecholamine concentrations, gastroesophageal reflux related to the supine position, or retained airway secretions resulting from a depressed cough reflex. An increased incidence of asthmatic deaths after midnight and before morning may reflect this phenomenon.

Aspirin-Induced Asthma

Aspirin and most nonsteroidal antiinflammatory drugs (NSAIDs) precipitate acute bronchospasm in an estimated 8% to 20% of adult asthmatics.[7] Within 15 minutes to 4 hours after the ingestion of as little as 10 mg of aspirin, sensitive patients may experience worsening of airflow obstruction, nasal congestion, conjunctival injection, and rhinorrhea. Nasal polyps, although common among aspirin-sensitive asthmatics, are also often present in the absence of aspirin sensitivity. It is likely that aspirin triggers bronchoconstriction in susceptible asthmatic patients by blocking the cyclooxygenase-mediated conversion of arachidonic acid to prostaglandins, thus shunting arachidonic acid toward the formation of bronchoconstrictor leukotrienes. The high incidence of cross-sensitivity with other NSAIDs favors a mechanism that involves drug-induced inhibition of cyclooxygenase.

An estimated 5% of patients with asthma are sensitive to bisulfite and metabisulfite, which are used for preservatives and antioxidants by the food-processing industry. These substances are also present in a large number of medications including some bronchodilator solutions. In view of the sensitivity to derivatives of benzoic acid, there is a theoretical but unsubstantiated concern for the use of ester local anesthetics in these patients.

Occupational Asthma

Occupational asthma is the most prevalent occupational lung disease in the world, affecting 5% to 10% of the world's population.[8] In the United States it is estimated that 15% of newly diagnosed cases of asthma are due to occupational exposures. Because the treatment for occupational asthma is to remove the affected person from exposure to the causative agent, the potential economic implications are substantial. An estimated 250 agents can cause occupational asthma, with isocyanates being responsible for an estimated 10% of cases.[8] Causative agents may be IgE-dependent (longer latency period between exposure and symptoms) and non-IgE-dependent (brief interval between exposure and symptoms). Chlorine and ammonia are the most common causes of occupational asthma without a significant latency period. Latex sensitivity in health care personnel may manifest as increasing expiratory obstruction to airflow during the normal workday in operating rooms (Fig. 14–3).[9]

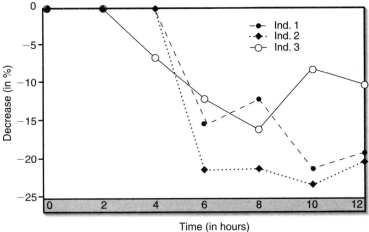

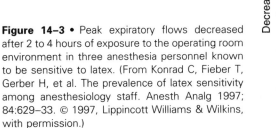

Figure 14–3 • Peak expiratory flows decreased after 2 to 4 hours of exposure to the operating room environment in three anesthesia personnel known to be sensitive to latex. (From Konrad C, Fieber T, Gerber H, et al. The prevalence of latex sensitivity among anesthesiology staff. Anesth Analg 1997; 84:629–33. © 1997, Lippincott Williams & Wilkins, with permission.)

Infectious Asthma

Infectious asthma is increased airway resistance caused by acute inflammatory disease of the bronchi. Causative agents may be viruses, bacteria, or *Mycoplasma* organisms. Eradication of the infectious organisms results in rapid subsidence of bronchoconstriction.

■ PHARMACOLOGIC THERAPY

In the past, treatment of asthma was directed at preventing and controling bronchospasm with bronchodilator drugs. Recognition of the consistent presence of airway inflammation in patients with asthma has resulted in changes in the routine pharmacologic therapy with emphasis on the use of corticosteroids for preventing and controlling bronchial inflammation.[10] In fact, bronchodilator therapy is unlikely to influence inflammatory changes in the airways and could mask underlying inflammation by relieving symptoms and allowing continued exposure to allergens.

Regular administration of antiinflammatory drugs, preferably inhaled corticosteroids, is recommended as the first line of therapy for treatment of clinically significant asthma.[10] Bronchodilator therapy with β_2-agonists is recommended only for pretreatment of exercise-induced asthma and for the symptomatic relief of acute exacerbations of asthma when antiinflammatory therapy is insufficient.

Conceptually, treatment of asthma is with drugs classified as antiinflammatory drugs (corticosteroids, cromolyn) and bronchodilators (β-adrenergic agonists, anticholinergics). Serial determinations of pulmonary function are useful for monitoring the response to treatment. When the FEV_1 returns to about 50% of normal, patients usually have minimal to no symptoms.

Antiinflammatory Drugs

Because chronic inflammation is central to the pathogenesis of asthma, it is logical to administer drugs such as corticosteroids and cromolyn to suppress inflammation.[10] These drugs are regarded as prophylactic therapy because they neither provide rapid bronchodilator effects nor evoke prompt relief of symptoms.

Corticosteroids

Corticosteroids are the most effective pharmacologic therapy for controlling the chronic symptoms of asthma and preventing exacerbations, including those in patients with only mild symptoms.[10] These drugs are preferentially administered by inhalation, as oral administration of corticosteroids is more likely to be associated with systemic side effects. Inhaled corticosteroids have antiinflammatory effects on the bronchial mucosa in patients with asthma. By decreasing airway inflammation, inhaled corticosteroids consistently reduce airway hyperresponsiveness in adults and children with asthma. The decrease in airway hyperresponsiveness may not be maximal until treatment has been given for several months. Corticosteroid preparations available for inhalation include beclomethasone, triamcinolone, flunisolide, fluticasone, and budesonide. Administration twice daily is a common therapeutic time frame. Regular administration of low-dose inhaled corticosteroids is associated with a decreased risk of death from asthma.[10]

Pharmacokinetics

A large proportion of the inhaled corticosteroid dose (80% to 90%) is deposited on the oropharynx and swallowed.[10] The swallowed drug is available for absorption into the systemic circulation followed by passage through the liver. About 10% to 20% of the inhaled drug enters the respiratory tract, where it is deposited in the airways and is available for absorption into the systemic circulation. Inhaled corticosteroids are highly lipophilic and rapidly enter airway cells where the most important effect is inhibition of transcription of the genes for the cytokines implicated in asthmatic inflammation.

Side Effects

Inhaled corticosteroids may produce local and systemic side effects. Local side effects include dysphonia (hoarseness), glossitis, pharyngitis, and oropharyngeal candidiasis especially in elderly patients. Dysphonia may reflect myopathy of the laryngeal muscles and is reversible when treatment is discontinued. The incidence of infections is not increased by inhaled corticosteroids. Systemic side effects of inhaled corticosteroids depend on the amount of the drug absorbed into the systemic circulation. Despite the known ability of corticosteroids to suppress the hypothalamic-pituitary-adrenal axis, there is evidence that inhaled corticosteroids in doses of 1500 μg per day or less in adults and 400 μg per day or less in children, have little if any effect on pituitary-adrenal function. There is no evidence that inhaled corticosteroids have metabolic effects, alter bone metabolism, or impair growth. Inhaled corticosteroids are safe to administer to parturients.

Cromolyn

Cromolyn acts as an inhibitor of inflammation apparently by inhibiting the release of chemical mediators from mast cells perhaps by membrane-stabilizing effects. The drug is administered by inhalation (metered-dose inhaler) and ideally is initiated about 7 days before allergen exposure and 10 to 20 minutes before exercise in patients with exercise-induced asthma. Cromolyn is not effective once bronchospasm is present. Side effects of cromolyn are unlikely. Nedocromil has an efficacy similar to that of cromolyn.

Leukotriene Inhibitors

Leukotriene inhibitor therapy is often effective in patients with mild to moderate asthma and may be added to or substituted for inhalational or oral antiinflammatory therapy. Leukotrienes play significant roles in asthma induced by exercise, allergens, and aspirin.

Bronchodilator Drugs

β-Adrenergic Agonists

β-Adrenergic agonists function as bronchodilators by stimulating β2-receptors on tracheobronchial smooth muscle with consequent activation of adenylate cyclase and increases in intracellular cyclic adenosine monophosphate (cAMP) concentrations. Conventional β2-agonists do not control asthma as effectively as inhaled corticosteroids, but the combination of these two classes of drugs may be efficacious. Among the β2-agonists available, albuterol is most commonly selected for treatment of acute bronchospasm. Using a metered-dose inhaler, the drug is delivered by two to three deep inhalations spaced 1 to 5 minutes apart. This dose may be repeated every 4 to 6 hours. Side effects, although minimal with inhaled delivery, reflect sympathetic nervous system stimulation and include tachycardia, cardiac dysrhythmias, and intracellular shifts of potassium. The use of β2-agonists and an increased risk of death or near-death from asthma has not been conclusively established as a drug-induced effect. A theoretical concern with chronic administration of β-agonists is the development of tolerance as a result of decreased numbers of β-receptors (down-regulation) in the cell membranes. Nevertheless, most evidence suggests that tolerance to the bronchodilator effects of β-agonists does not develop.

Anticholinergic Drugs

Anticholinergic drugs produce bronchodilation by blocking muscarinic receptors in airway smooth muscles, leading to decreases in vagal tone. Ipratropium is a synthetic derivative of atropine administered by metered-dose inhaler. The primary indication for ipratropium is treatment of bronchoconstriction in patients with COPD. In patients with asthma, ipratropium is less effective than β2-agonists. Compared with the prompt bronchodilator effects produced by β2-agonists, the onset of peak bronchodilator effect produced by ipratropium is 15 to 30 minutes, although the effect lasts 4 to 6 hours. The quaternary structure of ipratropium limits its systemic absorption and production of anticholinergic side effects.

▮ TREATMENT OF STATUS ASTHMATICUS

Status asthmaticus is defined as unresolving bronchospasm that, despite initial treatment, is considered life-threatening. The most effective emergency treatment of status asthmaticus is repeated administration of β2-agonists by inhalation using a metered-dose inhaler. There is no advantage of giving β2-agonists systemically. In patients younger than 45 years of age, β2-agonists can be administered every 15 to 20 minutes for up to three or four doses without adverse hemodynamic effects, although unpleasant sensations resulting from adrenergic overstimulation are likely. Intravenous corticosteroids are administered early in the treatment as it takes as long as 12 hours for a drug effect to occur. The two regimens of corticosteroids most commonly selected are (1) cortisol 2 mg/kg IV followed by 0.5 mg/kg/hr, and (2) methylprednisolone 60 to 125 mg IV every 6 hours. Supplemental oxygen is administered in the hope of maintaining arterial oxygen saturations higher than 95%. Empirical broad-spectrum antibiotic therapy is commonly initiated. There is only marginal benefit from vigorous hydration, inhaled saline mists, mucolytic therapy, and chest physiotherapy.

Measurements of lung function may be helpful for assessing the severity of the asthmatic attack and responses to treatment. Patients whose FEV1 or peak expiratory flow rates are decreased to 25% of normal or less are at risk for the development of hypercarbia. The presence of hypercarbia (PaCO2 higher than 50 mmHg) despite aggressive antiinflammatory and bronchodilator therapy may be a sign of impending respiratory fatigue that ultimately requires tracheal intubation and mechanical support of ventilation. Once tracheal intubation is performed, attention must be given to the pattern of ventilation. Because of the bronchoconstriction, high peak airway pressures may be required to deliver acceptable tidal volumes. In the operating room the anesthetic delivery circuit may exhibit too much compressible volume to make adequate ventilation possible in the presence of high resistance to ventilation. In the presence of low compressible volumes, little ventilation is wasted in the ventilator circuit. High gas flows allow shorter inspiratory time with adequate time for greater exhalation and lower positive end-expiratory pressure (auto-PEEP). The expiratory phase may have to be prolonged to allow exhalation and to prevent auto-PEEP. To prevent barotrauma, some recommend allowing hypercarbia to persist. When the FEV_1 or peak expiratory flow rates reach 50% of normal or higher, patients usually have minimal to no symptoms. At this point the frequency and intensity of bronchodilator therapy can be decreased.

When patients are resistant to therapy, it is likely that expiratory airflow obstruction is caused predominantly by edema and inflammation of the airways and by intraluminal secretions. Indeed, patients experiencing near-fatal exacerbations of asthma are at risk of asphyxia owing to the presence of mucus-plugged airways.[11] Under rare circumstances in which life-threatening status asthmaticus persists despite aggressive pharmacologic therapy, it may be acceptable to consider general anesthesia during attempts to produce bronchodilation. In this regard, halothane, enflurane, and isoflurane have been described as effective therapies in selected patients.[12, 13] Clearly, this hazardous approach is reserved for desperately ill patients and can be considered only when the potential benefits are judged to merit the risks.

▌ MANAGEMENT OF ANESTHESIA

Management of anesthesia for patients with asthma requires an understanding of the pathophysiology of the disease and the pharmacology of drugs being used for treatment.[5, 10] There is evidence that the frequency of perioperative bronchospasm and laryngospasm is infrequent in patients with asthma but no symptoms, whereas symptomatic patients are at increased risk for morbidity.[14, 15]

Preoperative Evaluation

Preoperative evaluation of patients with asthma requires an understanding of the severity of the disease and effectiveness of current pharmacologic management as well as the possible need to institute new therapy prior to surgery. The goal of preoperative evaluation is to formulate an anesthesia plan that prevents or blunts obstruction to expiratory airflow. Preoperative evaluation begins with a clinical history to elicit the severity and characteristics of the patient's asthma (Table 14–2).

The preoperative absence of wheezing during auscultation of the chest or complaints of dyspnea suggests that patients are not experiencing acute exacerbations of asthma. The observation that blood eosinophil counts may parallel the degree of airway inflammation and airway hyperreactivity provides an indirect preoperative assessment of the status of the disease. Performance of pulmonary function studies (especially FEV_1) before and after bronchodilator therapy may be indicated in patients with known bronchial asthma who are scheduled for major elective operations. Chest physiotherapy, systemic hydration, appropriate antibiotics, and bronchodilator therapy during the preoperative period often improve reversible components of asthma, as evidenced by pulmonary function tests. Comparison of a chest radiograph with a previous one is helpful for evaluating any change in the disease process. Measurement of arterial blood gases before undertaking elective surgery is indicated if there are any questions about the adequacy of ventilation or arterial oxygenation.

Preoperative Medication

No studies confirm a preferred drug or combination of drugs for use as preoperative medication in patients with asthma. In addition, there is no evidence that opioids, in doses used for preanesthesis medication, produce direct or reflex bronchoconstriction or stimulate release of vasoactive substances from mast cells. A more important consideration is the possible ventilatory depressant effects of opioids. The use of anticholinergic drugs should be individualized, remembering that these drugs can increase the viscosity of secretions, making it difficult to remove

---

Table 14–2 • Characteristics of the Patient's Asthma to be Evaluated Preoperatively

Age of onset
Known triggering events
Hospitalizations for asthma
Known allergies
Cough
Sputum (changes in color and characteristics)
Previous anesthetic history
Current medications

them from the airway. Furthermore, achievement of decreases in airway resistance by inhibition of postganglionic cholinergic receptors is unlikely with intramuscular doses of anticholinergic drugs used for preanesthetic medication. The administration of H_2-receptor antagonists to patients with asthma is questionable. This concern is based on evidence that histamine mediates bronchoconstriction by H_1-receptors, whereas bronchodilation is mediated by H_2-receptors. Conceivably, antagonism of H_2-receptors by antagonist drugs would unmask histamine-mediated H_1-receptor bronchoconstriction, leading to acute increases in airway resistance in patients with asthma.

Bronchodilator drugs used to treat asthma should be continued to the time of anesthesia induction. For example, cromolyn does not interact adversely with drugs used during anesthesia and thus can be safely continued during the immediate preoperative period. Supplementation with exogenous corticosteroids may be indicated before major surgery if hypothalamic-pituitary-adrenal suppression by drugs used to treat asthma is a possibility. Nevertheless, hypothalmic-pituitary-adrenal suppression as a result of inhaled corticosteroids to treat chronic asthma is unlikely.[10] The suggestion that routine preoperative corticosteroid therapy be administered to all patients with asthma to decrease perioperative morbidity is not supported by observations that perioperative complications are low even in untreated patients, especially those with inactive asthma.[14] Conversely, when the preoperative FEV_1 is less than 80%, a preoperative course of oral corticosteroids may be useful.

It should be kept in mind that a large number of adult asthmatic patients react adversely to aspirin or NSAIDs. For this reason, NSAIDs should be used cautiously during the postoperative period for the treatment of operative pain.[7]

Induction and Maintenance of Anesthesia

The goal during induction and maintenance of anesthesia in patients with asthma is to depress airway reflexes with anesthetic drugs to avoid bronchoconstriction of the patient's hyperreactive airways in response to mechanical stimulation. Stimuli that do not evoke airway responses in the absence of asthma can precipitate life-threatening bronchoconstriction in patients with asthma.

Regional Anesthesia

Regional anesthesia, by avoiding instrumentation of the airway and tracheal intubation is an attractive option when the operative site is superficial or on the extremities. Concerns about high sensory levels of anesthesia leading to sympathetic nervous system blockade and consequent bronchospasm seem unfounded. Nevertheless, it must be recognized that failed regional anesthesia and the subsequent need to induce general anesthesia is always a possibility.

General Anesthesia

When general anesthesia is selected, induction of anesthesia is most often accomplished with intravenous injection of short-acting drugs such as propofol, etomidate, or thiopental. The incidence of wheezing is higher in asthmatic patients receiving thiopental for induction of anesthesia than in similar asthmatic patients given propofol.[16] Indeed, respiratory resistance following tracheal intubation in healthy patients is lower after induction of anesthesia with propofol than after induction of anesthesia with thiopental or etomidate (Fig. 14–4).[17] The mechanism of propofol's relative bronchodilating effect is unknown. Based on these observations, propofol seems a logical selection for induction of anesthesia

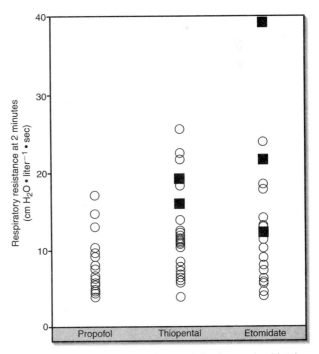

Figure 14–4 • Respiratory resistance following tracheal intubation was lowest in healthy patients receiving propofol. *Solid squares* represent patients in whom audible wheezing was present. (From Eames WO, Rooke GA, Wu RS-C, et al. Comparison of the effects of etomidate, propofol, and thiopental on respiratory resistance after tracheal intubation. Anesthesiology 1996;84:1307–11. © 1996, Lippincott Williams & Wilkins, with permission.)

in patients with asthma who are hemodynamically stable, especially when subsequent tracheal intubation or upper airway stimulation is anticipated. Alternatively, ketamine has sympathomimetic effects that may produce smooth muscle relaxation and contribute to decreased airway resistance especially in patients who are actively wheezing. Thiopental does not cause bronchospasm, but it is unlikely to suppress upper airway reflexes such that airway instrumentation may trigger bronchospasm. The presence of metabisulfites as preservatives in drugs has been alleged to cause bronchospasm in patients with hyperreactive airways. A generic formulation of propofol contains metabisulfites.

After unconsciousness is produced by intravenous induction drugs, the patient's lungs are often ventilated with gas mixtures containing volatile anesthetics. The goal is to establish a depth of anesthesia that depresses hyperreactive airway reflexes sufficiently to permit tracheal intubation without precipitating bronchospasm. Indeed, the one factor shown to precipitate bronchospasm in patients with asthma is introduction of a tracheal tube without previously establishing a sufficient depth of anesthesia to suppress airway reflexes.[18] It is often assumed that volatile anesthetics at comparable doses are equally effective bronchodilators. However, at doses less than 1.7 MAC, halothane has been shown to be a more effective bronchodilator than isoflurane in an animal model of histamine-induced bronchospasm (Fig. 14–5).[19] Additionally, the lesser pungency of halothane and sevoflurane (compared with isoflurane and desflurane) may make coughing less likely. This point is a consideration, as coughing

may trigger bronchospasm. Among the volatile drugs halothane is not ideal, as it sensitizes the myocardium to the cardiac dysrhythmic effects of catecholamines. However, it is not known if the effects of sevoflurane on the airways resemble those of halothane or isoflurane.

An alternative to administering volatile anesthetics to suppress airway reflexes before tracheal intubation may be the intravenous injection of lidocaine.[20] Lidocaine 1.5 mg/kg IV administered 1 to 3 minutes before direct laryngoscopy and tracheal intubation is useful for preventing reflex bronchoconstriction. The decision to administer intratracheal lidocaine just before placing the tube in the trachea must consider both the beneficial effect of topical anesthesia and the possible initiation of bronchospasm by placing of the solution into hyperreactive airways. Although data are not available to support a recommendation for the use of intratracheal lidocaine in patients with asthma, clinical experience suggests that, in the presence of adequate anesthesia, bronchospasm does not follow intratracheal administration of lidocaine. Despite the evidence that intravenous lidocaine causes bronchodilation, inhaled albuterol has been shown to blunt airway responses to tracheal intubation in asthmatic patients, whereas intravenous lidocaine did not.[21]

After tracheal intubation, it may be difficult to differentiate light anesthesia from bronchospasm as the cause of decreased pulmonary compliance. Administration of neuromuscular blocking drugs relieves the difficulty of ventilation due to light anesthesia but has no effect on bronchospasm.

Skeletal muscle relaxation during maintenance of anesthesia is often provided with nondepolarizing muscle relaxants. In this regard, drugs with limited ability to evoke the release of histamine are likely to be selected. For example, severe bronchospasm following administration of atracurium has been reported in patients with asthma.[22] Nevertheless, in large comparative studies, the incidence of bronchospasm following administration of atracurium or other nondepolarizing muscle relaxants is no different.[23] Although histamine release has been attributed to succinylcholine, there is no evidence that this drug is associated with the appearance of increased airway resistance when administered to patients with asthma.

Theoretically, antagonism of nondepolarizing neuromuscular blockade with anticholinesterase drugs could precipitate bronchospasm secondary to stimulation of postganglionic cholinergic receptors in airway smooth muscles. That bronchospasm does not predictably occur after administration of anticholinesterase drugs may reflect the protective ef-

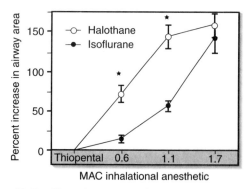

Figure 14–5 • Histamine-preconstricted airways were significantly more dilated ($p < 0.05$) in a dose-dependent manner by halothane than by isoflurane. At 1.7 MAC there was no difference in the amount of dilation in the airways between halothane and isoflurane. (From Brown RH, Zerhouni EA, Hirshman CA. Comparison of low concentrations of halothane and isoflurane as bronchodilators. Anesthesiology 1993;78:1097–1101. © 1993, Lippincott Williams & Wilkins, with permission.)

fects provided by the simultaneous administration of anticholinergic drugs.

Intraoperatively, the desirable level of arterial oxygenation and ventilation are best provided by mechanical ventilation of the patient's lungs. A slow inspiratory flow rate provides optimal distribution of ventilation relative to perfusion. Sufficient time for passive exhalation to occur is necessary to prevent air trapping in the presence of expiratory airflow obstruction characteristic of asthma. In this respect, positive end-expiratory pressure may not be ideal because of the likelihood that it impairs adequate exhalation in the presence of narrowed airways. Humidification and warming inspired gases would seem logical, particularly in patients with histories of exercise-induced asthma, in whom bronchospasm is presumed to be due to transmucosal loss of heat. Nevertheless, it must be appreciated that particulate humidification, as produced by ultrasonic nebulizers and pneumatic aerosols, can produce bronchospasm. Liberal intravenous administration of crystalloid solutions during the perioperative period is important for maintaining adequate hydration and ensuring the presence of less viscous secretions, which can be expelled more easily from the airways.

At the conclusion of anesthesia for elective surgery, it is prudent to remove the tracheal tube while anesthesia is still sufficient to suppress hyperreactive airway reflexes. When it is deemed unwise to extubate the trachea before patients are awake, it seems reasonable to attempt to minimize the likelihood of airway stimulation due to the tracheal tube. Therefore continuous intravenous infusions of lidocaine, 1 to 3 mg/kg/hr, may be useful.

Intraoperative Bronchospasm

Bronchospasm that occurs intraoperatively is usually due to factors other than acute asthmatic attacks (Table 14–3). Indeed, treatment with drugs appropriate for the management of bronchospasm caused by asthma should not be instituted until more likely causes of wheezing, such as mechanical obstruction to the breathing circuit and the patient's airway (including the tracheal tube), are considered. In this regard, fiberoptic bronchoscopy may be useful for ruling out mechanical obstructive causes of bronchospasm. Bronchospasm occurs intraoperatively in the presence of a patent anesthetic delivery system and tracheal tube but the absence of an acute exacerbation of asthma is treated locally by optimizing the depth of anesthesia with volatile anesthetics or instituting skeletal muscle paralysis. Bronchospasm due to asthma may respond to deepening the anesthesia with volatile anesthetics but not to skeletal muscle paralysis produced by administration of muscle relaxants. Should bronchospasm due to asthma persist despite adjusting the depth of anesthesia, the institution of β-agonist therapy should be considered. In this regard, albuterol may be delivered into the patient's airway by attaching the metered-dose inhaler to the anesthesia delivery system by a T-connector. The efficiency of the delivery can be improved by administering the drug through a small-bore catheter placed near the distal end of the tracheal tube.[24] Each actuation of the metered-dose inhaler delivers about 90 μg of albuterol. The effect of albuterol to attenuate bronchospasm is additive to the effects of volatile anesthetics.[25] When bronchospasm persists despite β_2-agonist therapy, the addition of corticosteroids to the treatment regimen may be considered recognizing that a minimum of 3 to 4 hours must pass before a therapeutic effect is apparent.

Emergency Surgery

The combination of emergency surgery and asthma introduces a conflict between protection of the airway in patients at risk for aspiration and the risk of triggering bronchospasm in the presence of light anesthesia. Awake tracheal intubation may stimulate laryngeal and tracheal reflexes that induce bronchospasm. Furthermore, there is often insufficient time to optimize bronchodilator therapy prior to surgery. Regional anesthesia may be preferable if the site of surgery is superficial or the extremities.

Table 14–3 • Differential Diagnosis of Intraoperative Bronchospasm and Wheezing

Mechanical obstruction of tracheal tube
  Kinking
  Secretions
  Overinflation of the tracheal tube cuff
Inadequate depth of anesthesia
  Active expiratory efforts
  Decreased functional residual capacity
Endobronchial intubation
Pulmonary aspiration
Pulmonary edema
Pulmonary embolus
Pneumothorax
Acute asthmatic attack

References

1. Busse WW, Lemanske RF. Asthma. N Engl J Med 2001; 344:350–62
2. Staton GW, Ingram RH. Asthma. Sci Am Med 2000;1–16
3. Asthma—United States, 1982–1992. MMWR Morb Mortal Wkly Rep 1995;43:952–9

4. McFadden ER, Warren EL. Observations on asthma mortality. Ann Intern Med 1997;127:142–9
5. Kingston HGG, Hirshman CA. Perioperative management of the patient with asthma. Anesth Analg 1984;63:844–55
6. McFadden ER, Gilbert IA. Exercise-induced asthma. N Engl J Med 1994;330:1362–7
7. Power I. Aspirin-induced asthma. Br J Anaesth 1993; 71:619–20
8. Chan-Yeung M, Malo J-L. Occupational asthma. N Engl J Med 1995;333:107–12
9. Konrad C, Fieber T, Gerber H, et al. The prevalence of latex sensitivity among anesthesiology staff. Anesth Analg 1997;84:629–33
10. Barnes PJ. Inhaled glucocorticoids for asthma. N Engl J Med 1995;332:868–75
11. Molfino NA, Nannine LJ, Martelli AN, et al. Respiratory arrest in near-fatal asthma. N Engl J Med 1991;324:285–8
12. Parnass SM, Feld JM, Chamberline WH, et al. Status asthmaticus treated with isoflurane and enflurane. Anesth Analg 1987;66:193–5
13. Schwartz SH. Treatment of status asthmaticus with halothane. JAMA 1984;151:2688–9
14. Warner DO, Warner MA, Barnes RD, et al. Perioperative respiratory complications in patients with asthma. Anesthesiology 1996;85:460–7
15. Bishop MJ, Cheney FW. Anesthesia for patients with asthma: low risk but not no risk. Anesthesiology 1996;85:455–6
16. Pizov R, Brown RH, Weiss YS, et al. Wheezing during induction of general anesthesia in patients with and without asthma: a randomized, blinded trial. Anesthesiology 1995; 82:1111–6
17. Eames WO, Rooke GA, Wu RS-C, et al. Comparison of the effects of etomidate, propofol, and thiopental on respiratory resistance after tracheal intubation. Anesthesiology 1996; 84:1307–11
18. Shnider SM, Papper EM. Anesthesia for the asthmatic patient. Anesthesiology 1961;22:886–92
19. Brown RH, Zerhouni EA, Hirshman CA. Comparison of low concentrations of halothane and isoflurane as bronchodilators. Anesthesiology 1993;78:1097–1101
20. Downes H, Berber N, Hirshman CA. I.V. lidocaine in reflex and allergic bronchoconstriction. Br J Anaesth 1980;52:873–8
21. Maslow AD, Regan MM, Israel E, et al. Inhaled albuterol, but not intravenous lidocaine, protects against intubation-induced bronchoconstriction in asthma. Anesthesiology 2000;93:1198–1204
22. Oh TE, Horton JM. Adverse reactions to atracurium. Br J Anaesth 1989;62:467–70
23. Lawson DH, Paice GM, Glavin RJ, et al. Atracurium—a post-marketing surveillance study: UK; study and discussion. Br J Anaesth 1989;62:596–600
24. Taylor RH, Lerman J. High-efficiency delivery of salbutamol with a metered-dose inhaler in narrow tracheal tubes and catheters. Anesthesiology 1991;74:360–3
25. Tobias JD, Hirshman CA. Attenuation of histamine-induced airway constriction by albuterol during halothane anesthesia. Anesthesiology 1990;72:105–10

15

Restrictive Lung Disease

Restrictive lung disease is characterized by decreases in total lung capacity, most often reflecting an intrinsic disease process that alters the elastic properties of the lungs, causing the lungs to stiffen (Table 15–1, Fig. 15–1). Intrinsic restrictive lung disease may be categorized as pulmonary edema and chronic intrinsic restrictive lung disease (Table 15–1). With pulmonary edema, water and solutes accumulate in the interstitial tissues of the lungs, causing these organs to become stiff. With chronic restrictive lung disease, changes in the elastic tissue elements of the lungs cause them to stiffen (Table 15–1). Destruction of the pulmonary vasculature by a disease process may result in pulmonary hypertension, ultimately leading to cor pulmonale (see Chapter 8). Chronic extrinsic restrictive lung disease may reflect disorders of the chest wall (obesity), intra-abdominal changes, and in a small group of patients neuromuscular disorders (Table 15–1). Disorders of the pleura and mediastinum may also contribute to restrictive lung disease (Table 15–1).

▊ PATHOPHYSIOLOGY

The lungs are enveloped by the thoracic cage, which consists of the parietal pleura, skeletal structures, and skeletal muscles.[1] The abdominal contents and abdominal wall function as part of the thoracic cage in that they influence the resting position and movement of the diaphragm. The respiratory pump apparatus consists of the rib cage and pumping musculature, including the intercostal muscles, diaphragm, and accessory muscles of respiration. Optimal pumping action requires structural integrity and the synchronized contraction of intercostal muscles and the diaphragm. Respiratory pump function may be

Table 15–1 • Causes of Restrictive Lung Disease

Acute intrinsic restrictive lung disease (pulmonary edema)
Acute respiratory distress syndrome
Aspiration
Neurogenic problems
Opioid overdose
High altitude
Reexpansion of collapsed lung
Upper airway obstruction (negative pressure)
Congestive heart failure

Chronic intrinsic restrictive lung disease
Sarcoidosis
Hypersensitivity pneumonitis
Eosinophilic granuloma
Alveolar proteinosis
Lymphangiomyomatosis
Drug-induced pulmonary fibrosis

Chronic extrinsic restrictive lung disease
Obesity
Ascites
Pregnancy
Deformities of the costovertebral skeletal structures
   Kyphoscoliosis
   Ankylosing spondylitis
Deformities of the sternum
Flail chest
Neuromuscular disorders
   Spinal cord transection
   Guillain-Barré syndrome
   Myasthenia gravis
   Eaton-Lambert syndrome
   Muscular dystrophies

Disorders of the pleura and mediastinum
Pleural effusion
Pneumothorax
Mediastinal mass
Pneumomediastinum

impaired by skeletal abnormalities, external mass imposed by obesity, neuromuscular disorders, or restriction of lung movement from pleural disease.

■ CLINICAL MANIFESTATIONS

Classic manifestations of restrictive lung disease include decreased vital capacity (normal is more than 70 ml/kg); but in contrast to obstructive airway disease, expiratory flow rates remain normal. Also, in contrast to patients with obstructive lung disease, the ratio of the forced exhaled volume in 1 second to the forced vital capacity (FEV_1/FVC) is preserved in the presence of restrictive lung disease. Patients with restrictive lung disease and respiratory pump dysfunction complain of dyspnea, reflecting the increased work of breathing necessary to expand the poorly compliant lungs. Severe restrictive lung disease causes tidal volumes to decrease and increases the proportion of wasted ventilation per breath. Despite a compensatory increase in the breathing frequency (rapid shallow breathing pattern minimizes the work of breathing), there is a subsequent decrease in alveolar ventilation that produces proportional increases in $PaCO_2$. Hypercarbia is often most severe during sleep because of loss of the conscious contribution to ventilatory drive. Hypercarbia and associated arterial hypoxemia cause vasoconstrictive pulmonary hypertension and cor pulmonale (see Chapter 8). Weakness of expiratory muscles from neuromuscular diseases may produce ineffective cough and result in recurring atelectasis or pneumonia.

Severe restrictive lung disease caused by disorders of the respiratory pump differs from alveolar and interstitial lung disease, in which ventilatory

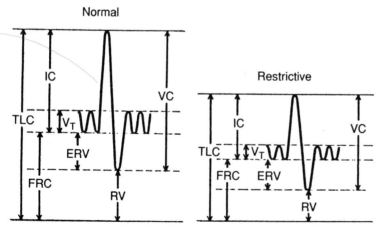

Figure 15–1 • Lung volumes in restrictive lung disease compared with normal values. In the presence of restrictive lung disease, TLC, FRC, RV, and VC are decreased. ERV, expiratory reserve volume; IC, inspiratory capacity; FRC, functional residual capacity; RV, residual volume; TLC, total lung capacity; VC, vital capacity, V_T, tidal volume.

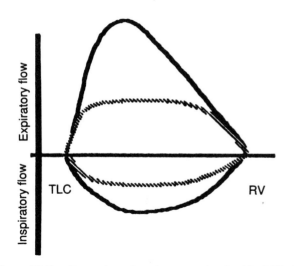

Figure 15–2 • Flow-volume loop in a normal patient (*solid line*) and in the presence of an intrathoracic (mediastinal) mass (*hatched line*). RV, residual volume; TLC, total lung capacity. (From Pullerits J, Holzman R. Anaesthesia for patients with mediastinal masses. Can J Anaesth 1989;36:681–8, with permission.)

abnormalities result from alterations in the lung parenchyma.[1] In this regard, changes in the elastic properties of the lungs can be quantitated by determining lung compliance, defined as the change in lung volume per unit change in pressure. Compliance is 0.1 to 0.2 L/cmH$_2$O in normal individuals, but it may be as low as 0.02 L/cmH$_2$O in patients with restrictive lung disease. Flow-volume curves are shifted downward and to the right in patients with increased lung stiffness (Fig. 15–2).[2] The diffusing capacity of the lungs for carbon monoxide is often decreased, attributable most often to an uneven ventilation-to-perfusion distribution rather than to impaired movement of gases across alveolar capillary membranes.

ACUTE INTRINSIC RESTRICTIVE LUNG DISEASE

Acute intrinsic restrictive lung disease is most often due to leakage of intravascular fluid into the interstitium of the lungs and into the alveoli. Clinically, leakage of fluid is characterized as pulmonary edema.

Clinical Manifestations of Pulmonary Edema

Acute pulmonary edema can be categorized as being caused by increased capillary pressure (hydrostatic

or cardiogenic edema) or by increased capillary permeability.[3] Pulmonary edema due to increased pulmonary capillary pressure or increased capillary permeability typically manifests as bilateral symmetrical opacities on chest radiographs.[3] A perihilar distribution ("butterfly pattern") of the lung opacity is common in the presence of acute pulmonary edema. However, this pattern of lung opacity is more commonly seen with increased capillary pressure (cardiogenic pulmonary edema) than with increased capillary permeability. On chest radiographs the presence of air bronchograms suggests permeability pulmonary edema. Cardiogenic pulmonary edema is characterized by extreme dyspnea, tachypnea and signs of sympathetic nervous system activation (systemic hypertension, tachycardia, diaphoresis) that may be more pronounced than in patients with capillary permeability pulmonary edema. Pulmonary edema caused by increased capillary permeability is characterized by high concentrations of protein in the edema fluid and evidence of secretory products due to an underlying inflammatory process. Diffuse alveolar damage is descriptive of increased permeability pulmonary edema typically associated with acute respiratory distress syndrome (see Chapter 16).

Acute Respiratory Distress Syndrome

Acute respiratory distress syndrome (ARDS) is characterized by diffuse pulmonary endothelial injury leading to pulmonary edema due to marked increases in pulmonary capillary permeability to water, solutes, and macromolecules (see Chapter 16). Most ARDS-related deaths are not caused by gas exchange failure but, rather, sepsis with multiple system organ failure. In addition to leading to multiple system organ failure, sepsis that complicates ARDS may also perpetuate and enhance lung injury.[3]

Posttraumatic Multiple Organ System Failure

The syndrome of multiple organ system failure may affect critically ill or injured patients.[4] It is characterized initially by a hyperdynamic, hypermetabolic state similar to sepsis. In most patients the lungs are the first organs to fail, followed progressively by the liver and then the kidneys. Failure of the gastrointestinal mucosa to act as a barrier to systemic access of luminal bacteria is common. Cardiac dysfunction manifests as ventricular wall motion abnormalities present on transesophageal echocardiography despite paradoxical increases in cardiac output. Central nervous system dysfunction may reflect effects of catabolic byproducts. Mortality approaches 100% if three or more organ systems become involved.

Aspiration Pneumonitis

Inhaled acidic gastric fluid is rapidly distributed throughout the lungs, leading to destruction of surfactant-producing cells and damage to the pulmonary capillary endothelium. As a result, atelectasis occurs and intravascular fluid leaks into the lungs, producing permeability pulmonary edema and a clinical picture similar to that of ARDS. Arterial hypoxemia is the most consistent clinical manifestation of aspiration pneumonitis. In addition, there may be tachypnea, bronchospasm, and pulmonary vascular vasoconstriction, with associated pulmonary hypertension. Chest radiographs may not demonstrate evidence of aspiration pneumonitis for 6 to 12 hours after the event. Evidence of aspiration, when it does appear, is most likely to manifest in the right lower lobe.

Assuming that a tracheal tube is placed promptly after inhalation of gastric fluid, it is reasonable to inject small volumes of saline (5 ml) through the tracheal tube. It must be appreciated, however, that gastric fluid is rapidly distributed to peripheral areas of the lungs and that lavage with large volumes of fluid could exaggerate this spread. Measurement of gastric fluid pH is useful, as it reflects the pH of the aspirated fluid. Measurement of tracheal aspirate pH is of doubtful value, as inhaled gastric fluid is likely to be rapidly diluted by airway secretions. Fiberoptic bronchoscopy may be performed if aspiration of solid materials is a possibility.

The most effective treatment of aspiration pneumonitis is delivery of supplemental inspired oxygen and institution of positive end-expiratory pressure. Inhalation of nebulized mists (metered-dose inhaler) containing β_2-agonists such as albuterol may effectively relieve bronchospasm. Although acid-injured lungs may be susceptible to bacterial infections, there is no evidence that antibiotics administered prophylactically decrease the incidence of infections or alter the outcome after aspiration of gastric fluid. The use of corticosteroids to treat aspiration pneumonitis is controversial. Despite the absence of confirmatory evidence that corticosteroids are beneficial, it is not uncommon for treatment of aspiration pneumonitis to include the empirical use of pharmacologic doses of methylprednisolone (30 mg/kg IV) or dexamethasone (1 mg/kg IV).

Hypoalbuminemia, resulting from extravasation of protein-containing fluids in the lungs, is logically treated with albumin solutions. This approach, however, must be tempered by the possibility that these solutions also leak across damaged pulmonary capillary endothelium and draw additional fluid into the lungs.

Neurogenic Pulmonary Edema

Neurogenic pulmonary edema develops in a small proportion of patients experiencing acute brain injury, especially in the medulla. Typically, this form of pulmonary edema occurs minutes to hours after central nervous system injury and may manifest during the perioperative period.[5] There is a massive outpouring of sympathetic nervous system impulses from the injured central nervous system, resulting in generalized vasoconstriction and a shift of blood volume into the pulmonary circulation. Presumably, increased pulmonary capillary pressures lead to transudation of fluid into the interstitial portions of the lungs and alveoli and a cardiogenic form of pulmonary edema. In addition, pulmonary hypertension and hypervolemia can injure blood vessels in the lungs.

The association of pulmonary edema with a recent central nervous system injury should suggest the diagnosis of neurogenic pulmonary edema. The principal differential diagnosis is aspiration pneumonitis; but unlike neurogenic pulmonary edema, chemical pneumonitis resulting from aspiration injury frequently persists for more than a few days and is often complicated by secondary bacterial infections. If the pulmonary process resolves promptly over a few days, the more likely diagnosis is neurogenic pulmonary edema.

Treatment of neurogenic pulmonary edema is directed at decreasing intracranial pressure and support of oxygenation and ventilation. Digitalis is not indicated, as cardiac function is normal in patients who develop neurogenic pulmonary edema. Diuretics should not be used in the absence of hypervolemia because of the risk of developing of hypovolemic hypotension, which could aggravate the central nervous system injury in the setting of increased intracranial pressure.

Drug-Induced Pulmonary Edema

Acute noncardiogenic pulmonary edema can occur after administration of a number of drugs, especially opioids (heroin) and cocaine. High permeability pulmonary edema is suggested by high protein concentrations in the pulmonary edema fluid. Cocaine may also cause pulmonary vasoconstriction, with acute myocardial ischemia or infarction, which could lead to pulmonary edema. As in patients with neurogenic pulmonary edema, the function of the left ventricle is likely to be normal. There is no evidence that naloxone speeds resolution of opioid-induced pulmonary edema. Treatment of patients who develop drug-induced pulmonary edema is supportive and may include tracheal intubation to protect the lungs against aspiration and to provide mechanical ventilation of the patient's lungs.

High-Altitude Pulmonary Edema

High-altitude pulmonary edema, which may occur at heights ranging from 2500 to 5000 meters, is influenced by the rate of ascent to that altitude. The onset of symptoms is often gradual but typically occurs within 48 to 96 hours at high altitude. Fulminant pulmonary edema may be preceded by the less severe symptoms of acute mountain sickness. The etiology of this high permeability pulmonary edema is presumed to be hypoxic pulmonary vasoconstriction, which increases pulmonary vascular pressures. Treatment is administration of oxygen and prompt descent from the high altitude. Inhalation of nitric oxide may improve arterial oxygenation.

Reexpansion of Collapsed Lung

Rapid expansion of a collapsed lung may lead to ipsilateral or occasionally bilateral pulmonary edema.[3] The risk of reexpansion pulmonary edema after evacuating a pneumothorax or pleural effusion is related to the amount of air or liquid in the plural space (more than 1 L), the duration of collapse (more than 24 hours), and the rapidity of reexpansion. High protein concentrations in edema fluids suggests that enhanced capillary membrane permeability is important in the development of pulmonary edema. Treatment of reexpansion pulmonary edema is supportive. There is no evidence that treatment with diuretics is beneficial.

Negative-Pressure Pulmonary Edema

Negative-pressure pulmonary edema may follow relief of acute upper airway obstruction ("postobstructive pulmonary edema") caused by postextubation laryngospasm, epiglottitis, tumors, obesity, hiccups, or obstructive sleep apnea in spontaneously breathing patients.[6-9] The time of onset of pulmonary edema after relief of airway obstruction ranges from a few minutes to as long as 2 to 3 hours. Subtle episodes of pulmonary edema due to prior upper airway obstruction may manifest as arterial oxygen desaturation detected by pulse oximetry. Tachypnea, cough, and failure to maintain arterial oxygen saturations above 95% are common presenting symptoms and may be confused with pulmonary aspiration or pulmonary embolism. It is possible that many cases of postoperative arterial oxygen desaturation are due to unrecognized negative-pressure pulmonary edema.

The pathogenesis of negative-pressure pulmonary edema is thought to be related to the development of highly negative intrapleural pressures caused by vigorous inspiratory efforts against an obstructed upper airway. Highly negative intrapleural pressures decrease the interstitial hydrostatic pressure, increase venous return, and impose increased afterload on the left ventricle. In addition, such negative pressure may lead to intense sympathetic nervous system activation, systemic hypertension, and central pooling of blood volume. These factors together can lead to acute pulmonary edema by increasing the transcapillary pressure gradients (negative-pressure pulmonary edema). Arterial hypoxemia and the associated sympathetic nervous system stimulation may further promote edema formation.

Maintenance of a patent upper airway and administration of supplemental oxygen are usually sufficient treatment, as this form of pulmonary edema is transient and self-limited. Aggressive interventions are not usually required, although mechanical ventilation of the patient's lungs may be needed for brief periods of time. Hemodynamic monitoring reveals normal left ventricular function as reflected by normal central venous pressures and pulmonary artery occlusion pressure. Radiographic evidence of pulmonary edema usually resolves within 12 to 24 hours.

CHRONIC INTRINSIC RESTRICTIVE LUNG DISEASE

Chronic intrinsic restrictive lung disease is characterized by changes in the intrinsic properties of the lungs, most often due to pulmonary fibrosis. Pulmonary hypertension and cor pulmonale are likely, as progressive pulmonary fibrosis results in the loss of pulmonary vasculature. Pneumothorax is common when pulmonary fibrosis is advanced. Dyspnea is prominent, and breathing is rapid and shallow. Examples of chronic intrinsic pulmonary disease include sarcoidosis, hypersensitivity pneumonitis, eosinophilic granuloma, and alveolar proteinosis.

Sarcoidosis

Sarcoidosis is a systemic granulomatous disorder that involves many tissues but has a marked predilection for the thoracic lymph nodes and lungs. Laryngeal sarcoid occurs in 1% to 5% of patients and may interfere with the passage of adult-size tracheal tubes.[10] Cor pulmonale owing to sarcoidosis may develop. Parotid gland, facial nerve, and optic nerve involvement are possible. Myocardial sarcoidosis, although rare, may manifest as heart block, cardiac dysrhythmias, or restrictive cardiomyopathy. Hepatic granulomas and splenomegaly are likely. Fever of unknown etiology is possible. Hypercalcemia is a rare but classic manifestation of sarcoidosis.

Mediastinoscopy is used to provide thoracic lymph node tissue for the diagnosis of sarcoidosis. The diffusion capacity for carbon monoxide across alveolar capillary membranes may be decreased, despite the presence of normal arterial blood gases. Angiotensin-converting enzyme activity is increased in these patients, but the significance of this change is not known. This enzyme is responsible for inactivating bradykinin and converting angiotensin I to angiotensin II. Corticosteroids are commonly administered as treatment for sarcoidosis associated with restrictive lung disease.

Hypersensitivity Pneumonitis

Hypersensitivity pneumonitis is characterized by diffuse interstitial granulomatous reactions in the lungs after inhalation of dust containing fungi, spores, or animal or vegetable material. Signs and symptoms of hypersensitivity pneumonitis include the onset of dyspnea and cough 4 to 6 hours after inhaling the antigens, followed by leukocytosis and eosinophilia. Arterial hypoxemia can occur despite hyperventilation. Chest radiographs show multiple pulmonary infiltrates. Repeated episodes of hypersensitivity pneumonitis lead to pulmonary fibrosis.

Eosinophilic Granuloma

Pulmonary fibrosis accompanies the disease process known as eosinophilic granuloma (histiocytosis X). Corticosteroids are beneficial if extensive pulmonary fibrotic changes have not already occurred.

Pulmonary Alveolar Proteinosis

Pulmonary alveolar proteinosis is a disease of unknown etiology characterized by the deposition of lipid-rich proteinaceous material in the alveoli. Dyspnea and arterial hypoxemia are typical clinical manifestations. This process may occur independently or in association with chemotherapy, acquired immunodeficiency syndrome (AIDS), or inhalation of mineral dusts. Although spontaneous remission may occur, treatment of severe cases consists of whole-lung lavage intended to remove alveolar material and improve macrophage function. Lung lavage in patients with co-existing arterial hypoxemia may decrease the level of oxygenation even further. Airway management during anesthesia for lung lavage includes placing a double-lumen endobronchial tube to optimize oxygenation during lavage.[11]

Lymphangiomyomatosis

Lymphangiomyomatosis is the proliferation of smooth muscle in abdominal and thoracic lymphatics, veins, and bronchioles that occurs in females of reproductive age.[12] Pulmonary function tests show restrictive and obstructive lung disease with decreases in diffusion capacity. It presents clinically as progressive dyspnea, hemoptysis, recurrent pneumothoraces, and ascites. The exclusive female distribution suggests a role for steroid hormone metabolism in the etiology. There is progressive deterioration in pulmonary function, with death generally occurring within 4 years.

CHRONIC EXTRINSIC RESTRICTIVE LUNG DISEASE

Chronic extrinsic restrictive lung disease is most often due to disorders of the thoracic cage (chest wall) that interfere with expansion of the lungs (Table 15–1). The lungs become compressed, and lung volumes are decreased. The work of breathing is increased owing to abnormal mechanical properties of the chest and increased airway resistance due to decreased lung volumes. Any thoracic deformity compresses the pulmonary vasculature and eventually leads to right ventricular dysfunction. Recurrent pulmonary infections resulting from poor cough dynamics may lead to the development of obstructive components of the lung disease.

Obesity

Obesity imposes a restrictive load on the thoracic cage directly by the weight that has been added to the rib cage and indirectly by the large abdominal panniculus, which impedes movement of the diaphragm when these individuals assume the supine position.[1] Functional residual capacity is decreased, and the likelihood of ventilation-to-perfusion mismatching with associated arterial hypoxemia is increased. Surprisingly, obesity causes little interference with lung function at rest, and the vital capacity and total lung capacity are likely to be normal. Obese patients may experience significant dyspnea during exercise because of the increased work required to move the weight of the chest and abdomen. The rapid shallow breathing pattern during exercise in morbidly obese patients reflects the combined effects of mass loading and diminished compliance of the respiratory system. Daytime hypercapnia may develop in morbidly obese patients, especially in the presence of obstructive sleep apnea.

Deformities of the Costovertebral Skeletal Structures

The two basic types of costovertebral skeletal deformity are scoliosis (lateral curvature with rotation of the vertebral column) and kyphosis (anterior flexion of the vertebral column), which are most commonly present in combination as kyphoscoliosis. Idiopathic kyphoscoliosis (accounts for 80% of cases) commonly begins during late childhood or early adolescence and may progress in severity during the years of rapid skeletal growth.[1] Mild to moderate kyphoscoliosis (scoliotic angle less than 60 degrees) is associated with minimal to mildly restrictive ventilatory defects. Dyspnea may occur during exercise; but as the skeletal deformity worsens, the vital capacity declines and dyspnea becomes a common complaint with even moderate exertion. Severe deformities (scoliotic angle more than 100 degrees) may lead to chronic alveolar hypoventilation, arterial hypoxemia, secondary erythrocytosis, pulmonary hypertension, and cor pulmonale. Respiratory failure is most likely in patients with kyphoscoliosis associated with a vital capacity less than 45% of the predicted value and a scoliotic angle of more than 110 degrees. In these patients compression of underlying lung tissue results in increased alveolar-to-arterial differences for oxygen. Patients with severe kyphoscoliosis are at increased risk for the development of pneumonia and hypoventilation induced by central nervous system depressant drugs. Supplemental oxygen therapy augmented by nocturnal ventilatory support may be useful.

Deformities of the Sternum

Deformities of the sternum and costochondral articulations are characterized by pectus excavatum (inward concavity of the lower sternum) and pectus carinatum (outward protuberance of the upper, middle, or lower sternum). In most patients with pectus excavatum, there are no significant functional limitations, as lung volumes and cardiovascular function are preserved. Surgical correction is indicated when the sternal deformity is accompanied by evidence of pulmonary restriction or cardiovascular dysfunction.

Flail Chest

Multiple rib fractures, especially when they occur in a parallel vertical orientation, can produce a flail chest characterized by paradoxical inward movement of the unstable portion of the thoracic cage as the remainder of the thoracic cage moves outward during inspiration.[1] The same portion of the chest then moves outward with exhalation. The pathophysiologic disturbances of a flail chest may also result from dehiscence of a median sternotomy, such as following cardiac surgery. Tidal volumes are diminished because the region of the lung associated with the chest wall abnormality paradoxically increases its volume during exhalation and deflates during inspiration. The result is progressive arterial hypoxemia and alveolar hypoventilation with associated increases in the $PaCO_2$. Treatment of flail chest is positive-pressure ventilation of the patient's lungs until definitive stabilization procedures can be accomplished or rib fractures stabilize.

Neuromuscular Disorders

Neuromuscular disorders that interfere with transfer of central nervous system output to skeletal muscles necessary for inspiration and exhalation can result in restrictive lung disease. In this regard, abnormalities of the spinal cord, peripheral nerves, neuromuscular junctions, or skeletal muscles may result in restrictive pulmonary defects characterized by an inability to generate normal respiratory pressures. In contrast to the mechanical disorders of the thoracic cage, in which an effective cough is typically preserved, expiratory muscle weakness characteristic of neuromuscular disorders prevents generation of sufficient expiratory velocities in the airways to provide forceful coughs. The extreme example is cervical spinal cord injury in which paralysis of abdominal and intercostal muscles severely decreases the ability to produce spontaneous coughing. Acute respiratory failure is a possibility, especially if atelectasis associated with pneumonia (caused by retained secretions due to an ineffective cough) occurs or depressant drugs are administered. Patients with neuromuscular disorders are somewhat dependent on the state of wakefulness to maintain ventilation. During sleep, arterial hypoxemia and hypercapnia may develop and contribute to the development of cor pulmonale. Vital capacity is an important indicator of the total impact of neuromuscular disorders on ventilation.

Diaphragmatic Paralysis

In the absence of respiratory complications, neuromuscular disorders rarely progress to the point of hypercapnic respiratory failure unless diaphragmatic weakness or paralysis is present. Thus quadriplegic patients who have preserved phrenic nerve and diaphragmatic function are unlikely to develop respiratory failure in the absence of pneumonia or administration of central nervous system depressant drugs. In the supine position, patients with diaphragmatic paralysis may develop a ventilatory pattern similar to that seen with a flail chest (abdominal contents push the diaphragm into the chest). In the upright posture these patients may experience significant increases in vital capacity and improved oxygenation and ventilation. Most cases of unilateral diaphragmatic paralysis are the result of neoplastic invasion of the phrenic nerve. In the absence of associated pleuropulmonary disease, most adult patients with unilateral diaphragmatic paralysis remain asymptomatic, with the defect being detected as an incidental finding on chest radiography. In contrast, infants are more dependent on bilateral diaphragm function for adequate respiratory pump function. In these patients and symptomatic adults, plication of the diaphragm may be necessary to prevent flail motion of the thoracic cage.

A transient form of diaphragmatic dysfunction may occur following abdominal surgery.[1] Lung volumes are decreased, and the alveolar-to-arterial difference for oxygen increases. At the same time, tidal volumes decrease, and breathing frequency increases. These changes may be caused by irritation of the diaphragm, which causes reflex inhibition of phrenic nerve activity. As a result of postoperative diaphragmatic dysfunction, atelectasis and arterial hypoxemia may occur. Incentive spirometry may alleviate these abnormalities.

Spinal Cord Transection

Breathing is maintained solely or predominantly by the diaphragm in quadriplegic patients (transection must be at or below C4 or the diaphragm is paralyzed). Because the diaphragm is active only during inspiration, cough, which requires activity by expiratory muscles, including those of the abdominal wall, is almost totally absent. Intercostal muscles are required to stabilize the upper rib cage against inward collapse when negative intrathoracic pressures are produced by descent of the diaphragm. Thus with diaphragmatic breathing there is a paradoxical inward motion of the upper thorax during inspiration. The result is a diminished tidal volume. When quadriplegic patients are placed in the upright position, the weight of the abdominal contents pulls on the diaphragm and the absence of abdominal tone results in less efficient function of the diaphragm. Abdominal binders serve to replace lost abdominal muscle tone and may be useful whenever tidal volumes decrease in the upright position. Quadriplegic patients have mild degrees of bronchial constriction caused by the parasympathetic tone from the uninjured vagus nerve that is unopposed by sympathetic nervous system activity from the spinal cord. Use of anticholinergic bronchodilating drugs reverse this abnormality. Respiratory failure almost never occurs in quadriplegic patients in the absence of complications such as pneumonia.

Guillain-Barré Syndrome

Respiratory insufficiency that requires mechanical support of ventilation occurs in 20% to 25% of patients with Guillain-Barré syndrome. Ventilatory support is needed, on average, for 2 months. A small number of patients have persistent skeletal muscle weakness and are susceptible to recurring episodes of respiratory failure in association with pulmonary infections.

Disorders of Neuromuscular Transmission

Myasthenia gravis is the most common of the disorders affecting neuromuscular transmission that may result in respiratory failure. The myasthenic (Eaton-Lambert) syndrome may be confused with myasthenia gravis. As with other paraneoplastic syndromes, there may be co-existing cerebral ataxia or carcinomatous neuropathy. Prolonged skeletal muscle paralysis or weakness may occur following prolonged administration of nondepolarizing neuromuscular blocking drugs, as administered to facilitate mechanical ventilation of the lungs.

Muscular Dystrophy

Patients with pseudohypertrophic (Duchenne's) dystrophy, myotonic dystrophy, and other forms of muscular dystrophy are predisposed to pulmonary complications and respiratory failure. Chronic alveolar hypoventilation caused by inspiratory muscle weakness may develop. Expiratory muscle weakness impairs cough, and accompanying weakness of the muscles of deglutition often leads to pulmonary aspiration of gastric contents. As with all neuromuscular syndromes, central nervous system depressant drugs should be avoided or administered in minimal doses when necessary. Nocturnal ventilation with noninvasive techniques such as nasal intermittent positive pressure or external negative-pressure ventilation may be useful.

DISORDERS OF THE PLEURA AND MEDIASTINUM

Disorders of the pleura and mediastinum may contribute to mechanical changes that interfere with optimal expansion of the lungs.

Pleural Fibrosis

Pleural fibrosis may follow hemothorax, empyema, or surgical pleurodesis for the treatment of recurrent pneumothoraces. Despite obliteration of the pleural space, the functional restrictive lung abnormalities are usually minor. Surgical decortication to remove thick fibrous pleura is technically difficult and is considered only if restrictive lung disease is symptomatic.

Pleural Effusion

Pleural effusion is most often confirmed by chest radiography. For example, blunting of the normal sharp costophrenic angle on lateral chest radiographs indicates the presence of at least 25 to 50 ml of pleural fluid. Larger amounts of fluid produce a characteristic homogeneous opacity that forms a concave meniscus with the chest wall. Ultrasonography and computed tomography are also useful for evaluating a pleural effusion. In patients with congestive heart failure, pleural fluid may collect in the interlobular fissures as an interlobular effusion. Various types of fluid may accumulate in the pleural space, including blood (hemothorax), pus (empyema), lipids (chylothorax), and serous liquid (hydrothorax). All these conditions present with identical radiographic appearances.

Treatment for pleural effusion is thoracentesis. Bloody pleural effusions are common in patients with malignant disease or injuries to the chest. The finding that pleural fluid is blood tinged is not diagnostically useful because 1 to 2 μl of blood added to 1000 ml of pleural fluid results in a sersanguineous appearance.

Pneumothorax

Pneumothorax is the presence of gas in the pleural space owing to disruption of the parietal pleura (external penetrating injury) or visceral pleura (tear in the lung parenchyma). Idiopathic spontaneous pneumothorax occurs most often in tall, thin males 10 to 30 years of age and rarely occurs in persons over age 40.[13] Smoking cigarettes increases the risk of primary spontaneous pneumothorax by as much as 20-fold. Most episodes of spontaneous pneumothorax occur while patients are at rest. Exercise or airline travel does not increase the likelihood of spontaneous pneumothorax. Patients with AIDS are at risk for the development of pneumothorax.

Signs and Symptoms

Dyspnea is always present with a pneumothorax and is usually severe, even in patients with a small pneumothorax. Most patients also have ipsilateral chest pain. Arterial hypoxemia and hypotension can be severe. The PaCO$_2$ may exceed 50 mmHg. Physical findings are often subtle, emphasizing the importance of considering this diagnosis whenever dyspnea and chest pain occur acutely. Tachycardia is the most common physical finding. In patients with a large pneumothorax, the findings on physical examination may include decreased movement of the chest wall, a hyperresonant percussion note, and decreased or absent breath sounds on the affected side.

Treatment

Treatment of a symptomatic pneumothorax is evacuation of air from the pleural space by aspiration with a small-bore plastic catheter (catheter over needle) that is removed after the pleural air is evacuated or placement of a chest tube attached to a one-way valve that allows patients to ambulate. Routine application of suction to the chest tube has not been shown to improve outcome.[13] When the pneumothorax is small (less than 15% of the hemithorax) and symptoms are absent, it is acceptable to observe the patient. Supplemental administration of oxygen accelerates by a factor of four the reabsorption of air by the pleura, which occurs at a rate of 2% per day in patients breathing room air.[13] Aspirating the pneumothorax followed by removing the catheter is successful in 70% of patients with a moderate-size primary spontaneous pneumothorax. Continued air leak from the lung requires placing a chest tube to treat the pneumothorax. Most air leaks resolve within 7 days. Complications of chest tube drainage include pain, pleural infection, hemorrhage, and pulmonary edema due to lung reexpansion. Persistent air leaks may require surgical intervention. Chemical pleurodesis with intrapleural instillation of a sclerosing agent has a low rate of success among patients with persistent air leaks. The exceptions are patients with AIDS in whom the installation of sclerosing agents through chest tubes is indicated even in the absence of an air leak, as the risk of recurrent pneumothorax is high. Video-assisted thoracoscopic surgery may offer a useful therapeutic option for patients who experience idiopathic spontaneous pneumothorax.

Tension Pneumothorax

Tension pneumothorax develops when gas enters the pleural space during inspiration and is prevented from escaping during exhalation. The result is a progressive increase in the amount of air trapped under increasing pressure (tension). Tension pneumothorax occurs in fewer than 2% of patients experiencing an idiopathic spontaneous pneumothorax, but it is a common manifestation of rib fractures or barotrauma in patients requiring mechanical ventilation of the lungs. Dyspnea is severe, and arterial hypoxemia and systemic hypotension are likely. Introduction of a small-bore plastic catheter (catheter over needle) into the second anterior intercostal space may be lifesaving.

Mediastinal Tumors

Contrast-enhanced computed tomography can distinguish between vascular structures, soft tissues, and calcifications as the cause of mediastinal widening. Lymphomas, thymomas, teratomas, and retrosternal goiters are common causes of an anterior mediastinal mass. Large mediastinal tumors may be associated with progressive airway obstruction, loss of lung volume, pulmonary artery or cardiac compression, and superior vena caval obstruction.[14]

Superior vena cava syndrome is a constellation of symptoms that develop in patients with mediastinal tumors, leading to obstruction of venous drainage in the upper thorax.[2] Increased venous pressure leads to: (1) dilation of collateral veins in the thorax and neck; (2) edema and cyanosis of the face, neck, and upper chest; (3) edema of the conjunctiva; and (4) evidence of increased intracranial pressure, including headache and altered mental status. Dyspnea is commonly associated with this syndrome.

Cancer accounts for nearly all cases of superior vena cava syndrome.

Acute Mediastinitis

Acute mediastinitis usually results from bacterial contamination after esophageal perforation. Symptoms include chest pain and fever. It is treated with broad-spectrum antibiotics and often surgical drainage.

Pneumomediastinum

Pneumomediastinum may follow tracheostomy and alveolar rupture, although it most often occurs independent of known causes. Spontaneous pneumomediastinum has been observed after recreational use of cocaine. Symptoms of retrosternal chest pain and dyspnea are typically abrupt in onset and usually follow exaggerated breathing efforts (cough, emesis, Valsalva maneuver). Subcutaneous emphysema may be extensive, including the neck, arms, abdomen, and in males the scrotum. Gas in the mediastinum may decompress into the pleural space, leading to pneumothorax, usually on the left. The diagnosis of pneumomediastinum is established with chest radiographs. Spontaneous pneumomediastinum resolves without specific therapy, although breathing supplemental concentrations of oxygen may accelerate the rate of gas resorption. In adults, only rarely does gas in the mediastinum create sufficient pressure to compress vascular structures; surgical decompression is rarely necessary.

Bronchogenic Cysts

Bronchogenic cysts are fluid- or air-filled cysts arising from the primitive foregut, lined with respiratory epithelium, and usually located adjacent to the tracheobronchial tree as mediastinal masses or in the pulmonary parenchyma.[15] These cysts may be asymptomatic, the focus of recurrent pulmonary infections, or a cause of life-threatening airway obstruction. Cysts located in the mediastinum are more likely to be filled with fluid and are usually not in direct communication with the airways. These masses cause symptoms of airway compression as they grow. Surgical excision usually requires an open thoractomy.

Theoretical concerns in patients with bronchogenic cysts include the hazards of nitrous oxide and use of positive-pressure ventilation. Nitrous oxide can diffuse into air-filled bronchogenic cysts and cause their expansion with associated life-threatening respiratory or cardiovascular compromise. Institution of positive pressure ventilation may have a ball-valve effect, particularly in cysts that extrinsically compress the tracheobronchial tree, resulting in air trapping. Despite these concerns, clinical experience confirms that nitrous oxide, muscle relaxant-induced skeletal paralysis, and positive pressure ventilation may be safely utilized in patients with bronchogenic cysts.[15]

▇ PREOPERATIVE PREPARATION

Preoperative preparation of patients with restrictive lung disease includes an assessment of the severity of the lung disease and treatment of the reversible components. A preoperative history of dyspnea that limits activity and that can be attributed to restrictive lung disease may be viewed as an indication for the performance of pulmonary function studies and the measurement of arterial blood gases. The most detailed assessment of flow-restrictive properties of the airways is obtained by analysis of flow-volume loops. For example, patients with restrictive lung disease show decreased peak flows and smaller total lung capacities and residual volumes compared with those in normal individuals (Fig. 15–2).[2] A decrease in the vital capacity to less than 15 ml/kg (normal about 70 mg/kg) or the presence of resting increases in the $PaCO_2$ suggests that these patients are at increased risk of developing exaggerated pulmonary dysfunction during the postoperative period. Interpretation of pulmonary function tests must consider the dependence of many of these tests on patient effort, as well as the role exerted by co-existing pain. Preoperative preparation also includes eradication of acute pulmonary infections, improved sputum clearance, treatment of cardiac dysfunction, exercises to improve the strength of skeletal muscles used for breathing, and training with respiratory therapy techniques that will be used postoperatively.

Preoperative evaluation of patients with mediastinal tumors includes chest radiography, flow-volume loops, computed tomography, and clinical evaluation of evidence of tracheobronchial compression (Fig. 15–2).[2] In general, the size of the mediastinal mass and the degree of tracheal compression can be established by computed tomography. The degree of tracheal compression found on computed tomography is a useful predictor of whether difficulty with the airway during anesthesia may be expected. Flexible fiberoptic bronchoscopy under topical anesthesia is an alternative method for evaluating airway obstruction. Nevertheless, the severity of preoperative pulmonary symptoms may bear no relation to the degree of respiratory compromise encountered during anesthesia. Indeed, a number of asymptomatic patients have developed unexpected airway obstruction during anesthesia.[2, 14, 16] For this reason, preoperative irradiation should be considered for patients whose mediastinal tumors are radiation-sensitive. In symptomatic patients requiring a diagnostic tissue biopsy, a local anesthetic technique should be considered. Patients may be asymptomatic while awake yet develop airway obstruction during anesthesia; this problem may reflect the effects of the supine position, including decreased gas volumes of the thorax owing to cephalad displacement of the diaphragm and increased central blood volume. Patients with mediastinal tumors compressing the pulmonary artery or atria may be relatively asymptomatic while awake; yet life-threatening arterial hypoxemia, hypotension, or cardiac arrest may develop during anesthesia.[17]

▇ MANAGEMENT OF ANESTHESIA

Restrictive lung disease unrelated to the presence of mediastinal tumors does not influence the choice of drugs used for induction or maintenance of anesthesia. The need to minimize ventilation depression, which may persist into the postoperative period, should be considered when selecting these drugs. A high index of suspicion for the presence of a pneumothorax and the need to avoid or discontinue nitrous oxide must be maintained. Regional anesthesia can be considered for peripheral operations, but it must be appreciated that sensory levels above T10 can be associated with impairment of the respiratory muscle activity necessary for patients with restrictive lung disease to maintain acceptable ventilation. Controlled ventilation of the lungs during the intraoperative period seems a prudent approach to facilitate optimal oxygenation and ventilation. Increased inflation pressures delivered from the ventilator may be necessary to inflate poorly compliant lungs. Mechanical ventilation of the lungs during the postoperative period is often required for patients with impaired pulmonary function documented preoperatively. Certainly, tracheal tubes must not be removed until patients have met established criteria for extubation (see Chapter 16). Restrictive lung disease contributes to postoperative pulmonary complications, as co-existing decreased lung volumes make it difficult to generate an effective cough to remove secretions from the airway.

The method selected for induction of anesthesia and tracheal intubation in the presence of mediastinal tumors depends on the preoperative assessment of the airway. External edema associated with superior vena cava syndrome may be accompanied by similar edema in the mouth and hypopharynx. If the edema due to venous obstruction is severe, it may be preferable to establish intravenous access in the legs rather than in the arms. Likewise, a central venous or pulmonary artery catheter can be inserted through the femoral vein, if necessary. Monitoring systemic blood pressure through an intra-arterial catheter is common. If patients must remain in the sitting position to achieve adequate ventilation, the anesthetic induction may proceed from this position using fiberoptic laryngoscopy to secure the airway. Topical airway anesthesia with or without sedation (midazolam, propofol, fentanyl) is useful for fiberoptic laryngoscopy. In very young patients, inhalation induction of anesthesia while maintaining spontaneous ventilation may be necessary. Should airway obstruction occur, placing patients in the lateral or prone positions may be life saving. Spontaneous ventilation and avoiding the use of muscle relaxants is recommended but is not likely to be possible during the maintenance of anesthesia. Acute worsening of superior vena cava syndrome may occur as a result of generous intraoperative fluid replacement. Drug-induced diuresis may decrease the tumor volume, but associated decreases in preload in patients with already compromised venous return may result in unacceptable hypotension. Surgical bleeding is likely to be increased in patients owing to increased central venous pressure. Postoperatively, reintubation of the trachea may be necessary because of increased airway obstruction owing to tumor swelling as a result of partial resection or biopsy after such diagnostic procedures as mediastinoscopy or bronchoscopy.

▌ DIAGNOSTIC TECHNIQUES

Fiberoptic bronchoscopy has replaced rigid scope bronchoscopy for visualizing the airways and for obtaining samples for culture, cytologic study, and histologic examination. Pneumothorax occurs in 5% to 10% of patients after transbronchial lung biopsies, emphasizing the need for chest radiograph after these procedures. Likewise, pneumothorax can be anticipated in 10% to 20% of patients after percutaneous needle biopsy of peripheral lung lesions. The principal contraindication to pleural biopsy is a coagulopathy. Pleuroscopy is direct visualization of the pleural surfaces through a fiberoptic scope introduced through an intercostal space into the pleural space. This procedure provides a means of avoiding an exploratory thoractomy to obtain a biopsy.

Mediastinoscopy is performed through small transverse incisions just above the suprasternal notch during general anesthesia. Blunt dissection along the pretracheal fascia is performed, permitting biopsy of paratracheal lymph nodes to the level of the carina. Complications include pneumothorax, mediastinal hemorrhage, venous air embolism, and injury to the recurrent laryngeal nerve leading to hoarseness and vocal cord paralysis. The mediastinoscope can also exert pressure against the right subclavian artery, causing loss of distal pulses in the right arm (erroneous diagnosis of cardiac arrest) or compression of the right carotid artery (postoperative neurologic deficits). Monitoring systemic blood pressure in the patient's left upper extremity avoids erroneous conclusions should the mediastinoscope compress the right subclavian artery.

References

1. Staton GW, Ingram RH. Disorders of the chest wall. Sci Am Med 1996;1–9
2. Pullerits J, Holzman R. Anaesthesia for patients with mediastinal masses. Can J Anaesth 1989;36:681–8
3. Staton GW, Ingram RH. Pulmonary edema. Sci Am Med 1997;1–10
4. DeCamp MM, Demling RH. Posttraumatic multisystem organ failure. JAMA 1988;260:530–4
5. Braude N, Ludgrove T. Neurogenic pulmonary oedema precipitated by induction of anaesthesia. Br J Anaesth 1989;62:101–3
6. Jacka MJ, Persuad SS. Negative-pressure pulmonary edema associated with saber-sheath trachea. Anesthesiology 1999;90:1209–10
7. Furuhashi-Yonaha A, Dohi S, Oshima T, et al. Acute pulmonary edema caused by impaired switching from nasal to oral breathing on the emergence from anesthesia. Anesthesiology 2000;92:1209–10
8. Lang SA, Duncan PG, Shephard DAE, et al. Pulmonary oedema associated with airway obstruction. Can J Anaesth 1990;37:210–8
9. Stuth EAE, Stucke AG, Berens RJ. Negative-pressure pulmonary edema in a child with hiccups during induction. Anesthesiology 2000;93:282–4
10. Willis MH, Harris MM. An unusual airway complication with sarcoidosis. Anesthesiology 1987;66:554–5
11. Spragg RG, Benumof JL, Alfrey DD. New method for performance of unilateral lung lavage. Anesthesiology 1982;57:535–8
12. Smith MB, Elwood RJ. Anesthetic management for oophorectomy in a patient with lymphangiomyomatosis. Anesthesiology 1989;70:548–50
13. Sahn SA, Heffner JE. Spontaneous pneumothorax. N Engl J Med 2000;342:868–74
14. John RE, Narang VPS. A boy with an anterior mediastinal mass. Anaesthesia 1988;144:1447–54
15. Birmingham PK, Uejima T, Luck SR. Anesthetic management of the patient with a bronchogenic cyst: a review of 24 cases. Anesth Analg 1993;76:879–83
16. Desoto H. Direct laryngoscopy as an aid to relieve airway obstruction in a patient with a mediastinal mass. Anesthesiology 1987;67:116–7
17. Levin H, Rursztein S, Heifetz M. Cardiac arrest in a child with mediastinal mass. Anesth Analg 1985;64:1129–30

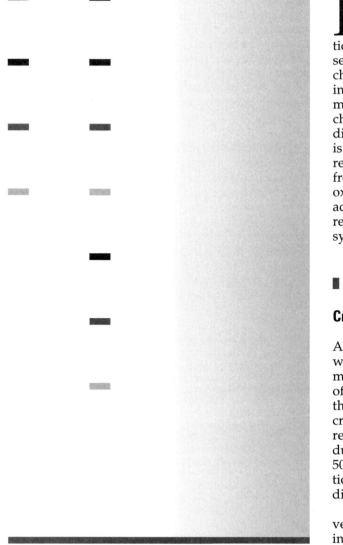

16

Acute Respiratory Failure

Respiratory failure is the inability of the patient's lungs to provide adequate arterial oxygenation with or without acceptable elimination of carbon dioxide. A variety of primary or secondary disorders of the airways, lung parenchyma, chest wall, and neural processes involved in breathing may be responsible for the development of respiratory failure, which may be acute, chronic, or acute and superimposed on a chronic disease process. Fatigue of the muscles of breathing is an important factor in the development of acute respiratory failure. Arterial hypoxemia resulting from right-to-left intracardiac shunts or low ambient oxygen concentrations are not considered causes of acute respiratory failure, as these defects do not represent disorders of the patient's respiratory system.

■ DIAGNOSIS

Criteria

Acute respiratory failure is considered to be present when the PaO_2 is less than 60 mmHg despite supplemental administration of oxygen and in the absence of a right-to-left intracardiac shunt. The $PaCO_2$ in the presence of acute respiratory failure can be increased, unchanged, or decreased depending on the relation of alveolar ventilation to metabolic production of carbon dioxide. A $PaCO_2$ higher than 50 mmHg in the absence of respiratory compensation for metabolic alkalosis is consistent with the diagnosis of acute respiratory failure.

The most likely explanations for a low PaO_2 are ventilation-to-perfusion mismatching, right-to-left intrapulmonary shunting, and alveolar hypoventilation. In the presence of increased $PaCO_2$, calculation of the alveolar-arterial difference for oxygen (A-aDO_2) is helpful for determining whether arterial hypoxemia is due to hypoventilation (respiratory muscle weakness, decreased ventilatory drive) or the combination of hypoventilation and ventilation-to-perfusion mismatching (chronic obstructive pulmonary disease). In the presence of pure alveolar hypoventilation A-aDO_2 is normal (no more than 15 mmHg), whereas A-aDO_2 is increased when arterial hypoxemia is due to ventilation-to-perfusion mismatching and/or right-to-left intrapulmonary shunting. Increasing the inspired concentrations of oxygen improves arterial oxygenation in all conditions except in the presence of significant (more than 30%) right-to-left intrapulmonary shunting.

Acute respiratory failure is distinguished from chronic respiratory failure on the basis of the relation of the $PaCO_2$ to arterial pH (pHa). For example, acute respiratory failure is typically accompanied by abrupt increases in the $PaCO_2$ and by corresponding decreases in pHa. Conversely, in the presence of chronic respiratory failure, pHa is usually between 7.35 and 7.45 despite an increased $PaCO_2$. This normal pHa reflects compensation, by virtue of renal tubular resorption of bicarbonate ions.

In addition to arterial hypoxemia, respiratory failure is usually accompanied by decreases in functional residual capacity (FRC) and lung compliance. There is often bilateral diffuse opacification of the lungs on chest radiographs. Pulmonary artery occlusion pressures are usually less than 15 mmHg despite the frequent presence of pulmonary edema (see Chapter 15). Increased pulmonary vascular resistance and pulmonary hypertension are likely to develop when respiratory failure persists.

Acute Respiratory Distress Syndrome

Arterial hypoxemia associated with acute lung injury characterized by diffuse alveolar damage (influx of protein-rich edema fluid into the alveoli as a consequence of increased permeability of the alveolar capillary membranes) and noncardiogenic pulmonary edema is designated the *acute respiratory distress syndrome* (ARDS).[1] Clinical disorders associated with the development of ARDS include direct lung injury (aspiration of gastric contents, pneumonia, pulmonary contusions) and indirect lung injury (sepsis, severe trauma with shock and multiple blood transfusions, cardiopulmonary bypass).

Arterial hypoxemia resistant to treatment with supplemental oxygen is a feature of ARDS. Radiographically, the findings are indistinguishable from those of cardiogenic pulmonary edema. Although acute lung injury and ARDS resolve completely in some patients after the acute phase, in others it progresses to fibrosing alveolitis with persistent arterial hypoxemia, increased alveolar deadspace, and further decreases in pulmonary compliance. Pulmonary hypertension owing to obliteration of the pulmonary capillary bed may be severe and lead to right ventricular failure. Pneumothorax is a possible complication. Recovery from ARDS is characterized by the gradual resolution of arterial hypoxemia and improved lung compliance. In most patients who survive ARDS, pulmonary function returns nearly to normal in 6 to 12 months.

▌ TREATMENT

Treatment of acute respiratory failure is directed at initiating specific therapies that support the oxygenation and ventilation functions of the lungs until they can recover from the insult responsible for pulmonary dysfunction (Table 16–1). The three principal goals in the management of acute respiratory failure are (1) correction of arterial hypoxemia, (2) removal of excess carbon dioxide, and (3) provision of a patent upper airway.

Supplemental Oxygen

Correction of arterial hypoxemia begins with providing sufficient supplemental inspired concentrations of oxygen to maintain the PaO_2 at 60 mmHg or higher (which results in arterial hemoglobin oxygen saturations of more than 90%) for acute arterial hypoxemia and 50 mmHg or higher for chronic arterial hypoxemia with hypercapnia. In the presence of chronic arterial hypoxemia and hypercapnia, the respiratory drive may be mediated in large part by

---

Table 16–1 • Treatment of Acute Respiratory Failure

Supplemental oxygen
Tracheal intubation
Mechanical support of ventilation (tidal volumes 6–8 ml/kg vs. 10–15 ml/kg)
Positive end-expiratory pressure
Optimize intravascular fluid volume
Drug-induced diuresis
Inotropic support of cardiac function
Glucocorticoids (?)
Removal of secretions
Control of infection
Nutritional support
Inhaled β-adrenergic agonists (?)

arterial hypoxemia; rapid normalization of the PaO_2 by overzealous administration of oxygen can result in depressed ventilation, further hypercapnia, and coma. It is also important to recognize that high inspired concentrations of oxygen may be toxic to the lungs.

Supplemental oxygen can be provided to spontaneously breathing patients using a nasal cannula, Venturi mask, nonrebreathing mask, or a T-piece attached to the free end of a tracheal tube. These devices seldom provide inspired oxygen concentrations higher than 50%, emphasizing the value of these methods for correcting the arterial hypoxemia that results from mild to moderate ventilation-to-perfusion mismatching. When these methods of supplemental oxygen delivery fail to maintain the PaO_2 above 60 mmHg, continuous positive airway pressure (CPAP) by face mask can be tried. CPAP serves to increase lung volumes by opening previously closed alveoli and thus decrease right-to-left intrapulmonary shunting. A disadvantage of this approach is that the tight mask fit required may increase the risk of aspiration should the patient vomit. Maintenance of the PaO_2 above about 80 mmHg is of little benefit, as hemoglobin saturation with oxygen is nearly 100% at this level. In some patients it is necessary to perform tracheal intubation and institute mechanical ventilation of the patient's lungs in an attempt to maintain acceptable arterial oxygenation and ventilation.

Mechanical Support of Ventilation

If adequate arterial oxygenation (PaO_2 at least 60 mmHg breathing 50% oxygen) cannot be provided by noninvasive means or if there is progressive hypoventilation and hypercarbia with associated respiratory acidosis, it is necessary to provide mechanical support of ventilation with devices that provide intermittent positive airway pressure.[2] All methods of delivering positive airway pressure in association with mechanical ventilation of the lungs require tracheal intubation. There are two types of positive-pressure ventilation: volume-cycled and pressure-cycled.

Volume-Cycled Ventilation

The more commonly used volume-cycled ventilation provides a fixed tidal volume, making inflation pressures the dependent variable. A pressure limit is set; and when inflation pressures exceed this value a pressure relief valve prevents further gas flow into the patient's lungs. This valve prevents the development of dangerously high peak airway and alveolar pressures and warns that a change in pulmonary compliance has occurred. Large increases in peak airway pressures may reflect worsening of pulmonary edema, development of a pneumothorax, kinking of the tracheal tube, or the presence of mucus plugs in the tracheal tube or large airways. In this regard, tidal volumes tend to be maintained despite these changes, which contrasts with pressure-cycled ventilators. The disadvantage of volume-cycled ventilators is the inability of these devices to compensate for the development of leaks in the delivery system. For example, a gas leak around the tracheal tube cuff could result in hypoventilation despite continued delivery of unchanged ventilatory volumes. The primary modalities of ventilation using volume-cycled ventilation are assist-control ventilation and synchronized intermittent mandatory ventilation (SIMV) (Fig. 16–1).[2]

Assist-Control Ventilation

In the assist-control mode, a breath is delivered at the preset tidal volume each time the patient creates a small negative airway pressure using inspiratory muscles. The preset respiratory rate ensures that patients receive a predetermined number of mechanically delivered breaths even if inspiratory efforts cease.

Synchronized Intermittent Mandatory Ventilation

The SIMV technique allows patients to breathe at spontaneous rates and tidal volumes while a certain minute ventilation is delivered from the ventilator. The gas delivery circuit is modified to provide sufficient gas flow for spontaneous breathing and to permit periodic mandatory breaths that are synchronous with the patient's inspiratory efforts. Theoretical advantages of SIMV compared with assist-control ventilation include continued use of muscles of respiration, lowering of the mean intrathoracic pressure, prevention of respiratory alkalosis, and improved patient–ventilator coordination.

Auto-Positive End-Expiratory Pressure

Airway obstruction can interfere with passive exhalation to the extent that exhalation of the preceding tidal volume is incomplete when the next mechanically delivered breath is delivered. As a result, positive airway pressure is maintained throughout the respiratory cycle. The positive end-expiratory pressure (PEEP) that results has been termed auto-PEEP or intrinsic PEEP.[2]

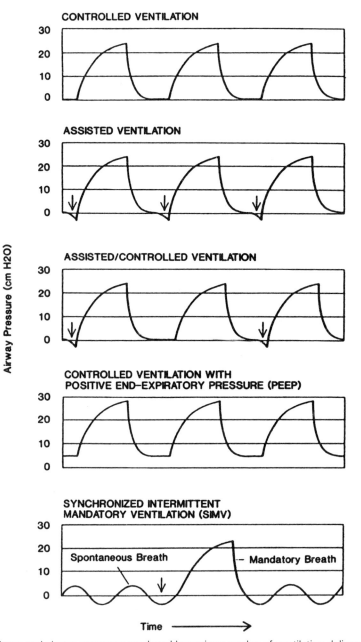

Figure 16–1 • Tidal volume and airway pressures produced by various modes of ventilation delivered through a tracheal tube. *Arrows* indicate initiation of a spontaneous breath by the patient, who triggers the ventilator to deliver a mechanically assisted breath.

Pressure-Cycled Ventilation

Pressure-cycled ventilation provides gas flow into the patient's airways until preset airway pressures are reached. With this airway pressure preset mode of ventilation, tidal volumes are the dependent variable and vary inversely with changes in airway resistance. Pressure-cycled ventilation is characterized by the continued delivery of constant delivered gas volumes until a preset time elapses or specific airway pressures are achieved.

MANAGEMENT OF PATIENTS RECEIVING MECHANICAL SUPPORT OF VENTILATION

Critically ill patients who require mechanical ventilation are often given continuous intravenous infusions of sedative drugs to treat anxiety and agitation and to facilitate coordination with ventilator-delivered breaths.[3] Inadequate sedation can lead to life-threatening problems such as self-extubation, acute deterioration in gas exchange, and barotrauma.[2] The need for skeletal muscle paralysis is decreased by the optimum use of sedation in mechanically ventilated patients. Nevertheless, when acceptable sedation without hemodynamic compromise cannot be achieved, it may be necessary to produce skeletal muscle paralysis to ensure acceptable ventilation and arterial oxygenation.

Sedation

Benzodiazepines (diazepam, lorazepam, midazolam) are the drugs most commonly selected to decrease anxiety and produce anterograde amnesia during mechanical ventilation of patients for the management of acute respiratory failure. New approaches to mechanical ventilation, often involving the use of permissive hypercapnia ($PaCO_2$ may reach 50 mmHg), can cause substantial discomfort, necessitating high levels of sedation. Analgesia, if needed, is provided by intravenous administration of opioids (morphine, fentanyl). The quality of sedation and depression of the patient's intrinsic respiratory drive and thus acceptance of mechanical ventilation, is enhanced by opioids administered in combination with benzodiazepines. Continuous intravenous infusion of drugs rather than intermittent injection provides a more constant and desirable level of drug effect. In this regard, daily interruption of intravenous sedative infusions and allowing patients to "awaken" may facilitate evaluation of the patient's mental status and ultimately shorten the period of mechanical ventilation.[3] For this reason, continuous intravenous infusions of propofol are uniquely attractive, as the brief context-sensitive half-time of this drug is not influenced by the duration of the infusion; and rapid awakening is predictable.[4] Likewise, prompt recovery from the opioid effects of remifentanil is not influenced by the duration of the intravenous drug infusion.

Paralysis

When sedation is inadequate or hypotension accompanies the administration of drugs utilized for sedation, the administration of nondepolarizing neuromuscular blocking drugs (pancuronium, vecuronium, rocuronium, atracurium, cisatracurium) to produce skeletal muscle paralysis may be necessary to permit optimal mechanical ventilation. The dependence of certain of these drugs on renal clearance (pancuronium, vecuronium, rocuronium) should be considered. Neuromuscular blocking drugs lack sedative and analgesic effects, emphasizing the need to administer appropriate drugs to provide these needed elements of patient comfort.[2] It is commonly recommended to use intermittent rather than continuous skeletal muscle paralysis so as periodically to be able to assess the adequacy of sedation and the need for ongoing paralysis. Monitoring of neuromuscular blockade with a peripheral nerve stimulator and titration of muscle relaxant doses such that a twitch response remains present is recommended. A risk of prolonged drug-induced skeletal muscle paralysis is accentuation of the diffuse polyneuropathy that may accompany critical illnesses (see "Critical Illness Myopathy").

COMPLICATIONS OF TRACHEAL INTUBATION AND MECHANICAL VENTILATION

Serious complications may accompany tracheal intubation and mechanical ventilation of the patient's lungs in an effort to prevent the morbidity and mortality associated with acute respiratory failure.[5–8]

Infection

In mechanically ventilated patients with acute respiratory failure, tracheal intubation is the single most important predisposing factor for developing nosocomial bacterial pneumonia ("ventilator-associated pneumonia").[5] The major pathogenic mechanism is microaspiration of contaminated secretions around the tracheal tube cuff. Diagnosis of pneumonia in the presence of acute respiratory failure may be difficult, as fever and pulmonary infiltrates may accompany acute respiratory failure.

Nosocomial sinusitis is strongly related to the presence of a nasotracheal tube. Treatment of nosocomial sinusitis includes antibiotics, replacement of nasal tubes with oral tubes, and use of decongestants and head elevation to facilitate drainage.

Alveolar Overdistension

Alveolar overdistension ("stretch") owing to delivery of large tidal volumes (10 to 12 ml/kg) and the associated high airway pressures (more than 50 cmH$_2$O) may result in alveolar rupture and alveolar hemorrhage.[1, 6-8] In the presence of acute respiratory failure and ARDS, a ventilator-delivered breath follows the path of least resistance and travels to normally aerated regions of the lungs, placing these alveoli at risk for overdistension. Subsequently, when end-expiratory pressure falls, these alveoli collapse and then reopen repeatedly, which could be responsible for ventilator-induced lung injury. In this regard, the traditional goal of mechanical ventilation designed to maintain the PaO$_2$ at 60 mmHg or higher utilizing increasing concentrations of oxygen and ventilator pressures may have to be reevaluated.[8] A more gentle form of mechanical ventilation creating tidal volumes of 5 to 8 ml/kg and airway pressures not exceeding 30 cmH$_2$O may be indicated for treating acute respiratory failure and ARDS.[7, 8] Use of this more gentle form of ventilation requires acceptance of some degree of hypercarbia and respiratory acidosis and often a PaO$_2$ of less than 60 mmHg.

Permissive hypercapnia (PaCO$_2$ as high as 80 mmHg) or controlled hypoventilation may accompany decreased tidal volumes and airway pressures designed to minimize or prevent alveolar overdistension. Increased respiratory drive associated with permissive hypercapnia causes discomfort, making sedation, skeletal muscle paralysis, or both necessary. Permissive hypercapnia is not recommended in patients with increased intracranial pressure, cardiac dysrhythmias, or pulmonary hypertension.

Barotrauma

Barotrauma may present as subcutaneous emphysema, pneumomediastinum, pulmonary interstitial emphysema, pneumoperitoneum, pneumopericardium, arterial gas embolism, or tension pneumothorax.[2] These examples of extra-alveolar air almost always reflect dissection or passage of air from overdistended and ruptured alveoli. Infections also increase the risk of barotrauma presumably by weakening pulmonary tissue. Tension pneumothorax is the most common life-threatening manifestation of ventilator-induced barotrauma. Hypotension, worsening arterial hypoxemia, and increased airway pressures suggest the presence of a tension pneumothorax.

Atelectasis

Atelectasis is a common cause of severe arterial hypoxemia that develops during mechanical ventila-

tion. Migration of the tracheal tube into the left or right mainstem bronchus or development of mucoid plugs should be considered when abrupt worsening of arterial oxygenation occurs in the absence of hypotension. Arterial hypoxemia due to atelectasis is not responsive to increased concentrations of delivered oxygen. Other causes of sudden increases in arterial hypoxemia in mechanically ventilated patients include tension pneumothorax and pulmonary embolism, but in contrast to atelectasis, these causes of decreased arterial oxygenation are also commonly accompanied by hypotension. Bronchoscopy is necessary to remove mucoid plugs, which are responsible for persistent atelectasis.

Critical Illness Myopathy

Patients who undergo mechanical ventilation for treatment of acute respiratory failure may be at risk for neuromuscular weakness that persists long after the cause of the respiratory failure has resolved. A common cause of diffuse skeletal muscle weakness is polyneuropathy of critical illness, an axonal disorder that occurs in the presence of sepsis and multiple system organ failure.[9] Phrenic nerve involvement may be associated with weakness that persists after the neuromuscular blocking drugs have been discontinued. Prolonged administration of nondepolarizing neuromuscular blocking drugs may contribute to the development of an acute myopathy, particularly in patients who undergo concomitant therapy with corticosteroids. The duration of drug-induced paralysis rather than the specific drug selected seems to be the most important determinant of persistent weakness. Decreased clearance of active metabolites of nondepolarizing neuromuscular blocking drugs owing to renal and/or hepatic dysfunction is also a consideration when persistent weakness follows prolonged intravenous infusion of these drugs.

▌CESSATION OF MECHANICAL SUPPORT ▌OF VENTILATION

Mechanical ventilatory support should be withdrawn once patients can maintain arterial oxygenation and carbon dioxide elimination without external assistance. When considering whether patients can be safely weaned from mechanical ventilation and tolerate tracheal extubation, it is important that patients be alert and cooperative and able to tolerate a trial of spontaneous ventilation without excessive tachypnea, tachycardia, or obvious respiratory distress. Arbitrary guidelines have been proposed for indicating the feasibility of discontinuing mechanical support of ventilation: (1) vital capacity more than 15 ml/kg; (2) A-aDO$_2$ less than 350 mmHg while breathing 100% oxygen; (3) PaO$_2$ more than 60 mmHg while breathing less than 50% oxygen; (4) maximal inspiratory pressures more than −20 cmH$_2$O with airway occlusion; (5) maintenance of normal pHa; (6) spontaneous breathing rates less than 20 breaths/min; and (7) deadspace ventilation/tidal volume (V$_D$/V$_T$) ratio less than 0.6. Breathing at rapid rates and low tidal volumes usually signify an inability to tolerate tracheal extubation. Ultimately, the decision to attempt withdrawal of mechanical ventilation is individualized, considering not only the status of pulmonary function but also co-existing abnormalities (anemia, hypokalemia, hypovolemia).

Removal of Ventilator Support

When a patient is considered ready for a trial of withdrawal from mechanical support of ventilation, three options may be considered: (1) SIMV, which allows spontaneous breathing and diminishing numbers of mandatory breaths per minute until patients are breathing unassisted; (2) intermittent trials with total removal of mechanical support while breathing through a T-piece; and (3) use of decreasing levels of pressure-support ventilation.[2] There does not seem to be any clear advantage to use of a T-piece or gradual reduction in the level of pressure support as methods for weaning. Gradual reductions in the number of machine-supported breaths in the SIMV mode appears to be the least effective method of weaning. Overall, correcting the underlying conditions responsible for needing mechanical support of ventilation seem to be more important for successful tracheal extubation than is the method of weaning.[10] Deterioration of arterial oxygenation after withdrawal of mechanical ventilation may reflect progressive alveolar collapse, which is responsive to treatment with CPAP (2.5 to 5.0 cmH$_2$O) rather than reinstitution of mechanical ventilation. Presumably, CPAP minimizes the decreases in FRC associated with cessation of positive airway pressure.

Several events may interfere with successful cessation of mechanical support of ventilation and tracheal extubation. Depressed ventilatory drive owing to respiratory alkalosis or persistent sedation may prevent successful tracheal extubation. Often failure to wean the patient from mechanical ventilation reflects an inability of the patient's muscles of respiration to perform the necessary level of ventilatory work. Excessive workload on the respiratory muscles imposed by excessive hyperinflation, voluminous airway secretions, bronchospasm, increased lung water, or increased carbon dioxide production from fever or parenteral nutrition greatly decreases the likelihood of successful tracheal extubation.[2] The use of sedatives may delay attempts to withdraw mechanical ventilatory support.

Tracheal Extubation

Tracheal extubation should be considered if patients tolerate 2 hours of spontaneous breathing during T-tube weaning or when an SIMV rate of 1 to 2 breaths/min is tolerated without deterioration of arterial blood gases, mental status, or cardiac function. For example, the PaO$_2$ should remain above 60 mmHg while breathing less than 50% oxygen. Likewise, the PaCO$_2$ should remain at less than 50 mmHg, and the pHa should remain above 7.30. Additional important criteria that may be considered before tracheal extubation include the need for less than 5 cmH$_2$O PEEP, spontaneous breathing rates of less than 30 breaths/min, and vital capacity of more than 15 ml/kg. These patients should also be alert with active laryngeal reflexes and the ability to generate an effective cough to clear secretions from the airways. Protective glottic closure function may be impaired following tracheal extubation, resulting in an increased risk of aspirating secretions and gastric contents.

Supplemental Oxygen

Supplemental oxygen is often needed after tracheal extubation. This need reflects the persistence of ventilation-to-perfusion mismatch. Weaning from supplemental oxygen is accomplished by gradual decreases in the inspired concentrations of oxygen, as guided by measurements of PaO$_2$ and monitoring the SpO$_2$ by pulse oximetry.

ACUTE RESPIRATORY FAILURE AND CHRONIC OBSTRUCTIVE PULMONARY DISEASE

Natural History

Patients with severe chronic obstructive pulmonary disease (COPD) often adapt to some degree of arterial hypoxemia and hypercarbia.[2] Acute deterioration in patients with COPD is most often triggered by events such as pneumonia, congestive heart failure, or increased metabolic production of carbon dioxide as produced by febrile states. The increasing arterial hypoxemia and hypercarbia that accompany these exacerbations of COPD lead to increasing dyspnea and alterations in consciousness that may be associated with retention of secretions and a further deterioration in gas exchange. The vicious cycle can be interrupted by treating the event that initiated the acute deterioration and providing support to improve gas exchange while the underlying precipitating event is resolved.

Treatment

Analysis of arterial blood gases is crucial for proper treatment of acute exacerbations of COPD.[2] Supplemental oxygen is administered to maintain the PaO_2 between 50 and 60 mmHg. A 10- to 15-mmHg increase in $PaCO_2$ above the normal value is common when oxygen is administered to patients with COPD, and it is considered acceptable assuming the pHa does not decrease below 7.2. Bronchopulmonary drainage is stimulated by encouragement to cough, administration of inhaled bronchodilators using metered-dose inhalers and systemic corticosteroids, and treatment of underlying infections with antibiotics. Acute exacerbations of COPD are often accompanied by persistent respiratory acidosis and excessive work of breathing.

Mechanical support of ventilation is considered when hypercarbia is sufficient to decrease the pHa below 7.2 or patients show signs of mental status deterioration or respiratory muscle fatigue. Tracheal intubation is performed when the patients demonstrate hemodynamic instability, somnolence occurs, or secretions cannot be cleared. When patients remain alert despite hypercarbia, delivery of positive-pressure ventilation via a tight-fitting face mask ("noninvasive ventilation") is an alternative to tracheal intubation. The most common method of noninvasive ventilation is to deliver a specified amount of inspiratory pressure (15 to 20 cmH_2O) combined with a low level of expiratory pressure (3 to 5 cmH_2O) to decrease the effort required to trigger the ventilator. Advantages of noninvasive ventilation are a lower risk of nosocomial infections, less antibiotic use, shorter length of stay in critical care units, decreased need for sedation, and decreased mortality.[11] A complication of noninvasive ventilation with a face mask is skin necrosis over the bridge of the patient's nose.

When tracheal intubation is required to treat acute exacerbations of COPD, the initial settings of the ventilator are likely to include tidal volumes of 10 ml/kg at breathing rates of 10 breaths/min. Patients with chronic hypercarbia should not have their $PaCO_2$ decreased abruptly to a normal range, as it can result in respiratory alkalosis and cardiac dysrhythmias. The goal is to adjust the ventilator to return the patient's $PaCO_2$ to prior baseline levels. Pulmonary hyperinflation with auto-PEEP occurs often in patients with COPD receiving mechanical ventilation especially if minute ventilation delivered by the ventilator is excessive for that patient. Excessive auto-PEEP increases the risk of barotrauma and may lead to erroneous interpretation of measurements from central venous pressure and pulmonary artery catheters. In addition, excessive auto-PEEP can increase the work of breathing and interfere with venous return, thereby decreasing cardiac output. Application of external PEEP equivalent to the level of auto-PEEP is indicated to allow the patient's inspiratory muscles of respiration to trigger mechanically delivered breaths more easily. In patients with COPD, external PEEP does not increase lung volumes or airway pressures so long as the level of applied external PEEP does not exceed the level of auto-PEEP.

ACUTE RESPIRATORY FAILURE IN PATIENTS WITH ACUTE LUNG INJURY AND ARDS

Acute respiratory failure characterized by profound arterial hypoxemia in the setting of diffuse alveolar damage with noncardiogenic pulmonary edema due to increased alveolar-capillary membrane permeability (ARDS) is associated with a high mortality rate.[1, 2] Death is most often attributed to sepsis or multiple organ system failure rather than primary respiratory causes, although improved survival using low tidal volumes indicates that some deaths can be directly related to lung injury.[1]

Epidemiology and Pathogenesis

Clinical disorders and risk factors associated with the development of ARDS include events associated with direct injury to the lungs and those that cause indirect injury to the lungs in the setting of a systemic process (Table 16–2).[1] Overall, sepsis is associated with the highest risk of progression of acute lung injury to ARDS. The acute or exudative phases of ARDS manifest as a rapid onset of respiratory failure accompanied by arterial hypoxemia refractory to treatment and radiographic findings indistinguishable from those of cardiogenic pulmonary edema. There is an influx of protein-rich edema fluid into the alveoli as a result of increased alveolar capillary membrane permeability. There is evidence of

Table 16–2 • Clinical Disorders Associated with Acute Lung Injury and Acute Respiratory Distress Syndrome

Direct lung injury
Pneumonia
Aspiration of gastric contents
Pulmonary contusion
Fat emboli
Near-drowning
Inhalational injury
Indirect lung injury
Sepsis
Trauma associated with shock
Multiple blood transfusions
Cardiopulmonary bypass
Drug overdose
Acute pancreatitis

neutrophil-mediated injury in acute lung injury and ARDS. Proinflammatory cytokines may be produced locally in the lungs. This acute phase may resolve completely or in some patients progress to fibrosing alveolitis with persistent arterial hypoxemia and decreased pulmonary compliance. The recovery or resolution phase of ARDS is characterized by gradual resolution of the arterial hypoxemia and improved lung compliance. Typically, the radiographic abnormalities resolve completely.

Treatment

Improved supportive care of patients with acute lung injury and ARDS may contribute to improved survival in these patients.[1] There should be a thorough search for any underlying causes of ARDS, with particular attention paid to the possibility of any treatable infection such as sepsis or pneumonia. Prevention or early treatment of nosocomial infections is critical. Adequate nutrition through the use of enteral feedings is preferred to parenteral nutrition, as this route does not introduce the risk of catheter-induced sepsis. Prevention of gastrointestinal bleeding and thromboembolism is important. At present, routine use of surfactant therapy or inhaled nitric oxide is not recommended for routine treatment of acute lung injury and ARDS.[1] In the future, strategies that hasten the resolution phase of ARDS, including maintenance of the ability to remove alveolar fluid to sustain improvements in arterial oxygenation, may become as important as traditional initial ventilator treatments.[1] In this regard, inhaled β-agonists may be of value in facilitating removal of pulmonary edema fluid from the alveoli, stimulating the secretion of surfactant, and even exerting

antiinflammatory effects, thereby helping to restore the vascular permeability of the lungs.[1]

Tracheal Intubation and Mechanical Ventilation

The initial steps in the treatment of patients with acute respiratory failure and ARDS who cannot be adequately oxygenated are tracheal intubation and mechanical support of ventilation with a volume-cycled ventilator. Inspired oxygen concentrations are adjusted to maintain the PaO_2 between 60 and 80 mmHg. A ventilation strategy using tidal volumes of 8 to 10 ml/kg (closer to the normal tidal volume of 6 to 8 ml/kg) is recommended.[1] The higher tidal volumes (12 to 15 ml/kg) utilized in the past for treatment of ARDS may be associated with decreased pulmonary compliance and can result in alveolar overdistension with resultant barotrauma.[1, 7, 8] The risk of barotrauma can be lessened by adjustment of tidal volumes such that increases in peak ("plateau") airway pressures do not exceed 35 to 40 cmH_2O. Tidal volume is determined by assessing lung mechanics rather than by measuring arterial blood gases.

Positive End-Expiratory Pressure

Application of PEEP is one of the most effective ways to improve arterial oxygenation in patients with ARDS.[2] PEEP acts to prevent alveolar collapse at end-expiration and thus increases lung volumes, improves ventilation-to-perfusion matching, and decreases the magnitude of right-to-left intrapulmonary shunting. Indeed, the best evidence of an effect of PEEP is an increase in FRC, probably as a result of recruiting collapsed alveoli. PEEP is unlikely to improve the PaO_2 when arterial hypoxemia is due to hypoventilation or is associated with a normal or even increased FRC. PEEP does not decrease the amount of extravascular lung water or prevent the formation of edema fluid in the lungs. Nevertheless, edema fluid is likely to be distributed to the interstitial lung regions, causing previously flooded alveoli to become ventilated.

Application of PEEP is indicated when high concentrations of delivered oxygen (more than 50%), as needed for prolonged periods of time to maintain an acceptable PaO_2, may introduce the risk of oxygen toxicity. It is possible that PEEP may decrease the shear stress associated with the opening and closing of alveoli in ARDS. The lowest level of PEEP required to achieve acceptable arterial oxygenation at nontoxic delivered concentrations of oxygen should be used because high levels of PEEP decrease cardiac output and increase the incidence of barotrauma. The level of PEEP that results in optimal pulmonary compliance is usually similar to the level associated with optimal arterial oxygenation. In this regard, PEEP is typically added in 2.5- to 5.0 cmH$_2$O increments until the PaO$_2$ is at least 60 mmHg with patients breathing less than 50% oxygen. Most patients show maximal improvement in arterial oxygen transport and pulmonary compliance with levels of PEEP below 15 cmH$_2$O. Excessive levels of PEEP can decrease the PaO$_2$ by overdistending open alveoli, thereby compressing the capillaries surrounding these alveoli and shunting more blood to collapsed alveoli.

An important adverse effect of PEEP is decreased cardiac output owing to interference with venous return and leftward displacement of the ventricular septum, which restricts filling of the left ventricle. It is conceivable that the improved PaO$_2$ produced by PEEP could be offset by decreased tissue blood flow due to decreases in cardiac output. The potential for PEEP to decrease cardiac output is exaggerated in the presence of decreased intravascular fluid volume or normal lungs, permitting maximal transmission of increased airway pressures. Replacement of intravascular fluid volume and administration of cardiac inotropes may offset the effects of PEEP on venous return and improve myocardial contractility. A pulmonary artery catheter is useful for monitoring the adequacy of intravascular fluid replacement, myocardial contractility, and tissue oxygenation [venous partial pressure of oxygen (PvO$_2$)] in patients being treated with PEEP. Measurement of pulmonary artery occlusion pressures is complicated by transmission of PEEP (intra-alveolar pressure) to the pulmonary capillaries, which is then erroneously interpreted as the pulmonary artery occlusion pressure.

Inverse-Ratio Ventilation

Inverse-ratio ventilation is characterized by inspiratory times that exceed the times permitted for exhalation. This is accomplished by adding an end-inspiratory pause to maintain the alveolar pressure briefly at the plateau level. As such, arterial oxygenation may be improved without increasing the minute ventilation or PEEP. Risks of inverse-ratio ventilation include barotrauma and hypotension due to development of auto-PEEP as the expiratory time is shortened. Although inverse-ratio ventilation may improve oxygenation in some patients with ARDS, prospective studies have not confirmed a benefit in most patients.[12]

Fluid and Hemodynamic Management

The rationale for restricting fluid administration to patients with acute lung injury and ARDS is to decrease the magnitude of the pulmonary edema. There is evidence that decreased left atrial pressures are associated with decreased formation of pulmonary edema fluid, although there is not total acceptance of this strategy.[1] Pulmonary artery occlusion pressures below 15 mmHg may reflect inadequate intravascular fluid volume. Urine outputs of 0.5 to 1.0 ml/kg/hr are consistent with an adequate cardiac output and intravascular fluid volume. Normally, a daily weight loss of 0.2 to 0.4 kg is anticipated in adult patients receiving conventional intravenous fluid therapy. A stable or increasing body weight implies excessive fluid administration. Drug-induced diuresis using furosemide is particularly effective in decreasing excessive accumulation of fluid in the lungs. Evidence of the beneficial effects of diuresis includes improved arterial oxygenation and resolution of pulmonary infiltrates on chest radiographs. Measurements of central venous pressure are probably not a reliable guide for monitoring intravascular fluid volume in patients with ARDS.

A reasonable goal is to maintain the intravascular fluid volume at the lowest level consistent with adequate organ perfusion as assessed by metabolic acid-base balance and renal function. If organ perfusion cannot be maintained after restoration of intravascular fluid volume, as in patients with septic shock, treatment with vasopressors is indicated to improve organ perfusion pressures in an attempt to normalize tissue oxygen delivery.

Corticosteroids

Despite the recognized role of inflammation in the acute lung injury associated with ARDS, the value of corticosteroids administered early in the course of the disease remains unproven.[1] Corticosteroids may have value in the treatment of the later fibrosing-alveolitis phase of ARDS or as rescue therapy in patients with severe ARDS that is not resolving.

Removal of Secretions

Optimal removal of secretions from the airways is facilitated by adequate systemic hydration and humidification of inspired gases. In addition, chest physiotherapy is important to enhance postural drainage of secretions and to stimulate effective coughing. Tracheal suction with sterile catheters is useful for stimulating active expiratory efforts and removing secretions from the airways. Fiberoptic bronchoscopy is indicated to remove the accumulated secretions, which are contributing to atelectasis.

Control of Infections

Control of infection using specific antibiotic therapy based on sputum cultures and sensitivity is a valuable adjunct to the management of ARDS. The use of prophylactic antibiotics without proven specificity for the infectious organisms, however, is not recommended, as this practice can lead to the overgrowth of resistant bacteria or fungi. Not uncommonly, the earliest evidence of infections in patients with ARDS is further deterioration of pulmonary function.

Nutritional Support

Nutritional support is important, as skeletal muscle weakness can interfere with the cessation of mechanical support of ventilation when acute respiratory failure is no longer present. Hypophosphatemia may contribute to skeletal muscle weakness and to the poor contractility of the diaphragm that may accompany acute respiratory failure and ARDS. Increased caloric intake, as associated with hyperalimentation, may increase the metabolic production of carbon dioxide, necessitating increases in alveolar ventilation that might not be possible without mechanical support of breathing.

Monitoring of Treatment

Monitoring the progress of the treatment of acute respiratory failure includes evaluation of pulmonary gas exchange (arterial and venous blood gases, pHa) and cardiac function (cardiac output, cardiac filling pressures, intrapulmonary shunt). A pulmonary artery catheter is useful for accomplishing many of these measurements.

Oxygen Exchange and Arterial Oxygenation

Adequacy of oxygen exchange across alveolar capillary membranes is reflected by the PaO_2. The efficacy of this exchange is paralleled by the differences between the calculated PaO_2 and measured PaO_2. Calculation of $A\text{-}aDO_2$ is useful for evaluating, the gas-exchange function of the lungs and for distinguishing among various mechanisms of arterial hypoxemia (Table 16–3).

Significant desaturation of arterial blood occurs only when the PaO_2 is less than 60 mmHg, which is the reason arterial hypoxemia is commonly defined as a PaO_2 less than 60 mmHg. Ventilation-to-perfusion mismatching, right-to-left intrapulmonary shunting, and hypoventilation are the principal causes of arterial hypoxemia (Table 16–4). Increasing the inspired oxygen concentration is likely to improve the PaO_2 in all these conditions, with the exception of a right-to-left intrapulmonary shunt, which exceeds 30% of the cardiac output.

Compensatory responses to arterial hypoxemia vary enormously among patients. As a guideline, these responses begin with acute decreases in PaO_2 below 60 mmHg; they are also present in chronic hypoxemia when the PaO_2 is less than 50 mmHg. Compensatory responses to acute arterial hypoxemia include (1) carotid body-induced increases in alveolar ventilation, (2) regional pulmonary artery vasoconstriction (hypoxic pulmonary vasoconstriction) to divert pulmonary blood flow away from hypoxic alveoli, and (3) increased sympathetic nervous system activity to enhance tissue oxygen delivery by an increased cardiac output. When arterial hypoxemia is chronic, increased erythrocyte mass enhances the oxygen-carrying capacity of the blood. Chronic arterial hypoxemia may be associated with somnolence and decreased renal function. When the PaO_2 is less than 30 mmHg, compensatory mechanisms fail and cell damage is likely.

Carbon Dioxide Elimination

The adequacy of alveolar ventilation relative to the metabolic production of carbon dioxide is reflected by the $PaCO_2$ (Table 16–3). The efficacy of carbon dioxide transfer across alveolar capillary membranes is reflected by the V_D/V_T. This ratio depicts areas in the lungs that receive adequate ventilation but inadequate or no pulmonary blood flow. Venti-

Table 16–3 • Mechanisms of Hypercarbia

Hypercarbia Mechanism	$PaCO_2$	V_D/V_T	$A\text{-}aDO_2$
Drug overdose	Increased	Normal	Normal
Restrictive lung disease (kyphoscoliosis)	Increased	Normal to increased	Normal to increased
Chronic obstructive pulmonary disease	Increased	Increased	Increased
Neuromuscular disease	Increased	Normal to increased	Normal to increased

Table 16–4 • Mechanisms of Arterial Hypoxemia

Hypoxemia Mechanism	PaO$_2$	PaCO$_2$	A-aDO$_2$	Response to Supplemental Oxygen
Low inspired oxygen concentration (altitude)	Decreased	Normal to decreased	Normal	Improved
Hypoventilation (drug overdose)	Decreased	Increased	Normal	Improved
Ventilation-to-perfusion mismatching (COPD, pneumonia)	Decreased	Normal to decreased	Increased	Improved
Right-to-left shunt (pulmonary edema)	Decreased	Normal to decreased	Increased	Poor to none
Diffusion impairment (pulmonary fibrosis)	Decreased	Normal to decreased	Increased	Improved

COPD, chronic obstructive pulmonary disease.

lation to these alveoli is described as "wasted ventilation." Normally, the V_D/V_T is less than 0.3 but may increase to 0.6 or more when there is an increase in wasted ventilation. An increased V_D/V_T occurs in the presence of acute respiratory failure, decreased cardiac output (e.g., due to anesthetic drugs or hypovolemia), and pulmonary embolism.

Hypercarbia is defined as PaCO$_2$ higher than 45 mmHg. Permissive hypercarbia is the strategy of allowing the PaCO$_2$ to increase to around 55 mmHg in spontaneously breathing patients, thereby avoiding or delaying the need for tracheal intubation. Symptoms of hypercarbia depend on the rate of increase and the ultimate level of increase in the PaCO$_2$. Acute increases in PaCO$_2$ are associated with increased cerebral blood flow and increased intracranial pressure. Extreme increases in the PaCO$_2$ to more than 80 mmHg may result in seizures and subsequent central nervous system depression.

Mixed Venous Partial Pressures of Oxygen

The mixed PvO$_2$ and the arterial-to-venous differences for oxygen (CaO$_2$ − CvO$_2$) reflect the overall adequacy of the oxygen transport system (cardiac output) relative to extraction of oxygen by tissues. For example, decreases in cardiac output that occur in the presence of unchanged tissue oxygen consumption cause the PvO$_2$ to decrease and the CaO$_2$ − CvO$_2$ to increase. These changes reflect the continued extraction of the same amount of oxygen by the tissues from a decreased tissue blood flow. A PvO$_2$ less than 30 mmHg or a CaO$_2$ − CvO$_2$ higher than 6 ml/dl indicates the need to increase the cardiac output to facilitate tissue oxygenation. A pulmonary artery catheter permits sampling of mixed venous blood through the distal port for use when measuring the PvO$_2$ and calculating the CvO$_2$.

Arterial pH

Measurements of pHa are necessary to detect acidemia or alkalemia. For example, metabolic acidosis predictably accompanies arterial hypoxemia and inadequate delivery of oxygen to tissues. Furthermore, acidemia due to respiratory or metabolic derangement is associated with cardiac dysrhythmias and with increased pulmonary vascular resistance due to constriction of the pulmonary vasculature.

Alkalemia, as reflected by increases in pHa, is most often associated with iatrogenic mechanical hyperventilation of the patient's lungs or with drug-induced diuresis leading to loss of chloride and potassium ions. As with acidemia, the incidence of cardiac dysrhythmias may be increased by metabolic or respiratory alkalosis. The presence of alkalemia in patients recovering from acute respiratory failure can delay or prevent successful weaning from mechanical support of ventilation because of compensatory hypoventilation by patients in attempts to restore total body carbon dioxide stores. The phenomenon known as posthyperventilation hypoxia reflects arterial hypoxemia due to hypoventilation that develops in the absence of administering supplemental oxygen to patients in whom previous mechanical hyperventilation of the lungs has led to depletion of carbon dioxide stores.

Intrapulmonary Shunt

Right-to-left intrapulmonary shunting of blood occurs when there is perfusion of alveoli that are not ventilated. The net effect is decreased PaO$_2$, reflecting dilution of oxygen in blood exposed to ventilated alveoli, with blood containing less oxygen coming from unventilated alveoli. Calculation of the shunt fraction provides a reliable assessment of ventilation-to-perfusion matching and serves as a useful estimate of the response to various therapeutic interventions during treatment of acute respiratory failure.

Physiologic shunt normally comprises 2% to 5% of the cardiac output. This degree of right-to-left intrapulmonary shunting reflects the passage of pulmonary arterial blood directly to the left side of the circulation through the bronchial and thebesian veins. It should be appreciated that determination of the shunt fraction in patients breathing less than 100% oxygen reflects the contribution of ventilation-to-perfusion mismatching and the right-to-left intrapulmonary shunt. Calculation of the shunt fraction from measurements obtained in patients breathing 100% oxygen eliminates the contribution of ventilation-to-perfusion mismatching.

LUNG TRANSPLANTATION

The four principal surgical approaches to lung transplantation are (1) single-lung transplantation, (2) bilateral sequential lung transplantation, (3) heart-lung transplantation, and (4) transplantation of lobes from living donors.[13, 14] The principal indications for a single-lung transplant in patients experiencing end-stage respiratory failure are chronic obstructive pulmonary disease (including emphysema due to α_1-antitrypsin deficiency), cystic fibrosis, idiopathic pulmonary fibrosis, and primary pulmonary hypertension. The presence of cor pulmonale is not an indication for heart-lung transplantation because recovery of right ventricular function is typically rapid and complete after replacing the lungs alone. In patients with pulmonary hypertension, high vascular resistance in the native lung requires the allograft to handle nearly the entire cardiac output, potentially causing exaggerated pulmonary edema due to reperfusion and poor allograft function during the immediate postoperative period. Bilateral sequential transplantation involves the sequential performance of two single-lung transplantations at one time. In the absence of marked pulmonary hypertension, cardiopulmonary bypass can usually be avoided by ventilating the contralateral lung during each implantation. The primary indications for double lung transplantation are cystic fibrosis and other forms of bronchiectasis. Immunosuppression is initiated during the immediate perioperative period and continued for the duration of the patient's life.

Management of Anesthesia

Management of anesthesia for lung transplantation invokes the principles followed when performing anesthesia for a pneumonectomy.[14–16] Physiologically, patients selected for lung transplantation most often demonstrate restrictive patterns of lung disease and a large A-aDO$_2$. Mild to moderate degrees of pulmonary hypertension and some degree of right heart failure are possible. The ability of the recipient's right ventricle to maintain a sufficient stroke volume in the presence of acute increases in pulmonary vascular resistance produced by clamping the pulmonary artery before pneumonectomy is evaluated preoperatively.

Scrupulous attention to asepsis is important, as these patients are immunosuppressed. Monitors include an intra-arterial and pulmonary artery catheter, pulse oximetry, and capnography. Pulmonary artery pressure monitoring is especially important in these patients. There are no uniquely recommended drugs for induction and maintenance of anesthesia and skeletal muscle paralysis. Drug-induced histamine release seems undesirable, whereas drug-induced bronchodilation appears useful.

Tracheal intubation is with a double-lumen endobronchial tube, and its proper placement is verified by fiberoptic bronchoscopy. Intraoperative problems may include arterial hypoxemia, especially when one-lung anesthesia is initiated, and pulmonary hypertension, when the pulmonary artery is clamped. When arterial hypoxemia accompanies one-lung ventilation, a trial of PEEP to the dependent ventilated lung is considered. Infusion of prostacyclin may be useful for controlling pulmonary hypertension. In extreme cases, support with partial cardiopulmonary bypass is required. Bronchospasm has been observed after heart-lung transplantation, even though the transplanted lung has been denervated.[15] Connection of the donor lung to the recipient is usually in the sequence of pulmonary veins to the recipient's left atrium, anastomosis of the pulmonary artery, and finally bronchial anastomosis, often with an omental wrap.

Postoperatively, mechanical support of ventilation is continued until it is appropriate to initiate the weaning process.[16] The principal causes of mortality are bronchial dehiscence or respiratory failure owing to sepsis or rejection. The denervated donor lung deprives patients of normal cough reflexes from the lower airways and predisposes to the development of pneumonia. In the absence of rejection pulmonary function tests are usually normal.

Physiologic Effects of Lung Transplantation

Single or bilateral lung transplantation in patients with end-stage respiratory failure often dramatically improves lung function with peak improvement usually achieved within 3 to 6 months postoperatively.[13] Arterial oxygenation rapidly returns to normal, and supplemental oxygen is no longer needed. For patients with pulmonary vascular disease, both single and bilateral lung transplantation result in immediate and sustained normalization of pulmonary vascular resistance and pulmonary arterial pressures. This is accompanied by prompt increases in cardiac output and more gradual remodeling of the right ventricle with decreases in ventricular wall thickness. Exercise capacity improves sufficiently to permit most lung transplant patients to resume an active lifestyle.

The innervation, lymphatics, and bronchial circulation are disrupted when the donor pneumonectomy is performed.[14] The principal effect of lung denervation is loss of the cough reflex, which places patients at risk for aspiration and pulmonary infections. Inhaled β_2-agonists produce bronchodilation. Mucociliary clearance is impaired during the early postoperative period. Lymphatic drainage disrupted by transection of the trachea and bronchi may be reestablished during the first 2 to 4 weeks postoperatively. Often blunted ventilatory responses to carbon dioxide persist even though pulmonary function improves. Denervation of the heart is also a consideration in patients undergoing heart-lung transplantation.

Complications of Lung Transplantation

Mild, transient pulmonary edema is a common feature of a newly transplanted lung.[13] However, in some patients pulmonary edema is sufficiently severe to cause a form of acute respiratory failure termed primary graft failure. The diagnosis is confirmed by infiltrates seen on chest radiographs and severe arterial hypoxemia during the first 72 hours postoperatively. Treatment is supportive and includes mechanical ventilation. Mortality is high.

Dehiscence of the bronchial anastomosis mandates immediate surgical correction or retransplantation. Anastomotic stenosis is the most common airway complication and typically occurs several weeks after transplantation. Evidence of the presence of clinically significant airway stenosis includes focal wheezing, recurrent lower respiratory tract infections, and suboptimal pulmonary function.

The rate of infection among lung-transplant patients is several times as high as that among recipients of other organs and is most likely related to exposure of the allograft to the external environment.[13] Bacterial infections of the lower respiratory tract are the most common manifestations of pulmonary infections. A ubiquitous organism acquired by inhalation is *Aspergillus*, which frequently colonizes the airways of lung-transplant recipients; clinical

infections develop in only a small number of these patients, however.

Acute rejection of the lung allograft is a common event, with the greatest incidence seen during the first 100 days following transplantation.[13] Clinical manifestations, which are nonspecific, include malaise, low grade fever, dyspnea, cough-impaired oxygenation, and leukocytosis. Transbronchial lung biopsies are needed for a definitive diagnosis. Treatment of acute rejection is with intravenous methylprednisolone. Most patients have a prompt clinical response, although histologic evidence of rejection may persist even in the absence of clinical symptoms.

Chronic rejection, a pervasive problem following lung transplantation, manifests histologically as bronchiolitis obliterans, a fibroproliferative process that targets the small airways and leads to submucosal fibrosis and luminal obliteration.[13] Bronchiolitis obliterans is uncommon during the first 6 months following transplantation, but its incidence exceeds 60% in patients who survive at least 5 years. The onset of this syndrome is insidious and is characterized by dyspnea, cough, and often colonization of the airways with *Pseudomonas aeruginosa*, which leads to recurrent bouts of purulent tracheobronchitis. The overall prognosis is poor. Retransplantation is the only definitive treatment for severe bronchiolitis obliterans.

Anesthetic Considerations in Lung Transplant Recipients

Anesthetic considerations for patients requiring surgery following lung transplantation should focus on (1) the function of the transplanted lung, (2) the possibility of rejection or infection in the transplanted lung, (3) the effect of immunosuppressive therapy on other organ systems and the effect of organ system dysfunction on the transplanted lung, (4) the disease in the native lung, and (5) the planned surgical procedure and its likely effects on the lungs.[14, 17]

Preoperative Evaluation

Evaluation before surgery includes eliciting a history of increasing dyspnea or the need for supplemental oxygen, auscultation of the lungs (normally clear), pulmonary function tests, arterial blood gases, and review of chest radiographs. If rejection or infection is suspected, elective surgery should be postponed. The side effects of immunosuppressive drugs are evaluated during the preoperative period. Systemic hypertension and renal dysfunction related to cyclosporine are present in many patients, and evidence of end-organ damage may be present.

Chronic Rejection

Because transplanted lungs may have ongoing rejection that can adversely affect pulmonary function, it may be recommended that spirometry be performed preoperatively. It is difficult to differentiate between chronic rejection and infection. If chronic rejection is occurring, the forced expiratory volume, vital capacity, and total lung capacity may decrease, and arterial blood gases may show increased alveolar-to-arterial oxygen gradients. Arterial hypoxemia and an increased A-aDO$_2$ occur, whereas carbon dioxide retention is rare. Obliterative bronchiolitis is a manifestation of chronic rejection and usually manifests as a nonproductive cough developing after the third month following transplantation. Symptoms can mimic upper respiratory tract infections and include fever and fatigue. Dyspnea occurs within months and is followed by a clinical course similar to that of COPD. Chest radiographs show peribronchial and interstitial infiltrates.

Preoperative Medication

Premedication is acceptable provided pulmonary function is adequate. Hypercarbia is common during the early posttransplant period, and increased sensitivity to opioids is a theoretical consideration. Antisialagogues are useful, as secretions can be excessive in these patients. Supplemental corticosteroids are a consideration especially for long, stressful surgical procedures. A major cause of morbidity and mortality in transplant recipients is infection. Prophylactic antibiotics are indicated, and strict sterile technique is needed for placement of intravascular catheters. Denervation of the lung seems to have limited effects on patterns of breathing. Increased bronchial responsiveness causing bronchoconstriction is common. Denervation ablates afferent sensations below the level of the tracheal anastomosis; patients with a tracheal anastomosis lose the cough reflex and are prone to retention of secretions and silent aspiration. Responses to carbon dioxide rebreathing are normal in these patients.

Choice of Anesthetic Technique

Because lung transplant recipients lack a cough reflex below the tracheal anastomosis level, they are unable to clear secretions unless they are awake. In view of the decreased cough reflex, the potential for bronchoconstriction, and the increased risk of pulmonary infections, it is recommended that re-gional anesthesia be selected in preference to general anesthesia and tracheal intubation. Epidural and spinal anesthesia are acceptable selections in lung transplant patients, keeping in mind that depression of intercostal muscle function may have special implications in these patients. Performing any nerve block carries a danger of introducing infection, emphasizing the importance of sterile technique in this high risk population. Fluid preloading may be a risk in patients with transplanted lungs, reflecting disruption of the lymphatic drainage in the transplanted lung causing interstitial fluid accumulation, particularly during the early posttransplantation period. For these reasons it has been suggested that the patients be treated with diuretics and limited crystalloid infusions.[17]

In heart-lung transplant recipients, fluid management may be a challenge, as the heart requires adequate preload to maintain cardiac output, and the lungs may have lower thresholds for developing pulmonary edema. In this regard, the value of invasive monitoring is balanced against the risk of infection. Transesophageal echocardiography may be useful for monitoring volume status and cardiac function. When an internal jugular catheter is in place, it is prudent to select the side of the native lung. The possibility of cardiac denervation is also a consideration in patients who have undergone double-lung transplantation with tracheal anastomosis. In addition to increased sensitivity to hypovolemia, these patients may develop intraoperative bradycardia that does not respond to atropine. In such cases epinephrine and/or isoproterenol may be required to increase the inherent heart rate.

An important goal of anesthetic management is prompt recovery of adequate respiratory function and early tracheal extubation. Volatile anesthetics are well tolerated, and nitrous oxide is acceptable in the absence of pneumothorax and bullous disease. Immunosuppressive drugs may interact with neuromuscular blocking drugs, and the impaired renal function caused by these drugs may prolong the effects of certain muscle relaxants. The effects of nondepolarizing neuromuscular blocking drugs are routinely antagonized pharmacologically, as even minimal residual drug-induced weakness can compromise ventilation in these patients. Likewise, careful assessment of the adequacy of ventilation is important before considering tracheal extubation.

Consideration should be given to the fact that these patients may have compromised upper airway protective reflexes, placing them at increased risk for aspiration of gastric contents.[16] When positioning a tracheal tube, it is best to place the cuff just beyond the vocal cords to minimize the risk of traumatizing the tracheal anastomosis. Accidental bronchial intubation of the native or transplanted lung must be avoided. If the surgical procedure requires a double-lumen endobronchial tube, it is preferable to place the endobronchial lumen in the native bronchus. Positive-pressure ventilation in the presence of a single-lung transplant may be complicated by differences in lung compliance between the native and transplanted lung. With emphysematous lung disease, the more compliant native lung may be preferentially ventilated and compress the transplanted lung. Nitrous oxide and PEEP are unlikely components of anesthetic management.

References

1. Ware LB, Matthay MA. The acute respiratory distress syndrome. N Engl J Med 2000;342:1334–49
2. Leatherman JW, Ingram RH. Respiratory failure. Sci Am Med 1998;1–9
3. Kress JP, Pohlman AS, O'Connor MF, et al. Daily interruption of sedative infusions in critically ill patients undergoing mechanical ventilation. N Engl J Med 2000;342:1471–7
4. Hughes MA, Glass PSA, Jacobs JR. Context-sensitive half-time in multicompartment pharmacokinetic models for intravenous anesthetic drugs. Anesthesiology 1992;76:334–41
5. Antonelli M, Conti G, Bufi M, et al. Noninvasive ventilation for treatment of acute respiratory failure in patients undergoing solid organ transplants: a randomized trial. JAMA 2000;283:235–41
6. Hudson LD. Progress in understanding ventilator-induced lung injury. JAMA 1999;282:77–8
7. The Acute Respiratory Distress Syndrome Network. Ventilation with lower tidal volumes as compared with traditional tidal volumes for acute lung injury and the acute respiratory distress syndrome. N Engl J Med 2000;342:1301–8
8. Tobin MJ. Culmination of an era in research on the acute respiratory distress syndrome. N Engl J Med 2000;342:1360–1
9. Chad DA, Lacomis D. Critically ill patients with newly acquired weakness: the clinicopathological spectrum. Ann Neurol 1994;35:257–62
10. Nava S, Ambrosino N, Clini E, et al. Noninvasive mechanical ventilation in the weaning of patients with respiratory failure due to chronic obstructive pulmonary disease. Ann Intern Med 1998;128:721–7
11. Girou E, Schortgen F, Delclaux C, et al. Association of noninvasive ventilation with nosocomial infections and survival in critically ill patients. JAMA 2000;284:2361–7
12. Lessard MR, Guerot E, Lorino H, et al. Effects of pressure-controlled ventilation with different I:E ratios versus volume-controlled ventilation on respiratory mechanics, gas exchange, and hemodynamics in patients with adult respiratory distress syndrome. Anesthesiology 1994;80:983–91
13. Arcasoy SM, Kotloff RM. Lung transplantation. N Engl J Med 1999;340:1081–91
14. Haddow GR. Anaesthesia for patients after lung transplantation. Can J Anaesth 1997;44:182–97
15. Casella ES, Humphrey LS. Bronchospasm after cardiopulmonary bypass in a heart-lung transplant recipient. Anesthesiology 1988;69:135–8
16. Smiley RM, Navedo AT, Kirby T, et al. Postoperative independent lung ventilation in a single-lung transplant patient. Anesthesiology 1991;74:1144–8
17. Kostopanagiotou G, Smyrniotis V, Arkadopoulos N, et al. Anesthetic and perioperative management of adult transplant recipients in nontransplant surgery. Anesth Analg 1999;89:613–22

17

Diseases of the Nervous System

Patients with diseases affecting the nervous system may undergo surgery as a result of the disease, whereas in others the need for surgery is unrelated to the nervous system disease. Regardless of the reason for surgery, co-existing nervous system diseases often have important implications when selecting anesthetic drugs, techniques, and monitors. In addition, concepts of cerebral protection and resuscitation may assume unique importance in these patients.

▌ INTRACRANIAL TUMORS

Intracranial (brain) tumors may be classified as primary tumors (those arising from the brain and its coverings) or metastatic tumors (Table 17–1).[1, 2] Astrocytomas and medulloblastomas are the most common primary brain tumors in children, whereas the most common brain tumors in adults are meningiomas, glioblastomas, pituitary adenomas, and metastatic tumors. Astrocytomas typically begin as slow-growing tumors in a cerebral hemisphere, and medulloblastomas most often arise in the cerebellum. Meningiomas are the most common benign brain tumors, accounting for about 15% of all primary brain tumors. Evidence of a hormonal component is enhanced meningioma growth during pregnancy. This tumor arises from arachnoidal cells, is slow growing, and may infiltrate the skull, with resultant evidence of osteoblastic activity on skull radiography. Glioblastomas are highly malignant, infiltrative intracranial tumors that most often arise in a cerebral hemisphere. The classification of pituitary adenomas as chromophobe, basophilic, or eosinophilic is based on the staining properties of granules present in the tumor cells. Nearly 80% of pituitary adenomas are classified as chromophobes.

Table 17–1 • Classification of Brain Tumors

Primary brain tumor
Histologically benign
Meningioma
Pituitary adenoma
Astrocytoma
Acoustic neuroma
Histologically malignant
Glioblastoma
Medulloblastoma
Metastatic brain tumor

These tumors rarely excrete hormones; rather, they produce panhypopituitarism by virtue of expanding and compressing normal anterior pituitary tissue. In addition, suprasellar extension of these adenomas characteristically produces bitemporal hemianopia owing to compression of the optic chiasm. Chromophobe adenomas may be part of an inherited syndrome, characterized by multiple endocrine neoplasia (see Chapter 22).

Metastatic brain tumors are most often from primary sites in the lungs or breasts. Malignant melanoma, hypernephroma, and carcinoma of the colon are also likely to spread to the brain. Metastatic brain tumor is the likely diagnosis when diagnostic tests indicate the presence of more than one lesion. Acoustic neuromas are benign tumors that grow from the nerve sheath of the vestibular nerve (cranial nerve VIII). Initial manifestations of acoustic neuromas are progressive unilateral sensorineural hearing loss and vertigo, followed by facial palsy and numbness due to compression of the facial nerve as the tumors fill the internal auditory meatus.

Causes

Ionizing radiation is the only unequivocal risk factor that has been identified for glial and meningeal neoplasms.[2] Radiation of the cranium, even at low doses, can increase the incidence of meningiomas by a factor of 10 and the incidence of glial tumors by factor of 3 to 7, with a latency period of 10 years to more than 20 years after exposure. No other environmental exposure or behavior has been clearly identified as a risk factor. The use of cellular telephones, exposure to high-tension wires, the use of hair dyes, head trauma, and dietary exposure to N-nitrosourea compounds have been alleged to increase the risk of brain tumors, but the data are conflicting and unconvincing.[2] Specifically, the use of handheld cellular telephones is not associated with the risk of brain cancer.[3, 4]

Diagnosis

Diagnosis of a brain tumor is based on classic symptoms (headache) and findings on the neurologic examination that are substantiated by specific diagnostic imaging techniques. The only test needed to diagnose a brain tumor is cranial magnetic resonance imaging. Magnetic resonance imaging with contrast agents improves visualization of certain intracranial tumors (meningiomas, acoustic neuromas) that are not well seen with computed tomography or that may be inconspicuous with enhanced magnetic resonance imaging. Computed tomography can miss structural lesions, particularly in the posterior fossa, or nonenhancing tumors such as low-grade gliomas.[2] Positron emission tomography and single photon emission computed tomography permit imaging not only of structures but also of some of the functional characteristics of the patient's brain including blood flow and locations of specific neurotransmitters. A vascular mass can be distinguished from a brain tumor on magnetic resonance imaging angiography. Patients with implanted metal devices (cardiac pacemakers, mechanical heart valves, intracranial metal clips) are not candidates for magnetic resonance imaging.

Treatment

Surgery is part of the initial management of virtually all brain tumors, as it quickly establishes the diagnosis and relieves symptoms due to the space-occupying intracranial mass. The operating microscope and intraoperative monitoring techniques, including evoked potential responses, facilitate optimal surgical removal of the tumor. Intraoperative monitoring of brain stem auditory evoked responses for resection of acoustic neuromas, visual evoked responses for parasellar tumors, and somatosensory evoked responses for parenchymal and brain stem lesions may be useful for guiding surgical resection. Intraoperative ultrasonography can establish the location of brain tumors for biopsy or resection. Surgery on areas of the cortex that control speech and motor function may be performed under local anesthesia with the use of stereotactic and stimulation techniques to provide precise tumor resection. Laser resection of brain tumors permits vaporization of tumor without manipulating the brain. Complete resection may be curative for benign tumors, and extensive resection of malignant tumors is likely to prolong survival.

Radiation therapy is particularly useful in the management of malignant brain tumors. Increased neurologic deficits during radiation treatment are probably due to cerebral edema, which usually responds to treatment with corticosteroids. Cardiorespiratory arrest has followed radiation of brain stem tumors.[5] Brachytherapy is the stereotactic implantation of radiation sources in tumors for 4 to 6 days. This treatment is most useful for prolonging survival of patients with glioblastomas. Radiation therapy is often avoided in children because of its potential long-term detrimental effects, which include developmental delay and panhypopituitarism. Chemotherapy, often combination therapy, is usually the initial treatment of brain tumors in children.

Signs and Symptoms

Increased intracranial pressure (ICP) is the most likely explanation for signs and symptoms caused by brain tumors. Symptoms of increased ICP are headache, nausea and vomiting, mental changes, and disturbances of consciousness. During the early stages of intracranial hypertension, it is common for symptoms to be most prominent during the early morning hours. Patients are awakened by dull headaches, followed by spontaneous vomiting after which symptoms subside. Presumably, increases in $PaCO_2$ and the associated cerebral vasodilation that accompanies sleep produces increases in intracranial contents that exceeds the limits of compensation, and ICP increases (Fig. 17–1). Progressive increases in ICP eventually result in unexplained fatigue and drowsiness. Papilledema is often accompanied by visual disturbances. Seizures occurring for the first time in adults without an apparent cause are presumed to be due to a brain tumor and are investigated with computed tomography and/or magnetic resonance imaging.

Systemic blood pressure may be increased in an attempt to maintain cerebral perfusion pressures in the presence of intracranial hypertension. As the systemic blood pressure increases, there are corresponding decreases in heart rate due to reflex activation of the carotid sinus by hypertension. Local tissue destruction by tumor infiltration or compression leads to symptoms determined by the areas of the brain involved. For example, mental and behavioral changes may be prominent in patients with intracranial tumors in the frontal cortex. Cerebral edema surrounds expanding intracranial tumors, particularly those with rapid growth rates. Edema may contribute to loss of neurologic function, creating the erroneous impression that the tumors are large and highly destructive. The presence of edema around intracranial tumors is thought to result from increased permeability of tumor capillaries, permit-

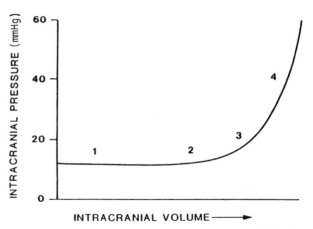

Figure 17–1 • Pressure–volume compliance curves depict the impact of increasing intracranial volume on intracranial pressure (ICP). As the intracranial volume increases from point 1 to 2, ICP does not increase because cerebrospinal fluid is shifted from the cranium into the spinal subarachnoid space. Patients with intracranial tumors, but between points 1 and 2 on the curve, are unlikely to manifest symptoms of increased ICP. Patients on the rising portion of the curve (point 3) can no longer compensate for increases in intracranial volume; the ICP begins to increase and is likely to be associated with clinical symptoms. Additional increases in intracranial volume at this point (point 3), as produced by anesthetic drug-induced increases in cereberal blood flow, can precipitate abrupt increases in ICP (point 4).

ting penetration of protein and fluid into adjacent normal brain tissue. This abnormal permeability is the basis for the lucency of tissues seen on computed tomography.

Intracranial tumors may result in displacement of the brain and compression of neural tissues at distant sites. The most common examples are supratentorial tumors, which lead to herniation of the uncus of the temporal lobes through the incisura of the tentorium. The oculomotor nerve becomes compressed at the tentorial notch, resulting in a dilated, unreactive homolateral pupil. Apnea and unconsciousness follow if the midbrain is compressed. Compression of the posterior cerebral artery against the edge of the tentorium may lead to infarction of the occipital lobe and contralateral hemianopia. Compression of the cerebral peduncle produces contralateral hemiplegia. A posterior fossa tumor leads to obstruction of the normal flow of cerebrospinal fluid (CSF), and the resulting increase in ICP predisposes to herniation of the cerebellar tonsils through the foramen magnum, manifesting as decreased levels of consciousness and slow breathing rates.

Management of Anesthesia

Management of anesthesia for resection of brain tumors requires an understanding of the pressure–

volume compliance relations of the brain, the methods available to monitor and decrease ICP, and the determinants of cerebral blood flow (CBF). The goals of perioperative anesthesia management are often based on keeping the ICP within the normal range and recognizing that autoregulation of CBF may be impaired. Hemodynamically stable induction and maintenance of anesthesia, minimal brain swelling to optimize surgical exposure, and rapid return to a level of consciousness that permits neurologic assessment are the principal objectives of anesthesia management for patients undergoing elective surgical resection of supratentorial tumors.[6]

Pressure–Volume Compliance Curves

Pressure–volume compliance curves reflect changes produced by expanding intracranial tumors (Fig. 17–1). These curves plot the changes in ICP that accompany alterations in intracranial volume produced by brain tumors. As tumors gradually enlarge, CSF in the cranium is shifted to the spinal subarachnoid space, preventing an increase in ICP above its normal value of about 15 mmHg. In addition, increased absorption of CSF attenuates the increase in ICP produced by expanding tumors. At this stage clinical symptoms suggesting an intracranial tumor are minimal. Eventually, a point is reached on the pressure–volume compliance curve at which even small increases in intracranial volume produced by the expanding tumor results in marked increases in ICP, and anesthetic drugs and techniques that affect cerebral blood volume can adversely and abruptly increase ICP.

Marked increases in ICP can interfere with adequate CBF. For example, cerebral perfusion pressure is determined by the difference between mean arterial pressure (MAP) and right atrial pressure. When the ICP is higher than the right atrial pressure, the cerebral perfusion pressure is determined by the difference between the MAP and the ICP. If cerebral perfusion pressure is substantially decreased in response to increased ICP, the systemic blood pressure shows a compensatory increase in an attempt to restore perfusion pressure and thus maintain CBF. Ultimately, this compensatory mechanism fails, producing cerebral ischemia.

Monitoring Intracranial Pressure

The importance of monitoring ICP (epidural or subdural placement of a transducer or intraventricular placement via a catheter positioned in a cerebral ventricle) in patients with space-occupying lesions is emphasized by the observation that alterations in ICP may not be accompanied by changes in the neurologic examination or the vital signs. The first evidence of hazardous increases in ICP in unresponsive patients may be sudden bilateral pupillary dilatation associated with herniation of the brain stem through the foramen magnum. Delay in the initiation of treatment to decrease ICP until these signs appear may be futile, as irreversible brain damage is likely.

A normal ICP wave is pulsatile and varies with the cardiac impulses and spontaneous breathing. The mean ICP should remain below 15 mmHg. Abrupt increases in ICP to as high as 100 mmHg observed during continuous monitoring are characterized as *plateau waves*. During this increase in ICP patients may become symptomatic, and spontaneous hyperventilation may occur. Events that can initiate abrupt increases in ICP include anxiety, painful stimulation, and induction of anesthesia. Indeed, in normal patients anxiety and painful stimulation can elicit substantial increases in oxygen uptake and CBF. In the presence of intracranial tumors, this increase in CBF can result in abrupt increases in ICP. For this reason, noxious stimuli should be avoided in patients with intracranial tumors, regardless of the level of consciousness. Hence the liberal use of analgesics to avoid or treat pain, even in unresponsive patients, may be recommended. Support of ventilation to avoid hypercarbia secondary to drug-induced depression of ventilation is necessary, especially when opioids are administered. Likewise, it is important to establish a depth of anesthesia that is sufficient to blunt the pressor responses to laryngoscopy and tracheal intubation or noxious surgical stimulation.

Methods to Decrease Intracranial Pressure

Methods to decrease ICP include posture, hyperventilation of the patient's lungs, CSF drainage, and administration of hyperosmotic drugs, diuretics, corticosteroids, and barbiturates. It is not possible to identify reliably the level of ICP than can interfere with regional CBF in individual patients. Therefore a frequent recommendation is to treat any sustained increase in ICP that exceeds 20 mmHg. Treatment may be indicated when the ICP is less than 20 mmHg if the appearance of occasional plateau waves suggests the presence of low intracranial compliance.

Posture

Posture is important for ensuring optimal venous drainage from the brain. For example, elevating the patient's head to about 30 degrees above heart level encourages venous outflow from the brain and lowers the ICP. Extreme flexion or rotation of the patient's head can obstruct the jugular veins and restrict venous outflow from the brain. The head-down position is avoided, as this position could increase the ICP.

Hyperventilation

Hyperventilation of the patient's lungs is an effective method for rapidly lowering the ICP. In adults a frequent recommendation is to maintain the $PaCO_2$ near 30 mmHg. Excessive lowering of the $PaCO_2$ can theoretically decrease CBF to the point that cerebral ischemia occurs. Nevertheless, there is no evidence that cerebral ischemia occurs when the $PaCO_2$ remains higher than 20 mmHg. Because no additional beneficial effect is demonstrable by lowering the $PaCO_2$ to extremely low levels, it seems reasonable to strive to achieve a $PaCO_2$ near 30 mmHg when treating increases in ICP. The duration of the efficacy of hyperventilation of the patient's lungs in decreasing ICP may be limited, as the beneficial effect of this intervention wanes after 6 to 12 hours. Rebound increases in ICP are a potential problem especially if normocapnia is not slowly restored.

It may be appropriate to initiate more aggressive hyperventilation of the lungs in children than is recommended for adults to maintain $PaCO_2$ levels between 20 and 25 mmHg. Presumably, increased therapeutic benefits of these lower $PaCO_2$ levels reflects the relatively high CBF that may be present in children, particularly in the presence of acute head injury. Moreover, hyperventilation of the lungs in children may result in more sustained CBF decreases than is possible in adults.

Cerebrospinal Fluid Drainage

Draining CSF from the lateral cerebral ventricles or the lumbar subarachnoid space decreases the intracranial volume and ICP. Lumbar drainage of CSF in patients with increased ICP is not recommended, as herniation of the cerebellum through the foramen magnum is a risk. Lumbar drainage of CSF is usually reserved for operations in which surgical exposure is difficult, such as surgery on the pituitary gland or an intracranial aneurysm.

Hyperosmotic Drugs

The use of hyperosmotic drugs such as mannitol is an important, effective method for decreasing ICP. These drugs produce transient increases in the osmolarity of plasma, which acts to draw water from tissues including the brain. The purpose of therapy with hyperosmotic drugs is not to dehydrate the patient but, rather, to draw fluid from the brain

along an osmotic gradient. As such, it is an error not to replace some of the intravascular fluid lost through the kidneys (see "Fluid Therapy"). Failure to replace intravascular fluid volume can result in hypotension and jeopardize maintenance of adequate cerebral perfusion pressures. Likewise, urinary losses of electrolytes, particularly potassium, may require careful monitoring and replacement. Moreover, an intact blood–brain barrier is necessary, so mannitol or urea can exert maximum beneficial effects on brain size. If the blood–brain barrier is disrupted, these drugs may cross into the brain, causing cerebral edema and increases in brain size. The brain eventually adapts to sustained increases in plasma osmolarity, such that chronic use of hyperosmotic drugs is likely to become less effective.

Mannitol is administered in doses of 0.25 to 1.0 g/kg IV over 15 to 30 minutes. There is little difference in ICP-lowering effects with this dose range, but higher doses may last longer. Smaller doses require less volume for intravenous administration and thus avoid the risk of serum hyperosmolarity. This dose range of mannitol results in removal of about 100 ml of water from the patient's brain. After administration, decreases in ICP are seen within 30 minutes, and maximum effects occur within 1 to 2 hours. Urine output can reach 1 to 2 L within 1 hour after initiating the administration of mannitol. Appropriate infusion of crystalloid and colloid solutions is often necessary to prevent adverse changes in the plasma concentrations of electrolytes and intravascular fluid volume due to the brisk drug-induced diuresis. Conversely, mannitol can initially increase the intravascular fluid volume, emphasizing the need to monitor carefully those patients who have limited cardiac reserve. Mannitol also has direct vascular vasodilating properties that can contribute to increased cerebral blood volume and ICP. The duration of hyperosmotic effects produced by mannitol is about 6 hours. Mannitol is not associated with a high incidence of rebound increases in ICP after this time. Furthermore, the incidence of venous thrombosis after administration of mannitol is low.

Diuretics

Diuretics, particularly furosemide, have been used in an attempt to promote decreases in ICP. Furosemide is particularly useful when there is evidence of increased vascular fluid volume and pulmonary edema. In this instance, promotion of diuresis and systemic dehydration may improve arterial oxygenation, with concomitant decreases in ICP. Furosemide, 1 mg/kg IV, may be more effective than mannitol for lowering elevated ICP; and unlike mannitol, it does not introduce the risk of altered plasma osmolarity.

Corticosteroids

Corticosteroids such as dexamethasone or methyl-prednisolone are effective in lowering increased ICP caused by the development of localized cerebral edema around brain tumors. The mechanism for the beneficial effects of corticosteroids is unknown but may involve stabilization of capillary membranes and/or decreased production of CSF. Patients with metastatic brain tumors or glioblastomas respond most favorably to corticosteroids with improved neurologic status and disappearance of headache often within 12 to 36 hours after initiating therapy. Pulmonary infections or gastrointestinal bleeding is not increased by short-term use of corticosteroids to decrease cerebral edema associated with brain tumors.

Barbiturates

Administration of barbiturates in high doses is particularly effective for treating increased ICP that develops after an acute head injury. This approach is especially useful when other, more traditional methods of treatment have failed (see "Traumatic Brain Injury").

Determinants of Cerebral Blood Flow

Determinants of CBF are the $PaCO_2$, PaO_2, arterial blood pressure and autoregulation, central venous pressure, and anesthetic drugs and techniques (Fig. 17–2). Cerebral blood vessels receive innervation

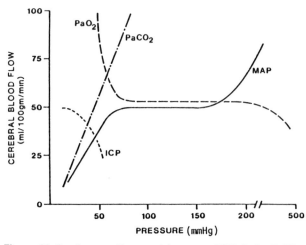

Figure 17–2 • Impact of intracranial pressure (ICP), PaO_2, $PaCO_2$, and mean arterial pressure (MAP) on cerebral blood flow.

from the autonomic nervous system, but the impact of this innervation on CBF is minimal. For example, it is estimated that neurogenic control can alter CBF by only 5% to 10%. Furthermore, stellate ganglion block does not predictably increase CBF.

Arterial Carbon Dioxide Partial Pressure

Variations in $PaCO_2$ produce corresponding changes in CBF (Fig. 17–2). As a guideline, CBF (normal about 50 ml/100 g/min) increases 1 ml/100 g/min for every 1 mmHg increase in the $PaCO_2$ above 40 mmHg. A similar decrease occurs during hypocarbia, such that CBF is decreased about 50% when the $PaCO_2$ is 20 mmHg. The impact of the $PaCO_2$ on CBF is mediated by variations in CSF pH around the walls of arterioles. Decreased CSF pH causes intense cerebral vasodilation, and increased CSF pH causes vasoconstriction. Corresponding changes in resistance to blood flow exerts predictable effects on CBF.

The ability of hypocapnia to decrease CBF and ICP is the basis for neuroanesthesia. Concern that cerebral hypoxia due to vasoconstriction can occur when the PCO_2 is lowered below 20 mmHg has not been substantiated. Nevertheless, because there is no evidence of an increased therapeutic benefit from lowering the $PaCO_2$ excessively, it seems reasonable to recommend maintaining the $PaCO_2$ values near 30 mmHg during anesthesia for removal of intracranial tumors. The long-term value of hypocapnia in decreasing ICP is offset by the return of CSF pH to normal, permitting increases in CBF despite decreases in $PaCO_2$. This adaptive change, which reflects active transport of bicarbonate ions into or from the CSF, requires about 6 hours to return the CSF pH to normal.

The influence of carbon dioxide on local CBF may be altered by acidosis, which often surrounds intracranial tumors. For example, acid metabolites from tumors diffuse into adjacent tissues, causing maximal vasodilation and increased blood flow around the tumor. These vessels have lost their responsiveness to carbon dioxide, and vasomotor paralysis is present. Increased blood flow in the area of brain tumors has been termed *luxury perfusion.*[7] When the $PaCO_2$ is allowed to increase, blood flow is shunted away from the tumor. This response reflects the vasodilation of normal vessels but no change in the vessels that have already been maximally dilated; thus the pressure gradient for blood flow is reversed. This phenomenon has been termed the *intracerebral steal syndrome.* Conversely, hypocapnia constricts normal vessels, whereas those manifesting vasomotor paralysis are not altered; the result is a change in the pressure gradient that favors flow to acidotic areas surrounding tumors. This response is referred to as the inverse steal, or *Robin Hood phenomenon*. The relative importance of these phenomena is unknown, but it is likely that their occurrence is infrequent. In the absence of regional CBF measurements, it is not known whether individual patients respond physiologically or paradoxically to alterations in $PaCO_2$. Therefore the prudent approach is to maintain a normal or modestly decreased $PaCO_2$ when the cerebral steal response is a consideration. If lowering the ICP is the goal, the common recommendation is to maintain the $PaCO_2$ near 30 mmHg. Inhaled anesthetics do not alter the responsiveness of the cerebral circulation to changes in $PaCO_2$.

Arterial Oxygen Partial Pressure

Decreased PaO_2 does not lead to significantly increased CBF until a threshold value of about 50 mmHg is reached (Fig. 17–2). Below this threshold there is abrupt cerebral vasodilation, and the CBF increases. Furthermore, the combination of arterial hypoxemia and hypercarbia exerts a synergistic effect, with increases in CBF that exceed the increase that would be produced by either factor alone.

Arterial Blood Pressure and Autoregulation

The ability of the brain to maintain CBF at constant levels, despite changes in MAP, is known as autoregulation (Fig. 17–2). Autoregulation is an active vascular response characterized by (1) arterial constriction when the distending blood pressure is increased and (2) arterial dilation in response to decreases in systemic blood pressure. The upper and lower limits of the MAP with maintenance of autoregulation have been defined. For example, in normotensive patients the lower limit of MAP associated with autoregulation is about 60 mmHg. Below this threshold the CBF decreases and becomes directly related to the MAP. Indeed, at a MAP of 40 to 55 mmHg, symptoms of cerebral ischemia may appear in the form of nausea, dizziness, and slow cerebration. Autoregulation of CBF also has an upper limit, above which the flow becomes directly proportional to the MAP. This upper limit of autoregulation in normotensive patients is a MAP of about 150 mmHg. Above this threshold the CBF increases, causing overdistension of the walls of the cerebral blood vessels. As a result, fluid is forced across vessel walls into the brain tissue, producing cerebral edema.

Autoregulation of CBF is altered in the presence of chronic hypertension. Specifically, the autoregulation curve is displaced to the right, such that a higher MAP is tolerated before CBF becomes pressure-dependent. The adaptation of cerebral vessels to increased blood pressure requires 1 to 2 months. Indeed, acute hypertension, as seen in children with glomerulonephritis or in patients with pregnancy-induced hypertension, often produces signs of central nervous system dysfunction at a MAP tolerated by patients who are chronically hypertensive. Likewise, acute hypertensive episodes associated with stimulation produced by direct laryngoscopy or surgery may cause a breakthrough of autoregulation. The lower limit of autoregulation is also shifted upward in chronically hypertensive patients, such that decreases in systemic blood pressure are not tolerated to the same low levels as in normotensive patients. After gradual decreases in systemic blood pressure due to antihypertensive drug therapy, however, the tolerance of the brain to hypotension may improve, as the autoregulation curve shifts back toward its original position.

Autoregulation of CBF may be lost or impaired in a variety of conditions, including the presence of intracranial tumors or head trauma and the administration of volatile anesthetics. The loss of autoregulation in the blood vessels surrounding intracranial tumors reflects acidosis leading to maximum vasodilation, such that blood flow becomes pressure-dependent.

Venous Blood Pressure

Venous blood pressure is usually low in supine or standing patients, such that the MAP is the predominant determinant of cerebral perfusion pressure. An increase in CBF can increase the pressure in cerebral veins owing to the rigid bony orifices surrounding the venous exits from the cranium. Furthermore, the rigidity of dural layers surrounding the intracranial venous sinuses may result in increased venous pressure when CBF is increased. Increases in central venous pressure are directly transmitted to intracranial veins. The impact of increased central venous pressure on cerebral perfusion pressure and ICP must be appreciated when considering the use of positive airway pressure during intracranial surgery or in patients with increased ICP. Indeed, the use of positive end-expiratory pressure may produce adverse increases in ICP and thus decrease cerebral perfusion pressure in patients with intracranial tumors. Increased venous pressure can also contribute to increased bleeding during intracranial surgery.

Anesthetic Drugs

Volatile anesthetics administered in concentrations higher than 0.6 MAC are often potent cerebral vasodilators that produce dose-dependent increases in CBF despite concomitant decreases in cerebral metabolic oxygen requirements. Normally, the tendency of ICP to increase in response to increases in CBF is prevented by displacement of CSF from the cranium. In patients with intracranial tumors, however, this compensatory mechanism may fail, such that drug-induced increases in CBF may produce abrupt increases in ICP. Like the volatile anesthetics, ketamine has been considered to be a cerebral vasodilator, although increases in CBF do not necessarily accompany administration of this drug when normocarbia is maintained.[8] In contrast to volatile anesthetics and possibly ketamine, barbiturates, etomidate, propofol, and opioids are classified as cerebral vasoconstrictors. Drugs that produce cerebral vasoconstriction predictably decrease CBF and ICP.

The institution of hyperventilation of the patient's lungs, simultaneous with the introduction of volatile anesthetics such as isoflurane into the inhaled gases, prevents increases in ICP that might accompany administration of these drugs at normocarbia to patients with brain tumors. Decreased cerebral metabolic oxygen requirements produced by volatile anesthetics may explain why CBF increases are minimal below 1.1 MAC. For example, decreased cerebral metabolism means that less carbon dioxide is produced, thereby opposing the cerebral vasodilating effects of volatile anesthetics. In contrast to volatile anesthetics, nitrous oxide has less effect on CBF, perhaps reflecting restriction of its dose to less than 1 MAC. For this reason, nitrous oxide is unlikely to increase ICP in patients with intracranial tumors maintained at normocarbia. In contrast to volatile anesthetics, nitrous oxide does not interfere with autoregulation of CBF. The administration of nitrous oxide during a craniotomy and after closure of the dura may contribute to the development of a tension pneumocephalus. Tension pneumocephalus reflects the entrance of nitrous oxide into the subdural air cavities.

Barbiturates, such as thiopental, are potent cerebral vasoconstrictors capable of decreasing CBF with associated decreases in a previously increased ICP. Decreases in CBF produced by barbiturates are even greater if hypocarbia is also present. Opioids, like barbiturates, are considered cerebral vasoconstrictors, assuming that opioid-induced ventilatory depression is not permitted to manifest as an increase in $PaCO_2$.

Administration of succinylcholine or nondepolarizing neuromuscular blocking drugs to patients with brain tumors is unlikely to alter the ICP. Nevertheless, drug-induced histamine release could theoretically produce cerebral vasodilation with associated increases in CBF and ICP.

Preoperative Evaluation

Preoperative evaluation of patients with intracranial tumors is directed toward establishing the presence or absence of increased ICP. Symptoms of increased ICP include nausea and vomiting, altered levels of consciousness, mydriasis and decreased reactivity of pupils to light, papilledema, bradycardia, systemic hypertension, and breathing disturbances. Evidence of midline shifts (more than 0.5 cm) on computed tomography suggests the presence of increased ICP.

Preoperative Medication

Preoperative medication that produces sedation or ventilatory depression should be avoided in patients with intracranial tumors. Patients with intracranial pathology may be extremely sensitive to the central nervous system depressant effects of drugs such as opioids. Opioid-induced hypoventilation can lead to accumulation of carbon dioxide and resulting increases in ICP. Likewise, drug-induced sedation can mask alterations in the levels of consciousness that accompany intracranial hypertension. Considering all the potential adverse effects of preoperative medication, it is an inescapable conclusion that pharmacologic premedication should be used sparingly, if at all, in patients with intracranial tumors. Certainly no preoperative depressant drugs should be administered to patients with depressed levels of consciousness. In alert adult patients with intracranial tumors, oral administration of benzodiazepines can provide anxiety relief without introducing the risk of ventilatory depression. Decisions to administer anticholinergic drugs or H_2-receptor antagonists are not influenced by the presence or absence of increased ICP.

Induction of Anesthesia

Induction of anesthesia is achieved with drugs (thiopental, etomidate, propofol) that produce a rapid, reliable onset of unconsciousness with minimal effects on CBF. The intravenous induction drug is often followed by large doses [three times the median effective dose (ED_{95})] of a nondepolarizing muscle relaxant to facilitate tracheal intubation. Administration of succinylcholine may be associated with modest, transient increases in ICP of unclear clinical significance. Mechanical hyperventilation of the patient's lungs is initiated with the goal of decreasing the $PaCO_2$ to near 30 mmHg. An adequate depth of anesthesia and profound skeletal muscle paralysis are necessary, as perception of noxious stimulation can abruptly increase the cerebral metabolic oxygen requirements, CBF, and ICP.

Direct laryngoscopy for tracheal intubation is accomplished during profound skeletal muscle paralysis as confirmed by the absence of electrically evoked responses delivered from a peripheral nerve stimulator. Administration of additional doses of intravenous induction drugs and/or potent short-acting opioids before initiation of direct laryngoscopy may blunt pressor responses to this painful stimulation. In addition, lidocaine, 1.5 mg/kg IV, administered about 1 minute before beginning direct laryngoscopy may be effective in attenuating the increases in systemic blood pressure and ICP that can accompany tracheal intubation (Fig. 17–3).[9]

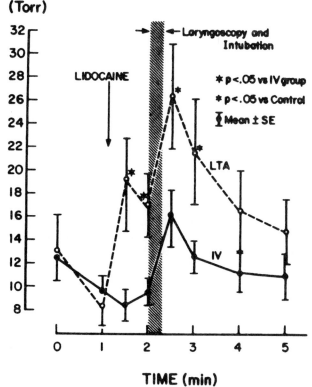

Figure 17–3 • Intravenous (IV) administration of lidocaine was more effective than laryngotracheal administration (LTA) of lidocaine in preventing increases in intracranial pressure (ICP) during laryngoscopy and tracheal intubation of patients with intracranial tumors. (From Hamill JF, Bedford RF, Weaver DC, et al. Lidocaine before endotracheal intubation: intravenous or laryngotracheal? Anesthesiology 1981;55:578–81, with permission.)

Abrupt, sustained increases in systemic blood pressure in the absence of autoregulation in areas of intracranial pathology may be accompanied by cerebral edema and undesirable increases in CBF and ICP. Sustained hypotension is also avoided, as brain ischemia can occur in the presence of decreased cerebral perfusion pressure and impaired autoregulation. Skeletal muscle responses during tracheal intubation reflect inadequate drug-induced skeletal muscle paralysis and may be associated with further increases in ICP that parallel increases in venous pressure. Following tracheal intubation, the patient's lungs are ventilated at a rate and tidal volume that maintain the $PaCO_2$ near 30 mmHg. Positive end-expiratory pressure is not likely to be utilized, as it could impair cerebral venous drainage, leading to increased ICP.

Maintenance of Anesthesia

Maintenance of anesthesia in patients undergoing surgical resection of supratentorial brain tumors is often achieved with combinations of drugs including nitrous oxide, volatile anesthetics (often isoflurane), opioids, and propofol. Although modest cerebrovascular differences can be demonstrated among different combinations of drugs, there is no evidence that effects on ICP and short-term patient outcome are significantly influenced by the choice.[6] Neuroprotection against focal ischemic effects provided by volatile anesthetics, although demonstrated in animals receiving isoflurane, is of questionable significance in patients.[10]

Some would question the wisdom of using nitrous oxide in situations in which the risk of venous air embolism is increased, as in operations performed with patients in the sitting position. Nevertheless, the incidence and severity of venous air embolism has not been documented to be influenced by the inclusion of nitrous oxide in the inhaled gases being delivered to patients in the sitting position.[11] Volatile anesthetics such as isoflurane are administered with caution because of the potential for these drugs to increase CBF and to interfere with its autoregulation. However, low concentrations of volatile anesthetics (0.6 MAC) may be useful for preventing or treating increases in systemic blood pressure related to noxious surgical stimulation. In addition to lowering systemic blood pressure, administration of volatile anesthetics increases the depth of anesthesia and decreases the likelihood that painful stimulation could increase CBF and ICP. Use of volatile anesthetics is typically accompanied by hyperventilation of the patient's lungs to maintain the $PaCO_2$ near 30 mmHg. Administration of peripheral vasodilating drugs, such as nitroprusside or nitroglycerin, may increase CBF and ICP despite accompanying decreases in systemic blood pressure. For this reason, selecting peripheral vasodilating drugs to treat intraoperative hypertension must be done cautiously.

Spontaneous movement by patients undergoing surgical resection of brain tumors must be prevented. Such movement could result in dangerous increases in ICP, excessive bleeding into the operative site, and bulging of the brain into the operative site, making surgical exposure difficult. Therefore, in addition to adequate depths of anesthesia, skeletal muscle paralysis is typically maintained during intracranial surgery.

Fluid Therapy

Selection of appropriate crystalloid infusions for administration to patients with brain tumors is important to minimize the risk of adversely influencing the ICP. For example, glucose-in-water solutions are rapidly distributed throughout body water; and if blood glucose concentrations decrease more rapidly than brain glucose concentrations, brain water becomes relatively hyperosmolar, and brain tissues accumulate water. Furthermore, metabolism of glucose in the brain leaves free water in excess. Hypertonic salt solutions such as 5% glucose in lactated Ringer's solution are appropriate fluid selections. These solutions initially tend to decrease brain water by increasing the osmolarity of plasma. Regardless of the crystalloid solutions selected, any solution administered in large amounts can increase brain water and ICP in patients with brain tumors. Therefore the rate of fluid infusion probably should not exceed 1 to 3 ml/kg/hr during the perioperative period. Intravascular fluid volume depletion due to blood loss during surgery should be corrected with packed red blood cells, whole blood, or colloid solutions—not with large volumes of balanced salt solutions.

Monitoring

Continuous monitoring of systemic blood pressure via a catheter placed in a peripheral artery is useful for rapid detection of undesirable changes in cerebral perfusion pressure. Capnography is useful for guiding ventilation to achieve desired degrees of hyperventilation and serving as a monitor to detect venous air embolism (see "Venous Air Embolism"). A continuous monitor of ICP, although not routine, is of obvious value. Nasopharyngeal or esophageal temperature is monitored as unexpected changes in the patient's body temperature are possible. A

bladder catheter is necessary if drug-induced diuresis is planned during the perioperative period.

Placing a catheter in the right atrium is helpful for guiding the rate of intravenous fluid infusions. Furthermore, this catheter may be important for aspirating air from the chambers of the heart should venous air embolism occur (see "Venous Air Embolism"). The anatomic position of this catheter may be confirmed by chest radiography, by the configuration of the P waves on the electrocardiogram (ECG) using a saline-filled catheter as a unipolar lead, or by the transduced pressure waveforms. The impracticality of obtaining a chest radiograph in the operating room and the electroshock hazard of recording the ECG from a saline-filled catheter are disadvantages of these approaches. Therefore observation of the phasic pressure waveforms recorded from the catheter seems the most acceptable method for confirming the central venous location of the catheter. An additional approach is to advance the catheter until right ventricular pressure waveforms are observed and then withdraw the catheter until the pressure traces reflect atrial pressure waveforms. It is common to consider placing a central venous catheter or a pulmonary artery catheter whenever the risk of venous air embolism is thought to be increased.[12]

A peripheral nerve stimulator is helpful for monitoring the persistence of drug-induced skeletal muscle weakness or paralysis. If paresis or paralysis of an upper extremity is associated with the brain tumor, it is important to appreciate the presence of resistance (decreased sensitivity) to the effects of nondepolarizing muscle relaxants in the paretic extremity, compared with the normal extremity (Fig. 17-4).[13] Therefore monitoring skeletal muscle paralysis with the leads of the peripheral nerve stimulator placed on the paretic arm may be misleading. For example, the evoked response may be erroneously interpreted as inadequate skeletal muscle paralysis. Likewise, at the conclusion of surgery the same response could be assumed to reflect recovery from the effects of the muscle relaxant when substantial neuromuscular blockade persists. Resistance of the skeletal muscles in a paralyzed or paretic extremity to muscle relaxants may reflect the proliferation of acetylcholine-responsive extrajunctional cholinergic receptor sites that can occur within 48 to 72 hours after denervation (see "Chronic Spinal Cord Transection").

Monitoring to detect a venous air embolism with a Doppler transducer may be utilized in patients undergoing intracranial operations. The transducer is placed to the right of the sternum, between the third and sixth intercostal spaces. Correct positioning is verified by rapid injection of 5 to 10 ml of

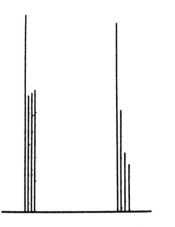

PARETIC   NORMAL

Figure 17–4 • Train-of-four ratio recorded from the paretic extremity (0.6) is higher than that from the normal arm (0.3), reflecting resistance of the paretic arm to the effects of nondepolarizing muscle relaxants. (From Moorthy SS, Hilgenberg JC. Resistance to nondepolarizing muscle relaxants in paretic upper extremities of patients with residual hemiplegia. Anesth Analg 1980;59:624–7, with permission.)

crystalloid solution into the right atrial catheter. Turbulence created by this rapid injection of fluid creates a signal ("roaring sound") similar to that caused by air. Amounts of air as small as 0.25 ml can be detected by the Doppler transducer. Air is detected as a change in the signal from the transducer because the air–blood interface is a much better acoustic reflector than erythrocytes alone. In addition, audible sounds from the transducer may provide early warning of changes in the heart rate or cardiac rhythm.

Monitoring the ECG is necessary to detect cardiac dysrhythmias related to the presence of intracranial tumors or from surgical stimulation of vital medullary centers. Abnormalities on the ECG can indicate the effects of intracranial tumors related to increased sympathetic nervous system activity and increased ICP. More importantly, alterations in heart rate and cardiac rhythm may reflect surgical retraction or manipulation of the brain stem or cranial nerves. Indeed, the cardiovascular centers, respiratory control areas, and nuclei of the lower cranial nerves lie in close proximity in the brain stem. Manipulation of the brain stem may produce systemic hypertension and bradycardia or hypotension and tachycardia. Cardiac dysrhythmias range from acute sinus dysrhythmias to ventricular premature beats or ventricular tachycardia.

Patient Position

Craniotomy to remove a supratentorial tumor is usually performed in the supine position with the patient's head elevated 10 to 15 degrees to facilitate cerebral venous drainage. Excessive flexion or rotation of the head should be avoided, as these positions can impair jugular vein patency and impede cerebral venous outflow. Macroglossia is a potentially lethal postoperative complication that has been attributed to venous obstruction due to excessive flexion of the neck when patients are placed in the sitting position.[14]

The sitting position is often used for exploration of the posterior cranial fossa, which may be necessary to resect intracranial tumors, clip aneurysms, decompress cranial nerves, or implant electrodes for cerebellar stimulation. Advantages of the sitting position are excellent surgical exposure and facilitation of cerebral venous and CSF drainage, thereby minimizing blood loss and increasing the ICP. These advantages are offset by the decreases in systemic blood pressure and cardiac output produced by this posture and the potential hazard of venous air embolism. For these reasons the lateral or prone position may be selected as an alternative. If the sitting position is used, it is mandatory to maintain a high index of suspicion for venous air embolism (see "Venous Air Embolism"). A serious postoperative complication after posterior fossa craniotomy is apnea due to hematoma formation. Cranial nerve injuries involving innervation to the pharynx and larynx could make these patients vulnerable to pulmonary aspiration.

Venous Air Embolism

Venous air embolism is a potential hazard whenever the operative site is above the level of the patient's heart, such that pressures in the veins are subatmospheric.[15] Although this complication is most often associated with neurosurgical procedures, venous air embolism may also occur during operations involving the neck, thorax, abdomen, and pelvis and during open heart procedures, repair of liver and vena cava lacerations, total hip replacement, and vaginal delivery associated with placenta previa. Patients undergoing intracranial surgery are at increased risk not only because the operative site is usually above the level of the patient's heart but also because veins in the skull may not collapse owing to their attachment to bone or dura. Indeed, the cut edge of bone, including burr holes, constituting the skull is a common site for the entry of air into veins held open by bone.[16]

Pathophysiology

The precise mechanism by which venous air embolism leads to cardiovascular collapse is undetermined. Presumably, when air enters the right ventricle there is interference with blood flow into the pulmonary artery. Pulmonary edema and reflex bronchoconstriction may result from the movement of air into the pulmonary circulation. Death is usually secondary to acute cor pulmonale and cardiovascular collapse, as well as to arterial hypoxemia from obstruction to right ventricular ejection into the pulmonary artery.

Air can probably pass through pulmonary vessels in small amounts to reach the coronary and cerebral circulations; large quantities of air can travel directly to the systemic circulation through right-to-left intracardiac shunts created by a patent foramen ovale (detectable in about 30% of the population). Fatal cerebral arterial gas embolism caused by venous air has occurred even in the absence of detectable shunt mechanisms or intracardiac defects.[15] Various anesthetic drugs may diminish the ability of the pulmonary circulation to filter out air emboli and thus facilitate the passage of venous air emboli to the arterial circulation.[17] Use of the sitting position inherently predisposes neurosurgical patients to paradoxical air embolism, as the normal interatrial pressure gradient frequently becomes reversed in this position.[18] When the likelihood of venous air embolism is increased, it is useful, but not mandatory, to place a right atrial catheter before beginning surgery (see "Monitoring"). Death due to paradoxical air embolism results from obstruction of the coronary arteries by air, leading to myocardial ischemia and ventricular fibrillation. Neurologic damage may follow air embolism to the brain.

Detection

Early detection of venous air embolism is important for successful treatment of this complication. A Doppler transducer placed over the right heart is the most sensitive indicator of intracardiac air. Indeed, the small amount of air detected by the transducer is often not clinically significant. In this regard the transducer does not provide information as to the volume of air that has entered the venous circulation. Transesophageal echocardiography is also useful for detecting intracardiac air resulting from venous air embolism. A sudden decrease in the end-tidal PCO_2 may reflect increased deadspace due to continued ventilation of alveoli that are no longer perfused because of obstruction of their vascular supply by air. An increase in right atrial and pulmonary artery pressures reflects acute cor pulmonale and correlates with abrupt decreases in the end-tidal PCO_2. Although these changes are less sensitive indicators of the presence of air than the Doppler transducer, they reflect the size of the venous air

embolism. Increased end-tidal nitrogen concentrations may reflect the occurrence of a venous air embolism. Changes in end-tidal nitrogen concentrations often precede decreased end-tidal PCO_2 or increased pulmonary artery pressures.[19] During controlled ventilation of the lungs, sudden attempts by patients to initiate spontaneous breaths ("gasp reflex") may be the first indication of the occurrence of venous air embolism. Hypotension, tachycardia, cardiac dysrhythmias, and cyanosis are late signs of venous air embolism. Certainly detection of the characteristic "millwheel" murmur, as heard through an esophageal stethoscope, is a late sign of catastrophic venous air embolism.

Treatment

A change in the signal from the Doppler transducer should alert the surgeon to identify and occlude sites of venous air entry by irrigating the operative site with fluid and applying occlusive material to all bone edges. Aspiration of air should be attempted through the right atrial catheter. The ideal location of the right atrial catheter tip is controversial, but evidence suggests that superior vena cava locations (junction of the superior vena cava with the right atrium) are preferable, as this position appears to provide the most rapid aspiration of air.[20] Right atrial multiorifice catheters permit aspiration of larger amounts of air than do single-orifice catheters. Because of its small lumen size and slow speed of blood return, a pulmonary artery catheter is not uniquely useful for aspirating air, but it may provide additional evidence that venous air embolism has occurred by virtue of increased pulmonary artery pressures. Nitrous oxide is promptly discontinued to avoid increasing the size of the venous air bubbles (Fig. 17–5).[21] Indeed, elimination of nitrous oxide from the inhaled gases after detecting a venous air embolism often results in decreased pulmonary artery pressure. At the same time oxygen is substituted for nitrous oxide, it may be helpful to apply positive end-expiratory pressure to increase venous pressure. Despite the logic of this maneuver, the prophylactic use of positive end-expiratory pressure has not been found to be of value in the prevention of venous air embolism. The notion has been raised that positive end-expiratory pressure increases right atrial pressure more than left atrial pressure, predisposing patients with probe-patent foramen ovales to paradoxical air embolism. Nevertheless, levels of positive end-expiratory pressure up to 10 cmH$_2$O probably do not alter the interatrial pressure differences in sitting neurosurgical patients and therefore do not increase the risk of paradoxical air embolism in these patients.[22] Extreme hypotension may re-

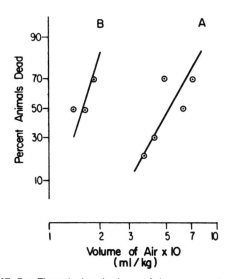

Figure 17-5 • The calculated volume of air necessary to produce death in 50% of animals was greater during administration of halothane alone (*A*) compared with halothane-nitrous oxide (*B*). Presumably, the rapid passage of nitrous oxide into air bubbles, with resultant expansion of the air bubbles, was responsible for the increased lethal effects of venous air embolism in the presence of nitrous oxide. (From Munson ES, Merrick HC. Effect of nitrous oxide on venous air embolism. Anesthesiology 1966;27: 783–7, with permission.)

quire the support of perfusion pressure with sympathomimetic drugs. Likewise, marked decreases in cardiac output may require infusion of β-agonists such as dopamine or dobutamine. Bronchospasm is treated with β_2-agonists by aerosol (metered-dose inhaler) or the intravenous route. The traditional admonition to treat venous air embolism by placing the patient in the lateral position with the right chest uppermost is rarely possible or safe during intracranial operations. It is likely that valuable time, better spent aspirating air and supporting circulation, could be lost attempting to attain this position.

After successful treatment of venous air embolism, the surgical procedure can be resumed. However, the decision to reinstitute administration of nitrous oxide must be individualized. If it is decided not to use nitrous oxide, maintenance of an adequate depth of anesthesia probably requires administration of volatile anesthetics. If nitrous oxide is added to the inhaled gases, it is possible that residual air in the circulation could again produce symptoms. Indeed, increased pulmonary artery pressure after resumption of breathing nitrous oxide should be viewed as evidence that residual air persists in the patient's circulation despite apparent successful treatment of venous air embolism.[12] Transfer of patients to a hyperbaric chamber in an attempt to decrease the size of air bubbles and to improve blood flow in the brain is likely to be helpful only if the transfer can be accomplished within 8 hours.

Postoperative Management

Ideally, the effects of anesthetics and muscle relaxants are dissipated or pharmacologically reversed at the conclusion of intracranial surgery. This facilitates monitoring the neurologic status and recognizing any adverse effects of the surgery. It is important to prevent any reaction to the tracheal tube as patients are awakening. Lidocaine, 0.5 to 1.5 mg/kg IV, may be administered to attenuate the initial responses to the continued presence of the tracheal tube as the patient awakens. It must be appreciated, however, that this local anesthetic can produce central nervous system depression and reduce the activity of protective upper airway reflexes. If a patient was alert preoperatively, it may be reasonable to place a nasal airway during anesthesia and remove the tracheal tube at the conclusion of surgery to avoid potentially adverse reactions to the tube. Conversely, if consciousness was depressed preoperatively, it may be best to delay tracheal extubation until it can be confirmed that airway reflexes are present and spontaneous ventilation is sufficient to prevent accumulation of carbon dioxide. Decreases in body temperature during anesthesia and surgery to less than 34°C must be considered as possible causes of slow postoperative awakening. It may be inappropriate to remove the tracheal tube in the presence of hypothermia, regardless of the preoperative mental status.

■ CEREBROVASCULAR DISORDERS

Cerebrovascular disorders ("stroke") are characterized by sudden neurologic deficits due to ischemic (80%) or hemorrhagic (20%) events (Table 17–2).[23, 24] Ischemic stroke is described by the area of the brain affected and the etiologic mechanisms. Hemorrhagic stroke is classified as intracerebral (15%) or subarachnoid. A transient ischemic attack (TIA) is a sudden vascular-related focal neurologic deficit that resolves promptly (within 24 hours). TIA is not considered a separate entity but, rather, evidence of an impending ischemic stroke.

Stroke is the leading cause of disability and the third leading cause of death in the United States.[23] The pathogenesis of stroke may differ among ethnic groups. Extracranial carotid artery disease and cardioembolism more commonly cause ischemic stroke in non-Hispanic whites, whereas intracranial thromboembolic disease is more common in African-Americans. Women have lower stroke rates

Table 17–2 • Characteristics of Stroke Subtypes

Parameter	Systemic Hypoperfusion	Embolism	Thrombosis	Subarachnoid Hemorrhage	Intracerebral Hemorrhage
Risk factors	Hypotension Hemorrhage Cardiac arrest	Smoking Ischemic heart disease Peripheral vascular disease Diabetes mellitus White men	Smoking Ischemic heart disease Peripheral vascular disease Diabetes mellitus White men	Often absent Hypertension Coagulopathy Drugs Trauma	Hypertension Coagulopathy Drugs Trauma
Onset	Parallels risk factors	Sudden	Often preceded by a TIA	Sudden, often during exertion	Gradually progressive
Signs and symptoms	Pallor Diaphoresis Hypotension	Headache	Headache	Headache Vomiting Transient loss of consciousness	Headache Vomiting Decreased level of consciousness Seizures
Imaging	CT (black) MRI	CT (black) MRI	CT (black) MRI	CT (white) MRI	CT (white) MRI

CT, computed tomography; MRI, magnetic resonance imaging; TIA, transient ischemic attack.
Adapted from: Caplan LR. Diagnosis and treatment of ischemic stroke. JAMA 1991;266:2413–8.

than men at all ages except 75 years and older, when stroke rates are at their highest. Overall, the decrease in stroke-related mortality has inexplicably slowed over the past several decades.[23]

Cerebrovascular Anatomy

Blood supply to the brain (20% of the cardiac output) is via two pairs of vessels: the internal carotid arteries and the vertebral arteries (Fig. 17–6). These vessels join on the surface of the brain to form the intracranial vessels (anterior cerebral artery, middle cerebral artery, posterior cerebral artery) and the circle of Willis. Occlusion of specific arteries results in predictable clinical neurologic deficits (Table 17–3). Isolated infarction of the anterior cerebral artery is uncommon. Clinical neurologic deficits following middle cerebral artery occlusion are extensive, reflecting the large areas of the brain supplied by this artery and its branches. The two major branches of the vertebral arteries are arteries to the spinal cord and the posteroinferior cerebellar artery to the inferior cerebellum and lateral medulla. The two vertebral arteries then unite to form the basilar artery. Occlusion of the vertebral arteries or basilar artery results in signs and symptoms that depend on the level of the infarction (Table 17–3). The basilar artery terminates by dividing into two posterior cerebral arteries, which supply the medial temporal lobe, occipital lobe, and parts of the thalamus. After the circle of Willis, vessels branch repeatedly and ultimately become end arteries. If occluded, even

these penetrating vessels can cause typical clinical neurologic deficits (motor hemiparesis, sensory loss, clumsy hand-dysarthria syndrome, ataxic hemiparesis).

Initial Evaluation

Patients who present with the sudden onset of neurologic dysfunction or describe neurologic signs and symptoms evolving over minutes to hours are most likely experiencing a stroke. Most of these patients have an ischemic stroke rather than a hemorrhagic stroke. It is important to recognize that stroke represents a medical emergency, and that the patient's prognosis often depends on the time elapsed from the onset of symptoms to thrombolytic intervention. Patients who receive early treatment to restore cerebral perfusion and to maximize neuronal protection have better outcomes.

Distinguishing Hemorrhage from Ischemia

The brain should first be imaged with noncontrast computed tomography, which reliably distinguishes acute intracerebral hemorrhage from ischemia.[23] This distinction is important, as treatment of hemorrhagic stroke is substantially different from that of ischemic stroke. Computed tomography is relatively insensitive to ischemic changes (hyperdense vessels, loss of gray matter–white matter boundaries) during the first few hours after a stroke. The ability to identify at-risk cerebral tissue has con-

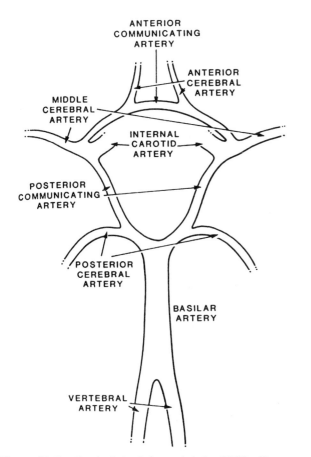

Figure 17–6 • Cerebral circulation and circle of Willis. The cerebral blood supply is from the vertebral arteries (arising from the subclavian arteries) and the internal carotid arteries (arising from the common carotid arteries).

Table 17–3 • Clinical Features of Cerebrovascular Occlusive Syndromes

Occluded Artery	Clinical Features
Anterior cerebral artery	Contralateral leg weakness
Middle cerebral artery	Contralateral hemiparesis and hemisensory deficit (face and arm more than leg)
	Aphasia (dominant hemisphere)
	Contralateral visual field defect
Posterior cerebral artery	Contralateral visual field defect
	Contralateral hemiparesis
Penetrating arteries	Contralateral hemiparesis
	Contralateral hemisensory
Basilar artery	Oculomotor deficits and/or ataxia with "crossed" sensory and motor deficits
Vertebral artery	Lower cranial nerve deficits and/or ataxia with crossed sensory deficits

Adapted from: Morgenstern LB, Kasner SE. Cerebrovascular disorders. Sci Am Med 2000:1–15.

natively, transcranial Doppler ultrasonography can provide indirect evidence of major vascular occlusion and offers the advantage of real-time bedside monitoring in patients undergoing thrombolytic therapy.[23]

Acute Ischemic Stroke

Acute ischemic stroke most likely reflects cardioembolism (atrial fibrillation, ventricular akinesis following myocardial infarction, dilated cardiomyopathy, valvular heart disease), large-vessel atherothromboembolism (atherosclerotic narrowing especially at major arterial branches such as the carotid bifurcation in the neck), and small-vessel occlusive disease (lacunar infarction). Patients with long-standing diabetes mellitus or systemic hypertension are most likely to experience acute ischemic stroke due to small-vessel occlusive disease. Echocardiography is useful for evaluating the patient's cardiac status and events that could result in cardioembolism. The extracranial carotid circulation and intracranial circulation can be visualized by angiography (computed tomography or magnetic resonance) or carotid ultrasonography. Transcranial Doppler imaging can help detect intracranial stenosis.

siderable clinical relevance because viable tissue (up to 17 hours after stroke) may be salvaged by specific therapeutic interventions. Diffusion-weighted imaging (DWI) reveals changes in infarcted tissues hours before conventional computed tomography or magnetic resonance imaging. Hyperintensity on DWI is predictive of the extent of infarction and areas of cytotoxic edema. Perfusion-weighted imaging demonstrates regionally decreased cerebral blood flow. The difference between the perfusion defect and the diffusion defect may represent salvageable tissue, which is the target of therapy.

Define Vascular Lesion

Conventional angiography demonstrates acute occlusion or an embolus lodged at a vascular bifurcation. The vasculature can also be visualized noninvasively utilizing computed tomography angiography and magnetic resonance angiography. Alter-

Risk Factors

Systemic hypertension is the most significant risk factor for acute ischemic stroke.[25] Adequate treatment of systolic or diastolic hypertension (to below 140/90 mmHg) dramatically reduces the risk of first stroke. Cigarette smoking substantially increases the risk of acute ischemic stroke. Hyperlipidemia appears to be an independent risk factor for the occurrence of acute ischemic stroke, and treatment of patients with evidence of coronary artery disease with statin drugs is associated with decreased risk of stroke. Diabetes mellitus is a well recognized risk factor for stroke. Excessive alcohol consumption (more than six drinks daily) seems to increase the risk of stroke, whereas moderate alcohol consumption (one or two drinks daily) may be protective. An increased homocysteine level is an independent risk factor for the development of stroke.

Carotid Endarterectomy

Surgical treatment of symptomatic or asymptomatic carotid artery stenosis greatly decreases the risk of stroke, especially in men with a stenosis diameter of more than 70%.[23, 26] Natural history studies show a high rate of stroke in patients with asymptomatic carotid stenosis of 75% or more; and 80% of carotid atherothrombotic strokes occur without warning symptoms.[26] Data from transcranial Doppler and duplex ultrasonography studies suggests that a carotid artery stenosis with a residual luminal diameter of 1.5 mm (70% to 75% stenosis) represents a point at which a pressure drop across the stenosis (hemodynamically significant stenosis) is likely to occur. At this point, if collateral cerebral blood flow through the ophthalmic artery or circle of Willis is not adequate, low-flow TIAs and infarcts occur. Angioplasty and stenting may become alternatives to carotid endarterectomy.

Preoperative Evaluation

In addition to the neurologic evaluation, these patients should be examined for cardiovascular and renal disease. Predictably, patients with cerebrovascular occlusive disease have occlusive disease in other arteries. For example, ischemic heart disease is a major cause of morbidity and mortality following carotid endarterectomy. Chronic essential hypertension is a common finding. It is useful to establish the range of normal arterial blood pressures for patients preoperatively so as to provide rational guidelines for acceptable perfusion pressures during anesthesia and surgery. The effect of changes in the patient's head position on cerebral function are ascertained, as extreme head rotation, flexion, or extension in patients with co-existing vertebral artery disease could lead to angulation and compression of the artery. Recognition of this response preoperatively allows hazardous head positions (especially hyperextension) to be avoided when patients are unconscious during general anesthesia, particularly during direct laryngoscopy for tracheal intubation. Palpation of the carotid artery is not recommended, as this maneuver could displace fragments of the occlusive intravascular lesion, causing cerebral embolism.

Management of Anesthesia

No clear advantages have been demonstrated for performing carotid endarterectomy under regional (cervical plexus block) or general anesthesia.[27, 28] Regional anesthesia permits patients to remain awake so the neurologic status can be assessed during carotid artery cross-clamping. However, perioperative strokes are more likely to be embolic than low flow in origin. The principal disadvantage of regional anesthesia is the need for patient cooperation. Systemic blood pressure lability may be greater in patients undergoing carotid endarterectomy with general anesthesia, whereas a drug-induced decrease in the cerebral metabolic oxygen requirement may provide some degree of cerebral protection. No anesthetic drug can be recommended for production of general anesthesia. The goals during general anesthesia are to maintain hemodynamic stability and permit prompt emergence, allowing rapid assessment of neurologic status.

Maintenance of adequate systemic blood pressure is important during carotid endarterectomy, as autoregulation may be lost in these patients. Vasopressors such as phenylephrine may be needed to maintain perfusion pressure during cross-clamping of the carotid artery. Some patients become hypertensive during carotid artery cross-clamping and require intravenous administration of vasodilators such as nitroglycerin. Surgical manipulation of the carotid sinus may cause marked alterations in heart rate and systemic blood pressure. It is generally accepted that changes in regional CBF associated with changes in the $PaCO_2$ in these patients are unpredictable, and maintenance of normocarbia is recommended. When the surgeon's practice is not to use a carotid shunt, administration of thiopental, 5 mg/kg IV, prior to cross-clamping the carotid artery is a consideration.

Monitoring often includes an intra-arterial catheter and, in patients with poor left ventricular function (coronary artery disease or a recent myocardial infarction), a pulmonary artery catheter or use of transesophageal echocardiography. No special central nervous system monitoring is required in patients undergoing carotid endarterectomy with regional anesthesia. When general anesthesia is utilized, it is common to monitor brain function during cross-clamping of the carotid artery, although a difference in stroke rate with or without shunting has not been demonstrated. The 16-channel electroencephalogram is the most sensitive indicator of inadequate cerebral perfusion during carotid cross-clamping, and intraoperative neurologic complications correlate with the electroencephalographic changes of cerebral ischemia. Somatosensory evoked potential monitoring, which is useful for monitoring cerebral perfusion during carotid cross-clamping, has a sensitivity similar to that of electroencephalography.[29] Stump pressures (internal carotid back-pressure) below 25 mmHg or above 50 mmHg are useful indicators of the adequacy of cerebral perfusion, although intermediate values are of questionable sensitivity and specificity. Transcranial Doppler, a noninvasive monitor, is valuable for determining the need for shunt placement; it provides a method for prompt recognition of shunt malfunction and management of postoperative hyperperfusion.

Postoperative Management and Complications

Following tracheal extubation, patients are observed for cardiac (blood pressure changes, myocardial ischemia or infarction), airway obstruction (hematoma formation), and neurologic complications (thrombosis, intracerebral hemorrhage).[30] Significant soft tissue edema of the neck may occur following carotid endarterectomy resulting in airway obstruction.[31]

Systemic hypertension is frequently observed during the immediate postoperative period, occurring most commonly in patients with co-existing essential hypertension. Systemic blood pressure is often increased maximally 2 to 3 hours after surgery and may persist for 24 hours. Systemic blood pressure must be lowered to normal ranges to avoid the hazards of cerebral edema and myocardial ischemia. Indeed, the incidence of neurologic defects is increased threefold in patients who become hypertensive postoperatively. Continuous intravenous infusions of nitroprusside are an acceptable treatment to lower the patient's blood pressure acutely. When systemic hypertension persists, longer-acting drugs such as hydralazine or labetalol are options. The mechanism of systemic hypertension is not known but may reflect increased intravascular fluid volume, altered activity of the carotid sinus, or loss of carotid sinus function due to denervation during carotid endarterectomy surgery. Likewise, hypotension can be explained on the basis of increased afferent nerve activity perceived by a carotid sinus previously shielded by an atheromatous plaque. Treatment of hypotension is with vasopressors such as phenylephrine, infusion of crystalloid solutions, and infiltration of the tissues surrounding the carotid sinus with local anesthetic-containing solutions.

Medical Management of Acute Ischemic Stroke

Management of the stroke patient's airway, oxygenation, ventilation, systemic blood pressure, blood glucose concentrations, and body temperature and institution of heparin prophylaxis are part of the initial global medical management.[23] In the most critically ill stroke patients, cerebral edema and increased ICP may complicate the clinical course. The expanding infarction may cause focal and diffuse effects that typically peak 2 to 5 days following the event. Large hemispheric strokes may be characterized by the malignant middle cerebral artery (MCA) syndrome in which the edematous infarcted tissue causes compression of the anterior and posterior cerebral arteries, resulting in secondary infarctions. Similarly, infarction of the cerebellum may result in basilar artery compression and brain stem ischemia. Mortality rates for both MCA syndrome and infarction of the cerebellum approach 80%.

Surgical decompression has a potential role in a small number of stroke patients. Craniotomy with cerebellar resection is a lifesaving intervention for acute cerebellar stoke by virtue of preventing secondary brain stem and vascular compression. The malignant MCA syndrome may be similarly amenable to hemicraniectomy.[23]

Respiratory Function

Respiratory function must be evaluated promptly in all stroke patients. Ventilatory drive is usually intact except after medullary or massive hemispheric infarction. The ability to protect the lungs against aspiration may be impaired in the acute setting, necessitating tracheal intubation. In most patients however, supplemental oxygen administration is sufficient to maintain arterial oxygen saturation above 95%.

Systemic Blood Pressure

Maintenance of adequate systemic blood pressure is critically important as blood flow to ischemic regions is dependent on cerebral perfusion pressure, which is the difference between the MAP and the ICP. Systemic hypertension is common at the time of initial stroke presentation. Rapid lowering of systemic blood pressure could impair CBF and worsen the ischemic injury. Increased systemic blood pressure often gradually decreases during the first few days following the acute stroke. Antihypertensive drug therapy (small intravenous doses of labetalol) may be utilized when necessary to maintain the systemic blood pressure below 185/110 mmHg.

Appropriate intravascular volume replacement in patients with acute stroke improves cardiac output and cerebral perfusion. Hypervolemic hemodilution may be considered in attempts to increase CBF while decreasing blood viscosity without causing significant decreases in oxygen delivery.

Blood Glucose Concentrations

Hyperglycemia appears to parallel the poor outcome in patients experiencing acute ischemic stroke. Glucose may be metabolized to lactic acid, resulting in acidosis and increased tissue injury. Normalization of blood glucose concentrations is recommended, and administration of parenteral glucose is minimized.

Body Temperature

Based on animal data, hypothermia may improve outcome following acute ischemic stroke in patients reflecting decreases in neuronal oxygen demands, cerebral edema, and neurotransmitter toxicity. Even mild increases in body temperature are known to be deleterious, and normothermia should be maintained in acute ischemic stroke patients with antipyretics or cooling blankets.

Heparin Prophylaxis

Prophylaxis for deep vein thrombosis is initiated early in the treatment of patients experiencing acute ischemic stroke. Heparin, 5000 units subcutaneously every 12 hours, is the most common intervention. Patients with acute hemorrhage who cannot be given heparin are treated with pneumatic compression stockings.

Pharmacologic Treatment of Acute Ischemic Stroke

Aspirin is often recommended as initial therapy for acute stroke patients and for the prevention of recurrent strokes. Intravenous recombinant tissue plasminogen activator (rt-PA) is utilized in patients who meet specific eligibility requirements if treatment

can be initiated within 3 hours of the onset of acute symptoms.[32] Direct infusion of thrombolytic drugs (prourokinase) into occluded blood vessels is a potential alternative or adjunctive therapy to intravenous rt-PA. Despite advances in the treatment of acute ischemic stroke, most patients have residual neurologic dysfunction. The initial stroke severity is a strong predictor of outcome, and early evidence of recovery is a good prognostic sign.

Man-in-the-Barrel Syndrome

Man-in-the-barrel syndrome, characterized by bilateral upper extremity paresis with intact motor function in the lower extremities, most often follows an episode of hypotension that causes global cerebral hypoperfusion.[33] Patients are unable to move either arm in response to a stimulus, making it appear as if the upper body is confined in a barrel. The clinical picture is presumed to reflect watershed ischemia or infarction of the border zone between the anterior cerebral artery and posterior cerebral artery following a period of global hypoperfusion. Cortical blindness may also result from watershed ischemia.

Acute Hemorrhagic Stroke

Acute hemorrhagic stroke may manifest as intracerebral hemorrhage or subarachnoid hemorrhage.

Intracerebral Hemorrhage

Intracerebral hemorrhage accounts for 11% of stroke mortality and notably affects African-Americans.[23] Acute hemorrhagic stroke cannot be reliably distinguished from ischemic stroke based on clinical criteria alone. Noncontrast computed tomography imaging is needed to detect the presence of blood. The estimated volume of blood and the level of consciousness are the two most reliable predictors of outcome. Patients with intracerebral hemorrhage often deteriorate clinically as cerebral edema worsens during the 24 to 48 hours following the acute bleed. Late hematoma evacuation is ineffective in decreasing mortality, whereas the efficacy of earlier surgical evacuation of the hematoma to decrease surrounding ischemic tissue injury and edema remains unclear.[23] In addition to surgery there are other strategies to control ICP (see "Methods to Decrease Intracranial Pressure"). Intraventricular hemorrhage is a particularly ominous complication, and prompt ventricular drainage should be performed for any signs of hydrocephalus. Sedation (propofol infusion) with or without drug-induced skeletal muscle paralysis is often helpful for managing patients who require tracheal intubation. An ICP monitor is often recommended for patients who are obtunded (Glasgow Coma Scale score less than 9).[23] Systemic blood pressure management in patients who experience intracerebral hemorrhage is controversial, as there is concern about decreasing cerebral perfusion pressure in those with increased ICP. In patients with co-existing essential hypertension, a goal may be to keep the MAP below 130 mmHg.

Subarachnoid Hemorrhage

Spontaneous subarachnoid hemorrhage most commonly results from aneurysms of the circle of Willis, often involving the anterior and posterior communicating arteries (Fig. 17–6).[23, 34] Systemic hypertension and cigarette smoking are risk factors for aneurysmal rupture. A family history in first-degree relatives of patients with subarachnoid hemorrhage is a risk factor for the presence of intracranial aneurysms, but routine screening is not recommended. The risk of aneurysm rupture depends on the size of the aneurysm with a 6% risk of rupture of aneurysms at least 25 mm in diameter during the first year.

Diagnosis

The diagnosis of subarachnoid hemorrhage is based on the clinical symptoms ("worst headache of my life") and computed tomography demonstration of subarachnoid blood. Magnetic resonance imaging is not sensitive for detecting acute hemorrhage, although this technique may be useful for demonstrating subacute or chronic subarachnoid hemorrhage after computed tomography findings have returned to normal. In addition to severe headache, the rapid onset of photophobia, stiff neck, decreased level of consciousness, and focal neurologic changes suggest subarachnoid hemorrhage. Establishing the diagnosis promptly followed by clipping the aneurysm can decrease morbidity and mortality.

Changes on the ECG are common following subarachnoid hemorrhage (inversion of T waves and ST segment depression). These changes are most often noted within 48 hours following hemorrhage and have been attributed to catecholamine release. The same catecholamine release that may result in cardiac dysrhythmias may be responsible for producing pulmonary edema.

Treatment

Treatment of subarachnoid hemorrhage involves localizing the aneurysm with cerebral angiography and surgically excluding the aneurysmal sac from the intracranial circulation while preserving the parent artery within the first 72 hours after bleeding.[23, 34] In this regard, placing a clip across the neck of the intracranial aneurysm is the most definitive treatment. Endovascular techniques consisting of placing soft metallic coils in the lumen of the aneurysm may serve as an alternative to surgical therapy.[34]

Surgery is often delayed in patients with severe symptoms (coma); and other options, including interventional radiologic procedures, may be utilized. Before proceeding with surgery, patients are often kept mildly sedated and given stool softeners to decrease the risk of rebleeding. Anticonvulsants are administered should seizure activity manifest. Systemic blood pressure is controlled, recognizing that hypertension is related to rebleeding; but at the same time blood pressure may act to tamponade the bleeding. Hydrocephalus is common after subarachnoid hemorrhage and is treated with ventricular drainage. Any change in mental status is promptly evaluated by computed tomography to look for signs of hydrocephalus.

Following aneurysm clipping, the goal is to prevent vasospasm ("intracranial arterial narrowing").[34] The cause of vasospasm is not known but is related to the amount of subarachnoid blood seen on computed tomography. Vasospasm occurs 3 to 15 days after subarachnoid hemorrhage. For this reason, daily transcranial Doppler examinations are performed, and "triple H" therapy (hypertension, hypervolemia, hemodilution) is initiated at the first sign of vasospasm. In this regard colloid and crystalloid therapy is utilized, and pressor support may be needed. Nimodipine, a calcium channel blocker, has been shown to improve outcome when initiated on the first day and continued for 21 days after subarachnoid hemorrhage, presumably reflecting a protective effect against the development of vasospasm.

Management of Anesthesia

The goals of anesthesia during intracranial aneurysm surgery are to limit the risks of aneurysm rupture, prevent cerebral ischemia, and facilitate surgical exposure. Cerebral angiography demonstrates the size and location of the intracranial aneurysm, which subsequently guides the patient's intraoperative positioning. Patients presenting for intracranial aneurysm surgery often manifest hypovolemia, which could exacerbate cerebral vasospasm and associated cerebral ischemia. Hyponatremia may accompany vasospasm and hypovolemia.

Induction of Anesthesia. The goal during induction of anesthesia is to prevent increases in the transmural pressure of the aneurysmal sac (MAP − ICP), which could increase the risk of aneurysmal rupture while maintaining an adequate cerebral perfusion pressure (MAP − ICP), so as to prevent cerebral ischemia. Patients with increased ICP prior to surgery represent a challenge, as they may not tolerate a MAP decrease to protect against aneurysm rupture without the risk of developing cerebral ischemia.

Monitoring the systemic blood pressure via an intra-arterial catheter is desirable to observe the adequacy of systemic blood pressure control during direct laryngoscopy. Prophylaxis against systemic hypertension during direct laryngoscopy may be achieved by prior intravenous administration of nitroprusside (1 to 2 μg/kg 15 to 30 seconds before initiating direct laryngoscopy), lidocaine, or short-acting opioids (fentanyl, sufentanil, remifentanil). Loss of consciousness is achieved with intravenous administration of thiopental, propofol, or etomidate. Nondepolarizing neuromuscular blocking drugs are most often selected to facilitate tracheal intubation.

Placing a central venous pressure catheter is useful, considering the likely presence of hypovolemia, the large intraoperative fluid shifts associated with osmotic and loop diuretics, the potential for intraoperative aneurysm rupture, and the need for fluid resuscitation. A pulmonary artery catheter may be considered when patients have known coronary artery disease. Electrophysiologic monitoring (electroencephalography, somatosensory evoked potentials) may be helpful, but their complexity limits routine use.

Maintenance of Anesthesia. The goals of anesthesia maintenance include providing a depth of anesthesia appropriate to the level of surgical stimulation, facilitating surgical exposure through optimal brain relaxation, maintaining cerebral perfusion pressure, reducing transmural pressure in the aneurysm during clipping of the aneurysm, and prompt awakening to permit neurologic assessment. Drugs and fluid must be immediately available to manage resuscitation should the aneurysm rupture intraoperatively. Most commonly, aneurysm rupture occurs during the late stages of surgical dissection, and anesthetic management consists of aggressive volume resuscitation to maintain normovolemia combined with controlled hypotension (nitroprusside) to permit the neurosurgeon to gain control of the aneurysm. If a temporary clip is used to gain control of a ruptured aneurysm, systemic blood pressure is returned to a normal level to improve collateral blood flow.

Anesthesia is most often maintained with volatile anesthetics (isoflurane, desflurane, sevoflurane), which may be supplemented with intermittent (fentanyl) or continuous infusion of opioids (remifentanil). Alternatively, a total intravenous anesthetic maintenance technique (propofol and fentanyl) can be utilized. Nitrous oxide is a potent cerebral vasodilator, and its use provides little benefit during maintenance of anesthesia.

In view of the trend for earlier surgical intervention in patients with subarachnoid hemorrhage due to rupture of intracranial aneurysms, it is predictable that many patients will manifest intraoperative brain edema. For this reason, optimization of brain relaxation is an important part of anesthetic maintenance. Combinations of lumbar CSF drainage, mild hyperventilation of the patient's lungs, administration of loop and/or osmotic diuretics, and proper patient positioning to facilitate cerebral venous drainage optimize surgical exposure. Intraoperative fluid administration is guided by blood loss, urine output, and measurement of cardiac filling pressures. Normovolemia or modest hypervolemia is the goal, which is best achieved by intravenous administration of balanced salt solutions. Intravenous solutions containing glucose are not recommended for fear of exacerbating focal and global cerebral ischemia.[35]

Controlled Hypotension. Traditionally, drug-induced controlled hypotension has been utilized to decrease transmural pressure in the aneurysm, thereby decreasing the risk of aneurysm rupture during microscopic isolation and clipping. However, the use of controlled hypotension has diminished based on the impairment of autoregulation that follows subarachnoid hemorrhage, the unpredictable cerebrovascular responses to drug-induced hypotension, and the risk of global ischemia. Alternatively, regional controlled hypotension produced by placing a vascular clamp on the parent artery supplying the aneurysm provides protection against aneurysm rupture without the risk of global cerebral ischemia.[36] Ideally, temporary occlusion of the parent artery does not exceed 10 minutes; but if longer periods of occlusion are needed, administration of metabolic suppressants (thiopental) and/or mild hypothermia may provide protection against regional cerebral ischemia and infarction.

Level of Drug-Induced Controlled Hypotension. Safe levels of drug-induced controlled hypotension can be estimated on the basis of predicted CBF, limits of autoregulation of CBF, and the $PaCO_2$.

For example, in normotensive patients MAP 90 mmHg), CBF is about 50 ml/100 g/min. There is no evidence of cerebral ischemia on the electroencephalogram when CBF remains above 25 ml/100 g/min. Assuming that CBF decreases linearly below perfusion pressures of 60 mmHg, blood flow to the brain would be decreased to 25 ml/100 g/min when cerebral perfusion pressure corresponds to a MAP of about 45 mmHg, provided the central venous pressure is 10 mmHg (cerebral perfusion pressure equals mean arterial pressure minus central venous pressure or ICP, whichever is higher). CBF is also decreased about 1 ml for each 1 mmHg decrease in $PaCO_2$. Therefore it is probably important to maintain the $PaCO_2$ at about 35 mmHg during controlled hypotension. On the basis of these concepts, safe cerebral perfusion pressures during controlled hypotension would be produced by a MAP of about 50 mmHg, which corresponds to systolic blood pressures of 60 to 70 mmHg. It should also be appreciated that patients safely tolerate a MAP of less than 50 mmHg for the short period of time needed to clip an intracranial aneurysm. Tolerance to low perfusion pressures is also improved by the zero ICP when the dura is open. Conversely, hypotension produced by hemorrhage is not as well tolerated as similar decreases in systemic blood pressure produced by vasodilating drugs. Presumably, the development of cerebral ischemia during hemorrhagic hypotension reflects sympathetic nervous system discharge, leading to increased cerebral metabolic oxygen requirements.

An alternative to these calculations as a guideline for safe levels of controlled hypotension is to decrease the MAP no more than 30 to 40 mmHg below the patient's normal awake level. This guideline assumes a central venous pressure (or ICP) of 10 mmHg or less and a $PaCO_2$ near 35 mmHg.

When drug-induced controlled hypotension is considered for hypertensive patients, it is important to appreciate the likely rightward shift of the curve for autoregulation of CBF. The lower limit of 60 mmHg assumed for autoregulation in normotensive patients MAP 90 mmHg) should be adjusted upward by an equal amount for each 1 mmHg that the MAP exceeds 90 mmHg. Therefore the lower limit of autoregulation would be 85 mmHg in chronically hypertensive patients with a MAP of 115 mmHg. This lower limit of autoregulation of CBF, and not 60 mmHg, is utilized when estimating safe levels of drug-induced controlled hypotension.

Monitoring Systemic Blood Pressure During Drug-Induced Controlled Hypotension. The need for accurate monitoring of systemic blood pressure

includes strict attention to accurate calibration of the transducer used to measure arterial blood pressure and to proper positioning of the transducer relative to the patient's heart level. With respect to positioning the transducer, a useful guideline is that systolic blood pressure decreases about 0.7 mmHg for each centimeter the patient's head is above the level of the heart. Therefore recording the MAP from a transducer positioned at the patient's heart level would not accurately reflect the perfusion pressure at the brain if the patient's head was elevated above the heart level. For example, when the patient's head is positioned 20 cm above heart level during surgery, the cerebral perfusion pressure is about 14 mmHg less than the MAP present at heart level. If drug-induced controlled hypotension was produced to a MAP of 50 mmHg, as recorded from a transducer at the heart level, the actual perfusion pressure at the patient's brain would be about 36 mmHg. A useful approach during drug-induced controlled hypotension is to place the transducer for measuring arterial blood pressure at the same height as the circle of Willis (level of the patient's external auditory canal).

Emergence from Anesthesia. Prompt emergence from the effects of anesthesia at the conclusion of the surgical procedure is desirable for immediate neurologic evaluation of the patient. The use of short-acting inhaled and injected anesthetic drugs facilitates achieving this goal. Incremental doses of antihypertensive drugs such as labetalol or esmolol may be needed as the patient emerges from anesthesia. In some patients, systolic blood pressures up to 180 mmHg may be tolerated and appropriate for decreasing the risk of vasospasm. Lidocaine may be administered intravenously to suppress airway reflexes and the associated responses to the presence of a tracheal tube. Tracheal extubation is acceptable in patients who are awake with adequate spontaneous ventilation and protective upper airway reflexes. Patients who were obtunded preoperatively are likely to require continued tracheal intubation and support of ventilation during the postoperative period. Likewise, patients who experience intraoperative rupture of intracranial aneurysms may recover slowly and benefit from postoperative airway and ventilation support.

The neurologic status is assessed at frequent time intervals in the postanesthesia care unit or intensive care unit. Occasionally, patients manifest delayed emergence following intracranial aneurysm resection, and it may be difficult to distinguish between drug-induced and surgical causes of this response. However, the appearance of any new focal deficit should raise suspicion of a surgical cause of delayed emergence, as anesthetic drugs would be expected to cause global effects. Unequal pupils that were not present preoperatively are also likely to reflect a surgical event. Computed tomography or angiography may be necessary when the patient does not awaken promptly during the postoperative period. Successful surgical therapy may be followed by delayed deficits due to cerebral vasospasm requiring aggressive therapy (hypertension, hypervolemia, hemodilution).

▌ TRAUMATIC BRAIN INJURY

Traumatic brain injury most often follows motor vehicle accidents and is the leading cause of disability and death in young adults in the United States. Brain injury may be caused by several types of head trauma, including the more typical closed head injury (rapid acceleration or deceleration causes the brain to strike the interior of the skull), a direct impact to the head, and penetrating injuries such as by bullets or foreign objects. Associated injuries including cervical spine injury and thoracoabdominal trauma frequently accompany acute head injury.

Treatment

Initial management of acute head injury patients includes immobilization of the cervical spine, establishment of a patent upper airway, and protection of the patient's lungs from aspiration of gastric contents. The most useful diagnostic procedure, in terms of simplicity and rapidity, is computed tomography, which should be performed as soon as possible. In this regard, computed tomography has greatly facilitated identification of epidural or subdural hematomas. Routine computed tomography may not be needed in patients with minor head trauma who meet the following criteria: no headache or vomiting, less than 60 years of age, no intoxication, no deficits in short-term memory, no physical evidence of trauma above the clavicles, and no seizures.[37]

It is not unusual for patients with traumatic brain injury who initially are stable and awake or in light coma to deteriorate suddenly. Delayed hematoma formation or expanding contusions that are amenable to surgery are often responsible for these changes. Uncontrolled brain swelling that may not respond to conventional management may also cause sudden neurologic deterioration. Delayed secondary injury at the cellular level is an important

contributor to brain swelling and subsequent irreversible brain damage.

The Glasgow Coma Scale score provides a reproducible method for assessing the seriousness of brain injury (scores less than 8 points indicate severe injury) and for following the patient's neurologic status (Table 17–4). Patients with scores less than 8 are by definition in coma, and about 50% of these patients die or remain in vegetative states. The patient's age and type of head injury are important determinants of outcome in the presence of low scores. For example, patients with acute subdural hematomas have a poorer prognosis than patients with diffuse brain contusion injury. Mortality in children with severe head injury is lower than adults.

Perioperative Management

Perioperative management of patients with acute head trauma, such as following motor vehicle accidents, must consider the risks of secondary injury in these patients due to cerebral ischemia. CBF is usually initially decreased and then gradually increases with time. CBF can also decrease during the hyperemic phase due to vasospasm. Factors contributing to poor outcome in head injury patients are increased ICP and systolic blood pressures less than 80 mmHg. Normal autoregulation of CBF is often impaired in patients with acute head injury, and carbon dioxide reactivity is usually preserved. Control of increased ICP with mannitol or furosemide is indicated, and in some patients craniectomy is necessary. Hyperventilation, although effective in

Table 17–4 • Glasgow Coma Scale

Response	Score
Eye opening	
Spontaneous	4
To speech	3
To pain	2
Nil	1
Best motor response	
Obeys	6
Localizes	5
Withdraws (flexion)	4
Abnormal flexion	3
Extensor response	2
Nil	1
Verbal responses	
Oriented	5
Confused conversation	4
Inappropriate words	3
Incomprehensible sounds	2
Nil	1

controlling ICP, may cause cerebral ischemia in head injury patients and for this reason it is a common recommendation not to decrease the $PaCO_2$ below 30 mmHg. A small subset of head injury patients may benefit from drug-induced coma using barbiturates. Hypothermia decreases cerebral metabolic oxygen requirements, cerebral blood volume, and CBF; and it may also be cerebroprotective. Nevertheless, treatment with hypothermia, with the body temperature reaching 33°C within 8 hours after injury, is not effective in improving outcomes in patients with severe head trauma.[38] Administration of hypertonic saline and mannitol may decrease CSF production. Associated lung injuries may impair oxygenation and ventilation in these patients and necessitate mechanical support of ventilation. Coagulopathy occurs in head injury patients and may be enhanced by hypothermia and the need for massive blood transfusions. Replacement of clotting factors may be necessary.

Management of Anesthesia

Management of anesthesia includes efforts to optimize cerebral perfusion pressures, minimize the occurrence of cerebral ischemia, and avoid drugs and techniques that could increase the ICP. Cerebral perfusion pressures are maintained above 70 mmHg if possible, and hyperventilation is not used unless it is needed as a temporizing measure to control the ICP. During surgical evacuation of acute epidural or subdural hematomas, systemic blood pressure may decrease precipitously at the time of surgical decompression and require aggressive fluid resuscitation. Patients with severe head injury may experience impaired oxygenation and ventilation that complicates the intraoperative period. The use of positive end-expiratory pressure to improve oxygenation must be balanced against the potential risks of increasing the ICP. Adequate fluid resuscitation and replacement are important during the intraoperative period. Although administration of colloids may have theoretical advantages for decreasing cerebral edema following head trauma, their use in critically ill patients may be associated with increased mortality. Hypertonic crystalloid solutions, such as 3% saline, increase the plasma osmotic pressure and thus remove water from the brain's interstitial space. Hypotonic crystalloid solutions are avoided, as they decrease plasma osmotic pressure and increase cerebral edema even in normal brains.

Induction and Maintenance of Anesthesia

In hemodynamically stable patients, rapid induction of anesthesia with intravenous induction drugs and facilitation of tracheal intubation with nondepolarizing muscle relaxants is acceptable. Maintenance of anesthesia often includes continuous infusions of intravenous drugs, keeping in mind the goal to optimize cerebral perfusion pressures and prevent increases in ICP. Low doses of volatile anesthetics may be added to the intravenous drug infusions, whereas nitrous oxide is likely to be avoided. Among the volatile anesthetics, sevoflurane may be unique in not impairing cerebral autoregulation.[39, 40] If acute brain swelling develops, correctable causes such as hypercarbia, arterial hypoxemia, systemic hypertension, and venous obstruction must be considered and corrected if present. Intra-arterial monitoring of systemic blood pressure is helpful, whereas time constraints may limit the use of central venous pressure or pulmonary artery catheter monitoring.

Postoperative Period

During the postoperative period, it is common to maintain skeletal muscle paralysis to facilitate mechanical ventilation of the patient's lungs. Continuous monitoring of ICP is likely to be maintained.

Epidural Hematoma

Epidural hematoma results from arterial bleeding into the space between the skull and dura. The cause is usually rupture of a meningeal artery associated with a skull fracture. Classically, patients experience loss of consciousness in association with head injury, followed by return of consciousness and a variable lucid period. Hemiparesis, mydriasis, and bradycardia then suddenly develop a few hours after the head injury, reflecting uncal herniation and brain stem compression. If an epidural hematoma is suspected on computed tomography, the treatment is prompt placement of burr holes at the site of the skull fracture.

Subdural Hematoma

Subdural hematoma results from lacerated or torn bridging veins that bleed into the space between the dura and arachnoid. Examination of CSF reveals clear fluid as it represents subarachnoid fluid. Diagnosis of subdural hematoma is confirmed by computed tomography. Head trauma is the most common cause of subdural hematomas. Patients may view the causative head trauma as trivial, and it may have been forgotten by the patient. Trivial head injury associated with formation of a subdural hematoma is most likely to occur in elderly patients. Occasionally, subdural hematoma formation is spontaneous, as in patients on hemodialysis or those being treated with anticoagulants.

Signs and symptoms of a subdural hematoma characteristically evolve gradually over several days (in contrast to epidural hematomas) because the hematoma that results is due to slow venous bleeding. Headache is a universal complaint of patients with subdural hematomas. Drowsiness and obtundation are characteristic findings, but the magnitude of these changes may fluctuate from hour to hour. Lateralizing neurologic signs eventually occur, manifesting as hemiparesis, hemianopsia, and language disturbances. Elderly patients may have unexplained progressive dementia.

Conservative medical management of subdural hematomas may be acceptable for patients whose condition stabilizes. Nevertheless, the most likely treatment is surgical evacuation of the clot, as the prognosis is poor if coma develops.

DEGENERATIVE DISEASES OF THE NERVOUS SYSTEM

Degenerative diseases of the nervous system may reflect defects in the development of the neural tube, which might not result in symptoms until adulthood. Often a hereditary pattern is responsible for these disorders. Pathologic processes may be diffuse or may involve only those neurons that are anatomically and functionally related.

Aqueductal Stenosis

Aqueductal stenosis is caused by congenital narrowing of the cerebral aqueduct that connects the third and fourth ventricles. Obstructive hydrocephalus can develop during infancy, when the narrowing is severe. Lesser degrees of obstruction result in slowly progressive hydrocephalus, which may not be evident until adulthood. Symptoms of aqueductal stenosis are the same as those seen with increased ICP. Seizure disorders are present in about one-third of these patients. Computed tomography confirms the presence of obstructive hydrocephalus. Aqueductal stenosis sufficient to produce signs of hydrocephalus and increased ICP is treated by ventricular shunting. Management of anesthesia for the creation of a cerebral ventricular shunt must consider the likely presence of increased ICP in these patients.

Arnold-Chiari Malformation

Arnold-Chiari malformation consists of downward displacement of the tonsillar portion of the cerebellum and caudad portion of the medulla through the foramen magnum into the upper cervical spinal canal. Cerebellar herniation results in the formation of arachnoidal adhesions, leading to obstruction of CSF flow from the fourth cerebral ventricle. This obstruction can lead to hydrocephalus and increased ICP. In addition, there is progressive entrapment of cranial nerves and torsion of the brain stem.

Signs and symptoms of Arnold-Chiari malformation appear at any age. The most common complaint is an occipital headache, often extending into the shoulders and arms, with corresponding cutaneous dysesthesias. Pain is aggravated by coughing or moving the head. Visual disturbances, intermittent vertigo, and ataxia are prominent symptoms. Signs of syringomyelia are present in about 50% of patients with this disorder.

Treatment of Arnold-Chiari malformation consists of surgical decompression by freeing adhesions and enlarging the foramen magnum. Management of anesthesia must consider the possibility of associated increases in ICP.

Syringomyelia

Syringomyelia is chronic, slowly progressive degeneration of the spinal cord, leading to cavitation. Presumably, this degeneration reflects an abnormality of embryologic development associated with obstruction to the outflow of CSF from the fourth cerebral ventricle. The pressure of the CSF is directed into the central canal of the spinal cord, which eventually leads to cyst formation.

Signs and symptoms of syringomyelia usually begin during the third or fourth decade of life. Early complaints are those of dissociated sensory impairment in the upper extremities, reflecting destruction of crossing fibers that convey the sensation of pain and temperature. As cavitation of the spinal cord progresses, destruction of lower motor neurons ensues, with the development of skeletal muscle weakness and wasting with areflexia. Thoracic scoliosis may result from weakness of paravertebral muscles. Extension of the cavitation process cephalad into the medulla results in syringobulbia characterized by paralysis of the palate, tongue, and vocal cords and loss of sensation over the face. Magnetic resonance imaging is the preferred diagnostic procedure.

No known treatment is effective in arresting the progressive degeneration of the spinal cord or medulla. Surgical procedures designed to restore normal CSF flow or to plug the central cavity have not been predictably effective.

Management of anesthesia in patients with syringomyelia or syringobulbia should consider the neurologic deficits associated with this disease. Thoracic scoliosis can contribute to ventilation-to-perfusion mismatching. The presence of lower motor neuron disease leading to skeletal muscle wasting suggests the possibility that hyperkalemia could develop after administration of succinylcholine. Likewise, co-existing skeletal muscle weakness could be associated with exaggerated responses to nondepolarizing muscle relaxants. Body temperature is often monitored, as thermal regulation may be impaired. Selection of drugs for induction and maintenance of anesthesia is not influenced by this disease. The possible presence of decreased or absent protective airway reflexes should be considered when contemplating removal of the tracheal tube during the postoperative period.

Amyotrophic Lateral Sclerosis

Amyotrophic lateral sclerosis (ALS) is a degenerative disease of motor ganglia in the anterior horn of the spinal cord and spinal pyramidal tracts. It most commonly afflicts men 40 to 60 years of age. When the degenerative process is limited to the motor cortex the disease is designated primary lateral sclerosis; limitation to the brain stem nuclei is known as pseudobulbar palsy. Werdnig-Hoffmann disease resembles ALS, except that manifestations of this disease occur during the first 3 years of life. Although the cause of ALS is unknown, occasionally a genetic pattern is present. A viral etiology is also a consideration.

Signs and symptoms of ALS reflect upper and lower motor neuron dysfunction. Frequent initial manifestations include skeletal muscle atrophy, weakness, and fasciculations, often beginning in the intrinsic muscles of the hands. With time, atrophy and weakness involve most of the patient's skeletal muscles, including the tongue, pharynx, larynx, and chest. Early symptoms of bulbar involvement include fasciculations of the tongue and dysphagia leading to pulmonary aspiration. For reasons that are not clear the ocular muscles are spared. Evidence of autonomic nervous system dysfunction in these patients manifests as orthostatic hypotension and resting tachycardia. Inability to control emotional responses is characteristic. Complaints of cramping and aching sensations, particularly in the legs, are common. Carcinoma of the lung has been associated with ALS. Plasma creatine kinase concentrations are

normal, distinguishing this disease from chronic polymyositis. ALS has no known treatment, and death is likely within 6 years after the onset of clinical symptoms, usually due to respiratory failure.

General anesthesia in patients with ALS may be associated with exaggerated ventilatory depression. In this regard, patients with lower motor neuron diseases such as ALS are vulnerable to hyperkalemia following administration of succinylcholine. Furthermore, these patients may show prolonged responses to nondepolarizing muscle relaxants.[41] Indeed, changes of ALS, as displayed on the electromyogram, resemble those of myasthenia gravis. Bulbar involvement with dysfunction of pharyngeal muscles may predispose to pulmonary aspiration. There is no evidence that specific anesthetic drugs or combinations of drugs are best for patients with this disease. Regional anesthesia is likely to be avoided for fear of exacerbating the disease. Nevertheless, epidural anesthesia has been successfully administered to patients with ALS without neurologic exacerbation or impairment of pulmonary function.[42, 43]

Tuberous Sclerosis

Tuberous sclerosis (Bourneville's disease) is an autosomal dominant disease characterized by mental retardation, seizures, and facial angiofibromas.[44] Pathologically, tuberous sclerosis can be viewed as a condition where a constellation of benign hamartomatous proliferative lesions and malformations (hamartias) occur in virtually every organ of the body. Brain lesions resulting from tuberous sclerosis include cortical tubers and giant cell astrocytomas. Cardiac rhabdomyoma, although rare, is the commonest benign cardiac tumor associated with tuberous sclerosis. Echocardiography and magnetic resonance imaging are useful for detecting cardiac tumors. An association of Wolff-Parkinson-White syndrome with tuberous sclerosis has been described. Renal involvement in tuberous sclerosis in the form of angiomyolipomas and cysts may result in renal failure. Oral lesions such as nodular tumors, fibromas, or papillomas may be present on the tongue, palate, pharynx, and larynx. The prognosis of patients with tuberous sclerosis depends on the organ systems involved, ranging from no symptoms to life-threatening complications.

Management of anesthesia in patients with tuberous sclerosis considers the likely presence of mental retardation and treatment of seizures with antiepileptic drugs. Upper airway abnormalities are determined preoperatively. Cardiac involvement may be associated with intraoperative cardiac dysrhythmias. Impaired renal function may have implications when selecting drugs that depend on renal clearance mechanisms. Although experience is limited, these patients seem to respond normally to inhaled and injected drugs, including opioids.[44]

Friedreich's Ataxia

Friedreich's ataxia is an autosomal recessive inherited condition characterized by degeneration of the spinocerebellar and pyramidal tracts. Cardiomyopathy is present in 10% to 50% of patients with this disease. Kyphoscoliosis, producing a steady deterioration of pulmonary function, is present in nearly 80% of affected patients. Ataxia is the typical presenting symptom. Dysarthria, nystagmus, skeletal muscle weakness and spasticity, and diabetes mellitus may be present. Friedreich's ataxia is usually fatal by early adulthood, often due to cardiac failure.

Management of anesthesia for Friedreich's ataxia is as described for ALS. In addition, the potential for exaggerated negative inotropic effects of anesthetic drugs in the presence of cardiomyopathy should be considered. Although experience is limited, the response to muscle relaxants seems normal.[45] Kyphoscoliosis may make epidural anesthesia technically difficult, whereas spinal anesthesia has been used successfully.[46] The likelihood of postoperative ventilatory failure may be increased, especially in the presence of kyphoscoliosis.

Parkinson's Disease

Parkinson's disease is a neurodegenerative disorder of unknown cause.[47] Increasing age is the single most important risk factor in the development of this disease. There is a characteristic loss of dopaminergic fibers normally present in the basal ganglia. As a result of the degeneration of these fibers, dopamine levels are depleted in basal ganglia. Dopamine is presumed to inhibit the rate of firing of the neurons that control the extrapyramidal motor system. Depletion of dopamine results in diminished inhibition of the extrapyramidal motor system and unopposed actions of acetylcholine.

Signs and Symptoms

The classic triad of major signs of Parkinson's disease is made up of skeletal muscle tremor, rigidity, and akinesia.[47] Skeletal muscle rigidity first appears in the proximal muscles of the neck. The earliest manifestations may be loss of associated arm swings when walking and absence of head rotation when turning the body. Facial immobility is characterized by infrequent blinking and by a paucity of emotional responses. Tremors are characterized as rhythmic, alternating flexion and extension of the thumbs and other digits at a rate of four or five movements per second ("pill-rolling tremor"). Tremors are most prominent in resting limbs but tend to disappear during the course of voluntary movement. Seborrhea, oily skin, pupillary abnormalities, diaphragmatic spasms, and oculogyric crises are frequent. Dementia and depression are often present.

Treatment

Treatment of Parkinson's disease is designed to increase the concentration of dopamine in the basal ganglia or to decrease the neuronal effects of acetylcholine.[47, 48] Drugs such as anticholinergics, amantadine, and monoamine oxidase inhibitors (selegiline) provide only mild to moderate benefit in these patients. Replacement therapy with the dopamine precursor levodopa combined with a decarboxylase inhibitor (prevents peripheral conversion of levodopa to dopamine and optimizes the amount of levodopa available to enter the central nervous system) is the standard medical treatment for Parkinson's disease. Indeed, levodopa is the most effective treatment for Parkinson's disease, and early treatment with this drug prolongs life. Levodopa is also associated with a number of side effects including dyskinesias (most serious side effect, developing in 80% of patients after 1 year of treatment) and psychiatric disturbances (agitation, hallucinations, mania, paranoia). Increased myocardial contractility and heart rate in treated patients may reflect increased levels of dopamine converted from levodopa. Orthostatic hypotension may be prominent in treated patients. Gastrointestinal side effects of levodopa therapy include nausea and vomiting, most likely reflecting stimulation of the chemoreceptor trigger zone by dopamine.

Surgical treatment of Parkinson's disease is reserved for disabling and medically refractory symptoms. Interventions at the thalamic nucleus may transiently relieve tremor. Pallidotomy is associated with significant improvement in levodopa-induced dyskinesias, although the improvement may be short-lived. Fetal tissue transplantation for treatment of Parkinson's disease is based on the demonstration that implanted embryonic dopaminergic neurons can survive in recipients.[48]

Management of Anesthesia

Management of anesthesia in patients with Parkinson's disease is based on an understanding of the treatment of this disease and the associated potential adverse drug effects. The elimination half-time of levodopa and the dopamine it produces is brief, so interruption of therapy for more than 6 to 12 hours can result in an abrupt loss of therapeutic effects derived from this drug.[49] The abrupt withdrawal of levodopa can lead to skeletal muscle rigidity, which interferes with maintaining adequate ventilation. In this regard, levodopa therapy should be continued during the perioperative period including the usual morning dose on the day of surgery. Oral levodopa can be administered about 20 minutes before inducing anesthesia and may be repeated intraoperatively and postoperatively. Alternatively, enteral administration of levodopa during the perioperative period may minimize the likelihood of exacerbations.[50]

The possibility of orthostatic hypotension, cardiac dysrhythmias, and even systemic hypertension must be considered during administration of anesthesia to patients being treated with levodopa. When selecting the drugs to be administered as preoperative medication, including antiemetics and anesthetics, one must consider the ability of butyrophenones (droperidol) to antagonize the effects of dopamine in the basal ganglia. An acute dystonic reaction following administration of alfentanil has been speculated to reflect opioid-induced decreases in central dopaminergic transmission.[51] Use of ketamine is questionable because of the possible provocation of exaggerated sympathetic nervous system responses. Nevertheless, ketamine has been administered safely to patients treated with levodopa. Decreased intravascular fluid volume may manifest as lowered systemic blood pressures during the induction of anesthesia, a situation that requires aggressive administration of crystalloid or colloid solutions. The choice of muscle relaxants does not seem to be influenced by the presence of Parkinson's disease.

Hallervorden-Spatz Disease

Hallervorden-Spatz disease is a rare autosomal recessive disorder of the basal ganglia. It follows a slowly progressive course from its onset during late childhood to death in about 10 years. No specific laboratory tests are diagnostic for this condition, and no effective treatment is known. Dementia and dystonia with torticollis, as well as scoliosis, are commonly present. Dystonic posturing is likely to disappear with the induction of anesthesia, although skeletal muscle contractures and bony changes may accompany the chronic forms of the disease, leading to immobility of the temporomandibular joint and cervical spine, even in the presence

of deep general anesthesia or drug-induced skeletal muscle paralysis.

Management of anesthesia must consider the possibility of being unable to position these patients optimally for tracheal intubation following the induction of anesthesia.[52] Noxious stimulation, as produced by attempted awake tracheal intubation, can intensify dystonia. For these reasons, induction of anesthesia may be achieved by inhalation and maintenance of spontaneous ventilation. Administration of succinylcholine is questionable, as skeletal muscle wasting and diffuse axonal changes in the brain, which may involve the upper motor neurons, could accentuate the release of potassium. Any required skeletal muscle relaxation is probably best provided by increased concentrations of volatile anesthetics or administration of nondepolarizing neuromuscular blocking drugs. Emergence from anesthesia is predictably accompanied by return of dystonic posturing.

Polyglucosan Body Disease

Polyglucosan body disease is a rare neurologic disorder characterized by progressive involvement of the upper and lower motor neurons, sensory loss predominantly in the legs, early neurogenic bladder, and in some individuals dementia.[53] Pathologically, there is an accumulation of intra-axonal polyglucosan bodies (glucose polymers) in the central and peripheral nervous systems. Experience is too limited to make recommendations regarding management of anesthesia, although uneventful general anesthesia without the use of muscle relaxants has been described.[53] Selection of regional anesthesia may be influenced by the presence of co-existing neurologic deficits.

Huntington's Chorea

Huntington's chorea is a premature degenerative disease of the central nervous system characterized by marked atrophy of the caudate nucleus and, to a lesser degree, the putamen and globus pallidus.[54] Biochemical abnormalities include deficiencies of acetylcholine in the basal ganglia and its synthesizing enzyme choline acetyltransferase and γ-aminobutyric acid (GABA). Selective loss of GABA may decrease inhibition of the dopamine nigrostriatal system. This disease is transmitted as an autosomal dominant trait, but its delayed appearance until 35 to 40 years of age interferes with effective genetic counseling.

Manifestations of Huntington's chorea consist of progressive dementia combined with choreoathetosis. Chorea is usually considered the first sign of Huntington's chorea, although behavioral changes (depression, dementia) may precede the onset of involuntary movement by several years. Involvement of the pharyngeal muscles makes these patients susceptible to pulmonary aspiration. The disease progresses over several years, and accompanying mental depression makes suicide a frequent cause of death. The duration of Huntington's chorea from its onset to the patient's death averages 17 years.

Treatment of Huntington's chorea is symptomatic and is directed at decreasing the choreiform movements. Haloperidol may be administered to control the chorea and emotional lability associated with the disease. The most useful therapy for controlling involuntary movements is with drugs that interfere with the neurotransmitter effects of dopamine. Butyrophenones may be helpful in this regard.

Experience with the management of anesthesia in patients with Huntington's chorea is too limited to recommend specific anesthetic drugs or techniques. Preoperative sedation utilizing butyrophenones such as droperidol may be helpful in controlling choreiform movements. The increased likelihood of pulmonary aspiration must be considered if pharyngeal muscles are involved. Nitrous oxide combined with opioids and droperidol may be a useful approach in view of the possible antagonism of dopamine by droperidol. Nevertheless, the use of nitrous oxide and volatile anesthetics such as sevoflurane is also acceptable.[55] Thiopental, succinylcholine, and mivacurium have been administered without adverse effects. Decreased plasma cholinesterase activity, with prolonged responses to succinylcholine, has been observed. Likewise, it has been suggested that these patients may be sensitive to the effects of nondepolarizing muscle relaxants.[56]

Olivopontocerebellar Degeneration

Olivopontocerebellar degeneration is a diverse group of diseases related by a common loss of neurons in the inferior olives, ventral pons, and cerebellar cortex. Cerebellar disturbances are the most common features and can progress from an ataxic gait to static and kinetic motion disorders. Dysarthria is common. Dysphagia often results in repeated choking and regurgitation. Laryngeal paralysis has been observed. As the disease progresses, abnormal movements, ocular motion disturbances (ophthalmoplegia), urinary incontinence, and mental deterioration may occur. Huntington's chorea and Friedreich's ataxia are closely related disorders. Regional anesthesia has been safely utilized for labor and delivery.[57] It is useful to document neurologic deficits before performing regional anesthesia. If general anesthesia is needed, it is prudent to avoid succinylcholine and to titrate doses of nondepolarizing muscle relaxants. These patients may be at high risk for aspiration of gastric contents.

Strumpell's Disease

Strumpell's disease (hereditary or familial spastic paraparesis) is a genetically determined neurodegenerative disorder manifesting as spastic paresis and sensory deficits predominantly of the lower limbs. Degenerative changes are present in the corticospinal and spinocerebellar tracts. General anesthesia is associated with the risk of aspiration, prolonged responses to nondepolarizing muscle relaxants, and hyperkalemic responses to succinylcholine.[58] The use of regional anesthesia has generally been discouraged in patients with central nervous system diseases owing to the theoretical risk of exacerbating the disease process. There is no evidence that this notion is valid, and epidural anesthesia has been used safely in patients with Strumpell's disease.[58]

Isaacs Syndrome

Isaacs syndrome is a rare peripheral motor neuron disorder. Involuntary continuous muscle fiber activity may cause stiffness, delayed relaxation of affected skeletal muscles, and continuous fine vibrating skeletal muscle movements (myokymia).[59] Patients affected by this syndrome may also experience ataxia, staggering and reeling, and an inability to coordinate voluntary muscle movements. The cause of Isaacs syndrome is not known but may reflect the presence of autoantibodies to peripheral potassium channels. In this regard, this syndrome may be associated with thymoma, myasthenia gravis, and the Eaton-Lambert syndrome. Treatment options include phenytoin, acetazolamide, or carbamazepine. Abnormal skeletal muscle discharges may be abolished by succinylcholine, epidural anesthesia, and spinal anesthesia, whereas there is increased sensitivity to nondepolarizing muscle relaxants. Epidural anesthesia has been administered for labor and delivery without incident.[59]

Spasmodic Torticollis

Spasmodic torticollis is thought to result from disturbances of basal ganglia function. The most common mode of presentation is spasmodic contraction of nuchal muscles, which may progress to involvement of limb and girdle muscles. Hypertrophy of the sternocleidomastoid muscles may be present. Spasm may involve the muscles of the vertebral column, leading to lordosis, scoliosis, and impaired ventilation. Treatment is not particularly effective, but a bilateral anterior rhizotomy at C1 and C3, with a subarachnoid section of the spinal accessory nerve, may be attempted. This operation may cause postoperative paralysis of the diaphragm, resulting in respiratory distress. There are no known problems relative to the selection of anesthetic drugs, but spasm of nuchal muscles can interfere with maintenance of a patent upper airway before institution of skeletal muscle paralysis. Furthermore, awake tracheal intubation may be necessary if chronic skeletal muscle spasm has led to fixation of the cervical vertebrae. Sudden appearance of torticollis after the induction of anesthesia has been reported; and administration of diphenhydramine, 25 to 50 mg IV, produces dramatic reversal of drug-induced torticollis.[60]

Shy-Drager Syndrome

Shy-Drager syndrome is characterized by autonomic nervous system dysfunction in association with widespread parenchymatous degeneration in the central nervous system and spinal cord. Although the primary defect is loss of neuronal cells, an element of sympathetic nervous system dysfunction can result from depletion of norepinephrine from peripheral efferent nerve endings. Idiopathic orthostatic hypotension, rather than Shy-Drager syndrome, is thought to be present when autonomic nervous system dysfunction occurs in the absence of central nervous system degeneration.

Signs and Symptoms

Signs and symptoms of Shy-Drager syndrome are related to dysfunction of the autonomic nervous system, as manifested by orthostatic hypotension, urinary retention, bowel dysfunction, diminished sweating, and sexual impotence. Postural hypotension is often severe enough to produce syncope. Plasma norepinephrine concentrations fail to show a normal increase after standing or exercise. Sweating may be absent, pupillary reflexes sluggish, and control of breathing abnormal. Further evidence of autonomic nervous system dysfunction is failure of baroreceptor reflexes to produce increases in heart rate or vasoconstriction in response to hypotension.

Symptoms of Parkinson's disease often develop in these patients.

Treatment

Treatment of orthostatic hypotension is symptomatic and includes head-up tilt at night, elastic stockings, high sodium diet to expand the intravascular fluid volume, and administration of α-agonists.[61] Death usually occurs within 8 years of the diagnosis, most often due to cerebral ischemia from prolonged hypotension. Theoretically, orthostatic hypotension can be lessened by treatment with selective α_2-agonists such as yohimbine, which would facilitate continued release of norepinephrine from postganglionic nerve endings. Levodopa is administered to decrease symptoms of Parkinson's disease.

Management of Anesthesia

Management of anesthesia is based on understanding the impact of decreased autonomic nervous system activity on the cardiovascular responses to such events as changes in body position, positive airway pressure, and acute blood loss, as well as the effects produced by administration of negative inotropic anesthetic drugs. Preoperative evaluation may elicit signs of autonomic nervous system dysfunction such as orthostatic hypotension and the absence of beat-to-beat variability in heart rate associated with deep breathing.

Despite the obvious vulnerability of these patients to events likely to occur during the perioperative period, clinical experience has shown that most patients tolerate general and regional anesthesia without undue risk.[61, 62] The key to the management of these patients is continuous monitoring of the systemic blood pressure and prompt correction of hypotension by infusion of crystalloid or colloid solutions. Continuous measurement of systemic blood pressure and cardiac filling pressures is useful for guiding the rate of intravenous fluid infusions. If vasopressors are needed, it should be appreciated that these patients may exhibit exaggerated responses to drugs that act by provoking the release of norepinephrine. Presumably, these excessive responses reflect denervation hypersensitivity. An appropriate choice for treating hypotension pharmacologically is a direct-acting vasopressor such as phenylephrine. Even the dose of phenylephrine should be initially decreased until the response of the individual patient can be confirmed. A continuous infusion of phenylephrine, 0.5 to 1.5 μg/kg/min IV, may be used to maintain systemic blood pressure in affected patients during general anesthesia.[61] The risk of hypotension after administering spinal or epidural anesthesia detracts from the use of these techniques in affected patients, although safe use of spinal anesthesia has been described.[62] Excessive decreases in cardiac output due to myocardial depression from volatile anesthetics can result in exaggerated hypotension. This is because compensatory responses such as vasoconstriction or tachycardia are unlikely in view of absent carotid sinus activity. Likewise, positive-pressure ventilation of the patient's lungs and acute blood loss may increase sympathetic nervous system activity. Bradycardia, which contributes to hypotension, is best treated with atropine. Signs of deep anesthesia may be less apparent in these patients because of decreased responses of the sympathetic nervous system to noxious stimulation. Induction of anesthesia with diazepam and fentanyl, pancuronium for skeletal muscle paralysis, and low doses of volatile anesthetic drugs combined with nitrous oxide has been described in these patients. Administration of muscle relaxants with minimal to absent effects on the systemic circulation represents an alternative to pancuronium. Thiopental, as used for induction of anesthesia, might provoke exaggerated decreases in systemic blood pressure if the rate of intravenous administration is rapid or if the patient's intravascular fluid volume is decreased. Conversely, the possibility of accentuated systemic blood pressure increases following administration of ketamine is a theoretical possibility.

Orthostatic Intolerance Syndrome

Orthostatic intolerance syndrome (postural tachycardia syndrome, hyperadrenergic orthostatic tachycardia) is a chronic idiopathic disorder of primary autonomic system failure characterized by episodic or postural tachycardia that occurs independent of alterations in the systemic blood pressure.[63] This syndrome is most often observed in young women. Symptoms often include palpitations, tremulousness, light-headedness, fatigue, and syncope. The pathophysiology of the orthostatic intolerance syndrome is unclear, although possible explanations include enhanced sensitivity of β_1-adrenergic receptors, hypovolemia, excessive venous pooling during standing, primary dysautonomia, and lower extremity sympathetic nervous system denervation.[64]

Medical treatment of patients with orthostatic intolerance syndrome includes attempts to increase the intravascular fluid volume (increased sodium and water intake, administration of mineralocorticoids) to increase venous return. Long-term administration of α_1-adrenergic agonists (phenylephrine, norepinephrine, midodrine) may compensate for

decreased sympathetic nervous system activity in the patient's lower extremities and blunt heart rate responses to standing by activating baroreceptor reflexes.

Management of anesthesia in patients with orthostatic intolerance syndrome includes preoperative administration of crystalloid solutions to expand the patient's intravascular fluid volume. Low-dose phenylephrine infusions may be cautiously administered recognizing that lower extremity sympathetic nervous system denervation may cause up-regulation of α_1-adrenergic receptors and contribute to receptor hypersensitivity. The combination of volume expansion and low-dose phenylephrine infusions should augment peripheral vascular tone, maintain systemic blood pressure, and decrease autonomic nervous system lability in the presence of vasodilating anesthetic drugs (volatile anesthetics) or techniques (epidural or spinal anesthesia). Postoperative pain management may utilize neuraxial opioids.

Chronic Fatigue Syndrome

Chronic fatigue syndrome is a relatively common condition of unclear origin.[65] Clinical features (headaches, myalgias, insomnia) resemble disorders referred to in the past as neurasthenia, neuromyasthenia, effort syndrome, or myalgic encephalopathy. It is estimated that chronic fatigue syndrome affects as many as 400 per 100,000 adults.[65] There is a potential for prolonged illness and substantial impairment of function in individuals who experience chronic fatigue syndrome. No pharmacologic therapy has been found to be consistently effective.

Chronic fatigue is recognized as a feature of autonomic nervous system dysfunction. There may be a relation between chronic fatigue syndrome and neurally mediated hypotension (vasovagal hypotension). Related forms of chronic orthostatic intolerance have been described in those with chronic fatigue syndrome.[65]

Harlequin Syndrome

Harlequin syndrome is characterized by unilateral cutaneous color changes, flushing, and diaphoresis, which seem to be due to dysfunction of the autonomic nervous system.[66] These changes often occur over the face. Vasomotor instability may be present.

Congenital Insensitivity to Pain

Congenital insensitivity to pain with anhidrosis is a rare heredity disorder that leads to self-mutilation and defective thermoregulation. Plasma concentrations of catecholamines may be decreased, and autonomic nervous system dysfunction may be present. Skeletal muscle weakness and joint laxity are characteristic. Management of anesthesia includes giving preoperative medication to relieve apprehension in patients who are often mentally retarded, monitoring body temperature, and avoiding joint extension.[67] Use of anticholinergic drugs is questionable considering the presence of anhidrosis and potential autonomic nervous system dysfunction. Indeed, systemic hypertension and tachycardia have been described following intravenous administration of scopolamine.[68]

Progressive Blindness

Degenerative diseases of the central nervous system limited to the optic nerve and retina include Leber's optic atrophy, retinitis pigmentosa, and the Kearns-Sayer syndrome. The most common cause of blindness during the postoperative period is ischemic optic neuropathy.[69] Other causes of postoperative visual defects are cortical blindness, retinal artery occlusion, and ophthalmic venous obstruction.

Leber's Optic Atrophy

Leber's optic atrophy is characterized by degeneration of the retina and atrophy of the optic nerves culminating in blindness. This disease is transmitted as a sex-linked autosomal recessive trait. Because the defect responsible for optic atrophy is most likely related to an abnormality of cyanide metabolism, these patients should probably not be given nitroprusside.

Retinitis Pigmentosa

Retinitis pigmentosa describes a genetically and clinically heterogeneous group of inherited retinopathies characterized by degeneration of the retina. These debilitating disorders collectively represent the most frequent forms of human visual handicap, with an estimated prevalence of about 1 in 3000. Mutations responsible for retinitis pigmentosa occur in genes responsible for encoding transmembranous proteins of the outer optic disc. Examination of the retina shows areas of pigmentation, particularly in the peripheral regions. Vision is lost from the periphery of the retina toward the center until total blindness develops.

Kearns-Sayer Syndrome

Kearns-Sayer syndrome is characterized by retinitis pigmentosa associated with progressive external ophthalmoplegia, typically manifesting before 20 years of age. Cardiac conduction abnormalities, ranging from bundle branch block to third-degree atrioventricular heart block, are common. Third-degree atrioventricular heart block can occur abruptly, leading to sudden death. Generalized degeneration of the central nervous system has been observed. This finding and the often increased concentrations of protein in the CSF suggest a viral etiology for this syndrome. Although Kearns-Sayer syndrome is rare, it is possible these patients will require anesthesia for placement of artificial external cardiac pacemakers.

Management of anesthesia requires a high index of suspicion and prior preparation to treat third-degree atrioventricular heart block should this cardiac conduction abnormality occur during the perioperative period. Such preparation includes prompt availability of isoproterenol for intravenous infusion as a chemical cardiac pacemaker to maintain an acceptable heart rate until an external artificial cardiac pacemaker can be placed. Experience is too limited to recommend specific drugs for induction and maintenance of anesthesia. Presumably, the response to succinylcholine and nondepolarizing muscle relaxants is not altered, as this disease does not involve the neuromuscular junctions.[70]

Ischemic Optic Neuropathy

Ischemic optic neuropathy should be suspected in patients who complain of visual loss during the first postoperative week.[69] If ischemic optic neuropathy is suspected during the postoperative period, urgent ophthalmologic consultation should be obtained to establish the diagnosis and determine the treatment. Visual losses due to ischemic optic neuropathy are categorized as anterior ischemic optic neuropathy and posterior ischemic optic neuropathy because these parts of the optic nerve have different blood supplies, differing predisposing factors for infarction, and variable clinical pictures.[69]

Anterior Ischemic Optic Neuropathy

The visual loss associated with anterior ischemic optic neuropathy is due to infarction at watershed zones between the areas of distribution of the small branches of the short posterior ciliary arteries. The usual presentation of anterior ischemic optic neuropathy comprises sudden, painless, monocular visual deficits varying in severity from slight decreases in visual acuity to blindness. Asymptomatic optic disk swelling may be the earliest sign of anterior ischemic optic neuropathy. A congenitally small optic disk is often present. The prognosis varies, but the most common sequence is little recovery of visual function. Drug therapy including retrobulbar steroids and antiplatelet drugs has not been shown to be effective.

The nonarteritic form of anterior ischemic optic neuropathy is more likely than the arteritic form to manifest during the postoperative period and is usually attributed to decreased oxygen delivery to the optic disk in association with hypotension and/or anemia. This form of visual loss has been associated with hemorrhagic hypotension (gastrointestinal hemorrhage), anemia, cardiac surgery, head and neck surgery, cardiac arrest, and hemodialysis; and it may occur spontaneously. Arteritic anterior ischemic optic neuropathy, which is less common than the nonarteritic form, is associated with inflammation and thrombosis of the short posterior ciliary arteries. The diagnosis is confirmed by demonstration of giant cell arteritis on the biopsy of the temporal artery. Treatment for arteritic anterior ischemic optic neuropathy is high-dose steroids to prevent progression and protect the contralateral eye.

Posterior Ischemic Optic Neuropathy

Posterior ischemic optic neuropathy presents as acute loss of vision and visual field defects similar to anterior ischemic optic neuropathy. It is presumed to be caused by decreased oxygen delivery to the posterior portion of the optic nerve between the optic foramen and the central retinal artery's point of entry. Spontaneous occurrence is less frequent than for anterior ischemic optic neuropathy. A symptom-free period often precedes the loss of vision, and there may be no abnormal ophthalmoscopic findings initially, reflecting retrobulbar involvement of the optic nerve. Mild disc edema is present after a few days, and computed tomography of the patient's orbits may reveal enlargement of the intraorbital optic nerve.

The etiology of postoperative ischemic optic neuropathy appears to be multifactorial and may include hypotension, anemia, congenital absence of the central retinal artery, altered optic disc anatomy, air embolism, venous obstruction, and infection.[71] Postoperative ischemic optic neuropathy has been described following prolonged spine surgery performed in the prone position, cardiac surgery, radical neck dissection, and hip arthroplasty.[72] Nonsurgical events associated with posterior ischemic optic neuropathy include cardiac arrest, treatment of malignant hypertension, blunt trauma, and severe anemia, such as is due to gastrointestinal hemorrhage.

Cortical Blindness

Cortical blindness may follow profound hypotension, such as cardiac arrest that results in hypoperfu-

sion and infarction of watershed areas in the parietal or occipital lobes.[69, 73] This form of blindness has been observed following diverse surgical procedures (cardiac surgery, craniotomy, laryngectomy, cesarean section) and may also result from air or particulate emboli during cardiopulmonary bypass. Cortical blindness is characterized by loss of visual sensation with retention of pupillary reactions to light and normal funduscopic examinations. Patients may not be aware of vision loss, which usually improves with time. Computed tomography or magnetic resonance imaging abnormalities in the parietal or occipital lobes confirm the diagnosis.

Retinal Artery Occlusion

Central retinal artery occlusion presents as painless monocular blindness and occlusion of a branch of the retinal artery that results in limited visual field defects or blurred vision. Visual field defects are often severe initially but, unlike ischemic optic neuropathy, improve with time. Ophthalmoscopic examination reveals a pale edematous retina. Unlike ischemic optic neuropathy, central retinal artery occlusion is often caused by emboli from an ulcerated atherosclerotic plaque of the ipsilateral carotid artery. Most retinal artery occlusions due to emboli during open heart surgery resolve promptly. Vasospasm or thrombosis may also cause central retinal artery occlusion following radical neck surgery complicated by hemorrhage and hypotension and after intranasal injection of α-adrenergic agonists.[69] Stellate ganglion block improves vision in some of these patients.

Ophthalmic Venous Obstruction

Obstruction of venous drainage from the eyes may occur intraoperatively when patient positioning results in external pressure on the orbits. The prone position and use of headrests during neurosurgical procedures require careful attention to ensure that the patient's orbits are free from external compression. Ophthalmoscopic examination reveals engorgement of the veins and edema of the macula.

Transmissible Spongiform Encephalopathies

Epidemiology

Human transmissible spongiform encephalopathies are Creutzfeldt-Jakob disease, kuru, Gerstmann-Straussler-Scheinker disease (cerebellar ataxia, spastic paraparesis), and fatal familial insomnia (progressive insomnia, dysautonomia, dementia).[74, 75] These noninflammatory diseases of the central nervous system are caused by transmissible slow infectious pathogens known as *prions*. Prions differ from viruses in that they lack RNA and DNA and fail to produce a detectable immune reaction. Inactivation of prions is reliably achieved by steam sterilization, ethylene oxide sterilization, and soaking in sodium hypochlorite. Transmissible spongiform encephalopathies are diagnosed on the basis of clinical and neuropathologic findings (diffuse or focally clustered small, round vacuoles that may become confluent). Familial progressive subcortical gliosis and some inherited thalamic dementias may also be spongiform encephalopathies. Bovine spongiform encephalopathy ("mad cow disease") is a transmissible spongiform encephalopathy that occurs in animals. Infectivity has not been detected in skeletal muscles, milk, or blood.[73]

Creutzfeldt-Jakob Disease

Creutzfeldt-Jakob disease is the most common transmissible spongiform encephalopathy, with an estimated incidence of one case per million worldwide.[63] About 10% to 15% of persons with Creutzfeldt-Jakob disease have a family history consistent with autosomal dominant inheritance of the disease. The incubation period is measured in months to years. The disease develops by an abnormal prion protein thought to act as a neurotransmitter accumulating in the central nervous system. This prion protein is encoded by a specific gene, and sporadic and random mutations may result in variants of Creutzfeldt-Jakob disease. Rapidly progressive dementia with ataxia and myoclonus suggests the diagnosis, although confirmation may require cerebral brain biopsy because there are no reliable diagnostic tests. Alzheimer's disease poses the most difficult differential diagnosis. In contrast to toxic and metabolic disorders, myoclonus is rarely present at the onset of Creutzfeldt-Jakob disease; and seizures, when they occur, are a late phenomenon. No vaccines or treatments are effective.

Universal precautions, as utilized for patients with hepatitis B or human immunodeficiency virus (HIV) infection, are recommended when caring for patients with Creutzfeldt-Jakob disease, but other precautions (such as isolation) are not necessary.[74] Handling CSF calls for special precautions (double gloves, protective glasses, specimen labeled infectious), as this fluid has been the only body fluid shown to result in transmission to primates. Biopsies and autopsies require similar precautions, although the risk is less than that created by similar procedures in those who are seropositive for hepatitis B

virus or HIV. Nevertheless, the main risk of transmitting Creutzfeldt-Jakob disease is during cerebral biopsy for diagnostic confirmation of the disease. Instruments should be disposable or should be decontaminated by soaking in sodium hypochlorite or autoclaving.

Human-to-human transmission has occurred inadvertently in association with surgical procedures (corneal transplant, stereotactic procedures with previously used electrodes, contaminated neurosurgical instruments including human cadaveric dura mater transplants). Transmission has been attributed to treatment with growth hormone and gonadotropic hormones. Injection or transplantation of human tissues may result in transmission of infectious prions, whereas the hazards of transmission through human blood are debatable (not observed in hemophiliacs).[74] Nevertheless, transfusion of blood from individuals known to be infected is not recommended.

Management of anesthesia includes the use of universal precautions, disposable equipment, and sterilization of any reusable equipment (laryngoscope blades) utilizing sodium hypochlorite.[76] Surgery in patients known or suspected to be infected may be better performed at the end of the day to allow thorough cleansing of equipment and the operating room before the next use. Personnel involved in the anesthesia and operation are kept to a minimum, and they should wear protective gowns, gloves, and face masks with transparent protective visors to protect the eyes.

Adrenoleukodystrophies

Adrenoleukodystrophies are genetic disorders caused by defective degradation of peroxisomes that lead to central nervous system demyelination and primary adrenal insufficiency.[77, 78] Typically, these diseases present during the first year of life with skeletal muscle spasticity, arrest of motor development, and gait disturbances. Because of their progressive nature, afflicted children often require anesthesia during diagnostic imaging procedures or surgical procedures intended to correct the sequelae of their disease.

Management of anesthesia may be influenced by the presence of hypotonia, impaired adrenal gland function, gastroesophageal reflux, and liver function abnormalities.[78, 79] Preoperative medication is not recommended, as the risk of upper airway obstruction is increased in the presence of co-existing hypotonia involving the pharyngeal muscles and copious oral secretions. Preoperative corticosteroid coverage is recommended. Induction of anesthesia and tracheal intubation requires that one consider the risk of aspiration in these patients. Use of muscle relaxants and the dose selected is influenced by the presence of hypotonia. The possibility of hyperkalemia is a consideration should succinylcholine be selected for administration to these patients. Anesthetic drugs known to decrease seizure thresholds are logical selections, as is avoidance of drugs known to have a potential to produce hepatotoxicity. Chronic treatment of these patients with anticonvulsants could induce enzyme induction manifesting as unexpected dose requirements for certain drugs.

Leigh Syndrome

Leigh syndrome is a progressive neurodegenerative disease (subacute necrotizing encephalomyelopathy) that develops during infancy or childhood. It is characterized by developmental delay, nervous system dysfunction (seizures, peripheral neuropathies, optic atrophy, altered temperature regulation), and respiratory abnormalities (aspiration, wheezing, dyspnea, hypoventilation, apnea).[80] With progression of the disease, central hypoventilation and apnea become more frequent. Increased serum lactate and pyruvate concentrations are often present, presumably reflecting a pyruvate dehydrogenase enzyme defect. Acute exacerbations may follow intercurrent illnesses and surgical procedures.

Management of anesthesia considers the need to maintain normoventilation and avoid infusion of crystalloid solutions containing lactate to avoid any iatrogenic contribution of co-existing metabolic acidosis.[80] Iatrogenic respiratory alkalosis due to intraoperative hyperventilation of the lungs could result in inhibition of pyruvate dehydrogenase and accumulation of lactic acid. Swallowing difficulties and the propensity to aspiration may influence the management of induction and emergence from anesthesia. Experience is too limited to recommend specific drugs or techniques, although volatile drugs, barbiturates, opioids, and muscle relaxants have been administered to these patients. Respiratory failure has been observed following anesthesia and surgery. In this regard, avoiding elective operations in patients with co-existing respiratory symptoms is recommended.

Rett Syndrome

Rett syndrome is a progressive neurologic disease that manifests exclusively in females as dementia, autistic behavior, stereotyped hand movements, and an abnormality of breathing control that results in frequent episodes of apnea and arterial hypoxemia. During the chronic phase there is diffuse and progressive skeletal muscle wasting; survival beyond 30 years of age is unlikely. The incidence of this syndrome may be as high as 25% among severely retarded females. In view of skeletal muscle weakness and wasting, the likelihood of pulmonary aspiration, release of excessive amounts of potassium after administration of succinylcholine, and the need for mechanical support of ventilation are considerations in the management of anesthesia.[81] Vasomotor disturbances and unexpected hypothermia may occur during anesthesia.

Sotos Syndrome

Sotos syndrome (cerebral giantism) is the association of mental retardation and macrocephaly. This syndrome is inherited as an autosomal dominant trait. Rapid skeletal growth may account for the high incidence of scoliosis in these patients and the likely need for corrective spinal surgery. Considerations in the management of anesthesia include the anatomic characteristics of the facies, which may make management of the patient's airway difficult, and severe mental retardation, which impairs the ability of these patients to cooperate during the perioperative period. In this regard, aggressive behavior may contraindicate the use of a "wakeup test" during corrective spinal surgery for correction of scoliosis, emphasizing the potential value of somatosensory evoked potential monitoring.[82] The choice of drugs for maintenance of anesthesia may be influenced by the decision to used evoked potential monitoring and the likely impact of anesthetic drugs on interpretation of this monitor.

Fragile X Syndrome

Fragile X syndrome, a common cause of mental retardation, is inherited as an X-linked dominant disorder.[83] Developmental delay (speech and language) and mental retardation are the most significant clinical features. A diagnosis of fragile X syndrome should be considered in any child with developmental delay and/or mental retardation. Adult male patients generally exhibit a long, narrow face with moderately increased head circumference. Prominence of the mandible and forehead, with particularly large, mildly dysmorphic ears are typical. Mental retardation in female patients is usually milder than that in affected males.

Menkes Syndrome

Menkes syndrome is an X-linked recessive disorder of copper absorption and metabolism. Defective processing of copper results in abnormalities of many enzymes, manifesting as dysfunction of multiple organ systems. The onset is generally within the first 2 months of life with progressive cerebral degeneration; death usually occurs by 3 years of age owing to intractable seizures or pneumonia. Affected children often require anesthetic care during diagnostic procedures such as magnetic resonance imaging.

The major anesthetic implications of this syndrome are related to the disease's effects on the central nervous system. Seizures often require multiple anticonvulsant drugs for control.[84] Preoperative measurement of plasma anticonvulsant concentrations with adjustments to ensure therapeutic levels may be indicated. Progressive central nervous system deterioration may be accompanied by gastroesophageal reflux, poor pharyngeal muscle control, and recurrent aspiration. Defective collagen formation similar to that of Ehler-Danlos syndrome may be associated with perioperative hemorrhage. Experience is too limited to recommend specific anesthetic drugs. The choice of muscle relaxants is likely to exclude succinylcholine, although there is no evidence to support this practice.

Stiff-Person Syndrome

Stiff-person syndrome (previously stiff-man syndrome) is a rare central nervous system disease characterized by persistent, painful skeletal muscle contractions resembling tetanus. Unlike tetanus, however, trismus does not accompany stiff-person syndrome. Skeletal muscle rigidity may interfere with adequate ventilation; when severe, it has resulted in disruption of skeletal muscles, fractures of long bones, and bending of internal orthopedic appliances. Electromyography reveals continuous motor unit activity in the affected skeletal muscles that is indistinguishable from voluntary contractions. The congenital form of stiff-person syndrome, known as stiff-baby syndrome, is inherited as an autosomal dominant trait. Stiff-person syndrome may reflect the development of antibodies against the enzyme glutamic acid decarboxylase, which is responsible for synthesis of the inhibitory neurotransmitter GABA.[85] Successful pharmacologic treatment of this syndrome is based on enhancement of central GABA neurotransmitter activity with benzodiazepine drugs such as diazepam. Diazepam decreases spasticity by activating GABA receptors in the spinal cord. Intrathecal baclofen has been administered to decrease spasticity by activating GABA receptors in the dorsal horn of the spinal cord.

Experience with anesthesia in these patients is too limited to make recommendations, although facilitatory effects of certain anesthetics on the GABA system (propofol, etomidate, thiopental) may contribute to postoperative hypotonicity.[86] If possible, avoidance of muscle relaxants is recommended.

Von Hippel-Lindau Disease

Von Hippel-Lindau disease is familial, transmitted by an autosomal dominant gene with variable penetrance.[87] It is characterized by retinal angiomas, hemangioblastomas, and central nervous system (cerebellar) and visceral tumors. Although benign, these tumors can cause symptoms secondary to pressure on surrounding structures or by virtue of hemorrhage. The incidence of pheochromocytoma, renal cysts, and renal cell carcinoma is increased in the presence of this syndrome. These patients may require intracranial surgery for resection of hemangioblastomas.

Management of anesthesia in patients with von Hippel-Lindau disease must consider the possible presence of pheochromocytomas.[88–90] Preoperative treatment with antihypertensive drugs is indicated when the presence of pheochromocytoma is recognized (see Chapter 22). The possibility of spinal cord hemangioblastomas may limit the use of spinal anesthesia, although use of epidural anesthesia has been described for cesarean section.[87] Exaggerated systemic hypertension, especially during direct laryngoscopy, or sudden changes in the intensity of surgical stimulation may require intervention with labetalol, nitroprusside, or esmolol (or a combination of these drugs).

Painful Legs and Moving Toes Syndrome

Painful legs and moving toes syndrome occurs after peripheral nerve injuries, neuropathy, or trauma.[91] The pain is diffuse, intractable, aching, and deep. Movements consist of writhing motions in the toes that cannot be initiated voluntarily. Derangement of the peripheral or central nervous system after nerve or tissue damage is a possible explanation. Relief of symptoms provided by lumbar sympathetic ganglion block suggests a role for the autonomic nervous system in the etiology of this syndrome.[91]

Kallmann Syndrome

Kallmann syndrome is an inherited disorder characterized by hypogonadism and anosmia.[92] In addition, affected individuals may manifest sensorineural deafness, cerebellar ataxia, spastic paraplegia, and mental retardation.

Multiple Sclerosis

Multiple sclerosis is an autoimmune disease affecting the central nervous system that seems to occur in genetically susceptible persons after an environmental exposure.[93–95] Although both genetic predisposition (twins) and environmental or infectious exposures contribute to the causation of multiple sclerosis, there is no clear understanding of the immunopathogenic processes that determine the sites of tissue damage in the central nervous system, the variations in natural history, or the severity of disability caused by the disease.[93] It is twice as common in women than in men. In women with multiple sclerosis, the rate of relapse decreases during pregnancy, especially in the third trimester, and increases during the first 3 months postpartum.[96] Exposure to viral illnesses and infections may trigger relapses. Pathologically, multiple sclerosis is characterized by diverse combinations of inflammation, demyelination, and axonal damage in the central nervous system. The loss of myelin covering the axons is followed by formation of demyelinative plaques. Peripheral nerves are not affected by multiple sclerosis.

Signs and Symptoms

Clinical manifestations of multiple sclerosis reflect its multifocal involvement. Its course may be subacute, with relapses followed by remissions, or chronic and progressive. Manifestations of multiple sclerosis reflect sites of demyelination in the central nervous system and spinal cord. For example, inflammation of the optic nerves (optic neuritis) causes visual disturbances; involvement of the cerebellum leads to gait disturbances; and lesions of the spinal cord cause limb paresthesias and weakness as well as urinary incontinence and sexual impotence. Optic neuritis is characterized by diminished visual acuity and defective pupillary reaction to light. Ascending spastic paresis of the skeletal muscles is often prominent. Demyelination of the pathways in the brain stem that coordinate eye movements causes paresis of the medial rectus muscle on lateral conjugate gaze. Nystagmus is seen in the abducted eye. Intramedullary disease of the cervical cord is suggested by an electrical sensation that runs down the back into the legs in response to flexion of the neck (Lhermitte's sign). Typically, symptoms develop over the course of a few days, remain stable for a few weeks, and then improve. Because remyelination in the central nervous system probably does not occur, remission of symptoms most likely results from correction of transient chemical and physiologic disturbances that have interfered with nerve conduction in the absence of complete demyelination. There is an increased incidence of seizure disorders in patients with multiple sclerosis.

The course of multiple sclerosis is characterized by exacerbations and remissions of symptoms at unpredictable intervals over a period of several years. Residual symptoms eventually persist during remissions, leading to severe disability from visual failure, ataxia, spastic skeletal muscle weakness, and urinary incontinence. Nevertheless, the disease in some patients remains benign, with infrequent, mild episodes of demyelination, followed by prolonged, occasionally permanent remissions. The onset of multiple sclerosis after 35 years of age is most likely to be associated with slow progression.

Diagnosis

The diagnosis of multiple sclerosis can be established with different degrees of confidence as probable or definite on the basis of clinical features alone or clinical features in combination with oligoclonal abnormalities of immunoglobulins in CSF, prolonged latency of evoked potentials reflecting slowing of nerve conduction due to demyelination, and signal changes in white matter seen on cranial magnetic resonance imaging. Indeed, magnetic resonance imaging is a sensitive marker of the pathologic process (demyelinative plaques) associated with multiple sclerosis.

Devic's disease (neuromyelitis optica) is a variant of multiple sclerosis. It affects the optic nerves (optic neuritis) and cervical spinal cord (transverse myelitis).

Treatment

No treatment is curative for multiple sclerosis.[95]

Corticosteroids, the principal treatment for acute relapses of multiple sclerosis,[94] have immunomodulatory and antiinflammatory effects that restore the blood–brain barrier, decrease edema, and possibly improve axonal conduction. Treatment with corticosteroids shortens the duration of the relapse and accelerates recovery; but whether the overall degree of recovery or progression of the disease is altered is not known.

Interferon-β is the treatment of choice for patients with relapsing-remitting multiple sclerosis. The most common side effect of interferon-β therapy is transient influenza-like symptoms for 24 to 48 hours after the injection. Slight increases in serum aminotransferase concentrations, leukopenia, or anemia may be present; and co-existing depression may be exaggerated.

Glatiramer acetate is a mixture of random synthetic polypeptides synthesized to mimic myelin basic protein. This drug is an alternative to interferon-β and may be most useful for patients who become resistant to interferon-β treatment owing to serum interferon-β-neutralizing activity.

Azathioprine is a purine analogue that depresses both cell-mediated and humoral immunity. Treatment with this drug may decrease the rate of relapses in multiple sclerosis but has no effect on the progression of disability. Azathioprine is considered when patients do not respond to therapy with interferon-β or glatiramer acetate. Treatment with azathioprine may be helpful in patients with Devic's disease.

Low-dose *methotrexate* is nontoxic and inhibits both cell-mediated and humoral immunity as a result of its antiinflammatory effects. Patients with secondary progressive multiple sclerosis may benefit most from treatment with this drug.

Management of Anesthesia

Management of anesthesia in patients with multiple sclerosis must consider the impact of surgical stress on the natural progression of the disease. For example, regardless of the anesthetic technique or drugs selected for use during the perioperative period, it is likely that symptoms of multiple sclerosis will be exacerbated during the postoperative period. In this regard, any increase in body temperature (as little as 1°C) that follows surgery may be more likely than drugs to be responsible for exacerbations of multiple sclerosis during the postoperative period. It is possible that increased body temperature results in complete block of conduction in demyelinated nerves. Furthermore, the unpredictable cycle of exacerbations and remissions of this disease could lead to erroneous conclusions that there are cause-and-effect relations between an exacerbation of the clinical manifestations of multiple sclerosis with drugs or events present during the perioperative period.

The changing and unpredictable neurologic picture in patients with multiple sclerosis during the perioperative period must be appreciated when selecting regional anesthetic techniques. Indeed, spinal anesthesia has been implicated in postoperative exacerbations of multiple sclerosis, whereas exacerbations of the disease after epidural anesthesia or peripheral nerve blocks have not been described.[97] The mechanism by which spinal anesthesia might be more likely than epidural anesthesia to exacerbate the clinical manifestations of multiple sclerosis is unknown but might reflect local anesthetic neurotoxicity. It is speculated that the lack of a protective nerve sheath around the spinal cord and the demyelination associated with multiple sclerosis renders the spinal cord of these patients more susceptible to potential neurotoxic effects of local anesthetics. Epidural anesthesia may be less of a risk than spinal anesthesia because the concentrations of local anesthetics in the white matter of the spinal cord is three to four times lower after epidural anesthesia than after spinal anesthesia. Nevertheless, both epidural and spinal anesthesia have been utilized in parturients with multiple sclerosis.[98, 99]

General anesthesia is most often chosen for anesthesia management in patients with multiple sclerosis. There are no unique interactions between multiple sclerosis and the drugs used to provide general anesthesia, and there is no evidence to support recommendations for a specific inhaled or injected anesthetic drug. When selecting muscle relaxants one should consider the possibility of exaggerated release of potassium following administration of succinylcholine to these patients. Prolonged responses to the paralyzing effects of nondepolarizing muscle relaxants would be consistent with co-exisitng skeletal muscle weakness ("myasthenia-like") and decreased skeletal muscle mass. Conversely, resistance to the effects of nondepolarizing muscle relaxants has been observed, perhaps reflecting proliferation of extrajunctional cholinergic receptors characteristic of upper motor neuron lesions.[100]

Corticosteroid supplementation during the perioperative period may be indicated in patients being treated chronically with these drugs. Efforts must be made during the perioperative period to recognize and prevent even modest increases in body temperature (more than 1°C), as this change might lead to deterioration of nerve tissue at sites of demyelination. Neurologic evaluation during the postoperative period may be useful for detecting evidence of exacerbation of multiple sclerosis.

Postpolio Sequelae

Postpolio sequelae manifest as fatigue, skeletal muscle weakness, joint pain, cold intolerance, and swallowing, sleep, and breathing problems that presumably reflect neurologic damage from the original polio virus infection. Polio virus may damage the reticular activating system, accounting for the exquisite sensitivity these individuals may exhibit to sedative effects of anesthetics with delayed awakening from anesthesia. Sensitivity to muscle relaxants is predictable. Severe back pain following surgery may be due to co-existing skeletal muscle atrophy and scoliosis. Postoperative shivering may be profound, as these individuals are highly sensitive to cold. Postoperative pain sensitivity seems to be increased and is presumed to be related to polio virus damage to endogenous opioid-secreting cells in the brain and spinal cord. Same-day surgery may not be an appropriate selection for postpolio patients.

■ CRANIAL MONONEUROPATHIES

Idiopathic Facial Paralysis (Bell's Palsy)

Idiopathic facial paralysis is characterized by the rapid onset of motor weakness or paralysis of all the facial muscles innervated by the facial nerve.[101] Often the onset is first noted on arising in the morning and looking into a mirror. Additional symptoms can include the loss of taste sensation over the anterior two-thirds of the tongue, as well as hyperacusis and diminished salivation and lacrimation. The absence of cutaneous sensory loss emphasizes that the facial nerve is a motor nerve. The cause of idiopathic facial paralysis is presumed to be inflammation and edema of the facial nerve, most often in the facial canal of the temporal bone. A viral inflammatory mechanism (perhaps herpes simplex virus) may be the cause. Indeed, the onset of this cranial mononeuropathy is often preceded by a viral prodrome. During pregnancy there is an increased incidence of idiopathic facial paralysis. The presence of idiopathic facial paralysis does not influence the choice of technique or the management of anesthesia.[101]

Spontaneous recovery usually occurs over about 12 weeks. If no recovery is seen within 16 to 20 weeks, the clinical signs and symptoms are probably not due to idiopathic facial paralysis. Prednisone, 1 mg/kg PO each day for 5 to 10 days, depending on the degree of facial nerve paralysis, dramatically relieves pain and decreases the number of patients experiencing complete denervation of the facial nerve. The patient's eye should be covered on the affected side to protect the cornea.

Surgical decompression of the facial nerve may be needed for persistent or severe cases of idiopathic facial paralysis or for facial paralysis secondary to trauma. Trauma to the facial nerve can reflect stretch injury produced by excessive traction on the angle of the mandible during maintenance of the upper airway in unconscious patients.[102] Uveoparotid fever (Heerfordt syndrome) is a variant of sarcoidosis characterized by bilateral anterior uveitis, parotitis, and mild pyrexia, as well as the presence of facial nerve paralysis in 50% to 70% of patients. Facial nerve paralysis associated with uveoparotid fever appearing during the postoperative period may be erroneously attributed to mechanical pressure over the nerve during general anesthesia.[103]

Facial nerve palsy associated with placement of an extradural blood patch for treatment of postdural puncture headaches has been described.[104] Sudden increases in ICP caused by placing the epidural blood patch were speculated to have transiently compromised the blood flow to the facial nerve.

Melkersson-Rosenthal Syndrome

Melkersson-Rosenthal syndrome is characterized by recurrent episodes of facial nerve palsy, orofacial edema, and the presence of a furrowed tongue.[105] Life-threatening upper airway obstruction due to edema of the larynx may occur in these patients, necessitating permanent tracheostomy. The cause of this syndrome is unknown, and there is no effective treatment.

Trigeminal Neuralgia (Tic Douloureux)

Trigeminal neuralgia is characterized by the sudden onset of brief but intense unilateral facial pain triggered by local sensory stimuli to the affected side of the face. Trigeminal neuralgia can be diagnosed based on purely clinical signs and symptoms. Patients report brief, stabbing pain or clusters of stabbing pains in the face or mouth that are restricted to one or more divisions of the trigeminal nerve, most often the mandibular division. Trigeminal neuralgia most often develops in otherwise healthy individuals during late middle age. The appearance of this neuralgia at an earlier age should arouse suspicion of multiple sclerosis. Although the pathophysiology of the pain associated with trigeminal neuralgia is uncertain, vascular compression of the trigeminal root is an important contributing factor.[106]

The treatment of choice for patients with trigeminal neuralgia is the anticonvulsant drug carbamazepine.[106] Phenytoin is less effective but is selected for patients who do not respond to carbamazepine. Other drugs to consider include GABA receptor agonists such as baclofen. Although the efficacy of surgical therapy (selective radiofrequency destruction of trigeminal nerve fibers, transection of the sensory root of the trigeminal nerve, microsurgical decompression of the trigeminal nerve) is not documented, it is accepted that surgery usually relieves the pain promptly. Hence it is recommended for individuals who develop pain refractory to drug therapy.

There are no special considerations for management of anesthesia in patients with trigeminal neuralgia. Patients undergoing surgical therapy for trigeminal neuralgia, however, may experience significant increases in systemic blood pressure during destruction of nerve fibers, necessitating treatment with nitroprusside. The potential enzyme-inducing effects of anticonvulsant drugs must be considered when predicting drug effects. Carbamazepine can cause altered hepatic function, leukopenia, and thrombocytopenia.

Myofascial Pain Dysfunction Syndrome

Myofascial pain dysfunction syndrome is often misdiagnosed ("the great impostor"), resulting in unnecessary and ineffective treatment.[107] Misdiagnosis as trigeminal neuralgia is possible, especially when pain appears in trigeminal nerve distributions. Patients with trigeminal neuralgia, however, do not typically exhibit masticatory trigger points. Myofascial pain typically arises from trigger points in taut bands of skeletal muscles that are painful to compression and give rise to characteristic tenderness, referred pain, and autonomic phenomena. Trigger points arise from cycles of sustained sarcomere contractions, increased metabolic activity, and ischemia. Nociceptor sensitization and sarcomere contractures are maintained by local release of substances such as lactate, bradykinin, prostaglandins, and substance P.

Glossopharyngeal Neuralgia

Glossopharyngeal neuralgia is characterized by episodes of intense pain in the throat, neck, tongue, and ear. Swallowing, chewing, coughing, or talking can trigger the pain. This neuralgia may also be associated with severe bradycardia and syncope, presumably reflecting activation of the motor nucleus of the vagus nerve. Hypotension, seizures due to cerebral ischemia, and even cardiac arrest may manifest in some patients.

Diagnosis

Glossopharyngeal neuralgia is usually idiopathic but has been described in patients with cerebellopontine angle vascular anomalies and tumors, vertebral and carotid artery occlusive disease, arachnoiditis, and extracranial tumors arising in the area

of the pharynx, larynx, and tonsils. The presence of glossopharyngeal neuralgia is supported by the occurrence of pain in the distribution of the glossopharyngeal nerve, the presence of a site in the oropharynx that reproduces the symptoms when stimulated, and relief of pain by topical anesthesia of the oropharynx.

In the absence of pain, cardiac symptoms associated with glossopharyngeal neuralgia may be confused with sick sinus syndrome or carotid sinus syndrome. Sick sinus syndrome can be discounted by the absence of characteristic changes on the electrocardiogram. Failure of carotid sinus massage to produce cardiac symptoms rules out the presence of carotid sinus hypersensitivity. Glossopharyngeal nerve block is useful for differentiating glossopharyngeal neuralgia from atypical trigeminal neuralgia. This nerve block does not differentiate glossopharyngeal neuralgia from the carotid sinus syndrome, as afferent pathways of both syndromes are mediated by the glossopharyngeal nerve. Topical anesthesia of the oropharynx anesthetizes receptors in the trigger area responsible for initiating glossopharyngeal neuralgia, distinguishing this response from the carotid sinus syndrome.

Treatment

Treatment of glossopharyngeal neuralgia associated with cardiac symptoms should be aggressive, as sudden death is a risk. Cardiovascular symptoms are treated with atropine, isoproterenol, an artificial external cardiac pacemaker, or a combination of these modalities. Pain associated with this syndrome is managed by chronic administration of anticonvulsant drugs such as carbamazepine or phenytoin. Topical anesthesia of the pharyngeal or oral mucosa or a glossopharyngeal nerve block effectively eliminates pain but only for the duration of the local anesthetic effect. Prevention of cardiovascular symptoms and provision of predictable pain relief are achieved by intracranial surgical section of the glossopharyngeal nerve and the upper two roots of the vagus nerve. Although permanent pain relief after repeated glossopharyngeal nerve blocks is possible, this neuralgia is sufficiently life-threatening to justify intracranial transection of the nerve in patients not responsive to medical therapy.

Management of Anesthesia

Preoperative evaluation of patients with glossopharyngeal neuralgia is directed at assessing the patient's intravascular fluid volume and cardiac status.[108] Hypovolemia may be present, as these patients avoid oral intake and its associated pharyngeal stimulation in attempts to avoid triggering the pain attacks. Furthermore, drooling and loss of saliva can contribute to decreased intravascular fluid volume. A preoperative history of syncope or documented bradycardia, concurrent with the episodes of pain, introduces the possible need for prompt introduction of noninvasive transcutaneous cardiac pacing or placement of a prophylactic transvenous artificial cardiac pacemaker before the induction of anesthesia. Continuous monitoring of the ECG and of systemic blood pressure via an intra-arterial catheter is useful. Topical anesthesia of the oropharynx with lidocaine is helpful for preventing bradycardia and hypotension, which may occur in response to the triggering of this syndrome during direct laryngoscopy for tracheal intubation. Furthermore, intravenous administration of atropine or glycopyrrolate just before initiating laryngoscopy may be recommended.

Cardiovascular changes in the response to surgical manipulation and intracranial section of glossopharyngeal and vagal nerve roots should be expected. For example, bradycardia and hypotension are likely during manipulation of the vagus nerve. Anticholinergic drugs are promptly available to treat vagal-mediated responses. Systemic hypertension, tachycardia, and ventricular premature beats may occur after surgical transection of the glossopharyngeal nerve and the upper two roots of the vagus nerve. These events may reflect the sudden loss of sensory input from the carotid sinus. Systemic hypertension is usually transient but persists in some patients into the postoperative period. Persistence of systemic hypertension is due to increased sympathetic nervous system activity. Administration of hydralazine during the postoperative period is useful for treating systemic hypertension. Experience is too limited to permit recommendations for specific anesthetic drugs or muscle relaxants.[108] The possibility of the development of vocal cord paralysis following transection of the vagus nerve should be considered if airway obstruction occurs following tracheal extubation.

Vestibular Neuronitis

Vestibular neuronitis is characterized by vertigo, vomiting, and gait disturbances. These symptoms are thought to reflect irritation of the vestibular portion of cranial nerve VIII. The absence of hearing loss distinguishes vestibular neuronitis from endolymphatic hydrops (Meniere's disease). Vestibular neuronitis is a benign condition for which no specific treatment is necessary.

Metastatic Cancer

Cranial nerve palsy may reflect compression or infiltration of the nerve by leukemia or lymphomas. Metastatic disease from the breast or lung may invade the trigeminal nerve, causing numbness of the chin or cheek. Similar metastatic invasion of the hypoglossal nerve produces atrophy of the tongue.

Mobius Syndrome

Mobius syndrome is a rare congenital dysplasia of the cranial nerves. The spinal accessory and facial nerves are most often affected, resulting in esotropia or partial facial paralysis. Occasionally, involvement of other cranial nerves is manifested as difficulty with mastication, swallowing, and coughing, often leading to aspiration and recurrent pneumonia.

■ PERIPHERAL NEUROPATHIES

The etiology of peripheral neuropathies may reflect hereditary, inflammatory, or nerve ischemia (stretch or compression) mechanisms. Diseases, especially diabetes mellitus, are associated with the development of peripheral neuropathies. The positioning of patients during surgery may increase the risk of peripheral nerve damage even when acceptable positioning and padding techniques are followed.[109, 110] In this regard, certain patients, particularly those with diabetes mellitus, seem to be most vulnerable to postoperative peripheral nerve injury.

Inherited Peripheral Neuropathies

Charcot-Marie-Tooth disease type 1A (CMT1A) and hereditary neuropathy with liability to pressure palsies (HNPP) are autosomal dominant, inherited primary demyelinating peripheral neuropathies that appear to result from a reciprocal DNA duplication/deletion gene on chromosome 17p that encodes a myelin protein.[111] These inherited peripheral neuropathies are a common, heterogeneous group of disorders that often remain undiagnosed. The significance of unrecognized inherited peripheral neuropathies in the development of postoperative peripheral nerve dysfunction attributed to positioning during the operative period is not known.

Charcot-Marie-Tooth Disease

The most common inherited cause of chronic motor and sensory peripheral neuropathy, CMT1A (peroneal muscle disease) has an estimated incidence of 1 in 2500 individuals.[111] This autosomal dominant disorder manifests as distal skeletal muscle weakness, wasting, and loss of tendon reflexes, which usually become evident by the middle teenage years. Classically, this neuropathy is described as being restricted to the lower one-third of the legs, producing foot deformities (high pedal arches and talipes) and peroneal muscle atrophy ("stork-leg" appearance).[112] The disease may slowly progress to include wasting of the quadriceps muscles and the muscles of the hands and forearms. Mild to moderate stocking-glove sensory loss occurs in many patients. Pregnancy may be associated with exacerbations of CMT1A.

Treatment of CMT1A is limited to supportive measures, including splints, tendon transfers, and various arthrodeses. Although life-span is not decreased, many individuals with CMT1A experience long-term disability. Use of epidural anesthesia for labor has been described.[113]

Management of anesthesia in patients with CMT1A is influenced by concerns about the responses to neuromuscular blocking drugs, the potential for development of malignant hyperthermia, and the possibility of postoperative respiratory failure.[112-115] Cardiac manifestations attributed to this neuropathy-including conduction disturbances (atrial flutter) and cardiomyopathy, have not been consistent observations. Patients with CMT1A do not seem to be susceptible to malignant hyperthermia, and the responses to neuromuscular blocking drugs seem to be predictable. It appears reasonable to avoid succinylcholine based on theoretical concerns about exaggerated potassium release following administration of this drug to individuals with neuromuscular diseases. Nevertheless, succinylcholine has been used safely in these patients without producing hyperkalemia or triggering malignant hyperthermia.[114]

Hereditary Neuropathy with Liability to Pressure Palsies

The disorder known as HNPP (familial recurrent polyneuropathy, tomaculous neuropathy) is characterized by periodic and recurrent episodes of focal demyelinating neuropathy following minor trauma or compression to peripheral nerves.[94] The onset is typically during adolescence, manifesting as numbness, skeletal muscle weakness, and atrophy. Pathologic changes observed in peripheral nerves of individuals with HNPP include segmental demyelination and tomaculous ("sausage-like") formations. Carpal tunnel syndrome and other entrapment neuropathies are frequent manifestations of HNPP. Un-

derexpression or deletion of the gene necessary for the production of peripheral myelin protein may be the genetic defect present in affected patients. The presence of HNPP deletion should be suspected in any family showing dominantly inherited pressure palsies and those with multiple members affected with carpal tunnel syndrome or other entrapment neuropathies. Early diagnosis of HNPP allows preventive measures to be taken to avoid nerve pressure or trauma in areas such as the elbows, wrists, and head of the fibula in the legs.

Inflammatory-Immune Peripheral Neuropathies

Peripheral neuropathies have been attributed to immune mechanisms or viral infection of nerve roots.

Brachial Plexus Neuropathy

Brachial plexus neuropathy (idiopathic brachial neuritis, Parsonage-Turner syndrome, shoulder-girdle syndrome) is characterized by the acute onset of severe pain in the upper arm with its maximum intensity at the onset of the neuropathy. As the pain diminishes there is the appearance of a patchy paresis or paralysis of the skeletal muscles of the shoulder girdle and arm innervated by individual branches of the brachial plexus.[116-118] Skeletal muscle wasting usually involving the shoulder girdle is common. Brachial plexus neuropathy is more common on the right, although the involvement and pain are bilateral in 10% to 30% of afflicted individuals, with both sides becoming involved simultaneously or sequentially. Although this neuropathy seems to have a predilection for the upper trunks of the brachial plexus (axillary, suprascapular, long thoracic nerves), it may involve a variety of nerves in the upper extremity. An estimated 70% of afflicted individuals manifest involvement of the axillary nerve.

Diagnosis of brachial plexus neuropathy and demonstration of the multifocal pattern of denervation is best demonstrated by electrodiagnostic studies including electromyography (fibrillations) and slowing of nerve conduction velocity studies. Skeletal muscles most often affected, in decreasing order, are the deltoid, supraspinatus, infraspinatus, serratus anterior, biceps, and triceps. The diaphragm may also be affected. Sensory disturbances occur in most patients but tend to be minimal and generally resolve with time. The incidence of this neuropathy is two to three times higher in males than females. Overall, recovery may take 24 to 36 months but is nearly always complete. The annual incidence of brachial plexus neuropathy is an estimated 1.64 cases per 100,000 population.[119]

Nerve biopsy of affected individuals suggests that these brachial plexopathies have an inflammatory-immune pathogenesis.[120] Antibody titers for immunoglobulins M and G were shown to be increased in one reported case.[117] Autoimmune neuropathies may occur during the postoperative period independent of the site of surgery.[116–119] It is possible that the stress of surgery activates an unidentified dormant virus in the nerve roots, a circumstance similar to the onset of herpes zoster after surgery. In addition to surgery, trauma, strenuous exercise, and pregnancy may be inciting events for the development of brachial plexus neuropathy. A hereditary form of this peripheral neuropathy has also been described.[118]

Postherpetic Neuralgia

Postherpetic neuralgia is characterized by severe burning and lancinating pain. It is typically accompanied by allodynia (pain provoked by nonnoxious stimuli) and continues more than 1 month after the onset of the herpes eruption.[121] The risk of postherpetic neuralgia increases with age. Pain associated with acute herpes zoster and postherpetic neuralgia is neuropathic and results from injury to the peripheral nerves and altered central nervous system signal processing.

Herpes zoster is caused by reactivation of the dormant virus that was seeded in sensory nerves during an earlier clinical course of varicella. This reactivation typically emerges as a rash in one or two adjacent dermatomes, with ophthalmic, cervical, and thoracic involvement being most common. Lesions progress from discrete patches or erythema to grouped vesicles that pustulate and crust in 7 to 10 days but may take 30 days to heal with anesthetic scars, changes in skin pigmentation, and persistent pain. Pain (deep aching or burning) is the most common symptom of herpes zoster often preceding the skin eruption by days to weeks. Occasionally it is the only symptom. The incidence of herpes zoster infection is increased in adults with HIV infection or cancer and children with leukemia.

Many approaches have been proposed to treat the pain of acute herpes zoster, prevent its progression to postherpetic neuralgia, and alleviate postherpetic neuralgia.[121] Aspirin and other mild analgesics are commonly used. Ibuprofen is ineffective, and neuropathic pain is usually less responsive than nonneuropathic pain to opioids. Tricyclic antidepressant drugs such as amitriptyline are important components of therapy for postherpetic neuralgia. Anticonvulsant drugs can decrease the lancinating component of the neuropathic pain. Intrathecal lumbar administration of methylprednisolone, 60 mg, is an effective treatment for postherpetic neuralgia.[122]

Corticosteroids may speed resolution of the acute neuritis, but there is no evidence these drugs influence the likely development of postherpetic neuralgia. Likewise, the ability of antiviral drugs to prevent postherpetic neuralgia is uncertain. Nevertheless, antiviral drugs initiated within 72 hours after the appearance of the herpes zoster rash reduce the magnitude of the acute pain.

Guillain-Barré Syndrome (Acute Idiopathic Polyneuritis)

Guillain-Barré syndrome is characterized by sudden onset of skeletal muscle weakness or paralysis that typically manifests initially in the legs and spreads cephalad over the ensuing days to involve skeletal muscles of the arms, trunk, and face. With the virtual elimination of poliomyelitis, this syndrome has become the most common cause of acute generalized paralysis, with an annual incidence of 0.75 to 2.0 cases per 100,000 population.[123] Bulbar involvement most frequently manifests as bilateral facial paralysis. Difficulty swallowing due to pharyngeal muscle weakness and impaired ventilation due to intercostal muscle paralysis are the most serious symptoms. Because of lower motor neuron involvement, paralysis is flaccid, and corresponding tendon reflexes are diminished. Sensory disturbances occur as paresthesias, most prominently in the distal part of the extremities; they generally precede the onset of paralysis. Pain often exists in the form of headache, backache, or tenderness of skeletal muscles to deep pressure.

Autonomic nervous system dysfunction is a prominent finding in patients with Guillain-Barré syndrome. Wide fluctuations in systemic blood pressure, sudden profuse diaphoresis, peripheral vasoconstriction, resting tachycardia, and cardiac conduction abnormalities on the ECG reflect alterations in the level of autonomic nervous system activity. Orthostatic hypotension may be so severe that elevating the patient's head on a pillow leads to syncope. Thromboembolism occurs with increased frequency. Sudden death associated with this disease is most likely due to autonomic nervous system dysfunction. A rare complication of Guillain-Barré syndrome is increased ICP.

Complete spontaneous recovery from acute idiopathic polyneuritis can occur within a few weeks, when segmental demyelination is the predominant pathologic change. Axonal degeneration, however, as shown by electromyography, may result in slower recovery over several months, with some degree of permanent weakness remaining. The mortality rate associated with Guillain-Barré syndrome is 3% to 8%, and death is most often due to sepsis, acute respiratory failure, pulmonary embolism, and in rare cases cardiac arrest, perhaps related to autonomic nervous system dysfunction.

Diagnosis

The diagnosis of Guillain-Barré syndrome is based on clinical signs and symptoms (Table 17–5),[123] supported by findings of increased protein concentrations in the CSF, although cell counts remain within a normal range. Support of a viral etiology is based on the observation that this syndrome develops after respiratory or gastrointestinal infections in about one-half of patients.

Treatment

Treatment of Guillain-Barré syndrome is mainly symptomatic. The vital capacity is monitored; and when it drops to less than 15 ml/kg, mechanical support of the patient's ventilation is considered. Arterial blood gas measurements help guide the adequacy of ventilation. Pharyngeal muscle weakness, even in the absence of ventilatory failure, may require that a cuffed tracheal tube be placed to protect the patient's lungs from aspiration of secretions and gastric fluid. Autonomic nervous system dysfunction may require treatment of systemic hypertension or hypotension. Corticosteroids are not considered useful therapy for this syndrome. Plasma exchange or infusion of gamma globulin may be of benefit in some patients.

Table 17–5 • Diagnostic Criteria for Guillain-Barré Syndrome

Features required for diagnosis
  Progressive bilateral weakness in legs and arms
  Areflexia
Features strongly supporting the diagnosis
  Progression of symptoms over several days
  Symmetry of symptoms
  Mild sensory symptoms or signs (sensory level makes diagnosis doubtful)
  Cranial nerve involvement (especially bilateral facial weakness)
  Spontaneous weakness beginning 2–4 weeks after progression ceases
  Autonomic nervous system dysfunction
  Absence of fever at onset
  Increased concentrations of protein in the cerebrospinal fluid

---

Management of Anesthesia

Altered function of the autonomic nervous system and the presence of lower motor neuron lesions are the two key considerations for management of anesthesia in patients with Guillain-Barré syndrome. Compensatory cardiovascular responses may be absent, resulting in profound hypotension in response to changes in posture, blood loss, or positive airway pressure. Conversely, noxious stimulation, such as during direct laryngoscopy, could manifest as exaggerated increases in systemic blood pressure, reflecting the labile activity of the autonomic nervous system in these patients. In view of these unpredictable changes in systemic blood pressure, it seems prudent to monitor the systemic blood pressure continuously with an intra-arterial catheter. Exaggerated responses to indirect-acting vasopressors should be considered when selecting these drugs, rather than intravenous infusion of fluids, to treat hypotension.

Succinylcholine should not be administered to these patients, as there is a risk of excessive potassium release from denervated skeletal muscles. A nondepolarizing muscle relaxant with minimal circulatory effects seems to be a better choice than pancuronium. Even if spontaneous ventilation is present preoperatively, it is likely that depression from anesthetic drugs will necessitate mechanical ventilation of the patient's lungs during surgery. Certainly, continued support of ventilation is likely to be necessary during the postoperative period.

Entrapment Neuropathies

Entrapment neuropathies occur at anatomic sites where peripheral nerves pass through narrow passages (median nerve and carpal tunnel at the wrist, ulnar nerve and cubital tunnel at the elbow), making compression a possibility. Peripheral nerves are probably more sensitive to compressive (ischemic) injury in patients who also have generalized polyneuropathies. For example, compressive neuropathies are more common in patients with diabetes mellitus or hereditary peripheral neuropathies. A peripheral nerve may also be more susceptible to compression if the same fibers have been partially damaged proximally ("double crush hypothesis"). In this regard, spinal nerve root compression (cervical radiculopathy) may increase the vulnerability of nerve fibers at distal sites for entrapment such as the carpal tunnel at the wrist. Alternatively, osteoarthritis may explain symptoms attributed to the double crush phenomenon. Peripheral nerve damage resulting from compression depends on the severity of the compression and the anatomy of the nerve. In most instances the outermost nerve fibers are more vulnerable to ischemia from compression than the fibers lying more deeply in the bundle of the nerve. Differing damage to fascicles in the peripheral nerve makes it difficult to localize the site of nerve injury precisely. Nerve conduction studies are useful for localizing the site of compression. Focal demyelination of nerve fibers causes slowing or blocking of nerve impulse conduction through the damaged area. Electromyography studies are adjuncts to nerve conduction studies, showing the presence of denervation impulses and ultimately reinnervation of muscle fibers by surviving axons.

Carpal Tunnel Syndrome

Compression of the median nerve between the transverse carpal ligament forming the roof of the carpal tunnel and the carpal bones at the wrist is the most common entrapment neuropathy. This compression neuropathy most often occurs in otherwise healthy women (three times more frequent in women than men) and is often bilateral, although the dominant hand is typically involved initially.[124, 125] Patients describe repeated episodes of pain and paresthesias in the wrist and hand following the distribution of the median nerve (thumb, index and middle fingers) often occurring during sleep or upon waking. Pain often spreads to the fingers, arm, and shoulder; and patients frequently describe involvement of all the fingers. Population-based studies reveal that about 3% of adults have symptomatic electrodiagnostically confirmed carpal tunnel syndrome.[125]

The cause of carpal tunnel syndrome is often unknown, although afflicted individuals may engage in occupations that require repetitive movements of the hands and fingers. Nerve conduction studies are the definitive method for confirming the diagnosis of carpal tunnel syndrome. Intraoperatively, patients may accumulate significant amounts of third space fluid, and the resulting increased tissue pressure may be sufficient to cause compression of peripheral nerves in previously asymptomatic patients. In patients manifesting numbness and tingling of the digits for the first time during the postoperative period, subsequent neurologic examination often confirmed the presence of preexisting carpal tunnel syndrome that was asymptomatic during the preoperative evaluation.[110] Pregnancy and associated peripheral edema may be associated with the initial manifestations of carpal tunnel syndrome. Cervical radiculopathy may produce similar symptoms, although these patients rarely experience bilateral pain.

Immobilizing the wrist with a splint is a common treatment for carpal tunnel syndrome that is likely to be transient (pregnancy) or due to a medically treatable disease (hypothyroidism, acromegaly). Injection of corticosteroids into the carpal tunnel may relieve symptoms but is seldom curative. Definitive treatment of carpal tunnel syndrome is decompression of the median nerve by surgical division of the transverse carpal ligament.

Cubital Tunnel Entrapment Syndrome

Compression of the ulnar nerve after it passes through the condylar groove and enters the cubital tunnel may result in clinical symptoms considered typical of ulnar nerve neuropathy. It may be difficult to differentiate clinical symptoms of ulnar nerve neuropathy due to compression in the condylar groove from symptoms that occur as a result of entrapment in the cubital tunnel. Treatment of cubital tunnel entrapment syndrome by tunnel decompression and transposition of the nerve may be helpful for relieving symptoms but may also make symptoms worse, perhaps by interfering with the nerve's blood supply.

Meralgia Paresthetica

Entrapment of the lateral femoral cutaneous nerve as it passes under the inguinal ligament can provoke burning pain over the anterolateral aspect of the thigh. Hypalgesia and hypesthesia are present in the involved areas. Obesity and tight belts can contribute to the development of entrapment neuropathy. Pain relief can be obtained by weight loss, removing the mechanical pressure produced by clothing, and blocking the lateral femoral cutaneous nerve using local anesthetics.

Diseases Associated with Peripheral Neuropathies

Diabetes Mellitus

Diabetes mellitus is commonly associated with peripheral polyneuropathies, with the incidence increasing with the duration of the disease and perhaps the degree of hypoinsulinemia.[126] Up to 7.5% of patients with non-insulin-dependent diabetes mellitus have clinical neuropathy at the time of diagnosis. Electromyograms may show evidence of denervation, and nerve conduction velocity is likely to be slowed. The most common neuropathy is a distal, symmetrical and predominantly sensory neuropathy. The principal manifestations are unpleasant tingling, numbness, burning, and aching in the lower extremities, skeletal muscle weakness, and distal sensory loss. Occasionally, an isolated sciatic neuropathy suggests the presence of a herniated intervertebral disk. Sciatic neuropathy in patients with diabetes mellitus is not associated with pain in response to straight-leg raising, serving to distinguish this peripheral neuropathy from lumbar disc disease. Discomfort is prominent at night and is often relieved by walking. Symptoms often progress and may extend to the upper extremities. Impotence, urinary retention, gastroparesis, resting tachycardia, and postural hypotension are common and reflect autonomic nervous system dysfunction. For reasons that are not understood, peripheral nerves of patients with diabetes mellitus are more vulnerable to ischemia due to compression or stretch injury, such as may occur during intraoperative and postoperative positioning, despite accepted padding and positioning during these periods.

Alcohol Abuse

Polyneuropathy of chronic alcoholism is nearly always associated with nutritional deficiencies. Presumably, vitamin deficiencies are contributing factors in the pathogenesis of alcoholic neuropathy. Symptoms characteristically begin in the lower extremities, with pain and numbness in the feet. Weakness and tenderness of the intrinsic muscles of the feet, absent Achilles tendon reflexes, and hypalgesia in a stocking-glove distribution are early manifestations. Restoration of a proper diet, abstinence from alcohol, and multivitamin therapy promote slow but predictable resolution of the neuropathy.

Vitamin B₁₂ Deficiency

The earliest neurologic symptoms of vitamin B_{12} deficiency resemble the neuropathy typically seen in patients who abuse alcohol. Paresthesias in the legs with sensory loss in a stocking distribution and absent Achilles tendon reflexes are characteristic findings. Similar neurologic findings have been reported in dentists who are chronically exposed to nitrous oxide and in individuals who chronically inhale nitrous oxide for nonmedical purposes (see Chapter 29). Nitrous oxide is known to inactivate certain vitamin B_{12}-dependent enzymes, which could lead to a deficiency of this essential vitamin.

Uremia

Distal polyneuropathy with sensory and motor components often occurs in the extremities of patients with chronic renal failure. Symptoms tend to be more prominent in the legs than in the arms. Presumably, metabolic abnormalities are responsible for axonal degeneration and segmental demyelination, which accompany the neuropathy. Slowing of nerve conduction has been correlated with increased plasma concentrations of parathyroid hormone and myoinositol, a component of myelin. Improved nerve conduction velocity often occurs within a few days after renal transplantation. Hemodialysis does not appear to be equally effective for reversing the polyneuropathy.

Cancer

Peripheral sensory and motor neuropathies occur in patients with a variety of malignancies, especially those involving the lung, ovary, and breast. Polyneuropathy that develops in elderly patients should always arouse suspicion of undiagnosed cancer. Myasthenic (Eaton-Lambert) syndrome is characteristically observed in patients with carcinoma of the lung. This syndrome, however, is an abnormality of the neuromuscular junction rather than of the nerves. Invasion of the lower trunks of the brachial plexus by tumors in the apex of the lungs (Pancoast syndrome) produces arm pain, paresthesias, and weakness of the hands and arms.

Collagen Vascular Diseases

Collagen vascular diseases are commonly associated with peripheral neuropathies. The most common conditions are systemic lupus erythematosus, polyarteritis nodosa, rheumatoid arthritis, and scleroderma. Detection of multiple mononeuropathies suggests vasculitis of nerve trunks and should stimulate a search for the presence of collagen vascular diseases.

Sarcoidosis

Polyneuropathy is a frequent finding in patients with sarcoidosis. Unilateral or bilateral facial nerve paralysis may result from sarcoid involvement of this nerve in the parotid gland.

Refsum's Disease

Refsum's disease is a multisystem disorder that manifests as polyneuropathies, ichthyosis, deafness, retinitis pigmentosa, cardiomyopathy, and cerebellar ataxia. Metabolic defects responsible for this disease reflect a failure to oxidize phytic acid, a fatty acid that subsequently accumulates in excessive concentrations.

■ SPINAL CORD TRANSECTION

Spinal cord transection is the description of damage to the spinal cord manifesting acutely as paralysis of the lower extremities (paraplegia) or all the extremities (quadriplegia). Associated medical problems accompany the early and late phases of spinal cord transection (Table 17–6).[127] Anatomically, the spinal cord is not divided, but the effect physiologically is the same as if it were transected. Spinal cord transection above the level of C2 to C4 is incompatible with survival, as innervation to the diaphragm is likely to be destroyed. The most common cause of spinal cord transection is trauma associated with motor vehicle or diving accidents resulting in fracture dislocation of cervical vertebrae. The most frequent nontraumatic cause of spinal cord transection is multiple sclerosis. Occasionally, rheumatoid arthritis of the spine results in spontaneous dislocation of the C1 vertebra on the C2 vertebra, producing progressive quadriparesis or sudden quadriplegia.

Unstable Cervical Spine Injuries

The mobility of the cervical spine makes it vulnerable to injury, especially hyperextension injury, during impact accidents. In this regard, it is estimated that cervical spine injury occurs in 1.5% to 3.0% of all major trauma victims.

Diagnosis

Cervical spine radiographs are obtained from nearly all patients who present with blunt trauma for fear of missing occult cervical spine injuries. Nevertheless, the probability of cervical spine injury is minimal in patients who meet the following five criteria: no midline cervical spine tenderness; no focal neurologic deficits; normal sensorium; no intoxication; and no painful distracting injury.[128] Patients who meet these criteria do not require routine imaging studies to rule out occult cervical spine injury.

An estimated two-thirds of trauma patients have multiple injuries that can interfere with cervical spine evaluation, which is ideally accomplished with computed tomography or magnetic resonance imaging. Nevertheless, routine computed tomography or magnetic resonance imaging may not be practical considering the risk of transporting unstable patients. For this reason, standard radiographic views (anteroposterior, lateral, open mouth) of the patient's cervical spine are often relied on to evaluate the presence of cervical spine injury and associated instability. Alignment of the vertebrae (lateral view), fractures (all views), and evaluation of disc and soft tissue spaces are analyzed on the radiologic examination. The sensitivity of plain radiographs is less than 100%, and the likelihood of cervical spine injury must be interpreted in conjunction with other clinical symptoms and risk factors. If there is any doubt, it may be prudent to treat all acute cervical spinal injuries as potentially unstable.

Treatment

Treatment of cervical fracture dislocation entails immediate immobilization to limit neck flexion and extension. Soft neck collars have almost no effect on limiting neck flexion, and neck extension is only modestly limited. Hard neck collars limit neck flexion and extension by about 25%. Immobilization and traction as provided by halo-thoracic devices are most effective in preventing cervical spine movement. Manual in-line stabilization (the assistant's hands are placed on each side of the patient's face with the fingertips resting on the mastoid process with downward pressure against the firm table surface to hold the head immobile in a neutral position) has been recommended to help minimize cervical spine flexion and extension during direct laryngoscopy for tracheal intubation.

Table 17–6 • Early and Late Complications in Patients with Spinal Cord Injury

Complication	Incidence (%)
2 Years after injury	
Urinary tract infection	59
Skeletal muscle spasticity	38
Chills and fever	19
Decubitus ulcer	16
Autonomic hyperreflexia	8
Skeletal muscle contractures	6
Heterotopic ossification	3
Pneumonia	3
Renal dysfunction	2
Postoperative wound infection	2
30 Years after injury	
Decubitus ulcers	17
Skeletal muscle or joint pain	16
Gastrointestinal dysfunction	14
Cardiovascular dysfunction	14
Urinary tract infection	14
Infectious disease or cancer	11
Visual or hearing disorders	10
Urinary retention	8
Male genitourinary dysfunction	7
Renal calculi	6

Adapted from: Ditunno JF, Formal CS. Chronic spinal cord injury. N Engl J Med 1994;330:550–6.

Direct Laryngoscopy and Tracheal Intubation

The key principle when performing direct laryngoscopy for tracheal intubation is to minimize neck movements during the procedure.[129] The fear of possible spinal cord compression from an unstable cervical spine injury must not prevent necessary airway intervention for avoiding arterial hypoxemia and alveolar hypoventilation. Extensive clinical experience seems to support the use of direct laryngoscopy for orotracheal intubation provided (1) maneuvers are taken to stabilize the head during the procedure (avoiding hyperextension of the patient's neck) and (2) evaluation of the patient's airway did not suggest the likelihood of technical difficulty.[130–132] In fact, direct laryngoscopy produces minimal movement below C3. However, cervical spine movement during direct laryngoscopy is likely to be concentrated at the occipito-atlanto-axial area, suggesting an increased risk of spinal cord injury in vulnerable patients. Topical anesthesia and awake fiberoptic laryngoscopy for tracheal intubation is an alternative if patients are cooperative and airway trauma does not preclude visualization with the fiberscope.

In addition to mechanical deformation of the spinal cord produced by movement of the neck in the presence of cervical spine injury, there is perhaps an even greater risk of compromise of the blood supply to the spinal cord produced by neck flexion that elongates the cord, with resultant narrowing of the longitudinal blood vessels. In fact, maintenance of perfusion pressure may be more important than positioning for preventing spinal cord injury in the presence of cervical spine injury.[133, 134]

Pathophysiology of Spinal Cord Injury

Spinal cord transection initially produces flaccid paralysis, with total absence of sensation below the level of the spinal cord injury. In addition, there is loss of temperature regulation and spinal cord reflexes below the level of the injury. Decreased systemic blood pressure and bradycardia are common. Abnormalities on the ECG are frequent during the acute phase of spinal cord transection and include ventricular premature beats and ST-T wave changes suggestive of myocardial ischemia. This phase, which occurs after acute spinal cord transection, is known as *spinal shock* and typically lasts 1 to 3 weeks. During this period the major cause of morbidity and mortality is alveolar hypoventilation combined with an inability to protect the airway and to clear bronchial secretions. Aspiration of gastric fluid or contents, as well as pneumonia and pulmonary embolism, are constant threats during spinal shock.

Sequelae of the chronic stage that jeopardize the patient's well-being include impaired alveolar ventilation, cardiovascular instability manifesting as autonomic hyperreflexia, chronic pulmonary and/or genitourinary tract infections, anemia, and altered thermoregulation. Chronic urinary tract infections reflect the patient's inability to empty the bladder completely, and they predispose to renal calculus formation. Renal failure may occur and is a common cause of death in patients with chronic spinal cord transection. Prolonged immobility leads to osteoporosis, skeletal muscle atrophy, and the development of decubitus ulcers. Pathologic fractures can occur when moving these patients. Pressure points should be well protected and padded to minimize the likelihood of trauma to the skin and the development of decubitus ulcers.

Mental depression and pain are very real problems after spinal cord surgery. Nerve root pain is localized at or near the level of the transection. Visceral pain is produced by distension of the bladder or bowel. Phantom body pain can occur in areas of complete sensory loss. As a result of mental depression or the presence of pain, these patients may be ingesting drugs that require consideration when planning anesthesia management.

Skeletal Muscle Spasticity

Several weeks after acute spinal cord transection the spinal cord reflexes gradually return, and patients enter a chronic stage characterized by overactivity of the sympathetic nervous system and involuntary skeletal muscle spasms. Baclofen, which potentiates the inhibitory effects of GABA, is useful for treating spasticity. Abrupt cessation of baclofen therapy, as may occur with hospitalization for unrelated problems, may result in dramatic withdrawal reactions including seizures. Diazepam and other benzodiazepines also facilitate the inhibitory effects of GABA. Spasticity refractory to pharmacologic suppression may necessitate surgical treatment (dorsal rhizotomy or myelotomy) or implantation of a spinal cord stimulator or subarachnoid baclofen pump.

Ventilation and Oxygenation

Spontaneous ventilation is not possible if the level of spinal cord transection results in paralysis of the diaphragm. Spinal cord transection between C2 and C4 may result in apnea due to denervation of the diaphragm. When function of the diaphragm is intact, the tidal volume is likely to remain adequate. Nevertheless, the ability to cough and clear secretions from the airway is often impaired because of decreased expiratory reserve volume. Indeed, acute

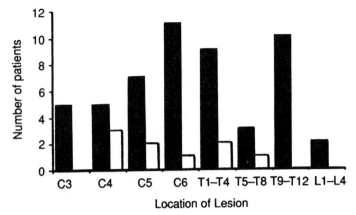

Figure 17–7 • Autonomic hyperreflexia did not occur in any patient with a spinal cord transection below T9 and undergoing extracorporeal shock-wave lithotripsy. *Shaded bars* represent the number of patients with spinal cord transections (n = 52); *open bars* represent the patients developing autonomic hyperreflexia (n = 9). (From Stowe DF, Bernstein JS, Madsen KE, et al. Autonomic hyperreflexia in spinal cord injured patients during extracorporeal shock wave lithotripsy. Anesth Analg 1989;68:788–91.)

spinal cord transection at the cervical level is accompanied by marked decreases in vital capacity. Furthermore, arterial hypoxemia is a consistent early finding during the period following cervical spinal cord injury. Tracheobronchial suctioning has been associated with bradycardia and cardiac arrest in these patients, emphasizing the importance of establishing optimal arterial oxygenation before undertaking this procedure.

Autonomic Hyperreflexia

Autonomic hyperreflexia appears following spinal shock and in association with return of spinal cord reflexes.[135-137] This reflex response can be initiated by cutaneous or visceral stimulation below the level of spinal cord transection. Distension of a hollow viscus, such as the bladder or rectum, is a common stimulus. The incidence of autonomic hyperreflexia depends on the level of spinal cord transection. For example, about 85% of patients with spinal cord transections above T6 exhibit this reflex, and it is unlikely to be associated with spinal cord transections below T10 (Fig. 17–7).[135] Surgery is a particularly potent stimulus to the development of autonomic hyperreflexia, and even patients with no history of this response may be at risk during operative procedures.

Mechanism

Stimulation below the level of spinal cord transection initiates afferent impulses that enter the spinal cord below that level (Fig. 17–8). These impulses elicit reflex sympathetic nervous system activity over the splanchnic outflow tract. In neurologically intact patients, this outflow is modulated by inhibitory impulses from higher centers in the central nervous system. In the presence of spinal cord transection, however, this outflow is isolated from inhibitory impulses, so generalized vasoconstriction persists below the level of the spinal cord injury. Vasoconstriction results in an increase in systemic blood pressure, which is then perceived by the carotid sinus. Subsequent activation of the carotid sinus results in decreased efferent sympathetic nervous system activity from the central nervous system, manifesting as a predominance of parasympathetic nervous system activity at the heart and peripheral vasculature. Such predominance cannot be produced below the level of the spinal cord transection, however, as this part of the body remains neurologically isolated. Therefore vasoconstriction persists below the level of the transection. If the level of the transection is above the level of splanch-

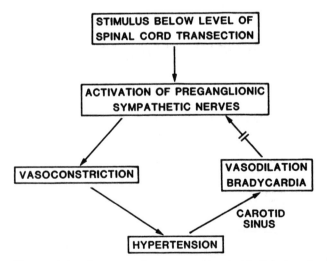

Figure 17–8 • Sequence of events associated with clinical manifestations of autonomic hyperreflexia. Because the afferent impulses that produce vasodilation cannot reach the neurologically isolated portion of the spinal cord, vasoconstriction develops below the level of the spinal cord transection, resulting in systemic hypertension.

nic nerve outflow (T4 to T6), vasodilation in the neurologically intact portion of the body is insufficient to offset the effects of vasoconstriction, as reflected by persistent systemic hypertension.

Signs and Symptoms

Systemic hypertension and bradycardia are the hallmarks of autonomic hyperreflexia. Stimulation of the carotid sinus due to systemic hypertension manifests as bradycardia and cutaneous vasodilation above the level of the spinal cord transection. Systemic hypertension persists, as vasodilation cannot occur below the level of injury. Nasal stuffiness reflects vasodilation. Patients may complain of headache and blurred vision as evidence of severe hypertension. Precipitous increases in systemic blood pressure can result in cerebral, retinal, or subarachnoid hemorrhages as well as increased operative blood loss. Loss of consciousness and seizures may occur. Cardiac dysrhythmias are often present. Pulmonary edema reflects acute left ventricular failure due to increased afterload produced by increases in systemic blood pressure.

Treatment

Treatment of autonomic hyperreflexia includes administration of peripheral vasodilating drugs such as nitroprusside. Anesthesia provided by inhaled drugs or regional anesthesia may also be helpful for controlling systemic hypertension.[136] Institution of epidural anesthesia has been described for the treatment of autonomic hyperreflexia provoked by uterine contractions.[137] Failure of epidural anesthesia to be as effective as spinal anesthesia in preventing autonomic hyperreflexia may be due to sparing of the sacral segments, which may occur in patients receiving epidural anesthesia.

Management of Anesthesia

Management of anesthesia in patients with spinal cord transections is largely determined by the acute or chronic nature of the injury. Regardless of the duration of spinal cord transection, institution of preoperative hydration may be helpful for preventing hypotension during induction and maintenance of anesthesia in these patients.

Acute Spinal Cord Injury

Patients with acute spinal cord transections may require special precautions during airway management (see "Direct Laryngoscopy and Tracheal Intu-
bation"). Topical anesthesia and awake fiberoptic laryngoscopy for tracheal intubation is an alternative to rapid-sequence induction of anesthesia with intravenous anesthetics and a muscle relaxant. When the cervical spine is unstable or there is a high index of suspicion for the presence of cervical spine injury, it is important to proceed carefully, as hyperextension of the patient's neck during direct laryngoscopy could further damage the spinal cord. Nevertheless, there is no evidence of increased neurologic morbidity after elective or emergency orotracheal intubation of anesthetized or awake patients who have an unstable cervical spine.[134] All factors considered, airway management during induction of anesthesia in the presence of cervical spine injury should be dictated by common sense, not by dogmatic approaches. Certainly, clinical experience in the airway management of these patients during anesthesia supports the safety of a variety of techniques.[127, 130–132, 134]

The absence of compensatory responses of the sympathetic nervous system makes these patients particularly likely to exhibit extreme decreases in systemic blood pressure in response to acute changes in body posture, blood loss, or positive airway pressure. Liberal intravenous infusion of crystalloid solutions may be necessary to replete the intravascular volume, which has been abruptly increased by vasodilation. Likewise, acute blood loss should be replaced promptly in these patients. Breathing is best managed by mechanical ventilation of the patient's lungs, as abdominal and intercostal muscle paralysis, combined with general anesthesia, mitigates against maintenance of adequate spontaneous ventilation. Hypothermia is avoided, as these patients tend to become poikilothermic below the level of the spinal cord transection. Anesthesia is maintained with drugs that ensure central nervous system sedation and facilitate tolerance of the tracheal tube. Nitrous oxide combined with volatile or injected drugs is satisfactory for this purpose. Arterial hypoxemia is common following spinal cord injury, emphasizing the likely need for increased delivered concentrations of oxygen to maintain acceptable oxygenation as evidenced by pulse oximetry.

The need for muscle relaxants is dictated by the operative site and the level of spinal cord transection. If muscle relaxants are necessary, the sympathomimetic effects of pancuronium makes this drug an attractive choice. Succinylcholine is unlikely to provoke excessive release of potassium during the first few hours after spinal cord transection. Nevertheless, it seems reasonable to avoid the use of this drug except in rare instances where it is the only drug capable of producing sufficiently rapid onset of action.

Chronic Spinal Cord Transection

The critical objective during management of anesthesia for patients with chronic transection of the spinal cord is prevention of autonomic hyperreflexia. Surgery is an intense stimulus for its development, emphasizing that patients who have a negative history for this reflex response are vulnerable to its occurrence during surgery. General anesthesia, which includes volatile drugs, prevents this response. Epidural and spinal anesthesia are also effective, but it may be technically difficult to perform regional anesthesia in patients with spinal cord injury. Furthermore, controlling the level of anesthesia is not easy. Nevertheless, spinal anesthesia seems particularly effective in preventing autonomic hyperreflexia.[136] The exception may be patients undergoing extracorporeal shock wave lithotripsy in whom autonomic nervous system hyperreflexia may occur even in the presence of general or spinal anesthesia.[135]

Epidural anesthesia has been reported to be occasionally ineffective for preventing systemic hypertension during urologic endoscopic procedures in patients with spinal cord injury.[132] This ineffectiveness may reflect occasional inadequate sacral analgesia produced by lumbar epidural placement of local anesthetic solutions. Nevertheless, epidural anesthesia has also been reported to prevent autonomic hyperreflexia during labor and delivery.[138] Blocking afferent pathways with topical local anesthetics applied to the urethra, as for a cystoscopic procedure, often does not prevent autonomic hyperreflexia, as this form of anesthesia does not block the bladder muscle proprioceptors, which are stimulated by bladder distension. Regardless of the technique selected for anesthesia, drugs such as nitroprusside must be readily available to treat precipitous systemic hypertension. Occasionally, administration of nitroprusside, 1 to 2 μg/kg IV, is needed to provide prompt decreases in dangerously increased systemic blood pressures. Persistence of systemic hypertension requires continuous intravenous infusions of nitroprusside. It is also important to appreciate that autonomic hyperreflexia may manifest postoperatively when the effects of the anesthetic drugs begin to wane.

When general anesthesia is selected, administration of muscle relaxants may be necessary to facilitate tracheal intubation and prevent reflex skeletal muscle spasms in response to surgical stimulation. Nondepolarizing muscle relaxants are used for this purpose, as succinylcholine is likely to provoke excessive potassium release from cells into the systemic circulation, particularly during the first 6 months following spinal cord transection. All factors considered, it seems reasonable to avoid the use of succinylcholine in patients with a spinal cord transection that occurred more than 24 hours earlier. The duration of susceptibility to the hyperkalemic effects of succinylcholine is unknown, but the risk is probably decreased after 3 to 6 months.

■ SEIZURE DISORDERS

Seizures are caused by transient, paroxysmal, and synchronous discharge of groups of neurons in the brain.[139, 140] Seizure is one of the most common neurologic disorders and may occur at any age, with more than 10% of the population experiencing seizures at some time during their life. Clinical manifestations of seizures depend on the location and number of neurons involved in the seizure discharge and its duration. Transient abnormalities of brain function, such as hypoglycemia, hyponatremia, and drug toxicity, typically result in a single seizure; treatment of the underlying disorder usually is curative. Conversely, epilepsy is defined as recurrent seizures resulting from congenital or acquired (cerebral scarring) factors; it affects approximately 0.6% of the population.[140] Classification of epileptic seizures into three major categories (partial, generalized, unclassified) is based on clinical symptoms and electroencephalographic criteria (Table 17–7). Magnetic resonance imaging is the preferred method for studying brain structure in patients with epilepsy.

Treatment

Treatment of seizures may be pharmacologic or surgical.

Pharmacologic Treatment

Seizures are treated initially with antiepileptic drugs starting with a single drug and achieving seizure control by increasing the dosage as necessary. Drug

---

Table 17–7 • Classification of Epileptic Seizures

Partial (focal and local) seizures
    Simple partial seizures (consciousness not impaired)
    Complex partial seizures (consciousness impaired)
    Partial seizures evolving to generalized seizures (tonic, clonic, tonic-clonic)
Generalized seizures (convulsive or nonconvulsive)
    Absence seizures
    Myoclonic seizures
    Clonic seizures
    Tonic seizures
    Clonic-tonic seizures
    Atonic seizures
Unclassified epileptic seizures

combinations may be considered when monotherapy fails. Changes in drug dosage are guided by the patient's clinical response rather than by serum drug concentrations. Monitoring serum drug levels is usually not necessary for patients who are experiencing adequate seizure control. Effective antiepileptic drugs appear to decrease neuronal excitability or enhance neuronal inhibition. The most commonly utilized antiepileptic drugs are carbamazepine, ethosuximide, gabapentin, lamotrigine, phenobarbital, phenytoin, primidone, topiramate, tiagabine, and valproate. Drugs effective for the treatment of partial seizures are carbamazepine, phenytoin, and valproate. Generalized seizure disorders can be managed with carbamazepine, phenytoin, valproate, barbiturates, gabapentin, or lamotrigine. Generalized nonseizure disorders can be treated with ethosuximide or valproate.

Except for gabapentin, all of the useful antiepileptic drugs are metabolized in the liver before undergoing renal excretion. Carbamazepine, phenytoin, and barbiturates cause enzyme induction, and long-term treatment with these drugs can alter the rate of their own metabolism and that of other drugs. Pharmacokinetic drug interactions are considerations in patients being treated with antiepileptic drugs.

Dose-dependent neurologic toxic effects are the most common adverse responses evoked by antiepileptic drugs. For example, carbamazepine may cause diplopia and sedation. All antiepileptic drugs can cause depression of cerebral function with symptoms of sedation. Persistent or fluctuation ataxia may reflect toxic effects of drugs on the cerebellum. Long-term use of these drugs is associated with dyskinesias of the tongue, face, and limbs. Mild sensory neuropathy is present in up to 15% of treated patients. Altered peripheral nerve function is thought to be an effect of antiepileptic drugs on folate metabolism. On rare occasions the initial exposure to valproate causes coma.

Valproate produces hepatic failure in about one in every 10,000 patients. The mechanism of this hepatotoxicity is unknown but may reflect idiosyncratic hypersensitivity reactions. Pancreatitis has been observed during valproate therapy. Adverse hematologic reactions associated with antiepileptic drugs range from mild anemia to aplastic anemia. Dose-related leukopenia is not infrequent in patients treated with carbamazepine. Valproate may depress the level of circulating platelets. Rashes occurring in response to antiepileptic drugs are relatively common. Antiepileptic drugs may cause systemic lupus erythematosus, scleroderma, and Sjögren's syndrome. Hyponatremia is a dose-related side effect of carbamazepine, but this electrolyte abnormality is rarely clinically significant. Phenytoin-induced acceleration of metabolism of endogenous or exogenous hormones may include birth control pills, leading to unexpected failure of these drugs. The results of thyroid function tests are altered by phenytoin.

Surgical Treatment

Surgical treatment of seizure disorders is a consideration in patients who do not respond to antiepileptic drugs. The seizure focus is first located by electrocorticography and information obtained from magnetic resonance imaging studies. The most commonly performed surgical operation for the treatment of epilepsy is temporal lobe lobectomy. Permanent hemiparesis is a potential adverse effect of this surgery.

Status Epilepticus

Status epilepticus is a life-threatening condition that manifests as continuous seizure activity or two or more seizures occurring in sequence without recovery of consciousness between the seizures.[141]

Treatment

The goal of treatment of status epilepticus is prompt pharmacologic suppression of seizure activity combined with support of the patient's airway, ventilation, circulation, and establishment of intravenous access (Fig. 17–9).[141] Hypoglycemia is excluded or corrected by intravenous administration of 50 ml of 50% glucose. Tracheal intubation, may be needed to protect the patient's lungs from aspiration and to optimize delivery of oxygen and adequate removal of carbon dioxide. Administration of short-acting nondepolarizing neuromuscular blocking drugs may be needed to facilitate tracheal intubation, whereas the short duration of the drug allows confirmation that seizure activity is suppressed. Monitoring arterial blood gases and pH may be useful for confirming the adequacy of oxygenation and ventilation and following the course of metabolic acidosis that invariably accompanies ongoing seizure activity. Intravenous administration of sodium bicarbonate is needed only in extreme cases. Hyperthermia occurs frequently during status epilepticus and necessitates active cooling.

Management of Anesthesia

Management of anesthesia in patients with seizure disorders includes consideration of the impact of antiepileptic drugs on organ function, coagulation,

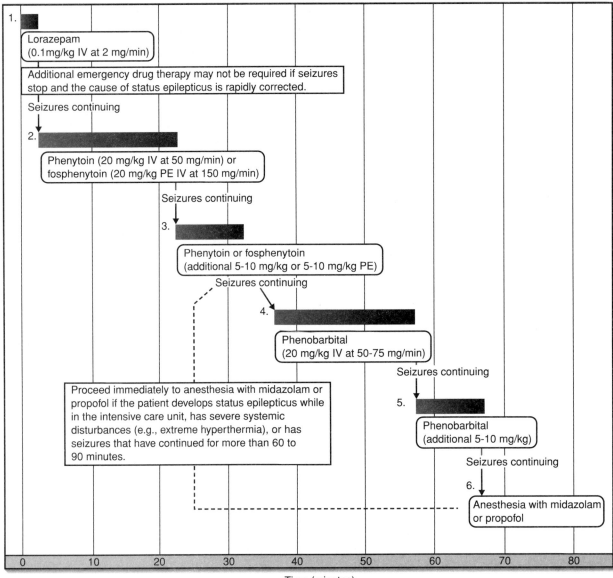

Figure 17–9 • Algorithm for pharmacologic management of status epilepticus. *Horizontal bars* indicate the approximate duration of drug infusions. PE, phenytoin equivalents. (From Lowenstein DH, Alldredge BK. Status epilepticus. N Engl J Med 1998;338:970–6. Copyright 1998 Massachusetts Medical Society, with permission.)

and response to anesthetic drugs. Known adverse effects of these drugs are evaluated with appropriate preoperative tests. Co-existing sedation produced by antiepileptic drugs may have additive effects with anesthetic drugs, whereas drug-induced enzyme induction could alter responses to other drugs or even contribute to organ toxicity.

When selecting drugs for induction and maintenance of anesthesia, one must consider the effects of these drugs on central nervous system electrical activity. For example, methohexital can activate epi-

leptic foci and has been recommended as a method for delineating these foci in patients undergoing surgical treatment of epilepsy.[142] The ability of ketamine to elicit seizure activity in patients with known seizure disorders and in those with no known central nervous system disease has not been a consistent observation. Seizures and opisthotonos have been observed following propofol anesthesia, suggesting caution when administering this drug to patients with known seizure disorders.[143] Nevertheless, this has not been a common or predictable occurrence following administration of propofol. When selecting muscle relaxants, the central nervous system-stimulating effects of laudanosine, a metabolite of atracurium and cisatracurium, may merit consideration.

Most inhaled anesthetics, including nitrous oxide, have been reported to produce seizure activity. The presence of halogen atoms is an important determinant of the convulsant properties of volatile anesthetics, with fluorine being incriminated as epileptogenic. Nevertheless, seizure activity is rare after administration of volatile anesthetics such as isoflurane, desflurane, and sevoflurane. Sevoflurane has stronger epileptogenic properties than isoflurane, but nitrous oxide or hyperventilation counteracts this specific epileptogenic property.[144] Enflurane is unique among the volatile anesthetics for evoking seizure activity evidenced on the electroencephalogram, making this drug an unlikely choice for patients with known seizure disorders.

In view of the availability of drugs that do not lower the patient's seizure threshold, it seems reasonable to avoid administering potentially epileptogenic drugs to patients with epilepsy. In this regard, thiobarbiturates, opioids, and benzodiazepines do not lower seizure thresholds or predispose to seizure activity. Isoflurane, desflurane, and sevoflurane seem to be acceptable choices in patients with seizure disorders. Regardless of the drugs used for anesthesia, it is important to maintain treatment with the existing antiepileptic drugs throughout the perioperative period.

■ HEADACHES

Headache is one of the most common symptoms described by patients. In most individuals the cause of headache is benign, and no treatment other than symptomatic measures is required. Occasionally, headache is a symptom of central nervous system disease. Perioperative caffeine withdrawal syndrome may manifest as postoperative headache in susceptible patients.[145]

Migraine Headaches

Migraine headaches are disorders of youth, occurring most often in women 20 to 35 years of age. A family history of migraine headache is present in about 60% of patients, and the incidence of systemic hypertension, stroke, and ischemic heart disease is increased. The onset of migraine headaches during middle age or their accentuation by maneuvers that increase ICP (coughing, bending over) suggests a focal intracranial tumor.

Signs and Symptoms

Signs and symptoms of migraine headache (abdominal pain, vertigo, motion sickness) commonly begin during childhood, but the actual headache may not be experienced until years later. Classic migraine headache begins with a prodrome characterized by neurologic symptoms suggestive of cerebral ischemia. Visual blurring and tingling paresthesias of the face and arms are frequent. After about 30 minutes these symptoms wane, followed by an intense (pounding) unilateral headache. Nausea and vomiting may occur. Typically, migraine headaches subside in about 6 hours.

The common migraine headache differs from the classic migraine headache in that the prodromal signs are absent and the headache is often protracted and may be present on awakening. A small number of patients manifest symptoms (vertigo, diplopia, ataxia) characterized as basilar artery migraine. Ophthalmic migraine is characterized by headache and ocular paralysis (ptosis due to oculomotor nerve involvement), presumably reflecting compression of the cranial nerve by an edematous carotid or basilar artery. The traditional explanation for migraine headaches is initial vasoconstriction, causing the prodromal phase of brain ischemia, followed by secondary extracranial vasodilation manifesting as headache. However, there is no evidence of an initial increase in CBF to support this hypothesis. A more likely explanation of the initiating event seems to be neuronal changes characterized by spreading inhibition of cortical neurons (similar to seizure activity). Abnormal serotoninergic transmission may be involved in the development of migraine headaches. Indeed, migraine headaches can be triggered by drugs that release serotonin.

Treatment

β-Adrenergic antagonists are the most commonly prescribed drugs for prophylaxis. Calcium channel blockers are used to decrease the frequency of migraine attacks. Divalproex is an antiepileptic drug that may be an effective prophylactic agent. Antidepressants may have effects on serotonin and possible analgesic effects. Sumatriptan, a selective agonist of a subpopulation of serotonin receptors (type 1D), is an effective treatment for migraine and cluster headaches. Methysergide is thought to block the inflammatory and vasoconstricting effects of serotonin but because of potential side effects is used only on selected patients. There are no known unique hazards of anesthetic drugs when administered to these patients.

Cluster Headaches

Cluster headaches (histamine cephalgia, atypical facial neuralgia) are vasodilating headaches that typically awaken patients at night by their excruciating unilateral pain often involving the temporal or malar regions. Maximum intensity of pain is reached at about 20 to 30 minutes, followed by the disappearance of symptoms over the next 1 to 2 hours. Visual disturbances or paresthesias typical of migraine headaches are absent, but ptosis and miosis may occur. Attacks occur in clusters, followed by long symptom-free intervals. Middle-aged men are most often affected.

Headaches Associated with Increased Intracranial Pressure

Headaches may be the initial manifestations of increased ICP due to intracranial tumors, abscesses, or hematomas. Commonly, headaches associated with increased ICP occur during the early morning hours, often awakening the patient. Presumably, this timing reflects decreased alveolar ventilation during physiologic sleep, leading to increases in $PaCO_2$ and corresponding increases in CBF. Spontaneous vomiting may accompany headaches. The headaches may be provoked by coughing, which leads to increased ICP by impeding venous outflow from the brain.

Headaches Associated with Benign Intracranial Hypertension

Benign intracranial hypertension (pseudotumor cerebri) is defined as a syndrome characterized by increased ICP above 20 mmHg, normal composition of CBF, normal sensorium, and absence of local intracranial lesions.[146] Computed tomography indicates a normal or even small cerebral ventricular system. Headaches and bilateral visual disturbances typically occur in obese women with menstrual irregularities. Symptoms of benign intracranial hypertension may be exaggerated during pregnancy. This syndrome may also occur after withdrawal of corticosteroid therapy or following initiation of treatment for hypothyroidism. No identifiable cause of increased ICP is found in most patients. The condition is self-limited, and the prognosis is excellent.

Treatment

Treatment of benign intracranial hypertension includes removal of 20 to 40 ml of CSF via a needle or catheter placed in the lumbar subarachnoid space as well as administration of acetazolamide to decrease formation of CSF and dexamethasone to decrease cerebral edema. The principal indication for treatment is loss of visual acuity. Initial treatment is often repeated lumbar puncture to remove CSF, which also facilitates measurement of the ICP. Furthermore, continued leakage of CSF through the dural puncture site may be therapeutic. Lumbar puncture is not advisable in patients with increased ICP secondary to space-occupying lesions. In such patients lumbar puncture could lead to herniation of the cerebellar tonsils and pressure on the medulla oblongata. In patients with benign intracranial hypertension, the presence of uniform swelling of the brain plus the normal position of the cerebellar tonsils prevents herniation and compression of the brain stem. Chronic administration of acetazolamide can result in acidemia, presumably reflecting inhibition of hydrogen ion secretion by renal tubules. Surgical therapy, most often a lumboperitoneal shunt, is indicated only after medical therapy has failed and the patient's vision has began to deteriorate.

Management of Anesthesia

Management of anesthesia in patients with benign intracranial hypertension who are undergoing lumboperitoneal shunt placement incorporates the same principles outlined for removal of intracranial tumors. Spinal anesthesia may be beneficial in parturients, as continued leakage of CSF is acceptable.[146] When lumboperitoneal shunts are present, a skull radiograph is helpful for localizing the point of entry into the subarachnoid space before performing lumbar puncture. Furthermore, there is a theoretical possibility that injection of local anesthetic solutions into the subarachnoid space could escape into the peritoneal cavity, resulting in inadequate anesthesia. Therefore general anesthesia may be a more logical choice in the presence of lumboperitoneal shunts.

■ INTERVERTEBRAL DISC HERNIATION

The intervertebral disc is composed of a compressible nucleus pulposus surrounded by a fibrocartilaginous annulus fibrosis. The disc acts as a shock absorber between vertebral bodies. Trauma or degenerative changes lead to changes in the intervertebral disc. Nerve root compression results when the nucleus pulposus protrudes through the posterolateral aspect of the annulus fibrosis. Occasionally, central protrusion of the discs occurs. There are signs of spinal cord compression if protrusion is into the cervical or thoracic regions, whereas signs of cauda equina compression appear if protrusion is into the lumbar region. Low back pain ranks second only to upper respiratory tract disease as a reason for office visits to physicians.[147] An estimated 70% of adults experience low back pain at some time. Among chronic conditions, low back pain is the most common cause for limitation of activity in patients younger than 45 years of age. Primary or metastatic cancer is the most common systemic disease affecting the vertebral bodies, although it accounts for fewer than 1% of all episodes of low back pain. Computed tomography confirms the diagnosis and the location of intervertebral disc herniation.

Cervical Disc Disease

Lateral protrusion of a cervical disc usually occurs at the C5-6 or C6-7 intervertebral spaces. Protrusion can be secondary to trauma or occur spontaneously. Pain starting in the neck that radiates to the shoulder and down the outer aspect of the arm into the thumb is characteristic of C5-6 disc protrusion. The biceps reflex is decreased, and the biceps muscle is weak. Pain in the scapula, triceps region, and middle and index fingers reflects protrusion at the C6-7 intervertebral space. Symptoms are commonly aggravated by coughing. The same symptoms can be due to osteophytes that compress nerve roots in the intervertebral foramina.

Initial treatment of cervical disc protrusion is with traction. Surgical decompression is necessary if symptoms do not abate with conservative treatment.

Lumbar Disc Disease

The most common site for lumbar disc protrusion is the L4-5 and L5-S1 intervertebral spaces. Both sites produce low back pain, which radiates down the posterior and lateral aspects of the thighs and calves ("sciatica"). Sensory loss and skeletal muscle weakness correspond to compression of the L5 or S1 nerve roots. A history of trauma, often viewed as trivial, is usually associated with the sudden back pain that signals disc protrusion. Back pain is aggravated by coughing or stretching the sciatic nerve, as produced by straight-leg raising. These mechanical signs help distinguish protrusion from peripheral

nerve disorders, such as may accompany diabetes mellitus, which are not accompanied by these signs.

Treatment of acute lumbar disc protrusion has historically included bed rest and the use of centrally acting muscle relaxants. In patients without neuromotor deficits the clinical outcome after 2 days of bed rest is similar to that in those with neuromotor deficits after longer periods of bed rest.[148] Among patients with acute low back pain, continuing ordinary activities within the limits permitted by the pain leads to more rapid recovery than either bed rest or back-mobilizing exercises.[149] When neurologic symptoms persist despite conservative medical management, surgical laminectomy or microdiscectomy can be considered to decompress the affected nerve roots. An alternative to surgery may be to place corticosteroid-containing solutions (triamcinolone, methylprednisolone) in the epidural space. Corticosteroids may decrease the inflammation and edema produced by compression of the nerve roots. Suppression of the hypothalamic-pituitary-adrenal axis is a consideration in treated patients.[150] Exogenous corticosteroid coverage may be indicated should these patients undergo surgery. Although epidural steroid injections may result in short-term alleviation of symptoms due to sciatica, this treatment offers no significant functional benefit nor does it decrease the need for surgery.[151]

Degenerative Vertebral Column Disease

Spinal spondylosis, spondylolisthesis, and stenosis are forms of degenerative vertebral column disease. It is not uncommon for more than one of these degenerative changes in the spine to occur concomitantly, leading to more rapid progression of neurologic symptoms and the need for surgical intervention.

Cervical spondylosis is a common disorder that leads to osteophyte formation and degenerative disc disease. There is narrowing of the spinal canal and compression of the spinal cord by transverse osteophytes, in addition to nerve root compression by bony spurs in the intervertebral foramina. Spinal cord dysfunction may also reflect ischemic infarction secondary to bony compression of the spinal arteries. Symptoms typically develop insidiously after about 50 years of age. Neck pain and radicular pain in the arms and shoulders are accompanied by sensory loss and skeletal muscle wasting. Later, sensory and motor signs appear in the legs, producing an unsteady gait. Sphincter disturbances are uncommon. Radiographs of the spine often demonstrate osteoarthritic changes, but these changes correlate poorly with neurologic symptoms. Surgery may be necessary to arrest progression of the symptoms.

Spina Bifida Occulta

Spina bifida occulta (incomplete formation of a single lamina in the lumbosacral spine without other abnormalities) is present in an estimated 20% of individuals.[151] The diagnosis is an incidental finding on radiologic examination. Because there are no underlying abnormalities, an increased risk with spinal anesthesia is not expected, and large numbers of these patients have received spinal anesthesia safely. However, a variant of spina bifida occulta known as occult *spinal dysraphism* exists wherein the bony defect may involve more than one lamina. A significant number of these defects are associated with a tethered spinal cord (cord ending below the L2-3 interspace) which may be responsible for progressive neurologic symptoms. Up to 50% of individuals with a tethered spinal cord have cutaneous manifestations overlying the anomaly, including tufts of hair, hyperpigmented areas, cutaneous lipomas, and skin dimples. Performance of spinal anesthesia in patients with a tethered spinal cord may increase the risk of lacerating vessels on the surface of the spinal cord, with subsequent formation of spinal hematomas.[152]

■ SLEEP DISORDERS

The three principal sleep-related complaints for which patients seek medical attention are excessive daytime somnolence, insomnia, and abnormal movements ("restless legs syndrome") or behavior during sleep. Excessive daytime somnolence may reflect obstructive sleep apnea syndrome, central sleep apnea syndrome, or narcolepsy (see Chapter 23). Insomnia may be idiopathic or associated with psychiatric disorders, stress, pain, or drug and alcohol abuse.[153] Chronic insomnia is associated with an increased incidence of motor vehicle accidents, increased alcohol consumption, and daytime sleepiness. Air travel across time zones ("jet lag") is often associated with insomnia. Treatment of transient insomnia is with intermediate-acting benzodiazepines such as temazepam. Hypnotic medications are not recommended for treatment of chronic insomnia. Sedative-antidepressants such as trazodone are used for insomnia associated with depression. Surgery is associated with postoperative sleep disturbances, which may result in postoperative cerebral dysfunction and confusion (see Chapter 33).[154]

Narcolepsy

Narcolepsy is a distinct neurologic disorder characterized by an uncontrollable urge to sleep and by abnormalities of rapid eye movement (REM) sleep.[155] This sleep disorder is estimated to occur in approximately 1 in 4000 persons in the United States, and about 30% of afflicted individuals have a positive family history, emphasizing the genetic predisposition for this disease. In some patients narcoleptic sleep attacks are associated with sleep apnea. Abnormalities of monoaminergic and cholinergic functioning in the brain are likely to be present. Cataplexy, the sudden loss of postural tone leading to collapse can accompany narcolepsy.

Treatment

Methylphenidate and dextroamphetamine are used as stimulants to prevent narcolepsy, whereas tricyclic antidepressants are considered the primary treatment for cataplexy. Pemoline is a central nervous system stimulant that facilitates presynaptic release of dopamine and inhibits its reuptake.[156] Unlike other stimulants, pemoline has minimal peripheral sympathomimetic effects. This drug is utilized in the treatment of narcolepsy and attention hyperactivity disorders. Increases in serum liver transaminase concentrations may occur, as may seizures, exacerbation of Tourette's syndrome, and tics.

Management of Anesthesia

Anesthetic implications in patients with narcolepsy include possible increased sensitivity to anesthetic drugs, increased risk of postoperative apnea, and interactions with treatment medications.[157] Theoretically, prolonged emergence and postoperative hypersomnia following general anesthesia are possibilities. Avoidance of preoperative sedatives and continuation of medical therapy for narcolepsy throughout the perioperative period should decrease the likelihood of excessive somnolence. Opioids administered intraoperatively may be avoided in consideration of the possible increased incidence of postoperative apnea. Short-acting intravenous induction drugs (propofol) and inhaled drugs (nitrous oxide, desflurane, sevoflurane) are attractive choices in patients with narcolepsy. Vasodilation and hypotension during general anesthesia has been attributed to treatment with pemoline.[156] Regional anesthesia is an acceptable option, although cataleptic attacks have been described in patients with narcolepsy receiving spinal anesthesia.[157]

Postoperative Sleep Disturbances

Changes in early postoperative sleep patterns are characterized by decreases in total sleep time, elimination of REM sleep, and increased amounts of non-REM sleep.[154] Postoperative sleep disturbances may contribute to the development of altered mental (cognitive) function, postoperative episodic arterial hypoxemia, and hemodynamic instability. Elderly patients may be particularly vulnerable to postoperative cognitive dysfunction, perhaps reflecting disruption of normal sleep patterns. Increased postoperative sympathetic nervous system activity and increased circulating plasma catecholamine concentrations may contribute to postoperative sleep disturbances by maintaining wakefulness.

Postoperative rebound of REM sleep during the middle of the first postoperative week may contribute to the development of sleep-disordered breathing and nocturnal arterial hypoxemia.[154] Arterial hypoxemia associated with postoperative sleep disturbances may result in myocardial ischemia, cardiac dysrhythmias, and hemodynamic instability. Impaired mental function with a peak incidence during the middle of the first postoperative week may reflect the effects of arterial hypoxemia associated with sleep disturbances. Postoperative mental dysfunction is especially common in elderly patients (see Chapter 33).

Postoperative pain is the most common cause of nighttime awakenings, and provision of analgesia is the most effective intervention to improve sleep. Noise levels in intensive care units may interfere with sleep patterns. The magnitude and duration of the surgical procedure determines the degree of postoperative sleep disturbances, suggesting that a decrease in the surgical stress response as associated with minimally invasive surgical techniques may be helpful.[154] Likewise, stress reduction provided by continuous neural blockade utilizing local anesthetics might improve postoperative sleep patterns. Because morphine may disrupt normal sleep patterns, there may be value in providing postoperative analgesia with local anesthetics and maximizing the opioid-sparing effects provided by nonsteroidal antiinflammatory drugs. Noise, nocturnal nursing procedures, calorie deprivation, and increased ambient temperatures are known to disrupt normal sleep patterns, and they can be minimized during the postoperative period. Sedative drugs with minimal effects on further decreasing REM sleep seem desirable.

Factitious Disorder as a Cause for Failure to Awaken

Although factitious disorders ("hysteria") are rarely the cause of delayed emergence, patient unwillingness to awaken following general anesthesia is a recognized phenomenon and, by necessity, is a diagnosis of exclusion.[158] After ruling out physiologic causes for delayed awakening following general anesthesia (residual effects of anesthetic drugs, inadequate antagonism of neuromuscular blocking drugs, hypoglycemia, electrolyte abnormalities, impaired oxygenation, impaired ventilation, hypothermia, organic cerebral insults), the possibility of a factitious disorder must be considered. The best known factitious disorder is Munchausen syndrome, a condition in which patients are sociopathic impostors who, purposefully and consciously, attempt to mislead those involved in their health care.

Circadian Rhythms and Sleep

Disturbances in circadian rhythms (jet lag, changes in work hours, blindness) often result in sleep disturbances. Melatonin is involved in circadian rhythms, and its secretion by the hypothalamus is synchronized to a 24 hour period largely by cues from the light–dark cycle. Normally, melatonin is produced during periods of darkness. Use of melatonin to treat circadian rhythm sleep disorders requires careful synchronization and timing for best results.[159] Claims of the effectiveness of using melatonin to manage jet lag have been exaggerated.

ABNORMAL PATTERNS OF BREATHING

Irregular breathing patterns may reflect an abnormality at a specific site in the central nervous system (Table 17–8). Ataxic breathing is characterized by a completely random pattern of tidal volumes that results from disruption of medullary neural pathways by trauma, hemorrhage, or extrinsic compression. Mechanical ventilation of the patient's lungs may be necessary if apnea occurs. Apnea may occur in response to the administration of sedative drugs or opioids. Lesions in the pons may result in apneustic breathing characterized by prolonged end-inspiratory pauses maintained for as long as 30 seconds. Occlusion of the basilar artery leading to pontine infarction is a common cause of apneustic breathing. Cheyne-Stokes breathing is characterized by breaths of progressively increasing and then decreasing volume (crescendo-decrescendo pattern),

Table 17–8 • Abnormal Patterns of Breathing

Abnormality	Pattern	Site of Lesion
Ataxic (Biot's breathing)	Unpredictable sequence of breaths varying in rate and tidal volume	Medulla
Apneustic breathing	Repetitive gasps and prolonged pauses at full inspiration	Pons
Cheyne-Stokes breathing	Cyclic crescendo-decrescendo tidal volume pattern interrupted by apnea	Cerebral hemispheres Congestive heart failure
Central neurogenic hypoventilation	Hypocarbia	Cerebral thrombosis or embolism
Posthyperventilation apnea	Awake apnea following moderate decreases in $PaCO_2$	Frontal lobes

followed by periods of apnea lasting 15 to 20 seconds. Arterial blood gases typically also fluctuate in cyclic patterns. This pattern of breathing may reflect brain damage (cerebral hemispheres or basal ganglia) due to arterial hypoxemia or may accompany congestive heart failure. In the presence of congestive heart failure, the delay in circulation time from the pulmonary capillaries to the carotid bodies is presumed to be responsible for Cheyne-Stokes breathing. Central neurogenic hyperventilation is most often due to acute neurologic insults as associated with cerebral thrombosis or cerebral embolism. Hyperventilation is spontaneous and may be so severe the $PaCO_2$ is decreased to less than 20 mmHg. Posthyperventilation apnea occurs in patients with frontal lobe disease after a sequence of five deep breaths that lowers the $PaCO_2$ by about 10 mmHg. Breathing in such individuals resumes when apnea is of sufficient duration to return the $PaCO_2$ to levels present before hyperventilation. In normal patients the same sequence of voluntary deep breaths does not produce apnea despite similar decreases in $PaCO_2$, reflecting the presence of a voluntary stimulus to breathe.

ACUTE MOUNTAIN SICKNESS

Acute mountain sickness is characterized by headache, fatigue, and anorexia, most likely due to the cerebral edema that accompanies rapid ascent to high altitudes. Symptoms are rare below 2240 meters elevation and common above 3660 meters. The onset of acute mountain sickness may not occur until 8 to 24 hours after ascent; symptoms usually subside within 2 to 4 days. Severe cases of cerebral edema may be accompanied by ataxia, obtundation, and coma. Computed tomography of the brain confirms the presence of cerebral edema, which probably is caused by increased CBF (vasogenic edema) and cellular swelling related to hypoxia (cytotoxic edema). Prompt descent from high altitude and oxygen therapy are the principal treatments. Furosemide is avoided, as diuresis may result in orthostatic hypotension.

DISORDERS INVOLVING THE AUDITORY PROCESSES

Vertigo is the cardinal symptom of vestibular dysfunction and may be accompanied by nausea, vomiting, nystagmus, postural instability, and autonomic nervous system stimulation. Vestibular neuritis is associated with disabling vertigo that usually resolves within about 1 week. Infarction of the inferior cerebellum may simulate vestibular neuritis. As many as 25% of patients with risk factors for stroke (systemic hypertension, smoking, diabetes mellitus, atrial fibrillation) who present with severe vertigo, nystagmus, and postural instability have an infarction of the inferior cerebellum.[160] Acoustic neuromas may initially present as vertigo. Abrupt onset of vertigo after rapid changes in head position is characteristic of benign positional vertigo, which usually lasts less than 60 seconds. Hypoglycemia must be eliminated as a cause of vertigo.

Meniere's Disease (Endolymphatic Hydrops)

Meniere's disease is a disorder of the membranous labyrinth of the inner ear characterized by the triad of hearing loss, tinnitus, and vertigo. This disease occurs most often in individuals 30 to 60 years of age; and in most patients the etiology is unknown. The pathognomonic feature of Meniere's disease is distension of the endolymphatic system of the inner ear. Treatment of Meniere's disease is surgical if bed rest and sedation with benzodiazepines are not effective. Surgical therapy is a labyrinthectomy or transection of the vestibular nerve, requiring craniotomy.

Nitrous Oxide and Middle Ear Dynamics

The middle ear is an air-filled cavity bounded by the tympanic membrane and the inner ear. During inhalation of nitrous oxide, middle ear pressures may increase, reflecting passage of nitrous oxide into the noncompliant confines of the middle ear. Under normal conditions this pressure buildup in the middle ear is passively vented through the eustachian tubes into the nasopharynx. Narrowing of the eustachian tubes by acute inflammation or the presence of scar tissue, as is likely after an adenoidectomy, impairs the ability of the middle ear to vent passively any pressure increases produced by nitrous oxide. Excessive middle ear pressures could jeopardize the integrity of the tympanic membrane. The presence of bright red blood in the external auditory canal (evidence of tympanic membrane rupture) has been described during administration of nitrous oxide even in the absence of middle ear disease.[161] Disruption of previous middle ear reconstructive surgery has also been observed when nitrous oxide is administered at a later date for operative procedures not involving the middle ear.[162] Manifestations of this disruption are the postoperative recurrence of hearing loss in previously operated ears. Administration of nitrous oxide during tympanoplasty may result in displacement of freshly placed grafts, reflecting the presence of air bubbles containing nitrous oxide in the middle ear. Postoperative nausea and vomiting could also be due to increased middle ear pressures that persist after administration of nitrous oxide.

Absorption of nitrous oxide after discontinuing inhalation of this drug can also exert deleterious effects on the middle ear. For example, rapid resorption of nitrous oxide can result in negative pressures in the middle ear, causing rupture of the tympanic membranes. Transient hearing impairment after administration of nitrous oxide to previously normal patients most likely reflects negative pressures in the middle ear. Serous otitis can also be a manifestation of these negative pressures.

The potential adverse effect of nitrous oxide on the middle ear poses questions as to the wisdom of administering this drug to patients with narrowing of the eustachian tubes (due to acute inflammation or chronic scarring from prior surgery). Indeed, a preoperative history of previous middle ear surgery introduces this concern, although it is undeniable that many patients with a history of middle ear surgery have been exposed to nitrous oxide on later occasions without subsequent detectable detrimental effects on their hearing.

GLOMUS TUMORS OF THE HEAD AND NECK

Glomus tumors are paragangliomas, which are of neural crest origin outside the adrenal medulla.[163] These tumors arise in the head and neck from neuroendocrine tissue that lies along the carotid artery, aorta, glossopharyngeal nerve, and middle ear. When a glomus tumor is present, it is likely a second craniocervical paraganglioma; usually a carotid body tumor also exists. These tumors are rarely malignant.

Signs and Symptoms

Tumor location determines signs and symptoms, which most often reflect middle ear and cranial nerve invasion. Unilateral pulsatile tinnitus, conductive hearing loss, aural fullness, and a bluish red mass behind the tympanic membrane are characteristic of middle ear involvement, whereas facial paralysis, dysphonia, hearing loss, and pain typify cranial nerve invasion. Recurrent aspiration, dysphagia, and upper airway obstruction may also accompany cranial nerve involvement. Invasion of the posterior fossa may obstruct the aqueduct of Sylvius, causing hydrocephalus. It is common for glomus jugulare tumors to invade the internal jugular vein; finger-like projections may extend to the right atrium. Occasionally, glomus jugulare tumors secrete norepinephrine, producing symptoms that mimic pheochromocytoma.

Treatment

Small glomus tumors are most often treated with radiation. Surgery is recommended if bony destruction is present. Preoperative determination of serum catecholamine concentrations may be used to recognize patients likely to respond as if a pheochromocytoma were present. Administration of phenoxybenzamine or prazosin may be utilized preoperatively in patients with increased serum catecholamine concentrations. Surgical excision may be preceded by radiation or embolization to decrease the vascularity of the tumor.

Management of Anesthesia

Management of anesthesia is a formidable challenge in these patients.[163] Anesthetic risks include catecholamine secretion, producing symptoms resembling pheochromocytomas; serotonin secretion, producing symptoms of carcinoid syndrome; aspiration after tumor resection; impaired gastric emptying; increased ICP; threat of venous air embolism; and massive blood loss. Intraoperatively, histamine and bradykinin released during surgical manipulation can cause profound hypotension. Cranial nerve deficits may be present preoperatively (vagus, glossopharyngeal, hypoglossal nerves), or they may occur as a result of tumor resection. Impaired sensory and motor function, especially of the vagus nerve, increase the risk of postoperative aspiration, especially if postoperative ileus occurs owing to increased cholecystokinin levels. Airway obstruction is a risk after cranial nerve injury. Unilateral vocal cord paralysis, which in adults usually does not result in complete airway obstruction, can produce airway obstruction in combination with airway edema or laryngeal distortion.

Invasive arterial and venous pressure monitoring is indicated; and urinary output is monitored after placing a Foley catheter. An internal jugular vein involved by tumor should not be cannulated for placing a right atrial or pulmonary artery catheter. Hypothermia is likely, especially with prolonged surgery, emphasizing the usefulness of warming inhaled gases and infused fluids. Drugs and techniques designed to control ICP may be necessary. Controlled hypotension minimizes blood loss and may facilitate surgical excision of the tumor.

Venous air embolism is a risk, especially if the internal jugular vein is opened to remove the tumor. It is also a risk if excision of a tumor that has invaded temporal bone results in exposure of veins that cannot collapse because of bony attachments. As a precaution, mechanical ventilation of the patient's lungs may be useful; and addition of skeletal muscle paralysis minimizes the possibility of a gasp reflex. Appropriate monitors for detecting venous air embolism are indicated when venous air embolism is considered a risk (see "Venous Air Embolism"). Sudden, unexplained cardiovascular collapse and death during resection of these tumors may reflect the presence of a venous air embolism and/or tumor emboli. If the surgeon finds it necessary to identify the facial nerve, avoidance of profound skeletal muscle paralysis (maintain visible twitch response) is useful. The choice of anesthetic drugs is not uniquely influenced by the presence of glomus jugulare tumors, although the potential adverse effects of nitrous oxide should be promptly appreciated if venous air embolism occurs.

■ CAROTID SINUS SYNDROME

Carotid sinus syndrome is an uncommon entity caused by exaggeration of normal activity of the baroreceptors in response to mechanical stimulation. For example, stimulation of the carotid sinus by external massage, which in normal individuals produces modest decreases in heart rate and systemic blood pressure, can produce syncope in those exhibiting carotid sinus syndrome. There is an increased incidence of peripheral vascular disease in these individuals. Carotid sinus syndrome is a recognized complication of carotid endarterectomy.

Two distinct cardiovascular responses may be noted in the presence of carotid sinus hypersensitivity. In about 80% of affected individuals, a cardioinhibitory reflex is mediated by the vagus nerve, producing profound bradycardia. In about 10% of affected individuals, a vasodepressor reflex is mediated by inhibition of sympathetic nervous system vasomotor tone, with resultant decreases in systemic vascular resistance and profound hypotension. The remaining 10% of individuals exhibit components of both reflexes.

Treatment

Treatment of carotid sinus syndrome may consist of administering drugs, placing a permanent demand artificial cardiac pacemaker, or ablation of the carotid sinus. Use of anticholinergic drugs and vasopressors is limited by their side effects and is rarely effective in patients with vasodepressor or mixed forms of carotid sinus hypersensitivity. Because most patients have the cardioinhibitory type of carotid sinus syndrome, implantation of an artificial cardiac pacemaker is the usual initial treatment. Ablation of the carotid sinus may be attempted in patients in whom the vasodepressor reflex response is refractory to cardiac pacing. Glossopharyngeal nerve block may be an alternative therapy in patients refractory to artificial cardiac pacing or drug therapy.[164]

Management of Anesthesia

Management of anesthesia in patients with carotid sinus syndrome is often complicated by hypotension, bradycardia, and cardiac dysrhythmias.[164] Infiltration of a local anesthetic-containing solution around the carotid sinus before dissection usually improves hemodynamic stability but may also interfere with determining the completeness of the ablation. Drugs such as atropine, isoproterenol, and epinephrine should be readily available to treat bradycardia, heart block, and hypotension.

▉ NEUROFIBROMATOSIS

Neurofibromatosis is due to an autosomal dominant mutation that is not limited to racial or ethnic origin. Both genders are affected with equal frequency and severity. Expressivity is variable, but penetrance of the trait is virtually 100%. Manifestations are classified as classic (vonRecklinghausen's disease), acoustic, and segmental neurofibromatosis.

Signs and Symptoms

The diversity of clinical features of neurofibromatosis emphasizes the protean nature of this disease (Table 17–9). One feature common to all patients is progression of the disease with time. Manifestations of neurofibromatosis are likely to worsen during pregnancy.

Café au Lait Spots

Café au lait spots (abnormal cutaneous pigmentation) are present in more than 99% of affected individuals; six or more spots larger than 1.5 cm in diameter are considered diagnostic of neurofibromatosis. Café au lait spots are usually present at birth and continue to increase in number and size during the first decade of life; they vary in size from 1 mm to more than 15 cm. Distribution of spots is random, except for disproportionately small numbers on the face. Other than an adverse cosmetic effect, café au lait spots pose no threat to health.

Table 17–9 • Manifestations of Neurofibromatosis

Café au lait spots
Neurofibromas (cutaneous, neural, vascular)
Intracranial tumor
Spinal cord tumor
Pseudarthrosis
Kyphoscoliosis
Short stature
Cancer
Endocrine abnormalities
Learning disability
Seizures
Congenital heart disease (pulmonic stenosis)

Watson Syndrome

Watson syndrome is a rare genetic disorder with an autosomal dominant mode of inheritance. Its most consistent clinical features are café au lait spots, short stature, mental retardation, and pulmonic valvular stenosis. Obstruction to right ventricular outflow results in both increased right ventricular work and pressures with compensatory concentric right ventricular hypertrophy. Increases in cardiac output associated with labor and delivery may result in acute right ventricular heart failure. Maintenance of adequate preload, a normal heart rate, and avoiding decreases in afterload and myocardial contractility are important considerations when planning anesthesia management. Ketamine analgesia and epidural anesthesia for cesarean section have been described.[165]

Neurofibromas

Neurofibromas virtually always involve the skin, but they can also occur in the deeper peripheral nerves and nerve roots and in or on viscera or blood vessels innervated by the autonomic nervous system. These neurofibromas may be nodular and discrete or diffuse with extensive interdigitations into surrounding tissues. Although neurofibromas are histologically benign, functional compromise and cosmetic disfigurement may result. The patient's airway may be compromised when neurofibromas develop in the laryngeal, cervical, or mediastinal regions. Neurofibromas may be highly vascular. Pregnancy or puberty can lead to increases in the number and size of neurofibromas.

Intracranial Tumors

Intracranial tumors occur in 5% to 10% of patients with neurofibromatosis, accounting for a major portion of the morbidity and mortality associated with this disease. Computed tomography to rule out the presence of intracranial tumors is indicated when the diagnosis of neurofibromatosis is considered. The bilateral presence of acoustic neuromas in patients with café au lait spots establishes the diagnosis of acoustic neurofibromatosis.

Orthopedic Abnormalities

Congenital pseudoarthrosis is commonly due to neurofibromatosis. The tibia is involved most often, with the radius the second most frequent site. Ordinarily, only a single site is involved in any one patient. The severity of pseudoarthrosis ranges from an asymptomatic radiologic presentation to the need for amputation. Kyphoscoliosis occurs in about 2% of patients afflicted with neurofibromatosis. Cervical and thoracic vertebrae are most often involved. Paravertebral neurofibromas are often present; but their role, if any, in the development of kyphoscoliosis is not defined. Untreated, kyphoscoliosis progresses, leading to cardiorespiratory and neurologic compromise. Short stature is a recognized feature of neurofibromatosis.

Cancer

There is an increased incidence of cancer in patients with neurofibromatosis. Associated cancers include neurofibrosarcoma, malignant schwannoma, Wilms' tumor, rhabdomyosarcoma, and leukemia. Other cancers, including neuroblastoma, medullary thyroid carcinoma, and pancreatic adenocarcinoma, are less often associated with neurofibromatosis.

Endocrine Disease

It is a misconception that neurofibromatosis entails diffuse endocrine dysfunction. Associated endocrine disorders, however, include pheochromocytomas, disturbances in reaching puberty, medullary thyroid carcinoma, and hyperparathyroidism. Pheochromocytomas occur with a frequency of probably less than 1% and are virtually unknown in children with neurofibromatosis.

Intellectual Function

Intellectual impairment occurs in about 40% of patients with neurofibromatosis. Mental retardation is less frequent than is impairment classified as learning disability. The intellectual handicap is usually apparent by school age and does not progress with time. Major and minor seizures are known complications of neurofibromatosis. Seizures may be idiopathic or may reflect the presence of intracranial tumors.

Treatment

Treatment of neurofibromatosis consists of symptomatic drug therapy (antihistamines for pruritus, antiepileptic drugs) and appropriately timed surgery. Surgical removal of cutaneous neurofibromas is reserved for those that are particularly disfiguring or functionally compromising. Progressive kyphoscoliosis is best treated with surgical stabilization.

Surgery is indicated for symptoms due to nervous system involvement by neurofibromas or to associated endocrine dysfunction.

Management of Anesthesia

Management of anesthesia for patients with neurofibromatosis includes consideration of the multiple clinical presentations of the disease.[166] Although rare, the possible presence of pheochromocytomas is a consideration during the preoperative evaluation. Signs of increased ICP may reflect the presence of expanding intracranial tumors. Airway patency may be jeopardized by expanding laryngeal neurofibromas. Patients with neurofibromatosis and scoliosis are also likely to have cervical spine defects that could influence positioning for direct laryngoscopy and the subsequent surgical procedure. Responses to muscle relaxants are monitored, as these patients have been described as both sensitive and resistant to succinylcholine and sensitive to nondepolarizing muscle relaxants.[167] Selection of regional anesthesia must recognize the possible future development of neurofibromas involving the spinal cord. Nevertheless, epidural analgesia is an effective method for producing analgesia during labor and delivery.[168]

References

1. Black PM. Brain tumors. N Engl J Med 1991;324:1471–6
2. DeAngelis LM. Brain tumors. N Engl J Med 2001;344:114–23
3. Inskip PD, Tarone RE, Hatch EE, et al. Cellular-telephone use and brain tumors. N Engl J Med 2001;344:79–86
4. Muscat JE, Malkin MG, Thompson S, et al. Handheld cellular telephone use and risk of brain cancer. JAMA 2000;284:3001–7
5. Brose WG, Samuels SI, Steinberg GK. Cardiorespiratory arrest following initiation of cranial irradiation for treatment of a brain-stem tumor. Anesthesiology 1989;71:450–1
6 Todd MM, Warner DS, Sokoll MD, et al. A prospective, comparative trial of three anesthetics for elective supratentorial craniotomy: propofol/fentanyl, isoflurane/nitrous oxide, and fentanyl/nitrous oxide. Anesthesiology 1993;78:1005–20
7. Lassen NA, Christensen MS. Physiology of cerebral blood flow. Br J Anaesth 1976;48:719–34
8. Mayberg TS, Lam AM, Matta BF, et al. Ketamine does not increase cerebral blood flow velocity and intracranial pressure during isoflurane-nitrous oxide anesthesia in humans. Anesthesiology 1993;78:288–94
9. Hamill JF, Bedford RF, Weaver DC, et al. Lidocaine before endotracheal intubation: intravenous or laryngotracheal? Anesthesiology 1981;55:578–81
10. Warner DS. Isoflurane neuroprotection: a passing fantasy, again? Anesthesiology 2000;92:1226–8
11. Losasso TJ, Black S, Muzzi DA, et al. Fifty percent nitrous oxide does not increase the risk of venous air embolism in

neurosurgical patients operated upon in the sitting position. Anesthesiology 1992;77:21–30

12. Marshall WK, Bedford RF. Use of a pulmonary-artery catheter for detection and treatment of venous air embolism: a prospective study in man. Anesthesiology 1980;52:131–4

13. Moorthy SS, Hilgenberg JC. Resistance to nondepolarizing muscle relaxants in paretic upper extremities of patients with residual hemiplegia. Anesth Analg 1980;59:624–7

14. Lam AM, Vavilala MS. Macroglossia: compartment syndrome of the tongue? Anesthesiology 2000;92:1832–5

15. Muth CM, Shank ES. Gas embolism. N Engl J Med 2000; 342:476–82

16. Edelman JD, Wingard DW. Air embolism arising from burr holes. Anesthesiology 1980;53:167–8

17. Katz J, Leiman BC, Butler BD. Effects of inhalation anaesthetics on filtration of venous gas emboli by the pulmonary vasculature. Br J Anaesth 1988;61:200–5

18. Perkins-Pearson NAK, Marshall WK, Bedford RF. Atrial pressures in the seated position: implications for paradoxical air embolism. Anesthesiology 1982;57:493–7

19. Matjasko J, Petrozza P, Mackenzie CF. Sensitivity of end-tidal nitrogen in venous air embolism detection in dogs. Anesthesiology 1985;63:418–25

20. Bunegin L, Albin MS, Helsel PE, et al. Positioning the right atrial catheter: a model for reappraisal. Anesthesiology 1981;55:343–8

21. Munson ES, Merrick HC. Effect of nitrous oxide on venous air embolism. Anesthesiology 1966;27:783–7

22. Zasslow MA, Pearl RG, Larson CP, et al. PEEP does not affect left atrial–right atrial pressure difference in neurosurgical patients. Anesthesiology 1988;68:760–3.

23. Morgenstern LB, Kasner SE. Cerebrovascular disorders. Sci Am Med 2000;1–15

24. Qureshi A, Tuhrim S, Broderick JP, et al. Spontaneous intracerebral hemorrhage. N Engl J Med 2001;344:1450–60

25. Bronner LL, Kanter DS, Manson JE. Primary prevention of stroke. N Engl J Med 1995;333:1392–1400

26. Kistler JP, Furie KL. Carotid endarterectomy revisited. N Engl J Med 2000;342:1743–5

27. Lam AM, Manninen PH, Ferguson GG, et al. Electrophysiologic function during carotid endarterectomy: a comparison of somatosensory evoked potentials and conventional electroencephalogram. Anesthesiology 1991;75:15–22

28. Garrioch MA, Fitch W. Anaesthesia for carotid artery surgery. Br J Anaesth 1993;71:569–79

29. Cantelmo NL, Babikian VL, Samaraweera RN, et al. Cerebral microembolism and ischemic changes associated with carotid endarterectomy. J Vasc Surg 1998;27:1024–30

30. Self DD, Bryson GL, Sullivan PJ. Risk factors for postcarotid endarterectomy hematoma formation. Can J Anesth 1999; 46:635–40

31. Carmichael FJ, McGuire GP, Wong DT, et al. Computed tomographic analysis of airway dimensions after carotid endarterectomy. Anesth Analg 1996;83:12–7

32. Brott T, Bogousslavsky J. Treatment of acute ischemic stroke. N Engl J Med 2000;343:710–22

33. Wahl CC. "Man-in-the-barrel" syndrome after endoscopic sinus surgery. Anesth Analg 1998;87:1196–8

34. Schievink WI. Intracranial aneurysms. N Engl J Med 1995; 336:28–40

35. Lam AM, Winn HR, Cullen BF, et al. Hyperglycemia and neurologic outcome in patients with head injury. J Neurosurg 1991;75:545–51

36. Lavine SD, Masri LS, Levy ML, et al. Temporary occlusion of the middle cerebral artery in intracranial aneurysm surgery: time limitation and advantage of brain protection. J Neurosurg 1997;87:917–24

37. Haydel MJ, Preston CA, Mills TJ, et al. Indications for computed tomography in patients with minor head injury. N Engl J Med 2000;343:100–5

38. Clifton GL, Miller ER, Choi SC, et al. Lack of effect of induction of hypothermia after acute brain injury. N Engl J Med 2001;344:556–63

39. Cho S, Fujigaki T, Uchiyama Y, et al. Effects of sevoflurane with and without nitrous oxide on human cerebral circulation: transcranial Doppler study. Anesthesiology 1996;85: 755–61

40. Gupta S, Heath K, Matta BF. Effect of incremental doses of sevoflurane on cerebral pressure autoregulation in humans. Br J Anaesth 1997;79:469–75

41. Rosenbaum KJ, Neigh JL, Stobel GE. Sensitivity to nondepolarizing muscle relaxants in amyotrophic lateral sclerosis: report of two cases. Anesthesiology 1971;35:38–41

42. Kochi T, Oka T, Mizuguchi T. Epidural anesthesia for patients with amyotrophic lateral sclerosis. Anesth Analg 1989;68:410–2

43. Hara K, Sakura S, Saito Y, et al. Epidural anesthesia and pulmonary function in a patient with amyotrophic lateral sclerosis. Anesth Analg 1996;83:878–9

44. Lee JJ, Imrie M, Taylor V. Anaesthesia and tuberous sclerosis. Br J Anaesth 1994;73:421–5

45. Bird TM, Strunin L. Hypotensive anesthesia for a patient with Freidreich's ataxia and cardiomyopathy. Anesthesiology 1984;60:377–80

46. Kubal K, Pasricha SK, Bhargava M. Spinal anesthesia in a patient with Freidreich's ataxia. Anesth Analg 1991;72:257–8

47. Lang AE, Lozano AM. Parkinson's disease. N Engl J Med 1998;339:1044–53,1130–43

48. Freeman TB, Vawter DE, Leaverton PE, et al. Use of placebo surgery in controlled trials of a cellular-based therapy for Parkinson's disease. N Engl J Med 1999;341:988–92

49. Reed AP, Han DG. Intraoperative exacerbation of Parkinson's disease. Anesth Analg 1992;75:850–3

50. Furuya R, Hirai A, Andoh T, et al. Successful perioperative management of a patient with Parkinson's disease by enteral levodopa administration under propofol anesthesia. Anesthesiology 1998;89:261–3

51. Mets B. Acute dystonia after alfentanil in untreated Parkinson's disease. Anesth Analg 1991;72:557–8

52. Roy RC, McLain S, Wise A, et al. Anesthesia management of a patient with Hallervorden- Spatz disease. Anesthesiology 1983;58:382–4

53. Inoue S, Ishii R, Fukuda H, et al. Sevoflurane anaesthesia for a patient with adult polyglucosan body disease. Can J Anaesth 1996;43:1257–9

54. Martin JB, Gusella JF. Huntington's disease: pathogenesis and management. N Engl J Med 1986;315:1267–76

55. Nagele P, Hammerle AF. Sevoflurane and mivacurium in a patient with Huntington's chorea. Br J Anaesth 2000; 85:320–1

56. Lamont AMS. Brief report: anaesthesia and Huntington's chorea. Anaesth Intensive Care 1979;7:189–90

57. Tsen LC, Smith TJ, Camann WR. Anesthetic management of a parturient with olivopontocerebellar degeneration. Anesth Analg 1997;85:1071–3

58. McTiernan CM, Haagenvik B. Strumpell's disease in a patient presenting for cesarean section. Can J Anaesth 1999; 46:679–82

59. Morgan PJ. Peripartum management of a patient with Isaacs' syndrome. Can J Anaesth 1997;44:1174–7

60. Stemp LI, Taswell C. Spastic torticollis during general anesthesia: case report and review of receptor mechanisms. Anesthesiology 1991;75:365–6

61. Osborne PJ, Lee LW. Idiopathic orthostatic hypotension, midodrine, and anaesthesia. Can J Anaesth 1991;38:499–501

62. Niquille M, VanGessel E, Gamulin Z. Continuous spinal anesthesia for hip surgery in a patient with Shy-Drager syndrome. Anesth Analg 1998;87:396–9

63. Mchaourab A, Mazzeo AJ, May JA, et al. Perioperative considerations in a patient with orthostatic intolerance syndrome. Anesthesiology 2000;93:571–3

64. Jacob G, Costa F, Shannon JR, et al. The neuropathic postural tachycardia syndrome. N Engl J Med 2000;343:1008–14

65. Rowe PC, Calkins H, DeBusk K, et al. Fludrocortisone acetate to treat neurally mediated hypotension in chronic fatigue syndrome. JAMA 2001;285:52–9

66. Turco GR, Farber NE. Postoperative autonomic deficit: a case of harlequin syndrome. Anesthesiology 1996;85:1197–9

67. Mitaka C, Tsunoda Y, Kikawa Y, et al. Anesthetic management of congenital insensitivity to pain with anhydrosis. Anesthesiology 1985;63:328–9

68. Kashtan HI, Heyneker TJ, Morell RC. Atypical response to scopolamine in a patient with type IV hereditary sensory and autonomic neuropathy. Anesthesiology 1992;76:140–2

69. Williams EL, Hart WM, Tempelhoff R. Postoperative ischemic optic neuropathy. Anesth Analg 1995;80:1018–29

70. D'Ambra MN, Dedrick D, Savarese JJ. Kearns-Sayer syndrome and pancuronium-succinylcholine-induced neuromuscular blockade. Anesthesiology 1979;51:343–5

71. Brown RH, Schauble JF, Miller NR. Anemia and hypotension as contributors to perioperative loss of vision. Anesthesiology 1994;80:222–6

72. Myers MA, Hamilton SR, Bogosian AJ, et al. Visual loss as a complication of spine surgery: a review of 37 cases. Spine 1997;22:1325–9

73. Borromeo CJ, Blike GT, Wiley CW, et al. Cortical blindness in a preeclamptic patient after a cesarean delivery complicated by hypotension. Anesth Analg 2000;91:609–11

74. Johnson RT, Gibbs CJ. Creutzfeldt-Jakob disease and related spongiform encephalopathies. N Engl J Med 1998;339:1994–2004

75. Haywood AM. Transmissible spongiform encephalopathies. N Engl J Med 1997;337:1821–8

76. Hernandez-Palazon J, Martinez-Lage JF, Tortosa JA, et al. Anaesthetic management in patients suspected of, or at risk of, having Creutzfeldt-Jakob disease. Br J Anaesth 1998;80:516–8

77. Kindopp AS, Ashbury T. Anaesthetic management of an adult patient with X-linked adrenoleukodystrophy. Can J Anaesth 1998;45:990–2

78. Schwartz RE, Stayer SA, Pasquariello CA, et al. Anaesthesia for the patient with neonatal adrenoleukodystrophy. Can J Anaesth 1994;41:56–8

79. Tobias JD. Anaesthetic considerations for the child with leukodystrophy. Can J Anaesth 1992;39:394–7

80. Shenkman Z, Krihevski I, Elpeleg ON, et al. Anaesthetic management of a patient with Leigh's syndrome. Can J Anaesth 1997;44:1091–5

81. Maguire D, Bachman C. Anaesthesia and Rett syndrome: a case report. Can J Anaesth 1989;36:478–81

82. Suresh D. Posterior spinal fusion in Sotos' syndrome. Br J Anaesth 1991;66:782–3

83. Warren ST, Nelson DL. Advances in molecular analysis of fragile X syndrome. JAMA 1994;271:536–42

84. Tobias JD. Anaesthetic considerations in the child with Menkes' syndrome. Can J Anaesth 1992;39:712–5

85. Layzer RB. Stiff-man syndrome: an autoimmune disease? N Engl J Med 1988;318:1060–3

86. Johnson JO, Miller KA. Anesthetic implications in stiff-person syndrome. Anesth Analg 1995;80:612–3

87. Neumann HPH, Berger DP, Sigmund G, et al. Pheochromocytomas, multiple endocrine neoplasia type 2, and Von Hippel-Lindau disease. N Engl J Med 1993;329:1531–8

88. Wang A, Sinatra RS. Epidural anesthesia for cesarean section in a patient with von Hippel-Lindau disease and multiple sclerosis. Anesth Analg 1999;88:1083–4

89. Mugawar M, Rajender Y, Purohit AK, et al. Anesthetic management of von Hippel-Lindau syndrome for excision of cerebellar hemangioblastoma and pheochromocytoma surgery. Anesth Analg 1998;86:673–4

90. Joffe D, Robbins R, Benjamin A. Caesarean section and phaeochromocytoma resection in a patient with Von Hippel Lindau disease. Can J Anaesth 1993;40:870–4

91. Shime N, Sugimoto E. Lumbar sympathetic ganglion block in a patient with painful legs and moving toes syndrome. Anesth Analg 1998;86:1056–7

92. Rugarli EI, Ballabio A. Kallman syndrome: from genetics to neurobiology. JAMA 1993;270:2713–6

93. Whitaker JN. Effects of pregnancy and delivery on disease activity in multiple sclerosis. N Engl J Med 1998;349:339–40

94. Rudick RA, Cohen JA, Weinstock-Guttman B, et al. Management of multiple sclerosis. N Engl J Med 1997;337:1604–11

95. Noseworthy JH, Lucchinetti C, Rodriquez M, et al. Multiple sclerosis. N Engl J Med 2000;343:938–52

96. Confavreux C, Hurtchinson M, Hours MM, et al. Rate of pregnancy-related relapse in multiple sclerosis. N Engl J Med 1998;339:285–91

97. Crawford JS, James FM, Nolte H, et al. Regional anaesthesia for patients with chronic neurological disease and similar conditions. Anaesthesia 1981;365:821–8

98. Warren TM, Datta S, Ostheimer GW. Lumbar epidural anesthesia in a patient with multiple sclerosis. Anesth Analg 1982;61:1022–3

99. Wang A, Sinatra RS. Epidural anesthesia for cesarean section in a patient with von Hippel-Lindau disease and multiple sclerosis. Anesth Analg 1999;88:1083–4

100. Brett RS, Schmidt JH, Gage JS, et al. Measurement of acetylcholine receptor concentration in skeletal muscle from a patient with multiple sclerosis and resistance to atracurium. Anesthesiology 1987;66:837–9

101. Dorsey DL, Camann WR. Obstetric anesthesia in patients with idiopathic facial paralysis (Bell's palsy): a 10-year survey. Anesth Analg 1993;77:81–3

102. Nightingale PJ, Longreen A. Iatrogenic facial nerve paresis. Anesthesiology 1982;37:322–3

103. Vagadia H. Facial paresis after general anesthesia: report of an unusual case: Heerfordt's syndrome. Anesthesiology 1986;64:513–4

104. Lowe DM, McCullough AM. 7th Nerve palsy after extradural blood patch. Br J Anaesth 1990;65:721–2

105. Jayamaha JEL. Respiratory obstruction in a patient with Melkersson-Rosenthal syndrome. Anesth Analg 1993;77:395–7

106. Fields HL. Treatment of trigeminal neuralgia. N Engl J Med 1996;334:1125–6

107. Dunteman ED, Swarm RA. Atypical facial "neuralgia." Anesth Analg 1995;80:188–90

108. Rao NL, Drupin BR. Glossopharyngeal neuralgia with syncope: anesthetic considerations. Anesthesiology 1981;54:426–8

109. Practice Advisory for the Prevention of Perioperative Peripheral Neuropathies: a report by the American Society of Anesthesiologists Task Force on Prevention of Perioperative Peripheral Neuropathies. Anesthesiology 2000;92:1168–82

110. Warner MA, Warner DO, Matsumoto JY, et al. Ulnar neuropathy in surgical patients. Anesthesiology 1999;90:54–9

111. Lupski JR, Chance PF, Garcia CA. Inherited primary peripheral neuropathies: molecular genetics and clinical implications of CMT1A and HNPP. JAMA 1993;270:2326–30

112. Greenberg RS, Parker SD. Anesthetic management for the child with Charcot-Marie-Tooth disease. Anesth Analg 1992;74:305–7

113. Scull T, Weeks S. Epidural analgesia for labour in a patient with Charcot-Marie-Tooth disease. Can J Anaesth 1996;43:1150–2

114. Antognini JF. Anaesthesia for Charcot-Marie-Tooth disease: a review of 86 cases. Can J Anaesth 1992;39:398–400

115. Pogson D, Telfer J, Wimbush S. Prolonged vecuronium neuromuscular blockade associated with Charcot-Marie-Tooth neuropathy. Br J Anaesth 2000;85:914–7

116. Eggers KA, Asai T. Postoperative brachial plexus neuropathy after total knee replacement under spinal anesthesia. Br J Anaesth 1995;75:642–4

117. Fibuch EE, Mertz J, Geller B. Postoperative onset of idiopathic brachial neuritis. Anesthesiology 1996;84:455–8

118. Horlocker TT, O'Driscoll SW, Dinapoli RP. Recurring brachial plexus neuropathy in a diabetic patient after shoulder surgery and continuous interscalene block. Anesth Analg 2000;91:688–90

119. Malamut RI, Marques W, England JD, et al. Postoperative idiopathic brachial neuritis. Muscle Nerve 1994;17:320–4

120. Suarez GA, Giannini C, Bosch EP, et al. Immune brachial plexus neuropathy: suggestive evidence for an inflammatory-immune pathogenesis. Neurology 1996;46:559–61

121. Kost RG, Straus SE. Postherpetic neuralgia: pathogenesis, treatment, and prevention. N Engl J Med 1996;335:32–44

122. Kotani N, Kushikata T, Hashimoto H, et al. Intrathecal methylprednisolone for intractable postherpetic neuralgia. N Engl J Med 2000;343:1514–9

123. Ropper AH. The Guillain-Barré syndrome. N Engl J Med 1992;326:1130–6

124. Atroshi I, Gummesson C, Johnsson R, et al. Prevalence of carpal tunnel syndrome in a general population. JAMA 1999;282:153–8

125. D'Arcy CA, McGee S. Does this patient have carpal tunnel syndrome? JAMA 2000;283:3110–7

126. Paartanen J, Niskanen L, Lehtinen J, et al. Natural history of peripheral neuropathy in patients with non-insulin-dependent diabetes mellitus. N Engl J Med 1995;333:89–94

127. Ditunno JF, Formal CS. Chronic spinal cord injury. N Engl J Med 1994;330:550–6

128. Hoffman JR, Mower WR, Wolfson AB, et al. Validity of set of clinical criteria to rule out injury to the cervical spine in patients with blunt trauma. N Engl J Med 2000;343:94–9

129. Hastings RH, Marks JD. Airway management for trauma patients with cervical spine injuries. Anesth Analg 1991;73:471–82

130. Suderman VS, Crosby ET, Lui A. Elective oral tracheal intubation in cervical spine-injured adults. Can J Anaesth 1991;38:785–9

131. Meschino A, Devitt JH, Kock J-P, et al. The safety of awake tracheal intubation in cervical spine surgery. Can J Anaesth 1992;39:114–7

132. Crosby ET, Lui A. The adult cervical spine: implications for airway management. Can J Anaesth 1990;37:77–93.

133. Calder I. Spinal cord injury in patients with undiagnosed cervical spine fractures. Anesthesiology 1998;88:1411

134. McLeod ADM, Calder I. Spinal cord injury and direct laryngoscopy—the legend lives on. Br J Anaesth 2000;84:705–9

135. Stowe DF, Bernstein JS, Madsen KE, et al. Autonomic hyperreflexia in spinal cord injured patients during extracorporeal shock wave lithotripsy. Anesth Analg 1989;68:788–91

136. Lambert DH, Deane RS, Mazuzan JE. Anesthesia and the control of systemic blood pressure in patients with spinal cord injury. Anesth Analg 1982;61:344–8

137. Ravindran RS, Cummins DF, Smith IE. Experience with the use of nitroprusside and subsequent epidural analgesia in a pregnant quadriplegic patient. Anesth Analg 1981;60:1–3

138. Kobayashi A, Mizobe T, Tojo H, et al. Autonomic hyperreflexia during labour. Can J Anaesth 1995;42:1134–6

139. Browne TR, Holmes GL. Epilepsy. N Engl J Med 2001;344:1145–51

140. Devinsky O. Patients with refractory seizures. N Engl J Med 1999;340:1565–70

141. Lowenstein DH, Alldredge BK. Status epilepticus. N Engl J Med 1998;338:970–6

142. Ford EW, Morrell F, Whisler WW. Methohexital anesthesia in the surgical treatment of uncontrollable epilepsy. Anesth Analg 1982;56:464–7

143. DeFriez CB, Wong HC. Seizures and opisthotonos after propofol anesthesia. Anesth Analg 1992;75:630–2

144. Iimima T, Nakamura Z, Iwao Y, et al. The epileptogenic properties of the volatile anesthetics sevoflurane and isoflurane in patients with epilepsy. Anesth Analg 2000;91:989–95

145. Fennelly M, Galletly DC, Purdie GI. Is caffeine withdrawal the mechanism of postoperative headache? Anesth Analg 1991;72:446–53

146. Abouleish E, Ali V, Tang RA. Benign intracranial hypertension and anesthesia for cesarean section. Anesthesiology 1985;63:705–7

147. Deyo RA, Ranville J, Kent DL. What can the history and physical examination tell us about low back pain. JAMA 1992;268:760–5

148. Deyo RA, Diehl AK, Rosenthal M. How may days of bed rest for acute low back pain? N Engl J Med 1986;315:1064–70

149. Malmivaara A, Hakkinen U, Aro T, et al. The treatment of acute low back pain-bed rest, exercises, or ordinary activity. N Engl J Med 1995;332:351–5

150. Kay J, Findling JW, Raff H. Epidural triamcinolone suppresses the pituitary-adrenal axis in human subjects. Anesth Analg 1994;79:501–5

151. Carette S, Leclaire R, Marcoux S, et al. Epidural corticosteroid injections for sciatica due to herniated nucleus pulposus. N Engl J Med 1997;336:1634–40

152. Wood GG, Jacka MJ. Spinal hematoma following spinal anesthesia in a patient with spinal bifida occulta. Anesthesiology 1997;87:983–4

153. Kupfer DJ, Reynolds CF. Management of insomnia. N Engl J Med 1997;336:341–6

154. Rosenberg-Adamsen S, Kehlet H, Dodds C, et al. Postoperative sleep disturbances: mechanisms and clinical implications. Br J Anaesth 1996;76:552–9

155. Aldrech MS. Narcolepsy. N Engl J Med 1990;323:389–95

156. Bohringer CH, Jahr JS, Rowell S, et al. Severe hypotension in a patient receiving pemoline during general anesthesia. Anesth Analg 2000;91:1131–3

157. Mesa A, Diaz AP, Frosth M. Narcolepsy and anesthesia. Anesthesiology 2000;92:1194–6

158. Albrecht RF, Wagner SR, Leicht CH, et al. Factitious disorder as a cause of failure to awaken after general anesthesia. Anesthesiology 1995;83:201–4

159. Arendt J. Melatonin, circadian rhythms, and sleep. N Engl J Med 2000;343:1114–6

160. Hotson JR, Baloh RW. Acute vestibular syndrome. N Engl J Med 1998;339:680–5

161. White PF. Spontaneous rupture of the tympanic membrane occurring in the absence of middle ear disease. Anesthesiology 1983;59:368–9

162. Perreault L, Normandin N, Plamondon L, et al. Tympanic membrane rupture after anesthesia with nitrous oxide. Anesthesiology 1982;57:325–6

163. Jensen NF. Glomus tumors of the head and neck: anesthetic considerations. Anesth Analg 1994;78:112–9

164. Kodama K, Seo N, Murayama T, et al. Glossopharyngeal nerve block for carotid sinus syndrome. Anesth Analg 1992;75:1036–7

165. Conway JB, Posner M. Anaesthesia for caesarean section in a patient with Watson's syndrome. Can J Anaesth 1994; 41:1113–6

166. Yamashita M, Matsuki A, Oyama R. Anaesthetic considerations in vonRecklinghausen's disease (multiple neurofibromatosis). Anaesthesia 1977;26:177–8

167. Baraka A. Myasthenia response to muscle relaxants in von-Recklinghausen's disease. Br J Anaesth 1974;46:701–3

168. Dounas M, Mercier FJ, Lhuissier C, et al. Epidural analgesia for labour in a parturient with neurofibromatosis. Can J Anaesth 1995;42:420–4

18

Diseases of the Liver and Biliary Tract

Diseases of the liver and biliary tract can be categorized as parenchymal liver disease (acute and chronic hepatitis, cirrhosis of the liver) and cholestasis with or without obstruction of the extrahepatic biliary pathway.

■ ACUTE HEPATITIS

Acute hepatitis is most often due to a virus, although hepatitis can also be caused by drugs and toxins.[1] Classic acute viral hepatitis is caused by one of five viruses: hepatitis A virus (HAV), hepatitis B virus (HBV), hepatitis C virus (HCV), hepatitis D virus (HDV), or hepatitis E virus (HEV). In the United States approximately 50% of reported cases of acute viral hepatitis in adults are classified as HBV infection, 30% as HAV infection, and 20% as HCV infections. Chronic infection may follow HBV, HCV, and HDV infections. Viruses that cause systemic illnesses and also affect the liver include cytomegalovirus and Epstein-Barr virus.

Viral Hepatitis

All five types of viral hepatitis are similar and cannot be distinguished reliably by clinical features or routine laboratory tests (Table 18–1).[1] Infections may be asymptomatic or may cause nonspecific flu-like symptoms; some patients develop jaundice. The diagnostic laboratory abnormality associated with acute hepatitis is a markedly increased aminotransferase level. The specific etiology of viral hepatitis is determined by serologic testing.

Table 18–1 • Characteristic Features of Viral Hepatitis

Parameter	Type A	Type B	Type C	Type D
Mode of transmission	Fecal-oral Sewage-contaminated shellfish	Percutaneous Sexual	Percutaneous	Percutaneous
Incubation period	20–37 days	60–110 days	35–70 days	60–110 days
Results of serum antigen and antibody tests	IgM early and IgG appears during convalescence	HBsAg and anti-HBc early and persists in carriers	Anti-HVC in 6 weeks to 9 months	Anti-HVD late and may be short-lived
Immunity	Antibodies in 45%	Antibodies in 5%–15%	Unknown	Protected if immune to type B
Course	Does not progress to chronic liver disease	Chronic liver disease develops in 1%–5% of adults and 80%–90% of children	Chronic liver disease develops in 85%	Co-infection with type B
Prevention after exposure	Pooled gamma globulin	Hepatitis B immune globulin Hepatitis B vaccine	Unknown	Unknown
Mortality	< 0.2%	0.3%–1.5%	Unknown	Acute icteric hepatitis: 2%–20%

IgM, IgG, immunoglobulin M and G; HBsAg, hepatitis B surface antigen; HBc, hepatitis B core; HVC, hepatitis virus C; HVD, hepatitis virus D. Adapted from: Keefe EB. Acute hepatitis. Sci Am Med 1999;1–9.

Classification

Hepatitis A

Hepatitis A virus is a picornavirus similar to poliovirus and rhinovirus.[1] Shed virus is present in the serum and stool of patients with hepatitis A. The antigenic composition of HAV is such that immune globulin and hepatitis A vaccine provide protection. Immunoglobulin M (IgM) antibodies to hepatitis A are detectable at the onset of the clinical illness and usually disappear within 60 to 120 days. Immunoglobulin G (IgG) antibodies achieve high titers during convalescence and persist indefinitely, thereby conferring immunity. Nearly one-half of the U.S. population has a high concentration of serum antibodies to HAV.[1]

Hepatitis A is highly contagious, being transmitted via food that has been contaminated by feces-soiled hands of infected persons. Ingestion of sewage-contaminated shellfish has resulted in epidemics of hepatitis A. Hepatitis A may be sexually transmitted in homosexual men and is a common disease among intravenous drug abusers. Viremia is present for several days prior to the onset of clinical symptoms, but transmission by serum or blood products seldom occurs. The virus is shed in the stool for 14 to 21 days before the onset of jaundice. Although patients may continue to shed virus for the first 7 to 14 days of the clinical illness, they are usually no longer infectious 21 days after the onset.

Hepatitis B

Hepatitis B is transmitted primarily through percutaneous inoculation of infected serum or blood products. HBV is present in the serum and body secretions of most patients early in the course of acute hepatitis B. The most common mode of transmission in homosexual men is by oral or genital contact with asymptomatic bleeding lesions in the rectal mucosa. Hepatitis B may also be transmitted to the fetus during pregnancy. The surface coat of the hepatitis B surface virion is composed of a polypeptide that acts as the major hepatitis B surface antigen (HBsAg). A large proportion of the population has serum antibodies to HBsAg (anti-HBs), which confers immunity to hepatitis B.

Hepatitis C

Hepatitis C virus is transmitted by parenteral routes including blood transfusions, occupational exposures to blood or blood products, and intravenous drug abuse. In this regard, hepatitis C is the most common chronic blood-borne infection in the United States.[2] Shared percutaneous exposures (toothbrushes, razors) are possible routes of transmission. The ability to screen for HCV has essentially eliminated HCV as a cause of posttransfusion hepatitis. The rate of perinatal infection in babies born from mothers with HCV infection is low. Recipients of organs from donors with antibodies to HCV have a high likelihood of becoming infected with HCV.

Hepatitis C has emerged as the predominant liver disease in the United States. Progression of chronic hepatitis C to cirrhosis may be slow, but end-stage liver disease due to HCV-associated cirrhosis is the most common indication for liver transplantation, and HCV-associated cirrhosis is responsible for an increasing incidence of hepatocellular cancers.

Hepatitis D

Hepatitis D occurs only in patients with hepatitis B and is transmitted via the percutaneous route. Simultaneous infection with HBV and HDV may produce more severe acute hepatitis than that caused by HBV alone.

Diagnosis

The diagnosis of viral hepatitis is dependent on the appearance of clinical signs and symptoms, laboratory findings, serologic assays, and in some patients a liver biopsy.

Signs and Symptoms

The onset of viral hepatitis may be gradual or sudden and most often manifests as dark urine, fatigue, anorexia, and nausea (Table 18–2).[1] Low grade fever is common. Right upper quadrant pain is less common than generalized abdominal discomfort. About one-half of patients complain of myalgias or arthralgias (especially those with hepatitis B). Many of the initial symptoms abate when jaundice develops. Hepatomegaly and splenomegaly may be present. When hepatitis is severe, there is evidence of acute liver failure including confusion, asterixis, peripheral edema, and ascites.

Table 18–2 • Incidence of Symptoms in Acute Viral Hepatitis

Symptom	Incidence (%)
Dark urine	94
Fatigue	91
Anorexia	90
Nausea	87
Fever	76
Emesis	71
Headache	70
Abdominal discomfort	65
Light-colored stools	52
Pruritus	42

Adapted from: Keefe EB. Acute hepatitis. Sci Am Med 1999;1–9.

Aminotransferase Concentrations

Serum aminotransferase concentrations [aspartate aminotransferase (AST), alanine aminotransferase (ALT)] are sensitive indicators of liver cell injury seen with viral hepatitis.[3] AST and ALT concentrations increase 7 to 14 days before the appearance of jaundice and begin to decrease shortly after the jaundice develops. The degree of aminotransferase increase does not necessarily parallel the severity of the hepatitis, but concentrations less than 500 IU/L usually reflect mild hepatitis.[1]

Laboratory Tests

Anemia and lymphocytosis are typically present. Serum bilirubin concentrations usually do not exceed 20 mg/dl. Severe acute hepatitis may impair the hepatocyte's synthetic capacity, resulting in decreased serum albumin concentrations and prolonged prothrombin times. Alkaline phosphatase is not increased unless cholestasis develops at a later phase of the acute hepatitis. Increased gamma globulin concentrations suggest chronic active hepatitis rather than acute viral hepatitis.

Serologic Measurements

Serologic measurements are used to identify each type of viral hepatitis.[1] The IgM antibody to HAV appears early in the course of the disease and is specific for acute hepatitis A. The antibody persists for about 120 days and is then replaced by IgG anti-HAV, which confers lasting immunity to future HAV infection.

HBsAg is present in the serum of patients as early as 7 to 14 days after infection with HAV and may persist for several months. The antibody to HBsAg usually appears in the blood 60 to 240 days after infection, at which time HBsAg is usually no longer detectable. Antibody to the core antigen of HBV (anti-HBc) appears promptly after infection and persists indefinitely. High titers of IgM anti-HBc may be the only marker of acute hepatitis B if HBsAg is no longer detectable. Detection of HBsAg indicates that HBV is actively replicating, and the blood of these individuals is highly infectious.

Detection of antibodies to HCV (anti-HCV) is the most reliable way to diagnose acute and chronic hepatitis C. The detection of HCV RNA confirms the presence of viremia. Hepatitis D virus infection is diagnosed by detecting anti-HDV with HBsAg (co-infection).

Liver Biopsy

Liver biopsy is not generally necessary to confirm the diagnosis of acute hepatitis, as serologic measurements are sufficient. Spotty necrosis of hepatocytes and inflammatory cell reactions are the typical histologic findings. Liver biopsy performed late in the course of acute infectious hepatitis reveals evidence of hepatic cell regeneration. With severe hepatitis, necrotic zones link portal areas to one another or to central areas; or they may involve whole lobules (bridging necrosis).[1] Sometimes late in the course of severe acute viral hepatitis the histologic picture may be difficult to distinguish from that of chronic active hepatitis.

Clinical Course

Hepatitis typically produces symptoms for 7 to 14 days before the appearance of dark urine and jaundice.[1] As jaundice increases, the appetite begins to return and malaise decreases. Serum bilirubin concentrations increase for 10 to 14 days and then decrease during the next 14 to 28 days. Aminotransferase concentrations usually begin to decrease just before peak jaundice occurs and then decrease rapidly. The clinical course is typically uneventful and the return to normal liver function is complete.

In a small percentage of patients, especially elderly patients or those with HBV or HCV, acute viral hepatitis runs a protracted course, with full recovery taking as long as 12 months. Rarely, acute viral hepatitis results in fulminant liver failure and death. Some patients never fully recover from the initial acute viral hepatitis, and chronic hepatitis develops. Chronic hepatitis does not occur after hepatitis A but develops in 1% to 5% of patients infected with HBV and in 85% of patients infected with HCV.[1] The development of cirrhosis and primary hepatocellular carcinoma in patients with chronic hepatitis C is a risk, although it does not occur in most patients, and in others decades may pass before these adverse effects occur. Unusual but life-threatening complications of acute hepatitis include aplastic anemia, hemolytic anemia, hypoglycemia, and polyarteritis.

Treatment

Treatment of acute viral hepatitis is symptomatic, with restriction of physical activity to a degree comfortable for the patient. Nausea and vomiting may be so severe as to require intravenous fluid and electrolyte replacement. Abstinence from alcohol during acute viral hepatitis is recommended, although alcohol has not been shown to affect the patient with viral hepatitis adversely. Acute hepatitis C is usually asymptomatic; but when chronic hepatitis C is recognized, administration of interferon combined with ribavirin is considered the treatment of choice.[4] Liver transplantation is a consideration when patients develop encephalopathy and associated coagulation abnormalities.

Prevention

Prevention of viral hepatitis includes avoidance of exposure to the virus, passive immunization with gamma globulin, and active immunization with specific vaccines. Pooled gamma globulin administered intramuscularly as soon as possible after known exposure dramatically decreases the incidence of hepatitis A. Administration of gamma globulin more than 14 days after exposure to HAV is not protective. Individuals exposed to HBV by percutaneous or mucous membrane routes should receive hepatitis B immune globulin and hepatitis B vaccine within 24 hours. The value of prophylactic gamma globulin for hepatitis C is not known.

Hepatitis B Vaccine

Hepatitis B vaccines are highly effective in inducing antibody to HBV and preventing HBV infection in infants, children, and adults. The vaccine is recommended for individuals at increased risk for HBV infection, including health care workers with frequent exposure to blood products, homosexual men, intravenous drug abusers, recipients of certain blood products, and infants born to HBsAg-positive mothers. After successful vaccination, titers of antibody to HBsAg begin to decline; and in 5 years 20% to 30% of patients lack protective antibody levels. These persons respond promptly to a booster dose of vaccine. Vaccination is of no value in HBV carriers, but it has no adverse effects if administered to these individuals.

Hepatitis A Vaccine

An inactivated hepatitis A vaccine is highly effective in eliciting an antibody response. Compared with short-term protection afforded by immune globulin, inactivated HAV vaccine probably provides protection for 5 to 10 years or longer. Travelers to endemic regions, neonatal intensive care workers, food handlers, children in daycare centers, and military personnel represent high risk groups for hepatitis A. Hepatitis A vaccine is safe and effective in patients with viral liver disease.

Additional Viruses that Cause Hepatitis

In addition to the classic hepatitis viruses, acute hepatitis may be due to viruses that cause systemic illness and also affect the liver.

Cytomegalovirus

Cytomegalovirus (CMV) is a herpesvirus that is ubiquitous.[1] Approximately 80% of adults have serum complement-fixation reactivity for CMV. This virus can produce a disease similar to infectious mononucleosis but without adenopathy or tonsillopharyngeal involvement. Liver dysfunction caused by CMV may mimic common forms of viral hepatitis, but it is usually mild and does not progress to chronic liver disease. Diagnosis requires demonstration of the virus following inoculation of an appropriate tissue culture.

Epstein-Barr Virus

Epstein-Barr virus (EBV) usually produces mild hepatitis associated with nausea and vomiting.[1] Jaundice occurs in 10% to 20% of patients. Serum aminotransferase concentrations are moderately increased. In most instances, the hepatitis is part of the typical clinical syndrome of infectious mononucleosis. In rare instances hepatic dysfunction is severe and may be fatal, especially in immunosuppressed patients. EBV appears to be transmitted during oral-oral contact through infected saliva but may also be transmitted parenterally. The incubation period is about 28 days. An increase in the titer of specific antibodies to EBV confirms the diagnosis.

Drug-Induced Hepatitis

Many drugs (analgesics, volatile anesthetics, antibiotics, antihypertensives, anticonvulsants, tranquilizers) can cause hepatitis indistinguishable histologically from acute viral hepatitis. These idiosyncratic drug reactions are rare, unpredictable, and not dose-dependent. Clinical signs of liver dysfunction usually occur 2 to 6 weeks after the initiation of drug therapy but can occur as early as the first day or as late as 6 months. Failure to discontinue the offending drug promptly may result in progressive hepatitis and death. The disease progresses in some patients despite withdrawal of the drug.

Acetaminophen Overdose

Acetaminophen overdose (usually associated with a suicide attempt) produces profound hepatocellular necrosis in most persons. Cell injury occurs because the liver produces toxic metabolites that are usually rendered harmless by conjugation with glutathione. When the drug dose is high, hepatic glutathione stores are depleted and the toxic metabolites accumulate and destroy liver cells. Oral N-acetylcysteine

given within 8 hours of an acetaminophen overdose decreases the hepatotoxicity. Acetaminophen can also cause hepatotoxicity in normal clinical doses if hepatic glutathione levels are decreased as a result of alcohol abuse with malnutrition (Tylenol-alcohol syndrome).

Volatile Anesthetics

Volatile anesthetics may produce mild, self-limiting postoperative liver dysfunction that likely reflects anesthetic-induced alterations in hepatic oxygen delivery relative to demand, resulting in inadequate hepatocyte oxygenation.[5-7] The cytosolic liver enzyme α-glutathione S-transferase (α-GST) is a more sensitive marker of hepatocellular damage than conventional liver enzyme markers (aminotransferases).[7] Any anesthetic that decreases hepatic blood flow could interfere with adequate hepatocyte oxygenation. Indeed, α-GST concentrations increase transiently after administration of isoflurane, desflurane, and sevoflurane.[8]

Immune-Mediated Hepatotoxicity

A rare but life-threatening form of hepatic dysfunction following administration of volatile anesthetics (most often *halothane hepatitis*) may reflect an immune-mediated hepatotoxicity in genetically susceptible patients. The most compelling evidence for an immune-mediated mechanism is the presence of circulating IgG antibodies in the majority of patients with the diagnosis of halothane hepatitis.[9, 10] These antibodies are directed against liver microsomal proteins on the surfaces of hepatocytes that have been covalently modified by the reactive oxidative trifluoroacetyl halide metabolite of halothane to form neoantigens. The acetylation of liver proteins, in effect, changes these proteins from self to nonself (neoantigens), resulting in the formation of antibodies against this new protein and a form of autoimmune hepatitis. To detect the IgG anti-trifluoroacetyl antibodies, synthetic trifluoroacetylated rabbit serum albumin is used as the antigen in the enzyme-linked immunosorbent assay. The anti-trifluoroacetyl antibody testing procedure is highly specific, as antibodies do not appear after other forms of liver disease or in the presence of drugs other than certain volatile anesthetics. It is presumed that the subsequent antigen-antibody interactions are responsible for the rare (estimated to occur in 1 in 10,000 to 1 in 30,000 adult patients receiving halothane) liver injury characterized as halothane hepatitis.

Like halothane, the fluorinated volatile anesthetics enflurane, isoflurane, and desflurane may form trifluoroacetyl metabolites, resulting in cross-sensitivity with halothane. The incidence of hepatitis after these anesthetics, however, is much lower than after halothane because the degree of anesthetic metabolism is substantially less.[11] It is possible that genetically susceptible patients could become sensitized to one volatile anesthetic (most likely halothane) and experience drug-induced hepatitis later in life when exposed to anesthetics such as isoflurane or desflurane, which are considered unlikely to cause liver damage. Indeed, suspected isoflurane hepatitis with associated anti-trifluoroacetyl IgG antibodies has been described in a patient with a history of halothane hepatitis (Fig. 18–1).[12]

The chemical structure of sevoflurane is such that it does not undergo metabolism to trifluoroacetylated metabolites. Therefore, unlike all the other fluorinated volatile anesthetics, sevoflurane would not be expected to produce immune-mediated hepatotoxicity or to cause cross-sensitivity in patients previously exposed to halothane.

Differential Diagnosis of Postoperative Hepatic Dysfunction

When postoperative hepatic dysfunction occurs, a predetermined approach, including serial liver function tests and a search for extrahepatic causes of hepatic dysfunction, facilitates the differential diagnosis. The causes of hepatic dysfunction can be categorized as prehepatic, intrahepatic (hepatocellular), or posthepatic (cholestatic) based on repeated measurements of the serum concentrations of bilirubin, aminotransferases, and alkaline phosphatase (Table 18–3). The causes of postoperative hepatic dysfunction are most likely multifactorial and difficult to confirm. When postoperative hepatic dysfunction occurs, the following steps may be helpful for determining the etiology rather than assuming that the history of an anesthetic establishes a cause-and-effect relation between hepatic dysfunction and the volatile anesthetic.

1. Review all drugs administered (analgesics, antibiotics, over-the-counter preparations), as every drug, regardless of how innocuous it may seem, must be considered a potential cause of hepatocyte injury. Administration of catecholamines or sympathomimetics may evoke splanchnic vasoconstriction sufficient to interfere with adequate hepatic blood flow and hepatocyte oxygenation.

2. Check for sources of sepsis. The development of jaundice is common in patients with severe infection.

3. Evaluate the possibility of increased exogenous bilirubin loads. A 500 ml transfusion of fresh whole blood contains 250 mg of bilirubin. This bilirubin load increases as the age of the transfused blood increases. Patients with normal hepatic function can be given large amounts of blood without appreciable increases in their bilirubin concentration. This response may be different in patients with co-existing hepatic disease.

4. Rule out occult hematomas. Resorption of large hematomas may produce hyperbilirubinemia for several days. Furthermore, patients with Gilbert syndrome have limited ability to conjugate bilirubin, and even small increases in bilirubin load may lead to jaundice (see "Gilbert Syndrome").

5. Rule out hemolysis. Decreases in hematocrit or increases in the reticulocyte count may reflect erythrocyte hemolysis.

6. Review perioperative records. Evidence of hypotension, arterial hypoxemia, hypoventilation, and hypovolemia must be considered possible etiologic factors for postoperative hepatic dysfunction.

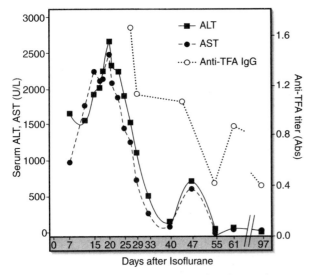

Figure 18–1 • Time course of postoperative changes in serum aminotransferase concentrations (ALT, AST) and anti-trifluoroacetyl immunoglobulin antibodies (anti-TFA IgG) in a patient following surgery and anesthesia that included isoflurane. (From Gunaratnam NT, Benson J, Gandolfi AJ, et al. Suspected isoflurane hepatitis in an obese patient with a history of halothane hepatitis. Anesthesiology 1995;83:1361–4. © 1995, Lippincott Williams & Wilkins, with permission.)

Table 18–3 • Liver Function Tests and Differential Diagnosis

Hepatic Dysfunction	Bilirubin	Aminotransferase Enzymes	Alkaline Phosphatase	Causes
Prehepatic	Increased unconjugated fraction	Normal	Normal	Hemolysis Hematoma resorption Bilirubin overload from whole blood
Intrahepatic (hepatocellular)	Increased conjugated fraction	Markedly increased	Normal to slightly increased	Viral Drugs Sepsis Hypoxemia Cirrhosis
Posthepatic (cholestatic)	Increased conjugated fraction	Normal to slightly increased	Markedly increased	Stones Sepsis

7. Consider extrahepatic abnormalities (congestive heart failure, respiratory failure, pulmonary embolism, renal insufficiency) as possible causes of postoperative hepatic dysfunction.

8. Consider the possibility of benign postoperative intrahepatic cholestasis (associated with extensive, prolonged surgery often with hypotension, arterial hypoxemia, and massive blood transfusions) (see "Benign Postoperative Intrahepatic Cholestasis").

9. Consider the possibility of immune-mediated hepatotoxicity. This is a diagnosis of exclusion based on the clinical history of a recent anesthetic that included a volatile anesthetic. It may be possible to confirm the diagnosis by documenting the presence of circulating anti-trifluoroacetyl antibodies.[9]

CHRONIC HEPATITIS

Chronic hepatitis encompasses an etiologically diverse group of diseases characterized by long-term elevation of liver chemistries and evidence of hepatocyte inflammation on liver biopsy.[13, 14] Chronic hepatitis is generally defined as disease that has lasted 6 months or longer. The most common diseases that cause chronic hepatitis are autoimmune hepatitis and chronic viral hepatitis (HBV with or without co-infection with HDV or infection with HCV). In addition, chronic hepatitis may be caused by drugs, Wilson's disease, α_1-antitrypsin deficiency, or the early stages of primary biliary cirrhosis and primary sclerosing cholangitis.

Signs and Symptoms

Signs and symptoms of chronic hepatitis are diverse, ranging from asymptomatic disease characterized by mildly increased serum aminotransferase concentrations to rapidly progressive illness with fulminant hepatic failure. The most common symptoms of chronic hepatitis are fatigue, malaise, and mild abdominal pain. Extrahepatic manifestations of chronic hepatitis are common and include arthralgias, arthritis, glomerulonephritis, skin rashes, amenorrhea, and thyroiditis.

Laboratory Tests

The ALT and AST concentrations are characteristically increased in patients with chronic hepatitis, and serum bilirubin concentrations are typically normal in patients with chronic viral hepatitis but increased in patients with autoimmune hepatitis. A characteristic feature of autoimmune hepatitis, but not of chronic viral hepatitis, is increased serum gamma globulin concentrations. With the most severe forms of chronic hepatitis, hepatic synthetic function is impaired, as reflected by decreased serum albumin concentrations and prolonged prothrombin times. Imaging studies of the abdomen reveal variable degrees of hepatomegaly with or without splenomegaly. The specific etiology of chronic hepatitis can usually be determined by clinical evaluation combined with immunologic and serologic testing, but liver biopsy helps confirm the presence of certain diseases (Wilson's disease or α_1-antitrypsin deficiency).

Autoimmune Hepatitis

Autoimmune hepatitis is characterized by a wide spectrum of clinical symptoms and immunoserologic manifestations. Hypergammaglobulinemia, increased serum aminotransferase concentrations to three to ten times normal, and the presence of antinuclear antibody are characteristic. Other autoimmune diseases may be present concurrently. Treatment with corticosteroids prolongs the survival rate. Nevertheless, treatment with corticosteroids for longer than 18 months is associated with diabetes mellitus, systemic hypertension, psychosis, infections, or osteoporosis in more than 50% of patients. Relapse occurs in nearly 50% of patients when corticosteroids are discontinued. The distinction between autoimmune hepatitis and chronic hepatitis C may be difficult but is important because autoimmune hepatitis responds to immunosuppressive drugs, although it may be exacerbated by treatment with interferon. Hepatitis C infection can be excluded in nearly all of these patients by the absence of anti-HCV antibodies.

Chronic Hepatitis B

Chronic hepatitis B is present in 5% of the world's population, and an estimated 0.2% to 0.5% of the U.S. population are chronic carriers of HBsAg.[14] In patients with chronic HBV infection, HBsAg remains detectable for more than 6 months. Persons who continue to test positive for HBsAg but who are asymptomatic and have normal serum aminotransferase concentrations are termed HBsAg carriers. Other chronically infected HBsAg-positive individuals who have clinical or laboratory evidence of chronic hepatic disease (increased serum aminotransferase levels) are diagnosed with chronic hepatitis B.

Age at the time of the initial HBV infection is the major determinant of chronicity (90% of infected neonates become chronic carriers). Another important risk factor for the development of chronic hepatitis B is the presence of intrinsic or iatrogenic immunosuppression. Women are more likely than men to clear HBsAg, and as a result men are the predominant HBsAg carriers. Persistent HBV infection is an important risk factor for development of hepatocellular carcinoma.

The goal of treatment of chronic hepatitis B is to eradicate HBV infection and prevent the development of cirrhosis or hepatocellular cancer. Although available therapies cannot achieve these goals, they can suppress HBV replication and lead to improvement in the clinical, biochemical, and histologic features of chronic hepatitis B. For example, treatment with interferon results in loss of HBV replication in about 40% of patients, resolution of symptoms of cirrhosis in about one-third of affected patients, and prolongation of life.[14] Lamivudine therapy may dramatically suppress HBV replication. Liver transplantation can be performed for liver failure associated with chronic hepatitis B, but HBV infects the allograft in nearly all recipients. For this reason antiviral prophylaxis is initiated intraoperatively.

Chronic Hepatitis C

Chronic HCV infection follows acute HCV infection in 85% of patients, and an estimated 1.8% of the population in the United States are carriers for HCV.[6] Therefore chronic HCV infection is more prevalent than chronic hepatitis B, which affects 0.2% to 0.5% of the population.

The diagnosis of chronic hepatitis C is typically based on persistently or intermittently increased serum aminotransferase concentrations in association with the presence of anti-HCV antibodies. The natural history of chronic hepatitis C spans several decades, progressing insidiously with the ultimate development of cirrhosis after about 30 years. Factors associated with an increased rate of progression to cirrhosis include age older than 40 years at the time of initial infection, daily alcohol consumption exceeding 50 g, and male gender.

Interferon normalizes or reduces serum ALT concentrations and decreases inflammation, as indicated by liver biopsy, in about one-half of patients with chronic hepatitis C. Relapse is common when interferon therapy is stopped. In this regard, long-term therapy with the lowest dose of interferon necessary to maintain remission may be a useful approach. The high relapse rate in interferon-treated patients suggests that interferon suppresses viral replication rather than eradicating or curing HCV infection. A combination of interferon with other antiviral drugs such as ribavirin may be more effective than interferon alone. Chronic hepatitis C with liver failure is one of the most common indications for liver transplantation. Although hepatitis C virus reinfects the allograft, the subsequent illness is usually mild and rarely progresses to liver failure.

Less Common Causes of Chronic Hepatitis

Several liver diseases must be distinguished from autoimmune and chronic viral hepatitis as causes of chronic hepatitis.[14] In most instances, these diseases can be identified on the basis of clinical, biochemical, and histologic evidence.

Drug-induced chronic hepatitis is seen in a small but important group of patients.[14] Methyldopa, trazodone, and isoniazid are recognized causes of drug-induced chronic hepatitis. In addition, occasional patients treated with sulfonamides, acetaminophen, aspirin, and phenytoin have been reported to develop drug-induced chronic hepatitis. Treatment is discontinuation of the suspected drug as soon as chronic hepatitis is diagnosed or suspected. If the chronic hepatitis is due to the drug, liver function abnormalities and the clinical course usually improve.

In the absence of associated neurologic symptoms, *Wilson's disease* mimics chronic hepatitis. The diagnosis is confirmed by liver biopsy and determination of hepatic copper content. Specific treatment is with penicillamine.

α_1-*Antitrypsin deficiency* is associated with mildly active progressive liver disease that progresses to cirrhosis. Liver disease due to α_1-antitrypsin deficiency can be differentiated from chronic hepatitis by decreased α_1-globulin on protein electrophoresis and by specific serum assays for α_1-antitrypsin.

Primary biliary cirrhosis may be indistinguishable from chronic viral hepatitis on liver biopsy. Characteristic hyperpigmentation, pruritus, and extreme increases in serum alkaline phosphatase concentrations are helpful for the differential diagnosis.

Primary sclerosing cholangitis can mimic chronic viral hepatitis. Marked increases in serum alkaline phosphatase concentrations and accompanying inflammatory bowel disease distinguish this illness from chronic viral hepatitis.

■ CIRRHOSIS OF THE LIVER

Cirrhosis of the liver is the sequela of a large variety of chronic, progressive liver diseases that are most often the result of excessive alcohol ingestion and chronic viral hepatitis due to HBV or HCV.[15] Cirrhosis is present when scarring of the liver results in disruption of the liver's normal architecture and regenerating nodules of parenchyma appear. The pattern of scarring seldom permits determination of the specific etiology, but associated histologic features may point to it.

Diagnosis

Percutaneous liver biopsy can unequivocally establish the diagnosis of cirrhosis of the liver. Guidelines for the performance of a liver biopsy in patients with suspected cirrhosis include an international normalized ratio (INR) for the prothrombin time no more than 1.5, a partial thromboplastin time no more than 10 seconds longer than control, and platelet counts higher than 50,000 cells/mm³. Computed tomography, magnetic resonance imaging, or hepatic ultrasonography with Doppler flow studies may reveal findings consistent with cirrhosis (sple-

nomegaly, ascites, irregular liver surface). Upper gastrointestinal endoscopy often establishes the presence of esophagogastric varices.

Signs and Symptoms

Fatigue and malaise are common with all forms of cirrhosis, but these nonspecific symptoms are present with almost all forms of acute and chronic liver disease.[15] Characteristic but nondiagnostic physical findings of cirrhosis include palmar erythema and spider nevi, gynecomastia, testicular atrophy, and evidence of portal hypertension (splenomegaly, ascites). Decreased hepatic blood flow resulting from increased intrahepatic resistance to flow through the portal vein (portal hypertension) reflects the fibrotic processes associated with cirrhosis. This increased resistance results in decreases in the proportion of hepatic blood flow delivered through the portal vein and to increases in the contribution to total hepatic blood flow from the hepatic artery. The cirrhotic liver is often enlarged, and the left lobe is typically palpable below the xiphoid process. Decreased serum albumin concentrations and prolonged prothrombin times are characteristic of cirrhosis. Increased serum aminotransferases and alkaline phosphatase concentrations are common.[3]

Specific Forms of Cirrhosis

Specific forms of cirrhosis include alcoholic cirrhosis, postnecrotic cirrhosis, primary biliary cirrhosis, hemochromatosis, Wilson's disease, α_1-antitrypsin deficiency, cirrhosis associated with jejunoileal bypass, and nonalcoholic steatohepatitis.[15]

Alcoholic Cirrhosis

Alcoholic cirrhosis is directly attributable to chronic ingestion of large quantities of alcohol. Women may develop alcoholic cirrhosis after consumption of lesser amounts of alcohol than is necessary to cause cirrhosis in men. Daily alcohol consumption of about 50 g (three to four drinks) a day for 10 to 15 years is associated with alcoholic liver disease in women, whereas consumption of 80 g (five to six drinks) is required for alcoholic cirrhosis to develop in men. The development of alcoholic cirrhosis does not require concomitant malnutrition, although this condition is almost invariably present (substitution of alcohol for normal dietary calories).

The diagnosis of alcohol abuse can be difficult because many patients conceal information about their alcohol use. However, the diagnosis of alcoholic cirrhosis is supported by an AST/ALT ratio of at least 2:1.[3] This increased ratio reflects the low serum activity of ALT in patients with an alcoholic liver due to an alcohol-related deficiency of pyridoxal 5-phosphate. In fact, the ALT concentration may be normal in patients with severe alcoholic liver disease. Alkaline phosphatase concentrations are often moderately increased. Decreased serum albumin concentrations (less than 3.5 g/dl) and prolonged prothrombin times are common.

The only effective therapy for patients with alcoholic liver disease is cessation of alcohol ingestion. Vigorous nutritional support may enhance survival. There is no convincing evidence that corticosteroids, propylthiouracil, or colchicine are efficacious treatments for alcoholic liver disease.

Postnecrotic Cirrhosis

Postnecrotic cirrhosis is characterized by a shrunken liver containing regenerating nodules. The most common causes of this condition are chronic viral hepatitis and autoimmune hepatitis, although the etiology in many patients is unknown (cryptogenic hepatitis). The distinguishing clinical features of postnecrotic cirrhosis are its predominance in women and increased serum concentrations of gamma globulin. Postnecrotic cirrhosis seems to progress insidiously even when the disease seems to be clinically inactive. The usual cause of death is gastrointestinal bleeding or hepatic failure. Primary liver cell cancer develops in about 10% to 15% of patients who have postnecrotic cirrhosis. Treatment is supportive and symptomatic, although corticosteroids may be administered when the disease is associated with autoimmune hepatitis.

Primary Biliary Cirrhosis

Primary biliary cirrhosis most often occurs in women 30 to 50 years of age.[16] The presence of serum autoantibodies and an association with bile duct lesions that resemble those present in chronic graft-versus-host disease suggest a role of immune mechanisms in the pathogenesis of this disease. There may even be a genetic predisposition to the development of primary biliary cirrhosis.

Presenting complaints are fatigue and generalized pruritus. Jaundice may not develop for 5 to 10 years after the onset of pruritus. Osteoporosis is common and may be associated with bone pain and spontaneous fractures. Alkaline phosphatase concentrations are increased, as are serum cholesterol and IgM concentrations. Concomitant diseases include renal tubular acidosis, CREST syndrome (calcinosis, Raynaud's phenomenon, esophageal dysmotility,

sclerodactyly, telangiectasia), and Sjögren's syndrome. Carcinoma of the pancreas, common bile duct obstruction, and chronic pericholangitis secondary to inflammatory disease may mimic primary biliary cirrhosis.

Treatment includes administration of a hydrophilic bile acid, ursodiol, which is presumed to decrease the concentration of potentially toxic endogenous hydrophobic bile acids. Corticosteroids do not alter the course of primary biliary cirrhosis and may exacerbate pruritus. Cholestyramine may alleviate the pruritus. Fat-soluble vitamin supplements are recommended, as malabsorption of fat-soluble vitamins occurs in patients with primary biliary cirrhosis.

Hemochromatosis

Hemochromatosis occurs when large amounts of iron are deposited in hepatocytes, resulting in hepatic scarring and cirrhosis.[17] The disease occurs 10 times more often in men than in women. Iron deposits in the pancreas and heart muscle are associated with the development of diabetes mellitus and congestive heart failure, respectively. There is bronze discoloration of the skin, and hepatosplenomegaly is likely. Signs of portal hypertension eventually develop in most patients. Primary liver cell cancer occurs in about 15% to 20% of patients.

Laboratory evaluation reveals an increase in serum iron and ferritin concentrations. Computed tomography and magnetic resonance imaging may demonstrate iron overload and primary hemochromatosis. The diagnosis of hemochromatosis can be confirmed only by liver biopsy (hemosiderin granules in hepatocytes and bile duct cells) because increased serum iron and ferritin concentrations also often accompany alcoholic liver disease, acute viral hepatitis, and chronic active hepatitis. Mild increases in the serum alkaline phosphatase and aminotransferase concentrations are common, but jaundice is unusual.

Treatment is removal of excess iron by phlebotomy. If patients are identified before cirrhosis develops and total body iron depletion is successfully accomplished, life expectancy approaches normal. Treated patients with cirrhosis are at increased risk of developing primary hepatocellular carcinoma even after total body iron stores are normalized. Normalization of total body iron stores is associated with decreases in signs of liver and cardiac disease, but endocrine abnormalities and arthropathy are likely to persist.

Wilson's Disease

Wilson's disease (hepatolenticular degeneration) is an autosomal recessive disorder due to a defect in the gene that codes for copper binding.[3] The subsequent excretion of copper into bile is defective, leading to total body accumulation of copper. Neurologic dysfunction (tremors, gait disturbances, slurring of speech) and hepatic dysfunction (fatigue, jaundice, ascites, splenomegaly, gastroesophageal varices) develop. Associated hemolytic anemia is a clue to the diagnosis, but the pathognomonic sign is the Kayser-Fleischer ring, a thin brown crescent of pigmentation at the periphery of the cornea. The distinguishing laboratory findings are decreased serum ceruloplasmin concentrations and increased urinary copper excretion.

Treatment of Wilson's disease is with trientine or penicillamine, chelating drugs that bind copper, thereby promoting urinary excretion. Penicillamine may be associated with nausea, vomiting, leukopenia, and thrombocytopenia, which may progress to aplastic anemia. Pyridoxine is administered weekly to offset the pyridoxine antagonist effects of penicillamine.

α_1-Antitrypsin Deficiency

Homozygous α_1-antitrypsin deficiency is associated with a rare syndrome of progressive cirrhosis.[3, 15] Adult patients usually have accompanying pulmonary emphysema. The presence of hepatomegaly, mild derangements in liver function tests, and the absence of α_1-antitrypsin on protein electrophoresis makes the diagnosis likely. Many of the affected patients also have evidence of hepatitis B or hepatitis C infection.

Cirrhosis Associated with Jejunoileal Bypass

Increased hepatic fat accumulation occurs in virtually all patients during the rapid weight loss period following jejunoileal bypass surgery, an operation that is no longer performed. The liver becomes enlarged and progressive hepatic dysfunction occurs. Treatment is reanastomosis of the bowel to prevent potentially fatal consequences.

Nonalcoholic Steatohepatitis

Nonalcoholic steatohepatitis is fat accumulation in the liver leading to cirrhosis. It is more common in women and is associated with obesity, hyperlipidemia, and diabetes mellitus.[3] Hepatomegaly may be marked, but evidence of hepatic dysfunction is mild. The mechanism of hepatic damage is not known, although the onset of the disorder often follows poor control of diabetes mellitus or rapid weight loss. Disease progression is gradual, and no specific therapy other than weight loss is available.

Complications of Cirrhosis

Hepatic and extrahepatic complications of hepatic cirrhosis, especially alcoholic cirrhosis, develop predictably in patients afflicted with progressive liver scarring (Table 18–4). Acute hepatic failure is characterized by the increased expression of these complications.

Portal Vein Hypertension

Portal vein hypertension typically does not develop until several years after the first attack of alcoholic hepatitis, followed by progressive scarring of the liver. The resulting elevated resistance to blood flow through the portal vein system, combined with hypoalbuminemia and increased secretion of antidiuretic hormone, contributes to the development of ascites. The most striking finding on physical examination is the presence of hepatomegaly with or without ascites.

Gastroesophageal Varices

Gastroesophageal varices are massively dilated submucosal veins that permit passage of splanchnic venous blood from the high-pressure portal venous system to the low-pressure azygos and hemiazgous thoracic veins. It is important to recognize that not all patients with cirrhosis of the liver develop esophageal varices, and not all patients with varices bleed from them. When bleeding does occur, variceal hemorrhage is usually from the distal esophagus or proximal stomach, and often it is hemodynamically significant. Bleeding esophageal varices are most reliably identified by upper gastrointestinal endoscopy.

Table 18–4 • Complications of Cirrhosis of the Liver

Portal vein hypertension
Varices
Ascites
Hyperdynamic circulation
Cardiomyopathy
Anemia
Coagulopathy
Arterial hypoxemia
Hepatorenal syndrome
Hypoglycemia
Duodenal ulcer
Gallstones
Spontaneous bacterial peritonitis
Hepatic encephalopathy
Primary hepatocellular carcinoma

Endoscopic therapy with variceal banding, ligation, or sclerotherapy (injection of a sclerosing substance into the esophageal varices) is the initial treatment for immediate control of esophageal variceal bleeding.[15] Banding or sclerotherapy is also effective for long-term control of recurrent esophageal variceal hemorrhage. Tracheal intubation may be performed to prevent pulmonary aspiration and to facilitate endoscopic evaluation of the bleeding site. Complications of sclerotherapy include esophageal ulceration, pleural effusion, and esophageal stricture and perforation. Respiratory distress may occur 24 to 48 hours after sclerotherapy. Bleeding from gastric varices is less common in patients with cirrhosis but more difficult to treat effectively.

If variceal bleeding persists or recurs and is life-threatening, balloon tamponade provided by insertion of a Sengstaken-Blakemore tube stops the bleeding in most patients. This treatment, which may require prior tracheal intubation, is associated with significant morbidity and is seldom utilized. Intra-arterial infusion of vasopressin does not improve overall survival and requires specialized angiographic experience. When vasopressin is administered, adjunctive therapy with nitroglycerin should be applied to minimize side effects related to peripheral vasoconstriction and tissue ischemia. Intravenous infusion of somatostatin or its analogue octreotide may be more effective than vasopressin and has a lower risk of side effects. Placing a transjugular intrahepatic portosystemic shunt is a possible intervention when bleeding from esophageal varices is refractory to endoscopic therapy. Hepatic encephalopathy develops in some patients following this procedure and is refractory to medical therapy.

Recurrent or continued bleeding from esophageal varices may indicate the need for a portosystemic shunt. This operation has a mortality rate of about 40% when performed as an emergency, whereas the mortality is substantially less when esophageal bleeding is controlled and the operation is performed electively. Portosystemic shunts may not prolong survival, but they do prevent subsequent variceal bleeding. The shunt procedure used is the one with which the surgeon is most experienced. A distal splenorenal shunt with concomitant gastro-esophageal devascularization selectively decompresses esophageal varices while maintaining mesenteric blood flow to the liver. The incidence of postoperative hepatic encephalopathy seems to be less when a distal splenorenal shunt is performed compared with conventional shunts.

Propranolol produces sustained decreases in portal venous pressures in patients with cirrhosis. Because the first episode of variceal bleeding can result in significant morbidity and mortality, there is interest in the prophylactic value of propranolol for preventing bleeding from esophageal varices.

Ascites

Ascites is a common sequela of many forms of cirrhosis, manifesting as a fluid wave across the abdomen on physical examination or right-sided pleural effusion. Factors that contribute to the formation of ascites include portal vein hypertension, decreased serum albumin concentrations with subsequent loss of oncotic pressure in the vascular system, and renal retention of sodium.

Drug-induced diuresis with the aldosterone antagonist spironolactone is an effective treatment for removing ascitic fluid. Maximum diuresis of ascitic fluid should not exceed 1 L daily for a daily weight loss of 0.5 to 1.0 kg. More rapid diuresis leads to possible hypovolemia and associated azotemia. Spironolactone tends to prevent renal excretion of potassium, which is desirable in patients with cirrhosis but prohibits use of the drug in patients with renal insufficiency. Long term treatment with spironolactone produces gynecomastia in some patients.

Ascites that does not respond to diuretic therapy may be treated by placing a LeVeen shunt that routes ascitic fluid subcutaneously from the peritoneal cavity to the internal jugular vein through a one-way valve. Complications of shunt placement include peritonitis, rupture of esophageal varices, and disseminated intravascular coagulation. These complications limit the use of this shunt. Placing a transjugular intrahepatic portosystemic shunt may be considered in patients with refractory ascites. Large-volume paracentesis (4 to 6 L daily) is an alternative to diuretic therapy in some patients. Administration of intravenous albumin after each tap decreases the likelihood of renal insufficiency and hyponatremia induced by paracentesis.

Spontaneous Bacterial Peritonitis

Spontaneous bacterial peritonitis (fever, leukocytosis, abdominal pain, decreased bowel sounds) may develop in patients with far-advanced cirrhosis and ascitic fluid that contains low concentrations of protein (opsonic activity is proportional to the level of ascitic fluid protein). Ascitic fluid should be analyzed whenever the condition of a patient with ascites deteriorates suddenly. The ascitic fluid is often turbid because of leukocytosis and bacterial growth. Presumably, hematogenous seeding of the ascitic fluid, which functions as an ideal bacterial culture medium, serves as a major route of infection. Cirrhosis likely facilitates the process by permitting enteric organisms to enter the systemic circulation via the portosystemic collaterals, thereby bypassing the major reticuloendothelial system in the liver. Despite antibiotic therapy the mortality associated with spontaneous bacterial peritonitis is about 50%.

Hepatorenal Syndrome

The hepatorenal syndrome is renal failure associated with cirrhosis of the liver (see Chapter 19). When this syndrome develops, the outcome is usually fatal. Typically, patients are deeply jaundiced, are moribund, and exhibit tense ascites, hypoalbuminemia, and hypoprothrombinemia. The pathogenesis of hepatorenal syndrome is uncertain, but decreased renal blood flow and glomerular filtration rate often precede the onset of the syndrome by several months.

Malnutrition

Almost all patients with cirrhosis of the liver have protein-calorie malnutrition, which leads to salt and water retention, defective immune responses, and delayed recovery of liver function.[15] In some critically ill patients, nutritional supplementation must be provided parenterally.

Systemic Circulation

Hepatic cirrhosis is often associated with a hyperdynamic circulation characterized by an increased cardiac output that is presumed to be due to vasodilating substances, such as glucagon, increased intravascular fluid volume, decreased viscosity of blood secondary to anemia, and arteriovenous communications, especially in the lungs. Conversely, cardiomyopathy manifesting as congestive heart failure can occur in patients with alcoholic cirrhosis. Megaloblastic anemia is frequent and is probably due to antagonism of folate by alcohol, rather than dietary deficiencies. Thrombocytopenia is likely; accumulation of fibrin degradation products may reflect the presence of disseminated intravascular coagulation or the inability of the diseased liver to clear these substances from the circulation.

Arterial Hypoxemia

Despite the frequent presence of hyperventilation due to accumulation of ammonia, PaO_2 values of 60 to 70 mmHg are common in patients with cirrhosis of the liver. A possible explanation for unanticipated low PaO_2 values is impaired movement of the diaphragm owing to accumulation of ascitic fluid. In addition, right-to-left intrapulmonary shunts may develop in the presence of portal vein hypertension,

leading to arterial hypoxemia. Likewise, many patients with hepatic cirrhosis smoke cigarettes, and chronic obstructive airway disease is likely. Arterial hypoxemia may be due to pneumonia, a frequent occurrence in alcoholic patients. Vulnerability to the development of pneumonia may reflect the ability of alcohol to inhibit the phagocytic activity normally present in the lungs. As a result, bacteria inhaled into the respiratory tract are more likely to lead to pneumonia. Indeed, most lung abscesses are found in chronic alcoholic patients. Also, regurgitation of gastric contents is made more likely by alcohol-induced decreases in lower esophageal sphincter tone.

Hypoglycemia

Hypoglycemia is a constant threat in patients with hepatic cirrhosis, especially in those who abuse alcohol. This may reflect glycogen depletion due to malnourishment plus alcohol-induced glycogenolysis and interference with gluconeogenesis. The liver is responsible for clearing lactic acid from the systemic circulation and subsequently converting lactate to glucose by gluconeogenesis. Severe hepatic cirrhosis may impair this function, contributing not only to hypoglycemia but to the development of metabolic acidosis as well.

Duodenal Ulcer

Duodenal ulcer disease is more common in patients with hepatic cirrhosis. Bleeding from duodenal ulcers, like that from gastroesophageal varices, contributes to anemia and presents increased ammonia loads to the gastrointestinal tract, which may aggravate hepatic encephalopathy. Gastrointestinal bleeding due to a duodenal ulcer is differentiated from variceal bleeding utilizing upper gastrointestinal endoscopy.

Gallstones

The incidence of gallstones is increased in patients with hepatic cirrhosis, presumably reflecting chronic increases in the bilirubin load caused by persistent hemolytic anemia and splenomegaly. The presence of gallstones complicates the differential diagnosis if jaundice occurs.

Impaired Immune Defense

Alcohol ingestion suppresses immune defense mechanisms, rendering alcoholic patients vulnerable to bacterial and viral infections, tuberculosis, and the development of cancer. In this regard, the patient using alcohol in excess, either episodically or on a regular basis, should be viewed as immunocompromised (see ''Spontaneous Bacterial Peritonitis'').

Hepatic Encephalopathy

The diagnosis of hepatic encephalopathy depends on documentation of mental obtundation, asterixis (flapping motion of hands at the wrists caused by intermittent loss of extensor tone), and fetor hepaticus (feculent-fruity odor of the breath). Asterixis may also develop in patients with uremia or severe pulmonary disease. Slowing or flattening of the waves on the electroencephalogram verifies encephalopathy. The cause of hepatic encephalopathy is multifactorial; and in most instances a precipitating event (gastrointestinal hemorrhage, electrolyte abnormalities such as hyponatremia, acid-base disorders, arterial hypoxemia, sepsis, injudicious use of diuretics or sedatives, creation of a portosystemic shunt) can be identified.

Treatment of hepatic encephalopathy is removal of any precipitating cause, especially sedative medications. Standard therapy includes dietary protein restriction to decrease production of endogenous nitrogenous substances such as ammonia. Lactulose is as effective as neomycin in decreasing plasma ammonia concentrations. Presumably lactulose decreases intraluminal pH in the gastrointestinal tract, causing ammonia to be protonated to ammonium, which is poorly absorbed and excreted in the feces. Liver transplantation has improved the prognosis for almost all forms of end-stage liver disease. Contraindications to liver transplantation include acquired immunodeficiency syndrome (AIDS), extrahepatic malignancy, sepsis, advanced cardiopulmonary disease, and active alcohol or other substance abuse.

Management of Anesthesia

It is estimated that 5% to 10% of all patients with cirrhosis of the liver undergo surgery during the last 2 years of life. Almost half of all trauma beds are occupied by patients who were injured while under the influence of alcohol.[18] In patients who abuse alcohol, the preoperative presence of ascites, sepsis, and chronic obstructive pulmonary disease are associated with increased postoperative morbidity and mortality.[19, 20] Postoperative morbidity is increased, especially with respect to the development of pneumonia, bleeding, sepsis, poor wound healing, and further deterioration of liver function. The pathogenic mechanisms of these complications often includes subclinical cardiorespiratory insufficiency and immune incompetence.[20] The complications of alcohol withdrawal syndrome may be fatal (see Chapter 30).

Preoperative Preparation

Preoperative criteria may correlate with the surgical risk and the postoperative outcome of patients with cirrhosis of the liver undergoing major surgery (Table 18–5).[21] Identifying co-existing problems that could be optimally and appropriately managed preoperatively (cardiorespiratory function, coagulation status, renal function, intravascular fluid volume, electrolyte balance, nutrition) may decrease the morbidity and mortality associated with elective surgery in patients with severe preoperative liver disease.[22] Coagulation status should be evaluated preoperatively and parenteral vitamin K administered if prothrombin times are prolonged. Failure of parenteral vitamin K to improve synthesis of prothrombin suggests the presence of severe hepatocellular disease. Conversely, impaired prothrombin production due to biliary obstruction and the absence of bile salts to facilitate gastrointestinal absorption of vitamin K is promptly reversed by parenteral vitamin K therapy. Thrombocytopenia, which often accompanies severe liver disease, may require treatment preoperatively. Hypoglycemia is a possibility, and administration of glucose solutions is a consideration during the perioperative period. That hydration with crystalloid solutions is adequate is evidenced by establishment of preoperative diuresis. It is important to

Table 18–5 • Prediction of Surgical Risk Based on Preoperative Evaluation

Parameter	Minimal	Modest	Marked
Bilirubin (mg/dl)	< 2	2–3	> 3
Albumin (g/dl)	> 3.5	3.0–3.5	< 3
Prothrombin time (seconds prolonged)	1–4	4–6	> 6
Encephalopathy	None	Moderate	Severe
Nutrition	Excellent	Good	Poor
Ascites	None	Moderate	Marked

Adapted from: Strunin I. Preoperative assessment of the patient with liver dysfunction. Br J Anaesth 1978;50:25–34.

remember that hepatic blood flow is predictably decreased in patients with cirrhosis of the liver, and any further decreases due to anesthetic-induced depression of cardiac output or systemic blood pressure could jeopardize hepatocyte oxygenation.

Chronic alcohol ingestion has been demonstrated to increase anesthetic requirements for isoflurane in animals (Fig. 18–2).[23] The most likely explanation for this increase is a cross-tolerance between depressant drugs. Accelerated metabolism of drugs in the presence of alcohol-induced microsomal enzyme stimulation might alter the amount of inhaled anesthetic needed to achieve given partial pressures but would not alter the partial pressures required to produce anesthesia. Surprisingly, thiopental dose requirements have not been shown to be increased in sober alcoholic patients (Fig. 18–3).[24] In contrast to resistance to depressant drugs, alcohol-induced cardiomyopathy could make these patients unusually sensitive to the cardiac depressant effects of volatile anesthetics. There may be decreased responsiveness

to catecholamines, manifesting as impaired tolerance to acute surgical blood loss. Likewise, decreased protein binding of drugs in the presence of decreased serum albumin concentrations would increase the pharmacologically active fractions of injected drugs available to act at peripheral receptors. Severely jaundiced patients (serum bilirubin concentrations higher than 8 mg/dl) are more likely to develop acute renal failure and sepsis postoperatively, emphasizing the possible value of establishing diuresis with mannitol preoperatively and initiating antibiotic therapy.

Intraoperative Management

Optimal anesthetic drug choices or techniques in the presence of liver disease are unknown. It is important to remember, however, that a constant feature of chronic liver disease is decreased hepatic blood flow owing to increased resistance to flow through the portal vein. As a result, hepatic blood

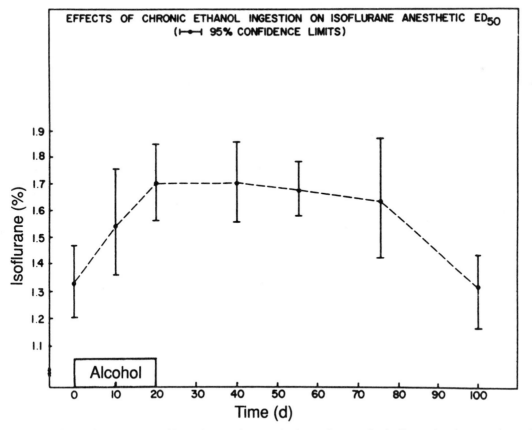

Figure 18–2 • Effect of chronic alcohol ingestion on the anesthetic requirement for isoflurane in mice was determined during and after exposure to alcohol. Isoflurane anesthetic requirements on days 20, 40, 55 and 75 were significantly increased above the control value ($P < 0.05$). (From Johnstone RE, Kulp RA, Smith TC. Effects of acute and chronic ethanol administration on isoflurane requirements in mice. Anesth Analg 1975;54:177–81, with permission.)

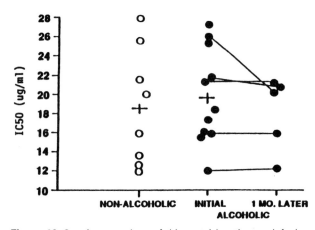

Figure 18–3 • Average dose of thiopental (continuous infusion of 100 mg/min IV) needed to produce a brief period of isoelectric activity on the electroencephalogram is no different in nonalcoholic and alcoholic patients. (From Swerdlow BN, Holley FO, Maitre PO, et al. Chronic alcohol intake does not change thiopental anesthetic requirement, pharmacokinetics, or pharmacodynamics. Anesthesiology 1990;72:455–61, with permission.)

flow and hepatocyte oxygenation are more dependent on hepatic artery blood flow than in normal patients. The hepatic artery may provide more than 50% of the oxygen supply by vasodilating during periods of decreased portal vein blood flow ("reciprocity of blood flow").[19] The portal venous system is essentially a passive vascular system such that intraoperative decreases in systemic blood pressure and cardiac output, as produced by volatile anesthetics, can result in decreases in portal vein blood flow. Surgical manipulation in the splanchnic vascular bed may also decrease portal vein blood flow. Hepatic blood flow and presumably hepatocyte oxygenation seem to be well maintained during administration of isoflurane, desflurane, and sevoflurane but not halothane (Fig. 18–4).[25, 26] Nevertheless, the hepatic artery's ability to vasodilate in response to decreases in portal vein blood flow is blunted by volatile anesthetics (especially halothane) and high anesthetic concentrations. Furthermore, in the presence of cirrhosis, the reciprocal relation between the hepatic artery and the portal vein blood flow is not well maintained. It is prudent to limit the doses of volatile anesthetics (combined with nitrous oxide and/or opioids) to minimize the likelihood of persistent mean arterial pressure decreases, as intraoperative hypotension may be associated with increased postoperative morbidity and mortality.[19] Injected anesthetic drugs may serve as valuable adjuncts to nitrous oxide with or without volatile anesthetics, but it must be appreciated that cumulative drug effects are likely if liver disease is severe enough to slow metabolism. Regardless of the drugs

selected for anesthesia, postoperative liver dysfunction is likely to be exaggerated in patients with chronic liver disease, presumably owing to the detrimental nonspecific effects of anesthetic drugs and to stress-induced activation of the sympathetic nervous system on hepatocyte oxygenation. Regional anesthesia is useful in patients with advanced liver disease, assuming that the coagulation status is acceptable.

Muscle Relaxants

The role of the liver in the clearance of muscle relaxants is considered when selecting these drugs for administration to patients with cirrhosis of the liver. Succinylcholine or mivacurium are acceptable, although severe liver disease may decrease plasma cholinesterase activity and prolong the duration of action of these drugs (Fig. 18–5).[27] The increased volume of distribution that accompanies cirrhosis may result in the need for larger initial doses of nondepolarizing muscle relaxants to produce the

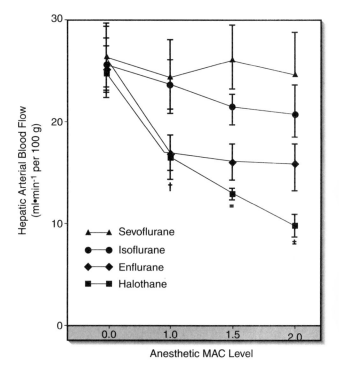

Figure 18–4 • In animal models, hepatic blood flow is better maintained during administration of sevoflurane, desflurane, and isoflurane than during administration of halothane. (Data from Frink EJ, Morgan SE, Coetzee A, et al. The effects of sevoflurane, halothane, enflurane, and isoflurane on hepatic blood flow and oxygenation in chronically instrumented dogs. Anesthesiology 1992;76:85–90; Eger EI. Desflurane (Suprane®): A Compendium and Reference. Nutley, NJ: Anaquest, 1993;1–119.)

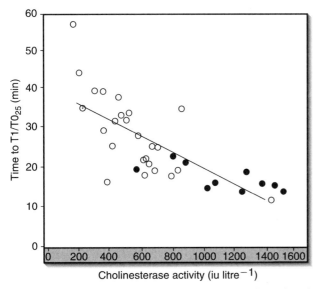

Figure 18–5 • Recovery from neuromuscular blockade produced by mivacurium is prolonged in patients with decreased cholinesterase activity as may be associated with cirrhosis of the liver (*open circles*). *Solid circles* represent normal patients, whereas the *circle with a dot* represents a heterozygous patient. (From Devlin JC, Head-Rapson AG, Parker CJR, et al. Pharmacodynamics of mivacurium chloride in patients with hepatic cirrhosis. Br J Anaesth 1993;71:227–31. © The Board of Management and Trustees of the British Journal of Anaesthesia. Reproduced by permission of Oxford Unviersity Press/British Journal of Anaesthesia.)

required plasma concentrations, but the resulting neuromuscular blockade may be prolonged if these drugs depend on hepatic clearance mechanisms. Indeed, the elimination half-time of pancuronium is prolonged owing to decreased hepatic clearance of this drug in patients with cirrhosis.[28] Hepatic dysfunction does not alter the elimination half-time of atracurium, and the same is presumed to be true for cisatracurium.[29] The elimination half-time of vecuronium in the presence of hepatic dysfunction or biliary tract obstruction is not increased until the dose exceeds 0.1 mg/kg, consistent with the dependence of this drug on hepatic clearance mechanisms (Fig. 18–6).[30–32] Altered protein binding of muscle relaxants in patients with hepatic cirrhosis is probably insignificant as a mechanism of altered responses in these patients. All factors considered, short-acting muscle relaxants (mivacurium) and intermediate-acting muscle relaxants (atracurium, cisatracurium) seem to be attractive choices for producing skeletal muscle relaxation in patients with severe liver disease.

Monitoring

Monitoring intraoperative arterial blood gases, pH, and urine output and providing exogenous glucose

are important principles. Arterial hypoxemia may be exaggerated intraoperatively if drugs used for anesthesia produce vasodilation of co-existing portosystemic and intrapulmonary shunts.[33] Intravenous infusions of glucose during the perioperative period are important, not only to prevent hypoglycemia but to decrease the likelihood of deposition of potentially harmful lipid-soluble metabolic products of volatile anesthetics in hepatocytes. Repeated blood glucose determinations may be helpful, especially during prolonged surgical procedures. When blood replacement is necessary, it is logical to administer the stored blood as slowly as possible to compensate for decreased clearance of citrate by the diseased liver. Fluid administration must be care-

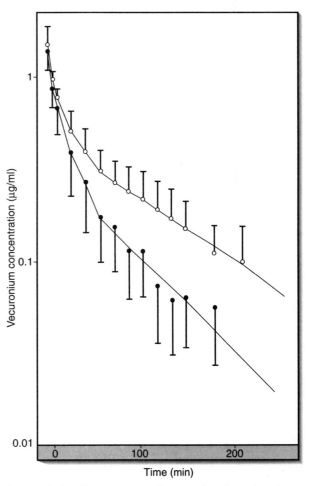

Figure 18–6 • Disappearance of vecuronium from the plasma of patients with cirrhosis of the liver (*open circles*) and control patients (*solid circles*) after a single bolus dose of 0.2 mg/kg IV. (From Lebrault C, Berger JL, D'Hollander AA, et al. Pharmacokinetics and pharmacodynamics of vecuronium (OR NC45) in patients with cirrhosis. Anesthesiology 1985;62:601–5. © 1985, Lippincott Williams & Wilkins, with permission.)

fully titrated in patients with cirrhosis of the liver. In this regard, it may be necessary to monitor cardiac filling pressures with a central venous or pulmonary artery catheter. Intraoperative maintenance of urine output, particularly in patients with co-existing jaundice, is a common goal to decrease the likelihood of postoperative acute renal failure. Mannitol may be necessary to establish diuresis. A practical point is avoidance of unnecessary esophageal instrumentation (stethoscope, gastric tube) in patients with known esophageal varices. The need for invasive intraoperative monitoring is determined by the extent and urgency of the surgery. Management of anesthesia for surgical creation of a portocaval shunt includes monitoring systemic arterial and cardiac filling pressures.

Postoperative Management

Regardless of the drugs selected for anesthesia, postoperative liver dysfunction is likely to be exaggerated in patients with chronic liver disease, presumably owing to detrimental nonspecific effects of anesthetic drugs on hepatic blood flow. Cholestasis is another possible cause of postoperative jaundice. Sepsis is a consideration when postoperative liver dysfunction manifests. Manifestations of alcohol withdrawal syndrome usually appear 48 to 72 hours after cessation of drinking and represent a life-threatening medical emergency (see Chapter 30).

Sober Alcoholic Patients

Management of anesthesia in sober patients with alcohol-induced cirrhosis of the liver is based on an understanding of the pathophysiologic changes associated with chronic liver disease. Postoperative morbidity and mortality are increased in patients with a history of alcohol abuse.[18-20]

Intoxicated Alcoholic Patients

In contrast to chronic but sober alcoholic patients, the acutely intoxicated patient requires less anesthetic because there is an additive depressant effect of the alcohol and anesthetics. Acutely intoxicated patients are also ill-equipped to withstand stress and acute surgical blood loss. Furthermore, alcohol tends to decrease the tolerance of the brain to hypoxia. Intoxicated patients may be more vulnerable to regurgitation of gastric contents, as alcohol slows gastric emptying and decreases the tone of the lower esophageal sphincter. Surgical bleeding may reflect alcohol-induced interference with platelet aggregation. Alcohol, even in moderate doses, causes increased plasma concentrations of catecholamines,

most likely reflecting inhibition of neurotransmitter uptake back into the presynaptic nerve endings. It is unknown whether the development of intraoperative cardiac dysrhythmias is influenced by this phenomenon.

◼ IDIOPATHIC HYPERBILIRUBINEMIA

Hyperbilirubinemia may occur in the absence of hemolysis or overt hepatobiliary disease. Unconjugated hyperbilirubinemia is present if there are defects before the conjugation steps in hepatocytes. These conjugation steps render bilirubin water soluble and are under the control of the hepatic enzyme glucuronyl transferase. If the defect in transport occurs after conjugation, conjugated bilirubin reenters the systemic circulation to produce conjugated hyperbilirubinemia.

Gilbert Syndrome

The most common example of idiopathic hyperbilirubinemia (present in varying degrees in 5% to 10% of the population) is Gilbert syndrome, inherited as an autosomal dominant trait with variable penetrance. The primary defect is decreased bilirubin uptake by hepatocytes, resulting in increased plasma concentrations of unconjugated bilirubin. Plasma bilirubin concentrations seldom exceed 5 mg/dl.

Crigler-Najjar Syndrome

Crigler-Najjar syndrome is a rare form of severe unconjugated hyperbilirubinemia beginning at birth and caused by decreased or absent glucuronyl transferase enzyme.[34] Children who lack this enzyme are jaundiced at birth; kernicterus develops, with plasma bilirubin concentrations close to 30 mg/dl. These children seldom survive to adulthood. When some enzyme activity is present, plasma bilirubin concentrations average 15 mg/dl, and jaundice is less severe. In these less severely afflicted patients, chronic phenobarbital therapy may decrease jaundice by stimulating enzymatic activity of glucuronyl transferase. Plasmapheresis and phototherapy represent temporary, alternative treatments. Liver transplantation is a consideration in these patients.

Bilirubin phototherapy lights should be available for anesthetic management of children with this syndrome.[35] Fasting should be minimized because this stress is known to increase plasma concentrations of bilirubin. Morphine is metabolized by a glucuronyl transferase enzyme system different from that deficient in Crigler-Najjar syndrome. For this reason, morphine can be safely administered to these patients. Barbiturates, inhaled anesthetics, and muscle relaxants are acceptable choices in these patients.

Dubin-Johnson Syndrome

Dubin-Johnson syndrome is due to decreased ability to transport organic ions from hepatocytes into the biliary system, resulting in conjugated hyperbilirubinemia. Inheritance of this syndrome is autosomal recessive.

Alagille Syndrome

Alagille syndrome (arteriohepatic dysplasia) is an autosomal dominant disease characterized by intrahepatic cholestasis.[36] Associated abnormalities include pulmonary artery stenosis, butterfly vertebrae, growth retardation, renal dysfunction, ocular abnormalities, and typical facial features. Refractory pruritus may be associated with cholestasis. Liver transplantation is indicated in the patients who progress to cirrhosis of the liver.

Benign Postoperative Intrahepatic Cholestasis

Benign postoperative intrahepatic cholestasis may occur when surgery is prolonged, especially if it is complicated by hypotension, arterial hypoxemia, and the need for blood transfusions.[37] Patients who experience these responses are often elderly. Jaundice, in association with conjugated hyperbilirubinemia, is usually apparent within 24 to 48 hours and may persist for 14 to 28 days. Liver function tests other than plasma bilirubin concentrations are usually normal or only mildly deranged. The prognosis depends on the underlying surgical or medical conditions.

Progressive Familial Intrahepatic Cholestasis (Byler's Disease)

Progressive familial intrahepatic cholestasis is a rare genetically determined metabolic disease that manifests during the first few months of life and progresses to end-stage hepatic cirrhosis before adulthood.[38] Pruritus may be severe. The precise metabolic defects responsible for this disease have not been identified. Liver transplantation is the only curative treatment for this disorder. Management of anesthesia in patients with progressive familial intrahepatic cirrhosis is influenced by malnutrition, portal hypertension, coagulation abnormalities, hypoalbuminemia, and chronic arterial hypoxemia.[38]

ACUTE LIVER FAILURE

Acute liver failure is characterized by altered mental status (hepatic encephalopathy) and impaired coagulation in the clinical setting of acute hepatic disease.[39] Fulminant hepatic failure is present when hepatic encephalopathy develops within 8 weeks of the onset of clinical illness. Viral hepatitis and drug-induced liver injury account for most patients who develop acute liver failure (Table 18–6).

Signs and Symptoms

Regardless of the cause, acute liver failure presents with clinical features that distinguish it from chronic hepatic insufficiency.[39] Typically, nonspecific symptoms such as malaise or nausea develop in a previously healthy individual, followed by jaundice, rapid onset of altered mental status, and coma. The progression of symptoms is rapid, with previously healthy patients becoming comatose in 2 to 10 days. Altered mentation and prolonged prothrombin times are the hallmarks of acute liver failure. Sup-

Table 18–6 • Causes of Acute Liver Failure

Viral hepatitis
Drug-induced
  Acetaminophen
  Idiosyncratic reactions
    Volatile anesthetics (especially halothane)
    Isoniazid
    Phenytoin
    Sulfonamides
    Propylthiouracil
    Amiodarone
Toxins
  Carbon tetrachloride
  Mushrooms
Vascular events
  Ischemia
  Veno-occlusive disease (Budd-Chiari syndrome)
Miscellaneous
  Acute fatty liver of pregnancy
  Wilson syndrome
  Reye syndrome

Adapted from: Lee WM. Acute liver failure. N Engl J Med 1993;329: 1862–72.

portive laboratory findings include increased serum aminotransferase concentrations, hypoglycemia, and evidence of respiratory alkalosis. The onset of hepatic encephalopathy is often abrupt and may precede the appearance of jaundice. Cerebral edema is often present, manifesting as systemic hypertension and bradycardia. Hypotension and decreased systemic vascular resistance are common, and oliguric renal failure (hepatorenal syndrome) occurs in most patients. These patients are at increased risk for the development of bacterial and fungal infections.

Acute fatty liver of pregnancy is characterized by accumulation of microscopic fat in hepatocytes.[40] About one-half of patients have evidence of pregnancy-induced hypertension, and many have laboratory results characteristic of the HELLP syndrome (see Chapter 31). Symptoms of acute fatty liver of pregnancy typically begin during the third trimester. The initial manifestations are nonspecific (nausea and vomiting, right upper quadrant pain, viral-like syndrome with malaise and anorexia) followed in 7 to 14 days by the appearance of jaundice. Treatment is prompt termination of pregnancy. Untreated, acute fatty liver of pregnancy typically progresses to acute liver failure and death.

Treatment

There are no specific treatments of proven efficacy for managing acute liver failure.[39] Efforts to elucidate the cause are important, as antidotes must be administered early for acetaminophen or mushroom poisoning. Glucose is indicated in the presence of hypoglycemia. Pulmonary artery catheter monitoring may be helpful for the management of intravascular fluid volume replacement. Conventional pressor treatment for hypotension with inotropes is relatively ineffective, and use of vasopressors may improve the mean arterial pressure but further impair peripheral oxygen delivery. Cerebral edema may require aggressive interventions in the hope of preventing cerebral herniation. When survival seems unlikely (prothrombin times longer than 100 seconds), the only curative treatment is liver transplantation.

Management of Anesthesia

Only surgery intended to correct life-threatening situations should be considered in patients with acute liver failure. Preoperative correction of coagulation abnormalities with fresh frozen plasma may be indicated. Depressant or sedative drugs are not required. Nitrous oxide may be sufficient to provide analgesia and total amnesia in these critically ill patients. Intravenous anesthetics may produce prolonged effects in the absence of normal rates of hepatic metabolism. Muscle relaxants are appropriate for facilitating operative exposure and the management of ventilation. When choosing a muscle relaxant one must consider the impact of decreased hepatic function and the often associated renal dysfunction. Because the plasma half-time of cholinesterase is 14 days, it is unlikely that acute liver failure would be associated with prolonged responses to succinylcholine or mivacurium.

Provision of exogenous glucose is important; and during long operations plasma glucose measurements to confirm the absence of hypoglycemia are prudent. Blood should be warmed and administered at as slow a rate as is practical to minimize the likelihood of citrate intoxication. The use of fresh whole blood optimizes delivery of coagulation factors and minimizes the ammonia load. Monitoring the arterial blood gases, pH, and electrolytes is helpful, as these patients are vulnerable to the development of arterial hypoxemia, metabolic acidosis, and decreased potassium, calcium, and magnesium concentrations. Hypotension and its potential adverse effects on hepatic blood flow and hepatocyte oxygenation must be appreciated. Urine output is maintained with intravenous infusions of crystalloid or colloid solutions and, if necessary, mannitol. Invasive monitoring, including systemic arterial and pulmonary artery catheters, is helpful for guiding perioperative management. These patients are vulnerable to infections, emphasizing the importance of aseptic techniques during insertion of intravascular catheters. Institution of lactulose therapy during the preoperative period decreases the ammonia load and helps prevent the development of hepatic encephalopathy.

▌ LIVER TRANSPLANTATION

Liver transplantation is the only curative therapy for patients in liver failure, such as that due to end-stage liver disease associated with cirrhosis of the liver. Hepatoma, biliary tract tumors, and genetically determined metabolic disturbances may also be treated with liver transplantation.

Management of Anesthesia

Candidates for liver transplantation may present with severe multiple system organ dysfunction. Many of the physiologic derangements (coagulation defects) are not correctable until after successful liver transplantation. The likely presence of hepatitis A, B, or C in recipients must be considered by the health care providers.

For induction of anesthesia one may have to consider the presence of ascites and its associated slowing of gastric emptying. Anesthesia is maintained by drugs that preserve the splanchnic circulation (opioids, isoflurane, desflurane, sevoflurane) combined with muscle relaxants (atracurium, cisatracurium) that are not dependent on hepatic clearance mechanisms. Nitrous oxide is usually avoided based on concerns regarding bowel distension and the ability of this gas to increase the size of air bubbles (air emboli) that may enter the circulation. Fluid warming devices and rapid infusion systems designed to deliver prewarmed fluids or blood products at rates exceeding 1 L/min are routinely employed. Invasive monitoring of systemic blood pressure and cardiac filling pressures and placing large-bore intravenous catheters to optimize fluid replacement are important parts of anesthetic management. Monitoring the systemic blood pressure via the radial artery is preferred over infradiaphragmatic sites because the abdominal aorta may be cross-clamped during hepatic arterial anastomosis. Clamping the suprahepatic inferior vena cava dictates placement of venous access catheters above the diaphragm. Removing the native liver followed by placing the donor liver is characterized as the preanhepatic, anhepatic, and neohepatic phases.[41]

The *preanhepatic phase* involves mobilizing and removing the native liver. Cardiovascular instability due to hemorrhage, venous pooling due to sudden decreases in intra-abdominal pressure, and impaired venous return due to surgical retraction are possible during this phase. Hypocalcemia, hyperkalemia, and metabolic acidosis may occur. Oliguria is common during the preanhepatic phase.

The *anhepatic stage* begins when the native liver is removed after transecting its blood supply (hepatic artery and portal vein). To avoid unacceptable decreases in venous return and cardiac output as well as venous congestion during occlusion of the inferior vena cava, a venovenous bypass system may be utilized. Support of the cardiac output with inotropes may be needed during this phase. Placement of the donor liver is likely to require vigorous retraction near the diaphragm, leading to possible compromise of ventilation and oxygenation. Because of the lack of liver metabolic function during the anhepatic phase, citrate intoxication from rapid transfusion is more likely, and calcium is administered to prevent hypocalcemia.

The *neohepatic phase* begins with reanastomosis of the major vascular structures. Before removing the vascular clamps, the allograft is flushed to remove air, debris, and preservative solutions. Despite this step, subsequent unclamping can cause release of large loads of potassium and metabolic acids. Cardiac dysrhythmias and hypotension may require pharmacologic intervention at this time. Once the allograft begins to function, hemodynamic and metabolic stability are gradually restored and urine output increases. Clotting parameters usually normalize with the administration of specific coagulation factors. Postoperative support of the recipient's ventilation and oxygenation is likely to be required.

Anesthetic Considerations

Potential adverse effects (systemic hypertension, anemia, thrombocytopenia) and drug interactions related to chronic immunosuppressant therapy are considered when planning the management of anesthesia in liver transplant recipients. Liver function tests return to normal following successful liver transplantation.[42] Recovery of drug metabolism capacity occurs soon after reperfusion of the graft. Renal dysfunction is common in liver transplant recipients, and renal excretion of drugs is an important consideration. Liver transplantation results in reversal of the hyperdynamic circulatory state that characterizes liver failure. Oxygenation improves following successful liver transplantation, although prior intrapulmonary shunts may persist and contribute to ventilation-to-perfusion abnormalities.

Normal physiologic mechanisms that protect hepatic blood flow are blunted after liver transplantation. The liver is normally an important source of blood volume in shock states via a vasoconstrictive response, and this mechanism may be impaired after liver transplantation. There is no evidence of increased risks of developing hepatitis after the administration of volatile anesthetics to liver transplant recipients.[42] Hepatic arterial thrombosis has been attributed to overtransfusion of blood products leading to hemoconcentration. For this reason, liver transplant recipients may benefit from maintaining the hematocrit near 30% during the postoperative period.

■ DISEASES OF THE BILIARY TRACT

Cholelithiasis and inflammatory biliary tract disease constitute major health problems in the United States, with an estimated 10% of adults older than 40 years of age having gallstones.[43, 44] The prevalence of gallstones is significantly higher in women than men. Furthermore, the prevalence increases with aging, obesity, rapid weight loss, and pregnancy. Gallstone formation is most likely related to abnormalities in the physicochemical aspects of the various components of bile. Approximately 90% of gallstones are radiolucent, composed primarily of hydrophobic cholesterol molecules. The remaining gallstones are usually radiopaque and are typically composed of calcium bilirubinate. These gallstones develop most often in patients with cirrhosis of the liver or hemolytic anemia.

Cholelithiasis and Cholecystitis

Patients who have stones in the gallbladder or biliary tree exhibit symptoms that range from acute disease to chronic symptomatic or silent disease.[33] Obstruction of the cystic duct or common bile duct by a gallstone that has migrated from the gallbladder may cause acute inflammation.

Acute Cholecystitis

Obstruction of the cystic duct, which is nearly always due to a gallstone, produces acute inflammation of the gallbladder. Cholelithiasis is present in 95% of patients with acute cholecystitis.

Signs and Symptoms

Signs and symptoms of acute cholecystitis include nausea, vomiting, fever (38°C to 39°C), severe abdominal pain, and right upper quadrant tenderness. Severe pain, which begins in the mid-epigastrium, moves to the right upper abdomen, and may radiate around the sides to the back or directly through to the back to the area between the scapulae, caused by a stone lodging in a duct is designated *biliary colic*. This pain is extraordinarily intense and usually begins abruptly and subsides gradually. Patients may notice dark urine and scleral icterus. Most jaundiced patients have stones in the common bile duct at the time of surgery. Laboratory tests commonly demonstrate peripheral leukocytosis, and serum amylase concentrations are often increased.

Diagnosis

Ultrasonography, which is noninvasive, is the diagnostic procedure utilized in patients with suspected gallstones and acute cholecystitis. In addition to detecting gallstones, ultrasonography can be used to identify other causes of right upper quadrant pain, such as an abscess or a malignancy, and it may reveal biliary duct obstruction. Radionuclide scanning is the most accurate test for diagnosing acute cholecystitis (radiolabeled material enters the common bile duct but not the gallbladder). Gallstones may be detected by computed tomography and magnetic resonance imaging, but these techniques are more expensive and less sensitive than ultrasonography.

Differential Diagnosis

Acute pancreatitis may be nearly impossible to distinguish from acute cholecystitis (Table 18–7). Patients with penetrating duodenal ulcers may experience severe epigastric pain, and free air may be evident on plain films of the abdomen if the ulcer has perforated. Acute appendicitis may produce symptoms similar to those of acute cholecystitis, particularly if the appendix is located retrocecally. Acute pyelonephritis of the right kidney may produce anterior pain similar to the pain that occurs with acute cholecystitis. Pneumonia or infarction in the right lung may cause upper abdominal pain similar to that of acute cholecystitis.

Treatment

Patients with a clinical diagnosis of acute cholecystitis are treated with intravenous fluids and electrolytes and administration of opioids to manage the pain. Febrile patients with leukocytosis are treated with antibiotics. Surgery is typically considered when the patient's condition has stabilized. Laparoscopic cholecystectomy has almost completely replaced open cholecystectomy, resulting in less postoperative pain and more rapid convalescence.[44] In about 5% of patients laparoscopic cholecystectomy must be converted to an open cholecystectomy because inflammation obscures the anatomy. Cholangiography can be performed during laparoscopic surgery. However, because patients with acute cholecystitis may have common duct stones, it is recommended that preoperative endoscopic retrograde cholangiopancreatography (ERCP) be performed. If endoscopic common duct stone removal is not pos-

Table 18–7 • Differential Diagnosis of Acute Cholecystitis

Acute viral hepatitis
Alcoholic hepatitis
Penetrating duodenal ulcer
Appendicitis
Pyelonephritis
Right lower lobe pneumonia
Pancreatitis
Acute myocardial infarction

sible, the operative procedure of choice is open cholecystectomy with common bile duct exploration and stone removal. Some patients (septic shock, peritonitis, pancreatitis, portal venous hypertension, clotting abnormalities) are not candidates for laparoscopic cholecystectomy and should undergo open cholecystectomy or cholecystostomy. Ultrasound-guided percutaneous puncture and aspiration of the gallbladder may be as effective as open cholecystostomy.

Complications

The principal complications of acute cholecystitis are related to severe inflammation and necrosis of the gallbladder.[43] Localized perforation and abscess formation are likely when symptoms persist for several days. Free perforation occurs in 1% to 2% of patients with acute cholecystitis and is associated with 30% mortality. Severe abdominal pain lasting longer than 7 days may be the result of empyema of the gallbladder. Mortality approaches 25% and is most often due to sepsis. Gallstone ileus results from obstruction of the small bowel at some point, usually at the ileocecal valve, by a large gallstone.

Management of Anesthesia

Anesthetic considerations for laparoscopic cholecystectomy are similar to those for other laparoscopic procedures.[43, 45] Insufflation of the abdominal cavity (pneumoperitoneum) with carbon dioxide introduced through a needle placed through a supraumbilical incision results in increased intra-abdominal pressure that may interfere with the adequacy of spontaneous ventilation and venous return. Indeed, changes in cardiovascular function due to insufflation of the abdomen are characterized by immediate decreases in venous return and cardiac output and increases in mean arterial pressure and systemic vascular resistance.[45] During the next few minutes there is partial restoration of cardiac output and systemic vascular resistance, but systemic blood pressure and heart rate are likely to remain unchanged. This pattern of cardiovascular responses is likely the result of an interaction between increased abdominal pressures, neurohumoral responses, and absorbed carbon dioxide.[44]

During laparoscopic cholecystectomy, placing patients in the reverse Trendelenburg position favors movement of abdominal contents away from the operative site and may improve ventilation. Mechanical ventilation of the lungs is recommended to prevent atelectasis and to ensure adequate ventilation in the presence of increased intra-abdominal pressures and to offset the effects of systemic ab-

sorption of carbon dioxide used to create the pneumoperitoneum. High intra-abdominal pressures may increase the risk of passive reflux of gastric contents. Clearly, tracheal intubation with a cuffed tube minimizes the risk of pulmonary aspiration should reflux occur. Venous carbon dioxide embolism may be responsible for cardiovascular collapse in the operating room or during the immediate postoperative period.[46] Capnography is important for recognizing a carbon dioxide embolism and the onset of cardiac dysrhythmias owing to hypercarbia. Intraoperative decompression of the stomach with a nasogastric or orogastric tube may decrease the risk of visceral puncture during needle insertion to produce the pneumoperitoneum. As with all laparoscopic procedures, careful observation for accidental injury to abdominal structures and blood vessels is important. The loss of hemostasis or injury to the hepatic artery or liver may require prompt intervention with an open laparotomy. There is no evidence that nitrous oxide (70%) expands bowel gas or interferes with surgical working conditions during laparoscopic cholecystectomy.[47] Subcutaneous emphysema associated with pneumomediastinum, pneumothorax, and pneumoscrotum as well as inappropriate antidiuretic hormone secretion have been observed in patients undergoing laparoscopic cholecystectomy.[48,49]

The use of opioids for anesthesia is controversial based on the known ability of these drugs to cause spasm of the choledochoduodenal sphincter (sphincter of Oddi) and subsequent choledochoduodenal hypertension (Fig. 18–7).[8] Despite these concerns, opioids have been used in many instances without adverse effects, emphasizing that not all patients respond to opioids with choledochoduodenal sphincter spasm. Indeed, it has been suggested that the incidence of opioid-induced sphincter spasm is so low (fewer than 3% of patients) that this response should not influence the selection of these drugs.[50] Furthermore, should opioid-induced sphincter spasm occur, it is possible to antagonize this effect with intravenous administration of naloxone (which may also antagonize desirable analgesic effects) or glucagon. Glucagon predictably produces hyperglycemia and in awake patients is likely to be associated with vomiting. Nitroglycerin 10 μg/min IV may be effective in treating spasm of the sphincter of Oddi.[51] Emergency surgery for acute cholecystitis or common bile duct obstruction associated with vomiting may necessitate volume and electrolyte replacement. Many of these patients have ileus and should be considered at increased risk for pulmonary aspiration of gastric contents. Compared with open cholecystectomy, postoperative pain after

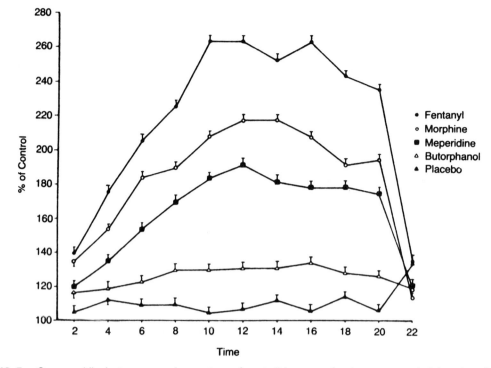

Figure 18–7 • Common bile duct pressures (percentage of control) increase after intravenous administration of an opioid agonist but not after injection of the opioid antagonist naloxone (placebo). Butorphanol, an opioid agonist-antagonist produces only modest increases in common bile duct pressures. (From Radnay P, Duncalf D, Nakakovic M, et al. Common bile duct pressure changes after fentanyl, morphine, meperidine, butorphanol, and naloxone. Anesth Analg 1984;63:441–4, with permission.)

laparoscopic cholecystectomy is much less, and the likelihood of pulmonary complications is decreased.

Chronic Cholecystitis

Chronic cholelithiasis is usually accompanied by evidence of chronic cholecystitis.[52] The wall of the gallbladder is often thickened, fibrotic, and rigid, thereby preventing normal contraction and expansion. Chronic cholecystitis typically follows a series of acute cholecystitis attacks.

Signs and Symptoms

Signs and symptoms are often nonspecific and include complaints of flatulence, heartburn, and postprandial distress. Findings on physical examination are normal. Results of routine laboratory tests are usually normal, although occasionally serum alkaline phosphatase concentrations are modestly increased.

Diagnosis

Ultrasonography is used to diagnose chronic cholecystitis. When the ultrasonogram is nondiagnostic, oral cholecystography may be utilized. Failure of the contrast dye to cause opacification is highly suggestive of chronic cholecystitis and cholelithiasis. ERCP may reveal gallstones in patients with biliary tract pain but normal oral cholecystograms and ultrasonograms. Computed tomography and magnetic resonance imaging may also detect gallstones, but these techniques are unlikely to demonstrate stones not detected by ultrasonography.

Treatment

Elective cholecystectomy is indicated for patients who have symptomatic gallstones and chronic cholecystitis. Recurrent pain is to be expected in these patients if cholecystectomy is not performed. Alternative forms of therapy for cholelithiasis include oral dissolution therapy and extracorporeal biliary lithotripsy.

Oral Dissolution Therapy. Ursodiol (ursodeoxycholic acid) administered orally for 6 to 12 months results in dissolution of up to 90% of cholesterol stones that are floating in a normally functioning gallbladder (accounts for about 15% of symptomatic patients).[44] Recurrence of cholesterol stones after discontinuation of ursodiol is common. Cholesterol stones can be rapidly dissolved by infusing methyl *tert*-butyl ether through a transhepatic catheter directly into the gallbladder. Overall, dissolution therapy has limited value except in patients who are poor candidates for surgery.

Extracorporeal Biliary Lithotripsy. Fragmentation of stones in the gallbladder or common bile duct may be produced by carefully focused shock waves.[44] The administration of ursodiol after fragmentation of stones increases the percentage of patients who are free of gallbladder stones several months after lithotripsy. The success of laparoscopic cholecystectomy limits the usefulness of lithotripsy for the treatment of biliary stones.

Choledocholithiasis

Choledocholithiasis is the lodgement of stones in the common bile duct after passage from the gallbladder and through the cystic duct.[53] Stones typically lodge at the point of insertion of the duct into the ampulla of Vater.

Signs and Symptoms

Patients with choledocholithiasis may present with signs of cholangitis (fever, shaking chills, jaundice, right upper quadrant pain) or jaundice alone and a history of pain suggestive of cholecystitis. Not all stones obstruct the common duct but, rather, pass into the duodenum or into a pancreatic duct resulting in acute pancreatitis. Serum bilirubin and alkaline phosphatase concentrations typically increase markedly and abruptly when the stone obstructs the common bile duct.[3] Aminotransferase concentrations are usually only modestly increased.

Diagnosis

Ultrasonography may reveal a dilated common bile duct, although this finding is not present in as many as 40% of patients with proven cholelithiasis.[52] Computed tomography is no more sensitive than ultrasonography. Cholescintigraphy may reveal common bile duct obstruction. The biliary tract can be visualized radiographically utilizing ERCP or percutaneous transhepatic cholangiography.

Differential Diagnosis

Acute obstruction of the common bile duct by a stone may clinically resemble ureterolithiasis because of the similarities in location and severity of pain. Liver function tests easily distinguish these two conditions. Acute inflammation of the head of the pancreas may produce obstruction of the common bile duct. Computed tomography or ERCP helps distinguish pancreatitis from choledocholithiasis. Symptoms of an acute myocardial infarction or viral hepatitis may produce abdominal pain that mimics biliary tract disease. The epigastric pain may be similar to that in patients with pancreatic carcinoma. In contrast to choledocholithiasis, liver function tests are not likely to be altered. Likewise, acute intermittent porphyria can cause severe abdominal pain, but alkaline phosphatase and bilirubin concentrations are unchanged.

Treatment

Endoscopic sphincterotomy is the initial treatment for the patient with choledocholithiasis. ERCP can be used to identify the cause of common bile duct obstruction and can also be used to remove a stone or place a stent. Operative exploration of the common bile duct is reserved for the few patients in whom endoscopic sphincterotomy is unsuccessful. Sphincterotomy is also the recommended treatment for patients with retained bile duct stones after gallbladder or biliary tract surgery. If nonsurgical treatment fails, surgical exploration of the biliary tract is necessary.

References

1. Keefe EB. Acute hepatitis. Sci Am Med 1999;1–9
2. Koff RS. Nonresponse to interferon in chronic hepatitis C. JAMA 2001;285:212–4
3. Pratt DS, Kaplan MK. Evaluation of abnormal liver-enzyme results in asymptomatic patients. N Engl J Med 2000;342:1266–71
4. Schafer DF, Sorrell MF. Conquering hepatitis C, step by step. N Engl J Med 2000;343:1723–4
5. Elliott RH, Strunin L. Hepatotoxicity of volatile anaesthetics. Br J Anaesth 1993;70:339–48
6. Suttner SW, Schmidt CC, Boldt J, et al. Low-flow desflurane and sevoflurane anesthesia minimally affect hepatic integrity and function in elderly patients. Anesth Analg 2000;91:206–12
7. Tiainen P, Lindgren L, Rosenberg PH. Changes in hepatocellular integrity during and after desflurane or isoflurane anaesthesia in patients undergoing breast surgery. Br J Anaesth 1998;80:906–22
8. Radnay PA, Duncalf D, Novakovic M, et al. Common bile duct pressure changes after fentanyl, morphine, meperidine, butorphanol, and naloxone. Anesth Analg 1984;63:441–4
9. Martin JL, Kenna JG, Pohl LR. Antibody assays for the detection of patients sensitized to halothane. Anesth Analg 1990;70:154–9
10. Munro HM, Snider SJ, Magee JC. Halothane-associated hepatitis in a 6-year old boy: evidence for native liver regeneration

following failed treatment with auxiliary liver transplantation. Anesthesiology 1998;89:524–7

11. Njoku D, Laster MJ, Gong DH, et al. Biotransformation of halothane, enflurane, isoflurane, and desflurane to trifluoroacetylated liver proteins: association between protein acylation and hepatic injury. Anesth Analg 1997;84:173–8

12. Gunaratnam NT, Benson J, Gandolfi AJ, et al. Suspected isoflurane hepatitis in an obese patient with a history of halothane hepatitis. Anesthesiology 1995;83:1361–4

13. Hoofnagle JH, DiBisceglie AM. The treatment of chronic viral hepatitis. N Engl J Med 1997;336:347–55

14. Keefe EB. Chronic hepatitis. Sci Am Med 1998;1–8

15. Keefe EB. Cirrhosis of the liver. Sci Am Med 1998;1–12

16. Kaplan MM. Primary biliary cirrhosis. N Engl J Med 1996; 335:1570–80

17. Rouault TA. Hereditary hemochromatosis. JAMA 1993; 269:3152–4

18. Spies CD, Rommelspacher H. Alcohol withdrawal in the surgical patient: prevention and treatment. Anesth Analg 1999;88:946–54

19. Ziser A, Plevak DJ, Wiesner RH, et al. Morbidity and mortality in cirrhotic patients undergoing anesthesia and surgery. Anesthesiology 1999;90:42–53

20. Tonneen H, Kehlet H. Preoperative alcoholism and postoperative morbidity. Br J Surg 1999;86:869–74

21. Strunin L. Preoperative assessment of the patient with liver dysfunction. Br J Anaesth 1978;50:25–34

22. Patel T. Surgery in the patient with liver disease. May Clin Proc 1999;74:593–9

23. Johnstone RE, Kulp RA, Smith TC. Effects of acute and chronic ethanol administration on isoflurane requirement in mice. Anesth Analg 1975;54:277–81

24. Swerdlow BN, Holley FO, Maitre PO, et al. Chronic alcohol intake does not change thiopental anesthetic requirement, pharmacokinetics, or pharmacodynamics. Anesthesiology 1990;72:455–61

25. Frink EJ, Morgan SE, Coetzee A, et al. The effects of sevoflurane, halothane, enflurane, and isoflurane on hepatic blood flow and oxygenation in chronically instrumented greyhound dogs. Anesthesiology 1992;76:5–10

26. Eger EI. Desflurane (Suprane®): A Compendium and Reference. Nutley, NJ: Anaquest, 1993;1–119.

27. Devlin JC, Head-Rapson AG, Parker CJR, et al. Pharmacodynamics of mivacurium chloride in patients with hepatic cirrhosis. Br J Anaesth 1993;71:227–31

28. Duvaldestin P, Agoston S, Henzel D, et al. Pancuronium pharmacokinetics in patients with liver cirrhosis. Br J Anaesth 1978;50:1131–6

29. Parker CJR, Hunter JM. Pharmacokinetics of atracurium and laudanosine in patients with hepatic cirrhosis. Br J Anaesth 1989;62:177–83

30. Lebrault C, Berger JL, D'Hollander AA, et al. Pharmacokinetics and pharmacodynamics of vecuronium (ORG NC45) inpatients with cirrhosis. Anesthesiology 1985;62:601–5

31. Arden JR, Lynam DP, Castagnoli KP, et al. Vecuronium in alcoholic liver disease: a pharmacokinetic and pharmacodynamic analysis. Anesthesiology 1988;68:771–6

32. Lebrault C, Duvaldestin P, Henzel D, et al. Pharmacokinetics and pharmacodynamics of vecuronium in patients with cholestasis. Br J Anaesth 1986;58:983–7

33. Kaplan JA, Bitner RL, Dripps RD. Hypoxia, hyperdynamic circulation, and the hazards of general anesthesia in patients with hepatic cirrhosis. Anesthesiology 1971;35:427–31

34. Fox IF, Chowdhury JR, Kaufman SS, et al. Treatment of the Crigler-Najjar syndrome type 1 with hepatocyte transplantation. N Engl J Med 1998;338:1422–6

35. Prager MC, Johnson KL, Ascher NL, et al. Anesthetic care of patients with Crigler-Najjar syndrome. Anesth Analg 1992; 74:162–4

36. Png K, Veyckemans F, De Kock M, et al. Hemodynamic changes in patients with Alagille's syndrome during orthotopic liver transplantation. Anesth Analg 1999;89:1137–42

37. LaMont JT, Isselbacher KJ. Postoperative jaundice. N Engl J Med 1973;288:305–7

38. Muller G, Veyckemans F, Carlier M, et al. Anaesthetic considerations in progressive familial intrahepatic cholestasis (Byler's disease). Can J Anaesth 1995;42:1126–33

39. Lee WM. Acute liver failure. N Engl J Med 1993;329:1862–72

40. Knox TA, Olans LB. Liver disease in pregnancy. N Engl J Med 1996;335:569–76

41. Catron EG, Plevak DR, Kranner PW, et al. Perioperative care of the liver transplant patient. Anesth Analg 1994;78:382–99

42. Kostopanagiotou G, Smyrniotis V, Arkadopoulos N, et al. Anesthetic and perioperative management of adult transplant recipients in nontransplant surgery. Anesth Analg 1999; 89:613–22

43. Marco PA, Yeo CJ, Rock P. Anesthesia for the patient undergoing laparoscopic cholecystectomy. Anesthesiology 1990;73: 1268–70

44. Johnston DE, Kaplan M. Pathogenesis and treatment of gallstones. N Engl J Med 1993;328:412–21

45. Wahba RWM, Beiquee F, Kleiman SJ. Cardiopulmonary function and laparoscopic cholecystectomy. Can J Anaesth 1995; 42:51–63

46. Clark CC, Weeks DB, Gusdon JP. Venous carbon dioxide embolism during laparoscopy. Anesth Analg 1977;56:650–2

47. Taylor E, Feinstein R, White PF, et al. Anesthesia for laparoscopic cholecystectomy; is nitrous oxide contraindicated? Anesthesiology 1992;76:541–3

48. Hasel R, Arora SK, Hickey DR. Intraoperative complications of laparoscopic cholecystectomy. Can J Anaesth 1993;40: 459–64

49. Cornforth BM. SIADH following laparoscopic cholecystectomy. Can J Anaesth 1998;45:223–5

50. Jones RM, Detmer M, Hill AB, Bjoraker DE. Incidence of choledochoduodenal sphincter spasm during fentanyl-supplemented anesthesia. Anesth Analg 1981;60:638–40

51. Toyoyama H, Kariya N, Hase I, et al. The use of intravenous nitroglycerin in a case of spasm of the sphincter of Oddi during laparoscopic cholecystectomy. Anesthesiology 2001; 94:708–9

52. Keefe EB. Gallstones and biliary tract disease. Sci Am Med 1998;1–9

19

Diseases of the Gastrointestinal System

T he principal function of the gastrointestinal tract is to provide the body with a continual supply of water, nutrients, and electrolytes. Each division of the gastrointestinal tract is adapted for specific functions, such as passage of food in the esophagus, storage of food in the stomach, and digestion and absorption of nutrients in the small intestines and proximal colon.

■ ESOPHAGEAL DISEASES

Dysphagia is the classic symptom produced at some stage with all disorders of the esophagus. Barium contrast examination is recommended for patients with dysphagia. After the barium contrast study, esophagoscopy permits direct viewing of the esophagus as well as recovery of biopsy and cytology specimens.

Diffuse Esophageal Spasm

Diffuse esophageal spasm occurs most often in elderly patients. It is most likely due to an alteration in the innervation of the esophagus by the autonomic nervous system. Pain produced by esophageal spasm may mimic angina pectoris. Indeed, some patients respond favorably to treatment with nitroglycerin. Nifedipine and isosorbide, which decrease lower esophageal sphincter (LES) pressure, may also relieve pain produced by esophageal spasm.

Chronic Peptic Esophagitis

Chronic peptic esophagitis is caused by reflux of acidic gastric fluid into the esophagus, producing retrosternal discomfort ("heartburn") relieved by oral administration of antacids. Reflux esophagitis is a common clinical problem, with more than one-third of healthy adults experiencing symptoms of heartburn at least once every 30 days. Normally, the LES exerts a relatively high resting pressure in the terminal 1 to 2 cm of the esophagus; this pressure tends to protect against spontaneous gastroesophageal reflux. The underlying defect leading to esophagitis seems to be a decrease in the resting tone of the LES. Indeed, patients with reflux esophagitis often manifest decreased LES pressures (average 13 mmHg versus 29 mmHg in normal patients).[1]

Collagen vascular diseases (scleroderma, dermatomyositis, polymyositis) may involve the esophagus and predispose to reflux esophagitis and, in some patients, the development of esophageal strictures. Tablets often remain in the esophagus for 5 minutes or longer when swallowed with a small volume of water (15 ml). Preferably, tablets are swallowed with at least 100 ml of water, with patients remaining upright for at least 90 seconds to ensure that ingested drugs pass promptly into the stomach. Unless these precautions are taken, drugs such as aspirin may produce irritation of the esophageal mucosa. Esophageal infections owing to *Candida albicans* are potential risks in immunosuppressed patients, typically developing several weeks after organ transplantation. Symptoms include dysphagia and retrosternal pain. Esophagoscopy is useful for documenting inflammation.

Treatment

Treatment of reflux esophagitis is initially with oral antacids and avoidance of substances (fat, chocolate, alcohol, nicotine) that decrease LES pressure. Administration of H_2-receptor antagonists may promote healing in these patients. Persistent, severe symptoms may be relieved by a surgical procedure designed to create a valve mechanism by wrapping a gastric pouch around the distal esophagus (Nissen fundoplication). Alternatively, an antrectomy with Roux-en-Y duodenal diversion or placement of a C-shaped plastic prosthesis (Angelchick valve) around the distal esophagus may be beneficial. Patients with chronic esophagitis are at risk for the development of strictures at the distal esophagus, requiring treatment with tapered dilators.

Management of Anesthesia

Preoperative evaluation of patients with chronic peptic esophagitis logically involves the exclusion of pneumonia, as may be evident on chest radiographs. The decision to include anticholinergic drugs in the preoperative medication must be balanced against the known ability of these drugs to decrease LES tone.[2] Theoretically, anticholinergic drugs, by decreasing LES pressure, could increase the likelihood of silent regurgitation and the possibility of pulmonary aspiration. This potential adverse effect of anticholinergic drugs has not been documented. Furthermore, decreases in the pH of esophageal fluid as evidence of gastric reflux during tracheal intubation and after tracheal extubation are unlikely, assuming the absence of upper airway obstruction or patient movement in response to the presence of the tracheal tube.[3,4] In this regard, the incidence of postoperative symptoms attributable to pulmonary aspiration is minimal when adult or pediatric patients undergo elective operations.[5–7] For these reasons, it does not seem justifiable to avoid anticholinergic drugs in the preoperative medication solely because a patient is known to experience reflux esophagitis. Routine pretreatment of patients with H_2-receptor antagonists or metoclopramide is not recommended.[8] Succinylcholine increases LES pressure, but the barrier pressure (LES pressure minus gastric pressure) is unchanged, as fasciculations are associated with increased gastric pressure.

Hiatus Hernia

Hiatus hernia is protrusion of a portion of the stomach through the hiatus of the diaphragm and into the thoracic cavity. The sliding type of hiatus hernia, formed by movement of the upper stomach through an enlarged hiatus, can be identified in about 30% of patients undergoing upper gastrointestinal radiographic examination. Because hiatus hernia and reflux esophagitis frequently co-exist by chance, they have been erroneously considered to have a cause-and-effect relation. Based on the assumption that the hiatus hernia predisposes to the development of peptic esophagitis, surgical repair of the hernia may be recommended. Nevertheless, most patients with hiatus hernia do not have symptoms of reflux esophagitis, emphasizing the importance of the integrity of the LES. Oral antacids or therapy with H_2-antagonists is not necessary for patients with hiatus hernia in the absence of symptoms of reflux esophagitis.

Esophageal Diverticula

Esophageal diverticula are classified according to their location as Zenker's diverticulum (upper esophagus), traction diverticulum (mid-esophagus), and epiphrenic diverticulum (near the

LES). Regurgitation of previously ingested food from a Zenker's diverticulum may predispose patients to pulmonary aspiration, even in the absence of recent food intake. Surgical excision of this diverticulum may be performed in two stages, with initial mobilization of the pouch followed by complete excision after granulation tissue has formed.

■ PEPTIC ULCER DISEASE

Peptic ulcer disease describes focal defects (ulcerations) in the gastrointestinal mucosa (esophagus, stomach, duodenum) that are associated with the presence of hydrochloric acid and pepsin in the gastric fluid.[9, 10] Regardless of the peptic ulcer's location [most commonly the duodenal bulb or distal stomach (antrum)], the pathology is similar.

Pathogenesis

Risk factors for the development of peptic ulcers are unclear. Peptic ulcers require the presence of hydrochloric acid and pepsin, but only rarely is this sufficient to produce an ulcer. In most patients there must be other predisposing factors. In this regard, infection with *Helicobacter pylori* is causally related to most duodenal and gastric ulcers. The second most common cause of peptic ulcers is use of nonsteroidal antiinflammatory drugs (NSAIDs). Many idiopathic peptic ulcers are subsequently determined to represent unrecognized NSAID use or false-negative tests for *H. pylori*. Emotional stress also appears to be a risk factor for the development of peptic ulcers. Alcohol can cause hemorrhagic gastritis but does not cause peptic ulcers. Rarely, peptic ulcers are due to an endocrine tumor (gastrinoma) of the pancreas or duodenum.

H. pylori Ulcers

Gastric infection with *H. pylori* and the resultant diffuse superficial active gastritis are necessary for the development of most duodenal ulcers and, to a somewhat lesser extent, the development of gastric ulcers. Although *H. pylori* appears to be the most important risk factor for duodenal and gastric ulcers, the mere presence of *H. pylori* in the stomach is not sufficient to cause peptic ulcers. Cure of *H. pylori* infection with antimicrobial therapy decreases the incidence of peptic ulcer recurrence.

NSAID-Induced Ulcers

The ulcerogenicity of NSAIDs is well established; and unlike *H. pylori*-related ulcers, which occur more often in the duodenal bulb, NSAID-induced ulcers typically occur in the stomach. Oral or parenteral NSAIDs are ulcerogenic in humans by virtue of their ability to inhibit cyclooxygenase-1 (COX-1), the rate-limiting enzyme step in the synthesis of gastrointestinal prostaglandins. These prostaglandins normally protect the gastrointestinal mucosa from damage by maintaining mucosal blood flow and increasing mucosal secretion of mucus and bicarbonate. Buffering of aspirin has no effect on decreasing gastrointestinal injury, but enteric coating appears to decrease the severity of the injury. The greatest risk for NSAID-induced ulcers is early in the course of treatment (7 to 30 days after initiation), with the risk declining thereafter. Selective COX-2 inhibitors are as effective as COX-1 inhibitors but evoke fewer gastrointestinal side effects. Although corticosteroids are not ulcerogenic, they may impair healing of an existing ulcer; and when administered with NSAIDs, the risk of ulcer formation is increased.

Acute Stress Ulcers

Acute gastroduodenal erosions and ulcers are common in patients with serious illnesses (trauma including head injury and burn injury, septic shock, respiratory failure requiring mechanical ventilation) and those who have undergone major surgical procedures. Unlike peptic ulcers, stress ulcers are typically asymptomatic. Approximately 10% to 25% of patients with acute stress ulcers experience painless upper gastrointestinal bleeding.[10] This bleeding may manifest as dark ("coffee ground") or bloody nasogastric aspirate, decreasing hematocrit, increasing transfusion requirements, or unexplained hypotension. The pathogenesis of acute stress ulcers is not well understood, but the common factor seems to be tissue hypoxia as precipitated by mucosal vasoconstriction and ischemia. Systemic hypoxemia, metabolic acidosis, anemia, and decreased cardiac output are viewed as contributing factors.

Gastrinoma

Gastrinoma (Zollinger-Ellison syndrome) is a gastrin-secreting tumor that develops in the pancreas or duodenum and accounts for approximately 0.1% of all peptic ulcers.[11] Release of gastrin stimulates histamine release and production of hydrochloric acid. Intractable abdominal pain, diarrhea, and multiple gastric ulcers are present. Plasma gastrin concentrations higher than 100 pg/ml in patients with duodenal ulcers confirms the diagnosis of Zollinger-Ellison syndrome. Hypergastrinemia results in a continuous high rate of pepsin and hydrochloric acid secretion even under fasting conditions. An estimated 20% to 30% of patients with gastrinomas have other features suggesting multiple endocrine neoplasia type 1 (MEN 1) syndrome (parathyroid adenoma with hypercalcemia and renal stones, pituitary adenoma).

Incidence

Peptic ulcer disease in the United States affects 10% of men and 4% of women at some time in their lives.[10] Recurrence of peptic ulcer is common such that the prevalence greatly exceeds the incidence. Eradication of *H. pylori* from the stomach and duodenum, especially in patients who smoke, greatly decreases the risk of recurrences of peptic ulcer disease.

Diagnosis

The diagnosis of peptic ulcer disease is suggested by clinical signs and symptoms. Ultimately, the diagnosis of peptic ulcer depends on endoscopy or surgery. The differential diagnosis of peptic ulcer disease includes nonulcer dyspepsia and gastric cancer (see "Chronic Peptic Esophagitis" and Chapter 28).

Signs and Symptoms

Peptic ulcers produce a variety of signs and symptoms, but none is specific for the disease. It is not possible to distinguish symptoms of duodenal ulcers from those of gastric ulcers. Patients often complain of mild to moderate epigastric pain that is typically relieved by food or antacids. Severe pain or a rapid increase in pain suggests an ulcer complication (perforation of the ulcer) or another diagnosis (acute pancreatitis). Likewise, the presence of repeated vomiting suggests an ulcer complication (gastric outlet obstruction) or another diagnosis (intestinal obstruction). Peptic ulcer is the most common cause of acute upper gastrointestinal bleeding (hematemesis, melena). Placing a nasogastric tube with return of grossly bloody aspirate confirms the likelihood of a bleeding peptic ulcer. During the first few hours following acute hemorrhage from a peptic ulcer, the hemoglobin concentration does not completely reflect the severity of the blood loss until compensatory hemodilution occurs or until intravenous fluids are administered. Thus the heart rate and systemic blood pressure in the supine and upright positions may be better initial indicators of the extent of blood loss than the hemoglobin concentra-

tions. Patients with bleeding peptic ulcers typically manifest azotemia with the serum blood urea nitrogen concentration/creatinine ratio exceeding 20:1, resulting from digestion and intestinal absorption of nitrogenous components in concert with decreased renal perfusion.[10] Anemia is likely with chronic hemorrhage from peptic ulcers.

Abdominal tenderness or rigidity, leukocytosis, and absence of bowel sounds suggest ulcer perforation with peritonitis. Upright chest radiographs may show free peritoneal air (typically below the right hemidiaphragm) in the presence of peptic ulcer perforation. Abdominal distension with associated hypokalemic, hypochloremic metabolic alkalosis suggests gastric outlet obstruction. Gastric distension is likely to be present on radiographs of the abdomen or computed tomography scan.

Endoscopy

Endoscopy is the most accurate method for confirming the clinical diagnosis of peptic ulcer disease and the presence of associated bleeding or intestinal obstruction. When bleeding is suspected, it is recommended that the stomach be emptied with a large-bore tube before initiating endoscopy to decrease the possibility of pulmonary aspiration and improve endoscopic visualization of mucosal lesions. Most patients require local pharyngeal anesthesia and conscious sedation produced with intravenous drugs such as midazolam. Biopsy specimens obtained during endoscopy are utilized to determine the presence of *H. pylori* and exclude the presence of malignancy. An alternative, noninvasive method for detecting *H. pylori* infection is the urea breath test, which is based on the fact that these organisms contain abundant amounts of urease, which splits urea into carbon dioxide and ammonia. The most serious complications of endoscopy are depression of ventilation, perforation of the gastrointestinal tract, and bleeding.

Surgery

In certain patients the diagnosis of peptic ulcer is not confirmed until surgery is performed. These patients include those who present with an "acute abdomen" in whom a perforated ulcer is diagnosed only at exploratory laparotomy and those in whom upper gastrointestinal bleeding makes visualization by endoscopy difficult.

Treatment

The goals of treating peptic ulcer disease are to relieve symptoms, promote healing of the ulcer, prevent ulcer recurrence, and decrease the likelihood of ulcer-related complications. In this regard it is important to eradicate infection with *H. pylori* (90% of patients with duodenal ulcers are infected) and to discontinue treatment with NSAIDs.[9] Antimicrobial therapy is usually empirical and utilizes combinations of drugs including bismuth subsalicylate, metronidazole, clarithromycin, tetracycline, and amoxicillin. One week of treatment with bismuth subsalicylate, metronidazole, and tetracycline achieves an 85% to 90% cure of *H. pylori* infection.[9] In addition, antacids and proton-pump inhibitors (omeprazole) are useful for suppressing the growth of *H. pylori*. The most common cause of recurrent ulceration in patients treated for *H. pylori*-related duodenal ulcer is failure to eradicate the organism. Peptic ulcers due to treatment with NSAIDs are treated by discontinuing the drug (if possible) and administration of antisecretory drugs (H_2-receptor antagonists, proton pump inhibitors) for 4 to 8 weeks. Most duodenal ulcers, regardless of cause, heal after 8 weeks of proton pump inhibitors or H_2-receptor antagonist therapy. Sucralfate is an alternative drug, but its mechanism of action is uncertain. Antacids can also heal duodenal ulcers but are rarely used as primary therapy because of their inconvenience. Antacids are often prescribed "as needed" to relieve ulcer symptoms.

Zollinger-Ellison Syndrome

Patients with duodenal ulcers as part of the Zollinger-Ellison syndrome are treated initially with proton pump inhibitors, such as omeprazole, followed by a maintenance dose guided by gastric acid measurements. Curative surgical resection of the gastrinoma is indicated in the absence of evidence of MEN 1 syndrome and metastatic disease.[12]

Management of anesthesia for surgical excision of a gastrinoma takes into account the presence of gastric hypersecretion and the likely presence of large gastric fluid volumes at the time of anesthesia induction. Esophageal reflux is common in these patients despite the ability of gastrin to increase LES tone. Depletion of intravascular fluid volume and electrolyte imbalance (hypokalemia, metabolic alkalosis) may accompany profuse watery diarrhea. Associated endocrine abnormalities (MEN 1 syndrome) could also influence the management of anesthesia in these patients.

Antacid prophylaxis with proton pump inhibitors and H_2-receptor antagonists is maintained until surgery. A preoperative coagulation screen and liver function tests may be recommended, as alterations in fat absorption could influence clotting factors and hepatic function may be impaired by liver metasta-

ses.[11] Intravenous administration of ranitidine is useful for preventing gastric acid hypersecretion during surgery. A nasogastric tube is placed preoperatively.

Bleeding Ulcers

The first priority in patients with suspected upper gastrointestinal bleeding from peptic ulcers is stabilization with intravascular fluid volume replacement guided by appropriate hemodynamic monitoring especially if co-existing heart disease is present. Once the patient is clinically stable, diagnostic upper gastrointestinal endoscopy is performed and any identifiable bleeding site treated (injection of epinephrine or saline, thermal application). Endoscopic therapy controls bleeding in approximately 90% of patients. Following endoscopic treatment of bleeding, infusion of omeprazole decreases the risk of recurrent bleeding.[13] Surgery to control bleeding from peptic ulcers is needed only if endoscopic treatment is not effective.

Perforated Ulcers

When a perforated peptic ulcer is confirmed or highly suspected, patients are rendered NPO; nasogastric suction is instituted, electrolyte disturbances are determined, and treatment with intravenous fluids and broad-spectrum antibiotics is initiated. Exploratory laparotomy for closure of the perforation utilizing a patch of omentum is performed when the patient is stabilized. Many perforated ulcers are associated with NSAID therapy, and an estimated 10% of perforated gastric ulcers are malignant. Mortality associated with perforated peptic ulcers reflects the advanced age of the patients and co-existing medical conditions such as cardiac, pulmonary, and liver disease.

Obstructing Ulcers

Endoscopic diagnosis of gastrointestinal obstruction due to peptic ulcer disease is followed by rendering patients NPO and instituting nasogastric suction and treatment with intravenous fluids, electrolytes, and H_2-receptor antagonists. Gastric outlet obstruction may resolve over 5 to 14 days as edema subsides during healing of the ulcer. Conversely, obstruction due to scarring from previous ulcers is unlikely to resolve with medical management. Evidence of healing and resolution of gastric outlet obstruction is passage of saline from the stomach following administration of 750 ml saline as a test. Parenteral hyperalimentation is a consideration during the period when ulcer healing is occurring. Endoscopic therapy using balloon dilatation to dilate a stenotic pylorus under fluoroscopic guidance is an option for patients whose gastrointestinal obstruction does not resolve with conservative medical management. Endoscopic balloon dilatation is a temporizing measure and rarely obviates the need for surgery. Gastrointestinal obstruction that recurs after endoscopic therapy is an indication for surgical drainage procedures such as pyloroplasty, gastroenterostomy, or resection plus gastroenterostomy. Pyloroplasty and gastroenterostomy are typically combined with a vagotomy to decrease the likelihood of recurrent ulceration.

Acute Stress Ulcers

Treatment of bleeding acute stress ulcers includes intravascular fluid replacement and attempts to treat the underlying associated disease. Endoscopic therapy is not usually curative because multiple bleeding sites are typically present. The role of intravenous antisecretory drugs in treating bleeding stress ulcers is unproven.[10] Surgical resection (gastrectomy) for continuous bleeding is associated with high mortality.

Patients at high risk of developing bleeding acute stress ulcers (multiple organ system failure plus mechanical ventilation) should be treated with prophylactic intragastric or oral antacids or sucralfate or with intravenous H_2-receptor antagonists or proton pump inhibitors by continuous intravenous infusion.[13] The goal of prophylactic therapy is to maintain the gastric fluid pH above 4.

■ IRRITABLE BOWEL SYNDROME

Patients with irritable bowel syndrome (spastic or mucous colitis) often complain of generalized bowel discomfort, usually confined to the left lower quadrant. There may be constipation; but more commonly the frequency of stools is increased, and the feces are covered with mucus. Many patients have associated symptoms of vasomotor instability, including tachycardia, hyperventilation, fatigue, diaphoresis, and headaches. Air trapped in the splenic flexure may produce pain in the left shoulder, radiating down the left arm ("splenic flexure syndrome"). Despite the frequent occurrence of irritable bowel syndrome, there is no known etiologic agent or structural or biochemical defect. This syndrome appears to be an intense intra-abdominal response to emotional stress.

■ INFLAMMATORY BOWEL DISEASE

Ulcerative colitis and Crohn's disease represent inflammatory bowel diseases that have different manifestations, prognoses, and treatments (Table 19–1). Inflammatory bowel diseases are the second most common chronic inflammatory disorders after rheumatoid arthritis. The diagnosis of ulcerative colitis and Crohn's disease and the differentiation between them are based on nonspecific clinical and histologic patterns often obscured by intercurrent infections or iatrogenic events or that are altered by medications or surgery.[14]

Ulcerative Colitis

Ulcerative colitis is an inflammatory disease of the colonic mucosa that primarily affects the rectum and distal colon. The cause of this disease is unknown, and remissions followed by exacerbations are common. There is a definite clustering of this disease in certain ethnic groups; it is most common among those of Jewish origin. Women, usually between the ages of 25 and 45 years, are affected most often. Most patients have mild disease characterized by intermittent diarrhea and cramping abdominal pain. Fatigue, low grade fever, and weight loss occur during exacerbations of the disease.

Complications

Severe ulcerative colitis is associated with complications classified as colonic and extracolonic (Table

Table 19–1 • Comparative Features of Ulcerative Colitis and Crohn's Disease

Feature	Ulcerative Colitis	Crohn's Disease
Acute toxicity	Common	Rare
Stools	Bloody and watery	Watery
Perirectal involvement	Occurs in 10%–20%, but usually self-limiting	Rectocutaneous fistulas in 50%
Extracolonic complications	Common	Common
Carcinoma of the colon	Incidence 5% after 10 years	Incidence 1% but unrelated to extent or duration of the disease
Treatment	Proctocolectomy is curative	Recurrence likely despite surgical resection

19–1). Toxic megacolon manifests as the sudden onset of fever, tachycardia, dehydration, and dilation of the colon. Intestinal perforation is associated with rebound pain, except when high doses of corticosteroids mask the symptoms. Apparently because of the presence of chronic inflammation produced by ulcerative colitis, patients are at increased risk for the development of carcinoma of the colon. Elective colectomy is considered when epithelial dysplasia is discovered during colonoscopic surveillance, especially when the duration of the disease exceeds 8 years. Arthritis tends to be restricted to large joints and is most often present when the colitis is clinically active. Patients with ulcerative colitis have an increased incidence of ankylosing spondylitis. Liver disease manifests most often as fatty liver infiltration or pericholangitis with jaundice and increased serum alkaline phosphatase concentrations.

Treatment

Sulfazalazine and 5-aminosalicylic acid (mesalamine) analogues are most commonly used to treat mild to moderately severe ulcerative colitis. Corticosteroid treatment is indicated primarily for short-term induction of a remission of ulcerative colitis. Oral budesonide is as effective as prednisolone for inducing remissions, and it causes less adrenal suppression.[15] The efficacy of long-term administration of low doses of corticosteroids as maintenance therapy or to prevent relapses is not supported by controlled trials.[14] Nevertheless, dependence on corticosteroids is often encountered in patients with ulcerative colitis. Sulfazalazine is not as effective as corticosteroids for inducing remissions in patients with moderate to severe inflammatory bowel disease. Acute exacerbations may require hospitalization to replace electrolytes and intravascular fluid volume. The only curative treatment is protocolectomy with ileostomy. About 25% of patients with ulcerative colitis undergo this procedure during the first 5 years of the disease.

Immunomodulatory drugs such as azathioprine and mercaptopurine are appropriate for long-term treatment of some patients with ulcerative colitis.[14] Pancreatitis occurs in as many as 15% of patients treated with these drugs, and bone marrow depression manifesting as neutropenia is a possible risk. This treatment is most likely to be considered in patients who become dependent on corticosteroids or who do not manifest therapeutic responses to aminosalicylate treatment. Continuous intravenous infusions of cyclosporine have been effective in acute, severe cases of inflammatory bowel disease. Risks of cyclosporine therapy include nephrotoxicity and neurotoxic effects manifesting as seizures.

Nutritional therapy in patients with ulcerative colitis may be considered in attempts to reduce symptoms and to provide adequate nutrition to compensate for reduced caloric intake and increased colonic losses. Nevertheless, neither an elemental diet nor total parenteral nutrition decreases the inflammation associated with ulcerative colitis.

Crohn's Disease

Crohn's disease is characterized by ileal and colonic involvement (granulomatous ileocolitis) in about 50% of patients; the remainder are equally divided between those with disease restricted to the small intestine (regional enteritis) and those with disease confined to the colon. The cause of Crohn's disease is unknown; the peak incidence is about 30 years of age.

Complications

There is chronic inflammation of all layers of the bowel, often leading to the development of fistulas between the diseased intestinal loops and adjacent structures. Rectal fissures, rectocutaneous fistulas, or perirectal abscesses occur in as many as 50% of patients. Extracolonic complications include arthritis and iritis. Renal stones and gallstones containing calcium oxalate are common, especially if the distal ileum is involved, reflecting increased colonic absorption of oxalate. Anemia is likely and may be due to chronic hemorrhage, iron deficiency, vitamin B_{12} deficiency, or folate deficiency. Decreased plasma albumin concentrations reflect protein loss through diseased bowel mucosa. Distinction from ulcerative colitis is important, as Crohn's disease is infrequently associated with cancer, and recurrences after surgical resection are common (20% to 80% within 5 years).

Treatment

Treatment of Crohn's disease is similar to that described for ulcerative colitis.[14, 15] In contrast to the results in patients with ulcerative colitis, elemental diets and total parenteral nutrition with bowel rest improve the symptoms, inflammatory sequelae, and nutritional status in patients with Crohn's disease.[14] Hyperalimentation may be indicated if weight loss and malnutrition are prominent. An estimated 60% of patients require surgery because of drug failure or the development of complications such as intra-abdominal fistulas.

Pseudomembranous Enterocolitis

Pseudomembranous enterocolitis is attributable to unknown causes, although it is often associated with antibiotic therapy (especially clindamycin and lincomycin), bowel obstruction, uremia, congestive heart failure, and intestinal ischemia. Clinical manifestations include fever, watery diarrhea, dehydration, hypotension, cardiac dysrhythmias, skeletal muscle weakness, intestinal ileus, and metabolic acidosis.

Management of Anesthesia

Surgical treatment of inflammatory bowel disease most often involves resection of varying lengths and portions of the gastrointestinal tract. Management of anesthesia requires preoperative evaluation of intravascular fluid volume and electrolyte status and assessment of the colonic and extracolonic complications (anemia, arthritis, liver disease) that may be associated with the inflammatory bowel process (Table 19–2). Underlying liver disease may influence the choice of volatile anesthetics and muscle relaxants. In the presence of bowel distension, administration of nitrous oxide may be limited or avoided. The need to provide additional corticosteroids during the perioperative period is introduced when these drugs have been used as part of the medical therapy. Adverse effects associated with hyperalimentation must be appreciated (see Chapter 23). Although reversal of nondepolarizing muscle relaxants with anticholinesterase drugs increases gastrointestinal intraluminal pressure, there is no evidence it results in a risk of colon suture line dehiscence (Fig. 19–1).[16–18]

Table 19–2 • Complications Associated with Ulcerative Colitis

Complication	Incidence (%)
Colonic	
Toxic megacolon	1–3
Intestinal perforation	3
Carcinoma of the colon	2.5
Hemorrhage	4
Stricture	10
Extracolonic	
Erythema nodosum	3
Iritis	5–10
Ankylosing arthritis	5–10
Fatty liver infiltration	40
Pericholangitis	30–50
Cirrhosis of the liver	3

■ CARCINOID TUMORS

General Considerations

Carcinoid tumors arise from enterochromaffin tissues and are typically found in the gastrointestinal tract (stomach, appendix, jejenum, ileum, colon, rectum), although they may also occur in the bronchi and lungs.[11, 19] Carcinoid cells secrete a variety of amine and neuropeptide hormones including serotonin, histamine, prostaglandins, corticotropin, and kallikrein (generates kinins including bradykinin) (Table 19–3).[11] Bronchial carcinoids can produce an excess of corticotrophic hormone and growth hormone-releasing factor, and they may present as Cushing syndrome or acromegaly. Tumor location is identified by computed tomography, magnetic resonance imaging, and ultrasound imaging. Patients in whom metastatic disease is suspected should be evaluated with abdominal computed tomography. Measurements of the serotonin metabolite 5-hydroxyindoleacetic acid in a 24-hour urine collection may be useful for confirming the diagnosis. Symptomatic tumors are treated with somatostatin analogues and surgery.[11, 19]

Carcinoid Syndrome

Carcinoid syndrome is present when systemic effects of carcinoid tumor secretions result in clinical symptoms reflecting metastases to the liver or release of reactive products from tumors in the lungs. Generally, release of secretory products from tumors in the gastrointestinal tract does not produce clinical symptoms, as these products are destroyed in the liver before reaching the systemic circulation. An estimated 18% of patients with carcinoid tumors develop carcinoid syndrome.

Signs and Symptoms

Signs and symptoms of carcinoid syndrome are due to the release of vasoactive substances from the carcinoid tumor (Table 19–3).[11] The most common features of carcinoid syndrome are episodic cutaneous flushing involving principally the face and neck, diarrhea due to gastrointestinal hypermotility, and asthma. Flushing may be precipitated by alcohol ingestion, certain foods, and circulating catecholamines and may be associated with hypotension and bronchospasm, suggesting a role for bradykinins. Bronchoconstriction and hypotension may be resistant to treatment and so be life-threatening. Acute cardiorespiratory events (supraventricular tachydysrhythmias, systemic hypertension, hypotension)

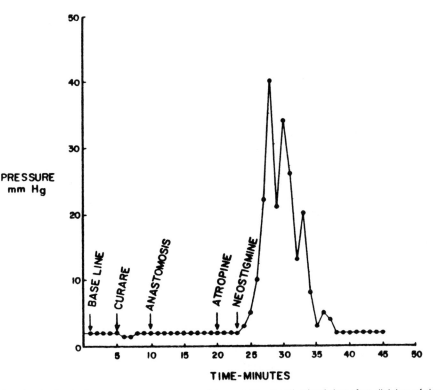

Figure 19–1 • Intraluminal colonic pressure was measured in a single anesthetized dog after division of the colon and a standard two-layer anastomosis. There was no evidence that the neostigmine-induced increase in intracolonic pressure caused disruption of the freshly completed bowel anastomosis. (From Yellin YE, Newman J, Donovan AJ. Neostigmine-induced hyperperistalsis: effects of security of colonic anastomoses. Arch Surg 1973;106:779–81, with permission.)

are most common following embolization of liver metastases or surgical manipulation of the tumor.

Right-sided valve distortion from metastases may occur, whereas valves on the left side of the heart are usually spared, perhaps reflecting the ability of pulmonary parenchymal cells to inactivate vasoactive substances. Echocardiography can confirm the presence of right ventricular dysfunction, tricuspid regurgitation (most common), and pulmonic stenosis. Nevertheless, left-sided heart disease occurs in about 10% of patients with carcinoid syndrome.[20] The preponderance of lesions in the right side of the heart suggests that carcinoid heart disease is related to factors (possibly serotonin) secreted into the hepatic vein by liver metastases. It is of interest that the anorexic drugs fenfluramine and dexfenfluramine appear to interfere with normal serotonin metabolism and have been associated with valvular lesions identical to those seen with carcinoid heart disease.

Hyperglycemia most likely reflects the ability of serotonin to mimic the metabolic effects of epinephrine and to stimulate glycogenolysis and gluconeogenesis. Pellegra dermatitis and hypoalbuminemia may reflect diversion of tryptophan from the production of protein to the synthesis of serotonin.

Table 19–3 • Signs and Symptoms of Carcinoid Syndrome

Episodic cutaneous flushing (kinins, histamine)
Diarrhea (serotonin, prostaglandins E and F)
Heart disease
   Tricuspid regurgitation and/or pulmonic stenosis
   Supraventricular tachydysrhythmias (serotonin)
Bronchoconstriction (serotonin, bradykinin, substance P)
Hypotension (kinins, histamine)
Hypertension (serotonin)
Abdominal pain (small bowel obstruction)
Hepatomegaly (metastases)
Hyperglycemia
Hypoalbuminemia (pellegra-like skin lesions due to niacin deficiency)

Treatment

Treatment of carcinoid syndrome is with the synthetic somatostatin analogue octreotide, which prevents the release of vasoactive products from carcinoid tumors.[11, 19, 20–22] High-dose corticosteroids have been advocated to inhibit bradykinin secretion, but the efficacy of these drugs has not been documented. Histamine receptor antagonists may be recommended based on the known ability of this mediator to cause bronchoconstriction. Cytotoxic chemotherapy has had only limited success in the treatment of metastatic carcinoid tumors. Definitive surgical resection of the tumor is the only curative procedure. In patients who are not candidates for hepatic resection of metastases, hepatic artery occlusion or embolization may be a useful palliative intervention. The development of right-sided heart failure in patients with carcinoid syndrome may be an indication for tricuspid or pulmonic valve replacement.

Management of Anesthesia

Anesthesia management focuses on preventing a carcinoid crisis, which may accompany stress, physical stimulation, or manipulation of the tumor.[20–22] Of greatest concern during anesthesia are the vasoactive and bronchoconstriction effects of carcinoid tumor products. In this regard, the continuation of preoperative therapy with octreotide, 50 to 500 μg every 8 hours, throughout the perioperative period is essential. Anesthetic premedication with benzodiazepines is recommended to allay preoperative anxiety. In addition, the preoperative medication includes subcutaneous octreotide (common dose is 50 to 150 μg). During surgery octreotide may be continued as an intravenous infusion at 100 μg/hr. Octreotide inhibits insulin release and may complicate blood glucose control in insulin-dependent diabetic patients. Inclusion of histamine receptor antagonists in the preoperative medication is a consideration. Likewise, drugs with a known potential to evoke histamine release (meperidine, mivacurium, atracurium), especially when administered at high doses, are often avoided. Drugs reported to produce a carcinoid crisis (bronchoconstriction, hypotension) include histamine, norepinephrine, epinephrine, and dopamine. Catecholamines may result in the release of serotonin (with associated vasoconstriction) or kallikrein (which activates bradykinins with associated vasodilation). If catecholamines such as epinephrine are needed, a recommended approach is administration of a small dose to evaluate the response. If there is a beneficial response, epinephrine can be continued as an intravenous infusion.

The occurrence of intraoperative carcinoid crisis manifesting as bronchospasm or hypotension is treated with intravenous administration of octreotide, 100 to 200 μg IV.[20–22] Epinephrine is not recommended for the treatment of bronchospasm or hypotension in patients experiencing a carcinoid crisis.

Intraoperative hypertension resulting from a carcinoid crisis is best treated with labetalol or ketanserin.[21] Octreotide may be administered prophylactically prior to predictable surgical manipulation of the carcinoid tumor.

Systemic hypertensive responses that may accompany direct laryngoscopy and tracheal intubation are minimized by administering short-acting opioids (fentanyl commonly) and intravenous induction drugs such as propofol or etomidate. Succinylcholine has been used without adverse effects, although hormone release theoretically could be stimulated by fasciculations and resulting increased intra-abdominal pressure. Nondepolarizing muscle relaxants are selected on the basis of their lack of potential to evoke histamine release. Volatile anesthetic drugs such as isoflurane, desflurane, and sevoflurane are acceptable, recognizing the need to provide cardiac stability. Ketamine is not a likely selection, as activation of the sympathetic nervous system and release of catecholamines may activate kallikreins. In view of the known ability of serotonin to cause sedation, there is the possibility that anesthetic requirements could be decreased and postoperative awakening delayed. Selection of regional anesthesia is controversial because treatment with catecholamines is not recommended. Nevertheless, epidural anesthesia has been utilized successfully in these patients and provides the advantage of postoperative pain relief.[11]

■ ACUTE PANCREATITIS

Acute pancreatitis is characterized as an inflammatory disorder of the pancreas in which normal pancreatic function is restored once the primary cause of the acute event is resolved.[23, 24] Pancreatic autodigestion is the most likely explanation for the pathogenesis of acute pancreatitis. The incidence of acute pancreatitis has increased 10-fold since the 1960s, perhaps reflecting increased alcohol abuse and/or improved diagnostic techniques.

Etiology

Gallstones and alcohol abuse are etiologic factors in 60% to 80% of patients with acute pancreatitis (Fig. 19–2).[24] Gallstones are believed to cause pancreatitis by transiently obstructing the ampulla of Vater, leading to pancreatic ductal hypertension. Acute pancreatitis is common in patients with acquired immunodeficiency syndrome (AIDS) and those with hyperparathyroidism and associated hypercalcemia. Trauma-induced acute pancreatitis is usually associated with blunt trauma rather than penetrat-

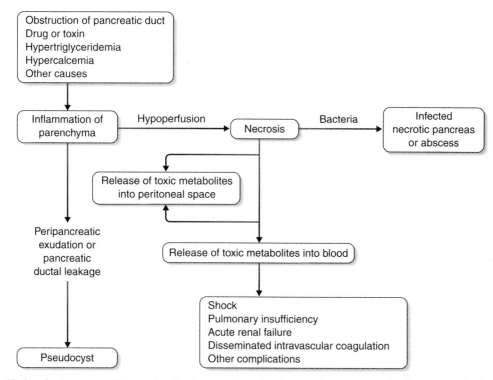

Figure 19-2 • Acute pancreatitis may be due to several mechanisms and progress to significant complications. (From Steinberg W, Tenner S. Acute pancreatitis. N Engl J Med 1994;330:1198–210. Copyright 1994 Massachusetts Medical Society, with permission.)

ing injury to the upper abdomen, reflecting compression of the pancreas against the spine. Postoperative pancreatitis has been described after abdominal and thoracic surgery, especially with the use of cardiopulmonary bypass. Clinical pancreatitis develops in 1% to 2% of patients following endoscopic retrograde cholangiopancreatography (ERCP).[23]

Signs and Symptoms

Excruciating, unrelenting mid-epigastric abdominal pain that radiates to the back occurs in almost every patient who develops acute pancreatitis. Patients find that sitting and leaning forward decreases the pain. Nausea and vomiting occur at the peak of the pain, and abdominal distension with ileus often develops. Dyspnea may reflect the presence of pleural effusions or ascites. Fever may appear despite the absence of an identifiable infection, and shock occurs in nearly half of these patients. Obtundation and psychosis may be present and often reflect delirium tremens associated with alcohol withdrawal. Development of tetany may reflect hypocalcemia. Occasionally, severe hemorrhagic pancreatitis leads

to hyperglycemia. Most patients with acute pancreatitis have a benign course.

Diagnosis

The hallmark of acute pancreatitis is increased serum amylase concentrations. Contrast-enhanced computed tomography is the best noninvasive test for documenting the morphologic changes associated with acute pancreatitis. ERCP is useful for evaluating traumatic pancreatitis (localization of injury) and severe gallstone pancreatitis (endoscopic drainage). The differential diagnosis of acute pancreatitis includes a perforated duodenal ulcer, acute cholecystitis, mesenteric ischemia, and bowel obstruction. Acute myocardial infarction may cause severe abdominal pain, but the serum amylase concentrations are usually not increased. Patients with pneumonia may present with severe epigastric pain and fever.

Complications

Nearly 25% of the patients who develop acute pancreatitis experience significant complications (Fig.

19–2).[24] Shock develops early in the course of severe acute pancreatitis and is a major risk factor for death. Sequestration of large volumes of fluid in the peripancreatic space, hemorrhage, and decreased systemic vascular resistance contribute to hypotension. Arterial hypoxemia is often present early in the course of the disease, and acute respiratory distress syndrome is seen in 20% of patients. Renal failure occurs in 25% of patients and is associated with a poor prognosis.[23] Gastrointestinal hemorrhage and coagulation defects from disseminated intravascular coagulation may occur. Pseudocyst formation occurs in 10% to 15% of patients and may be associated with acute hemorrhage. Pancreatic infection is a serious complication associated with more than 50% mortality. Acute pancreatitis is unlikely to lead to chronic pancreatitis unless complications such as pseudocysts or ductal strictures develop.[25]

Treatment

Aggressive intravenous fluid administration (up to 10 L of crystalloid) is necessary as significant hypovolemia occurs even in patients with mild pancreatitis. Colloid replacement may be necessary if there is significant bleeding or albumin loss into interstitial spaces. Oral intake is stopped on the presumption that it "rests" the pancreas. Further attempts to suppress pancreatic secretions with nasogastric suction or administration of H_2-receptor antagonists provide no additional benefit. Nasogastric suction is needed only to treat persistent vomiting or ileus. Opioids administered intravenously are likely to be necessary to manage the severe pain that accompanies acute pancreatitis. Prophylactic antibiotic therapy may be instituted in patients with necrotizing pancreatitis. Endoscopic removal of obstructing gallstones is indicated within the first 24 to 72 hours of the onset of symptoms to decrease the risk of cholangitis. Parenteral feeding is indicated if it is anticipated that patients will experience a protracted course.

■ CHRONIC PANCREATITIS

The true incidence of chronic pancreatitis is difficult to determine, as the disease may be clinically asymptomatic or abdominal pain is attributed to other causes.[25] The chronic inflammation characteristic of chronic pancreatitis leads to irreversible damage to the pancreas. The clinical course of chronic pancreatitis may consist of acute attacks or unrelenting progression of symptoms.[24]

Etiology

Chronic pancreatitis is most often due to chronic alcohol abuse, accounting for 80% to 90% of affected patients.[23] Alcohol-induced pancreatitis is most frequent among men and has a peak incidence between 35 and 45 years of age. Diets high in protein seem to predispose alcoholic patients to the development of chronic pancreatitis. Idiopathic chronic pancreatitis is the second most common form of this disease. Chronic pancreatitis occasionally occurs in association with cystic fibrosis or hyperparathyroidism (hypercalcemia) or as a hereditary disease transmitted by an autosomal dominant gene. Obstruction of the pancreatic duct can lead to chronic pancreatitis.

Signs and Symptoms

Chronic pancreatitis, often characterized by epigastric abdominal pain that radiates to the back and is often postprandial, is nevertheless painless in 10% to 30% of patients.[23] Steatorrhea is present when at least 90% of the pancreas is destroyed. Diabetes mellitus eventually manifests, although the development of ketoacidosis is uncommon. Pancreatic calcifications develop in most alcohol-induced chronic pancreatitis.

Diagnosis

The diagnosis of chronic pancreatitis may be based on the history of chronic alcohol abuse and demonstration of pancreatic calcifications. Patients who develop chronic pancreatitis are often thin and appear emaciated. Serum amylase concentrations are usually normal. Once exocrine secretions are decreased to the point that enzymes entering the duodenum are 10% to 20% of normal, maldigestion of proteins and fats is evident. An abdominal radiograph may reveal pancreatic calcifications. Ultrasonography is useful for documenting the presence of an enlarged pancreas or identifying a fluid-filled pseudocyst. Computed tomography in patients with chronic pancreatitis demonstrates dilated pancreatic ducts and changes in the size of the pancreas. ERCP is the most sensitive imaging test for detecting early changes in the pancreatic ducts caused by chronic pancreatitis.

Treatment

Treatment of chronic pancreatitis includes management of the patient's pain, malabsorption, and diabetes mellitus (develops in 30% to 40% of patients). Opioids may be required for adequate pain control, and in some patients celiac plexus block may be considered. An internal surgical drainage procedure (pancreaticojejunostomy) or endoscopic placement of stents and extraction of stones may be helpful in patients who are otherwise resistant to medical management of pain. Steatorrhea is treated by administration of an enzyme supplement (lipase) to permit fat digestion in the duodenum. Surgical resection and drainage of pancreatic pseudocysts is definitive therapy, although percutaneous cyst drainage is an alternative to surgery. Paracentesis, or thoracentesis, or both may be necessary when patients develop ascites or pleural effusions.

■ MALABSORPTION AND MALDIGESTION

Malabsorption of nutrients is reflected by impaired absorption of fat (steatorrhea), although other substances (iron, calcium, bile salts, specific amino acids, saccharides) may be selectively poorly absorbed in the absence of steatorrhea.[26] Steatorrhea is most likely due to small bowel disease, liver or biliary tract disease, or pancreatic exocrine insufficiency. Patients with small bowel disease may develop hypoalbuminemia due to a protein leak through diseased intestinal mucosa. Fat-soluble vitamin deficiencies (vitamins A, D, E, K), hypocalcemia, and hypomagnesemia may be present in patients with liver and biliary tract disease. Pancreatic exocrine insufficiency is characterized by massive excretion of fat in the patient's feces. Tests for malabsorption are based on measuring fecal fat excretion.

Gluten-Sensitive Enteropathy

Gluten-sensitive enteropathy (previously termed celiac disease in children or nontropical sprue in adults) is a disease of the small intestine resulting in malabsorption (steatorrhea), weight loss, abdominal pain, and fatigue. Diagnosis of this malabsorption syndrome is based on findings in the small bowel biopsy specimen. Treatment is removal of gluten (wheat, rye, barley) from the diet.

Small Bowel Resection

Massive small bowel resection (mesenteric ischemia, volvulus, Crohn's disease) may result in malabsorption if the small intestinal surface area that remains for absorption is decreased below critical levels. Clinical manifestations of the resulting "short bowel

syndrome'' include diarrhea, steatorrhea, trace element deficiencies, and electrolyte imbalance (hyponatremia, hypokalemia). Vitamins and minerals are added to the therapeutic replacement regimens. Total parenteral nutrition is needed only if multiple small feedings are not effective.

Postgastrectomy Steatorrhea

Extensive gastric surgery (resection of the antrum and a variable portion of the body of the stomach with a gastrojejunostomy) may result in malabsorption and steatorrhea. Because of the small stomach, these patients cannot eat large meals; and this situation in combination with steatorrhea often results in stabilization at a lower weight than preoperatively. Iron deficiency anemia is common, and folate deficiency may develop. Vitamin B_{12} deficiency is possible.

■ GASTROINTESTINAL BLEEDING

Gastrointestinal bleeding most often originates from the upper gastrointestinal tract (peptic ulcer) and is a common reason for hospital admission (Table 19–4).[27] Bleeding from the lower gastrointestinal tract (diverticulosis) accounts for 10% to 20% of all cases of gastrointestinal bleeding and primarily affects elderly patients (Table 19–4).[27]

Upper Gastrointestinal Bleeding

Patients with acute upper gastrointestinal bleeding may experience hypotension and tachycardia if

Table 19–4 • Causes of Upper and Lower Gastrointestinal Bleeding

Causes	Incidence (%)
Upper gastrointestinal bleeding	
Peptic ulcer	
Duodenal ulcer	36
Gastric ulcer	24
Mucosal erosive disease	
Gastritis	6
Esophagitis	6
Esophageal varices	6
Mallory-Weiss tear	3
Malignancy	2
Lower gastrointestinal bleeding	
Colonic diverticulosis	42
Colorectal malignancy	9
Ischemic colitis	9
Acute colitis of unknown causes	5
Hemorrhoids	5

Adapted from: Young HS. Gastrointestinal bleeding. Sci Am Med 1998;1–10.

blood loss exceeds about 25% of the total blood volume (1500 ml in adults). Most patients with evidence of acute hypovolemia (orthostatic hypotension characterized by decreases in systolic blood pressure of 10 to 20 mmHg and corresponding increases in heart rate) have hematocrits less than 30%. The hematocrit may be normal early in the course of acute hemorrhage because of the insufficient time for equilibration of the plasma volume. Melena usually indicates that bleeding has occurred at a site above the cecum. With upper gastrointestinal bleeding, the blood urea nitrogen (BUN) concentration is usually higher than 40 mg/dl because of the absorbed nitrogen load in the small intestine. A history of epigastric pain that precedes the passage of black stools by 1 to 2 weeks suggests peptic ulcer disease. Weight loss, anorexia, and chronic anemia may antedate acute bleeding from gastric cancer. Recurrent retching just before hematemesis is commonly described in patients with a Mallory-Weiss tear at the esophagogastric junction. Elderly individuals with esophageal variceal bleeding, those with malignancy, and those who develop bleeding after hospitalization for other co-morbid diseases have an acute mortality rate higher than 30%.[27] Multiple organ system failure, rather than hemorrhage, is the usual cause of death in these patients. Endoscopy following hemodynamic stabilization is the diagnostic procedure of choice in patients with acute upper gastrointestinal bleeding.

For patients with bleeding peptic ulcers, endoscopic coagulation (thermotherapy, injection with epinephrine or a sclerosant) is indicated when active bleeding is visible. Patients receiving anticoagulants can be safely treated with endoscopic coagulation. Perforation occurs in about 0.5% of patients undergoing endoscopic coagulation.[27] Ligation of bleeding esophageal varices by endoscopic ligation is as effective as sclerotherapy for controlling esophageal variceal bleeding. Transient bacteremia, aspiration pneumonia, and bacterial pneumonitis may occur in patients treated by endoscopic variceal ligation. A transjugular intrahepatic portosystemic shunt may be utilized in patients with esophageal variceal bleeding resistant to control by endoscopic coagulation or sclerotherapy, especially those awaiting liver transplantation. Surgical treatment of nonvariceal upper gastrointestinal bleeding (oversewing an ulcer, gastrectomy for diffuse hemorrhagic gastritis) is utilized in patients who continue to bleed despite optimal supportive therapy and in whom endoscopic coagulation is unsuccessful. Surgical creation of a portocaval shunt to manage bleeding esophageal varices may not be more effective than sclerotherapy and is associated with high morbidity and mortality.

Lower Gastrointestinal Bleeding

Lower gastrointestinal (colonic) bleeding usually occurs in elderly patients and typically presents as abrupt passage of bright red blood and clots. In contrast to those with upper gastrointestinal bleeding, the BUN concentrations are not likely to be significantly increased in these patients.

Sigmoidoscopy to exclude anorectal lesions is indicated as soon as patients are hemodynamically stable. Colonoscopy can be performed only after the bowel has been purged with polyethylene glycol solution. If bleeding is persistent and brisk, angiography and possibly embolic therapy may be attempted. Unlike patients with upper gastrointestinal bleeding, a significant number of patients with lower gastrointestinal bleeding (up to 15%) require surgical intervention to control the bleeding.[27] Death caused by gastrointestinal bleeding is increased among elderly patients, especially if the bleeding develops during hospitalization from another co-morbid disease.

Occult Gastrointestinal Bleeding

Occult gastrointestinal bleeding may present as unexplained iron deficiency anemia or as intermittent positive tests for blood in the patient's feces.[27] Peptic ulcer disease and colonic neoplasm are the most common causes of occult gastrointestinal bleeding. The site of occult bleeding is determined by upper gastrointestinal endoscopic examination or colonoscopy.

Gastrointestinal Bleeding in Critically Ill Patients

Routine use of prophylactic therapy (nasogastric infusion of antacids or sucralfate and administration of H_2-antagonists) to prevent upper gastrointestinal bleeding may not be necessary in all critically ill patients.[27] Risk factors for the development of gastrointestinal bleeding in critically ill patients include head injuries, burns covering more than 30% of the patient's body surface area, respiratory failure that requires mechanical ventilation of the patient's lungs, and coagulopathy. Propranolol may be efficacious prophylactically in patients with esophageal varices.

▪ DIVERTICULOSIS AND DIVERTICULITIS

Colonic diverticula, herniations of the mucosa and submucosa through the muscularis propria, occur most often in individuals who consume low-fiber diets.[28] It is estimated that 10% to 20% of individuals older than 50 years of age have diverticulosis. Diverticuli most often involve the sigmoid colon and rarely cause symptoms (abdominal pain). Among patients with known diverticulosis, only 10% to 25% develop acute diverticulitis. Patients with mild diverticulitis typically manifest with left-sided lower abdominal pain, low-grade fever, anorexia, and nausea without vomiting. Right-sided colonic diverticulitis is usually indistinguishable from appendicitis. Lower gastrointestinal bleeding is rarely associated with acute diverticulitis. Severe diverticulitis is characterized by development of a diverticular abscess that may rupture and produce purulent peritonitis. Fistula formation, when it occurs, is most commonly from the sigmoid colon to the bladder. Abdominal computed tomography is the most useful study for early evaluation of suspected diverticulitis.

Surgical treatment of acute diverticulitis, especially that associated with fistula formation, is resection of the diseased segment of colon. Before elective surgery, a barium enema is performed to define the extent of the diverticulosis. About 20% of patients hospitalized for diverticular bleeding require surgery to control bleeding.[28]

■ APPENDICITIS

Approximately 7% to 9% of the population require appendectomy during their lifetime.[28] The incidence of appendicitis peaks between 10 and 20 years of age, with 85% of cases occurring before 45 years of age. Appendicitis is generally caused by obstruction of the lumen of the appendix (lymphoid hyperplasia, fecaliths) followed by bacterial overgrowth distal to the obstruction. Continued inflammation and ischemia, if untreated, may result in gangrenous appendicitis, perforation, or both.

Signs and Symptoms

Pain is present in nearly all patients and initially is typically referred to the periumbilical or epigastric areas. Within 12 to 24 hours pain (tenderness) becomes more localized to the right lower quadrant and is exacerbated by coughing. Nevertheless, this classic sequential presentation of pain does not occur in all patients. Anorexia is present, but vomiting is unusual and if present suggests the presence of gastroenteritis or bowel obstruction. High fever suggests appendiceal perforation and development of peritonitis. The proximity of the inflammatory pro-

cess to the right psoas muscle results in pain when patients are asked to raise their right leg. Laboratory tests are nonspecific, and surgical intervention should not be delayed based on the absence of leukocytosis.

An atypical location of the appendix results in atypical signs and symptoms. For example, a retrocecal appendix is relatively shielded from the parietal peritoneum, and pain and tenderness are less intense. A pelvic appendix may produce symptoms more typical of bladder (dysuria) or rectal (tenesmus) inflammation. Third-trimester pregnancy displaces the appendix toward the right upper quadrant, causing pain that mimics acute cholecystitis or perforated peptic ulcer.

Treatment

Although there is evidence that appendicitis may resolve spontaneously, the recommended treatment is prompt surgical appendectomy. The decision to proceed with surgery is based primarily on the history and physical examination. A pregnancy test is performed in women of child-bearing age. Waiting for other tests is not recommended as any delay may increase the risk that perforation will occur. Acceptance of the need to minimize delay is associated with a 15% to 40% incidence of "negative appendectomy." Appendiceal computed tomography may decrease the incidence of negative appendectomy. Laparoscopic appendectomy may be particularly useful in women of childbearing age when gynecologic conditions cannot be excluded. Preoperative preparation consists of intravenous fluid administration and antibiotic therapy.

■ PERITONITIS

Peritonitis is a diffuse or localized inflammatory process that affects the peritoneal lining.[29] Acute peritonitis caused by bacteria is often associated with concurrent bacteremia. Spontaneous bacterial peritonitis may occur in patients with systemic lupus erythematosus and hepatic cirrhosis. The source of infection in these patients is presumed to be hematogenous. The diagnosis of spontaneous bacterial peritonitis is based on examination of ascitic fluid for bacteria and leukocytes. It is important to distinguish spontaneous bacterial pneumonitis from secondary peritonitis from intra-abdominal disease such as a perforated viscus (appendicitis, peptic ulcer, diverticulitis). In the absence of ascites, the peritoneum has a remarkable ability to wall off and localize infections (periappendiceal or pelvic abscess). Ultrasonography and computed tomography are the standard radiologic techniques for evaluating intra-abdominal abscesses. A subphrenic abscess may mimic right lower lobe pneumonia. As many as 60% of patients undergoing continuous ambulatory peritoneal dialysis develop peritonitis during the first year of treatment, with elderly patients being the most vulnerable.[29] Acute pancreatitis, perforated peptic ulcer, mesenteric artery occlusion, and acute cholecystitis may mimic bacterial peritonitis. In these patients, paracentesis is necessary to rule out bacterial peritonitis. Patients with spontaneous bacterial peritonitis or who are undergoing peritoneal dialysis are treated with antibiotics, whereas patients developing secondary peritonitis require antibiotic and surgical therapy.

■ ACUTE COLONIC PSEUDO-OBSTRUCTION

Acute colonic pseudo-obstruction (Ogilvie syndrome) refers to marked dilation of the colon in the absence of mechanical obstruction.[30] This event usually occurs in hospitalized patients over a period of several days and most of these patients have associated medical or surgical conditions (trauma, recent surgery, sepsis). It is speculated that sympathetic nervous system overactivity and/or parasympathetic nervous system suppression are responsible for the development of pseudo-obstruction. The diagnosis is based on abdominal radiographic evidence of colonic distension. When the colonic diameter increases or remains above a certain level (12 cm), colonoscopic decompression decreases the diameter of the cecum and presumably the risks of perforation. Repeated colonoscopy is often required, as the condition recurs. Alternatively, intravenous administration of neostigmine, 2 mg, may result in prompt evacuation of flatus or feces and decreased abdominal distension.[31]

References

1. Feldman M, Walker P, Green JL, et al. Life events, stress and psychosocial factors in men with peptic ulcer disease. Gastroenterology 1986;91:1370–8
2. Brock-Utne JG, Welman RS, Dimopoulos GE, et al. The effect of glycopyrrolate (Robinal) on the lower esophageal sphincter. Can Anaesth Soc J 1978;25:144–6
3. Hardy J-F, Lepage Y, Bonneville-Chouinard N. Occurrence of gastroesophageal reflux on induction of anaesthesia does not correlate with the volume of gastric contents. Can J Anaesth 1990;37:502–8
4. Illing L, Duncan PG, Yip R. Gastroesophageal reflux during anaesthesia. Can J Anaesth 1992;39:466–70
5. Warner MA, Warner ME, Weber JG. Clinical significance of pulmonary aspiration during the perioperative period. Anesthesiology 1993;78:56–62
6. Warner MA, Warner ME, Warner DO, et al. Perioperative pulmonary aspiration in infants and children. Anesthesiology 1999;90:66–71
7. Cote CJ. NPO after midnight for children: a reappraisal. Anesthesiology 1990;72:589–92
8. Practice guidelines for preoperative fasting and the use of pharmacologic agents to reduce the risk of pulmonary aspiration: application to healthy patients undergoing elective procedures; a report by the American Society of Anesthesiologists Task Force on Preoperative Fasting. Anesthesiology 1999;90:896–905
9. Soll A. Medical treatment of peptic ulcer disease: practice guidelines. JAMA 1996;275:622–9
10. Feldman M. Peptic ulcer diseases. Sci Am Med 2000;1–13
11. Holdcroft A. Hormones and the gut. Br J Anaesth 2000;85:58–68
12. Norton JA, Fraker DL, Alexander R, et al. Surgery to cure the Zollinger-Ellison syndrome. N Engl J Med 1999;341:635–44
13. Lau JY, Sung JJY, Lee KKC, et al. Effect of intravenous omeprazole on recurrent bleeding after endoscopic treatment of bleeding peptic ulcers. N Engl J Med 2000;343:310–6
14. Hanauer SB. Inflammatory bowel disease. N Engl J Med 1996;334:841–8
15. Bickston SJ, Cominelli F. Treatment of Crohn's disease at the turn of the century. N Engl J Med 1998;339:401–2
16. Yellin AE, Newman J, Conovan AJ. Neostigmine-induced hyperperistalsis: effects on security of colonic anastomoses. Arch Surg 1973;106:779–81
17. Aitkenhead AR. Anaesthesia and bowel surgery. Br J Anaesth 1984;56:95–101
18. Hunter AR. Colorectal surgery for cancer: the anaesthetist's contribution? Br J Anaesth 1986;58:825–6
19. Kulke MH, Mayer RJ. Carcinoid tumors. N Engl J Med 1999;340:858–68
20. Neustein SM, Cohen E. Anesthesia for aortic and mitral valve replacement in a patient with carcinoid heart disease. Anesthesiology 1995;82:1067–70
21. Quinlivan JK, Roberts WA. Intraoperative octreotide for refractory carcinoid-induced bronchospasm. Anesth Analg 1994;78:400–2
22. Veall GRQ, Peacock JE, Reilly CS. Review of the anaesthetic management of 21 patients undergoing laparotomy for carcinoid syndrome. Br J Anaesth 1994;72:335–41
23. Young HS. Diseases of the pancreas. Sci Am Med 1997;1–16
24. Steinberg W, Tenner S. Acute pancreatitis. N Engl J Med 1994;330:1198–1210
25. Steer ML, Waxman I, Freedman S. Chronic pancreatitis. N Engl J Med 1995;332:1482–9
26. Mansbach CM. Diseases producing malabsorption and maldigestion. Sci Am Med 1998;10–1
27. Young HS. Gastrointestinal bleeding. Sci Am Med 1998;1–10
28. Harford WV. Diverticulosis, diverticulitis, and appendicitis. Sci Am Med 1998;1–8
29. Simon HB, Swartz MN. Peritonitis and intra-abdominal abscesses. Sci Am Med 2000;1–7
30. Laine L. Management of acute colonic pseudo-obstruction. N Engl J Med 1999;341:137–41
31. Ponec RJ, Saunders MD, Kimmey MB. Neostigmine for the treatment of acute colonic pseudo-obstruction. N Engl J Med 1999;341:137–41

20

Renal Diseases

Essential physiologic functions of the kidneys include excretion of end-products of metabolism (urea), with retention of nutrients (amino acids, glucose) and control of electrolyte and hydrogen ion concentrations of body fluids. It has been estimated that 5% of the adult population of the United States have co-existing renal disease that could contribute to perioperative morbidity.[1]

CLINICAL ASSESSMENT OF RENAL FUNCTION

The kidneys perform many functions: filtering blood; removing nitrogenous wastes from the blood while preventing various solutes, proteins, and blood cells from being excreted; maintaining the proper balance of sodium and water; regulating acid-base balance; maintaining and regulating electrolyte homeostasis, bone metabolism, and erythropoiesis; and controlling systemic blood pressure.[2] Renal function can be evaluated preoperatively by laboratory tests that reflect the glomerular filtration rate (GFR) and renal tubular function (Table 20–1). Current laboratory tests of renal function are often nonspecific, insensitive (more than 50% of nephrons must be destroyed before test results change), or impractical to perform on a routine clinical basis (Table 20–2).[3] Furthermore, normal values for renal function tests established in healthy individuals may not be applicable during anesthesia.[4] Trends are more useful than a single laboratory measurement for evaluating renal function.

Glomerular Filtration Rate

The GFR is considered the best measure of renal function, as it parallels the various functions of the

Table 20–1 • Tests Used to Evaluate Renal Function

Test	Normal Value
Glomerular filtration rate	
Blood urea nitrogen	10–20 mg/dl
Serum creatinine	0.7–1.5 mg/dl (higher in males)
Creatinine clearance	110–150 ml/min
Proteinuria (albumin)	< 150 mg/day
Renal tubular function and/or integrity	
Urine specific gravity	1.003–1.030
Urine osmolality	38–1400 mOsm/L
Urine sodium excretion	< 40 mEq/L
Glucosuria	
Enzymuria	
N-Acetyl-β-glucoseaminidase	
α-Glutathione-S-transferase	
Factors that influence interpretation	
Dehydration	
Variable protein intake	
Gastrointestinal bleeding	
Catabolism	
Advanced age	
Skeletal muscle mass	
Accurate timed urine volume measurement	

nephrons. Alterations in GFR are associated with predictable changes in erythropoietic activity. Clinical manifestations of uremia generally appear when the GFR falls below 10 ml/min (normal 125 ml/min). Because many drugs are excreted by kidney filtration, dosage adjustments may be necessary to prevent cumulative effects when the GFR is decreased.

Blood Urea Nitrogen

Blood urea nitrogen (BUN) concentrations vary with the GFR. Nevertheless, the influence of dietary intake, co-existing disease, and intravascular fluid volume on BUN concentrations make it a potentially misleading test of renal function. For example, production of urea is increased by high-protein diets or gastrointestinal bleeding, resulting in increased BUN concentrations despite a normal GFR. Other causes of increased BUN concentrations despite a normal GFR include dehydration and increased catabolism, as occur during a febrile illness. Increased BUN concentrations in the presence of dehydration most likely reflect increased urea absorption owing to slow movement of fluid through the renal tubules. When the latter is responsible for increased BUN concentrations, the serum creatinine levels remain normal. BUN concentrations can remain normal in the presence of low-protein diets (hemodialysis patients) despite decreases in GFR. Even with these extraneous influences, BUN concentrations higher than 50 mg/dl almost always reflect a decreased GFR.

Table 20–2 • Stages of Chronic Renal Failure

Stage of Failure	Functioning Nephrons (% of total)	Glomerular Filtration Rate (ml/min)	Signs	Laboratory Abnormalities
Normal	100	125	None	None
Decreased renal reserve	40	50–80	None	None
Renal insufficiency	10–40	12–50	Nocturia	Increased blood urea nitrogen
				Increased serum creatinine
Renal failure	10	< 12	Uremia	Increased blood urea nitrogen
				Increased serum creatinine
				Anemia
				Hyperkalemia
				Increased bleeding time

Serum Creatinine

Serum creatinine levels can be used as an estimate of the GFR. Normal serum creatinine concentrations range from 0.6 to 1.0 mg/dl in women and 0.8 to 1.3 mg/dl in men, reflecting differences in skeletal muscle mass. A number of factors (accelerated creatinine production, decreased tubular secretion of creatinine, presence of chromogens in the blood) can increase serum creatinine concentrations without there being a concomitant decrease in GFR. A change in the serum creatinine concentrations from 0.6 mg/dl to 1.2 mg/dl reflects a decrease in the GFR of about 50%. The maintenance of normal serum creatinine concentrations in elderly patients with known decreases in GFR reflects decreased creatinine production owing to the decreased skeletal muscle mass that accompanies aging. In this regard, mild increases in serum creatinine concentrations suggest significant renal disease. Serum creatinine values are slow to reflect acute changes in renal function. For example, if acute renal failure occurs and the GFR decreases from 100 ml/min to 10 ml/min, serum creatinine values do not increase correspondingly for about 7 days.

Creatinine Clearance

Creatinine, an endogenous marker of renal filtration, is produced at a relatively constant rate by hepatic conversion of skeletal muscle creatine. Creatinine is freely filtered and is not reabsorbed. As a result, the creatinine clearance correlates with the GFR and is the most reliable measure of GFR. Creatinine clearance does not depend on corrections for age or the presence of a steady state. Preoperatively, patients with creatinine clearances between 10 and 25 ml/min must be considered at risk for developing prolonged or adverse responses to drugs (such as nondepolarizing muscle relaxants) that depend on renal excretion for their clearance from the plasma. The reliability of creatinine clearance is diminished by the variability in tubular secretion of creatinine and the inability of most patients to collect timed urine samples accurately.

Renal Tubular Function and Integrity

Renal tubular function is most often assessed by measuring the urine concentrating ability. The presence of proteinuria may reflect renal tubular damage. Enzymes present in the renal tubular cells (N-acetyl-β-glucose aminidase, α-glutathione-S-transferase) may be detectable in the urine following sevoflurane anesthesia presumably reflecting transient drug-induced tubular dysfunction that is not accompanied by changes in the BUN or serum creatinine concentrations.[5]

Urine Concentrating Ability

The diagnosis of renal tubular dysfunction is established by demonstrating that the kidneys do not produce appropriately concentrated urine in the presence of a physiologic stimulus for the release of antidiuretic hormone. In the absence of diuretic therapy or glycosuria, urine specific gravity higher than 1.018 suggests that the ability of renal tubules to concentrate urine is adequate. Treatment with diuretics or the presence of hypokalemia or hypercalcemia may interfere with the ability of renal tubules to concentrate urine. Although unlikely following the administration of sevoflurane, the inorganic fluoride resulting from metabolism of this anesthetic is capable of interfering with the urine concentrating ability of the renal tubules.

Proteinuria

Proteinuria (transient, orthostatic, persistent) is relatively common, being present in 5% to 10% of tested adults during screening examinations. Transient proteinuria may be associated with fever, congestive heart failure, seizure activity, pancreatitis, and exercise. This form of proteinuria resolves with treatment of the underlying illness. Orthostatic proteinuria occurs in up to 5% of adolescents while in the upright position and resolves when the recumbent position is assumed. Generally, orthostatic proteinuria resolves spontaneously and is not associated with any deterioration in renal function. Persistent proteinuria generally connotes significant renal disease. Microalbuminuria is the earliest sign of diabetic nephropathy. Severe proteinuria may result in hypoalbuminemia, with associated decreases in plasma oncotic pressures and decreased protein binding of drugs.

Urinary Sodium Excretion

Urinary sodium excretion exceeding 40 mEq/L reflects decreased ability of the renal tubules to conserve sodium. Damage to the renal tubules by hypoxia results in increased loss of sodium in the urine, and the urine osmolarity is likely to be less than 350 mOsm/L. Minimal urinary sodium excretion (less than 15 mEq/L) occurs when normally functioning renal tubules conserve sodium in the presence of hypovolemia, and the urine osmolarity is likely to exceed 500 mOsm/L. Drug-induced diuresis is also associated with increased urinary excretion of sodium.

Additional Diagnostic Tests

Urinalysis

Examination of the urine is useful for diagnosing urinary tract disease. Urinalysis is intended to detect the presence of protein, glucose, acetoacetate, blood, and leukocytes. The urine pH and solute concentrations (specific gravity) are determined, and sediment microscopy is used to examine for the presence of cells, casts, microorganisms, and crystals. Hematuria may be caused by bleeding anywhere between the glomerulus and urethra. Microhematuria may be benign (focal nephritis), or it may reflect glomerulonephritis, renal calculi, or cancer of the genitourinary tract. Joggers may experience hematuria presumably as a result of trauma to the urinary tract. Sickle cell disease is a consideration in African-Americans who exhibit hematuria. In the absence of proteinuria or red blood cell casts, glomerular disease as a cause of hematuria is unlikely. Red blood cell casts are pathognomonic of acute glomerulonephritis. White blood cell casts are most commonly seen with pyelonephritis.

Imaging Techniques of the Genitourinary Tract

A plain film of the kidneys, ureters, and bladder (KUB) and renal ultrasonography are the initial methods for assessing kidney size, structure, symmetry, cortical thickness, and the presence of hydronephrosis or nephrolithiasis.[2] Residual urine volume exceeding 100 ml can be detected by ultrasonography. Computed tomography provides useful information when ultrasonography is inconclusive. Magnetic resonance imaging has advantages over ultrasonography and computed tomography when evaluating renal anatomy, although calcifications are not demonstrated by this technique. In view of the known nephrotoxicity of large-volume radiocontrast procedures in patients with decreased renal function, noncontrast techniques such as KUB radiography and ultrasonography offer obvious advantages.

▪ CHRONIC RENAL FAILURE

Chronic renal failure is progressive, irreversible deterioration of renal function that results from a wide variety of diseases (Table 20–3).[6] Diabetes mellitus is the leading cause of end-stage renal disease followed closely by systemic hypertension. The clinical manifestations of chronic renal failure are typically independent of the initial insult that damaged the kidneys and, instead, reflect the overall inability of the kidneys to excrete nitrogenous waste products, regulate fluid and electrolyte balance, and secrete hormones. In most patients with chronic renal disease, regardless of the etiology, a decrease in the GFR to less than 25 ml/min is characterized by progressive deterioration in renal function that eventually leads to end-stage renal failure requiring dialysis or transplantation.

Pathogenesis

The pathogenesis of renal disease and its progression to renal failure is multifactorial.

Glomerular Hypertension, Hyperfiltration, Systemic Hypertension

Intrarenal hemodynamic changes (glomerular hypertension, glomerular hyperfiltration and permeability changes, glomerulosclerosis) are likely responsible for progression of renal disease. Systemic

---

Table 20–3 • Causes of Chronic Renal Failure

Glomerulopathies
 Primary glomerular disease
  Focal glomerulosclerosis
  Membranous nephropathy
  Immunoglobulin A nephropathy
  Membranoproliferative glomerulonephritis
 Glomerulopathies associated with systemic disease
  Diabetes mellitus
  Amyloidosis
  Postinfectious glomerulonephritis
  Systemic lupus erythematosus
  Wegener's granulomatosis
Tubulointerstitial disease
 Analgesic nephropathy
 Reflux nephropathy with pyelonephritis
 Myeloma kidney
 Sarcoidosis
Heredity disease
 Polycystic kidney disease
 Alport syndrome
 Medullary cystic disease
Systemic hypertension
Renal vascular disease
Obstructive uropathy
Human immunodeficiency virus

Adapted from: Tolkoff-Rubin NE, Pascual M. Chronic renal failure. Sci Am Med 1998;1–12.

hypertension may be a primary cause of renal failure and is also a major risk factor for progression of renal disease. Genetic factors may be important in determining if renal disease develops in hypertensive patients. For example, mild to moderate systemic hypertension alone is rarely associated with progressive loss of renal function. Decreases in glomerular hypertension and in systemic hypertension can be achieved by the administration of angiotensin-converting enzyme (ACE) inhibitors. In addition to beneficial effects on intraglomerular hemodynamics and systemic pressures, the renoprotective effects of ACE inhibitors manifest as reductions in proteinuria and slowing of the progression of glomerulosclerosis in patients with diabetic and nondiabetic nephropathy. Other antihypertensive drugs that lower the systemic pressure to similar degrees do not provide the renoprotective effects seen with ACE inhibitors.

Dietary Factors

In animal models, protein intake can influence the progression of renal disease. In nondiabetic patients with moderate renal insufficiency (GFR 25 to 55 ml/min), protein restriction has not been confirmed to have detectable beneficial effects.[6] Furthermore, there is no evidence in humans that restricting dietary phosphate or lipid intake slows the progression of renal disease.

Hyperglycemia

Strict control of blood glucose concentrations (attempts to maintain hemoglobin A_{1c} near normal) can delay the onset of proteinuria and slow the progression of nephropathy, neuropathy, and retinopathy.

Growth Factors

Growth factors, particularly transforming growth factor-β (TGFβ) may be important in the pathogenesis and progression of renal insufficiency.[6] Overexpression of TGFβ is capable of causing glomerular sclerosis and interstitial fibrosis by stimulating cellular proliferation and fibrogenesis. Angiotensin II may act as a growth factor that induces TGFβ expression in vascular smooth muscle cells. It is possible that the efficacy of ACE inhibitors in preventing the progression of renal failure may include downregulation of TGFβ and improved intraglomerular hemodynamics.

Adaptation to Chronic Renal Failure

The normally functioning kidneys precisely regulate the concentrations of solutes and water in the extracellular fluid despite large variations in daily dietary intake.[6] Patients with chronic renal disease can still excrete solute and water loads without altering their diet, even when the GFR has been significantly decreased. Hence patients with chronic renal failure may remain relatively asymptomatic until renal function is less than 10% of normal.

The kidneys demonstrate three stages of adaptation to progressive impairment of renal function.[6] The first pattern includes substances such as creatinine and urea, which are dependent largely on the GFR for their urinary excretion. As the GFR decreases the plasma concentrations of these substances begin to increase, but the increase is not directly proportional to the degree of GFR impairment. For example, early in the course of renal insufficiency there are minimal changes in serum creatinine concentrations despite more than 50% decreases in GFR. Beyond this point, however, when the renal reserve has been exhausted, even minimal further decreases in the GFR can result in significant increases in the serum creatinine and urea concentrations.

The second stage of adaptation to progressive renal impairment is seen with solutes such as potassium.[6] Serum potassium concentrations are maintained within normal limits until the decrease in GFR approaches 10% of normal, at which point hyperkalemia manifests. Normally, potassium is secreted by the distal renal tubules; and as nephrons are lost, the remaining nephrons increase their secretion of potassium through increased blood flow and increased sodium delivery to the collecting tubules. In addition, because aldosterone secretion increases in patients with renal failure, there is a greater loss of potassium through the gastrointestinal tract. This system of enhanced gastrointestinal secretion is an effective compensatory mechanism in the presence of normal dietary intake of potassium but can be easily overwhelmed by an acute exogenous potassium load (administration of potassium, such as during the perioperative period) or acute endogenous potassium load (hemolysis, tissue trauma such as that associated with surgery).

The third stage of adaptation is seen in sodium homeostasis and regulation of the extracellular fluid volume.[6] In contrast to the levels of other solutes, sodium balance remains intact despite progressive deterioration in renal function and variations in dietary intake. Nevertheless, the system can be overwhelmed by abruptly increased sodium intake (resulting in volume overload) or decreased sodium intake (sodium restriction during the perioperative period leading to extracellular volume depletion).

Approach to Patients with Chronic Renal Failure

Once patients have progressed to chronic renal failure, regardless of the underlying etiology, the function of the remaining nephrons inexorably deteriorates.[6] Measurements of serum creatinine and creatinine clearance provide a useful clinical index of the GFR and changes in renal function. An abrupt increase in the serum creatinine concentration is an indication of acute deterioration of the remaining renal function. Bilateral renovascular disease is suspected in any patient with refractory systemic hypertension and renal failure. Angiography confirms this suspicion, and renal function may be improved by angioplasty or surgical revascularization. In the absence of any reversible components that may be contributing to the progression of renal insufficiency, the approach to the patient includes attempts to prevent progression of the disease (control of hyperglycemia, management of systemic hypertension with ACE inhibitors) and management of the consequences of impaired renal function (Table 20–4).[6]

Uremic Syndrome

Uremic syndrome is a constellation of signs and symptoms (anorexia, nausea, vomiting, pruritus,

---

Table 20–4 • Manifestations of Chronic Renal Failure

Electrolyte imbalance
  Hyperkalemia
  Hypermagnesemia
  Hypocalcemia
Metabolic acidosis
Unpredictable intravascular fluid volume status
Anemia
  Increased cardiac output
  Oxyhemoglobin dissociation curve shifted to the right
Uremic coagulopathies
  Platelet dysfunction
Neurologic changes
  Encephalopathy
Cardiovascular changes
  Systemic hypertension
  Congestive heart failure
  Attenuated sympathetic nervous system activity due to treatment with antihypertensive drugs
Renal osteodystrophy
Pruritus

---

anemia, fatigue, coagulopathy) that reflect the kidney's progressive inability to perform its excretory, secretory, and regulatory functions.[6] Although it is questionable whether urea itself produces the signs and symptoms (except at high concentrations), the BUN concentration is a useful clinical indicator of the severity of the uremic syndrome and the patient's response to therapy. In contrast, the serum creatinine concentration, although a reliable measure of GFR, correlates poorly with uremic symptoms. Traditional treatment of the uremic syndrome is dietary protein restriction based on the presumption that a low-protein diet results in decreased protein catabolism and urea production.

Hyperkalemia

Patients in chronic renal failure can adapt by increasing their potassium secretion such that the development of hyperkalemia is more gradual and better tolerated until late in the course of the disease so long as the dietary intake of potassium is restricted and drugs [triamterene, spironolactone, nonsteroidal antiinflammatory drugs (NSAIDs), β-blockers, ACE inhibitors] that affect potassium homeostasis are avoided.[6] Any patient with chronic renal failure whose dietary intake of potassium exceeds the rate of excretion may become dangerously hyperkalemic. In addition, severe acidosis, acute infection with marked catabolism, acute hemolysis, marked hyperglycemia, or any superimposed complication leading to oliguria may result in the rapid development of life-threatening hyperkalemia.

Changes on the electrocardiogram (ECG) (peaked T waves, prolongation of the QRS complex and PR interval, heart block, ventricular fibrillation) are the best guide for when immediate therapy of hyperkalemia must be considered (Table 20–5).[6] If the serum potassium concentration is higher than 6.5 mEq/L or if electrocardiographic changes are present, immediate therapy should be instituted (Table 20–5).[6] Initial treatment of hyperkalemia should be directed at antagonizing the effects of potassium on the heart (intravenous calcium gluconate) and rapidly shifting potassium into cells (intravenous glucose, insulin, bicarbonate). Because these measures only temporarily control hyperkalemia, efforts to eliminate potassium from the body must be initiated simultaneously. Potassium can be removed by administering exchange resins. If these measures are not effective, emergency dialysis is indicated.

Metabolic Acidosis

The kidneys remove acid produced by the metabolism of dietary protein, and the pH is maintained

Table 20–5 • Treatment of Hyperkalemia

Treatment	Mechanism of Action	Onset of Effect	Duration of Action	Side Effects
Calcium gluconate (10–20 ml of a 10% solution IV)	Directly antagonizes effects of potassium on the heart	Immediate	Brief	Avoid if being treated with digitalis
Sodium bicarbonate (50–100 mEq IV)	Shifts potassium into cells	Prompt	Short	Possible sodium overload
Glucose (50 ml of a 50% solution) and regular insulin (10 units IV)	Shifts potassium into cells	Prompt	4–6 hours	Hyperglycemia Hypoglycemia
Ion exchange resin	Removes potassium from the body	1–2 hours		Sodium overload
Dialysis	Removes potassium from the body	Prompt		Requires vascular access

Adapted from: Tolkoff-Rubin NE, Pascual M. Chronic renal failure. Sci Am Med 1998;1–12.

in a normal range until the GFR decreases below 50 ml/min, at which point metabolic acidosis develops. Chronic metabolic acidosis (pH less than 7.3) produces symptoms of fatigue and lethargy, increases respiratory work and catecholamine responsiveness, stimulates protein degradation, and exacerbates renal osteodystrophy.

Treatment is with intravenous sodium bicarbonate, taking care not to correct the acidosis too rapidly, particularly if hypocalcemia is present. Acidosis depresses neuromuscular irritability and protects against the effects of hypocalcemia and signs of tetany. When the acidosis is corrected, the serum level of ionized calcium decreases as a result of increased protein binding of free calcium. Because the free ionized calcium concentration is critical for neuromuscular function, too rapid correction of the metabolic acidosis may precipitate seizures.[6]

Renal Osteodystrophy

Renal osteodystrophy is a complication of chronic renal failure, reflecting the complex interaction of secondary hyperparathyroidism and decreased vitamin D production by the kidneys.[6, 7] As the GFR declines there is a parallel decrease in phosphate clearance and an increase in the serum phosphate concentrations that results in reciprocal decreases in serum calcium concentrations. Hypocalcemia stimulates parathyroid hormone (PTH) secretion, which leads to bone resorption and calcium release. As a result of decreased renal production of vitamin D by the kidneys, intestinal absorption of calcium is impaired, which also leads to hypocalcemia, stimulation of PTH release, and bone resorption.

Hyperparathyroid bone disease is the most common form of uremic osteodystrophy. Radiographs demonstrate evidence of bone demineralization (clavicles, skull, middle phalanges of the middle and index fingers). Further evidence of bone resorption is the presence of increased serum alkaline phosphatase concentrations. The diagnosis of hyperparathyroidism is confirmed by documentation of increased serum PTH concentrations. Accumulation of aluminum in patients undergoing chronic renal dialysis, although decreasing in frequency, may result in bone pain, fractures, and weakness. Hyperparathyroidism seems to protect against aluminum-induced bone disease. Adynamic (aplastic) bone disease occurs in patients (often diabetics) with end-stage renal disease who are undergoing chronic renal dialysis and who do not have secondary hyperparathyroidism (after parathyroidectomy).

Treatment of renal osteodystrophy is intended to prevent skeletal complications by restricting dietary phosphate intake (antacids may be administered to bind phosphorus in the gastrointestinal tract), administration of oral calcium supplements, and vitamin D therapy. Magnesium-containing antacids introduce the risk of hypermagnesemia, whereas aluminum-containing antacids are equally undesirable. If aluminum toxicity is present, deferoxamine chelation therapy is helpful. Overzealous suppression of PTH by calcium and vitamin D may be undesirable, as PTH may be necessary to maintain bone mass in chronic renal failure patients. If medical therapies fail to control hypercalcemia and hyperparathyroidism, subtotal parathyroidectomy is often recommended.

Anemia

Anemia frequently accompanies chronic renal failure and is presumed to be responsible for many of the symptoms (fatigue, weakness, decreased exercise tolerance) characteristic of the uremic syndrome. This anemia is primarily due to decreased erythropoietin production by the kidneys. Excess PTH appears to contribute to anemia by replacing bone marrow with fibrous tissue.

Treatment of the anemia of chronic renal disease is with recombinant human erythropoietin (epoetin), eliminating the need for blood transfusions and avoiding the symptoms of anemia in most patients. Blood transfusions are avoided if possible, as the resultant sensitization to HLA antigens makes kidney transplantation less successful. The goal of erythropoietin therapy is to maintain the hematocrit between 36% to 40%.[7] Intermittent injections of parenteral iron are recommended to maximize the responses to erythropoietin. The development of systemic hypertension or exacerbation of co-existing systemic hypertension, necessitating further antihypertensive therapy, is a risk of erythropoietin administration.

Uremic Bleeding

Patients with chronic renal failure have an increased tendency to bleed despite the presence of normal laboratory coagulation studies (platelet count, prothrombin time, plasma thromboplastin time). The bleeding time is the screening test that best correlates with the tendency to bleed. Hemorrhagic episodes (gastrointestinal bleeding, epistaxis, hemorrhagic pericarditis, subdural hematoma) remain major factors contributing to the morbidity and mortality associated with anemia.[6]

Treatment of uremic bleeding may include the administration of cryoprecipitate to provide factor VIII–von Willebrand Factor (vWF) complex (risk of transmission of viral diseases) or administration of 1-desamino-8-D-arginine vasopressin (DDAVP, desmopressin) (Table 20–6).[6] DDAVP, an analogue of antidiuretic hormone, increases the circulating levels of factor VIII–vWF complex and decreases the bleeding time. In patients with uremia, the intravenous infusion or subcutaneous injection of DDAVP decreases prolonged bleeding and is particularly useful for preventing clinical hemorrhage when invasive procedures such as surgery are planned.[6] The maximal effect of DDAVP is present within 2 to 4 hours and lasts 6 to 8 hours. The effects of DDAVP appear to be attenuated by repeated doses. DDAVP may act by increasing or changing platelet membrane receptor binding of the factor VIII–vWF complex or by inducing the appearance of a more active complex.

Although cryoprecipitate and DDAVP can correct bleeding times so surgical procedures can be performed without excessive bleeding in patients with chronic renal failure, the effects of both drugs last for only a few hours. Conversely, conjugated estrogen administration may improve bleeding times for up to 14 days (Table 20–6).[6] It has also been observed that erythropoietin shortens bleeding times. It is of interest that prior to the availability of erythropoietin, it had been recognized that blood transfusions to increase the hematocrit to above 30% also corrected the bleeding times.

Neurologic Changes

Neurologic changes may be early manifestations of progressive renal insufficiency.[6, 7] Initially, symptoms may be mild (impaired abstract thinking, insomnia, irritability); but as renal disease progresses, more significant changes (increased deep tendon reflexes, seizures, obtundation, uremic encephalopathy, coma) may develop. A disabling complication of advanced chronic renal failure is development of a distal, symmetrical mixed motor and sensory polyneuropathy that may present as "restless legs syndrome" (inability to control activity of the lower extremities), paresthesias or hyperesthesias of the feet secondary to sensory neuropathy, or distal weakness of the lower extremities. The arms may also be affected, but the incidence is less than in the legs. Diabetic neuropathy may be superimposed on uremic peripheral neuropathy. Some aspects of uremic encephalopathy and the severity of peripheral neurologic symptoms may be improved by hemodialysis.

Table 20–6 • Treatment of Uremic Bleeding

Drug	Dosage	Onset of Effect	Peak Effect	Duration of Effect
Cryoprecipitate	10 units IV over 30 minutes	< 1 hour	4–12 hours	12–18 hours
DDAVP (desmopressin)	0.3 μg/kg IV or SC	< 1 hour	2–4 hours	6–8 hours
Conjugated estrogen	0.6 mg/kg/day IV for 5 days	6 hours	5–7 days	14 days

Adapted from: Tolkoff-Rubin NE, Pascual M. Chronic renal failure. Sci Am Med 1998;1–12.

Cardiovascular Changes

Systemic hypertension is the most significant risk factor accompanying chronic renal failure and contributes to the congestive heart failure, coronary artery disease, and cerebrovascular disease that occurs in these patients. Uncontrolled systemic hypertension speeds the progressive decrease in GFR. The pathogenesis of systemic hypertension in these patients reflects intravascular fluid volume expansion due to retention of sodium and water and activation of the renin-angiotensin-aldosterone system. Uremic pericarditis is common in patients with severe chronic renal failure. Cardiac ultrasonography determines the size of an associated pericardial effusion and its effect on myocardial contractility. Atrial cardiac dysrhythmias are common in the presence of uremic pericarditis.

Dialysis is the indicated treatment for patients who are hypertensive because of hypervolemia (remove volume to attain "dry weight") and those who develop uremic pericarditis. Dialysis is less likely to control systemic hypertension due to activation of the renin-angiotensin-aldosterone system. Increasing doses of antihypertensive drugs are recommended in these patients. ACE inhibitors are used cautiously in patients in whom the GFR is dependent on increased efferent arteriolar vasoconstriction (bilateral renal artery stenosis, transplanted kidney with unilateral stenosis), which is mediated by angiotensin II. Administration of ACE inhibitors to these patients can result in efferent arteriolar dilation and decreased GFR, which results in sudden deterioration in renal function.

Cardiac tamponade and hemodynamic instability associated with uremic pericarditis and effusion is an indication for prompt drainage of the effusion, often via placement of a percutaneous pericardial catheter. In occasional patients, surgical drainage with creation of a pericardial window or pericardiectomy is necessary. The development of hypotension unresponsive to intravascular fluid volume replacement may be an important clue that cardiac tamponade is present.

Hemodialysis

Hemodialysis is utilized for treating patients in whom chronic renal failure would otherwise result in the uremic syndrome.[7, 8] Objectives when caring for patients who are undergoing hemodialysis include adequate dialysis, ensuring adequate nutrition, maintaining vascular access, correcting hormonal deficiencies, minimizing hospitalizations, and prolonging life while enhancing its quality.

During hemodialysis, diffusion of solutes between the blood and dialysis solution results in removal of metabolic waste products and replenishment of body buffers.[8] The dose of dialysis, which depends on the length of treatment, the type of dialysis membrane, and solute clearance are the most important modifiable determinants of survival in patients with end-stage renal disease undergoing hemodialysis.[7] Inadequate dialysis shortens survival and leads to malnutrition, anemia, and functional impairment, resulting in frequent hospitalizations and increased cost of care (Table 20–7).[7] The annual mortality for patients on hemodialysis is near 25% and is most often attributed to cardiovascular causes or infection.

Vascular Access

A surgically created vascular access site is necessary for effective hemodialysis.[8] To preserve the blood vessels for vascular access, venipuncture should be avoided in the nondominant arm and the upper part of the dominant arm of patients with chronic renal failure. Despite the presence of coagulopathy in patients with uremia and the routine use of heparin during dialysis, thrombosis of the vascular access site is common. Native arteriovenous fistulas (cephalic vein anastomosed to the radial artery) are superior to polytetrafluoroethylene (PTFE) grafts as sites of vascular access because of their longer lifespan and lower incidence of thrombosis and infection. Native arteriovenous fistulas are the preferred vascular access sites in all patients undergoing hemodialysis. The most common access-related com-

Table 20–7 • Findings Suggestive of Inadequate Hemodialysis

Clinical
Anorexia, nausea, vomiting
Peripheral neuropathy
Poor nutritional status
Depressed sensorium
Pericarditis
Ascites
Minimal weight gain or weight loss between treatments
Fluid retention and systemic hypertension
Chemical
Decrease in blood urea nitrogen concentration during hemodialysis < 65%
Albumin concentration < 4 g/dl
Predialysis blood urea concentration < 50 mg/dl
Predialysis serum creatinine concentration < 5 mg/dl
Persistent anemia (hematocrit < 30%) despite erythropoietin therapy

Adapted from: Ifudu O. Care of patients undergoing hemodialysis. N Engl J Med 1998;339:1054–62.

plication is thrombosis due to intimal hyperplasia, which results in stenosis proximal to the venous anastomosis. Other complications related to access include infection, the formation of aneurysms, and ischemia of the arm. When dialysis is urgently required, vascular access is obtained with a double-lumen dialysis catheter most often utilizing the jugular or femoral vein.

Complications During Hemodialysis

Hypotension is the most common adverse event during hemodialysis and most likely reflects osmolar shifts and ultrafiltration-induced volume depletion.[8] Hypotensive episodes may reflect myocardial ischemia, cardiac dysrhythmias, or pericardial effusion with cardiac tamponade. Most hypotensive episodes are successfully treated by slowing the rate of ultrafiltration and/or administering intravenous saline.

Hypersensitivity reactions to the ethylene oxide used to sterilize the dialysis machine may occur as an adverse reaction to the specific membrane material, polyacrylonitrile. Reactions to polyacrylonitrile occur most commonly in patients receiving ACE inhibitors.[8] When blood comes in contact with the polyacrylonitrile membrane, the membrane's high negative surface charge stabilizes enzymes, which generate bradykinins. Normally, bradykinin is degraded by kinases, but ACE inhibitors block this response, and profound peripheral vasodilation and hypotension may occur.

Nutrition and Fluid Balance

During progressive renal failure, catabolism and anorexia lead to loss of lean body mass, but concomitant fluid retention masks weight loss and may even lead to weight gain.[7] There is no justification for stringent restriction of dietary potassium in patients undergoing hemodialysis. Patients with end-stage renal disease have decreased total body potassium and an inexplicable tolerance for hyperkalemia. The expected cardiac and neuromuscular responses to hyperkalemia are less pronounced in patients on hemodialysis than in those with normal renal function. Clearance of potassium by hemodialysis is efficient, and because most potassium is intracellular it is likely that hypokalemia will be suggested by a blood sample obtained soon after completion of hemodialysis and before transcellular equilibration has occurred. Water-soluble vitamins are removed by hemodialysis and should be replaced. Between treatments a weight gain of 3% to 4% of body mass in 2 days is appropriate.[7]

Cardiovascular Disease

Cardiovascular disease accounts for nearly 50% of all deaths in patients on hemodialysis.[7]

Ischemic Heart Disease

The increased incidence of ischemic heart disease and myocardial infarction among patients with end-stage renal disease is attributed to systemic hypertension, anemia, hyperlipidemia, hyperhomocysteinemia, accelerated atherosclerosis, and possibly impaired oxygen delivery to the myocardium due to uremic toxins. Chemical stress testing (dipyridamole or dobutamine), may be preferred to exercise stress testing, as patients in renal failure are often unable to exercise adequately. The baseline ECG may be altered by metabolic derangements. For unknown reasons, baseline serum creatine kinase concentrations are increased in nearly one-third of patients on hemodialysis. Because this increase is accounted for principally by the MM isoenzyme, the value of the MB fraction for diagnosis of an acute myocardial infarction remains intact. Medical management of ischemic heart disease in patients on hemodialysis is the same as for those with normal renal function. However, antianginal medications may predispose patients to hypotension during hemodialysis.

Congestive Heart Failure

Congestive heart failure in patients on hemodialysis is treated as in patients with normal renal function with the exception that diuretics are not administered. Protein-bound digoxin-like immunoreactive substances in the serum of patients on hemodialysis may interfere with the accuracy and interpretation of measurements of digoxin concentrations and the diagnosis of toxicity. Hemodialysis has beneficial effects on cardiac hemodynamics, as removal of fluid during hemodialysis provides symptomatic relief for patients in congestive heart failure.

Systemic Hypertension

Fluid retention during progressive renal failure is the most likely explanation for the presence of systemic hypertension in most patients who present for hemodialysis. Failure to distinguish essential hypertension from that due to fluid retention in the presence of end-stage renal disease may lead to the inappropriate and ineffective use of antihypertensive drugs. The appropriate management of systemic hypertension is gradual removal of fluid by hemodialysis to achieve an ideal postdialysis body weight. Patients with associated essential hypertension also require treatment with antihypertensive drugs.

Pericarditis

Pericarditis with pericardial effusion occurs infrequently in patients on hemodialysis and is often due to inadequate hemodialysis. Intensive heparin-free dialysis is the treatment for suspected uremic pericarditis. Persistent effusion despite intensive dialysis or early suspicion of infection is an indication for pericardiocentesis or pericardiotomy.

Bleeding Tendency

Bleeding due to altered platelet function is partially correctable by hemodialysis. Heparin-free dialysis or administration of DDAVP is often sufficient to correct a bleeding tendency.

Infection

Patients requiring hemodialysis have increased susceptibility to infection because of impaired phagocytosis and chemotaxis. Some of the factors resulting in impaired phagocytosis and chemotaxis may be partially reversed by hemodialysis. Some patients on hemodialysis have severe infection without a fever. Tuberculosis in patients on hemodialysis is usually extrapulmonary and often presents with atypical symptoms that mimic those of inadequate dialysis. Because anergy in response to skin testing is common, unexplained weight loss and anorexia, with or without persistent fever, should prompt further testing to rule out tuberculosis. All patients on hemodialysis are vaccinated against pneumococcus, and those who are not already immune receive hepatitis B vaccine. Malnutrition or inadequate dialysis may impair antibody response to vaccines.

Hepatitis B or C virus infection in patients on hemodialysis is often asymptomatic, and liver aminotransferase concentrations may not be increased. Patients with hepatitis B virus should undergo hemodialysis in isolation with a dedicated machine. A substantial proportion of patients on hemodialysis have antibodies to hepatitis C. Dose adjustments of drugs used to treat acquired immunodeficiency syndrome (AIDS) is not necessitated by hemodialysis. Furthermore, isolation of patients with AIDS or use of a dedicated hemodialysis machine is not necessary.[7]

Miscellaneous Considerations

Good glucose control, as evidenced by a glycosylated hemoglobin (HbA_{1c}) value less than 8% is important in patients with diabetes mellitus requiring hemodialysis, as hyperglycemia may result in hyperkalemia or excessive weight gain. Decreased catabolism of insulin in many patients on hemodialysis may result in decreased insulin requirements compared with needs prior to the initiation of hemodialysis. The presentation of diabetic ketoacidosis may be atypical with respiratory acidosis and alkalosis but without metabolic acidosis and hypovolemia.[7] Hypertriglyceridemia reflects diminished clearance in patients on hemodialysis. Depression is a potential risk in patients on hemodialysis and may be misdiagnosed as functional impairment due to renal failure. There is conflicting evidence on whether the risk of cancer is increased in patients on hemodialysis.

Peritoneal Dialysis

Peritoneal dialysis is simple to perform; it requires placing an anchored plastic catheter in the peritoneal cavity for infusion of a dialysis solution that remains in place for several hours.[8] During that time, diffusive solute transport occurs across the peritoneal membrane until fresh fluid is exchanged for the old fluid. Automated peritoneal dialysis, in which a mechanized cycler infuses and drains peritoneal dialysate at night is used in many patients. Peritoneal dialysis may be selected over hemodialysis for patients with congestive heart failure or unstable angina who may not tolerate the rapid fluid shifts or systemic blood pressure changes that may accompany hemodialysis. Peritoneal dialysis is also indicated for patients with extensive vascular disease that prevents placing a catheter for vascular access. In patients with diabetes, insulin can be infused with the dialysate with resultant precise regulation of blood glucose concentrations. The presence of abdominal hernias or adhesions may interfere with the ability to utilize peritoneal dialysis effectively. Peritonitis presenting as abdominal pain and fever is the most common serious complication of peritoneal dialysis. Treatment is with antibiotics, which may include cephalosporins, aminoglycosides, and vancomycin. Survival rates and annual costs are similar with peritoneal dialysis or hemodialysis, but hospitalization rates are higher among patients treated with peritoneal dialysis.

Drug Clearance in Patients Undergoing Dialysis

Patients who are undergoing dialysis may require special consideration with respect to drug dosing intervals, and they may require supplemental dosing with drugs that have been cleared by dialysis. When possible, scheduled doses of drugs are administered after completion of dialysis. Drug properties that influence clearance by dialysis include protein binding, water solubility, and molecular weight. In this regard, low-molecular-weight (less than 500 daltons), water-soluble non-protein-bound drugs are readily cleared by dialysis. Continuous renal replacement therapies, such as continuous venovenous hemofiltration, and continuous arteriovenous hemofiltration, efficiently remove drugs unless they are bound to protein.

Perioperative Hemodialysis

Patients should undergo adequate hemodialysis before elective surgery to minimize the likelihood of uremic bleeding, pulmonary edema, and impaired arterial oxygenation.[4] Depending on the planned surgery, the use of heparin may be avoided or minimized during preoperative hemodialysis. Urgent hemodialysis is not required after radiocontrast dye studies in those who are undergoing regular hemodialysis. Although these dyes can be removed by hemodialysis, the volume administered in most studies does not result in pulmonary edema in patients with adequate dialysis, and nephrotoxicity is not a concern in patients with end-stage renal disease. Meperidine is avoided for postoperative analgesia because its metabolites may accumulate in patients with renal failure and result in seizures.

▮ RENAL EFFECTS OF ANESTHETIC DRUGS

Volatile anesthetics produce similar dose-related decreases in renal blood flow, GFR, and urine output. These changes are not a result of the release of antidiuretic hormone but, rather, likely reflect the effects of volatile anesthetics on systemic blood pressure and cardiac output. Painful stimulation associated with the onset of surgery produces significant increases in circulating levels of antidiuretic hormone, which may contribute to subsequent decreased urine output. Preoperative hydration attenuates or abolishes the increase in antidiuretic hormone concentrations produced by surgical stimulation and many of the changes in renal function associated with the volatile anesthetics. Epidural or spinal anesthesia results in minimal changes in renal blood flow and GFR, assuming renal perfusion pressure is maintained. Anesthetic-induced depression of renal blood flow, GFR, and urine output is transient and usually clinically insignificant.

Fluoride-Induced Nephrotoxicity

Sevoflurane, but not desflurane or isoflurane, undergoes significant metabolism that results in production of inorganic fluoride. Despite the common view that fluoride-induced nephrotoxicity is a risk when the serum inorganic fluoride concentrations exceed $50 \mu mol/L$, there is no evidence that this peak value is a valid indicator of renal dysfunction. It has been postulated that intrarenal production of inorganic fluoride may be a more important factor than hepatic metabolism for the nephrotoxicity that causes increased serum fluoride concentrations, such as follows administration of sevoflurane.[9] This may explain why patients receiving sevoflurane may experience less renal dysfunction than patients receiving enflurane which often results in lower serum inorganic fluoride concentrations than those seen after sevoflurane use. Despite the absence of reported nephrotoxicity following administration of sevoflurane, there is evidence of transient impairment of renal concentrating ability and renal tubular injury (increased urinary excretion of β-N-acetylglucosaminidase) in patients receiving this anesthetic, whereas similar changes do not follow administration of desflurane.[5, 10] More conventional measurements of renal function (serum creatinine, BUN) do not indicate renal dysfunction. Concern that administration of sevoflurane to patients with preexisting renal disease could accentuate renal dysfunction has not been confirmed.[11]

Vinyl Halide Nephrotoxicity

Carbon dioxide absorbents (soda lime, Baralyme) react with sevoflurane to form a degradation product (compound A) that may be nephrotoxic in animals. Nevertheless, concentrations that occur in patients following administration of sevoflurane are far below the nephrotoxic levels in animals. Recommendations to deliver sevoflurane at a total gas flow of 1 L/min or higher are intended to minimize the accumulation of compound A in the breathing circuit.[10] Carbon dioxide absorbents that contain calcium hydroxide and calcium chloride do not result in formation of compound A when exposed to volatile anesthetics, including sevoflurane.

▮ MANAGEMENT OF ANESTHESIA IN PATIENTS WITH CHRONIC RENAL DISEASE

Management of anesthesia in patients with chronic renal disease requires an understanding of the pathologic changes that accompany renal disease and whether the renal disease is sufficient to require hemodialysis (see "Chronic Renal Failure").[11] An important assessment is whether the renal disease is stable, progressing, or diminishing. This information is obtained by monitoring the serum creatinine concentrations.

Preoperative Evaluation

Preoperative evaluation of patients with chronic renal disease includes consideration of concomitant drug therapy and evaluation of the changes deemed characteristic of chronic renal failure (Table 20–4).[6] Blood volume status may be estimated by comparing body weight before and after hemodialysis, monitoring of vital signs (orthostatic hypotension, tachycardia), and measuring atrial filling pressures. Diabetes mellitus is often present in these patients. Insulin replacement regimens may require attention. Signs of digitalis toxicity should be sought in treated patients, emphasizing the role of renal clearance for digitalis and other drugs.

Antihypertensive drug therapy is usually continued. Preoperative medication must be individualized, remembering that these patients may exhibit unexpected sensitivity to central nervous system depressant drugs. In addition to patients with preoperative renal dysfunction, it is important to recognize others who are at high risk for developing perioperative renal failure, even in the absence of co-existing renal disease (see "Risk Factors for Development of Acute Renal Failure"). Preservation of renal function intraoperatively depends on maintaining an adequate intravascular fluid volume and minimizing drug-induced cardiovascular depression.

Patients on hemodialysis should undergo dialysis during the 24 hours preceding elective surgery. Control of systemic hypertension is achieved with antihypertensive drugs and appropriate adjustment of intravascular fluid volume with hemodialysis. A common recommendation is that the serum potassium concentration should not exceed 5.5 mEq/L on the day of surgery.[12] Anemia is evaluated preoperatively, but the introduction of recombinant human erythropoietin therapy has decreased the number of patients in renal failure who present for elective surgery with a hematocrit less than 30%. The preoperative presence of a coagulopathy may be treated with DDAVP.

Induction of Anesthesia

Induction of anesthesia and tracheal intubation can be safely accomplished with intravenous drugs (propofol, etomidate, thiopental) plus a muscle relaxant such as succinylcholine, remembering that these patients may exhibit uremia-induced slowing of gastric emptying. Alternatively, if the possibility of increased gastric fluid volume does not mandate the rapid onset of skeletal muscle paralysis, administration of intermediate- or short-acting nondepolarizing neuromuscular blocking drugs that are independent of renal clearance mechanisms (mivacurium, atracurium, cisatracurium) is a consideration.[13] Logic suggests slow injection of induction drugs to minimize the likelihood of drug-induced decreases in systemic blood pressure. Regardless of blood volume status, these patients often respond to induction of anesthesia as if they were hypovolemic. The likelihood of hypotension during induction of anesthesia may be increased if sympathetic nervous system function is attenuated by antihypertensive drugs or uremia. Attenuated sympathetic nervous system activity impairs compensatory peripheral vasoconstriction; thus small decreases in blood volume, institution of positive-pressure ventilation of the patient's lungs, abrupt changes in body position, or drug-induced myocardial depression can result in an exaggerated decrease in systemic blood pressure. Patients being treated with ACE inhibitors may be at increased risk for experiencing intraoperative hypotension especially with acute surgical blood loss.

Exaggerated central nervous system effects of anesthetic induction drugs may reflect uremia-induced disruption of the blood–brain barrier. Furthermore, decreased protein binding of drugs may result in the availability of more unbound drug to act at receptor sites. Indeed, the amount of pharmacologically active unbound thiopental in plasma is increased in patients with chronic renal failure.

Potassium release following administration of succinylcholine is not exaggerated in patients with chronic renal failure, although there is a theoretical concern that those with extensive uremic neuropathies might be at increased risk. Likewise, caution is indicated when the preoperative serum potassium concentration is in the high-normal range, as this finding combined with maximum drug-induced potassium release (0.5 to 1.0 mEq/L) could result in dangerous hyperkalemia. It is important to recognize that small doses of nondepolarizing muscle relaxants administered before the injection of succinylcholine do not reliably attenuate the succinylcholine-induced release of potassium.

Maintenance of Anesthesia

In patients with chronic renal disease who are not dependent on hemodialysis or in those vulnerable to renal dysfunction because of advanced age or the need for major thoracic or abdominal vascular surgery, anesthesia is often maintained with nitrous oxide combined with isoflurane, desflurane, or short-acting opioids. Sevoflurane may be avoided because of concerns related to fluoride nephrotoxicity or production of compound A, although there is no evidence that patients with co-existing renal disease are at increased risk for renal dysfunction following administration of sevoflurane (see "Renal Effects of Anesthetic Drugs"). Isoflurane or desflurane combined with nitrous oxide provides sufficient potency to suppress excessive increases in systemic blood pressure due to surgical stimulation, to avoid the controversy related to fluoride nephrotoxicity, and to decrease the dose of nondepolarizing muscle relaxants needed to produce skeletal muscle relaxation. Total intravenous anesthesia with remifentanil, propofol, and cisatracurium has been recommended for patients with end-stage renal failure.[14]

Potent volatile anesthetics are useful for controlling intraoperative systemic hypertension and decreasing the doses of muscle relaxants needed for adequate surgical relaxation. The high incidence of associated liver disease in patients with chronic renal disease should be considered, however, when selecting these drugs. Furthermore, excessive depression of cardiac output is a potential hazard of volatile anesthetics. Decreases in tissue blood flow must be minimized in the presence of anemia to avoid jeopardizing oxygen delivery to the tissues. Opioids decrease the likelihood of cardiovascular depression and avoid the concern of hepatotoxicity or nephrotoxicity. Nevertheless, opioids do not reliably control intraoperative systemic blood pressure elevations. Furthermore, prolonged sedation and depression of ventilation from small doses of opioids have been described in anephric patients. Conceivably, pharmacologically active metabolites of opioids accumulate in the circulation and cerebrospinal fluid when renal function is absent.

When systemic hypertension does not respond to adjustments in the depth of anesthesia, it may be appropriate to administer vasodilators, such as hydralazine or nitroprusside. Cyanide produced from the breakdown of nitroprusside is unlikely to cause toxicity in these patients. Indeed, animal data have demonstrated resistance to the development of cyanide toxicity in the absence of renal function. The most likely explanation for this resistance is decreased renal excretion of thiosulfate, which serves as an endogenous sulfur donor and facilitates conversion of cyanide to thiocyanate.

Ventilation of the patient's lungs during general anesthesia should be designed to maintain normocapnia and minimize the effects of positive intrathoracic pressure on cardiac output. Hypoventilation with resulting respiratory acidosis is undesirable, as decreases in arterial pH can result in the transfer of potassium from cells into the circulation, accentuating hyperkalemia. Conversely, respiratory alkalosis from hyperventilation of the lungs shifts the oxyghemoglobin dissociation curve to the left and decreases oxygen availability to the tissues. This change is particularly undesirable in patients with anemia. Changes in cardiac output produced by positive-pressure ventilation of the lungs can be minimized by using a slow breathing rate to permit sufficient time for venous return during pauses between mechanical breaths.

Meticulous attention is needed for management of ventilation and intravenous fluid replacement. Normocapnia is desirable, as hyperventilation of the lungs with associated respiratory alkalosis adversely affects the position of the oxyghemoglobin dissociation curve, whereas respiratory acidosis from hypoventilation could result in acute increases in serum potassium concentrations. Monitoring the ECG is important for recognizing signs of hyperkalemia. Arteriovenous shunts must be carefully protected to ensure continued patency during the perioperative period.

Muscle Relaxants

Selection of nondepolarizing muscle relaxants for maintenance of skeletal muscle paralysis during surgery is influenced by the known clearance mechanisms of these drugs. Renal disease may slow excretion of vecuronium and rocuronium, whereas clearance of mivacurium, atracurium, and cisatracurium from plasma is independent of renal function. Renal failure may delay clearance of laudanosine, the principal metabolite of atracurium and cisatracurium. Laudanosine lacks effects at the neuromuscular junction, but at high plasma concentrations it may stimulate the central nervous system. Regardless of the nondepolarizing neuromuscular blocking drug selected, it seems prudent to decrease the initial dose of the drug and administer subsequent doses on the basis of the responses observed using a peripheral nerve stimulator.

The diagnosis of residual neuromuscular blockade after apparent reversal of nondepolarizing neuromuscular blockade with anticholinesterase drugs should be considered in anephric patients who manifest signs of skeletal muscle weakness during the early postoperative period. In normal patients whose neuromuscular blockade is adequately reversed with anticholinesterase drugs, neuromuscular blockade does not reappear because continued renal elimination of the neuromuscular blocking drug offsets waning effects of the anticholinesterase drug. Renal excretion accounts for about 50% of the clearance of neostigmine and about 75% of the elimination of edrophonium and pyridostigmine. As a result, the elimination half-time of these drugs is greatly prolonged by renal failure. Even in anephric patients, there is some protection because renal elimination of anticholinesterase drugs is delayed as long as, if not longer than, that of the nondepolarizing neuromuscular blocking drugs. Indeed, other explanations (antibiotics, acidosis, electrolyte imbalance, diuretics) should be considered when neuromuscular blockade persists or reappears in patients with renal dysfunction.

Fluid Management and Urine Output

Patients with severe renal dysfunction but not requiring hemodialysis and those without renal disease undergoing operations associated with a high incidence of postoperative renal failure may benefit from preoperative hydration with administration of balanced salt solutions, 10 to 20 ml/kg IV. Indeed, most patients come to the operating room with a contracted extracellular fluid volume unless corrective measures are taken. Lactated Ringer's solution (potassium 4 mEq/L) or other potassium-containing fluids should not be administered to anuric patients. Administration of balanced salt solutions, 3 to 5 ml/kg/hr IV, is often recommended to maintain acceptable urine output. Rapid infusion of balanced salt solutions (500 ml IV) should increase urine output in the presence of hypovolemia. Stimulation of urine output with osmotic (mannitol) or tubular (furosemide) diuretics in the absence of adequate intravascular fluid volume replacement is discouraged. Indeed, the most likely etiology of oliguria is an inadequate circulating fluid volume, which can only be further compromised by drug-induced diuresis. Furthermore, although administration of mannitol or furosemide predictably increases urine output, there is no evidence of corresponding improvements in the GFR. Likewise, intraoperative urine output has not been shown to be predictive of postoperative renal insufficiency after abdominal vascular surgery.

If fluid replacement does not restore urine output, a diagnosis of congestive heart failure may be considered. Dopamine, 0.5 to 3.0 μg/kg/min IV, increases renal blood flow, the GFR, and urine output in normovolemic patients by stimulating renal dopaminergic receptors. This drug-induced diuresis is associated with natriuresis and kaliuresis. Higher doses of dopamine (3 to 10 μg/kg/min IV) stimulate β-receptors, making this drug useful for treating oliguria due to congestive heart failure. Although not always possible, it is helpful for confirming the diagnosis of congestive heart failure and the beneficial responses to drugs with measurements obtained from a pulmonary artery catheter. Another consideration in the differential diagnosis of oliguria is mechanical obstruction of the urinary catheter or pooling of urine in the dome of the bladder in response to the head-down position.

Patients dependent on hemodialysis require special attention with respect to perioperative fluid management. An absence of renal function narrows the margin of safety between insufficient and excessive fluid administration to these patients. Noninvasive operations require replacement of only insensible water losses with 5% glucose in water (5 to 10 ml/kg IV). The small amount of urine output can be replaced with 0.45% sodium chloride. Thoracic or abdominal surgery can be associated with loss of significant intravascular fluid volume to the interstitial spaces. This loss is often replaced with balanced salt solutions or 5% albumin solutions. Blood transfusions may be considered if the oxygen-carrying capacity must be increased or if blood loss is excessive. Measuring the central venous pressure may be useful for guiding fluid replacement.

Monitoring

Minor surgical procedures can be monitored by noninvasive methods. Permanent vascular shunts should be protected, and their patency may be monitored with a Doppler sensor to confirm continued patency during the operative procedure.

Continuous monitoring of intra-arterial blood pressure is helpful when major operative procedures are being performed. A femoral or dorsalis pedis artery is often used, as patients may require the availability of arteries in the upper extremity for future placement of vascular shunts. Intravenous fluid replacement is guided by central venous pressure measurements and urine output. A pulmonary artery catheter is useful if interpretation of the central venous pressure measurements is questionable, as in the presence of co-existing chronic obstructive airway disease or left ventricular dysfunction. Furthermore, thermodilution cardiac output measurements and systemic vascular resistance calculations can be helpful in guiding doses of anesthetic drugs and recognizing the need for inotropic drugs, such as dopamine. Strict asepsis is mandatory when placing intravascular catheters, such as those used to measure systemic blood pressure or cardiac filling pressures.

Regional Anesthesia

Brachial plexus block is useful for placing the vascular shunts necessary for chronic hemodialysis. In addition to providing analgesia, this form of regional anesthesia abolishes vasospasm and provides optimal surgical conditions by producing maximal vascular vasodilation. The suggestion that the duration of brachial plexus anesthesia is shortened in patients with chronic renal failure has not been confirmed in controlled studies. Adequacy of coagulation should be considered and the presence of uremic neuropathies excluded before regional anesthesia is performed in these patients. Co-existing metabolic acidosis may decrease the seizure threshold for local anesthetics.

Postoperative Management

A diagnosis of recurarization should be considered in anephric patients who show signs of skeletal muscle weakness during the postoperative period. A weak hand grip or inability to maintain head lift and improvement after administration of edrophonium, 5 to 10 mg IV, confirms the diagnosis.

Systemic hypertension is a common problem during the postoperative period. Hemodialysis is useful if hypervolemia is the cause. Vasodilators (nitroprusside, hydralazine, labetalol) are helpful until excess fluid can be removed by hemodialysis.

Caution is indicated in the use of parenteral opioids for postoperative analgesia in view of a potential for exaggerated central nervous system depression and hypoventilation after administration of even small doses of opioids. Administration of naloxone may be necessary if the depression of ventilation is severe. Continuous monitoring of the ECG is helpful for detecting cardiac dysrhythmias, such as those related to hyperkalemia. Continuation of supplemental oxygen into the postoperative period is a consideration, especially if anemia is present.

◼ ACUTE RENAL FAILURE

Acute renal failure is characterized by deterioration of renal function over a period of hours to days, resulting in failure of the kidneys to excrete nitrogenous waste products and to maintain fluid and electrolyte homeostasis.[15, 16] Commonly used definitions of acute renal failure include increases in serum creatine concentrations of more than 0.5 mg/dl compared with the baseline value, a 50% decrease in the calculated creatinine clearance, or decreased renal function that results in the need for dialysis. Acute renal failure may be oliguric (urinary output less than 400 ml per day) or nonoliguric (urinary output more than 400 ml per day). Despite major advances in dialysis therapy and critical care, the mortality

rate among patients with severe acute renal failure (primarily ischemic in origin) requiring dialysis remains high and has not decreased greatly over the last 50 years.[16–18] This observation can be explained by the fact that, compared with patients 50 years ago, patients today are often elderly and have multiple co-existing diseases. When acute renal failure occurs in the setting of multiorgan failure, especially in patients with severe hypotension or respiratory failure, the mortality rate often exceeds 50%. The most common causes of death are sepsis, cardiovascular dysfunction, and pulmonary complications.

Etiology

The etiology of acute renal failure may be classified as prerenal, renal (intrinsic), and postrenal (obstructive) azotemia (Table 20–8, Fig. 20–1).[15, 16] Prerenal failure and intrinsic renal failure due to ischemia or nephrotoxins are responsible for most episodes of acute renal failure. Frequently encountered combinations of acute events that predispose to the development of acute renal failure include exposure to aminoglycoside antibiotics in the presence of sepsis, administration of radiographic contrast dyes in patients taking ACE inhibitors, or treatment with NSAIDs in the presence of congestive heart failure.

Table 20–8 • Causes of Acute Renal Failure

Prerenal azotemia (decreased renal blood flow)
  Absolute decrease in blood volume
    Acute hemorrhage
    Gastrointestinal fluid loss
    Trauma
    Surgery
    Burns
  Relative decrease in blood volume
    Sepsis
    Hepatic failure
    Allergic reaction
Renal azotemia (intrinsic)
  Acute glomerulonephritis (5% of cases)
  Interstitial nephritis (drugs, sepsis) (10% of cases)
  Acute tubular necrosis (85% of cases)
    Ischemia (50% of cases)
    Nephrotoxic drugs (antibiotics, anesthetic drugs?)
      (35% of cases)
    Solvents (carbon tetrachloride, ethylene glycol)
    Radiographic contrast dyes
    Myoglobinuria
Postrenal (obstructive)
  Upper urinary tract obstruction (ureteral)
  Lower urinary tract obstruction (bladder outlet)

Adapted from: Klahr S, Miller SB. Acute oliguria. N Engl J Med 1998;338:671–5; Thadhani R, Pascual M, Bonventre JV. Acute renal failure. N Engl J Med 1996;334:1148–69.

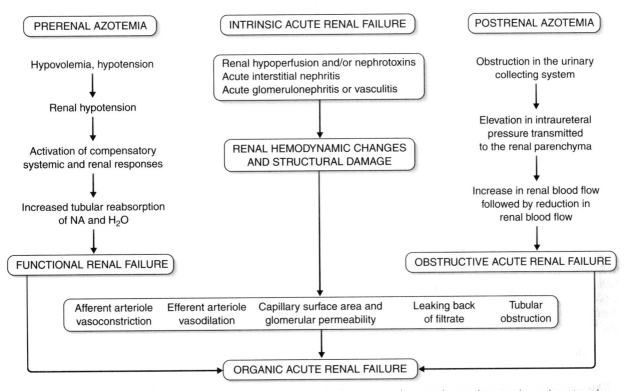

Figure 20–1 • Causes of acute renal failure can be categorized as prerenal azotemia, renal azotemia, and postrenal azotemia. Exclusion of prerenal and postrenal causes of acute renal failure make the most likely etiology a renal cause that is often associated with a high incidence of morbidity and mortality.

Prerenal Azotemia

Prerenal azotemia accounts for nearly half of hospital-acquired cases of acute renal failure. Sustained prerenal azotemia is the most common factor that predisposes patients to ischemia-induced acute tubular necrosis. Prerenal azotemia is rapidly reversible if the underlying cause (hypovolemia, congestive heart failure) is corrected. Elderly patients are uniquely susceptible to prerenal azotemia because of their predisposition to hypovolemia (poor fluid intake) and high incidence of renovascular disease. Among hospitalized patients, prerenal azotemia is often due to congestive heart failure, liver dysfunction, or septic shock. Renal blood flow may be a result of anesthetic drug-induced decreases in perfusion pressure particularly in the presence of hypovolemia associated with the intraoperative period.

Assessment of blood volume status, hemodynamics, and drug therapy may result in identification of potential prerenal causes of acute oliguria. Invasive monitoring (central venous pressure, pulmonary artery catheter) may be necessary to assess the intravascular fluid volume. Renal ultrasonography is the best diagnostic test for determining the presence of obstructive nephropathy. Urinary indices may help distinguish prerenal from intrinsic acute renal failure (Table 20–9).[15] The use of urinary indices is based on the assumption that the ability of renal tubules to reabsorb sodium and water is maintained in the presence of prerenal causes of acute renal failure, whereas these functions are impaired in the presence of tubulointerstitial disease or acute tubular necrosis. Blood and urine specimens for determination of urinary indices must be obtained before the administration of fluids, dopamine, mannitol, or other diuretic drugs.

Renal Azotemia

Intrinsic renal diseases that result in acute renal failure are categorized according to the primary site of injury (renal tubules, interstitium, glomerulus, renal vasculature). Injury to the renal tubules is most often due to ischemia or nephrotoxins (aminoglycoside antibiotics, radiographic contrast agents). Prerenal azotemia and ischemic tubular necrosis present as a continuum with the initial prerenal-induced decreases in renal blood flow leading to ischemia of the renal tubular cells. The principal functional de-

Table 20-9 • Characteristic Urinary Indices in Patients with Acute Oliguria Due to Prerenal or Renal Causes

Index	Prerenal Causes	Renal Causes
Urinary sodium concentration (mEq/L)	< 20	> 40
Fractional excretion of sodium (%)	< 1	> 1
Urine osmolarity (mOsm/L)	> 400	250–300
Urine creatinine/plasma creatinine	> 40	< 20
Urine/plasma osmolarity	> 1.5	< 1.1

Adapted from: Klahr S, Miller SB. Acute oliguria. N Engl J Med 1998;338:671–5.

rangements in patients with acute oliguria are sudden and profound decreases in GFR that are sufficient to cause acute renal failure manifesting as increased serum urea and creatinine concentrations, retention of sodium and water, and development of acidosis and hyperkalemia. Although most cases of ischemic acute renal failure are reversible if the underlying cause is corrected, irreversible cortical necrosis can occur if the ischemia is severe or prolonged. Ischemia and toxins often combine to cause acute renal failure in severely ill patients with conditions such as sepsis or AIDS. Acute renal failure due to acute interstitial nephritis is most often caused by allergic reactions to drugs.

Postrenal Azotemia

Acute renal failure occurs when urinary outflow tracts are obstructed, as with prostatic hypertrophy or cancer of the prostate or cervix. It is important to diagnose postrenal causes of acute renal failure promptly, as the potential for recovery often parallels the duration of the obstruction. Percutaneous nephrostomy can relieve the obstruction and may improve the outcome. Renal ultrasonography is the best diagnostic test for determining the presence of obstructive nephropathy.

Risk Factors for Development of Acute Renal Failure

Risk factors for the development of acute renal failure include co-existing renal disease, advanced age, congestive heart failure, symptomatic cardiovascular disease that is likely to be associated with renovascular disease, and major operative procedures (cardiopulmonary bypass, abdominal aneurysm resection).[1, 15, 17, 19] Sepsis and multiple organ system dysfunction due to trauma introduce the risk of acute renal failure. Iatrogenic components that predispose to acute renal failure include inadequate fluid replacement, delayed treatment of sepsis, and

administration of nephrotoxic drugs or dyes. The incidence of radiographic contrast dye-induced acute renal failure may approach 50% in patients with diabetes mellitus or co-existing renal disease.[20]

Appropriate hydration and optimal preservation of the intravascular fluid volume are essential to maintain adequate renal perfusion. It is also important to maintain adequate systemic blood pressure and cardiac output and to prevent peripheral vasoconstriction. Hypotension may result in inadequate renal perfusion and loss of renal autoregulation. Potentially nephrotoxic substances (NSAIDs, aminoglycosides, radiographic contrast dyes, ACE inhibitors, general anesthetics) are logically avoided in patients with prerenal oliguria, and diuretic therapy may be detrimental in these patients. Prophylactic administration of furosemide or mannitol prior to injection of radiographic contrast dyes may decrease renal function further rather than protect it. Conversely, prior administration of acetylcysteine, a thio-containing antioxidant that acts as a free radical scavenger, may provide protection against radiographic dye-induced nephropathy.[20]

Complications

Complications of acute renal failure may manifest in the central nervous system, cardiovascular system, and gastrointestinal system.[15] In addition, infections occur frequently in patients who develop acute renal failure and are leading causes of morbidity and mortality. Drugs known to be excreted by the kidneys (cephalosporins, digoxin, diazepam, propranolol) should be avoided or the doses adjusted in proportion to the decrease in renal function.

Neurologic complications of acute renal failure include confusion, asterixis, somnolence, and seizures. These changes may be ameliorated by dialysis.

Cardiovascular complications include systemic hypertension, congestive heart failure, and pulmonary edema principally as reflections of sodium and water retention. Hypotension is also commonly encountered. Cardiac dysrhythmias may occur. Pericarditis appears to be less common than in the past. The presence of systemic hypertension, congestive heart failure, or pulmonary edema suggests the need to decrease the intravascular fluid volume. Acute renal failure is accompanied by anemia with hematocrit values between 20% and 30%.

Gastrointestinal complications include anorexia, nausea, vomiting, and ileus. Gastrointestinal bleeding occurs in as many as one-third of patients who develop acute renal failure and may contribute to anemia in patients with acute renal failure. Administration of H_2-receptor antagonists may decrease the risk of gastrointestinal bleeding.

Primary sites of *infection* include the respiratory and urinary tracts and sites where breaks in normal anatomic barriers have occurred owing to indwelling catheters.[15] Impaired immune responses due to uremia may contribute to the increased likelihood of infections in patients who develop acute renal failure. Preventing infection requires frequently monitoring the body temperature, minimal use of instrumentation or devices that interrupt normal anatomic barriers, early ambulation, use of aseptic techniques, and careful skin and mouth care.

Management of Acute Renal Failure

Acute oliguric renal failure, especially that acquired in the hospital, is associated with high morbidity and mortality. In addition, the costs of caring for patients with acute renal failure are high.[17] A variety of therapies have shown promise in animal models only to show disappointing results in patients. Conversion from oliguric to nonoliguric renal failure has been considered beneficial, which is the rationale for administering diuretics or dopamine (selective renal vasodilator drug that causes natriuresis) to patients with acute oliguria. The presumed benefits of conversion to a nonoliguric state include less stringent restrictions on sodium and water intake, a decreased need for dialysis, and perhaps an improved prognosis.[15]

When acute oliguria occurs in hospitalized patients it is important to rule out prerenal or postrenal causes promptly and, when possible, to discontinue drugs with known nephrotoxic potential.[1] Management of acute oliguria during the perioperative period often begins with a fluid challenge (amount determined on an individual basis) especially if the patient is considered to be at risk for acute renal failure and is not hypervolemic (Fig. 20–2). Administration of a loop diuretic, furosemide 100 to 200 mg IV, is an acceptable consideration if the response to the fluid challenge is inadequate.[15] If the diuretic

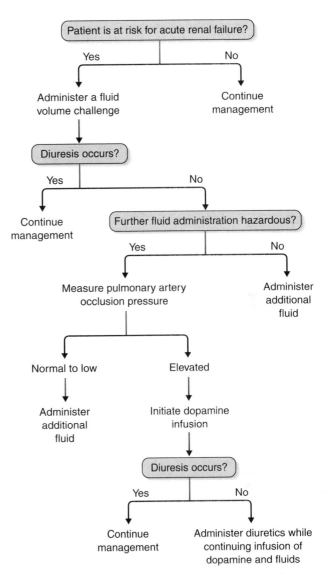

Figure 20–2 • Treatment algorithm for management of acute oliguria during the perioperative period.

evokes a response, it is important to monitor the intravascular fluid volume, electrolyte concentrations, and hemodynamic status. Diuretic therapy should not be continued if oliguria persists. The benefit of dopamine therapy, 1 to 3 μg/kg/min IV, as prophylaxis against the development of acute renal failure or for treatment of acute renal failure is controversial.[21] Expansion of extracellular fluid volume with crystalloids may be as effective as prophylactic administration of diuretics or dopamine in patients at high risk for developing acute renal failure. In selected patients to whom dopamine is administered, a diuretic response may be evident within the first 6 hours of therapy. If urinary output does not increase during this time, dopamine should be discontinued, as undesirable side effects (depression of the carotid body response to arterial hypoxemia, cardiac dysrhythmias) may occur.[22] Fenoldopam is a dopamine-1 agonist and α_2-agonist that is devoid of any activity at β-receptors. As such, fenoldopam is a vasodilator in many organs including the afferent and efferent renal vasculature. Administration of fenoldopam increases urine output and lowers excessively increased systolic blood pressure, but there is no evidence that it is a beneficial treatment for acute renal failure.

Dialysis

When the diagnosis of intrinsic acute renal failure is established, therapeutic interventions are confined to supportive care and institution of dialysis in an effort to normalize extracellular fluid volume and electrolyte concentrations and to control hyperkalemia and metabolic acidosis.[15] The appropriate frequency and duration of dialysis for acute renal failure have not been determined. It is possible that hypotension during dialysis could exacerbate the renal injury and slow the recovery of renal tubular cells. An alternative to intermittent dialysis and the associated risks of hypotension is continuous renal replacement therapy, which has the benefit of slow, controlled ultrafiltration with a marked decrease in the incidence of hypotension. The selection of dialysis membranes may also be important in patients with acute renal failure. Cellulose membranes may activate complement and lead to mobilization of leukocytes with adverse effects on patients.[15]

Protein Intake

Adequate protein and caloric intake is important in patients with acute oliguria.[15] Protein catabolism may be excessive in patients with acute renal failure, particularly those who are in shock or are septic. Increased protein catabolism may accelerate the rate of increase in serum potassium concentrations and the development of metabolic acidosis in patients with acute renal failure. A negative nitrogen balance may result in malnutrition and impaired immune defense mechanisms. Nutritional therapy, often in the form of total parenteral nutrition, should be initiated early in the treatment of acute renal failure.

▌ PRIMARY DISEASES OF THE KIDNEYS

A number of pathologic processes can primarily involve the kidneys or occur in association with dysfunction of other organ systems. Knowledge of the associated pathology and characteristics of the renal disease may be important when planning management of these patients during the perioperative period.

Glomerulonephritis

Acute glomerulonephritis is usually due to deposition of antigen-antibody complexes in the glomeruli. The source of antigens may be exogenous (poststreptococcal infection) or endogenous (collagen diseases). Clinical manifestations of glomerular diseases include hematuria, proteinuria, hypertension, edema, and increased plasma creatinine concentrations. Red blood cell casts are suggestive of glomerular disease, rather than of nonglomerular disease, such as nephrolithiasis or prostatic disease. Proteinuria reflects an increase in glomerular permeability. It is important to diagnose glomerulonephritis quickly, as prompt use of immunosuppressive drugs may be efficacious.

Nephrotic Syndrome

The nephrotic syndrome is defined by daily urinary protein excretion exceeding 3.5 g associated with sodium retention, hyperlipoproteinemia, and thromboembolic and infectious complications.[23] Diabetic nephropathy is the most common cause of nephrotic proteinuria. In the absence of diabetes, the most common cause of nephrotic syndrome in adults is membranous glomerulonephritis, which is frequently associated with neoplasia (carcinoma, sarcoma, lymphoma, leukemia). Human immunodeficiency virus (HIV) nephropathy typically causes nephrotic proteinuria and renal insufficiency, which may be the first clinical manifestation of AIDS. Pregnancy-induced hypertension is often associated with nephrotic syndrome.

Signs and Symptoms

Sodium retention and edema formation in patients with nephrotic syndrome have been presumed to reflect decreased plasma oncotic pressure with resultant hypovolemia. Increased tubular reabsorption of sodium was assumed to be a homeostatic response to hypovolemia. Nevertheless, there is evidence that the primary event is initial sodium retention by the kidneys that precedes proteinuria.[23] Increased sodium reabsorption by the distal renal tubules may be due to an inappropriately low natriuretic response to atrial natriuretic peptide. Patients with nephrotic syndrome may experience hypovolemia with associated orthostatic hypotension, tachycardia, peripheral vasoconstriction, and occasionally even acute renal failure in response to the administration of diuretics. The risk of acute renal failure is increased in elderly patients and those who receive NSAIDs. Infusion of albumin corrects the clinical signs of hypovolemia. Hyperlipidemia accompanies nephrotic syndrome and may be associated with an increased risk of vascular disease.

Thromboembolic Complications. Thromboembolic complications manifesting as renal vein thrombosis are major risks of the nephrotic syndrome, particularly in patients with membranous glomerulonephritis. Pulmonary embolism and deep vein thrombosis in other vascular beds are also hazards. Arterial thrombosis is less common than venous thrombosis, although the risk of acute myocardial infarction in these patients may be increased. Prophylactic administration of heparin and support stockings are utilized to protect against thromboembolic complications.

Infection. Pneumococcal peritonitis has been responsible for fatalities in children with nephrotic syndrome. Viral infections may be more likely in immunosuppressed patients, whereas susceptibility to bacterial infections seems to be related to decreased levels of immunoglobulin G.

Protein Binding. Plasma levels of vitamins and hormones may be decreased in patients with nephrotic syndrome as a result of proteinuria. Hypoalbuminemia decreases the available binding sites for drugs and increases the proportion of circulating free drug. In this regard, when plasma drug levels are monitored, low levels of highly protein-bound drugs do not necessarily indicate low therapeutic concentrations.

Treatment

Treatment of nephrotic syndrome is directed at managing edema and reducing proteinuria.

Nephrotic Edema. Generalized edema implies that total body sodium content is increased, and stimulation of a negative sodium balance by administering diuretics is enhanced by dietary decreases in sodium intake. Potent loop diuretics such as furosemide are needed to offset the kidney's avidity to retain sodium. In addition, thiazide diuretics or potassium-sparing diuretics may be added to decrease sodium reabsorption in the distal nephrons. The goal is to decrease edema slowly, as abrupt natriuresis may cause hypovolemia and even acute renal failure; it may also produce hemoconcentration, increasing the risk of thromboembolic complications. Administration of albumin solutions to expand the plasma volume is considered only if symptomatic hypovolemia is present. In particularly severe cases, plasma ultrafiltration may be considered.

Proteinuria. Proteinuria is a predictor of rapidly progressive renal failure, and its management is considered important in the prevention of acute renal failure. In addition to dietary protein restriction, the administration of ACE inhibitors often produces antiproteinuric effects. Blood pressure-lowering effects of ACE inhibitors are present within a few hours, but the antiproteinuric effect may take as long as 28 days to be maximal.[23] ACE inhibitors, by decreasing urinary protein losses, also decrease cholesterol and lipid concentrations.

Nonspecific Interventions. Idiopathic nephrotic syndrome often responds to treatment with corticosteroids. If the response to corticosteroids is not adequate, administration of cyclophosphamide, cyclosporine, or chlorambucil is a consideration.

Goodpasture Syndrome

Goodpasture syndrome is a combination of pulmonary hemorrhage and glomerulonephritis, occurring most often in young males. Antibodies account for renal lesions and apparently react also with similar antigens in the lungs, producing alveolitis, which results in hemoptysis. Typically, hemoptysis precedes clinical evidence of renal disease. The prognosis is poor, with no known effective therapy to prevent progression to renal failure usually within 1 year of the diagnosis.

Interstitial Nephritis

Interstitial nephritis has been observed as an allergic reaction to drugs, including sulfonamides, allopurinol, phenytoin, and diuretics. Other, less common causes include autoimmune diseases (lupus erythematosus) and infiltrative diseases (sarcoidosis). Patients exhibit decreased urine concentrating ability, proteinuria, and systemic hypertension. Renal failure due to acute interstitial nephritis is often reversible after withdrawal of the offending drug or treatment of the underlying disease. Corticosteroid therapy may be beneficial.

Hereditary Nephritis

Hereditary nephritis (Alport syndrome) is often accompanied by hearing loss and ocular abnormalities. Males are afflicted more often, with the disease culminating in systemic hypertension and renal failure. Drug therapy has not proven successful, although lowering the intraglomerular pressure with ACE inhibitors may offer some protection.

Polycystic Renal Disease

Polycystic renal disease is inherited as an autosomal dominant trait. The disease typically progresses slowly until renal failure occurs during middle age. Mild systemic hypertension and proteinuria are common. Decreased urine concentrating ability develops early in the course of the disease. Cysts may also be present in the liver and in the central nervous system as intracranial aneurysms. Hemodialysis or renal transplantation is eventually necessary in most of these patients.

Fanconi Syndrome

Fanconi syndrome results from inherited or acquired disturbances of proximal renal tubular function, causing hyperaminoaciduria, glycosuria, and hyperphosphaturia. There is renal loss of substances normally conserved by proximal renal tubules, including potassium, bicarbonate, and water. The symptoms of Fanconi syndrome, which reflect the abnormality of the renal tubules, include polyuria, polydipsia, metabolic acidosis due to loss of bicarbonate ions, and skeletal muscle weakness related to hypokalemia. Dwarfism and osteomalacia, reflecting loss of phosphate, is prominent in these patients. Presentation as vitamin D-resistant rickets is common. Management of anesthesia includes evaluation of fluid and electrolyte disorders characteristic of this syndrome and the recognition that left ventricular cardiac failure secondary to uremia is often present in the final stages.[24]

Bartter Syndrome

Bartter syndrome (congenital hypokalemic alkalosis) is characterized by hypokalemic, hypochloremic, metabolic alkalosis in the presence of increased circulating concentrations of renin and aldosterone and the paradoxical absence of systemic hypertension.[25] Clinical features that appear during infancy or childhood include anorexia, failure to thrive (most common presenting feature of early infancy), polyuria, polydipsia, and skeletal muscle weakness due to hypokalemia. This syndrome may be inherited as an autosomal recessive trait.

Pathogenesis

The pathogenesis of Bartter syndrome is unclear but is thought to be related to a defect in chloride reabsorption. This defect results in presentation of increased loads of sodium chloride to the distal renal tubules, where the sodium is reabsorbed in exchange for potassium, resulting in increased urinary potassium loss. Hyperaldosteronism manifests as hypokalemic alkalosis; and in some patients hypokalemia is further exaggerated by renal tubular defects in potassium conservation. Metabolic alkalosis further potentiates hypokalemia by stimulating the intracellular transfer of potassium. Increased arterial pH causes a shift of the oxyhemoglobin dissociation curve to the left with resultant increased oxygen binding to hemoglobin and less oxygen unloading at the tissues. Other adverse effects of metabolic alkalosis include decreased serum ionized calcium concentrations and increased susceptibility to seizures.

Juxtaglomerular cell hyperplasia is prominent, which may in part be due to hypovolemia caused by sodium wasting. Depletion of intravascular fluid volume is an important factor in maintaining metabolic alkalosis. In addition, hypokalemia and skeletal muscle weakness are often present when hypovolemia complicates metabolic alkalosis. Overproduction of prostaglandins is recognized as a secondary phenomenon that occurs with any condition of profound, prolonged potassium depletion. Prostaglandins, in turn, activate the renin-angiotensin-aldosterone system by increasing renin release and stimulating aldosterone synthesis.

Treatment

Treatment of Bartter syndrome includes supplemental potassium chloride to treat hypokalemia.[25, 26] Potassium replacement alone may be inadequate to correct symptomatic hypokalemia, and administration of potassium-sparing diuretics (spironolactone) is added. Metabolic alkalosis is treated by restoring the intravascular fluid volume. Serum chloride and bicarbonate concentrations may be used to guide the adequacy of fluid replacement and correction of metabolic alkalosis.

Management of Anesthesia

Acid-base and electrolyte abnormalities (hypokalemia, hypochloremia, metabolic alkalosis) that may accompany Bartter syndrome have implications for anesthesia management. Although chronic asymptomatic hypokalemia may be benign, it is often recommended that supplemental potassium be administered during the preoperative period in an attempt to increase serum potassium concentrations to near 2.5 mEq/L. Preoperative anxiety may contribute to hypokalemia, and anxiolytic preoperative premedication seems prudent. The impact of co-existing hypokalemia on the response to neuromuscular blocking drugs is a consideration, and monitoring with a peripheral nerve stimulator is encouraged. Hypokalemia may be associated with ileus and delayed gastric emptying due to smooth muscle weakness, introducing the risk of pulmonary aspiration. Cardiac dysrhythmias may reflect the effects of hypokalemia or cardiac electrical activity. Hyperventilation of the patient's lungs is avoided, as it could further potentiate metabolic alkalosis and hypokalemia. Resistance to vasopressors in these patients has been attributed to the effects of prostaglandins. Hemodynamic stability in the presence of anesthetic drugs, especially volatile anesthetics and regional anesthesia, may be influenced by co-existing hypovolemia and altered baroreceptor activity. A brisk diuresis with associated loss of potassium may occur during the perioperative period, requiring careful monitoring of acid-base and electrolyte status.

Nephrolithiasis

Although the pathogenesis of renal stones is poorly understood, several predisposing factors are recognized for the five major types of stones (Table 20–10).[27] Most stones are composed of calcium oxalate; and the causes of hypercalcemia (hyperparathyroidism, sarcoidosis, cancer) must be considered in these patients. Urinary tract infections with urea-splitting organisms that produce ammonia favors the formation of magnesium ammonium phosphate stones. Formation of uric acid stones is favored by a persistently acidic urine (pH less than 6.0) that decreases

the solubility of uric acid. About 50% of patients with uric acid stones have gout.

Stones in the renal pelvis are typically painless unless they are complicated by infection or obstruction. By contrast, renal stones passing down the ureter can produce intense flank pain, often radiating to the groin, associated with nausea and vomiting and mimicking an acute surgical abdomen. Hematuria is common during ureteral passage of stones, whereas ureteral obstruction may lead to signs and symptoms of renal failure.

Treatment

Treatment for renal stones depends on identifying the composition of the stone and correcting the predisposing factors, such as hyperparathyroidism, urinary tract infection, or gout. High fluid intake sufficient to maintain daily urine output at 2 to 3 L is often part of the therapy. Extracorporeal shockwave lithotripsy (ESWL) is a noninvasive treatment for renal stones that destroys the stones by shock waves. As an alternative to percutaneous nephrolithotomy, this approach has the advantages of being associated with low morbidity and being performed on an outpatient basis. Patients undergoing ESWL are placed in a hydraulically operated chair-lift support device and submerged in water (electrohydraulic lithotripsy) from the clavicles down in a large immersion tub. The water transmits the carefully focused shock wave to the patient. Alternatively, nonimmersion lithotriptors generate shock waves within a "shock tube" that is coupled to the patient's body with a water cushion, thereby eliminating the waterbath and the potential undesirable side effects associated with immersion. Contraindications to ESWL include pregnancy, morbid obesity, aortic aneurysm, and coagulopathy. The presence of an arti-

Table 20–10 • Composition and Characteristics of Renal Stones

Type of Stone	Incidence (%)	Radiographic Appearance	Etiology
Calcium oxalate	65	Opaque	Primary hyperparathyroidism Idiopathic hypercalciuria Hyperoxaluria Hyperuricosuria
Magnesium ammonium phosphate (struvite)	20	Opaque	Alkaline urine (usually due to chronic bacterial infection)
Calcium phosphate	7.5	Opaque	Renal tubular acidosis
Uric acid	5	Lucent	Acid urine Gout Hyperuricosuria
Cystine	1.5	Opaque	Cystinuria

ficial cardiac pacemaker does not prohibit treatment with lithotripsy.[28]

Placing patients in a waterbath during ESWL produces several physiologic changes. Immersion causes peripheral venous compression, resulting in increased central blood volume and central venous pressure. Despite the increase in central venous pressure, some patients experience hypotension due to vasodilation from the warm water. Hypotension may also occur during removal from the waterbath. In view of the physiologic changes, patients with severe heart disease may be at risk for developing congestive heart failure or myocardial ischemia when placed in the waterbath. For patients at risk of cardiovascular problems, immersion should be achieved in graded steps or consideration should be given to utilizing a nonimmersion lithotriptor.

Cardiac dysrhythmias may occur during immersion or emersion, presumably reflecting abrupt changes in the right atrial pressure as a result of rapid changes in venous return to the heart. To minimize the risk of initiating cardiac dysrhythmias, shock waves are triggered from the ECG to occur 20 ms after the R wave, ensuring that the shock wave is delivered to the kidney during the absolute refractory period of the heart.

Immersion lithotripsy increases the work of breathing, and breathing by awake patients often becomes shallow and rapid. Extrinsic pressure on the chest and abdomen results in decreased vital capacity and functional residual capacity. Patients with co-existing pulmonary disease may experience impaired ventilation and oxygenation during water immersion.

Water temperature in the immersion bath is maintained near body temperature to decrease the likelihood of alterations in temperature regulation. Renal parenchymal damage is presumed to be responsible for the hematuria that occurs in nearly all patients following ESWL. Pulmonary contusions and pancreatitis may occur as evidence of damage to surrounding organs by the shock waves. Flank pain may persist several days following ESWL, and petechiae and soft tissue swelling are common at the shock wave cutaneous entry site. Sepsis occurs in a small number of patients following ESWL.

Management of Anesthesia

The impact of the shock waves at the water–cutaneous interface is painful and necessitates general or regional anesthesia; alternatively, intravenous sedation and analgesia may be used (most useful for nonimmersion lithotripsy).[29, 30] Immobilization is important, as any movement may displace stones from the predetermined focus sites for the

shock waves. General anesthesia offers the advantages of controlling the patient's ventilation and avoiding the discomfort associated with immersion and exposure to the loud noise associated with operation of the lithotriptor. A disadvantage of general anesthesia is the need to position unconscious patients in the lithotriptor chair. The method for ventilating the patient's lungs during general anesthesia is a consideration, as movement of the diaphragm and abdominal contents could interfere with precise localization of the shock waves. There is no evidence, however, that high-frequency jet ventilation offers any advantage over conventional methods of mechanically ventilating the lungs, especially slow breathing rates that ensure long expiratory pauses.[31]

Regional anesthesia has the advantage that patients are awake and cooperative, simplifying the positioning in the lithotriptor chair. Spinal anesthesia may be associated with a higher incidence of hypotension than epidural anesthesia. Regional anesthetic techniques for ESWL require a T6 sensory level.

Intravenous sedation techniques (propofol, fentanyl) are especially useful for nonimmersion lithotripsy.[26, 32] Local anesthetic infiltration of the flank, topical local anesthetic cream, and intercostal nerve blocks may decrease analgesic requirements, although intravenous opioids are likely to be required to provide patient comfort.

Intravenous fluid administration is intended to maintain an adequate urine output for facilitating passage of disintegrated stones and to maintain the intravascular fluid volume and systemic blood pressure. Monitoring the body temperature is useful for detecting changes due to water immersion. Monitors, epidural catheter insertion sites, and vascular access sites are protected with water-impermeable dressings.

Renal Hypertension

Renal disease is the most common cause of secondary systemic hypertension. Accelerated or malignant hypertension is likely to be associated with renal disease. Furthermore, the appearance of systemic hypertension in young patients suggests the diagnosis of renal, rather than essential hypertension. Hypertension due to renal dysfunction reflects parenchymal disease of the kidneys or renovascular disease.

Chronic pyelonephritis and glomerulonephritis are parenchymal diseases often associated with systemic hypertension, particularly in younger patients. Less common forms of renal parenchymal disease that can cause systemic hypertension include diabetic nephropathy, cystic disease of the kidneys, and renal amyloidosis. Renovascular disease is characterized by atherosclerosis and accounts for only a small percentage of patients with systemic hypertension. However, the sudden onset of a marked increase in systemic blood pressure or the presence of hypertension before the age of 30 years should arouse suspicion of renovascular disease. A bruit may be audible on auscultation of the abdomen over the kidneys. Systemic hypertension due to renovascular disease does not respond well to treatment with antihypertensive drugs.

The mechanism that produces systemic hypertension in the presence of renal parenchymal or renovascular disease is not established. Stimulation of the renin-angiotensin-aldosterone system is a possible, but unproven, mechanism. Alternatively, the kidneys may function to some extent as antihypertensive organs, possibly producing substances with vasodepressor activity. Regardless of the mechanism, treatment of systemic hypertension due to renal parenchymal disease is usually with antihypertensive drugs, including β-adrenergic antagonist drugs, which inhibit the release of renin from the kidneys. Treatment of renovascular hypertension is with renal artery endarterectomy or nephrectomy.

Uric Acid Nephropathy

Acute uric acid nephropathy is distinct from gout. It occurs when uric acid crystals are precipitated in the renal collecting tubules or ureters, producing acute oliguric renal failure. This precipitation occurs when uric acid concentrations reach a saturation point in acidic urine. The condition is particularly likely to occur when uric acid production is greatly increased, as in patients with myeloproliferative disorders being treated for cancer with chemotherapeutic drugs. These patients are particularly vulnerable to uric acid nephropathy if they have good renal function and urine concentrating ability and then become dehydrated or acidotic because of decreased caloric intake.

Hepatorenal Syndrome

Acute oliguria manifesting in patients with decompensated cirrhosis of the liver is designated hepatorenal syndrome. Indeed, cirrhosis of the liver is associated with decreased GFR and renal blood flow preceding overt renal dysfunction by several weeks. The typical patient is deeply jaundiced and moribund; ascites, hypoalbuminemia, and hypoprothrombinemia are present. Renal failure in these pa-

tients may reflect hypovolemia caused by vigorous attempts to treat ascites. Treatment is directed at intravascular fluid volume replacement, remembering that saline and albumin may aggravate ascites. Therefore whole blood or packed red blood cells may be a more appropriate form of volume replacement. A peritoneal to venous shunt for the treatment of ascites may also be associated with improved renal function. In some patients, a circulating toxin may be responsible for extreme renal vasoconstriction and acute renal failure. Nevertheless, hemodialysis has not been reliable for eliminating suspected hepatic toxins.

There is an increased incidence of postoperative acute renal failure in patients with obstructive jaundice who undergo surgery. The cause of renal failure in these patients is unclear, but preoperative administration of mannitol may be recommended in the hope of providing some renoprotective effect.

■ RENAL TRANSPLANTATION

Candidates for renal transplantation are selected from patients with end-stage renal disease who are on established programs of chronic hemodialysis. In adults, the most common causes of end-stage renal failure are diabetes mellitus, glomerulonephritis, polycystic kidney disease, and systemic hypertension. Despite concerns about the recurrence of disease in the donor kidney, it has generally been only slowly progressive. The kidney must be removed from the donor and transplanted into the recipient promptly to minimize the potential for ischemic damage to the organ. A kidney from a cadaver donor can be preserved by perfusion at low temperatures for up to 48 hours, making its transplantation a semielective surgical procedure. Attempts are made to match human leukocyte antigens (HLA) and ABO blood groups between donor and recipient. Paradoxically, the presence of certain common shared HLA in blood administered to a potential transplant recipient has been observed to induce tolerance to donor antigens and thus improve graft survival.[21] The donor kidney is placed in the lower abdomen and receives its vascular supply from the iliac vessels. The ureter is anastomosed directly to the bladder. Immunosuppressive therapy is instituted during the perioperative period.

Management of Anesthesia

Management of anesthesia for renal transplantation invokes the same principles as are applied for patients with chronic renal failure. They include preoperative hemodialysis to optimize intravascular fluid volume and evaluation of coagulation, electrolyte status, and acid-base balance. Many of these patients are diabetics, emphasizing the need to monitor blood glucose concentrations during the perioperative period. In addition, strict asepsis must be adhered to during placement of intravascular catheters and tracheal intubation.

General Anesthesia

Although both regional and general anesthesia have been successfully utilized for renal transplantation, general anesthesia is most often selected. General anesthesia provides the advantage of mechanically maintaining the patient's ventilation, which may become compromised by surgical retraction in the area of the diaphragm. Drug selection is influenced by known side effects of anesthetic drugs (bowel distension from nitrous oxide, metabolism of sevoflurane to inorganic fluoride). Renal function after kidney transplantation is not predictably influenced by the volatile anesthetic administered. A common approach is to combine volatile anesthetics (isoflurane or desflurane) with nitrous oxide or short-acting opioids. Decreased cardiac output due to negative inotropic effects of volatile anesthetics is minimized to avoid jeopardizing the adequacy of tissue oxygen delivery, especially if anemia is present. To promote renal perfusion, a high normal systemic blood pressure is achieved by decreasing the depth of anesthesia, administering crystalloid solutions, infusing dopamine (3 μg/kg/min IV), or a combination of these measures. The selection of muscle relaxants is influenced by the dependence of many of these drugs on renal clearance. In this regard, atracurium, cisatracurium, and mivacurium are attractive selections, as their clearance from the plasma is independent of renal function. A newly transplanted but functioning kidney is able to clear neuromuscular blocking drugs and the anticholinesterase drugs used for their reversal at the same rate as normal patients.[33]

Central venous pressure monitoring is useful for guiding the rate and volume of crystalloid infusions. Optimal hydration during the intraoperative period is intended to optimize renal blood blood flow and improve early function of the transplanted kidney. Diuretics are often administered to facilitate urine formation by the newly transplanted kidney. In this regard, osmotic diuretics such as mannitol facilitate urine output and decrease excess tissue and intravascular fluid. Unlike the loop diuretic furosemide, mannitol does not depend on renal tubular concentrating mechanisms to produce diuresis.

When the vascular clamps are released, renal preservative solution from the transplanted kidney and venous drainage from the legs are also released into the circulation. These effluents contain potassium and acid metabolites but, in adults, seem to have minimal systemic effects. Nevertheless, cardiac arrest has been described after completion of the arterial anastomosis to the transplanted kidney and release of the vascular clamp.[34] This event is most likely due to sudden hyperkalemia caused by washout of the potassium-containing preservative solutions from the newly perfused kidney. Unclamping may also be followed by hypotension due to the abrupt addition of up to 300 ml to the capacity of the intravascular fluid space and the release of vasodilating chemicals from previously ischemic tissues. When hypotension results from this change, the treatment is most often intravenous infusion of fluids. Emergence from anesthesia is often accompanied by severe pain and systemic hypertension. Neuraxial opioids are a consideration for controlling the postoperative pain.

Regional Anesthesia

The advantages of regional anesthesia compared with general anesthesia are the absence of a need for tracheal intubation or administration of neuromuscular blocking drugs. These advantages are negated, however, if regional anesthesia must be extensively supplemented with injected or inhaled drugs. Furthermore, blockade of the peripheral sympathetic nervous system, as produced by regional anesthesia, can complicate control of systemic blood pressure, especially considering the unpredictable intravascular fluid volume status of many of these patients. The use of regional anesthesia, particularly epidural anesthesia, is controversial in the presence of abnormal coagulation.

Postoperative Complications

The newly transplanted kidney may suffer acute immunologic rejection, which manifests in the vasculature of the transplanted kidney. It can be so rapid that inadequate circulation is evident almost immediately after the blood supply to the kidney is established. The only treatment for this acute rejection reaction is removal of the transplanted kidney, especially if the rejection process is accompanied by disseminated intravascular coagulation. A hematoma also may arise in the graft postoperatively, causing vascular or ureteral obstruction.

Delayed signs of graft rejection include fever, local tenderness, and deterioration of urine output. Treatment with high doses of corticosteroids and antilymphocyte globulin may be helpful. The acute tubular necrosis that occurs in the transplanted kidney secondary to prolonged ischemia usually responds to hemodialysis. Cyclosporine toxicity may also cause acute renal failure. Ultrasonography and needle biopsy are performed to differentiate between the possible causes of kidney malfunction.

Opportunistic infections owing to chronic immunosuppression are common after renal transplantation. Long-term survival is unsatisfactory in renal transplant patients who are immunosuppressed and who also carry hepatitis B surface antigen. The frequency of cancer is 30 to 100 times higher in transplant recipients than in the general population, presumably reflecting the loss of protective effects due to immunosuppression. Large cell lymphoma is a well recognized complication of transplantation, occurring almost exclusively in patients with evidence of Epstein-Barr virus infections.

Anesthetic Considerations in Renal Transplant Recipients

Renal transplant recipients are often elderly with co-existing cardiovascular disease and diabetes mellitus.[35] The side effects of immunosuppressant drugs (systemic hypertension, lowered seizure thresholds, anemia, thrombocytopenia) must be considered when planning the management of anesthesia. Serum creatinine concentrations are likely to be normal in the presence of normally functioning renal transplants. Nevertheless, the GFR and renal blood flow are likely to be lower than those of healthy individuals, and the activity of drugs excreted by the kidneys may be prolonged. The presence of azotemia, proteinuria, and systemic hypertension may indicate chronic rejection of the kidney transplant. Drugs that are potentially nephrotoxic or dependent on renal clearance are avoided. Diuretics are administered only with careful evaluation of the patient's intravascular fluid volume status. Decreases in renal blood flow from hypovolemia are minimized. It is likely these patients will be receiving oral antihypertensive drugs.

■ BENIGN PROSTATIC HYPERPLASIA

Benign prostatic hyperplasia (BPH) is a nonmalignant enlargement of the prostate due to excessive cellular growth of both the glandular and stromal elements of the gland.[36] BPH is common worldwide in men over 40 years of age. The two components of BPH are a static component related to enlarge-

ment of the prostate and a dynamic component that reflects the tone of the smooth muscle in the prostate. α-Adrenergic receptors are present in the prostatic capsule and hyperplastic prostatic tissue. Transurethral resection of the prostate and open prostatectomy have been the traditional treatments for men with symptomatic BPH. Surgery, however, may be associated with intraoperative complications (bleeding, hypervolemia from systemic absorption of the irrigating fluid) and postoperative problems (retrograde ejaculation, impotence, urinary incontinence). As a result, alternative treatments are being developed, including medical management with androgen-deprivation drugs and minimally invasive surgical approaches.

Medical Therapy

The prostate gland is androgen-sensitive such that androgen deprivation decreases the size of the prostate and the resistance to outflow through the prostatic urethra. Finasteride, an orally effective inhibitor of 5 α-reductase, is moderately effective for symptomatic treatment of BPH by reducing the static component of this disease. Side effects of 5 α-reductase inhibitors are minimal. α-Adrenergic antagonists (terazosin, doxazosin, tamsulosin) are administered to block adrenergic receptors in hyperplastic prostatic tissue, the prostatic capsule, and the bladder neck so the smooth muscle tone (dynamic component of BPH) of these structures is decreased. As a result, resistance to urinary flow through the bladder neck and the prostatic urethra decreases, and urinary flow increases. These drugs may also have antihypertensive effects, whereas undesirable side effects include orthostatic hypotension.

Minimally Invasive Treatments

The most commonly utilized minimally invasive treatment of BPH is transurethral incision of the prostate.[36] This technique is effective in patients with bladder-outlet obstruction and enlarged prostates weighing 30 g or less and in whom the primary obstruction is located at the bladder neck. As the incisions are deepened the bladder neck and prostatic urethra "spring open," and the bladder outlet obstruction is relieved. Regional or general anesthesia is utilized for this surgical procedure. Other minimally invasive treatments for BPH include placement of prostatic stents (primarily in patients who are poor surgical risks), microwave therapy, and laser prostatectomy. Advantages of visual laser ablation of the prostate is a brief operating time (20 minutes or less) and the absence of perioperative hemorrhage.

Transurethral Resection of the Prostate

Definitive surgical treatment of BPH requires transurethral resection of the prostate (TURP). The surgical procedure is accompanied by absorption of non-electrolyte irrigating fluids (glycine, sorbitol, mannitol) used to distend the bladder and wash away blood and prostatic tissue. The irrigation fluid gains direct intravascular access through the prostatic venous plexus or is more slowly absorbed from the retroperitoneal and perivesical spaces. When irrigation fluid enters the intravascular space, the results are acute changes in intravascular fluid volume and plasma solute concentrations manifesting as cardiovascular and central nervous system complications known as the TURP syndrome (Fig. 20–3).[37] Despite the seemingly consistent etiology, TURP syndrome lacks a consistent and predictable presentation, making its diagnosis difficult. No consistent correlation has been found between the volume of fluid absorbed, the duration of TURP, and the weight of prostatic tissue removed. TURP syndrome may occur as quickly as 15 minutes after the resection begins or up to 24 hours postoperatively.

TURP Syndrome

The TURP syndrome is characterized by intravascular fluid volume shifts and plasma solute effects (Table 20–11).[37] Solute changes may alter neurologic function independent of volume-related effects. The risk of intravascular hemolysis is greatly reduced by use of osmotically active irrigating solutions rather than distilled water. Although monitoring serum sodium concentrations during TURP is common practice and is effective for assessing intravascular fluid absorption, there may be benefits from monitoring serum osmolality as well. Hypo-osmolality appears to be the principal factor that contributes to the neurologic and hypovolemic changes considered to reflect the TURP syndrome. Supportive care remains the most important therapeutic approach for managing cardiovascular, central nervous system, and renal complications of the TURP syndrome. The introduction of medical management and minimally invasive surgical procedures to treat BPH may decrease the risk of TURP syndrome in the future.

A disorder similar to TURP syndrome may occur in women undergoing endometrial ablation that utilizes irrigation fluids (saline, glycine, sorbitol) to improve surgical visualization.[37] When 32% dextran 70 irrigation is used, the major risk is a reaction to dextran, whereas hypo-osmolality is not a problem as this solution is hyperosmolar.

Intravascular Fluid Volume Expansion

Rapid intravascular fluid volume expansion due to systemic absorption of irrigating fluids (absorption rates may reach 200 ml/min) can cause systemic hypertension and reflex bradycardia. Patients with poor left ventricular function may develop pulmonary edema owing to this acute circulatory volume overload. Factors that influence the amount of irrigating solution absorbed include the intravesicular pressure, which is determined by the height of the irrigation bag above the prostatic sinuses (limit height to 40 cm above the prostate) and the number of prostatic sinuses opened (limit resection time to 1 hour and leave a rim of tissue on the capsule). If intravesical pressures are maintained below 15 cm H_2O, absorption of irrigating fluids is minimal.

The most widely used indicator of intravascular fluid volume gain is hyponatremia or the breath-alcohol level when ethanol is added as a marker to the irrigation fluid. Monitoring breath alcohol is noninvasive, sensitive (can detect absorption of as little as 100 to 150 ml during any 10-minute period), and more practical than frequent monitoring of serum sodium concentrations as a measure of the intensity of irrigating solution absorption (Fig. 20–4).[38] Before treating TURP syndrome with hypertonic saline, it is important to exclude the presence of hypervolemia with near-normal plasma sodium concentrations. Cardiovascular compromise and impaired arterial oxygenation due to pulmonary edema require aggressive intervention, which may include administration of inotropic drugs, diuretics, and even augmentation of intravascular fluid volume.

Intravascular Fluid Volume Loss

Perioperative hypotension during TURP is sometimes preceded by systemic hypertension. It is conceivable that hyponatremia in association with systemic hypertension can result in water flux along osmotic and hydrostatic pressure gradients out of the intravascular space and into the lungs with resultant pulmonary edema and hypovolemic shock. Sympathetic nervous system blockade produced by regional anesthesia could compound the hypotension, as could intraoperative endotoxemia, which is common during TURP.

Hyponatremia

Acute hyponatremia due to intravascular absorption of sodium-free irrigating fluids may cause con-

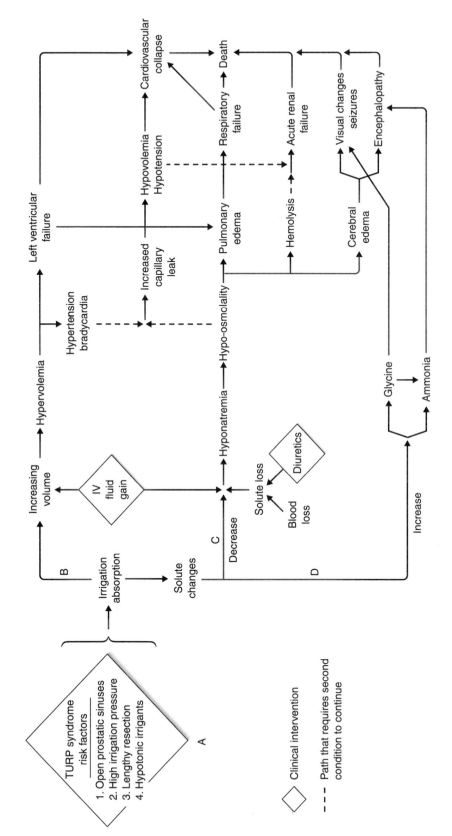

Figure 20–3 • Mechanisms and pathways that lead to transurethral resection of the prostate (TURP) syndrome. The initiating event is systemic absorption of the irrigating solution (A), which increases intravascular fluid volume (B) with its sequelae and decreases (C) or increases (D) solute concentrations. (From Gravenstein D. Transurethral resection of the prostate (TURP) syndrome: a review of the pathophysiology and management. Anesth Analg 1997;84:438–46. © 1997, Lippincott Williams & Wilkins, with permission.)

Table 20–11 • Signs and Symptoms of the Transurethral Resection of the Prostate Syndrome

Cardiopulmonary
  Hypertension
  Bradycardia
  Hypotension
  Increased central venous pressure
  Cardiac dysrhythmias
  Pulmonary edema
  Arterial hypoxemia
  Myocardial ischemia
  Shock
Hematologic and renal
  Hyponatremia
  Hypo-osmolality
  Metabolic acidosis
  Hyperammonemia
  Hyperglycinemia
  Hemolysis
  Acute renal failure
Central nervous system
  Nausea and vomiting
  Confusion and agitation
  Seizures
  Coma
  Blindness

Adapted from: Gravenstein D. Transurethral resection of the prostate (TURP) syndrome: a review of the pathophysiology and management. Anesth Analg 1997;84:438–46.

fusion, agitation, visual disturbances, pulmonary edema, cardiovascular collapse, and seizures. Changes in the ECG may accompany progressive decreases in serum sodium concentrations (Table 20–12). Spinal anesthesia associated with hypoten-

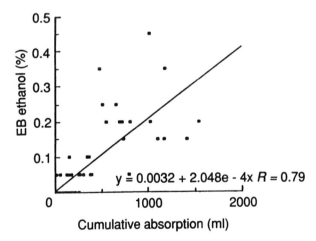

Figure 20–4 • Ethanol concentration in the exhaled gases (EB, ethanol) parallels the cumulative absorption of irrigating fluid. (From Hulten J, Sarma VJ, Hjertberg H, et al. Monitoring of irrigating fluid absorption during transuretheral prostatectomy. A study in anaesthetized patients using a 1% ethanol tag solution. Anaesthesia 1991;46:349–53 with permission.)

sion may cause nausea and vomiting indistinguishable from that caused by acute hyponatremia. Nevertheless, some hyponatremic patients show no signs of water intoxication, and it is possible that hyponatremia may not be the sole or even the primary cause of the neurologic manifestations of the TURP syndrome.[37]

Hypo-osmolality

Hypo-osmolality rather than hyponatremia is the crucial physiologic derangement leading to central nervous system dysfunction during TURP. This is predictable because the blood–brain barrier is essentially impermeable to sodium but freely permeable to water. Based on the Nernst equation, it is predicted that serum sodium concentrations should not contribute substantially to neuronal excitability independent of the serum osmolality.[11] Cerebral edema caused by acute hypo-osmolality can result in increased intracranial pressure with resultant bradycardia and hypertension.

Diuretics administered to treat hypervolemia during TURP may accentuate hyponatremia and hypo-osmolality. A patient's serum sodium concentration and osmolality may continue to decrease following TURP because of continued absorption of irrigating solutions from the perivesicular and retroperitoneal spaces. If the serum osmolality is near normal, no interventions to correct serum sodium concentrations are recommended for asymptomatic patients even in the presence of hyponatremia. The most feared complication of correcting hyponatremia is central pontine myelinolysis ("osmotic demyelination syndrome"), which has been observed after both rapid and slow correction of serum sodium concentrations in patients undergoing TURP. The safest treatment of hyponatremia and hypo-osmolality may be symptomatic, recognizing that the presence of symptoms is the single most important factor determining morbidity and mortality from hyponatremia.[37] Instituting treatment in the absence of symptoms risks too rapid correction because the correction rate is difficult to control. Serum osmolality should be monitored and corrected aggressively with hypertonic saline only until symptoms resolve substantially; then correction should be continued slowly (serum sodium concentrations increase 1.5 mEq/L/hr).[37]

Metabolic Acidosis

Mild metabolic acidosis has been observed in patients undergoing TURP.[39] Moderate irrigating solution absorption during TURP leads to metabolic acidosis ("TURP acidosis"), and this derangement

Table 20–12 • Manifestations of Acute Hyponatremia on the Electrocardiogram

Serum Sodium Concentration (mEq/L)	Electrocardiographic Manifestation	Central Nervous System Signs
120	Possible widening of QRS	Restlessness Confusion
115	Widened QRS Elevated ST segment	Nausea Somnolence
110	Ventricular tachycardia Ventricular fibrillation	Seizures Coma

could be more severe should irrigating solution absorption be more profound.

Hyperammonemia

Hyperammonemia is the result of the use of glycine-containing irrigation solutions with subsequent systemic absorption of glycine and its oxidative deamination to glyoxylic acid and ammonia. Alterations in central nervous system function may accompany hyperammonemia, but its role in the TURP syndrome remains unclear.[37] Endogenous arginine in the liver prevents hepatic release of ammonia and facilitates conversion of ammonia to urea. The time necessary to deplete endogenous arginine stores may be as brief as 12 hours, which approximates the preoperative fasting time. Prophylactic administration of intravenous arginine blunts the increase in serum ammonia concentrations associated with the presence of glycine in the systemic circulation.

Hyperglycinemia

Glycine is an inhibitory neurotransmitter similar to γ-aminobutyric acid (GABA) in the spinal cord and brain. Glycine is the most likely cause of visual disturbances including transient blindness during TURP syndrome, reflecting the role of glycine as an inhibitory neurotransmitter in the retina. Therefore glycine likely affects retina physiology independent of cerebral edema caused by hyponatremia and hypo-osmolality. Vision returns to normal within 24 hours as serum glycine concentrations approach normal. Reassurance that unimpaired vision will return is probably the best treatment. In addition to glycine, benzodiazepines, by their actions on GABA receptors, may mediate some compromise of vision through activation of the retinal GABA receptor.

Glycine may lead to encephalopathy and seizures via its ability to potentiate the effects of N-methyl-D-aspartate (NMDA), an excitatory neurotransmitter. Magnesium exerts a negative control on the NDMA receptor; and hypomagnesemia caused by dilution (due to systemic absorption of irrigating solutions during TURP or administration of loop diuretics) may increase the susceptibility to seizures. For this reason, a trial of magnesium therapy may be indicated in patients who develop seizures and in whom glycine-containing irrigating solutions were used.

Glycine may also exert toxic effects on the kidneys. Hyperoxaluria due to metabolism of glycine to oxalate and glycolate could compromise renal function in patients with co-existing renal disease as is often present in elderly patients undergoing TURP.

References

1. Byrick RJ, Rose DK. Pathophysiology and prevention of acute renal failure: the role of the anaesthetist. Can J Anaesth 1990;37:457–67
2. Swan SK. Approach to the patient with renal disease. Sci Am Med 1999;1–7
3. Kellen M, Aronson S, Roizen M, et al. Predictive and diagnostic tests of renal failure: a review. Anesth Analg 1994;78:134–42
4. Mazze RI. No evidence of sevoflurane-induced renal injury in volunteers. Anesth Analg 1998;86:228–35
5. Eger EI, Gong D, Koblin DD, et al. Dose-related biochemical markers of renal injury after sevoflurane versus desflurane anesthesia in volunteers. Anesth Analg 1997;85:1154–63
6. Tolkoff-Rubin NE, Pascal M. Chronic renal failure. Sci Am Med 1998;1–12
7. Ifudu O. Care of patients undergoing hemodialysis. N Engl J Med 1998;339:1054–62
8. Pastn S, Bailey J. Dialysis therapy. N Engl J Med 1998;338:1428–37
9. Kharasch ED, Hankins DC, Thummel KE. Human kidney methoxyflurane and sevoflurane metabolism: intrarenal fluoride production as a possible mechanism of methoxyflurane nephrotoxicity. Anesthesiology 1995;82:689–99
10. Bedford RF, Ives HE. The renal safety of sevoflurane. Anesth Analg 2000;90:505–8
11. Weir PH, Chung FF. Anaesthesia for patients with chronic renal disease. Can Anaesth Soc J 1984;31:486–90
12. Byrick RJ. Anesthesia and end-stage renal failure: is TIVA an advance? Can J Anesth 1999;46:621–5

13. Lien CA, Schmith VD, Belmont MR, et al. Pharmacokinetics of cisatracurium in patients receiving nitrous oxide/opioid/barbiturate anesthesia. Anesthesiology 1996;84:300–8

14. Dahaba AA, von Klobucar F, Rehak PH, et al. Total intravenous anesthesia with remifentanil, propofol, and cisatracurium in end-stage renal failure. Can J Anesth 1999;46:696–700

15. Klahr S, Miller SB. Acute oliguria. N Engl J Med 1998;338:671–5

16. Thadhani R, Pascual M, Bonventre JV. Acute renal failure. N Engl J Med 1996;334:1448–60

17. Turney JH. Acute renal failure: a dangerous condition. JAMA 1996;275:1517–27

18. Levy LM, Viscoli CM, Howritz RI. The effect of acute renal failure on mortality: a cohort analysis. JAMA 1996; 275:1489–94

19. Novis M, Aronson S, Roizen MF, et al. Association of preoperative risk factors with postoperative renal failure. Anesth Analg 1994;78:143–9

20. Safirstein R, Andrade L, Vieira JM. Acetylcysteine and nephrotoxic effects of radiographic contrast agents: a new use for an old drug. N Engl J Med 2000;343:310–2

21. VanTwuyver G, Mooijaart RJD, tenBerge IJM, et al. Pretransplantation blood transfusion revisited. N Engl J Med 1991;325:1210–3

22. Swan SK. Pharmacologic approach to renal insufficiency. Sci Am Med 2000;1–5

23. Orth SR, Ritz E. The nephrotic syndrome. N Engl J Med 1998;338:1202–11

24. Joel M, Rosales JK. Fanconi syndrome and anesthesia. Anesthesiology 1981;55:455–6

25. Kannan S, Delph Y, Moseley HSL. Anaesthetic management of a child with Bartter's syndrome. Can J Anaesth 1995;42:808–12

26. Nishikawa T, Dohi S. Baroreflex function in a patient with Bartter's syndrome. Can Anaesth Soc J 1985;32:646–50

27. Coe FL, Parks JH, Asplin JR. The pathogenesis and treatment of kidney stones. N Engl J Med 1992;327:1141–52

28. Long AL, Venditti FJ. Lithotripsy in a patient with an automatic implantable cardioverter defibrillator. Anesthesiology 1991;74:937–8

29. Zeitlin GL, Roth RA. Effect of three anesthetic techniques on the success of extracorporeal shock wave lithotripsy. Anesthesiology 1988;68:272–6

30. Monk TG, Boure B, White PF, et al. Comparison of intravenous sedative-analgesic techniques for outpatient immersion lithotripsy. Anesth Analg 1991;72:616–21

31. Perel A, Hoffman B, Podeh D, et al. High frequency positive pressure ventilation during general anesthesia for extracorporeal shock wave lithotripsy. Anesth Analg 1986;65:1231–4

32. Monk TG, Ding Y, White PF, et al. Effect of topical eutectic mixture of local anesthetics on pain response and analgesic requirement during lithotripsy procedures. Anesth Analg 1994;79:506–10

33. Cronnelly R, Stanski DR, Miller RD, et al. Pyridostigmine kinetics with and without renal function. Clin Pharmacol Ther 1980;28:78–81

34. Hirshman CA, Leon D, Edelstein G, et al. Risk of hyperkalemia in recipients of kidneys preserved with an intracellular electrolyte solution. Anesth Analg 1980;59:283–6

35. Kostopanagiotou G, Smyrniotis V, Arkadopoulos N, et al. Anesthetic and perioperative management of adult transplant recipients in nontransplant surgery. Anesth Analg 1999;89:613–22

36. Oesterling JE. Benign prostatic hyperplasia: medical and minimally invasive treatment options. N Engl J Med 1995; 332:99–110

37. Gravenstein D. Transuretheral resection of the prostate (TURP) syndrome: a review of the pathophysiology and management. Anesth Analg 1997;84:438–46

38. Hulten J, Sarma VJ, Hjertberg H, et al. Monitoring of irrigating fluid absorption during transurethral prostatectomy: a study of anaesthetized patients using a 1% ethanol tag solution. Anaesthesia 1991;46:349–53

39. Scheingraber S, Heitmann L, Weber W, et al. Are there acid-base changes during transurethral resection of the prostate (TURP)? Anesth Analg 2000;90:946–50

21

Water, Electrolyte, and Acid-Base Disturbances

Alterations of water and electrolyte content and distribution as well as acid-base disturbances can produce multiple organ system dysfunction during the perioperative period. For example, impairment of central nervous system, cardiac, and neuromuscular function is likely in the presence of water, electrolyte (sodium, potassium, calcium, magnesium), and acid-base disturbances. Furthermore, these disorders often accompany events associated with the perioperative period (Table 21–1). Management of patients manifesting water and electrolyte disturbances is based on an understanding of the distribution of total body water and electrolytes. Often the signs and symptoms of water and electrolyte disturbances are related more to the rate of change and less to the absolute change.

TOTAL BODY WATER AND ELECTROLYTE DISTURBANCES

Total body water content is categorized as intracellular fluid and extracellular fluid, according to the location of the water relative to cell membranes (Fig. 21–1). The body's main priority is to maintain intravascular fluid volume. Acute decreases in intravascular fluid volume, as occur with fluid deprivation during the preoperative period, blood loss, or surgical trauma resulting in tissue edema ("third-space loss"), elicits the release of antidiuretic hormone (ADH), renin, and possibly atrial natriuretic factor. These substances subsequently result in responses at the renal tubules that lead to restoration of intravascular fluid volume. The distribution and concentration of electrolytes differs greatly among fluid compartments for total body water (Table 21–2). The electrophysiology of excitable cells is dependent

Table 21–1 • Etiology of Water, Electrolyte, and Acid-Base Disturbances During the Perioperative Period

Disease states
 Endocrinopathies
 Nephropathies
 Gastroenteropathies
Drug therapy
 Diuretics
 Corticosteroids
Nasogastric suction
Surgery
 Transurethral resection of the prostate
 Translocation of body water due to tissue trauma
 Resection of portions of the gastrointestinal tract
Management of anesthesia
 Intravenous fluid administration
 Alveolar ventilation
 Hypothermia

on the intracellular and extracellular concentrations of sodium, potassium, and calcium. An inherent characteristic of excitable cells is their ability to maintain concentration gradients across their cell membranes. The resulting unequal distribution of ions (excess potassium inside and sodium outside) produces electrochemical differences across cell membranes. The electrophysiology of cells and the resulting action potentials are altered by changes in the concentrations of electrolytes.

Hyponatremia

Hyponatremia is defined as decreases in serum sodium concentrations below 136 mEq/L.[1] Plasma osmolarity may be low, high, or normal in the presence of hyponatremia. Hypotonicity can lead to cerebral edema. Hyponatremia frequently develops in hospitalized patients.

Causes of Dilutional Hyponatremia

Dilutional (hypotonic) hyponatremia, the most common form of hyponatremia, is caused by water retention. If water intake exceeds the ability of the kidneys to excrete water, dilution of body solutes results, causing hypo-osmolarity and hypotonicity of the plasma. Retention of water most often reflects the presence of conditions that impair renal excretion of water, and in only a small number of cases is hyponatremia due to excessive water intake (Table 21–3).[1] Hyperglycemia is the most common cause of translocational hyponatremia. An increase of 100 mg/dl in the serum glucose concentrations decreases serum sodium concentrations by about

1.7 mEq/L. Massive absorption of irrigant solutions that do not contain sodium (as used during transurethral resection of the prostate) can cause severe, symptomatic hyponatremia. The most common causes of severe hyponatremia in adults are treatment with thiazide diuretics and the postoperative state associated with inappropriate secretion of ADH. In infants and children the most common causes of hyponatremia are gastrointestinal fluid loss, ingestion of dilute formula, and accidental ingestion of excess water.

Hyponatremia in Hospitalized Patients

Hyponatremia that develops in hospitalized patients is largely preventable.[1] A defect of water excretion can be present on admission to the hospital, or it can develop or worsen during hospitalization as a result of factors that stimulate inappropriate secretion of ADH (postoperative state, drugs, organ failure). Even in the presence of such defects, however, development of dilutional hyponatremia is not likely so long as the intake of electrolyte-free water does not exceed the capacity for water excretion and insensible losses.

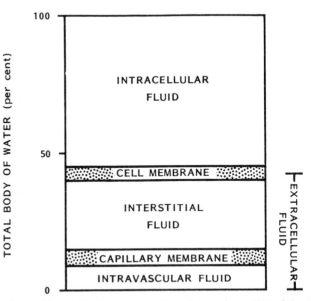

Figure 21–1 • Total body water (constitutes about 60% of the total body weight in kilograms or about 42 L in male adults and 35 L in female adults) is designated intracellular or extracellular fluid, depending on the location of water relative to cell membranes. Water in extracellular compartments is further subdivided as interstitial or intravascular (plasma) fluid, depending on its location relative to cell membranes. About 55% of total body water is intracellular, 37% is interstitial, and the remaining 8% is intravascular.

Table 21–2 • Approximate Composition of Extracellular and Intracellular Fluid*

Substance Assayed	Extracellular Fluid (mEq/L)		Intracellular Fluid (mEq/L)
	Intravascular	Interstitial	
Sodium	140	145	10
Potassium	5	4	150
Calcium	5	2.5	< 1
Magnesium	2	1.5	40
Chloride	103	115	4
Bicarbonate	28	30	10

* Total anion concentration consists of phosphates, sulfates, organic acids, and negatively charged sites on proteins.

Signs and Symptoms of Dilutional Hyponatremia

Patients with serum sodium concentrations higher than 125 mEq/L are usually asymptomatic, whereas those with lower values may have symptoms, especially if hyponatremia has developed rapidly. Complications of severe, rapidly developing hyponatremia include seizures, coma, respiratory arrest, brain stem herniation, permanent brain damage, and death. These complications may occur in euvolemic postoperative patients who develop excessive water retention. Dilutional hyponatremia causes water to enter the brain with resulting cerebral edema and increased intracranial pressure. Solutes subsequently leave the brain within hours, thereby ameliorating brain swelling. This brain adaptation is also the origin of the risk for osmotic demyelination. Although rare, osmotic demyelination can develop one to several days after aggressive treatment of hyponatremia, including water restriction.[1] Shrinkage of the brain triggers demyelination of pontine and extrapontine neurons and may result in quadriplegia, seizures, coma, and death. Hepatic failure, potassium depletion, and poor nutrition increase the risk of osmotic demyelination.

Treatment of Dilutional Hyponatremia

Treatment of dilutional hyponatremia balances the risks of serum hypotonicity and hypo-osmolarity with the hazards of therapy. The presence of symptoms and their severity largely determines the speed of correction of hyponatremia.[1] Although water restriction ameliorates all forms of hyponatremia, it is not the optimal therapy in all patients. Hyponatremia associated with hypovolemia requires correction of prevailing sodium deficits with saline. Conversely, saline is not appropriate for correcting hyponatremia due to inappropriate secretion of ADH. Hyponatremia due to hypothyroidism or adrenal insufficiency may mimic hyponatremia due to inappropriate secretion of ADH.[1] The presence of hyperkalemia suggests the possibility of adrenal insufficiency in these patients.

Symptomatic Dilutional Hyponatremia

Patients with symptomatic dilutional hyponatremia are treated with intravenous infusions of hypertonic saline (5% sodium chloride in water, which is equivalent to 855 mEq of sodium per liter). Hypertonic

Table 21–3 • Causes of Dilutional Hyponatremia Reflecting Impaired Renal Water Excretion

Decreased extracellular fluid volume
Renal sodium loss
  Thiazide diuretics
  Osmotic diuretics
  Adrenal insufficiency
  Ketonuria
Extrarenal sodium loss
  Vomiting
  Blood loss
  Fluid sequestration in "third spaces" (bowel obstruction, trauma, burns)
Increased extracellular fluid volume
Congestive heart failure
Cirrhosis of the liver
Renal failure (acute or chronic)
Pregnancy
Normal extracellular fluid volume
Syndrome of inappropriate antidiuretic hormone secretion
  Postoperative
  Pain
  Acute respiratory failure
  Positive-pressure ventilation
  Cancer (lungs, mediastinum)
  Stroke
  Intracranial hemorrhage
  Acute brain trauma
  Drugs (desmopressin, oxytocin, tricyclic antidepressants, serotonin reuptake inhibitors, opioids, cyclophosphamide, vincristine)
Thiazide diuretics
Adrenal insufficiency
Hypothyroidism

saline is usually combined with furosemide to limit treatment-induced expansion of the extracellular fluid volume. Electrolyte-free water is withheld from these patients. Correction of hyponatremia is at a rate and magnitude that reverses the manifestations of hypotonicity but not so rapid and large as to pose a risk of the development of osmotic demyelination. Relatively small increases in serum sodium concentrations (3 to 7 mEq/L) may be sufficient to reverse cerebral edema and stop seizure activity. Most cases of osmotic demyelination have occurred when the rate at which the serum sodium concentration increases exceeded 12 mEq/L daily. A target goal is to increase serum sodium concentrations 8 mEq/L daily. Cessation of life-threatening complications and achievement of serum sodium concentrations of 125 to 130 mEq/L are indications to slow the rate of serum sodium correction.

Asymptomatic Dilutional Hyponatremia

Asymptomatic dilutional hyponatremia that accompanies edematous states or the syndrome of inappropriate secretion of ADH is treated with restriction of daily water intake to less than 800 ml.[1] In the presence of congestive heart failure, treatment with angiotensin-converting enzyme inhibitors can increase excretion of electrolyte-free water and moderate the magnitude of hyponatremia. Loop but not thiazide diuretics augment excretion of electrolyte-free water, thereby permitting relaxation of fluid restriction.

Management of Anesthesia

Management of anesthesia considers the likely presence of renal, cardiac, or liver disease as the etiology of excess total body water and dilutional hyponatremia. Decreased excitability of cells due to hyponatremia could manifest as poor myocardial contractility and increased sensitivity to nondepolarizing muscle relaxants. Unexpected hypotension in the presence of cardiac depressant anesthetic drugs may reflect poor myocardial function in the presence of hyponatremia.

Hypernatremia

Hypernatremia is defined as increases in serum sodium concentrations above 145 mEq/L. Total body water deficit (dehydration) is the most likely cause of hypernatremia, as the kidneys closely regulate total body sodium content. As a result, accumulation of sodium is almost impossible unless there is impaired renal function. Nevertheless, impaired sodium excretion by the kidneys is common in the presence of congestive heart failure and cirrhosis of the liver with ascites.

Signs and Symptoms

Clinical manifestations of total body water deficit as a cause of hyponatremia reflect loss of water from all fluid compartments. When dehydration is severe, systemic blood pressure, venous pressure, and urine output are decreased, and heart rate is increased. Because both intracellular and extracellular fluid volumes are decreased, the hematocrit is unlikely to increase. Blood urea nitrogen and serum creatinine concentrations are likely to increase, as hypovolemia results in decreased renal blood flow and glomerular filtration rate. If the kidneys are functioning properly, the urine specific gravity is higher than 1.030. Peripheral edema is absent, emphasizing that decreases in total body water content are responsible for hypernatremia. Conversely, peripheral edema is the hallmark of hypernatremia due to total body excess of sodium. Interstitial fluid spaces, however, can expand by as much as 5 L in normal adults before edema is clinically detectable. Other features of total body sodium excess include ascites, pleural effusions, and increased intravascular fluid volumes manifesting as systemic hypertension.

Treatment

Hypernatremia Due to Total Body Water Deficit

Treatment for hypernatremia due to total body water deficit consists of administering electrolyte-free water on the basis of the measured decrease in body weight or, more commonly, the magnitude of the increase in serum sodium concentration. An acceptable approach is administration of 5% glucose in water, with the volume and rate of infusion guided by changes in systemic blood pressure, central venous pressure, urine output, and repeated determinations of the serum sodium concentration. It should be appreciated that brain water does not necessarily decrease to the same extent as total body water, particularly if dehydration is gradual. Thus if the total body water deficit is corrected too rapidly, the brain can take up excessive water, resulting in cerebral edema. To minimize the risk of cerebral edema, it is recommended that hypernatremia be corrected gradually at a maximum rate of 0.5 mEq/L/hr.[2]

Hypernatremia Due to Excess Total Body Sodium

Treatment for hypernatremia due to excess total body sodium is administration of diuretics to facilitate sodium excretion by the kidneys. Furosemide is often selected to treat hypernatremia associated with congestive heart failure, whereas spironolactone is useful to treat edema due to cirrhosis of the liver.

Management of Anesthesia

Management of anesthesia in the presence of hypernatremia due to total body water deficit is likely to be accompanied by hypotension, as drug-induced vasodilation unmasks hypovolemia. Positive-pressure ventilation of the patient's lungs may be associated with exaggerated decreases in the systemic blood pressure. A contracted intravascular fluid volume also results in a decreased volume of distribution for drugs such as nondepolarizing muscle relaxants, which are limited in their distribution principally to extracellular fluid. Conceivably, these patients would experience increased sensitivity to muscle relaxants. Measurements of cardiac filling pressures and urine output are helpful for guiding the volume and rate on intravenous fluid administration during the perioperative period. When hypernatremia is due to excess sodium concentrations, there are no specific recommendations for the management of anesthesia other than recognizing the presence of an increased intravascular fluid volume.

Hypokalemia

Hypokalemia is defined as decreases in serum potassium concentrations to less than 3.5 mEq/L.[3] Based on this definition, hypokalemia is found in more than 20% of hospitalized patients and 10% to 40% of patients treated with thiazide diuretics, making it the most common electrolyte disturbance seen clinically.

Diagnosis

Hypokalemia is rarely suspected on the basis of clinical presentation; rather, the diagnosis is made by measuring serum potassium concentrations. Chronic hypokalemia is likely to be associated with decreased total body potassium stores as well as decreases in serum potassium concentrations. In contrast, acute hypokalemia is usually due to intracellular translocation of potassium without changes in total body potassium content. It is important to remember that 98% of potassium is intracellular and is not measured by serum potassium determinations (Table 21–2). Furthermore, as extracellular potassium is lost, intracellular potassium crosses cell membranes along a concentration gradient and thus maintains a normal intracellular to extracellular potassium ratio. Enormous potassium deficits can exist despite only small decreases in the serum potassium concentrations. For example, it is estimated that chronic decreases of 1 mEq/L in the serum potassium concentration can reflect total body deficits of 600 to 800 mEq of potassium.

Causes

Hypokalemia is almost always the result of potassium depletion due to drug-induced losses of potassium (Table 21–4).[3] Less often, hypokalemia occurs as the result of abrupt shifts of potassium from extracellular to intracellular sites, inadequate potassium intake, or abnormal losses of potassium through the kidneys due to metabolic alkalosis or diarrhea (Table 21–4).[3]

Drug-Induced Abnormal Losses of Potassium

Diuretic therapy is the most common cause of hypokalemia. Both thiazide and loop diuretics block

---

Table 21–4 • Drug-Induced and Non-Drug-Induced Causes of Hypokalemia

Hypokalemia due to increased renal potassium loss
Thiazide diuretics
Loop diuretics
Mineralocorticoids
High-dose glucocorticoids
High-dose antibiotics (penicillin, nafcillin, ampicillin)
Drugs associated with magnesium depletion (aminoglycosides)
Surgical trauma
Hyperglycemia
Aldosteronism
Hypokalemia due to transcellular potassium shift
β-adrenergic agonists
Epinephrine
Decongestants (pseudoephedrine)
Bronchodilators (albuterol, terbutaline, ephedrine, isoproterenol)
Tocolytic drugs (ritodrine)
Verapamil overdose
Insulin overdose
Respiratory or metabolic alkalosis
Familial periodic paralysis
Hypercalcemia
Hypomagnesemia
Hypokalemia due to excessive gastrointestinal loss of potassium
Vomiting and diarrhea
Zollinger-Ellison syndrome
Jejunoileal bypass
Malabsorption
Chemotherapy
Nasogastric suction

Adapted from: Gennari JF. Hypokalemia. N Engl J Med 1998;339: 451–8.

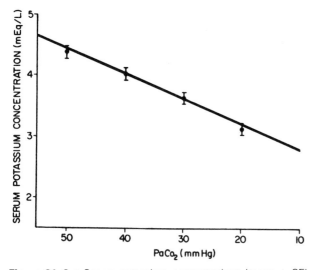

Figure 21–2 • Serum potassium concentrations (mean ± SE) are directly related to the PaCO$_2$. A 10 mmHg change in PaCO$_2$ results in corresponding changes in serum potassium concentrations of about 0.5 mEq/L. (From Edwards R, Winnie AP, Ramamurthy S. Acute hypocapneic hypokalemia: an iatrogenic anesthetic complication. Anesth Analg 1977;56:786–92, with permission.)

chloride-associated sodium reabsorption, creating favorable electrochemical gradients for potassium secretion. The degree of hypokalemia is directly related to the doses of thiazide diuretics and is greater when dietary sodium intake is higher. Diuretic-induced hypokalemia is often associated with metabolic alkalosis (bicarbonate concentrations 28 to 36 mEq/L). Other drugs that may increase renal potassium loss include fludrocortisone, an oral mineralocorticoid that promotes renal potassium excretion, and glucocorticoids, which also increase renal potassium excretion and can lower serum potassium concentrations 0.2 to 0.4 mEq/L. Large doses of laxatives cause excessive potassium losses in the stool and can produce hypokalemia.

Drug-Induced Transcellular Shifts of Potassium

Drugs with β_2-adrenergic activity (bronchodilators, inhibitors of uterine contractions, decongestants) can acutely decrease serum potassium concentrations. A standard dose of nebulized albuterol decreases the serum potassium concentration by 0.2 to 0.4 mEq/L, and a second dose administered within 1 hour can decrease it by nearly 1 mEq/L. This hypokalemia may be sustained for up to 4 hours. Intentional ingestion of excessive amounts of pseudoephedrine can cause severe hypokalemia. Ritodrine and terbutaline administered as uterine contraction inhibitors can decrease serum potassium

concentrations to as low as 2.5 mEq/L for 4 to 6 hours following intravenous administration.[4] Intentional ingestion of large amounts of verapamil can cause severe hypokalemia. Insulin, by virtue of stimulating movement of potassium into cells, is associated with transient decreases in serum potassium concentrations. Insulin-induced hypokalemia is not an important clinical problem, however, except in the case of intentional insulin overdose or during treatment of diabetic ketoacidosis.

Non-Drug-Induced Transcellular Shifts of Potassium

Hypokalemia without changes in total body potassium content occurs when potassium is acutely shifted from the extracellular fluid into cells to replace hydrogen ions, which have left cells to offset increased arterial pH (pHa). For example, serum potassium concentrations decrease approximately 0.5 mEq/L for each 10 mmHg decrease in the PaCO$_2$ (Fig. 21–2).[5] Hyperventilation of the patient's lungs during anesthesia and surgery is a common cause of acute hypokalemia due to changes in the distribution of potassium between cells and extracellular fluid.

The sympathetic nervous system modulates the distribution of potassium between intracellular and extracellular sites. In this regard, it has been observed that serum potassium concentrations measured in samples obtained immediately before the induction of anesthesia are often lower than the concentrations measured 1 to 3 days preoperatively (Fig. 21–3).[6] The most likely explanation for this

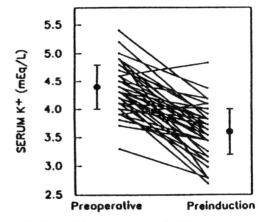

Figure 21–3 • Individual and mean (±SE) preoperative (measured 1 to 3 days before surgery) and preinduction serum potassium concentrations measured in adult patients. (From Kharasch ED, Bowdle A. Hypokalemia before induction of anesthesia and prevention by beta-2 adrenoceptor antagonism. Anesth Analg 1991;72:216–20, with permission.)

finding is stress-induced catecholamine release during the immediate preoperative period leading to β_2-adrenergic-mediated translocation of potassium into intracellular sites (Fig. 21–4).[7] The possible presence of acute stress-induced hypokalemia should be considered when interpreting serum potassium concentrations, as measured during the immediate preoperative period.

Nondrug Causes of Abnormal Losses of Potassium

Trauma, as produced by surgery, results in loss of potassium (50 mEq daily) in the urine for the first 2 days postoperatively. Potassium-free crystalloid solutions may exaggerate the clinical impact of this loss. In addition, large amounts of potassium are lost through the kidneys in the presence of acid-base disorders. Hypokalemia is an invariable consequence of metabolic alkalosis. Most often selective chloride depletion due to vomiting or nasogastric suction leads to increased renal loss of potassium. More rarely, metabolic alkalosis occurs independent of chloride depletion, as a result of systemic (primary hyperaldosteronism) or intrarenal abnormalities that augment sodium reabsorption in the distal nephrons. Hypokalemia is a cardinal feature of distal renal tubular acidosis. Magnesium depletion results in renal potassium wasting. Severe, often refractory hypokalemia due to renal potassium wasting occurs in patients with acute myelogenous or lymphoblastic leukemia. With uncontrolled dia-

betes mellitus, renal glucose loss causes osmotic diuresis and potassium excretion. With prolonged glycosuria, there is depletion of body stores or potassium, but hypokalemia is usually mild or absent because hypertonicity and insulin deficiency impede the entry of potassium into cells. The underlying potassium deficiency is rapidly unmasked when insulin is administered, and severe hypokalemia can develop, particularly in patients with diabetic keto-acidosis, unless aggressive replacement of potassium stores is undertaken at the same time.

Signs and Symptoms

Patients with hypokalemia often have no symptoms, particularly when serum potassium concentrations are between 3.0 and 3.5 mEq/L. The likelihood of symptoms appears to correlate with the rapidity of the decrease in serum potassium concentrations. In patients without underlying heart disease, abnormalities in cardiac conduction are unusual, even when serum potassium concentrations are below 3.0 mEq/L. In patients with ischemic heart disease, congestive heart failure, or left ventricular hypertrophy, however, even mild to moderate hypokalemia increases the likelihood of cardiac dysrhythmias. Chronic hypokalemia is associated with decreased myocardial contractility. Hypokalemia increases the dysrhythmogenic potential of digoxin. Potassium depletion and hypokalemia increase systolic and diastolic blood pressure when sodium intake is not restricted, presumably by promoting renal sodium

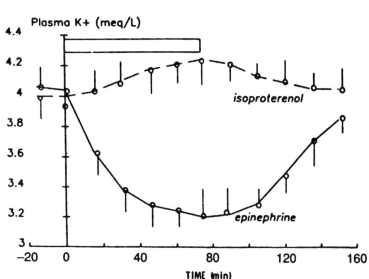

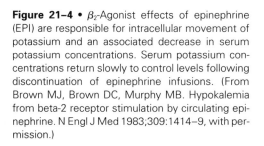

Figure 21–4 • β_2-Agonist effects of epinephrine (EPI) are responsible for intracellular movement of potassium and an associated decrease in serum potassium concentrations. Serum potassium concentrations return slowly to control levels following discontinuation of epinephrine infusions. (From Brown MJ, Brown DC, Murphy MB. Hypokalemia from beta-2 receptor stimulation by circulating epinephrine. N Engl J Med 1983;309:1414–9, with permission.)

retention. Orthostatic hypotension in the presence of hypokalemia may reflect autonomic nervous system dysfunction.

Skeletal muscle weakness, intestinal ileus, and abnormalities of cardiac electrical conduction that may accompany hypokalemia most likely reflect changes in the extracellular to intracellular potassium ratio. Skeletal muscle weakness is most prominent in the legs and rarely affects muscles innervated by cranial nerves. The kidneys often respond to potassium deficiency with decreased concentrating ability that may manifest clinically as polyuria. Metabolic alkalosis and extreme potassium deficits can result in hypokalemia.

Acute hypokalemia, as produced by hyperventilation of the patient's lungs is unlikely to produce significant alterations in cardiac conduction or myocardial contractility. In contrast, abrupt additional decreases in serum potassium concentrations in the presence of co-existing chronic hypokalemia are more likely to produce cardiac conduction and rhythm abnormalities than is the same degree of hypokalemia produced acutely but in the absence of co-existing total body potassium depletion. It is presumed that abrupt decreases in serum potassium concentrations exert more profound effects on electrochemical gradients for potassium in chronically hypokalemic patients.

Changes on the electrocardiogram (ECG) produced by hypokalemia characteristically reflect impaired cardiac conduction (Fig. 21–5).[8] Initially, U waves appear immediately after the T waves and, if erroneously considered as part of the T waves, result in calculation of falsely prolonged QT intervals. As hypokalemia becomes more severe, PR intervals are prolonged, ST segments are depressed, T waves are inverted, and prominent U waves are present. There is increased automaticity of the atria and ventricles, reflecting the more rapid rate of spontaneous depolarization, which occurs in the presence of hypokalemia. Ventricular fibrillation is a common terminal dysrhythmia in the presence of hypokalemia. Despite the commonly described characteristic changes on the ECG produced by hypokalemia, the extent to which these changes correlate with serum potassium concentrations or total body potassium deficits is controversial.

Treatment

Treatment of hypokalemia is based on potassium replacement. However, supplemental potassium administration is also the most important cause of severe hyperkalemia in patients who are hospitalized.[3] Treatment of serum potassium concentrations below 3.5 mEq/L in patients scheduled for cardiac surgery decreases the incidence of perioperative cardiac dysrhythmias.[9] The risk of treatment is highest with intravenous administration of potassium. When potassium is administered intravenously, the dose is 0.2 mEq/kg/hr (no more than 20 mEq/hr), and the patient's cardiac rhythm should be monitored continuously with the ECG. It must be appreciated that chronic hypokalemia is often associated with total body potassium deficits exceeding 500 mEq or even 1000 mEq. This finding emphasizes that total body potassium deficits cannot be totally corrected within the 12 to 24 hours preceding elective surgery. Nevertheless, intravenous infusions of potassium chloride, 0.2 mEq/kg/hr, during the few hours preceding surgery may be beneficial. It is presumed that even small amounts of potassium are helpful in normalizing the electrophysiology of cells. Repeat serum potassium concentration measurements every 12 to 24 hours are useful for guiding continued replacement and rates of intravenous infusion. When digitalis toxicity is suspected, potassium chloride can be administered as 0.5- to 1.0-mEq intravenous boluses every 3 to 5 minutes until the ECG reverts to normal. A practical point is to administer potassium chloride in a glucose-free solution; hyperglycemia would favor potassium entrance into cells, which would further exaggerate the degree of hypokalemia.

Oral potassium administration is safer than intravenous administration because potassium enters the systemic circulation more slowly. The safest way to minimize hypokalemia is to ensure adequate dietary potassium intake (bananas, oranges, cantaloupe, bran cereals, lima beans). Potassium in foods is almost entirely coupled with phosphate rather than chloride and therefore is not effective in repairing potassium loss associated with chloride depletion (diuretics, vomiting, nasogastric suction) unless chloride intake is also adequate. Salt substitutes contain approximately 12 mEq of potassium per gram as the chloride salt.

Typically, 40 to 100 mEq of supplemental potassium chloride is needed each day to maintain serum potassium concentrations near or within the normal range in patients receiving diuretics, and hypokalemia persists despite aggressive potassium replacement in approximately 10% of such patients.[3] A more effective way to restore serum potassium concentrations in these patients is to use a second diuretic drug that inhibits renal tubular secretion of potassium, such as amiloride, triamterene, or spironolactone. Although effective, these drugs can cause hyperkalemia, especially in patients with diabetes mellitus and renal insufficiency.

Regardless of the cause of hypokalemia, the ability to correct potassium deficiency is impaired when

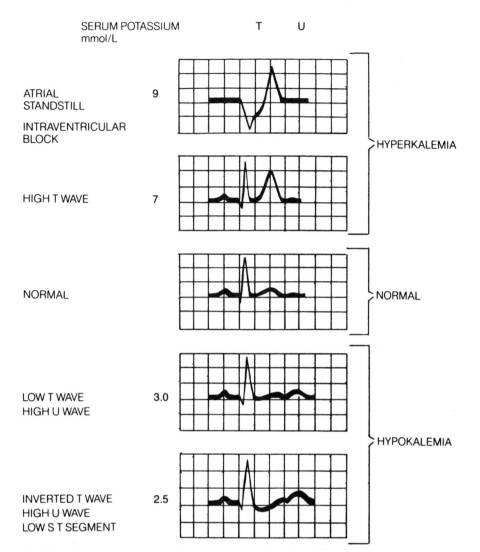

SERUM POTASSIUM mmol/L

Figure 21–5 • Manifestations on the electrocardiogram of changes in serum potassium concentrations. (From Goudsouzian NG, Karamanian A. The electrocardiogram. In: Physiology for the Anesthesiologist. Norwalk, CT: Appleton-Century-Crofts, 1977, p 37, with permission.)

magnesium deficiency is present, particularly when serum magnesium concentrations are less than 0.5 mEq/L. Magnesium repletion improves co-existing potassium deficits. For the chloride-sensitive form of metabolic alkalosis, administration of chloride corrects the metabolic alkalosis and allows repletion of body stores of potassium if potassium intake is adequate.

Management of Anesthesia

The advisability of proceeding with elective surgery in the presence of chronic serum potassium concentrations below 3.5 mEq/L is controversial.[10, 11] It is suggested that chronically hypokalemic patients are at increased risk for the development of cardiac dysrhythmias intraoperatively, especially if serum potassium concentrations are less than 3 mEq/L. Nevertheless, it is not possible to validate arbitrary serum potassium concentration values that are acceptable for elective surgery. Indeed, the incidence of intraoperative cardiac dysrhythmias is not increased in asymptomatic patients with chronic hypokalemia (2.6 to 3.5 mEq/L) undergoing elective operations.[10, 11] It is not possible to support the practice of routine preoperative potassium repletion in otherwise asymptomatic patients (with or without cardiovascular disease) solely on the basis of preoperative serum potassium concentrations.[10] It must be emphasized that adverse effects of hypokalemia are most likely when acute decreases in serum potassium concentrations are superimposed on co-existing chronic hypokalemia.

It seems logical to repeat serum potassium measurements and to obtain an ECG for evaluation of cardiac rhythm before the induction of anesthesia in patients considered at risk from the effects of hypokalemia. In this regard it is useful to recognize that the serum potassium concentrations measured just before induction of anesthesia are often lower than values measured 24 hours or more earlier (Fig. 21–3).[6] During surgery intravenous fluids should be selected to avoid glucose loads, as hyperglycemia can contribute to hypokalemia. The addition of 10 to 20 mEq of potassium chloride to each liter of intravenous fluid administered as maintenance replacement therapy is a consideration, but this approach must be weighed against the hazards of too rapid administration should infusion rates be accidentally increased during the perioperative period. Use of exogenous epinephrine should be discouraged, as β_2-agonist stimulation may shift potassium intracellularly and exaggerate co-existing hypokalemia (Fig. 21–4).[7] Furthermore, the potassium-depleted heart may be vulnerable to the dysrhythmogenic effects of catecholamines, digitalis, and calcium. Excessive hyperventilation of the patient's lungs is avoided. Continuous capnography and measurements of arterial blood gases and pHa are helpful for confirming the proper management of ventilation.

The potential for prolonged responses to nondepolarizing muscle relaxants is a consideration. A prudent approach is to decrease the initial muscle relaxant dose 30% to 50%. Administration of subsequent doses should be based on responses shown by a peripheral nerve stimulator. Nevertheless, chronic hypokalemia is likely to be associated with normal intracellular to extracellular potassium ratios such that responses to muscle relaxants are not altered.

No specific anesthetic drugs or techniques appear to be superior for use in hypokalemic patients. Nevertheless, it should be appreciated that chronic hypokalemia has been associated with decreased myocardial contractility and postural hypotension. Therefore patients with chronic hypokalemia might be unusually sensitive to the cardiac depressant effects of volatile anesthetics. Likewise, exaggerated systemic blood pressure decreases in response to positive-pressure ventilation of the patient's lungs or blood loss are likely in the presence of decreased sympathetic nervous system activity. The association of chronic hypokalemia with polyuria is considered when choosing anesthetics that are metabolized to inorganic fluoride. There is evidence that epinephrine included in local anesthetic solutions used to perform axillary blocks may be associated with evidence of hypokalemia on the ECG.[12] For this reason, it may be prudent to avoid inclusion of epinephrine in local anesthetic solutions administered to patients with co-existing hypokalemia.

It is important to monitor the ECG continuously during the intraoperative and postoperative periods for evidence of hypokalemia. Any new evidence of hypokalemia on the ECG requires prompt treatment with intravenous administration of potassium chloride, including consideration of the injection of 0.5 to 1.0 mEq IV boluses until the ECG reverts to normal.

Hyperkalemia

Hyperkalemia is defined as an increase in serum potassium concentration above 5.5 mEq/L.

Causes

The etiology of hyperkalemia is either an increase in total body potassium content or alterations in the distribution of potassium between intracellular and extracellular sites (Table 21–5).

Increased Total Body Potassium Content

Increased total body potassium content occurs when the kidneys are unable to excrete sufficient potassium to maintain the serum potassium concentrations below 5.5 mEq/L. Acute oliguric renal failure is the classic cause of hyperkalemia. In contrast, patients with chronic renal disease do not usually develop hyperkalemia until the glomerular filtration rate decreases to less than 15 ml/min. Patients

---

Table 21–5 • Causes of Hyperkalemia

Increased total body potassium content
  Acute oliguric renal failure
  Chronic renal disease
  Hypoaldosteronism
  Drugs that impair potassium excretion
    Triamterene
    Spironolactone
    Nonsteroidal antiinflammatory drugs
  Drugs that inhibit the renin-angiotensin-aldosterone system
  β-Antagonists
  Angiotensin-converting enzyme inhibitors
Altered transcellular potassium shift
  Succinylcholine
  Respiratory or metabolic acidosis
  Hemolysis
  Lysis of cells due to chemotherapy
  Iatrogenic bolus
Pseudohyperkalemia

with severe renal disease, but not requiring hemodialysis, may be vulnerable to hyperkalemia if they are challenged with exogenous potassium loads. This risk is a consideration when penicillin (1.7 mEq of potassium per 1 million units) or banked whole blood (about 1 mEq of potassium per liter for every day of storage) is administered to patients with chronic renal disease. Hypoaldosteronism favors potassium retention such that hyperkalemia can result. Likewise, diuretics such as spironolactone and triamterene, which act as aldosterone antagonists, can interfere with renal elimination of potassium.

Altered Distribution of Potassium

Altered distribution of potassium between intracellular and extracellular sites can result in hyperkalemia, even in the absence of changes in total body content of potassium. For example, the release of intracellular potassium and subsequent hyperkalemia following administration of succinylcholine to patients with burns, spinal cord transection, or skeletal muscle trauma is well recognized. Respiratory or metabolic acidosis favors passage of potassium from intracellular to extracellular locations. For example, a 0.1 unit decrease in pHa, as produced by a 10 mmHg increase in the $PaCO_2$, can increase serum potassium concentrations by about 0.5 mEq/L (Fig. 21–2).[5] Increased serum potassium concentrations can result from tumor lysis and release of intracellular constituents, including potassium. This response is most likely to occur in patients receiving cancer chemotherapeutic drugs for treatment of leukemia or lymphoma. Iatrogenic hyperkalemia has been attributed to poor mixing of potassium chloride added to plastic fluid containers, resulting in intravenous delivery of the added potassium chloride to the patient as a bolus.[13] The likelihood of inadequate mixing is minimal when potassium chloride is added to plastic containers being held in the inverted position, with the injection port uppermost.

Signs and Symptoms

Adverse effects of hyperkalemia are likely to accompany acute increases in serum potassium concentrations. In contrast, chronic hyperkalemia is more likely to be associated with normalization of gradients between intracellular and extracellular sites for potassium and subsequent return of resting membrane potentials to near-normal. Indeed, patients with chronic increases in serum potassium concentrations are often asymptomatic, which supports the notion that normalized potassium gradients across cell membranes is more important than the absolute serum potassium concentrations.

The most detrimental effect of hyperkalemia is on the cardiac conduction system. Characteristic changes produced on the ECG by hyperkalemia are prolongation of the PR intervals progressing to loss of P waves, widening of the QRS complexes, and peaking of the T waves (Fig. 21–5).[8] Ventricular tachycardia and ventricular fibrillation may occur, although the most likely cardiac event in the presence of hyperkalemia is cardiac standstill during diastole. The changes on the ECG due to hyperkalemia may be difficult to distinguish from idioventricular rhythm or acute myocardial infarction.

The appearance of abnormalities on the ECG depends on the serum potassium concentrations present as well as on the rapidity with which the concentrations increase. Cardiac conduction abnormalities are frequently present when serum potassium concentrations exceed 7.0 mEq/L. Nevertheless, these changes can manifest at even lower serum potassium concentrations if the increases are acute. Peaking of T waves on the ECG, although diagnostic, occurs in fewer than 25% of patients in the presence of hyperkalemia.

Hyperkalemia decreases the intracellular to extracellular potassium ratio, compromising neuromuscular function. Presumably, this is the explanation for the common presence of skeletal muscle weakness in these patients.

Treatment

Immediate treatment of hyperkalemia is indicated in the presence of abnormalities on the ECG or if serum potassium concentrations exceed 6.5 mEq/L (Table 21–6). Initial treatment of hyperkalemia is directed at antagonizing the adverse effects of potassium on the heart (intravenous calcium) and facilitating the movement of potassium from plasma into cells (intravenous glucose, insulin, bicarbonate, hyperventilation of the patient's lungs). Insulin is administered to ensure that glucose enters cells and carries potassium with it. Because these measures only redistribute potassium within the body to control hyperkalemia temporarily, efforts to facilitate potassium excretion (ion-exchange resins) may be initiated simultaneously. Dialysis is instituted if these measures are not promptly effective. If serum potassium concentrations are less than 6.5 mEq/L and there are no indications of cardiac toxicity on the ECG, treatment of hyperkalemia may be conservative, directed at correcting the underlying problem.

Management of Anesthesia

A common recommendation is that serum potassium concentrations should be below 5.5 mEq/L

Table 21-6 • Treatment of Hyperkalemia

Treatment	Dose	Mechanism	Onset	Duration
Calcium gluconate	10–20 ml of 10% solution IV	Direct antagonism	Rapid	15–30 minutes
Sodium bicarbonate	50–100 mEq IV	Intracellular shift	15–30 minutes	3–6 hours
Glucose and insulin	25–50 g with insulin 10–20 units IV	Intracellular shift	15–30 minutes	
Hyperventilation	PaCO$_2$ 25–30 mmHg	Intracellular shift	Rapid	
Kayexelate		Remove	1–3 hours	
Peritoneal dialysis		Remove	1–3 hours	
Hemodialysis		Remove	Rapid	

before subjecting patients to elective operations that require anesthesia. If this is not possible, it may be important to adjust anesthetic techniques to facilitate recognition of adverse effects of hyperkalemia intraoperatively and to minimize the likelihood of any additional increases in the serum potassium concentrations. Specifically, it is helpful to monitor the ECG continuously for any evidence of hyperkalemia. Ventilation of the patients' lungs is managed to maintain normocapnia. Any accumulation of carbon dioxide and concomitant respiratory acidosis could result in transfer of potassium from intracellular to extracellular sites. Metabolic acidosis due to unrecognized arterial hypoxemia or excessive depths of anesthesia could also contribute to increased extracellular distribution of potassium. Mild hyperventilation of the patient's lungs during the intraoperative period is a consideration, as a 10 mmHg decrease in the PaCO$_2$ decreases serum potassium concentrations by about 0.5 mEq/L (Fig. 21–2).[5] These goals may be facilitated by continuous capnography and periodically measuring arterial blood gases and pHa.

Possible altered responses to muscle relaxants are also considerations when hyperkalemia is present. Serum potassium concentrations may increase 0.3 to 0.5 mEq/L following administration of paralyzing doses of succinylcholine. The implications of this acute drug-induced intracellular release of potassium must be considered when the co-existing serum potassium concentration is also increased. Because there is no reliable method to prevent succinylcholine-induced potassium release, including pretreatment with nonparalyzing doses of nondepolarizing muscle relaxants, it may be best to avoid administering this drug to patients with co-existing hyperkalemia. Nevertheless, the institution of hyperventilation of the patient's lungs before administration of succinylcholine may provide some degree of protection. Responses to nondepolarizing muscle relaxants in the presence of hyperkalemia are unclear. The presence of skeletal muscle weakness preoperatively suggests the possibility of decreased muscle relaxant requirements intraoperatively. A practical approach is to titrate muscle relaxants until the desired effects are achieved, as evidenced by the responses evoked using a peripheral nerve stimulator.

Perioperative intravenous fluids must be selected with the realization that most solutions contain potassium (lactated Ringer's solution contains 4 mEq/L; Normosol-R contains 5 mEq/L). Drugs such as calcium and glucose-insulin are kept readily available to treat intraoperative manifestations of hyperkalemia. Unlike alterations in serum sodium concentrations, hyperkalemia is not associated with alterations in dose requirements for volatile anesthetics.[14]

Pseudohyperkalemia

Pseudohyperkalemia ("benign or spurious hyperkalemia") is characterized by increased serum potassium concentrations (as high as 7.0 mEq/L) owing to in vitro release of intracellular stores of this ion from leukocytes and platelets during the clotting or separation process.[15] This abnormal in vitro leakage of potassium from cells into the plasma may reflect an inherited trait and usually occurs only in patients with high leukocyte and/or platelet counts.[16] Clinically, pseudohyperkalemia is distinguished from hyperkalemia by measuring both plasma and serum concentrations of potassium. With pseudohyperkalemia only the serum concentrations are increased, and plasma levels remain normal. These patients are asymptomatic and lack detectable adrenal or renal abnormalities. Failure to recognize this syndrome could result in hypokalemia if aggressive pharmacologic attempts are instituted to lower serum potassium concentrations. Other causes of spurious hyperkalemia include hemolysis of blood samples used to measure serum potassium concentrations and perhaps the practice of repeatedly clenching and unclenching the hand

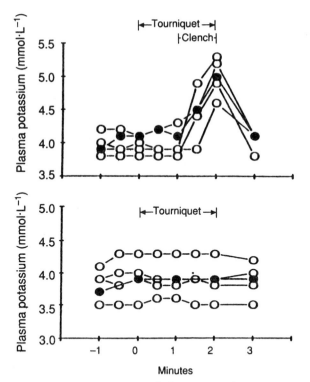

Figure 21-6 • Measurement of plasma potassium concentrations in venous blood samples obtained while the subject is clenching the hand ("making a fist") results in increased circulating concentrations of potassium compared with measurements in venous blood samples obtained when only a tourniquet is used. (From Don BR, Sebastian A, Cheitlin M, et al. Pseudohyperkalemia caused by fist clenching during phlebotomy. N Engl J Med 1990;322:1290–3, with permission.)

during venipuncture (Fig. 21–6).[17] Confirmation of the presence of pseudohyperkalemia preoperatively removes the concerns typically expressed about management of anesthesia in the presence of hyperkalemia.

Hypocalcemia

Hypocalcemia is defined as decreases in serum calcium concentrations below 4.5 mEq/L. The most common cause of hypocalcemia is decreased plasma albumin concentrations. Critically ill patients with low plasma albumin concentrations characteristically have low plasma calcium concentrations, but ionized calcium levels may be normal.[18] Other causes of hypocalcemia include acute pancreatitis, hypoparathyroidism (especially following thyroid surgery), decreased serum magnesium concentrations (malnutrition, sepsis, aminoglycoside administration), vitamin D deficiency, and renal failure.

Radiographic contrast media may contain calcium chelators that lower plasma calcium concentrations. Hyperventilation of the lungs may result in decreases in plasma ionized calcium concentrations due to alkalosis-induced increases in calcium binding to proteins. This mechanism can lead to acute ionized hypocalcemia in patients treated with sodium bicarbonate for the management of metabolic acidosis. Increased serum free fatty acid concentrations, as associated with total parenteral nutrition, may lower plasma ionized calcium concentrations. Hypocalcemia and hyperphosphatemia resulting from the use of hypertonic phosphate enemas (Fleet enema) have been associated with cardiac arrest during induction of anesthesia.[19]

Signs and Symptoms

Signs and symptoms of hypocalcemia reflect actions of calcium on the central nervous system, heart, and neuromuscular junctions. Numbness and circumoral paresthesias can progress to confusion and occasionally to seizures. Abrupt decreases in ionized calcium concentrations may be associated with hypotension and increased left ventricular filling pressures. QT intervals on the ECG can be prolonged, but this is not a consistent observation; therefore the QT interval is not a clinically reliable guide to the presence of hypocalcemia. Impaired neuromuscular function in the presence of hypocalcemia probably reflects the decreased presynaptic release of acetylcholine. Indeed, many patients with chronic hypocalcemia complain of skeletal muscle weakness and fatigue. Rapid decreases in plasma calcium concentrations, as can follow total parathyroidectomy, can produce skeletal muscle spasm manifesting as laryngospasm. Skeletal muscle spasm is most likely to occur when plasma calcium concentrations abruptly decrease below 3.5 mEq/L. In anesthetized or critically ill and unresponsive patients, the only evidence of hypocalcemia may be hypotension due to decreased myocardial contractility.[20]

Treatment

Initial treatment of hypocalcemia includes correction of any co-existing respiratory or metabolic alkalosis. An intravenous infusion of calcium is a consideration when there are clinical symptoms of hypocalcemia (hypotension, tetany) or when plasma calcium concentrations decrease below 3.5 mEq/L. Treatment consists mainly of intravenous administration of 10 ml of 10% calcium chloride (1.36 mEq/ml) or calcium gluconate (0.45 mEq/ml). Equal elemental calcium doses of calcium chloride (2.5 mg/

kg IV) or calcium gluconate (7.5 mg/kg IV) are equivalent in terms of their ability to increase the serum ionized calcium concentration.[21] Calcium should be administered until serum calcium concentrations approach 4 mEq/L or the ECG tracing returns to a normal pattern. Thiazide diuretics may be useful, as these drugs cause sodium depletion without proportional potassium excretion, thereby tending to increase serum calcium concentrations.

Management of Anesthesia

Management of anesthesia is intended to prevent further decreases in serum calcium concentrations and to recognize and treat adverse effects of hypocalcemia, particularly on the heart. For this reason, it may be important to monitor serum ionized calcium concentrations during the perioperative period in patients considered to be at risk for the development of hypocalcemia. During anesthesia and surgery it is important to appreciate that respiratory or metabolic alkalosis can rapidly decrease serum ionized calcium concentrations. This can occur during hyperventilation of the lungs or after intravenous administration of sodium bicarbonate to treat metabolic acidosis. Development of life-threatening hypocalcemia during general anesthesia has been observed in patients with renal insufficiency undergoing vascular surgery.[20]

Administration of whole blood containing citrate preservatives usually does not decrease serum calcium concentrations because calcium is rapidly mobilized from body stores. The ionized calcium concentrations can be decreased with rapid infusions of blood (500 ml every 5 to 10 minutes) or when metabolism or elimination of citrate is limited by hypothermia, cirrhosis of the liver, or renal dysfunction.[22] Although there is no evidence that co-existing hypocalcemia predisposes to citrate intoxication, it seems prudent to maintain a high index of suspicion when whole blood is administered.

Continuous monitoring of the ECG to facilitate recognition of changes characteristic of hypocalcemia is useful during the perioperative period. Intraoperative hypotension may reflect exaggerated cardiac depression produced by anesthetic drugs in the presence of decreased serum ionized calcium concentrations. Arterial blood gases, pHa, and serum ionized calcium concentration measurements are useful for guiding intraoperative management. The importance of serum albumin concentrations and administration of protein in intravenous maintenance and replacement fluids is a consideration when interpreting serum calcium concentrations. Administration of colloid solutions is particularly important in the presence of loss of intravascular fluid into tissues due to surgical trauma.

Responses to nondepolarizing muscle relaxants could be potentiated by hypocalcemia. Nevertheless, clinical experience is too limited to confirm this speculation. Theoretically, coagulation abnormalities could also accompany extreme decreases in serum calcium concentrations. Postoperatively, it is useful to recognize that sudden decreases in the serum calcium concentrations can produce skeletal muscle spasm, including laryngospasm.

Hypercalcemia

Hypercalcemia is defined as increases in serum calcium concentrations above 5.5 mEq/L. The most common causes of hypercalcemia are hyperparathyroidism and neoplastic disorders with bone metastases. Less common causes include pulmonary granulomatous diseases (sarcoidosis), vitamin D intoxication, and immobilization.

Signs and Symptoms

Signs and symptoms of hypercalcemia reflect actions of calcium on the central nervous system, heart, kidneys, gastrointestinal tract, and neuromuscular junctions. Early signs and symptoms include sedation and vomiting. Persistently increased serum calcium concentrations (7 to 8 mEq/L) can interfere with urine concentrating ability, resulting in polyuria. In addition, increased serum calcium concentrations can contribute to the formation of renal calculi, and oliguric renal failure can develop in advanced cases of hypercalcemia. When serum calcium concentrations exceed 8 mEq/L, cardiac conduction disturbances, characterized as prolonged PR intervals, wide QRS complexes, and shortened QT intervals may appear on the ECG tracing.

Treatment

Treatment of hypercalcemia is hydration with normal saline, 150 ml/hr.[23] Hydration lowers serum calcium concentrations by dilution, and sodium acts to inhibit renal tubular absorption of calcium. Diuresis produced with furosemide, 40 to 80 mg IV every 2 to 4 hours, minimizes the risk of overhydration and further facilitates renal elimination of calcium. Volume expansion precedes the administration of furosemide because drug-induced diuresis depends on delivery of calcium to the renal tubules. The goal is a daily urine output of 3 to 5 L. Thiazide diuretics are not administered for treatment of hypercalcemia, as these drugs may enhance renal tubular reabsorption of calcium. Ambulation is an important aspect of treatment, as it decreases calcium release from bone associated with immobilization.

Bisphosphonates such as disodium etidronate are the drugs of choice for treating life-threatening hypercalcemia. These drugs bind to hydroxyapatite in bones and act as potent inhibitors of osteoclastic bone resorption. The effectiveness of bisphosphonate allows surgery to be performed electively rather than emergently in unstable hypercalcemic patients. Hemodialysis can also be used to lower serum calcium concentrations promptly. Calcitonin is effective for prompt lowering of serum calcium concentrations, but the effects of this hormone are transient. Mithramycin inhibits osteoclastic activity of parathormone, producing prompt lowering of serum calcium concentrations. The toxic effects of mithramycin (thrombocytopenia, hepatotoxicity, nephrotoxicity) limit its use.

Management of Anesthesia

Management of anesthesia in the presence of hypercalcemia includes intravenous hydration with sodium-containing crystalloid solutions to stimulate urine output. Continuous monitoring of the ECG for evidence of adverse effects of calcium on the cardiac conduction system is useful. The choice of anesthetic drugs may be influenced by the presence of impaired urine concentrating ability and polyuria, which could be confused with fluoride-induced nephrotoxicity attributed to metabolism of certain volatile anesthetics. Theoretically, hyperventilation of the patient's lungs is undesirable, as respiratory alkalosis lowers serum potassium concentrations and leaves the actions of calcium unopposed. Nevertheless, by lowering the ionized calcium concentrations, alkalosis could be beneficial. Responses to nondepolarizing muscle relaxants are not well defined, but the preoperative existence of skeletal muscle weakness suggests decreased dose requirements for these drugs.

Hypomagnesemia

Hypomagnesemia is defined as decreases in serum magnesium concentrations below 1.5 mEq/L. Total body magnesium stores are about 2000 mEq, and most of this magnesium is distributed to intracellular sites (Table 21–2). Excretion of magnesium is via the gastrointestinal tract and kidneys. The most important physiologic effect of magnesium is regulation of the presynaptic release of acetylcholine.

Hypomagnesemia is associated with chronic alcoholism, malabsorption syndromes, hyperalimentation therapy without added magnesium, and protracted vomiting or diarrhea.[24] Hypokalemia that is resistant to treatment with potassium supplements may be caused by hypomagnesemia.

Signs and Symptoms

Signs and symptoms of hypomagnesemia are similar to those observed in patients with hypocalcemia. Indeed, both hypomagnesemia and hypocalcemia frequently present as combined electrolyte disorders. Predictable manifestations of hypomagnesemia include central nervous system irritability reflected by hyperreflexia and seizures, skeletal muscle spasms, and cardiac irritability. Hypomagnesemia can potentiate digitalis-induced cardiac dysrhythmias. Cardiac dysrhythmias attributed to diuretic-induced hypokalemia may in fact be due to hypomagnesemia.[25]

Treatment

Treatment of hypomagnesemia is with magnesium sulfate, 1 g IV, administered over 15 to 20 minutes. Systemic blood pressure, heart rate, and patellar reflexes should be monitored. Depression or disappearance of patellar reflexes is an indication to stop magnesium replacement therapy.

Management of Anesthesia

The importance of hypomagnesemia in the management of anesthesia is primarily related to associated disturbances such as alcoholism, malnutrition, and hypovolemia. Conceivably, decreased plasma magnesium concentrations could interfere with responses to muscle relaxants, but this possibility has not been studied.

Hypermagnesemia

Hypermagnesemia is defined as increases in serum magnesium concentrations above 2.5 mEq/L. The most common causes of hypermagnesemia are iatrogenic, including administration of magnesium sulfate to treat pregnancy-induced hypertension and excessive individual use of antacids or laxatives. Patients with chronic renal dysfunction are at increased risk of developing hypermagnesemia, as magnesium elimination depends on the glomerular filtration rate. Indeed, serum magnesium concentrations increase predictably when exogenous magnesium is administered to patients with glomerular filtration rates below 30 ml/min.

Signs and Symptoms

Hypermagnesemia can exert adverse effects on the central nervous system, heart, and neuromuscular junctions. Central nervous system depression is displayed as hyporeflexia plus sedation, which may progress to coma. Cardiac depression may be prominent. Skeletal muscle weakness, presumably reflecting decreased acetylcholine release secondary to increased magnesium levels, can be so severe as to impair ventilation. Indeed, the most common causes of death from hypermagnesemia are cardiac and ventilatory arrest.

Treatment

Signs and symptoms of hypermagnesemia can be temporarily reversed with intravenous administration of calcium. Elimination of magnesium can be facilitated by fluid loading and diuresis produced by diuretics. The definitive therapy for persistent and life-threatening hypermagnesemia requires peritoneal dialysis or hemodialysis.

Management of Anesthesia

Acidosis and dehydration must be prevented intraoperatively, as these events lead to increased serum magnesium concentrations. Therefore ventilation of the patient's lungs should be managed to ensure the absence of respiratory acidosis due to hypoventilation. Capnography, arterial blood gases, and pHa determinations are useful for guiding management of ventilation of the lungs and ensuring the absence of systemic acidosis. Intravenous fluid maintenance and replacement should be adjusted to maintain urine output. Stimulation of urine output with diuretics, such as furosemide, may be necessary.

Hypermagnesemia potentiates the actions of nondepolarizing and depolarizing muscle relaxants, emphasizing the importance of decreasing the initial doses of muscle relaxants. Subsequent doses are based on responses observed with a peripheral nerve stimulator.

It is conceivable that cardiac depression produced by anesthetic drugs could be exaggerated in the presence of hypermagnesemia. Furthermore, increased serum magnesium concentrations produce vasodilation, which might be further accentuated by drugs administered during anesthesia and surgery. These speculations remain undocumented, but it seems prudent to titrate doses of anesthetic drugs, maintaining a high index of suspicion for magnesium-anesthetic drug interactions should hypotension occur.

■ ACID-BASE DISTURBANCES

Acid-base homeostasis exerts major influences on enzyme function with subsequent effects on tissue and organ system function.[26] Deviations in pHa from the normal value of 7.4 can have adverse consequences and in some instances can be life-threatening. It is the condition that causes the change in pHa more than the actual pHa value that determines the patient's status and prognosis. In this regard, the management of serious acid-base disturbances always requires diagnosis and treatment of the underlying disease as well as any indicated interventions to treat changes in pHa.[26]

Classification

Acid-base disturbances are classified as respiratory or metabolic based on measurement of arterial hy-

Table 21–7 • Direction of Changes During Acute and Chronic Acid-Base Disturbances

Parameter	pHa	PaCO$_2$	HCO$_3$
Respiratory acidosis			
Acute	Moderate decrease	Marked increase	Slight increase
Chronic	Slight decrease	Marked increase	Moderate increase
Respiratory alkalosis			
Acute	Moderate increase	Marked decrease	Slight decrease
Chronic	Slight increase to no change	Marked decrease	Moderate decrease
Metabolic acidosis			
Acute	Moderate to marked decrease	Slight decrease	Marked decrease
Chronic	Slight decrease	Moderate decrease	Marked decrease
Metabolic alkalosis			
Acute	Marked increase	Moderate increase	Marked increase
Chronic	Marked increase	Moderate increase	Marked increase

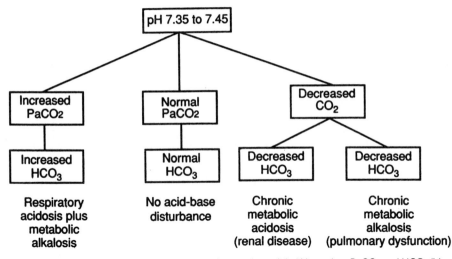

Figure 21–7 • Diagnostic approach to the interpretation of normal arterial pH based on $PaCO_2$ and HCO_3 (bicarbonate) concentrations.

drogen ion concentrations (pHa) and $PaCO_2$ and estimation of serum bicarbonate concentrations from a nomogram (Table 21–7). The first determination is whether the pHa is less than 7.35, higher than 7.45, or in between. A normal pHa may reflect the absence of an acid-base disturbance, a chronic disturbance with compensation, or a mixed acid-base disturbance (Fig. 21–7). If the pHa is less than 7.35, the diagnosis is either respiratory acidosis or metabolic acidosis (Fig. 21–8). If the pHa is higher than 7.45, the diagnosis is respiratory alkalosis or metabolic alkalosis, as determined by measuring the

$PaCO_2$ and calculating the serum bicarbonate concentration (Fig. 21–9). Once the nature of the acid-base disturbance has been established, the search for causes can be initiated and appropriate treatment instituted.

When the acid-base disturbance results principally from changes in alveolar ventilation, the designation is respiratory acidosis or alkalosis. By convention, $PaCO_2$ values above 45 mmHg are defined as representing alveolar hypoventilation, whereas alveolar hyperventilation is present when $PaCO_2$ values are below 35 mmHg. Alveolar hypoventila-

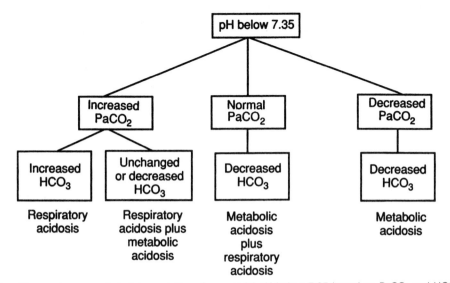

Figure 21–8 • Diagnostic approach to interpretation of an arterial pH below 7.35 based on $PaCO_2$ and HCO_3 (bicarbonate) concentrations.

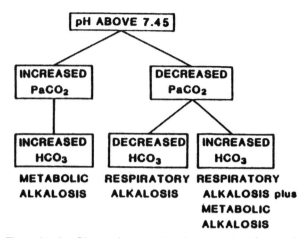

Figure 21–9 • Diagnostic approach to interpretation of an arterial pH above 7.45 based on PaCO₂ and HCO₃ (bicarbonate) concentrations.

tion is synonymous with respiratory acidosis, and alveolar hyperventilation is synonymous with respiratory alkalosis. Changes in pHa that are unrelated to primary alterations in $PaCO_2$ are designated metabolic acidosis or alkalosis.

Henderson-Hasselbalch Equation

Normal pHa is regulated over a narrow range of 7.35 to 7.45. In this regard, a normal pHa depends on maintenance of an optimal 20:1 ratio of bicarbonate to carbon dioxide concentrations (Henderson-Hasselbalch equation) (Table 21–8). Acid-base disturbances characterized by changes in serum bicarbonate concentrations are predictably accompanied by appropriate compensatory changes in $PaCO_2$ secondary to alterations in alveolar ventila-

---

Table 21–8 • Henderson-Hasselbalch Equation

$$pHa = pK + \log \frac{HCO_3}{0.03 \times PaCO_2}$$

where pHa = negative logarithm of the arterial concentration of hydrogen ions; pK = 6.1 at 37°C; HCO₃ = concentration of bicarbonate (mEq/L).

Substitution of average values for pHa (7.4) and PaCO₂ (40 mmHg) results in a calculated bicarbonate concentration of 24 mEq/L. Maintenance of a normal bicarbonate concentration relative to the concentration of carbon dioxide results in an optimal ratio of about 20:1 (24 mEq/L divided by 1.2). This optimal ratio of 20:1 permits maintenance of a relatively normal pHa despite deviations from normal in the bicarbonate concentration.

$$CO_2 + H_2O \rightleftarrows H_2CO_3 \rightleftarrows HCO_3^- + H^+$$

Figure 21–10 • Hydration of carbon dioxide results in H₂CO₃ (carbonic acid), which subsequently dissociates into HCO₃ (bicarbonate) and H⁺ (hydrogen) ions.

tion. If a 20:1 ratio is maintained, the pHa remains within the normal range, despite the presence of acid-base disturbances (Fig. 21–7). For example, respiratory acidosis or alkalosis is compensated for by renal-induced changes in serum bicarbonate concentrations that begin in 6 to 12 hours and serve to maintain a 20:1 ratio. After a few days, as a result of this renal compensation, the pHa in the presence of chronic respiratory acidosis or alkalosis is returned to normal despite persistent alterations in $PaCO_2$ (Table 21–7). Acid-base disturbances due to metabolic acidosis or alkalosis are compensated for by ventilation-induced changes in the $PaCO_2$ that tend to restore the 20:1 ratio and return the pHa toward normal (Table 21–7). In contrast to the renal compensatory mechanisms that restore pHa to normal in the presence of respiratory acidosis or alkalosis, ventilatory compensatory mechanisms only partially correct the pHa in the presence of metabolic acidosis or alkalosis.

Serum Bicarbonate Concentrations

Interpretation of nomogram-derived estimates of serum bicarbonate concentrations as a reflection of acid-base disturbances due to metabolic derangements requires an adjustment for the impact of alveolar ventilation. For example, an increase in $PaCO_2$ leads to hydration of carbon dioxide to carbonic acid with subsequent increases in serum bicarbonate concentrations (Fig. 21–10). Conversely, lowering the $PaCO_2$ reverses the direction of this reaction, resulting in decreases in serum bicarbonate concentrations. These changes are nearly linear and permit use of a guideline for clinical interpretation and adjustment of the estimated serum bicarbonate concentrations (Table 21–9). For example, using this

---

Table 21–9 • Impact of Ventilation on Serum Bicarbonate Concentrations

Change in PaCO₂ Equal to 10 mmHg	Change in Bicarbonate Concentration (from 24 mEq/L)
Acute increase	Increase 1 mEq/L
Chronic increase	Increase 3 mEq/L
Acute decrease	Decrease 2 mEq/L
Chronic decrease	Decrease 5 mEq/L

guideline, alveolar hypoventilation leading to acute increases in PaCO$_2$ up to 70 mmHg would result in normalized serum bicarbonate concentrations of 27 mEq/L, assuming a normal value of 24 mEq/L.

Signs and Symptoms

Major adverse consequences of severe systemic acidosis (pHa less than 7.2) can occur independently of whether the acidosis is of respiratory, metabolic, or mixed origin (Table 21–10).[26] The effects of acidosis are particularly detrimental to the cardiovascular system. Acidosis decreases myocardial contractility, although minimal clinical effects are present until the pHa decreases below 7.2, perhaps reflecting the effects of catecholamine release in response to acidosis.[27] When the pHa is less than 7.1, cardiac responsiveness to catecholamines decreases, and compensatory inotropic effects are diminished. Detrimental effects of acidosis may be accentuated in those with underlying left ventricular dysfunction or myocardial ischemia or in those in whom sympathetic nervous system activity is impaired, as by drug-induced β-adrenergic blockade or general anesthesia.

Major adverse consequences of severe systemic alkalosis (pHa above 7.60) reflect impairment of cerebral and coronary blood flow due to arteriolar vasoconstriction, an effect that is more pronounced in respiratory than metabolic alkalosis (Table 21–11).[26] Associated decreases in serum ionized calcium concentrations probably contribute to the neurologic abnormalities associated with systemic alkalosis. Alkalosis predisposes patients to refractory ventricular dysrhythmias, especially in patients with co-existing heart disease. Alkalosis depresses ventilation and can frustrate efforts to wean patients from mechanical ventilation.[26] Hypokalemia accompanies systemic alkalosis but is more prominent in the presence of metabolic alkalosis. Alkalosis stimulates anaerobic glycolysis and increases the production of lactic acid and ketoacids. Although alkalosis can decrease the release of oxygen to the tissues by tightening the binding of oxygen to hemoglobin, chronic alkalosis negates this effect by increasing the concentrations of 2,3-diphosphoglycerate in erythrocytes.

Respiratory Acidosis

Respiratory acidosis is present when decreases in alveolar ventilation result in increases in the PaCO$_2$ sufficient to decrease the pHa to less than 7.35 (Table 21–12). Carbonic acid resulting from dissolved carbon dioxide is considered a respiratory acid. The most likely cause of respiratory acidosis during the perioperative period is drug-induced depression of ventilation (opioids, general anesthetics). Respiratory acidosis may be complicated by metabolic aci-

---

Table 21–10 • Adverse Consequences of Severe Acidosis

Nervous system
  Obtundation
  Coma
Cardiovascular system
  Impaired myocardial contractility
  Decreased cardiac output
  Decreased arterial blood pressure
  Sensitization to reentrant cardiac dysrhythmias
  Decreased threshold for ventricular fibrillation
  Decreased responsiveness to catecholamines
Ventilation
  Hyperventilation
  Dyspnea
  Fatigue of muscles of breathing
Metabolism
  Hyperkalemia
  Insulin resistance
  Inhibition of anaerobic glycolysis

Adapted from: Adrogue HJ, Madias NE. Management of life-threatening acid-base disorders. N Engl J Med 1998;338:26–34.

Table 21–11 • Adverse Consequences of Alkalosis

Nervous system
  Decreased cerebral blood flow
  Seizures
  Lethargy
  Delirium
  Tetany
Cardiovascular system
  Arteriolar vasoconstriction
  Decreased coronary blood flow
  Decreased threshold for angina pectoris
  Predisposition to refractory supraventricular and
    ventricular cardiac dysrhythmias
Ventilation
  Hypoventilation
  Hypercarbia
  Arterial hypoxemia
Metabolism
  Hypokalemia
  Decreased serum ionized calcium concentrations
  Hypomagnesemia
  Hypophosphatemia
  Stimulation of anaerobic glycolysis and production of
    organic acids

Adapted from: Adrogue JH, Madias NE. Management of life-threatening acid-base disorders. N Engl J Med 1998;338:107–11.

Table 21–12 • Causes of Respiratory Acidosis

Drug-induced depression of ventilation (opioids, volatile anesthetics)
Permissive hypercapnia
Upper airway obstruction
Status asthmaticus
Restriction of ventilation (rib fractures with flail chest)
Disorders of neuromuscular function
Malignant hyperthermia
Hyperalimentation solutions

Table 21–13 • Causes of Respiratory Alkalosis

Iatrogenic (mechanical hyperventilation)
Decreased barometric pressure
Arterial hypoxemia
Central nervous system injury
Hepatic disease
Pregnancy
Salicylate overdose

dosis when renal perfusion is decreased to the extent that reabsorption mechanisms through the renal tubules are impaired (Fig. 21–8). For example, cardiac output and renal blood flow may be so decreased in patients with chronic obstructive pulmonary disease and cor pulmonale as to lead to metabolic acidosis.

Respiratory acidosis is treated by correcting the disorder responsible for hypoventilation. Mechanical ventilation of the patient's lungs is necessary when the increases in $PaCO_2$ are marked. It must be remembered that rapid lowering of chronically increased $PaCO_2$ levels by mechanical hyperventilation decreases body stores of carbon dioxide more rapidly than the kidneys can produce corresponding decreases in the serum bicarbonate concentrations. The resulting metabolic alkalosis can cause neuromuscular irritability and excitation of the central nervous system, manifesting as seizures. For this reason it is best to decrease the $PaCO_2$ slowly to permit sufficient time for renal tubular elimination of bicarbonate.

Metabolic alkalosis may also accompany respiratory acidosis when the body stores of chloride and potassium are decreased. For example, decreased serum chloride concentrations facilitate renal tubular reabsorption of bicarbonate, leading to metabolic alkalosis. Hypokalemia stimulates renal tubules to excrete hydrogen, which may produce metabolic alkalosis or aggravate a co-existing alkalosis due to chloride deficiency. Treatment of metabolic alkalosis associated with these electrolyte disturbances is with intravenous administration of potassium chloride.

Respiratory Alkalosis

Respiratory alkalosis is present when increases in alveolar ventilation result in decreases in $PaCO_2$ sufficient to increase the pHa to higher than 7.45 (Table 21–13). The most likely cause of acute respiratory alkalosis during the perioperative period is iatrogenic hyperventilation of the patient's lungs, as may occur during general anesthesia. Respiratory alkalosis occurs normally during pregnancy and on ascents to high altitudes.

Treatment of respiratory alkalosis is directed at correcting the underlying disorder responsible for alveolar hyperventilation. During anesthesia this is most often accomplished by adjusting the mechanical ventilator to decrease alveolar ventilation. Additional deadspace can be added to the breathing circuit to increase rebreathing of exhaled gases containing carbon dioxide. In selected patients it may be appropriate to add carbon dioxide from a metered source to the inspired gases in attempts to reestablish a more normal $PaCO_2$. The hypokalemia and hypochloremia that characterize respiratory alkalosis may also require treatment.

Metabolic Acidosis

Metabolic acidosis is characterized by decreased pHa owing to accumulation of nonvolatile acids, as is likely to accompany major organ system dysfunction, especially renal failure (Table 21–14). Decreased cardiac output and associated inadequate tissue oxygenation results in anaerobic metabolism and accumulation of lactic acid.[28] Severe diarrhea and loss of bicarbonate can lead to metabolic acidosis, especially in pediatric patients. Serum bicarbonate concentrations decrease owing to buffering of nonvolatile acids in the circulation.

Table 21–14 • Causes of Metabolic Acidosis

Lactic acidosis (inadequate tissue oxygenation)
Dilutional acidosis
Diabetic ketoacidosis
Renal failure
Hepatic failure
Methanol and ethylene glycol intoxication
Aspirin intoxication
Increased skeletal muscle activity
Cyanide poisoning
Carbon monoxide poisoning

Specific Disorders

Metabolic acidosis may reflect specific disorders leading to accumulation of organic acids (Table 21–14).[26]

Lactic acidosis is most often caused by tissue hypoxia due to circulatory failure.[26] The resultant acidosis compounds hemodynamic dysfunction, which further suppresses lactate consumption by the liver and kidneys, creating a vicious cycle. Improvements in tissue oxygenation may require administration of supplemental oxygen, mechanical support of ventilation, repletion of extracellular fluid volume, and administration of vasodilating and inotropic drugs such as dopamine or dobutamine. Specific interventions include administration of antibiotics for treatment of sepsis, operative intervention for trauma or tissue ischemia, and dialysis to remove specific toxins. In the presence of severe lactic acidosis, intravenous administration of sodium bicarbonate may be indicated. The prognosis of patients with lactic acidosis is poor if the underlying cause cannot be effectively managed.

Dilutional acidosis may occur when serum bicarbonate concentrations are diluted by expansion of the extracellular fluid volume due to administration of solutions (normal saline) that do not contain bicarbonate.[29, 30] Clinically, a hyperchloremic dilutional metabolic acidosis may accompany aggressive volume resuscitation with isotonic saline during intraoperative management of patients experiencing blood loss and/or extensive tissue dissection. Provision of sodium bicarbonate in the infused crystalloid solutions should prevent this complication. Measurement of serum lactic acid concentrations and calculation of the anion gap from sodium, chloride, and bicarbonate concentrations differentiates dilutional acidosis from acidosis due to inadequate tissue perfusion.

Treatment

Metabolic acidosis is treated by removing the cause of the accumulation of nonvolatile acids in the circulation. It has been common practice to treat acute metabolic acidosis with intravenous administration of sodium bicarbonate, especially if myocardial depression or cardiac dysrhythmias are present. A formula designed to calculate doses of sodium bicarbonate is based on the deviation of serum bicarbonate concentrations from normal, the percentage of body mass that exists as extracellular fluid, and the ideal body weight (Table 21–15). A useful approach is to administer about one-half the calculated dose of sodium bicarbonate, followed in about 30 minutes by repeat measurements of the pHa to evaluate the impact of treatment. It is important to appreciate that sodium bicarbonate administration results in endogenous carbon dioxide production (1 mEq/kg IV produces about 180 ml of carbon dioxide), necessitating increases in alveolar ventilation to prevent hypercarbia and worsening of the already existing acidosis. In addition, administration of sodium bicarbonate may result in hypernatremia and hyperosmolarity and contribute to extracellular volume overload, especially in patients with congestive heart failure and renal failure. For these reasons, alternatives to sodium bicarbonate, such as tromethamine [tris(hydroxymethyl)aminomethane (THAM)], have been proposed as treatments for metabolic acidosis.[27] THAM limits carbon dioxide production and increases intracellular and extracellular pH, but it has not been documented to be clinically more efficacious than bicarbonate. In fact, serious side effects, including hyperkalemia, hypoglycemia, ventilatory depression, and local tissue injury (should accidental extravasation occur), have markedly limited the usefulness of THAM.[26] Administration of sodium bicarbonate during cardiopulmonary resuscitation is considered less important than alveolar ventilation for correction of acidosis.

Metabolic Alkalosis

Metabolic alkalosis is characterized by the loss of nonvolatile acids from extracellular fluid (Table 21–16). For example, prolonged vomiting and nasogastric suction can result in the loss of hydrochloric

---

Table 21–15 • Calculation of the Dose of Sodium Bicarbonate to Treat Metabolic Acidosis

Sodium bicarbonate (mEq) = body weight (kg) × deviation of serum bicarbonate concentration from normal
× extracellular fluid volume as a fraction of body mass (0.2)

Evaluation of an 80 kg patient in hemorrhagic shock reveals the following: pHa 7.20, $PaCO_2$ 60 mmHg, and bicarbonate 16 mEq/L. The normalized serum bicarbonate concentration corrected for the increased $PaCO_2$ would be 26 mEq/L (see Table 21–9). The calculated dose of sodium bicarbonate to replace the bicarbonate deficit would be 160 mEq (80 kg × 10 mEq/L × 0.2). About one-half of this calculated dose of sodium bicarbonate should be administered intravenously followed by a repeat measurement of the pHa in about 30 minutes to evaluate the impact of therapy.

Table 21–16 • Causes of Metabolic Alkalosis

Hypovolemia
Vomiting
Nasogastric suction
Diuretic therapy
Iatrogenic
Hyperaldosteronism
Chloride-wasting diarrhea

acid, with subsequent metabolic alkalosis. Diuretics that inhibit renal tubular reabsorption of sodium and potassium lead to hypokalemia and an associated metabolic alkalosis. In the past, overzealous intravenous administration of sodium bicarbonate to treat metabolic acidosis during cardiopulmonary resuscitation has resulted in metabolic alkalosis.

Depletion of intravascular fluid volume is often the most important factor in maintaining metabolic alkalosis. Indeed, hypovolemia should be considered during the postoperative period in patients who develop metabolic alkalosis. Because loss of potassium often parallels loss of sodium, hypokalemia is frequently present when hypovolemia complicates metabolic alkalosis. Skeletal muscle weakness also accompanies hypokalemia. Urinary chloride excretion is usually less than 10 mEq/L in the presence of metabolic alkalosis associated with depletion of intravascular fluid volume.[31]

Treatment of metabolic alkalosis is directed at resolution of those events responsible for the acid-base derangement, as well as appropriate replacement of electrolytes. On occasion, intravenous infusion of hydrogen in the form of ammonium chloride or 0.1 N hydrochloric acid (no more than 0.2 mEq/kg/hr) is used to facilitate the return of pHa to near-normal levels. Administration of hydrochloric acid requires insertion of a central venous catheter, as injection through a peripheral vein can cause sclerosis of the vein.

References

1. Adrogue HJ, Madias NE. Hyponatremia. N Engl J Med 2000;342:1581–9
2. Ayxis JC, Krothapalli RK, Arieff AI. Treatment of symptomatic hyponatremia and its relation to brain damage: a prospective study. N Engl J Med 1987;317:1190–7
3. Gennari FJ. Hypokalemia. N Engl J Med 1998;339:451–8
4. Hurlbert BJ, Edelman JD, David K. Serum potassium levels during and after terbutaline. Anesth Analg 1981;60:723–5
5. Edwards R, Winnie AR, Ramamurthy S. Acute hypocapneic hypokalemia: an iatrogenic anesthetic complication. Anesth Analg 1977;56:786–92
6. Kharasch ED, Bowdle TA. Hypokalemia before induction of anesthesia and its prevention by beta-2 adrenoceptor antagonism. Anesth Analg 1991;72:216–20
7. Brown MJ, Brown DC, Murphy MB. Hypokalemia from beta-2 receptor stimulation by circulating epinephrine. N Engl J Med 1983;309:1414–9
8. Goudsouzian NG, Karamanian A. The electrocardiogram. In: Physiology for the Anesthesiologist. Norwalk, CT: Appleton-Centrury-Crofts, 1977;37
9. Wahr JA, Parks R, Boisvert D, et al. Preoperative serum potassium levels and perioperative outcomes in cardiac surgical patients. JAMA 1999;281:2203–10
10. Hirsch IA, Tomlinson DL, Slogoff S, et al. The overstated risk of preoperative hypokalemia. Anesth Analg 1988;67:131–6
11. Vitez TS, Soper LE, Wong KC, et al. Chronic hypokalemia and intraoperative dysrhythmias. Anesthesiology 1985;63:130–3
12. Toyoda Y, Kuboa Y, Kubota H, et al. Prevention of hypokalemia during axillary nerve block with 1% lidocaine and epinephrine 1:100,000. Anesthesiology 1988;69:109–2
13. Williams RP. Potassium overdosage: a potential hazard of nonrigid parenteral fluid containers. BMJ 1973;1:714–5
14. Tanifuji Y, Eger EI. Brain sodium, potassium, and osmolality: effects on anesthetic requirement. Anesth Analg 1978;57:404–10
15. Naidu R, Steg NL, MacEwen GD. Hyperkalemia: benign, hereditary autosomal trait. Anesthesiology 1982;56:226–8
16. Ho AM-H, Woo JCH, Kelton JG, et al. Spurious hyperkalemia associated with severe thrombocytosis and leukocytosis. Can J Anaesth 1991;38:613–5
17. Don BR, Sebastian A, Cheitlin M, et al. Pseudohyperkalemia caused by fist clenching during phlebotomy. N Engl J Med 1990;322:1290–2
18. Zaloga GP, Chernow B. Hypocalcemia in critical illness. JAMA 1986;256:1924–9
19. Reddy JC, Zwiren GT. Enema-induced hypocalcemia and hyperphosphatemia leading to cardiac arrest during induction of anesthesia in an outpatient surgery center. Anesthesiology 1983;59:578–9
20. Prielipp RC, Zaloga GP. Life-threatening hypocalcemia after abdominal aortic aneurysm repair in patients with renal insufficiency. Anesth Analg 1991;73:638–41
21. Cote CJ, Drop LJ, Daniels AL, et al. Calcium chloride versus calcium gluconate: comparison of ionization and cardiovascular effects in children and dogs. Anesthesiology 1987;66:465–70
22. Denlinger JK, Nahrwold ML, Gibbs PS, et al. Hypocalcemia during rapid blood transfusion in anesthetized man. Br J Anaesth 1976;48:995–1000
23. Bilezikian JP. Management of acute hypercalcemia. N Engl J Med 1992;326:1196–1203
24. James MFM. Clinical use of magnesium infusions in anesthesia. Anesth Analg 1992;74:129–36
25. Harris MNE, Crowther A, Jupp RA, et al. Magnesium and coronary revascularization. Br J Anaesth 1988;60:779–83
26. Adrogue HJ, Madias NE. Management of life-threatening acid-base disorders. N Engl J Med 1998;338:26–34, 107–11
27. Hindman BJ. Sodium bicarbonate in the treatment of subtypes of acute lactic acidosis: physiologic considerations. Anesthesiology 1990;72:1064–76
28. Mizock BA. Controversies in lactic acidosis: implications in critically ill patients. JAMA 1987;258:497–501
29. Mathes DD, Morell RC, Rohr MS. Dilutional acidosis: is it a real clinical entity? Anesthesiology 1997;86:501–3
30. Prough DS. Acidosis associated with perioperative saline administration: dilution or delusion? Anesthesiology 2000;93:1167–9
31. Sherman RA, Eisinger RP. The use (and misuse) of urinary sodium and chloride measurements. JAMA 1982;247:3121–4

22

Endocrine Diseases

Endocrine disease is characterized by overproduction or underproduction of single or multiple hormones. Alterations in the physiologic responses to stress or to changes in homeostatic mechanisms reflect the impact of excessive or deficient amounts of these hormones. An endocrine gland disorder may be the primary reason for surgery, or it may co-exist in patients requiring operations unrelated to endocrine gland dysfunction. The presence of unsuspected endocrine disease may be determined by seeking the answer to specific questions during the patient's preoperative evaluation (Table 22–1).

▌ DIABETES MELLITUS

Diabetes mellitus (diabetes) is characterized by metabolic dysregulation, most notably that of glucose metabolism, accompanied by predictable long-term vascular and neurologic complications.[1] The isolation of insulin in 1922 resulted in an effective treatment and converted an otherwise uniformly fatal disease to a chronic disease with significant morbidity (peripheral vascular disease, ischemic heart disease, renal disease, blindness, peripheral neuropathy).

Classification

Diabetes has several clinical forms, each of which has a distinct etiology, clinical presentation, and course (Table 22–2).[1]

Insulin-Dependent Diabetes Mellitus

Insulin-dependent diabetes mellitus (IDDM) occurs most often in patients younger than 20 years of age with a peak onset around the time of puberty. A relatively small percentage of new cases of IDDM first manifest in patients older than 50 years of age, and these patients are thin, prone to ketoacidosis, and share genetic and immunologic markers with IDDM patients whose disease begins in youth. The greatest incidence of IDDM is found in northern Europe (1 in every 150 Finns develop IDDM by 15 years of age), whereas it is less common in African-American and Asian populations. IDDM affects approximately 1 in every 250 persons in the United States. Loci on chromosome 6 may account for the major genetic component of IDDM.

Non-Insulin-Dependent Diabetes Mellitus

Non-insulin-dependent diabetes mellitus (NIDDM) is almost always associated with obesity, a sedentary lifestyle, and advancing age (most patients are older than 40 years of age). Compared with IDDM, NIDDM is a common disease with an incidence of 6.6% in the United States.[1] Approximately 50% of patients with NIDDM are unaware of their disease. Patients who develop NIDDM at a young age are often morbidly obese, are offspring of two parents with NIDDM, have a history of gestational diabetes mellitus, or are members of a racial group with a high incidence of the disease (Native Americans, African-Americans, Hispanic-Americans). The dramatic increase in the prevalence of NIDDM in the United States is commonly attributed to an aging population (18% of patients older than 65 years of age have NIDDM), obesity (nearly 90% of patients with NIDDM are obese), and sedentary lifestyle. Abdominal obesity, which reflects increased visceral fat (increased waist to hip ratio), is an important characteristic of NIDDM.

Gestational Diabetes

Gestational diabetes is defined as glucose intolerance that is first detected during pregnancy.[2] In this regard, glucose intolerance usually develops during the last trimester in 2% to 3% of pregnancies and resembles NIDDM. Maternal hyperglycemia is a risk factor for fetal morbidity, including congenital anomalies and stillbirth. Maternal morbidity is limited to an increased frequency of hypertensive disorders. These patients become glucose-tolerant following delivery, but nearly 50% develop NIDDM within 10 years.

Table 22–2 • Classification of Diabetes Mellitus

Class	Prevalence	Clinical Characteristics	Diagnostic Criteria
Insulin-dependent diabetes mellitus (IDDM, type I)	0.4%	Absolute insulin deficiency Usual onset in youth Ketosis-prone Anti-islet cell antibodies	Hyperglycemia Polyuria Polydipsia Weight loss
Non-insulin-dependent diabetes mellitus (NIDDM, type II)	6.6%	Insulin resistance often in the presence of adequate insulin secretion Usual onset after 40 years of age Ketosis-resistant Obese	Same as IDDM Fasting serum glucose >140 mg/dl Abnormal oral glucose tolerance test
Gestational diabetes mellitus	2%–3% of pregnancies	Glucose intolerance with usual onset at 24–30 weeks' gestation Increased perinatal complications Glucose intolerance corrects after delivery NIDDM develops in 30%–50% within 10 years	Abnormal oral glucose tolerance test
Secondary diabetes		Pancreatic disease Drugs (glucocorticoids) Acromegaly Cushing's disease	Same as IDDM

Secondary Diabetes

Secondary diabetes may be due to pancreatic destruction (recurrent pancreatitis, pancreatectomy, toxins) or drugs that result in insulin resistance (β-adrenergic antagonists, phenytoin). Maturity-onset diabetes of the young is a relatively rare form of diabetes in which affected individuals are not prone to ketosis. This disease most commonly develops in thin adolescents and is inherited as an autosomal dominant trait. Famine diabetes may be the most common form of diabetes mellitus in countries with limited food supplies. Malnutrition and carbohydrate-restricted diets are associated with decreased insulin secretion.

Pathogenesis

The pathogenesis of diabetes mellitus includes insulin deficiency, genetic factors, and insulin resistance.[1]

Absolute Insulin Deficiency

The IDDM form of the disease is characterized by an absolute insulin deficiency, making these patients dependent on exogenous insulin for survival.[1] IDDM characteristically has an abrupt clinical onset with symptoms of hyperglycemia (polyuria, polydipsia, weight loss, blurred vision) and subsequent ketoacidosis. Despite this abrupt onset, the natural history of IDDM is known to include a long asymptomatic preclinical period during which insulin-producing pancreatic beta islet cells are being progressively destroyed and anti-islet cell antibodies appear. Patients destined to develop IDDM can be identified by the appearance of anti-islet cell antibodies as long as 10 years before clinical symptoms develop. These antibodies are not cytotoxic and are probably markers of immune destruction. Clinical diabetes mellitus manifests when more than 90% of the beta islet cells have been destroyed.

Genetics and IDDM

Although IDDM is clearly an inherited disease, the pattern of inheritance is not clear.[1] It seems likely that environmental influences are superimposed on the heritable component of IDDM. Some HLA loci are associated with an increased risk of developing IDDM, whereas other loci appear to be protective. All of the genetic linkages are located on chromosome 6.

Insulin Resistance

Most patients with NIDDM do not manifest any abnormality in the structure of insulin receptors, and examination of the pancreas typically reveals only modestly decreased islet cell mass. Furthermore, circulating serum insulin concentrations may be normal or even increased. Insulin-mediated stimulation of tyrosine kinase, which is necessary for normal function of insulin receptors, is impaired in patients with NIDDM. This effect is reversible with improved control of blood glucose concentrations and probably does not entirely account for insulin resistance.

The principal sequela of insulin resistance is decreased skeletal muscle uptake of glucose.[1] This is consistent with the increased postprandial blood glucose concentrations seen in individuals with impaired glucose tolerance or early NIDDM because the major fraction of postprandial glucose disposal is by skeletal muscle uptake. Impaired glucose uptake by skeletal muscles may be due to abnormal glucose transporters, decreased glucose phosphorylation (the rate-limiting step of glucose metabolism in skeletal muscles), impaired glycogen synthesis, or relatively unsuppressed glycogenolysis or gluconeogenesis.

The demonstration of insulin resistance in most patients with NIDDM is not sufficient to explain the progression of impaired glucose tolerance to clinical diabetes mellitus. Indeed, many insulin-resistant persons, which includes most obese individuals, do not develop NIDDM. Most patients with insulin resistance do not develop diabetes because they can increase insulin secretion sufficiently to overcome the resistance. Patients who develop NIDDM are incapable of sustained increased insulin secretion, and demonstration of decreased serum insulin concentrations (previously increased) uniformly accompanies the transition to NIDDM.

A common feature of NIDDM is that both insulin resistance and insulin secretion are improved if fasting blood glucose concentrations are normalized by diet or drugs. The reversible effect of increased blood glucose concentrations on insulin resistance and secretion is termed *glucotoxicity*. In addition, a specific pattern of abdominal obesity, reflecting visceral fat deposition, is particularly related to the risk of developing NIDDM. Drugs such as glucocorticoids increase insulin resistance. Gestational diabetes develops in the setting of increased placental somatomammotropin (human placental lactogen), which increases insulin resistance.

Genetics and NIDDM

The NIDDM is an inherited disorder in which insulin resistance and abnormal insulin secretion play important pathogenic roles.[1] Impaired glucose tolerance precedes the development of NIDDM and is characterized by insulin resistance, which causes postprandial hyperglycemia because of decreased skeletal muscle uptake of glucose. Insulin resistance appears to be an inherited characteristic. Nevertheless, only 30% to 50% of patients with impaired glucose tolerance progress to NIDDM. The critical factor associated with progression from impaired glucose tolerance to NIDDM is a decrease in insulin secretion. It is not known if abnormal insulin secretion is acquired or is also inherited.

Metabolic Abnormalities

Insulin is the principal anabolic hormone in humans, producing myriad cellular effects by binding to specific high-affinity receptors. The insulin receptor has been isolated and its DNA sequence determined. Tyrosine kinase activity of the insulin receptor promotes autophosphorylation at several sites following insulin binding and is critical for mediating the activity of insulin receptors. There is no major abnormality in the insulin receptor or insulin action that is present in patients with IDDM. The predominant abnormality in patients with IDDM is insulin deficiency, which results in predictable metabolic abnormalities (Table 22–3). Although insulin deficiency is sufficient to explain these metabolic abnormalities, increased circulating concentrations of counterregulatory hormones (glucagon, epinephrine, norepinephrine, cortisol) serve to accentuate many of these abnormalities. For example, increased circulating concentrations of counterregulatory hormones promote ketogenesis. Because ketogenesis is more sensitive than hepatic glucose output to suppression by insulin, low circulating levels of insulin, as are present in patients with NIDDM, are typically associated with hyperglycemia but not with ketosis.

Table 22–3 • Metabolic Abnormalities Associated with Insulin Deficiency

Hyperglycemia (unrestrained hepatic glucose production due to glycogenolysis and gluconeogenesis plus decreased skeletal muscle uptake)
Increased serum fatty acid concentrations (lipolysis)
Increased serum ketone concentrations (unrestrained hepatic ketogenesis from free fatty acids)
Increased serum triglyceride concentrations (decreased lipoprotein lipase activity resulting in increased synthesis of very low density lipoproteins)
Decreased protein synthesis
Dehydration (glucose acts as an osmotic diuretic)

The complete destruction of insulin-producing beta cells predisposes patients with IDDM to labile blood glucose concentrations. Overall, blood glucose control is highly variable in IDDM because of the mismatch between insulin requirements and exogenous insulin delivery, which is characteristic of most insulin regimens. The most dramatic expression of metabolic instability in patients with IDDM is ketoacidosis. Ketoacidosis can be precipitated by interruption of exogenous insulin therapy or by a stress state with increased circulating concentrations of counterregulatory hormones and insufficient exogenous insulin delivery.

The metabolic consequences of partial insulin deficiency or insulin resistance characteristic of patients with NIDDM are predictable.[1] Hyperglycemia leads to dehydration and a hyperosmolar state. In contrast to patients with IDDM, patients with NIDDM are ketosis-resistant because their circulating insulin concentrations are usually sufficient to suppress ketogenesis. However, in the presence of extreme stress (sepsis, shock, myocardial infarction) even patients with NIDDM may develop ketoacidosis. More commonly, elderly patients with NIDDM are at risk for the development of hyperglycemic, hyperosmolar, nonketotic coma. This metabolic emergency develops in NIDDM patients who have become severely hyperglycemic because of stress or drugs (corticosteroids). Failure to replace water loss due to the osmotic diuresis induced by hyperglycemia results in further hyperosmolarity and ultimately leads to coma.

Metabolic lability tends to be less severe in patients with NIDDM than in those with IDDM. In patients with NIDDM, blood glucose concentrations tend to be lower before meals and then increase after meals as evidence of impaired glucose uptake into skeletal muscles and resistance to the effects of insulin. Fasting blood glucose concentrations and measurements of chronic hyperglycemia tend to be stable and reproducible in patients with NIDDM. Other metabolic abnormalities commonly associated with NIDDM include increased circulating concentrations of very low density lipoproteins, low density lipoproteins (atherogenic) (LDL), and triglycerides.

Clinical Presentation

The clinical presentation of IDDM is usually unmistakable. Special diagnostic tests other than blood glucose and possibly serum ketone and electrolyte assays are not required. Measurement of anti-islet cell antibodies and the response to an intravenous glucose tolerance test may increase the specificity of the diagnosis. Compared with IDDM, patients with NIDDM are more likely to have no or fewer clinical symptoms (as many as 50% of patients are undiagnosed), and the diagnosis may require measuring the fasting glucose concentration or performing an oral glucose tolerance test.

Management of IDDM

Management of IDDM requires delivery of exogenous insulin, self-monitoring by the patient, and lifestyle adaptations including diet and exercise. To facilitate matching insulin doses to meals and to prevent hypoglycemia, the IDDM patient should eat consistent, regular meals. The glycemic goals of therapy have been clarified by documentation that intensive exogenous insulin therapy intended to maintain normal blood glucose concentrations (hemoglobin A_{1c} levels less than 7.5%) decreases the development and progression of long-term diabetic complications (retinopathy, nephropathy, neuropathy).[3] In this regard, it may be necessary frequently to adjust the insulin regimen in response to frequent measurements (four to seven times daily) of blood glucose concentrations and to diet and exercise. It is not known if intensive therapy for achieving normoglycemia in patients with NIDDM has the same beneficial effects as demonstrated for patients with IDDM. However, the similarity between the complications of NIDDM and IDDM, as well as the similar relation between progression of retinopathy and presence of chronic hyperglycemia in both diseases suggests that intensive therapy should also be effective for NIDDM. The high exogenous insulin doses that may be required to treat patients with NIDDM may be atherogenic, which may influence the enthusiasm for implementation of intensive blood glucose control in these patients. The disadvantage of more intensive control of hyperglycemia is an increased incidence of symptomatic hypoglycemia. Intensive management of blood glucose concentrations is uniquely important in women with IDDM who are trying to conceive. Furthermore, during pregnancy management is particularly difficult because of changing insulin requirements.

Self-Monitoring

Development of insulin delivery systems and attempts to provide more precise control of blood glucose concentrations require accurate self-monitoring of the metabolic status. Glucose profiles in patients with IDDM are highly labile, and urine glucose tests cannot provide accurate information regarding blood glucose concentrations. In this regard, reagent strips and meters are available to make measurements more accurate. As the complexity of treatment regimens increases, patients must check their blood glucose concentrations more frequently, with adjustment of insulin doses based on these measurements. Testing the urine for ketones is indicated when unusually high blood glucose concentrations resulting from superimposed illness are present or patients develop nausea and vomiting, which may be symptoms of ketoacidosis.

Glycosylated Hemoglobin

The concentration of glycosylated hemoglobin (HbA_{1c}) reflects mean blood glucose concentrations over approximately 60 days. Increased amounts of glucose exposed to a target protein, such as hemoglobin, leads to increased covalent binding of glucose to the target protein (glycosylation). As such, measurement of HbA_{1c} provides the most accurate objective assessment of long-term blood glucose control and the efficacy of therapeutic interventions. The nondiabetic range for HbA_{1c} is less than 6.05%, and the goal of intensive therapy in patients with IDDM is to maintain the HbA_{1c} at less than 7.5%.

Insulin

Insulin formulations may be classified as rapid-acting, intermediate-acting, or long-acting (Table 22–4).[1] Human insulin is synthesized by modifying porcine insulin or by using recombinant methods. Despite the differences in amino acid sequences and the anti-insulin antibodies generated when bovine, porcine, or a combination of bovine and porcine insulin is administered, these insulins exhibit potency similar to that of human insulin and seldom cause immune-mediated reactions. Human insulins generally have a slightly faster onset (15 minutes versus 30 to 60 minutes for animal-derived regular insulins) and a shorter duration of action than corresponding animal species insulins. Fixed-ratio formulations of regular and intermediate-acting insulins are available but of limited usefulness in patients with IDDM and constantly changing insulin requirements. These fixed-ratio insulin combinations may be more useful in patients with NIDDM. Insulin delivery devices (implantable pumps, mechanical syringes) may be utilized to facilitate the frequent administration of regular insulin that is part of intensive treatment regimens. Similar metabolic results can be achieved with three or more daily subcutaneous injections of regular insulin.

Table 22–4 • Insulin Formulations*

Insulin Type	Onset (hr)	Duration (hr)	Peak (hr)	Other Characteristics
Rapid acting (regular, crystalline zinc insulin [CZI])	0.5–1.0	6–8	2–3	Subcutaneous injection does not produce a sharp peak CZI must be administered 30–60 minutes before meals
Very rapid acting (lispro)	0.25–0.50	4–6	1–2	As a recombinant human insulin, is more rapidly absorbed Administer 10–15 minutes before meals
Intermediate acting (Lente, NPH)	2–4	10–14	4–8	
Long-acting (Ultralente)	8–14	18–24	10–14	Because of long half-life, a new steady state is not achieved for 3–4 days after a change in dose

* All available in animal and human formulations except for lispro and Ultralente, which are available only as human (recombinant) preparations.
Adapted from: Nathan DM. Diabetes mellitus. Sci Am Med 1997;1–24.

Innovative and Experimental Treatments

Innovative and experimental treatments of IDDM include implantable insulin infusion pumps (dependent on reliable blood glucose concentration measurements), transplantation of isolated islets, and use of immunosuppressive drugs (azathioprine, cyclosporine, corticosteroids). Whole-organ pancreas transplantation may be successful in restoring normoglycemia, but this procedure requires chronic immunosuppression with cyclosporine, which may induce lesions in the native or transplanted kidneys and an increased incidence of infection and cancer.[4] For these reasons, pancreas transplantation is not currently preferred over less invasive treatments. Nevertheless, transplantation is superior to intensive insulin treatment with regard to blood glucose control based on HbA_{1c} levels. Intraportal pancreatic-islet cell transplantation is less invasive than pancreatic transplantation, and it may decrease or eliminate the need for immunosuppression while providing normal blood glucose homeostasis.

Management of NIDDM

The clinical goals of therapy for NIDDM are similar to those for IDDM, although the long-term benefits of strict blood glucose control are not as well established.[1] Many NIDDM patients can be treated with diet, which when successful decreases multiple cardiovascular risk factors and improves glucose tolerance. Typically, normoglycemia in NIDDM patients can be achieved with less complex drug regimens and a lower risk of ketoacidosis and hypoglycemia than in IDDM patients. Diet is the most important initial treatment of NIDDM, with weight loss being a major goal in the presence of obesity. In some patients, 5 to 10 kg weight loss is sufficient to "cure"

NIDDM. Exercise regimens in NIDDM patients are intended to aid in weight loss and increase insulin sensitivity. Because patients with NIDDM are at increased risk for cardiovascular disease, patients should be evaluated for evidence of ischemic heart disease before initiating therapy.

Monitoring patients with NIDDM is less demanding than monitoring patients with IDDM, as glucose profiles in NIDDM patients are relatively stable and the risk of hypoglycemia is less. Furthermore, the risk of ketoacidosis is low, and urine testing for ketones is not routinely required. Insulin- and sulfonylurea-treated NIDDM patients who are at risk for hypoglycemia should monitor their blood glucose concentrations initially or when doses are adjusted; after a satisfactory dose has been established, the stability of the blood glucose profile makes frequent testing unnecessary. NIDDM patients treated with diet alone do not need to monitor blood glucose concentrations routinely. Laboratory measurements of fasting blood glucose concentrations or HbA_{1c} every 3 to 6 months usually provides an accurate index of blood glucose concentrations in stable NIDDM patients.

Hypoglycemia Medications

Hypoglycemia medications may be necessary in NIDDM patients in whom dietary therapy fails, although drug therapy is more effective when there is continued attention to the diet (Table 22–5).[1]

Sulfonylureas

Sulfonylureas are oral medications that act primarily by stimulating endogenous insulin secretion (Table 22–6).[1] Although sulfonylureas decrease insulin resistance, this effect probably is not important for

Table 22–5 • Comparison of Insulin with Oral Hypoglycemic Drugs for the Treatment of NIDDM

Parameter	Insulin	Sulfonylurea	Metformin	Acarbose
Lowers HbA$_{1c}$	> 2%	1.5%–2.0%	1.5%–2.0%	0.5%–1.0%
Maximum daily dose	None	20–40 mg	25–50 mg	300 mg
Primary failure rate	None	10%–20%	10%–20%	10%–20%
Effect on lipids				
Triglycerides	Decreases	Decreases	Decreases	Decreases
Total cholesterol	Decreases	Minimal	Decreases	Minimal
HDL cholesterol	Increases	Minimal	Minimal	Minimal
Hypoglycemia	Rare but severe	Rare	No	No
Weight gain	Yes	No	No	No
May be combined with other antidiabetic medications	All	All	All	All

HbA$_{1c}$, hemoglobin A$_{1c}$; NIDDM, non-insulin-dependent diabetes mellitus; HDL, high density lipoprotein.
Adapted from: Nathan DM. Diabetes mellitus. Sci Am Med 1997;1–24.

their therapeutic efficacy. Sulfonylureas lower HbA$_{1c}$ by 1% to 2%. These drugs have no role in the treatment of IDDM and are usually not effective in nonobese patients. As many as 20% of NIDDM patients who begin sulfonylurea treatment fail to experience an adequate hypoglycemic response (primary failures), and each year an additional 5% to 10% of patients who initially responded begin to fail (secondary failures). Hypoglycemia secondary to sulfonylureas is infrequent, but when it does occur it is often more prolonged and more dangerous than hypoglycemia secondary to insulin. Hypoglycemia is more common in patients receiving second-generation sulfonylureas. Weight gain and an increased risk of cardiovascular mortality may result from treatment with these drugs.

Biguanides

Biguanides are useful in the management of NIDDM by virtue of their ability to decrease hyperglycemia (inhibit gluconeogenesis in the liver and kidneys, increase glucose uptake into skeletal muscles) with a low risk of hypoglycemia. In addition, these drugs decrease hypertriglyceridemia and hypercholesterolemia and may result in mild weight loss in obese patients. Lactic acidosis (serum lactate concentration higher than 5 mmol/L) is the most important adverse side effect of biguanides and was the reason these drugs were largely supplanted by sulfonylureas. Biguanides cause glucose to be metabolized anaerobically, and the resulting pyruvate is reduced to lactate, which is usually metabolized rapidly in the liver. Should hepatic metabolism fail or be overwhelmed, severe lactic acidosis and associated multiple organ dysfunction may occur.

Metformin is a biguanide that has a lower risk of causing lactic acidosis (5 to 9 cases per 100,000 treated patients) than the previously available biguanide, phenformin.[5] Nevertheless, lactic acidosis has been described following minor surgery in a patient receiving metformin.[6] The risk of lactic acidosis is increased in elderly patients (not recommended for treatment in patients older than 80 years of age) or

Table 22–6 • Classification of Sulfonylureas

Drug	Dose Range (mg)	Duration (hr)	Other Considerations
First generation			
Chlorpropamide	100–750	> 36	Disulfiram-like effects
			Prolonged hypoglycemia
			Hyponatremia
Tolbutamide	500–3000	6–12	Metabolized in liver
			Use in patients with renal insufficiency
Acetohexamide	250–1500	12–18	Metabolized in liver to active metabolites
Tolazamide	100–1000	12–24	
Second generation			
Glyburide	2.5–20.0	18–24	Fewer side effects than first-generation drugs
Glipizide	5–40	12–18	
Glimepiride	1–8	24	Administer once a day

Adapted from: Nathan DM. Diabetes mellitus. Sci Am Med 1997;1–24.

patients with decreased glomerular filtration rates, congestive heart failure, or shock.[5] In this regard, regular measurement of creatinine clearance in patients receiving metformin may be recommended, as this drug is dependent on renal clearance for its elimination. Other than hemodialysis, treatment of biguanide-induced lactic acidosis is symptomatic. Metformin may be used as monotherapy or in combination with sulfonylureas.

Glycoside Inhibitors

Acarbose is an α-glycoside inhibitor. This nonabsorbed drug acts like dietary fiber, decreasing the absorption of carbohydrate by competitively inhibiting the intestinal wall enzymes that convert polysaccharides to absorbable monosaccharides. The result is a blunted glycemic response during the postprandial period. The drug is less potent than the sulfonylureas and metformin in lowering the HbA_{1c} level but is effective in all patients, including those with IDDM. Acarbose can be used as monotherapy or in combination with other hypoglycemic drugs. When used as monotherapy, it is not associated with hypoglycemia or weight gain.

Insulinomimetics

Troglitazone is an insulinomimetic drug that lowers HbA_{1c} by 0.5% to 1.0% and improves triglyceride levels with less insulin and without significant weight gain or other serious side effects.

Insulin

Insulin is the most effective hypoglycemic drug and is always effective in NIDDM patients at some dose. Relatively high doses (50 to 100 units/day) are generally needed to produce normoglycemia in obese NIDDM patients. Insulin is typically selected for treatment after therapy with oral hypoglycemic drugs has failed. Insulin can be administered as an intermediate- or long-acting formulation in the morning or at bedtime. NIDDM patients who are not initially overweight and those who are profoundly hyperglycemic or develop ketosis should be started on insulin therapy initially. Because most NIDDM patients who are treated first with oral hypoglycemic drugs ultimately require insulin to maintain acceptable blood glucose concentrations, the oral hypoglycemic drugs can be viewed as a temporizing measure.[1] Combination therapy with a sulfonylurea and insulin may result in acceptable blood glucose concentrations with lower insulin doses. A potential advantage of using lower insulin doses is the concern that high doses may be atherogenic.

Complications

The most serious acute metabolic complication of diabetes mellitus is ketoacidosis. Late complications of diabetes may manifest as macrovascular events (coronary artery disease, cerebrovascular disease, peripheral vascular disease), microvascular events (retinopathy, nephropathy), and disorders of the nervous system (autonomic nervous system neuropathy, peripheral neuropathy).[7] The incidence of microvascular and neuropathic complications in IDDM and NIDDM diabetics is similar when adjusted for duration of disease and quality of blood glucose control. The cumulative lifetime incidence of proliferative retinopathy, proteinuria, and distal neuropathy is about 50% for both types of diabetes.[7] This implies that the primary causes of these complications is hyperglycemia, as the underlying metabolic pathology is different for IDDM and NIDDM. Macrovascular complications, as measured by the rates of coronary artery disease, cerebrovascular disease, and peripheral vascular disease, are similar for IDDM and NIDDM. Macrovascular sequelae, such as premature myocardial infarction, angina pectoris, or peripheral vascular insufficiency, may be the presenting symptoms in an undiagnosed diabetic.

Retinopathy and nephropathy are specific complications of diabetes, whereas macrovascular complications (cardiac, peripheral, and cerebrovascular disease) due to atherosclerosis also occur in nondiabetics, but the incidence is much greater in diabetic patients. Cardiomyopathy is not an uncommon problem in diabetics. The development of long-term complications in diabetic patients changes a relatively benign metabolic condition into a life-threatening disease. The clinical course for the IDDM population is likely to include visual impairment or blindness, renal failure, and vascular disorders. The major tissues affected by diabetes (retina, kidneys, nerves) are all freely permeable to glucose. That chronic hyperglycemia plays a role in diabetes-specific complications (perhaps due to glycosylation of membrane proteins) is supported by the observation that the incidence of these complications is greatly decreased by intensive management of blood glucose concentrations in IDDM patients and possibly in NIDDM patients.[3] Other than hyperglycemia, risk factors for the development of life-threatening complications include the duration of the diabetes, systemic hypertension and nephropathy, and possibly a genetic component. Hyperinsuli-

currence of cardiac disease in women independent of other risk factors). Development of nephropathy in IDDM or NIDDM patients confers an especially high risk of ischemic heart disease.

The incidence of peripheral vascular and cerebrovascular disease is increased in patients with diabetes. The combination of peripheral neuropathy and peripheral vascular disease results in a risk of amputation in the diabetic population that is significantly greater than that in the nondiabetic population.

Peripheral Neuropathy

The most common manifestation of peripheral neuropathy in diabetic patients is a symmetrical sensorimotor neuropathy that presents as numbness or tingling in the toes and feet, often at night. Nerve conduction abnormalities may precede the diagnosis of NIDDM, and the incidence of clinically detectable polyneuropathy increases progressively with the duration of NIDDM (Fig. 22–1).[14] Symptoms associated with peripheral neuropathy often abate as the neuropathy becomes more severe and hypoesthesia or anesthesia takes the place of paresthesias and dysesthesias. Insensitive feet become vulnerable to trauma, and neuropathic foot ulcers are a

common cause of gangrene and the need for amputation. In some patients peripheral neuropathies are painful, with dysesthesias interfering with sleep and normal activity. Tricyclic antidepressants, phenytoin, and carbamazepine are somewhat effective treatments. Intensive diabetic therapy is beneficial in the management of diabetic peripheral neuropathy. The intensity and extent of the functional and anatomic abnormalities of diabetic neuropathy parallel the degree and duration of hyperglycemia. Acute hyperglycemia decreases nerve function, and chronic hyperglycemia is associated with axonal degeneration and loss of myelinated and unmyelinated nerve fibers.[13, 14]

Other forms of diabetic peripheral neuropathy are mononeuropathies and entrapment syndromes. Mononeuropathies are generally asymmetrical, affect cranial or peripheral nerves, and are thought to be secondary to vascular occlusion leading to nerve infarcts. These isolated peripheral nerve lesions often occur at common sites for external pressure, such as the radial nerve in the upper arm or the common peroneal nerve at the head of the fibula. Entrapment syndromes (ulnar nerve at the cubital tunnel, median nerve at the carpal tunnel) occur more frequently in diabetics than nondiabetics. Segmental demyelination and vascular occlusion of nutrient arteries, especially to the cranial nerves, as well as the median and ulnar nerves of the arm are often involved. It is conceivable that unavoidable pressure on the extremities associated with positioning during anesthesia and surgery result in exacerbation of previously asymptomatic peripheral nerve entrapment. Indeed, diabetes mellitus is often present in patients who develop postoperative peripheral nerve injuries involving the arms or legs.[15, 16]

Autonomic Nervous System Neuropathy

Autonomic nervous system neuropathy reflects dysfunction of the autonomic nervous system and is estimated to be present in 20% to 40% of patients with long-standing diabetes mellitus (Table 22–9).[17, 18] The likelihood of autonomic nervous system neuropathy is even greater in the presence of systemic hypertension, renal failure, or peripheral sensory neuropathy. In fact, abnormal results of cardiovascular reflex tests (orthostatic hypotension, resting tachycardia, absent beat-to-beat variation in heart rate) may be present in patients before hyperglycemia characteristic of clinical diabetes is recognized.

Autonomic nervous system neuropathy may manifest in the cardiovascular system, gastrointestinal system, or genitourinary system. Hypoglycemic unawareness (blood glucose concentration less than

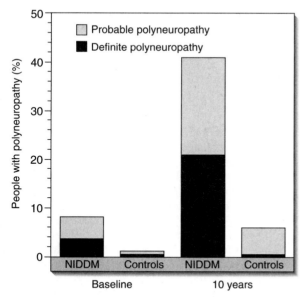

Figure 22–1 • Incidence of probable and definite polyneuropathy was greater in the presence of non-insulin-dependent diabetes mellitus (NIDDM) compared with nondiabetic controls. Over the next 10 years the incidence of neuropathy progressed at a more rapid rate in those with NIDDM than in nondiabetic controls. (From Partanen J, Niskanen L, Lehtinen J, et al. Natural history of peripheral neuropathy in patients with non-insulin-dependent diabetes mellitus. N Engl J Med 1995;333:89–94. Copyright 1995 Massachusetts Medical Society, with permission.)

Table 22–9 • Manifestations of Diabetic Autonomic Neuropathy

Resting tachycardia
Orthostatic hypotension
Absent beat-to-beat variation in heart rate with deep
  breathing
Cardiac dysrhythmias (QT abnormalities)
Sudden death syndrome
Gastroparesis
  Vomiting
  Diarrhea
  Abdominal distension
Bladder atony
Impotence
Asymptomatic hypoglycemia

50 mg/dl) reflects autonomic neuropathy and the absence of expected sympathetic nervous system responses (tachycardia, diaphoresis) to hypoglycemia. In addition, repeated episodes of hypoglycemia decrease the threshold at which hypoglycemic symptoms ("deconditioning") occur. Peripheral sympathetic nervous system denervation also results in increased arteriovenous shunting and decreased skin capillary blood flow as well as decreased sweating in the extremities. These changes contribute to the development of neuropathic foot problems in diabetic patients. Patients with autonomic nervous system neuropathy experience greater intraoperative core body temperature decreases than do nondiabetics, perhaps reflecting delayed onset of thermoregulatory vasoconstriction.[19]

Cardiovascular Manifestations

Cardiovascular manifestations of autonomic nervous system neuropathy include resting tachycardia, orthostatic hypotension, and decreased or absent beat-to-beat variation of the heart rate during voluntary deep breathing. The basic defect in orthostatic hypotension associated with diabetes is the lack of vasoconstriction due to sympathetic nervous system dysfunction. Plasma concentrations of norepinephrine increase less when diabetics with symptoms of orthostatic hypotension assume the standing position. Cardiac vagal denervation often occurs early and is reflected by the loss of variability in heart rate during deep breathing. The heart rate response to drugs such as atropine and propranolol is blunted in diabetics with evidence of autonomic nervous system neuropathy compared with nondiabetics.[20] Shortening of the QT interval on the electrocardiogram (ECG) in association with autonomic nervous system neuropathy may result in serious cardiac dysrhythmias. Autonomic nervous system neuropathy may interfere with control of breathing and make patients with diabetes more susceptible to depressant effects of drugs, as administered during anesthesia. Unexpected cardiac or respiratory arrest may occur in diabetics with autonomic nervous system neuropathy.[17, 21-24] The presence of autonomic nervous system neuropathy may prevent the development of angina pectoris and thus obscure the presence of ischemic heart disease.[14] Unexplained hypotension may be due to painless myocardial infarction in diabetics with autonomic nervous system neuropathy.

Sudden Death Syndrome

Autonomic nervous system neuropathy may manifest as sudden death syndrome. Indeed, once autonomic nervous system neuropathy develops, the prognosis is poor and mortality is increased.[25] Sudden death syndrome in diabetic patients with cardiac autonomic nervous system neuropathy may complicate the perioperative period, manifesting as sudden, unexpected profound bradycardia that is responsive only to intravenous administration of epinephrine.[23, 24, 26] The preoperative presence of abnormal autonomic nervous system function tests (respiratory variation in heart rate, blood pressure, heart rate response to standing) has been associated with an increased incidence of postoperative cardiorespiratory arrest.[27] Restoration of normoglycemia, as with a pancreatic transplant, does not reliably reverse manifestations of autonomic nervous system neuropathy.

Gastroparesis

Gastroparesis (delayed gastric emptying) is a manifestation of autonomic nervous system neuropathy with obvious risk implications for diabetic patients during the perioperative period (Fig. 22–2).[28] It is estimated that gastroparesis occurs in 20% to 30% of all diabetic patients, manifesting as nausea, vomiting, diarrhea, and abdominal distension. Symptoms may appear early in the disease and occur in patients with IDDM and NIDDM. Metoclopramide improves gastric emptying and decreases symptoms of gastroparesis. Genitourinary autonomic nervous system neuropathy causes impotence and hypotonia of the bladder, resulting in overflow incontinence.

Genitourinary Problems

Bladder dysfunction and impotence in men are manifestations of autonomic nervous system neuropathy.

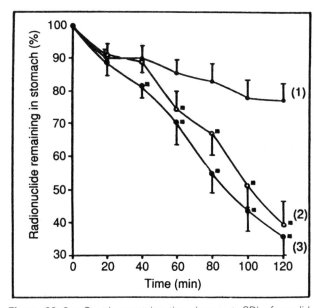

Figure 22–2 • Gastric emptying time (mean ± SD) of a solid test meal in patients with diabetes mellitus (1), diabetes mellitus and receiving metoclopramide 10 mg IV before the test meal (2), and no evidence of diabetes mellitus (3). (From Wright RA, Clemente R, Wathen R. Diabetic gastroparesis: an abnormality of gastric emptying of solids. Am J Med Sci 1985;289:240–2, with permission.)

Stiff Joint Syndrome

An estimated 30% to 40% of patients with IDDM show evidence of limited joint mobility, most often initially manifesting in the small joints of the digits and hands. An inability to approximate the palmar surfaces of the interphalangeal joints ("prayer sign") correlates with the presence of the stiff joint syndrome.[29] The atlanto-occipital joint may be involved, contributing to potential difficulty with tracheal intubation during laryngoscopy, although this difficulty is not predictably increased in patients with IDDM.[30] In addition to joint involvement, afflicted patients often have rapidly progressive microangiopathy (microalbuminuria, renal failure), nonfamilial short stature, and tight waxy skin. Glycosylation of tissue proteins due to chronic hyperglycemia seems to be responsible for this complication.

Diabetic Scleredema

Diabetic scleredema manifests as thickening and hardening of the skin characteristically over the back of the neck, shoulders, and upper back, although it can involve the hands, arms, and legs. The induration is nonpitting and usually symmetrical. It may develop after an acute infection in patients with poorly controlled diabetes, or it may occur with no known cause. In children with diabetes, associated findings may include carpal tunnel syndrome and limited mobility of the finger joints. A report of anterior spinal artery syndrome as a complication of epidural anesthesia in a patient with diabetic scleredema was attributed to restriction of arterial blood flow to the spinal cord. This problem was caused by a marked increase in epidural pressure, when a large volume of local anesthetic solution was placed in an epidural space containing noncompressible collagen.[31]

Management of Anesthesia

The principal goal in the management of anesthesia for diabetic patients undergoing elective surgery is to mimic normal metabolism as closely as possible by avoiding hypoglycemia, excessive hyperglycemia, ketoacidosis, and electrolyte disturbances.[7, 32, 33] Improved glycemic control has been shown to decrease perioperative morbidity and mortality in diabetic patients undergoing major surgery.[33] Hypoglycemia is prevented by ensuring an adequate supply of exogenous glucose. Hyperglycemia and associated ketoacidosis, dehydration, and electrolyte abnormalities are prevented by administering exogenous insulin. The goal for controlling blood glucose concentrations is to maintain levels well above that considered hypoglycemic but below levels at which the deleterious effects of hyperglycemia (hyperosmolarity, osmotic diuresis, electrolyte disturbances, impaired phagocyte function, impaired wound healing) become evident. In this regard, it is recommended that blood glucose concentrations be maintained between 120 and 180 mg/dl. Despite the technical ability to normalize blood glucose concentrations, there is no consensus on the optimal medical management of the diabetic patient's blood glucose concentration during the perioperative period.[32]

Preoperative Evaluation

It is recommended that diabetic patients be scheduled for surgery early in the day to limit the duration of preoperative fasting. The well controlled, diet-treated NIDDM patient does not require hospitalization or any special treatment (including insulin) before or during surgery. Likewise, patients with well controlled IDDM undergoing brief outpatient surgical procedures may not require any adjustment in the usual subcutaneous insulin regimen. If oral hypoglycemic drugs are being administered, they may be continued until the evening before surgery, remembering that these drugs may produce hypoglycemia several hours (as long as 36 hours with chlor-propamide) after their administration in the absence of caloric intake. An exception to the recommendation that oral hypoglycemic drugs be continued until the time of anesthesia induction in the patient being treated with metformin. Some have recommended that metformin be discontinued 2 days or more before elective surgery in view of the rare possibility that this drug may cause lactic acidosis.[6] When metformin is continued, it is recommended that patients be monitored for the development of lactic acidosis. Preadmission to the hospital is probably indicated only for patients with poorly controlled IDDM.

Preoperative evaluation and treatment of hyperglycemia, electrolyte disturbances, and ketoacidosis is important before proceeding with elective surgery. Measurement of HbA_{1c} is a practical means of estimating blood glucose concentrations during the several weeks before operation (approximately 60 days). Adequate blood glucose control is suggested by HbA_{1c} concentrations of less than 7.5%. Evidence of ischemic heart disease, cerebrovascular disease, or renal dysfunction should be sought. Indeed the most common cause of perioperative morbidity in diabetic patients is ischemic heart disease. Review of the ECG and a search for proteinuria may provide useful information about the patient with IDDM. Signs of peripheral neuropathy (which may influence the choice of regional anesthesia) and autonomic nervous system neuropathy are noted (Table 22–9). Patients with evidence of autonomic nervous system dysfunction may be at increased risk for aspiration on induction of anesthesia and intraoperative cardiovascular lability (hypotension requiring vasopressor therapy) (Fig. 22–3).[34] Evaluation of IDDM patients for evidence of limited joint mobility is important for predicting possible difficulty when performing direct laryngoscopy for tracheal intubation. The common presence of obesity in this patient population may influence the ease of tracheal intubation or performance of regional anesthetic techniques.

Exogenous Insulin

There is a consensus that IDDM patients undergoing major surgery should be treated with insulin, but the accepted route of administration (subcutaneous, intravenous) remains unsettled.[32, 35, 36] Furthermore, there is no evidence to confirm that close control of blood glucose concentrations during the relatively brief intraoperative period benefits diabetic patients. It seems that the most important factor in controlling the diabetic patient's blood glucose concentration during the perioperative period is not the

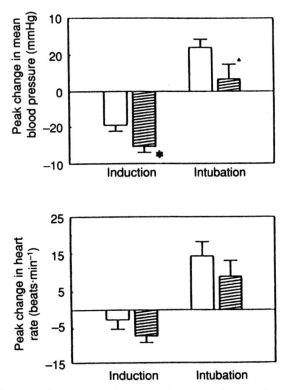

Figure 22–3 • Mean systemic blood pressure decreased more ($P < 0.05$) during induction of anesthesia, and the heart rate increased less ($P < 0.05$) during tracheal intubation in patients with diabetes mellitus (*cross-hatched bars*) and preoperative evidence of autonomic nervous system dysfunction compared with nondiabetic patients (*open bars*). (From Burgos LUG, Bert TJ, Asiddao C, et al. Increased intraoperative cardiovascular morbidity in diabetics with autonomic neuropathy. Anesthesiology 1989;70:591–7, with permission.)

method utilized for delivery of insulin but, rather, frequent measurement of blood glucose concentrations (as often as every 1 to 2 hours during major surgery and the early postoperative period).[36, 37] The use of commercially available blood glucose meters is recommended. On the basis of these measurements, blood glucose concentrations can be maintained at 100 to 200 mg/dl during the intraoperative period by intravenous administration of regular insulin (5 to 10 units IV if blood glucose concentrations are higher than 250 mg/dl) or increasing the rate of fluid infusion containing glucose (blood glucose concentrations less than 100 mg/dl).

A traditional, effective approach to insulin delivery for diabetic patients undergoing elective surgery is subcutaneous administration of one-fourth to one-half the usual daily intermediate-acting dose of insulin on the morning of surgery. If regular insulin is part of the morning schedule, the intermediate-acting insulin dose may be increased by 0.5 unit for each unit of regular insulin, remembering that the stress of anesthesia and surgery (increased circulating concentrations of catecholamines and cortisol) increases the need for insulin. It is common practice to initiate an intravenous infusion of glucose (5 to 10 g/hr) during the preoperative fasting period, along with the subcutaneous insulin, to minimize the likelihood of hypoglycemia. In addition, administration of potassium (2 mEq/L) is often included with glucose.

An alternative to subcutaneous delivery of insulin is the continuous intravenous infusion of a low dose of regular insulin.[32, 35] Intravenous insulin administration circumvents the unpredictable absorption of subcutaneous insulin, which may be exaggerated by changes in systemic blood pressure and cutaneous blood flow that might occur during the perioperative period. Although the insulin dose required for optimal control of the blood glucose concentration is unknown, the usual starting dose for the variable-rate intravenous infusion of regular insulin is 0.5 to 1.0 unit/hr (Table 22–10).[32] Cardiopulmonary bypass is associated with significant metabolic derangements and insulin resistance due to hypothermia. As a result, the continuous intravenous infusion rate of insulin may have to be increased to more than 10 units/hr to maintain euglycemic blood glucose concentrations.

Induction and Maintenance

The choice of drugs for induction and maintenance of anesthesia is less important than monitoring the blood glucose concentration and the treatment of potential physiologic derangements associated with diabetes. Rapid, accurate measurements of the blood glucose concentration with a blood glucose meter should be accomplished in the operating room. Tracheal intubation with a cuffed tracheal tube seems prudent in view of the potential for delayed gastric emptying in patients with autonomic nervous system neuropathy. Hyperglycemia during surgery most likely reflects increases in plasma concentrations of catecholamines and cortisol. In addition, volatile anesthetics may impair the release of insulin in response to the administration of glucose. Nevertheless, there is no evidence that maintenance of anesthesia with specific volatile anesthetics in diabetic patients is advantageous. Epidural and spinal anesthesia preserve glucose tolerance, presumably owing to inhibition of the catecholamine response to surgery. Systemic absorption of local anesthetics, such as following brachial plexus block, has been associated with presumed myocardial depression in diabetic patients.[34] The increased incidence of peripheral neuropathies is a consideration when choosing regional anesthetic techniques in diabetic patients. Conversely, there may be an increased risk of peripheral nerve injury in diabetic patients during the perioperative period despite applying accepted techniques of padding and positioning the patient's extremities. Monitoring the core body temperature seems prudent, as patients with diabetic autonomic nervous system neuropathy may be at risk for exaggerated intraoperative hypothermia.[19]

Episodes of bradycardia and hypotension that develop suddenly and that are unresponsive to intravenous administration of atropine and/or ephedrine have been described during maintenance of anesthesia in diabetic patients with preoperative evidence of cardiac autonomic nervous system neuropathy (orthostatic hypotension, resting tachycardia).[23–25, 34] Prompt intervention with intravenous administration of epinephrine may be the most effective therapy.

Table 22–10 • Continuous Intravenous Infusion of Regular Insulin During the Perioperative Period

1. Mix 50 units of regular insulin in 500 ml of normal saline (1 unit/hr = 10 ml/hr).
2. Initiate intravenous infusion at 0.5–1.0 unit/hr.
3. Measure blood glucose concentrations as necessary (every 1–2 hours) and adjust glucose infusion rate accordingly.

< 80 mg/dl	Turn intravenous infusion off for 30 minutes
	Administer 25 ml of 50% glucose
	Remeasure the blood glucose concentration in 30 minutes
80–120 mg/dl	Decrease insulin infusion rate by 0.3 unit/hr
120–180 mg/dl	No change in insulin infusion rate
180–220 mg/dl	Increase insulin infusion rate by 0.3 unit/hr
> 220 mg/dl	Increase insulin infusion rate by 0.5 unit/hr

4. Provide sufficient glucose (5–10 g/hr) and potassium (2–4 mEq/L).

Adapted from: Hirsh IB, Magill JOB, Cryer EG, et al. Perioperative management of surgical patients with diabetes mellitus. Anesthesiology 1991;74:346–59.

If diabetic patients are receiving adequate amounts of exogenous insulin, glucose, and potassium, any additional fluids administered during surgery for treatment of intraoperative blood loss need not contain glucose. Administration of lactated Ringer's solution to diabetic patients is controversial, as lactate is converted to glucose. For this reason, a higher insulin dose may be required for diabetic patients receiving lactated Ringer's solution during the perioperative period. Metoclopramide increases gastric motility and may be an effective postoperative antiemetic in diabetic patients with gastroparesis.

Emergency Surgery

The most common emergency operations performed in diabetic patients are appendectomy, incision and drainage procedures, and lower extremity amputation for ischemia or infection. In these situations it is useful to evaluate the patient's metabolic status (blood glucose concentrations, HbA$_{1c}$, electrolytes, pH, urine ketones) when preparing for anesthetic management. If diabetic ketoacidosis is present, surgery can be delayed for a short time to institute treatment with intravenous administration of regular insulin and replacement of potassium and intravascular fluid volume. In some patients treatment of diabetic ketoacidosis may result in the disappearance of abdominal pain and tenderness.[32] Placing a central venous pressure catheter may be helpful for guiding volume replacement therapy.

Hyperosmolar, Hyperglycemic Nonketotic Coma

Hyperosmolar, hyperglycemic nonketotic coma is associated with severe hyperglycemia (higher than 600 mg/dl) but by definition is not associated with ketoacidosis (Table 22–11). Volume depletion is severe (average fluid deficit is 25% of total body water), and the serum osmolarity is higher than

---

Table 22–11 • Hyperosmolar Hyperglycemic Nonketotic Coma

Hyperglycemia (> 600 mg/dl)
Hyperosmolarity (> 350 mOsm/L)
Normal pHa
Osmotic diuresis (hypokalemia)
Hypovolemia (hemoconcentration)
Central nervous system depression
Elderly

---

350 mOsm/kg. Precipitating factors in the development of hyperosmolar, hyperglycemic nonketotic coma include advanced age, sepsis, hyperalimentation using concentrated carbohydrate solutions, and drugs (corticosteroids). The presence of hyperglycemia and insulin resistance during cardiopulmonary bypass in patients with NIDDM render these patients vulnerable to the development of hyperosmolar, hyperglycemic nonketotic coma.[32]

Hyperglycemia stimulates osmotic diuresis, leading to dehydration, somnolence, and eventually coma. Treatment is directed at correcting hypovolemia and hyperosmolarity with the administration of hypotonic saline. A low-dose intravenous insulin infusion effectively lowers blood glucose concentrations to less than 300 mg/dl. After the initial episode is successfully treated, patients usually do not continue to require exogenous administration of insulin. Potassium supplementation may be required to replace that lost owing to osmotic diuresis. In contrast to diabetic ketoacidosis, mortality due to hyperosmolar, hyperglycemic nonketotic coma may approach 50%, perhaps reflecting the advanced age of many of the patients who develop this syndrome.

Anesthetic Considerations in Pancreas Transplant Recipients

Pancreatic transplantation effectively restores normal glucose metabolism, and pancreas transplant recipients do not require insulin to compensate for the stress response to surgery.[38] When urinary bladder-drained pancreatic grafts are utilized, recipients may experience chronic dysuria because of the presence of amylase in the urine. Urinary amylase levels are used for monitoring pancreatic graft function. Pancreatic ductal cells also secrete significant amounts of bicarbonate and water. Bicarbonate loss in the urine may cause dehydration and metabolic acidosis. It is presumed that these patients have ischemic heart disease. The effects of anesthesia on catecholamine responses to hypoglycemia following pancreas transplants are not documented, and recommendations for glucose management are not possible in these patients.

◼ HYPOGLYCEMIC DISORDERS

Hypoglycemic disorders may be categorized as drug-induced, fasting, or reactive.[10,39] The most common cause of clinical hypoglycemia is a relative excess of insulin in diabetic patients treated with exogenous insulin. Hypoglycemia associated with sulfonylurea therapy may be prolonged and result in death. Phenylbutazone and sulfonamide compounds can potentiate the effects of oral hypoglycemic drugs. Metformin is rarely a cause of hypoglycemia but when combined with a sulfonylurea may be associated with hypoglycemia. Aspirin overdose, alcohol abuse, and treatment with β-adrenergic blocking drugs may cause or contribute to clinical hypoglycemia. Factitious hypoglycemia due to surreptitious administration of insulin or sulfonylurea drugs is characterized by recurrent neuroglycopenia in association with increased circulating concentrations of insulin and suppressed levels of C-peptide (peptide chain released during endogenous cleavage of proinsulin to insulin but not produced by exogenous administration of insulin). Reactive hypoglycemia is characterized by hypoglycemia in response to a nutrient challenge. Forms of reactive hypoglycemia include alimentary hypoglycemia (sequela of gastric surgery in which delivery of nutrients to the small intestine results in poorly timed release of insulin), NIDDM-associated reactive hypoglycemia, and idiopathic causes.

Fasting hypoglycemia is characterized by an inability to maintain normal blood glucose concentrations in the postabsorptive or fasting state. Parturients tend to develop hypoglycemia more readily than nonpregnant women because they are in a state of "accelerated starvation," and the hypoglycemic counterregulatory hormone responses are blunted.[40] Prolonged labor, work of delivery, and fasting are contributing causes. Additionally, epidural analgesia inhibits hyperglycemic responses to pain and surgical stress, blocks sympathetic nervous system tone, and removes the autonomic control of both the adrenal medulla and the hepatic glycogenolytic systems. Indeed, severe hypoglycemia in nondiabetic parturients is a rare complication.[40]

Inappropriate insulin secretion by an insulinoma (incidence similar to that of pheochromocytoma) resulting in fasting hypoglycemia is suggested by hypoglycemia that follows an overnight fast in association with increased circulating concentrations of insulin.[39] An estimated 65% of patients with an insulinoma develop fasting hypoglycemia within the first 12 hours of fasting.[10] Endoscopic ultrasonography is useful for diagnosing these highly vascular tumors. More than 90% of insulinomas are solitary, are less than 2 cm in diameter, and can be cured by surgical excision.[10] When metastatic disease makes surgery an unacceptable treatment option, chemotherapy with streptozotocin, alone or in combination with other chemotherapeutic drugs, can sometimes decrease insulin secretion. To ameliorate hypoglycemia further in these patients, treatment with frequent feedings plus drugs such as corticosteroids, β-adrenergic agents, or phenytoin may be useful.

The principal challenge during anesthesia for surgical excision of an insulinoma is avoidance of hypoglycemia, as may occur during manipulation of the tumor.[41] Hyperglycemia may follow successful surgical removal of the tumor. A blood glucose meter is necessary to permit frequent measurements (about every 15 minutes) of blood glucose concentrations. Because evidence of hypoglycemia (systemic hypertension, tachycardia, diaphoresis) may be masked during anesthesia, it is probably prudent to include glucose in the intravenous fluids administered intraoperatively. The known ability of volatile anesthetics to inhibit the release of insulin is a theoretical advantage during surgical resection of an insulinoma, remembering that the efficacy of this effect is unproven in these patients.[11] The minimum blood glucose concentrations needed to maintain glucose transport across the blood–brain barrier and into brain cells is undefined. Some patients adapt to blood glucose concentrations as low as 40 mg/dl, whereas others may experience symptoms of neuroglycopenia when blood glucose levels are abruptly decreased from 300 mg/dl to 100 mg/dl.

THYROID GLAND DYSFUNCTION

Thyroid gland dysfunction reflects the overproduction or underproduction of triiodothyronine (T_3) and/or thyroxine (tetraiodothyronine, T_4).[42, 43] The regulation of serum thyroid hormone levels is complex and relies primarily on negative feedback mechanisms involving thyrotropin. The two physiologically active thyroid gland hormones (T_3 and T_4) act on cells through the adenylate cyclase system, producing changes in the speed of biochemical reactions, total body oxygen consumption, and energy (heat production).

Hyperthyroidism

Hyperthyroidism is estimated to affect approximately 2.0% of women and 0.2% of men. When hyperthyroidism is suspected, the diagnosis is confirmed by documenting the presence of decreased circulating concentrations of thyrotropin (thyroid-stimulating hormone) and increased circulating concentrations of T_4 in the plasma.[44] If the thyrotropin concentration is low but T_4 level is normal, the serum T_3 is measured, as the patient may have T_3 toxicosis. The presence of normal serum thyrotropin concentrations nearly always excludes the diagnosis of hy-

Table 22–12 • Causes of Hyperthyroidism

Cause	Pathogenesis
Common	
Graves' disease	Most common cause of hyperthyroidism
Iatrogenic	Second most common cause of hyperthyroidism
	Administration of thyroxine or triiodothyronine
Toxic nodular goiter	Nodules functioning independently of normal feedback regulation
Thyroiditis	Inflammation-induced release of thyroxine and triiodothyronine
Rare	
Neonatal hyperthyroidism	Transplacental passage of thyroid-stimulating antibodies
	Occurs transiently in infants born to mothers with Graves' disease
Inappropriate secretion of thyroid-stimulating hormone	Pituitary tumor
	Pituitary resistance to thyroxine and triiodothyronine
Exogenous iodide	Sources may include health food preparations, amiodarone, and radiograph contrast dyes
Factitious illness	
Very rare	
Thyroid cancer	
Choriocarcinoma	Tumor production of chorionic gonadotropin-stimulating thyroid

Adapted from: Franklyn JA. The management of hyperthyroidism. N Engl J Med 1994;330:1731–9.

perthyroidism. Diagnosing hyperthyroidism during pregnancy (which occurs in about 0.2% of parturients) is difficult, as estrogen-induced increases in T_4-binding globulins results in increased circulating T_4 concentrations.

Causes

Among the many possible causes of hyperthyroidism, Graves' disease (diffuse goiter and ophthalmopathy) is the most common explanation, occurring typically in women 20 to 40 years of age (Table 22–12).[44, 45] An autoimmune pathogenesis for Graves' disease is suggested by the presence of immunoglobulin G autoantibodies, such as long-acting thyroid stimulator, in the plasma, which mimics the effects of thyrotropin and produces effects for up to 12 hours, compared with 1 hour for normal thyrotropin. Passive transfer of antibody across the placenta may produce transient neonatal Graves' disease.

Signs and Symptoms

Signs and symptoms of hyperthyroidism reflect the impact of excessive amounts of T_3 and/or T_4 on the speed of biochemical reactions, total body oxygen consumption, and energy (heat) production (Table 22–13). Patients manifest anxiety and weight loss despite high calorie intake. Fatigue, diaphoresis, skeletal muscle weakness, and heat intolerance are characteristic. The appearance or worsening of angina pectoris or congestive heart failure or the un-

expected onset of congestive heart failure or atrial fibrillation may reflect undiagnosed hyperthyroidism, especially in elderly patients in whom increased amounts of thyroid hormones are sufficient to aggravate underlying heart disease.

Mild to moderate hyperthyroidism may be difficult to diagnose clinically during pregnancy, as many normal parturients experience tachycardia, heat intolerance, and emotional instability. With overt hyperthyroidism, a hyperdynamic circulation characterized by tachycardia, tachydysrhythmias, and increased cardiac output suggests excessive activity of the sympathetic nervous system and a compensatory attempt to eliminate excess heat. The sensitivity of β-receptors is increased in hyperthyroid patients. Adrenal cortex hyperplasia reflects increased production and utilization of cortisol. Ex-

Table 22–13 • Signs and Symptoms of Hyperthyroidism

Signs and Symptoms	Incidence (% of Patients)
Goiter	100
Tachycardia	100
Anxiety	99
Tremor	97
Heat intolerance	89
Fatigue	88
Weight loss	85
Eye signs	71
Skeletal muscle weakness	70
Atrial fibrillation	10

Table 22–14 • Medical Treatment of Hyperthyroidism

Drug	Mechanism of Action	Indications

Antithyroid drugs
  Propylthiouracil
  Methimazole
  Carbimazole
	Inhibit thyroid hormone synthesis	Initial therapy for Graves' disease

β-Adrenergic antagonists
  Propranolol
  Metoprolol
  Atenolol
  Nadolol
	Ameliorate action of T_3 and T_4 in tissues	Adjunctive therapy and may be only treatment needed for thyroiditis

Iodine-containing compounds
  Potassium iodide
  Lugol's solution
	Inhibit T_3 and T_4 release	Preparation for surgery
		Thyrotoxic crisis

Lithium	Inhibits T_3 and T_4 release	
Glucocorticoids	Ameliorates actions of T_3 and T_4 in tissues Immunosuppressive actions	Severe subacute thyroiditis Thyrotoxic crisis Graves' disease

T_3, triiodothyronine; T_4, thyroxine.
Adapted from: Franklyn JA. The management of hyperthyroidism. N Engl J Med 1994;330:1731–9.

ophthalmos is due to an infiltrative process that involves retrobulbar fat and the eyelids. Retrobulbar edema can be so severe that the optic nerve is compressed, with resultant blindness. Patients with hyperthyroidism may exhibit increased bone resorption and associated hypercalciuria.

Treatment

Treatment of hyperthyroidism includes administration of drugs (antithyroid drugs, β-adrenergic antagonists, inorganic iodine), radioiodine therapy, and surgical removal of a portion of the gland (subtotal thyroidectomy) (Table 22–14).[44] Regardless of the therapy, patients with hyperthyroidism are monitored frequently, usually with serum thyrotropin measurements (to determine if hypothyroidism develops) or T_4 measurements (to determine if hyperthyroidism recurs). Hyperthyroidism that develops during pregnancy often requires no treatment because it is mild or resolves spontaneously.

Antithyroid Drugs

The initial medical management of hyperthyroidism is usually with antithyroid drugs (methimazole, carbimazole, propylthiouracil). These drugs prevent synthesis of thyroid hormones by inhibiting oxidation of inorganic iodide and coupling of iodothyronines. Propylthiouracil also inhibits peripheral monodeiodination of T_4 to T_3. Graves' disease is most often initially treated with antithyroid drugs in the hope of inducing a remission or achieving euthyroidism before treatment with radioiodine or surgery. Parturients should be treated with propylthiouracil (among the antithyroid drugs, it crosses the placenta in the least amount), thereby minimizing the risk of goiter and hypothyroidism in the fetus. The fact that Graves' disease often remits during pregnancy facilitates the use of low doses of propylthiouracil. Conversely, the disease tends to exacerbate following delivery.

Serious side effects occur in approximately 0.3% of treated patients, although methimazole may be less likely than propylthiouracil to cause agranulocytosis (Table 22–15). Agranulocytosis (granulocyte count less than 500 cells/mm^3) is an idiosyncratic reaction to these drugs. Patients who are developing agranulocytosis often present with pharyngitis

Table 22–15 • Side Effects of Antithyroid Drugs

Rare and serious side effects
  Agranulocytosis
Very rare serious side effects
  Hepatitis (propylthiouracil)
  Cholestatic jaundice (methimazole)
  Thrombocytopenia
  Aplastic anemia
  Lupus-like syndrome
Common and minor side effects
  Pruritus
  Urticarial rash
  Arthralgia
  Fever
Uncommon and minor side effects
  Gastrointestinal distress
  Hypoglycemia due to insulin autoantibodies
  Abnormal taste sensation

Adapted from: Franklyn JA. The management of hyperthyroidism. N Engl J Med 1994;330:1771–9.

and/or fevers at which time the drug must be discontinued. Because agranulocytosis develops rapidly, routine measurements of the leukocyte count are of questionable value.[44] Propylthiouracil may cause modest, transient increases in aminotransferase concentrations, but this response does not mandate a change in therapy. Intraoperative bleeding attributed to drug-induced thrombocytopenia or hypoprothrombinemia has been described in patients being treated with propylthiouracil.[46] Hypothyroidism is a risk of antithyroid drug therapy and is the reason these patients may receive supplemental T_4.

β-Adrenergic Antagonists

β-Adrenergic antagonists (propranolol, nadolol, atenolol) are useful adjunctive therapies for patients with Graves' disease in that they ameliorate some of the signs and symptoms (tachycardia, anxiety, tremor) of hyperthyroidism more rapidly than can be achieved with administration of antithyroid drugs. Nadolol and atenolol have a longer duration of action than propranolol, which improves patient compliance by permitting a once-a-day dosing schedule. These drugs do not affect the synthesis and secretion of T_4 or T_3 and should not be used as single therapy except for brief periods before radioiodine or surgical therapy.[47] Caution is needed when administering these drugs to patients with hyperthyroidism-induced asthma or congestive heart failure.

Inorganic Iodine

Iodine administered in pharmacologic doses (Lugol's solution, 5% iodine, 10% potassium iodide in water) inhibits the release of T_4 and T_3 for a limited time (days to weeks) after which its antithyroid activity is lost. For this reason, inorganic iodine is used principally to prepare patients for surgery and to treat thyrotoxic crisis.

Radioiodine Therapy

Radioiodine therapy is often selected as the initial treatment for Graves' disease and is the treatment of choice for hyperthyroidism that recurs following therapy with antithyroid drugs. The objective of radioiodine therapy is to destroy sufficient thyroid tissue to cure hyperthyroidism. Patients treated with radioiodine are reliably rendered euthyroid without the possible associated risks of anesthesia and surgery.

Permanent hypothyroidism is the only important complication of radioiodine therapy, occurring in a significant number of treated patients.[44] The presence of hypothyroidism is likely if the serum thyrotropin concentrations are increased and the serum T_4 concentrations are normal (subclinical hypothyroidism). Occasionally, there is transient worsening of hyperthyroidism during the first 2 weeks after radioiodine therapy that is likely due to radiation thyroiditis. Radiation thyroiditis sufficient to cause a thyrotoxic crisis is rare. There is no relation between radioiodine therapy and thyroid cancer or the occurrence of congenital anomalies in the offspring of treated women. Pregnancy is an absolute contraindication to radioiodine therapy, as it may cause ablation of the fetal thyroid gland.

Subtotal Thyroidectomy

Subtotal thyroidectomy is appropriate treatment for Graves' disease only when radioiodine therapy is refused and for rare patients with large goiters causing tracheal compression or cosmetic concerns. Any patient with hyperthyroidism scheduled for elective subtotal thyroidectomy should first be rendered euthyroid with drugs (Table 22–16).[44, 48] In an emergency, patients can be prepared for surgery in less than 1 hour by intravenous administration of esmolol or propranolol.[49] The risk of intraoperative or postoperative thyrotoxic crisis in patients rendered euthyroid with drugs is nearly zero.

Damage to the recurrent laryngeal nerves, postoperative bleeding into the neck (resultant tracheal compression), and hypoparathyroidism are recognized but uncommon complications of subtotal thyroidectomy. Relapse of hyperthyroidism occurs in at least 10% of surgically treated patients, seen most often during the first 5 years after surgery. Permanent hypothyroidism occurs in 5% of patients during the first year following subtotal thyroidectomy, and nearly 50% are hypothyroid by 25 years.[44]

The most common *nerve injury* after subtotal thyroidectomy is damage to the abductor fibers of the

---

Table 22–16 • Treatments to Render Hyperthyroid Patients Euthyroid Prior to Surgery

Emergency surgery
    Esmolol 100–300 μg/kg/min IV until heart rate < 100 beats/min
Elective surgery
    Oral administration of a β-adrenergic antagonist (propranolol, nadolol, atenolol) until heart rate is < 100 beats/min
    Antithyroid drugs
    Antithyroid drug plus potassium iodide
    Potassium iodide plus a β-adrenergic receptor antagonist

recurrent laryngeal nerves. This type of nerve damage, when unilateral, is characterized by hoarseness and a paralyzed vocal cord that assumes an intermediate position. Bilateral recurrent nerve injury results in aphonia and paralyzed vocal cords, which can collapse together, producing total airway obstruction during inspiration. Selective injury of the adductor fibers of the recurrent laryngeal nerves leaves the adductor fibers unopposed and pulmonary aspiration a hazard. In view of the possibility of damage to these nerves, it may be useful to evaluate vocal cord movement at the conclusion of subtotal thyroidectomy surgery. This can be accomplished by asking the patient to phonate by saying "e."

Airway obstruction that occurs soon after tracheal extubation despite normal vocal cord function suggests the diagnosis of tracheomalacia, reflecting weakening of the tracheal rings by chronic pressure from a goiter. The appearance of airway obstruction during the early postoperative period, as in the post-anesthesia care unit, may be due to tracheal compression at the operative site by a hematoma. Prompt opening of the surgical closure site and evacuation of the hematoma may be a life-saving intervention.

Hypoparathyroidism resulting from accidental removal of the parathyroid glands rarely occurs after subtotal thyroidectomy. If damage to the parathyroid glands does occur, hypocalcemia typically develops 24 to 72 hours postoperatively but may manifest as early as 1 to 3 hours after surgery. Laryngeal muscles are the most sensitive to hypocalcemia, and inspiratory stridor progressing to laryngospasm may be the first indication of surgically induced hypoparathyroidism. Treatment consists of prompt intravenous administration of calcium until laryngeal stridor ceases.

Thyrotoxic Crisis (Thyroid Storm)

Thyrotoxic crisis is a medical emergency characterized by the abrupt appearance of clinical signs of hyperthyroidism (tachycardia, hyperthermia, agitation, skeletal muscle weakness, congestive heart failure, dehydration, shock) due to the abrupt release of T_4 and T_3 into the circulation.[44] Thyrotoxic crisis associated with surgery can occur intraoperatively but is more likely to occur 6 to 18 hours postoperatively. When thyroid storm occurs intraoperatively, it may mimic malignant hyperthermia.[50] Thyrotoxicosis factitia results when patients ingest levothyroxine (T_4) deliberately or accidentally.[51, 52] In this regard, the delayed conversion of levothyroxine to T_3 could result in manifestations of thyrotoxic crisis intraoperatively in patients who were clinically euthyroid prior to the induction of anesthesia.

Treatment of thyrotoxic crisis is with intravenous infusion of cooled crystalloid solutions and continuous intravenous infusion of esmolol to maintain the heart rate at an acceptable level (usually less than 100 beats/min).[48] When hypotension is persistent, the administration of cortisol, 100 to 200 mg IV, may be a consideration. Propylthiouracil is given in a dose of 100 mg every 6 hours by mouth or by nasogastric tube to take advantage of this drug's ability to inhibit extrathyroidal conversion of T_4 to T_3. Potassium iodide is also administered to block the release of T_4 and T_3. It is important to treat any suspected infection in these patients.

Management of Anesthesia

Elective surgery should be deferred until patients have been rendered euthyroid and the hyperdynamic cardiovascular system has been controlled with β-adrenergic antagonists, as evidenced by an acceptable resting heart rate (Table 22–16).[44, 48] Clearly, all drugs being administered to manage the hyperthyroid state should be continued through the perioperative period. When surgery cannot be delayed in symptomatic hyperthyroid patients, the continuous infusion of esmolol, 100 to 300 μg/kg/min IV, may be useful for controlling cardiovascular responses evoked by sympathetic nervous system stimulation.[48] Poor control of hyperthyroidism plus surgery or parturition are associated with an increased risk of developing thyrotoxic crisis.[53]

Preoperative Medication

Anxiety relief is often provided by oral administration of benzodiazepines. The use of anticholinergic drugs is not likely, as these drugs could interfere with the body's normal heat-regulating mechanisms and contribute to an increased heart rate. Evaluation of the upper airway for evidence of obstruction (goiter compressing on the trachea) is an important part of the preoperative preparation. In this regard, computed tomography may be helpful for evaluating the airway in selected patients.

Induction of Anesthesia

Induction of anesthesia may be acceptably achieved with several intravenous induction drugs. Thiopental is an attractive selection because its thiourea structure lends antithyroid activity to the drug. Nevertheless, it is unlikely that a significant antithyroid effect can be produced by an induction dose of thiopental. Ketamine is not a likely selection for induction of anesthesia because it can stimulate the sympathetic nervous system. Indeed, tachycardia and systemic hypertension have been described after administration of ketamine to euthyroid patients being treated with thyroid hormone replacement.[54] Assuming the absence of airway obstruction from an enlarged goiter, the administration of succinylcholine or nondepolarizing muscle relaxants that do not affect the cardiovascular system is useful for facilitating tracheal intubation.

Maintenance of Anesthesia

The goals during maintenance of anesthesia in hyperthyroid patients are to (1) avoid administration of drugs that stimulate the sympathetic nervous system and (2) provide sufficient anesthetic-induced sympathetic nervous system depression to prevent exaggerated responses to surgical stimulation. The possibility of organ toxicity owing to altered or accelerated drug metabolism in the presence of hyperthyroidism is a consideration when selecting volatile anesthetics. In an animal model rendered hyperthyroid, the administration of halothane, enflurane, and isoflurane was followed by evidence of hepatic centrilobular necrosis in some animals, with the greatest incidence (92%) occurring in animals exposed to halothane.[55] Nevertheless, liver function tests are not altered postoperatively in hyperthyroid patients undergoing surgery and anesthesia that includes a volatile anesthetic.[56] An undocumented but potential concern with sevoflurane is nephrotoxicity caused by increased production of fluoride owing to accelerated metabolism of this anesthetic. Despite experimental evidence of hepatic necrosis after exposure to the tested volatile anesthetics, the ability of potent volatile anesthetics such as isoflurane, desflurane, or sevoflurane to offset adverse sympathetic nervous system responses to surgical stimulation, yet not sensitize the heart to catecholamines, makes these drugs an attractive choice to combine with nitrous oxide. Nitrous oxide combined with short-acting opioids is an alternative to administering volatile anesthetics, but it has the disadvantage of not reliably suppressing sympathetic nervous system activity.

It is a clinical impression that anesthetic requirements (MAC) are increased in hyperthyroid patients, but a controlled animal study did not confirm this impression.[57] The discrepancy between clinical impression and objective data may reflect the impact of increased cardiac output, which is characteristic of hyperthyroidism, on the rate of increase of the alveolar partial pressure of inhaled anesthetics. For example, increased cardiac output accelerates the uptake of inhaled anesthetics, resulting in the need to increase the inspired (delivered) concentration of the anesthetic (perceived clinically as an increased anesthetic requirement) to achieve a brain partial pressure (MAC) similar to that seen with a lower inspired concentration in the euthyroid patient. Likewise, accelerated metabolism of volatile anesthetics does not alter the partial pressure of the drugs needed in the brain to produce the desired pharmacologic effects. Cerebral metabolic oxygen requirements may not be altered by thyroid gland dysfunction, which is also consistent with unchanged anesthetic requirements. Another factor that should be considered when evaluating anesthetic requirements in the presence of altered thyroid gland function is body temperature. For example, increases in body temperature, as could accompany thyrotoxic crisis, would be expected to increase MAC by about 5% for each degree the body temperature increases above 37°C.

Monitoring during maintenance of anesthesia in hyperthyroid patients is directed at early recognition of increased thyroid gland activity, suggesting the onset of thyrotoxic crisis. Constant monitoring of body temperature is useful; methods to lower body temperature, including a cooling mattress and cold crystalloid solutions for intravenous infusion, may be helpful. The ECG may show resting tachycardia and/or cardiac dysrhythmias indicating the need for intraoperative administration of β-adrenergic antagonists (continuous intravenous infusion of esmolol) or lidocaine. Patients with exophthalmos are susceptible to corneal ulceration and drying, emphasizing the need to protect the patient's eyes during the perioperative period.

The choice of muscle relaxants is influenced by the potential impact of these drugs on sympathetic nervous system activity. Pancuronium is not a likely selection in view of the ability of this drug to increase heart rate and thereby mimic sympathetic nervous system stimulation. Administration of muscle relaxants with minimal effects on the cardiovascular system is preferable. Conceivably, prolonged responses could occur when traditional doses of muscle relaxants are administered to patients with co-existing skeletal muscle weakness. For this reason, it may be prudent to decrease the initial dose of muscle relaxant and closely monitor the effect produced at the neuromuscular junction using a peripheral nerve stimulator. Antagonism of neuromuscular blockade with anticholinesterase drugs combined with anticholinergic drugs introduces a concern about drug-induced tachycardia. Although experience is too limited to make recommendations, it seems unwarranted to avoid pharmacologic antagonism of nondepolarizing muscle relaxants in hyperthyroid patients. Perhaps glycopyrrolate, which has fewer chronotropic effects than atropine, would be a more appropriate anticholinergic drug selection.

Treatment of hypotension with sympathomimetic drugs must consider the possibility of the exaggerated responsiveness of hyperthyroid patients to endogenous or exogenous catecholamines. For these reasons, decreased doses of direct-acting vasopressors, such as phenylephrine, may be a more logical choice than ephedrine, which acts in part by provoking the release of catecholamines.

Regional Anesthesia

Regional anesthesia with its associated blockade of the sympathetic nervous system is a potentially useful choice for hyperthyroid patients, assuming there is no evidence of high-output congestive heart failure. A continuous epidural anesthetic may be preferable to spinal anesthesia because of the slower onset of sympathetic nervous system blockade, making severe hypotension less likely. If hypotension occurs, decreased doses of phenylephrine are recommended, keeping in mind the possible hypersensitivity of these patients to sympathomimetic drugs. Epinephrine should not be added to local anesthetic solutions, as systemic absorption of this catecholamine could produce exaggerated circulatory responses. Increased anxiety and associated activation of the sympathetic nervous system can be treated in awake patients with intravenous administration of benzodiazepines such as midazolam.

Hypothyroidism

Hypothyroidism is a generic term for all conditions in which body tissues are exposed to decreased circulating concentrations of T_3 and T_4, a condition estimated to be present in 0.5% to 0.8% of the adult population.[58] The diagnosis of hypothyroidism is based on clinical signs and symptoms plus confirmation of decreased thyroid gland function, as demonstrated by appropriate tests. Subclinical hypothyroidism manifesting only as increased plasma thyrotropin concentrations is present in about 5% of the population, with a prevalence of 13.2% in otherwise healthy elderly patients, especially women.

Causes

The etiology of hypothyroidism is categorized as primary (destruction of the thyroid gland) or secondary (central nervous system dysfunction) (Table 22–17). Chronic thyroiditis (Hashimoto's thyroiditis) is the most common cause of hypothyroidism, manifesting as an autoimmune disease characterized by progressive destruction of the thyroid gland. The presence of other autoimmune diseases (myasthenia gravis, adrenal insufficiency, premature ovarian failure) should direct attention to the thyroid gland. Other causes of hypothyroidism are drug ablative therapy and hypothalamic or pituitary insufficiency. Hypogonadism that presents as amenorrhea or impotence almost invariably develops before pituitary hypothyroidism.

Signs and Symptoms

The onset of hypothyroidism in adult patients is insidious and may go unrecognized. Adults with diffuse enlargement of the thyroid gland should have antibody measurements to determine the presence of chronic thyroiditis and associated hypothyroidism. Characteristically, there is a generalized decrease in metabolic activity in hypothyroid patients. Lethargy is prominent, and intolerance to cold is likely to be present. Cardiovascular changes are often the earliest clinical manifestations of hypothyroidism.[59] Chronic hypothyroidism results in bradycardia, decreased stroke volume and myocardial contractility, decreased cardiac output, increased systemic vascular resistance, systemic hypertension, narrow pulse pressure, and increased circulating concentrations of catecholamines. Systemic hypertension, particularly diastolic hypertension, occurs in about 15% of hypothyroid patients, reflecting decreased thyroid hormone levels with resultant increased systemic vascular resistance and increased levels of circulating catecholamines. Systolic and diastolic myocardial function are impaired in patients with chronic hypothyroidism, with congestive heart failure occasionally occurring. Myocar-

Table 22–17 • Etiology of Hypothyroidism

Primary hypothyroidism
  Thyroid gland dysfunction
    Chronic thyroiditis (Hashimoto's thyroiditis)
    Previous subtotal thyroidectomy
    Previous radioiodine therapy
    Irradiation of the neck
  Thyroid hormone deficiency
    Antithyroid drugs
    Excess iodide (inhibits release)
    Dietary iodine deficiency
Secondary hypothyroidism
  Hypothalamic dysfunction
    Thyrotropin-releasing hormone deficiency
  Anterior pituitary dysfunction
    Thyrotropin hormone deficiency

dial depression associated with severe hypothyroidism may be refractory to the administration of catecholamines. Overt congestive heart failure is unlikely, however, and if present may indicate coexisting heart disease or an unrecognized myocardial infarction. Echocardiography reveals evidence of myocardial dysfunction. Patients with hypothyroidism are predisposed to pericardial effusion. The ECG may reveal low voltage and prolonged PR, QRS, and QT intervals due to pericardial effusion and/or primary myocardial dysfunction. Conduction abnormalities may predispose patients to ventricular tachycardia, particularly torsades de pointes. Cardiovascular dysfunction is minimal to absent in patients with subclinical hypothyroidism.

Thyroid hormone appears necessary for normal production of pulmonary surfactant. Chronic hypothyroidism is associated with pleural effusions, which may further impair pulmonary function. The ventilatory drive in response to hypoxia and hypercapnia is decreased in patients with severe hypothyroidism. The basal metabolic rate is decreased by about 50%, consistent with the hypothermia that occurs in some patients. Peripheral vasoconstriction is characterized by cool, dry skin. Presumably, vasoconstriction represents an attempt to minimize loss of body heat. There is often atrophy of the adrenal cortex and associated decreases in the production of cortisol. Inappropriate secretion of antidiuretic hormone by hypothyroid patients can result in hyponatremia owing to the impaired ability of renal tubules to excrete free water.

Treatment

Treatment of hypothyroidism consists of oral administration of T_4. Optimal therapy is characterized by the disappearance of all symptoms of hypothyroidism and normal serum thyrotropin concentrations. Patients with ischemic heart disease and hypothyroidism may not tolerate even modest amounts of T_4 without the development of angina pectoris. If angina pectoris appears or worsens during T_4 therapy, coronary angiography and revascularization surgery can be safely undertaken before adequate T_4 therapy is achieved. It is not unusual to encounter patients previously started on thyroid hormone replacement without convincing laboratory confirmation of hypothyroidism. Confirmation of the diagnosis may require discontinuing treatment for 5 weeks and measuring serum thyrotropin concentrations, which if increased verifies the initial diagnosis.

Myxedema Coma

Myxedema coma is a rare complication of hypothyroidism, manifesting as loss of deep tendon reflexes, spontaneous hypothermia, hypoventilation, cardiovascular collapse, coma, and death. Sepsis in elderly patients or exposure to cold may be an initiating event. Treatment is with intravenous administration of T_3 (exerts a physiologic effect within 6 hours) and cortisol if adrenal insufficiency is suspected. Digitalis, as used to treat congestive heart failure, is used sparingly because the hypothyroid patient's heart cannot easily perform increased myocardial contractile work. Fluid replacement is important, remembering that these patients may be vulnerable to water intoxication and hyponatremia.

Management of Anesthesia

Elective surgery should probably be deferred in patients with symptomatic hypothyroidism. Nevertheless, controlled clinical studies do not confirm an increased risk when patients with mild to moderate hypothyroidism undergo elective surgery. There are no controlled studies to support the position that hypothyroid patients are unusually sensitive to inhaled anesthetic drugs and opioids, have a prolonged recovery, or experience an increased incidence of cardiovascular complications. Considering the likely presence of subclinical hypothyroidism in many patients who undergo uneventful anesthesia and the lack of increased morbidity in patients with mild to moderate hypothyroidism, there is little evidence to support delaying elective surgery in these patients. Nevertheless, a high index of suspicion for possible adverse effects, including exaggerated cardiac and ventilatory effects of depressant drugs, still seems warranted (Table 22–18).[60]

Preoperative Preparation

Most patients with hypothyroidism are receiving thyroid hormone replacement therapy and are eu-

Table 22–18 • Possible Adverse Responses of Hypothyroid Patients During the Perioperative Period

Increased sensitivity to depressant drugs
Hypodynamic cardiovascular system
   Decreased heart rate
   Decreased cardiac output
Slow metabolism of drugs
Unresponsive baroreceptor reflexes
Impaired ventilatory responses to arterial hypoxemia or hypercarbia
Hypovolemia
Delayed gastric emptying time
Hyponatremia
Hypothermia
Anemia
Hypoglycemia
Adrenal insufficiency

thyroid at the time of surgery. These patients are not at increased risk of perioperative morbidity and do not require special treatment other than continuation of their chronic thyroid hormone replacement.[59] Because of the long half-life of T_4 (7 days), administration of T_4 on the morning of surgery is considered optional. Conversely, it may be prudent for patients receiving T_3 to take their usual dose on the day of surgery because of its relatively short half-life (1.5 days).

In contrast to euthyroid patients, controversy exists regarding the perioperative management of patients with mild clinical or laboratory evidence of hypothyroidism presenting for elective surgery.[59] There is no evidence that postponing surgery in this setting to allow thyroid replacement therapy improves the perioperative outcome. The greatest controversy surrounds the role of preoperative thyroid hormone replacement in patients with coronary or valvular heart disease. Theoretically, myocardial ischemia might be provoked or worsened after thyroid hormone replacement if myocardial oxygen delivery is fixed and thyroid hormone-mediated inotropic and chronotropic effects increase myocardial oxygen demand. Nevertheless, the available data suggest that symptoms of angina pectoris actually decrease with the initiation of thyroid hormone replacement therapy. Based on these data it may be prudent to initiate thyroid hormone replacement carefully in hypothyroid patients with ischemic heart disease prior to cardiac and noncardiac surgery.[59]

Preoperative Medication

Preoperative medication for hypothyroid patients should emphasize the value of the preoperative visit and resultant psychological support. Opioid premedication has been administered safely, but there is a historical concern that the depressant effects of these drugs may be exaggerated in hypothyroid patients. Supplemental cortisol may be considered if there is concern that surgical stress could unmask decreased adrenal function that may accompany hypothyroidism. In some patients it is better to administer sedative and anticholinergic drugs intravenously after the patient arrives in the operating room, so any unexpected effect may be promptly recognized and treated.

Induction of Anesthesia

Induction of anesthesia may be accomplished with intravenous administration of ketamine with the presumption that the inherent support of the cardiovascular system by this drug is beneficial. Thiopental has been used for induction of anesthesia in hypothyroid patients without apparent excessive cardiovascular depression.[60] Even ketamine, in the absence of an active sympathetic nervous system, may produce unexpected cardiovascular depression. There is, however, no evidence of decreased responsiveness of hypothyroid patients to exogenous catecholamines. In severely hypothyroid patients inhalation of nitrous oxide might be sufficient to produce unresponsiveness. Tracheal intubation is facilitated by muscle relaxation produced by succinylcholine or nondepolarizing muscle relaxants, keeping in mind that co-existing skeletal muscle weakness could be associated with an exaggerated drug effect.

Maintenance of Anesthesia

Maintenance of anesthesia for hypothyroid patients is often achieved by inhalation of nitrous oxide plus supplementation, if necessary, with short-acting opioids, benzodiazepines, or ketamine. Volatile anesthetics may not be recommended in overtly symptomatic hypothyroid patients for fear of inducing exaggerated cardiac depression. Furthermore, vasodilation produced by anesthetic drugs in the presence of hypovolemia and/or attenuated baroreceptor reflex responses could result in abrupt decreases in systemic blood pressure, suggesting increased sensitivity to the anesthetic drugs. Nevertheless, hypothyroidism does not seem to decrease significantly anesthetic requirements (MAC) for volatile anesthetics.[57] Failure of MAC to change may reflect maintenance of cerebral metabolic oxygen requirements independent of thyroid hormone activity.[60] The clinical impression that MAC is decreased likely reflects decreases in cardiac output that accelerate the establishment of an anesthetizing brain partial pressure of the anesthetic, manifesting as a rapid induction of anesthesia. Furthermore, decreases in body temperature below 37°C would be expected to decrease MAC for inhaled drugs and slow the hepatic metabolism and renal clearance of injected drugs.

Maintaining skeletal muscle paralysis to provide surgical working conditions while minimizing the dose of anesthetic drugs is an appropriate goal for management of hypothyroid patients. Furthermore, controlled ventilation of the lungs is recommended in view of the tendency for hypothyroid patients to hypoventilate in the presence of anesthetic drugs. Decreased production of carbon dioxide associated with a decreased metabolic rate could make hypothyroid patients vulnerable to excessive decreases in $PaCO_2$ during mechanical ventilation of the lungs. Because of mild cardiovascular stimulating effects, pancuronium may be selected for the production of skeletal muscle paralysis in hypothyroid patients. Conversely, intermediate- and short-acting nondepolarizing muscle relaxants are acceptable and less likely to produce prolonged neuromuscular blockade. Indeed, decreased skeletal muscle activity associated with hypothyroidism suggests the possibility of prolonged responses when traditional doses of muscle relaxants are administered to hypothyroid patients. Antagonism of nondepolarizing neuromuscular blockade with anticholinesterase drugs combined with anticholinergic drugs does not pose a known hazard to hypothyroid patients.

Monitoring hypothyroid patients during anesthesia is intended to facilitate prompt recognition of exaggerated cardiovascular depression (perhaps reflecting the onset of congestive heart failure) and detection of the onset of hypothermia. Continuous recording of systemic blood pressure with a catheter placed in a peripheral artery and measurement of cardiac filling pressures are useful for invasive operations that may be prolonged or associated with significant surgical blood loss. Measurement of central venous pressure is helpful for guiding the rate of intravenous fluid infusion. In addition, the glucose solutions used for intravenous fluid replacement should contain sodium to decrease the likelihood of hyponatremia caused by impaired clearance of free water in hypothyroid patients. Hypotension requiring treatment with infusion of fluids or administration of sympathomimetic drugs may introduce the risk of evoking congestive heart failure. For example, administration of α-adrenergic agonists, such as phenylephrine, could adversely increase systemic vascular resistance in the presence of a heart that cannot reliably increase its contractility. By contrast, drugs with β-agonist effects could result in cardiac dysrhythmias. A useful approach to the treatment of hypotension may therefore be small doses of ephedrine, 2.5 to 5.0 mg IV, administered while monitoring cardiac filling pressures and continuously observing the ECG. The possibility of acute adrenal insufficiency is a consideration when hypotension persists despite treatment with fluids and/or sympathomimetic drugs. Maintenance of body temperature is facilitated by increasing the temperature of the operating room, using a warming device placed over the patient, warming inhaled gases, and passing intravenous fluids through a warmer.

Postoperative Management

Recovery from the sedative effects of anesthetic drugs may be delayed in hypothyroid patients, resulting in the need for prolonged observation during the postoperative period. Prolonged postoperative somnolence and an inability to wean the patient from mechanical ventilatory support have been described in a previously undiagnosed hypothyroid patient (Fig. 22–4).[61] In another report, acute postoperative hypothyroidism manifested as hypothermia, delayed awakening, and hypoventilation despite documented normal thyroid function 1 month preoperatively.[62] This report emphasized that a severe nonthyroid illness (gastric ulcer perforation) can precipitate acute hypothyroidism in a vulnerable patient (thyroid adenoma removal 20 years previously). Tracheal extubation is deferred until hypothyroid patients are responding appropriately and the body temperature is near 37°C. Concern about possible increased sensitivity to the effects of opioids is a consideration in the management of postoperative pain, perhaps with emphasis on the use of nonopioid analgesics. Despite these concerns, comparing patients who have mild to moderate hypothyroidism with euthyroid patients fails to demonstrate any difference with respect to the lowest body temperature or systemic blood pressure intraoperatively, the incidence of cardiac dysrhythmias, the need for vasopressors, the time to tracheal extubation, and the need for postoperative ventilatory support.[63]

Regional Anesthesia

Regional anesthesia is an appropriate choice for hypothyroid patients provided the intravascular fluid

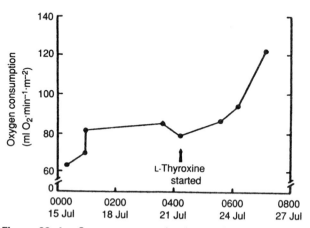

Figure 22–4 • Oxygen consumption in a patient with unsuspected hypothyroidism who underwent elective orthopedic surgery complicated by hypotension and the need for continued mechanical ventilation of the lungs during the postoperative period. Subsequent institution of thyroid replacement therapy restored the patient's vital signs and spontaneous ventilation to normal. (From Levelle JP, Jopling MW, Sklar GA. Perioperative hypothyroidism: an unusual postanesthetic diagnosis. Anesthesiology 1985;63:195–7, with permission.)

volume is maintained. Although supporting evidence is not available, theoretically the dose of local anesthetic necessary for a peripheral nerve block could be decreased. Furthermore, metabolism of amide local anesthetics that are absorbed into the systemic circulation could be slowed, possibly predisposing hypothyroid patients to the development of drug-induced systemic toxicity.

PARATHYROID GLAND DYSFUNCTION

The four parathyroid glands are located behind the upper and lower poles of the thyroid gland and produce a polypeptide hormone, parathormone.[64] Parathormone is released into the systemic circulation by a negative feedback mechanism that depends on the plasma calcium concentration. Hypocalcemia stimulates the release of parathormone, whereas hypercalcemia suppresses both the synthesis and release of this hormone. Parathormone maintains normal plasma calcium concentrations (4.5 to 5.5 mEq/L) by promoting the movement of calcium across three interfaces represented by the gastrointestinal tract, renal tubules, and bone.

Hyperparathyroidism

Hyperparathyroidism is present when the secretion of parathormone is increased. Serum calcium concentrations may be increased, decreased, or unchanged. Hyperparathyroidism is classified as primary, secondary, or ectopic.

Primary Hyperparathyroidism

Primary hyperparathyroidism results from excessive secretion of parathormone due to a benign parathyroid adenoma, carcinoma of a parathyroid gland, or hyperplasia of the parathyroid glands. A benign parathyroid adenoma is responsible for primary hyperparathyroidism in about 90% of patients; carcinoma of a parathyroid gland is responsible in fewer than 5% of affected patients. Hyperplasia usually involves all four parathyroid glands, although not all glands may be enlarged to the same degree. Hyperparathyroidism due to an adenoma or hyperplasia is the most common presenting symptom of multiple endocrine neoplasia type 1.

Diagnosis

Hypercalcemia (serum calcium concentration higher than 5.5 mEq/L and ionized calcium concentration higher than 2.5 mEq/L) is the hallmark of primary hyperparathyroidism. Primary hyperparathyroidism is the most common cause of hypercalcemia in the general population, whereas cancer is the most common cause in hospitalized patients. Modest increases in plasma calcium concentrations discovered incidentally in otherwise asymptomatic patients are most likely due to parathyroid adenomas, whereas marked hypercalcemia (higher than 7.5 mEq/L) is more likely due to cancer. Use of automated methods to measure serum calcium concentrations has detected primary hyperparathyroidism in a surprisingly large number of individuals, especially postmenopausal women. Patients in surgical intensive care units for prolonged periods of time may develop hypercalcemia, which may reflect increased secretion of parathormone in response to repeated episodes of hypocalcemia due to sepsis, shock, and blood transfusions. Urinary excretion of cyclic adenosine monophosphate is increased in patients with primary hyperparathyroidism. Measurement of serum parathormone concentrations is not always sufficiently reliable to confirm the diagnosis of primary hyperparathyroidism.

Signs and Symptoms

Hypercalcemia is responsible for the broad spectrum of signs and symptoms that accompany primary hyperparathyroidism and that affect multiple organ systems (Table 22–19). Symptoms due to hypercalcemia reflect changes in ionized calcium concentrations, which is the physiologically active form

Table 22–19 • Signs and Symptoms of Hypercalcemia Due to Hyperparathyroidism

Organ System	Signs and Symptoms
Neuromuscular	Skeletal muscle weakness
Renal	Polyuria and polydipsia
	Decreased glomerular filtration rate
	Kidney stones
Hematopoietic	Anemia
Cardiac	Prolonged PR interval
	Short QT interval
	Systemic hypertension
Gastrointestinal	Vomiting
	Abdominal pain
	Peptic ulcer
	Pancreatitis
Skeletal	Skeletal demineralization
	Collapse of vertebral bodies
	Pathologic fractures
Nervous system	Somnolence
	Decreased pain sensation
	Psychosis
Ocular	Calcifications (band keratopathy)
	Conjunctivitis

of calcium and represents about 45% of the total serum calcium concentration. Ionized serum calcium concentrations are dependent on arterial pH and the plasma albumin concentration. For this reason, it is preferable to measure ionized calcium concentrations directly using an ion-specific electrode.

Early signs and symptoms of primary hyperparathyroidism and associated hypercalcemia include sedation and vomiting. Skeletal muscle weakness and hypotonia is a frequent complaint and may be so severe as to suggest the presence of myasthenia gravis. Loss of skeletal muscle strength and mass is most notable in the proximal musculature of the lower extremities. This skeletal muscle weakness is a neuropathy (muscle biopsies resemble amyotrophic lateral sclerosis) and not a myopathy. The cause of the neuropathy is unclear, but it is not related to hypercalcemia; it is reversible, as skeletal muscle strength often improves following surgical removal of the excess parathormone-producing tissues.

Persistent increases in plasma calcium concentrations can interfere with urine concentrating ability, and polyuria results. Oliguric renal failure can occur in advanced cases of hypercalcemia. Renal stones, especially in the presence of polyuria and polydipsia must arouse suspicion of primary hyperparathyroidism. Increased serum chloride concentrations (higher than 102 mEq/L) are most likely due to the influence of parathormone on renal excretion of bicarbonate, producing a mild metabolic acidosis. Anemia, even in the absence of renal dysfunction, is a consequence of primary hyperparathyroidism. Peptic ulcer disease is frequent and may reflect potentiation of gastric acid secretion by calcium. Acute and chronic pancreatitis is associated with primary hyperparathyroidism. Even in the absence of peptic ulcer disease or pancreatitis, abdominal pain that often accompanies hypercalcemia can mimic an acute surgical abdomen.

Systemic hypertension is common, and the ECG may reveal prolonged PR intervals, whereas QT intervals are often shortened. When serum calcium concentrations exceed 8 mEq/L, cardiac conduction disturbances are likely. The classic skeletal consequence of primary hyperparathyroidism is osteitis fibrosa cystica. Radiographic evidence of skeletal involvement includes generalized osteopenia, subcortical bone resorption in the phalanges and distal ends of the clavicles, and the appearance of bone cysts. Bone pain and pathologic fractures may be present. There may be deficits of memory and cerebration, with or without personality changes or mood disturbances, including hallucinations. Loss of sensation for pain and vibration may occur.

Treatment

Primary hyperparathyroidism and the associated hypercalcemia are treated initially by medical means followed by definitive surgical removal of the diseased or abnormal portions of the parathyroid glands.

Medical Management. Saline infusion (150 ml/hr) is the basic treatment for all patients with symptomatic hypercalcemia. Intravascular fluid volume may be depleted by vomiting, polyuria, and urinary loss of sodium. The calcium-lowering effect of saline hydration alone is limited, and it is often necessary to add loop diuretics (furosemide 40 to 80 mg IV every 2 to 4 hours) to the therapeutic regimen but only after the intravascular fluid volume has been optimized. Central venous pressure monitoring may be useful for guiding fluid replacement in these patients. Loop diuretics inhibit sodium (and therefore calcium) reabsorption in the proximal loop of Henle. The goal is a daily urine output of 3 to 5 L. Addition of loop diuretics to saline hydration increases calcium excretion only if the saline infusion is adequate to restore the intravascular fluid volume necessary for delivery of calcium to the renal tubules. Thiazide diuretics are not administered for treatment of hypercalcemia, as these drugs may enhance renal tubular reabsorption of calcium.

Bisphosphonates such as disodium etidronate administered intravenously are the drugs of choice for treatment of life-threatening hypercalcemia.[65] These drugs bind to hydroxyapatite in bone and act as potent inhibitors of osteoclastic bone resorption. The effectiveness of bisphosphonates allows surgery to be performed under elective conditions rather than as an emergency in unstable hypercalcemic patients. Hemodialysis can also be used to lower serum calcium concentrations promptly, as can calcitonin, but the effects of this hormone are transient. Mithramycin inhibits osteoclastic activity of parathormone, producing prompt lowering of serum calcium concentrations. The toxic effects (thrombocytopenia, hepatotoxicity, nephrotoxicity) of mithramycin, however, limits its use.

Surgical Management. Definitive treatment of primary hyperparathyroidism is surgical removal of the diseased or abnormal portions of the parathyroid glands. Successful surgical treatment is reflected by normalization of serum calcium concentrations within 3 to 4 days and a decrease in the urinary excretion of cyclic adenosine monophosphate. Postoperatively, the first potential complication is hypocalcemic tetany. The hypomagnesemia that occurs postoperatively aggravates the hypocalcemia and renders it refractory to treatment. Acute arthritis may occur following parathyroidectomy. Hyperchloremic metabolic acidosis, in association with deterioration of renal function, may occur transiently after parathyroidectomy.

Management of Anesthesia

There is no evidence that specific anesthetic drugs or techniques are indicated in patients with primary hyperparathyroidism undergoing elective surgical treatment of the disease. Maintenance of hydration and urine output is important during the perioperative management of hypercalcemia. The existence of somnolence before induction of anesthesia introduces the possibility that intraoperative anesthetic requirements could be decreased. Ketamine is an unlikely selection in patients with co-existing personality changes attributed to chronic hypercalcemia. The possibility of co-existing renal dysfunction is a consideration when selecting sevoflurane, as impaired urine concentrating ability associated with polyuria and hypercalcemia could be confused with anesthetic-induced fluoride nephrotoxicity. Co-existing skeletal muscle weakness suggests the possibility of decreased requirements for muscle relaxants, whereas hypercalcemia might be expected to antagonize the effects of nondepolarizing muscle relaxants. Increased sensitivity to succinylcholine and resistance to atracurium have been described in a patient with hyperparathyroidism.[66] In view of the unpredictable response to muscle relaxants, it is probably important to decrease the initial dose of these drugs and to monitor the response produced at the neuromuscular junction using a peripheral nerve stimulator.[67] Monitoring the ECG for manifestations of adverse cardiac effects of hypercalcemia is often recommended, although there is evidence that the QT interval may not be a reliable index of changes in serum calcium concentrations during anesthesia.[68] Theoretically, hyperventilation of the lungs is undesirable, as respiratory alkalosis lowers serum potassium concentrations and leaves the actions of calcium unopposed. Nevertheless, by lowering ionized fractions of calcium, alkalosis could also be beneficial. Careful positioning of hyperparathyroid patients is necessary because of the likely presence of osteoporosis and the associated vulnerability to pathologic fractures.

Secondary Hyperparathyroidism

Secondary hyperparathyroidism reflects an appropriate compensatory response of the parathyroid glands to secrete more parathormone to counteract a disease process that produces hypocalcemia. For example, chronic renal disease impairs elimination of phosphorus and decreases hydroxylation of vitamin D, resulting in hypocalcemia and compensatory hyperplasia of the parathyroid glands with increased release of parathormone. Because secondary hyperparathyroidism is adaptive rather than autonomous, it seldom produces hypercalcemia. Treatment of secondary hyperparathyroidism is best directed at controlling the underlying disease, as is achieved by normalizing serum phosphate concentrations in patients with renal disease by administering an oral phosphate binder.

On occasion, transient hypercalcemia may follow otherwise successful renal transplantation. This response reflects the inability of previously hyperactive parathyroid glands to adapt quickly to normal renal excretion of calcium and phosphorus and to hydroxylation of vitamin D. The parathyroid glands usually return to normal size and function with time, although parathyroidectomy is occasionally necessary.

Ectopic Hyperparathyroidism

Ectopic hyperparathyroidism (humoral hypercalcemia of malignancy, pseudohyperparathyroidism) is due to secretion of parathormone (or a substance with similar endocrine effects) by tissues other than the parathyroid glands. Carcinoma of the lung, breast, pancreas, or kidney and lymphoproliferative disease are the most likely ectopic sites for parathormone secretion. Ectopic hyperparathyroidism is more likely than primary hyperparathyroidism to be associated with anemia and increased plasma alkaline phosphatase concentrations. A role for prostaglandins in the production of hypercalcemia in these patients is suggested by the calcium-lowering effects produced by indomethacin, which is an inhibitor of prostaglandin synthesis.

Hypoparathyroidism

Hypoparathyroidism is present when secretion of parathormone is absent or deficient or peripheral tissues are resistant to the effects of the hormone (Table 22–20). Absence or deficiency of parathormone is almost always iatrogenic, reflecting inadvertent removal of the parathyroid glands, as during thyroidectomy. Pseudohypoparathyroidism is a congenital disorder in which the release of parathormone is intact but the kidneys are unable to respond to the hormone. Affected patients manifest mental retardation, calcification of the basal ganglia, obe-

Table 22–20 • Etiology of Hypoparathyroidism

Decreased or absent parathormone
    Accidental removal of parathyroid glands during
        thyroidectomy
    Parathyroidectomy to treat hyperplasia
    Idiopathic (DiGeorge syndrome)
Resistance of peripheral tissues to effects of
      parathormone
    Congenital
      Pseudohypoparathyroidism
    Acquired
      Hypomagnesemia
      Chronic renal failure
      Malabsorption
      Anticonvulsive therapy (phenytoin)
Unknown
    Osteoblastic metastases
    Acute pancreatitis

sity, short stature, and short metacarpals and metatarsals.

Diagnosis

Measurement of serum calcium concentrations and the ionized fractions of calcium is the most valuable diagnostic indicator for hypoparathyroidism. In this regard, a serum calcium concentration less than 4.5 mEq/L and an ionized calcium concentration lower than 2.0 mEq/L are indicative of hypoparathyroidism.

Signs and Symptoms

Signs and symptoms of hypoparathyroidism depend on the rapidity of the onset of hypocalcemia.

Acute hypocalcemia, as can occur after accidental removal of the parathyroid glands during thyroidectomy, is likely to manifest as peroral paresthesias, restlessness, and neuromuscular irritability, as evidenced by a positive Chvostek sign or Trousseau sign. A positive Chvostek sign consists of facial muscle twitching produced by manual tapping over the area of the facial nerve at the angle of the mandible. The Chvostek sign is positive in the absence of hypocalcemia in 10% to 15% of patients. A positive Trousseau sign is carpopedal spasm produced by 3 minutes of limb ischemia produced by a tourniquet. Inspiratory stridor reflects neuromuscular irritability of the intrinsic laryngeal musculature.

Chronic hypocalcemia is associated with complaints of fatigue and skeletal muscle cramps that may be associated with a prolonged QT interval on the ECG. The QRS complex, PR interval, and cardiac rhythm usually remain normal. Neurologic changes include lethargy, cerebration deficits, and personal-

ity changes reminiscent of hyperparathyroidism. Chronic hypocalcemia is associated with formation of cataracts, calcification involving the subcutaneous tissues and basal ganglia, and thickening of the skull. Chronic renal failure is the most common cause of chronic hypocalcemia.

Treatment

Treatment of acute hypocalcemia consists of an infusion of calcium (10 ml of 10% calcium gluconate IV) until signs of neuromuscular irritability disappear. Correction of any co-existing respiratory or metabolic alkalosis is indicated. For treatment of hypoparathyroidism not complicated by symptomatic hypocalcemia, the approach is administration of oral calcium and vitamin D. An exogenous parathyroid hormone replacement preparation is not yet practical for clinical use. Thiazide diuretics may be useful, as these drugs cause sodium depletion without proportional potassium excretion, thereby tending to increase serum calcium concentrations.

Management of Anesthesia

Management of anesthesia in the presence of hypocalcemia is designed to prevent any further decreases in the serum calcium concentrations and to treat the adverse effects of hypocalcemia, particularly those on the heart. In this regard it is important to avoid iatrogenic hyperventilation of the patient's lungs. Administration of whole blood containing citrate usually does not decrease serum calcium concentrations because calcium is rapidly mobilized from body stores. The ionized calcium concentrations can be decreased, however, with rapid infusions of blood (500 ml every 5 to 10 minutes, as during cardiopulmonary bypass or liver transplantation) or when metabolism or elimination of citrate is impaired by hypothermia, cirrhosis of the liver, or renal dysfunction.

DiGeorge Syndrome

The DiGeorge syndrome (congenital thymic hypoplasia) is characterized by hypoplasia or aplasia of the parathyroid glands and thymus gland, resulting in secondary hypocalcemia and a propensity for the development of infections due to defects in cell-mediated immunity. Neonatal tetany is usually present. Associated anomalies are often vascular, including right aortic arch, persistent truncus arteriosus, and tetralogy of Fallot.

Micrognathia may interfere with adequate exposure of the glottic opening during direct laryngoscopy. Iatrogenic hyperventilation and associated respiratory alkalosis, as may occur during anesthesia, could accentuate co-existing hypocalcemia. The response to neuromuscular blocking drugs could be altered in the presence of hypocalcemia. Hemodynamic instability may occur if hypoparathyroid patients are made acutely hypocalcemic. Measurement of serum calcium concentrations, particularly the ionized fraction, is helpful for perioperative management of these patients.

■ ADRENAL GLAND DYSFUNCTION

The adrenal glands consist of the adrenal cortex and adrenal medulla. The body's adjustments to the upright posture and responses to stress, as produced by hemorrhage, sepsis, anesthesia, and surgery, are dependent on normal function of the adrenal glands. The adrenal cortex is responsible for the synthesis of three groups of hormones classified as glucocorticoids (cortisol essential for life), mineralocorticoids (aldosterone), and androgens. Corticotropin is secreted by the anterior pituitary gland in response to corticotropin-releasing hormone, which is synthesized in the hypothalamus and carried to the anterior pituitary in the portal blood. Corticotropin stimulates the adrenal cortex to produce cortisol. Maintenance of systemic blood pressure by cortisol reflects the importance of this hormone in facilitating conversion of norepinephrine to epinephrine in the adrenal medulla. Hyperglycemia in response to cortisol secretion reflects gluconeogenesis and inhibition of the peripheral use of glucose by cells. Retention of sodium and excretion of potassium are facilitated by cortisol. Antiinflammatory effects of cortisol and other glucocorticoids (cortisone, prednisone, methylprednisolone, dexamethasone, triamcinolone) are particularly apparent in the presence of high serum concentrations of these hormones. Aldosterone secretion is regulated by the renin-angiotensin system and the serum concentrations of potassium. Aldosterone regulates the extracellular fluid volume by promoting resorption of sodium by the renal tubules. In addition, aldosterone promotes renal tubular excretion of potassium. The adrenal medulla is a specialized part of the sympathetic nervous system that is capable of synthesizing norepinephrine and epinephrine. The only important disease process associated with the adrenal medulla is pheochromocytoma. Adrenal medulla insufficiency is not known to occur.

Hypercortisolism (Cushing Syndrome)

Cushing syndrome is categorized as corticotropin-dependent Cushing syndrome (inappropriately high plasma corticotropin concentrations stimulate the adrenal cortex to produce excessive amounts of cortisol) and corticotropin-independent Cushing syndrome (excessive production of cortisol by abnormal adrenocortical tissues causes the syndrome and suppresses secretion of corticotropin-releasing hormone and corticotropin).[69] The term Cushing's disease is reserved for Cushing syndrome caused by excessive secretion of corticotropin by pituitary corticotroph tumors (microadenomas). These microadenomas account for nearly 70% of patients with corticotropin-dependent Cushing syndrome. Acute ectopic corticotropin syndrome (rapid onset of systemic hypertension, edema, hypokalemia, glucose intolerance) is another form of corticotropin-dependent Cushing syndrome that is most often associated with small cell lung carcinoma. Benign or malignant adrenocortical tumors are the most common cause of corticotropin-independent Cushing syndrome.

Diagnosis

There are no pathognomonic signs or symptoms that confirm the diagnosis of Cushing syndrome. The most common symptom is the relatively sudden onset of weight gain, which is usually central and often accompanied by thickening of the facial fat, which rounds the facial contour (moon facies), and a florid complexion due to telangiectasias. Systemic hypertension, glucose intolerance, oligomenorrhea, or amenorrhea in premenopausal women, decreased libido in men, and spontaneous ecchymoses are frequent concomitant findings. Skeletal muscle wasting and weakness manifest as difficulty climbing stairs. Depression and insomnia are often present. The diagnosis of Cushing syndrome is confirmed by demonstrating cortisol hypersecretion based on 24-hour urinary secretion of cortisol. Determining whether a patient's hypercortisolism is corticotropin-dependent or corticotropin-independent requires reliable measurements of plasma corticotropin utilizing immunoradiometric assays. Because most patients with corticotropin-dependent Cushing syndrome have Cushing's disease, the goal is to identify the patients who have the less common ectopic corticotropin syndrome. The high-dose dexamethasone suppression test distinguishes Cushing's disease from the ectopic corticotropin syndrome (complete resistance present). Imaging procedures provide no information about adrenal cortex function and are useful only for determining the location of a tumor.

Treatment

The treatment of choice for patients with Cushing's disease is transsphenoidal microadenomectomy if a clearly circumscribed microadenoma can be identified and resected.[69] Alternatively, patients may undergo 85% to 90% resection of the anterior pituitary. Pituitary radiation and bilateral total adrenalectomy are necessary in some patients. Surgical removal of the adrenal glands is the treatment for adrenal adenoma or carcinoma.

Management of Anesthesia

Management of anesthesia for patients with hypercortisolism must consider the physiologic effects of excessive cortisol secretion (Table 22–21).[70] Preoperative evaluation of systemic blood pressure, electrolyte balance, and the blood glucose concentration are especially important. Osteoporosis is a consideration when positioning patients for the operative procedure.

The choice of drugs for preoperative medication, induction of anesthesia, and maintenance of anesthesia is not influenced by the presence of hypercortisolism. Etomidate may transiently decrease the synthesis and release of cortisol by the adrenal cortex, but a therapeutic role for this drug in the presence of hypercortisolism seems unlikely. Surgical stimulation predictably increases the release of cortisol from the adrenal cortex. It seems unlikely that this stress-induced release would produce a different effect from that in normal patients. Furthermore, attempts to decrease adrenal cortex activity with opioids, barbiturates, or volatile anesthetics are probably futile, as any drug-induced inhibition is likely overridden by surgical stimulation. Even regional anesthesia may not be effective in preventing increased cortisol secretion during surgery. Doses of muscle relaxants should probably be decreased initially in view of skeletal muscle weakness, which frequently accompanies hypercortisolism. In addition, the presence of hypokalemia could influence responses to nondepolarizing muscle relaxants. Mechanical ventilation of the patient's lungs during surgery is recommended, as skeletal muscle weakness, with or without co-existing hypokalemia, may decrease strength in the muscles of breathing. Regional anesthesia is acceptable, but the likely presence of osteoporosis, with possible vertebral body collapse, is a consideration.

Plasma cortisol concentrations decrease promptly after microadenomectomy or bilateral adrenalectomy, for which replacement therapy is recommended. In this regard, a continuous infusion of cortisol (100 mg daily IV) may be initiated intraoperatively. Likewise, patients with metastatic disease involving the adrenal glands may show development of acute adrenal insufficiency, suggesting the need to institute supplemental therapy. Transient diabetes insipidus and meningitis may occur after microadenomectomy.

Hypocortisolism (Addison's Disease)

Hypocortisolism may develop as a result of (1) destruction of the adrenal cortex by hemorrhage, cancer, or granulomatous disease; (2) prolonged exogenous administration of corticosteroids that suppresses the pituitary-adrenal axis; and (3) deficiency of corticotropin. Primary adrenal insufficiency (Addison's disease) reflects the absence of cortisol and aldosterone due to destruction of the adrenal cortex. The most common cause is adrenal hemorrhage in anticoagulated patients, but adrenal insufficiency can also develop as a result of sepsis or accidental or surgical trauma. The adrenal gland is the endocrine gland most often involved in patients who die from complications of acquired immunodeficiency syndrome (AIDS), although adrenal insufficiency is uncommon in these patients. Tuberculosis formerly was a leading cause of primary adrenal failure and is an important consideration in patients with a history of this infection.[71] Secondary adrenal insufficiency occurs in patients with panhypopituitarism that includes corticotropin deficiency. In contrast to primary adrenal insufficiency, manifestations of secondary adrenal insufficiency reflect the absence of cortisol, as aldosterone secretion remains normal. The definitive diagnosis of hypocortisolism requires measurement of plasma cortisol concentrations before and 1 hour after administration of corticotropin.

Signs and Symptoms

Primary adrenal insufficiency manifests as weight loss, skeletal muscle weakness, hypotension, and abdominal or back pain. Pain caused by hemorrhage into the adrenal cortex, as in the anticoagulated patient, may be the only clue to the onset of adrenal insufficiency. The clinical picture may be indistin-

Table 22–21 • Physiologic Effects of Excess Cortisol Secretion

Systemic hypertension
Hyperglycemia
Skeletal muscle weakness
Osteoporosis
Obesity
Menstrual disturbances
Poor wound healing
Susceptibility to infection

guishable from shock owing to loss of intravascular fluid volume. Blood urea nitrogen concentrations are likely to be increased owing to hypovolemia and decreased renal blood flow. Hyponatremia, hyperkalemia, hypoglycemia, and hemoconcentration are often present. A useful clue to the diagnosis of adrenal insufficiency is the presence of hyperpigmentation principally over the palmar surfaces and pressure points.

Secondary adrenal insufficiency is less likely than primary adrenal insufficiency to be associated with severe hypovolemia or electrolyte derangements, as aldosterone secretion is maintained. Panhypopituitarism, however, may be associated with symptoms due not only to the lack of corticotropin but of thyrotropin, gonadotropins, and growth hormone as well.

Treatment

Treatment of life-threatening hypocortisolism consists of administration of cortisol, 100 mg IV, followed by continuous infusion at 10 mg/hr IV. It is useful to obtain blood samples for analysis of plasma cortisol concentrations before initiating therapy, although a delay for more specific diagnostic testing is not recommended. Intravenous infusion of glucose in saline, colloid solutions, and in some cases whole blood is necessary to restore the intravascular fluid volume. Replacement therapy for chronic hypocortisolism is with administration of cortisone, 20 to 25 mg PO in the morning and 10 to 15 mg PO in the afternoon. In addition, a mineralocorticoid effect is provided with fludrocortisone, 0.05 to 0.10 mg PO daily.

Surgery and Suppression of the Pituitary Adrenal Axis

Corticosteroid supplementation should be provided for patients being treated for chronic hypocortisolism who undergo surgical procedures. This practice is based on the concern that these patients are more susceptible to cardiovascular collapse, as the release of additional endogenous cortisol in response to surgical stress is not likely. More controversial is the management of patients who display suppression of the pituitary-adrenal axis due to current or previous treatment with corticosteroids for treating a disease (asthma, rheumatoid arthritis) unrelated to any pathology in the anterior pituitary or adrenal cortex. The precise dose of corticosteroids or duration of therapy with corticosteroids that produce suppression of the pituitary-adrenal axis is unknown. Furthermore, recovery of normal pituitary-adrenal axis function may require as long as 12 months after discontinuation of therapy. Documentation of nor-

mal serum cortisol concentrations in treated patients does not confirm an intact pituitary-adrenal axis or the ability of the adrenal cortex to release cortisol in response to surgical stress. The intactness of this axis can be confirmed by the plasma cortisol response to corticotropin administered intravenously (serum cortisol concentrations double within 1 hour if the axis is intact), but this remains an impractical and infrequently performed preoperative test. Instead, the clinical approach is often to administer empirically a supplemental dose of corticosteroids during the perioperative period when surgery is planned in patients being treated with corticosteroids or in those who have been treated longer than 1 month during the 6 to 12 months preceding surgery. It should be appreciated that the original recommendations for supplemental corticosteroid dosages were excessive and based on anecdotal information.[72] Indeed, cause-and-effect relations between intraoperative hypotension and acute hypocortisolism in patients previously treated with corticosteroids have not been documented, and it is clear that the risk of acute adrenal failure during the perioperative period has been exaggerated.[73,74]

Steroid Coverage Based on Physiologic Responses to Stress

In view of the possible adverse influences of corticosteroids (delayed healing, increased susceptibility to infection, gastrointestinal hemorrhage, decreased glucose tolerance, unconfirmed risk of acute hypocortisolism during surgery), attempts have been made to rationalize corticosteroid supplementation for surgical patients considered to be at risk for the development of acute hypocortisolism and to define an appropriate but minimal effective dose. There is evidence that adrenalectomized animals undergoing subsequent surgery are adequately protected by physiologic replacement doses of corticosteroids.[75] A recommended regimen for corticosteroid supplementation during the perioperative period is administration of cortisol, 25 mg IV at induction of anesthesia, followed by a continuous infusion of cortisol, 100 mg IV during the next 24 hours.[76] This regimen maintains plasma cortisol concentrations above normal levels during major surgery in patients receiving chronic treatment with corticosteroids for management of medical diseases unrelated to chronic hypocortisolism and who show a subnormal response to the perioperative infusion of corticotropin (Fig. 22–5).[76] An alternative to this physiologic replacement regimen is administration of cortisol, 25 mg IV, every 4 hours.[73] These regimens provide a rational, physiologic approach to low-dose corticosteroid supplementation during the perioperative

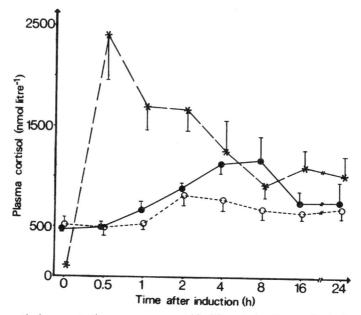

Figure 22–5 • Plasma cortisol concentrations were measured in (1) control patients who had never been treated with corticosteroids (*solid symbols*), (2) patients treated chronically with corticosteroids but showing a normal cortisol release response to corticotropin (*open symbols*), and (3) patients treated chronically with corticosteroids and showing a subnormal cortisol release response to corticotropin (*asterisks*). Only the latter patients were treated with supplemental corticosteroids (cortisol 25 mg IV after induction of anesthesia followed by a continuous infusion of 100 mg IV over the next 24 hours). This approach maintained plasma cortisol concentrations near or above that present in untreated patients. (From Symreng T, Karlberg BE, Kagedal B, et al. Physiological cortisol substitution on long-term steroid-treated patients undergoing major surgery. Br J Anaesth 1981;53:949–53, with permission.)

period for patients considered to be at risk for pituitary-adrenal axis suppression and who are scheduled for major surgery. In addition to this cortisol supplementation, patients receiving daily maintenance doses of corticosteroids should also receive this dose with the preoperative medication on the day of surgery. This maintenance dose should be continued postoperatively.

Continuation of corticosteroid supplementation into the postoperative period is based on the magnitude of surgical stress and the known corticosteroid production rates associated with this stress.[72] There are no data to support the practice of instituting increased maintenance doses preoperatively followed by gradual decreases over several days until the original maintenance dose is reached.[75] For minor surgical procedures and an uncomplicated postoperative course, patients can be returned to their preoperative treatment dose on the first postoperative day. For moderate surgical stress (total hip replacement, colon resection, open cholecystectomy) cortisol production rates suggest the need for supplemental cortisol, 50 to 75 mg for the first 1 to 2 days postoperatively. For major surgical stress (cardiopulmonary bypass, esophagectomy) the cortisol

supplemental dose is 100 to 150 mg for the first 2 to 3 days postoperatively. These recommendations are based on estimates that endogenous cortisol production produced by intense physiologic stress (burns) is 75 to 150 mg daily. It is known that after uncomplicated major surgery the serum cortisol concentrations decrease rapidly. Circulating serum cortisol concentrations are normal by 24 to 48 hours in most patients.

Management of Anesthesia

Management of anesthesia for patients with known hypocortisolism introduces no unique considerations other than provision of exogenous corticosteroid supplementation and a high index of suspicion for primary adrenal failure if unexplained intraoperative hypotension occurs. Despite the frequent suggestion that unexplained intraoperative hypotension and even death reflect unrecognized hypocortisolism, there is no evidence that primary adrenal insufficiency is a likely explanation for this response.[73,74] Selection of anesthetic drugs and muscle relaxants is not influenced by the presence of treated hypocortisolism, with the possible exception of etomidate. In this regard, etomidate has been shown to inhibit synthesis of cortisol transiently in normal patients. Typically, plasma cortisol concentrations increase during surgery in response to surgical stimulation, independent of the anesthetic drugs being administered.

Emergency surgery in the presence of untreated hypocortisolism should be rare. If surgery becomes necessary, however, perioperative management must include administration of supplemental corticosteroids and intravenous infusion of sodium-containing fluids. Minimal doses of anesthetic drugs should be administered, as these patients may be exquisitely sensitive to drug-induced myocardial depression. Invasive monitoring of systemic blood pressure and cardiac filling pressures is indicated. Plasma concentrations of glucose and electrolytes should be measured frequently during the perioperative period. In view of skeletal muscle weakness, the initial dose of muscle relaxant should be decreased and the response monitored using a peripheral nerve stimulator.

Primary Hyperaldosteronism (Conn Syndrome)

Primary aldosteronism (Conn syndrome) is present when there is excess secretion of aldosterone from a functional tumor (aldosteronoma) independent of a physiologic stimulus.[77] Aldosteronomas occur more often in women than in men and only rarely in children. Occasionally, primary aldosteronism is associated with pheochromocytoma, primary hyperparathyroidism, or acromegaly. Secondary hyperaldosteronism is present when increased circulating serum concentrations of renin, as associated with renovascular hypertension, stimulate the release of aldosterone. Aldosteronism associated with Bartter syndrome is not accompanied by systemic hypertension. The prevalence of primary aldosteronism in patients with essential hypertension appears to be less than 1%.[77]

Signs and Symptoms

Clinical signs and symptoms of primary aldosteronism are nonspecific, and some patients are completely asymptomatic.[77] Symptoms may reflect systemic hypertension (headache) or hypokalemia (polyuria, nocturia, skeletal muscle cramps, skeletal muscle weakness). Systemic hypertension (diastolic blood pressure often 100 to 125 mmHg) reflects aldosterone-induced sodium retention and the resulting increased extracellular fluid volume. This hypertension may be resistant to treatment. Aldoste-

rone promotes renal excretion of potassium, resulting in hypokalemic metabolic alkalosis. Increased urinary excretion of potassium (more than 30 mEq daily) in the presence of hypokalemia suggests primary aldosteronism. Hypokalemic nephropathy can result in polyuria and an inability to concentrate urine optimally.[78] Skeletal muscle weakness is presumed to reflect hypokalemia. Hypomagnesemia and abnormal glucose tolerance may be present.

Diagnosis

Spontaneous hypokalemia in patients with systemic hypertension is highly suggestive of aldosteronism. Plasma renin activity is suppressed in almost all patients with untreated primary aldosteronism and in many with essential hypertension; with secondary aldosteronism, however, the plasma renin activity is high. A plasma aldosterone concentration of less than 9.5 ng/dl at the end of a saline infusion rules out primary aldosteronism. A syndrome exhibiting all the features of hyperaldosteronism (systemic hypertension, hypokalemia, suppression of the renin-angiotensin system) may result from chronic ingestion of licorice.

Treatment

Initial treatment of hyperaldosteronism consists of supplemental potassium and administration of a competitive aldosterone antagonist, such as spironolactone. Skeletal muscle weakness due to hypokalemia may require treatment with potassium administered intravenously. Systemic hypertension may require treatment with antihypertensive drugs. Accentuation of hypokalemia due to drug-induced diuresis is decreased by using a potassium-sparing diuretic such as triamterene. Definitive treatment for an aldosterone-secreting tumor is surgical excision. Bilateral adrenalectomy may be necessary if multiple aldosterone-secreting tumors are found.

Management of Anesthesia

Management of anesthesia for the treatment of hyperaldosteronism is facilitated by preoperative correction of hypokalemia and treatment of systemic hypertension. Persistence of hypokalemia may modify responses to nondepolarizing muscle relaxants. Furthermore, it must be appreciated that intraoperative hyperventilation of the patient's lungs can decrease the plasma potassium concentration. Inhaled or injected drugs are acceptable for maintenance of anesthesia. The use of sevoflurane is questionable, however, if hypokalemic nephropathy and polyuria exist preoperatively.[78] Measurement of cardiac filling pressures through a right atrial or pulmonary artery catheter may be useful during surgery for adequate evaluation of the intravascular fluid volume and the response to intravenous infusion of fluids. Indeed, aggressive preoperative preparation can convert the excessive intravascular fluid volume status of these patients to unexpected hypovolemia, manifesting as hypotension in response to vasodilating anesthetic drugs, positive-pressure ventilation of the lungs, body position changes, or sudden surgical blood loss. The existence of orthostatic hypotension detected during the preoperative evaluation is a clue to the presence of unexpected hypovolemia in these patients. Acid-base status and plasma electrolyte concentrations should be measured frequently during the perioperative period. Supplementation with exogenous cortisol is probably unnecessary for surgical excision of a solitary adenoma in the adrenal cortex. Bilateral mobilization of the adrenal glands to excise multiple functional tumors, however, may introduce the need for exogenous administration of cortisol. A continuous intravenous infusion of cortisol, 100 mg every 24 hours, may be initiated on an empirical basis if transient hypocortisolism due to surgical manipulation is a consideration.

Hypoaldosteronism

Hyperkalemia in the absence of renal insufficiency suggests the presence of hypoaldosteronism.[79] Heart block secondary to hyperkalemia and orthostatic hypotension and hyponatremia may be present. Hyperkalemia is sometimes abruptly enhanced by hyperglycemia. Hyperchloremic metabolic acidosis is a predictable finding in the presence of hypoaldosteronism.

Isolated deficiency of aldosterone secretion may reflect (1) congenital deficiency of aldosterone synthetase or (2) hyporeninemia due to defects in the juxtaglomerular apparatus or treatment with angiotensin-converting enzyme inhibitors that leads to loss of angiotensin stimulation. Hyporeninemic hypoaldosteronism typically occurs in patients older than 45 years of age with chronic renal disease and/or diabetes mellitus. Indomethacin-induced prostaglandin deficiency is a reversible cause of this syndrome. Treatment of hypoaldosteronism includes liberal sodium intake and daily administration of fludrocortisone.

Pheochromocytoma

Pheochromocytoma is a catecholamine-secreting tumor that originates in the adrenal medulla or in chromaffin tissues along the paravertebral sympathetic chain, extending from the pelvis to the base of the skull.[80–82] More than 95% of all pheochromocytomas are found in the abdominal cavity, and about 90% originate in the adrenal medulla. An estimated 10% of these tumors involve both adrenal glands, and functional tumors in multiple sites are present in nearly 20% of patients, especially children. Fewer than 10% of pheochromocytomas are malignant. Pheochromocytomas typically occur in patients 30 to 50 years old, although about one-third of reported cases have been in children, principally males. Pheochromocytoma can also occur as part of an autosomal dominant multiglandular neoplastic syndrome, designated multiple endocrine neoplasia (MEN) (Table 22–22).[81, 83, 84] All patients with pheochromocytomas should be screened for MEN type 2 and von Hippel-Lindau disease.[84] Persons carrying the MEN 2 mutation are predisposed to develop medullary thyroid carcinoma, pheochromocytoma, and hyperparathyroidism (MEN 2A subtype) or mucosal neuromas and marfanoid habitus (MEN 2B subtype). Medullary thyroid carcinoma is the most common of the many rare disorders associated with pheochromocytoma. Although fewer than 0.1% of patients with systemic hypertension have a pheochromocytoma, nearly 50% of deaths in patients with unsuspected pheochromocytoma occur during unrelated anesthesia and surgery or parturition.[85] Pheochromocytoma and associated systemic hypertension and hypermetabolism may mimic other diseases, including malignant hyperthermia.[86]

Diagnosis

Computed tomography and magnetic resonance imaging provide accurate identification and localization of most pheochromocytomas (tumors as small as 1 cm), especially when the tumors are suprarenal.[82] Diagnosis of pheochromocytoma requires chemical confirmation of excessive catecholamine

Table 22–22 • Manifestations of Multiple Endocrine Neoplasia

Syndrome	Manifestations
MEN type 1A (Sipple syndrome)	Medullary thyroid cancer Parathyroid adenoma Pheochromocytoma
MEN type 2B	Medullary thyroid cancer Mucosal adenomas Marfan appearance Pheochromocytoma
von Hippel-Lindau syndrome	Hemangioblastoma involving the central nervous system Pheochromocytoma

release into the systemic circulation. Measurement of free norepinephrine in a 24-hour urine collection provides a more sensitive index of pheochromocytoma than do catecholamine metabolites (normetanephrine, metanephrine, vanillylmandelic acid).[82, 87] The presence of normotension despite increased plasma concentrations of catecholamines presumably reflects a decrease in the number of α-adrenergic receptors (down-regulation) in response to increased circulating concentrations of the neurotransmitter. Clonidine, 0.3 mg PO, suppresses plasma concentrations of catecholamines in hypertensive patients but not in patients with pheochromocytomas.[88] This response reflects the ability of clonidine to suppress an increase in serum catecholamine concentrations that result from neurogenic release but not from diffusion of excess catecholamines from pheochromocytomas into the systemic circulation.

Signs and Symptoms

The hallmark of pheochromocytoma is systemic hypertension associated with diaphoresis, headache, tremulousness, palpitations, and weight loss, especially in young to middle-aged adults. Only a small proportion, about 10% to 17% of those with pheochromocytomas, present with paroxysmal symptoms that reflect excessive secretion of catecholamines.[82] The triad of diaphoresis, tachycardia, and headache in hypertensive patients is highly suggestive of pheochromocytoma. Conversely, the absence of this triad virtually rules out its presence. Flushing is so rare that its presence casts doubt on the diagnosis of pheochromocytoma. Symptoms may last several minutes to hours and are often followed by fatigue.

Hyperglycemia reflects a predominance of α-adrenergic activity (inhibition of insulin release, glycogenolysis) over β-adrenergic effects (insulin release) produced by catecholamines secreted by pheochromocytomas. Enhanced coagulation may accompany chronic catecholamine excess. Orthostatic hypotension is a common finding and reflects decreases in intravascular fluid volume associated with sustained systemic hypertension. A hematocrit higher than 45% may reflect hypovolemia caused by chronic increases in systemic blood pressure. Nevertheless, there is evidence that patients with pheochromocytomas do not always develop hypovolemia.[89] Sustained increases in plasma catecholamine concentrations can result in focal necrosis of cardiac muscle and the development of dilated cardiomyopathy and congestive heart failure, which occurs in about one-third of patients.[82] Catecholamines can cause damage to the walls of small arteries, leading to the development of ischemic heart disease. Death resulting from a pheochromocytoma is often due to congestive heart failure, myocardial infarction, or intracerebral hemorrhage.

Treatment

Treatment of pheochromocytoma is surgical excision of the catecholamine-secreting tumor(s). Before surgery is scheduled, however, it is important to establish α-adrenergic blockade to stabilize the systemic blood pressure, expand the intravascular volume, and normalize myocardial performance. Most studies recommend that patients receive α-blockers (phenoxybenzamine 10 to 20 mg PO twice daily) for 10 to 14 days preoperatively.[90] Competitive α-antagonists (prazosin, labetalol) have not been as effective as phenoxybenzamine in controlling systemic blood pressure responses to massive release of catecholamines intraoperatively, as may occur with manipulation of the tumor. Presumably, irreversible alkylation of α-receptors by phenoxybenzamine, and not just competitive inhibition, is necessary to ensure that α-receptors do not respond to increased plasma concentrations of catecholamines caused by tumor manipulation.[81]

α-Adrenergic blockade attenuates or prevents catecholamine-induced vasoconstriction and may lead to decreased systemic blood pressure. Return to normotension facilitates an increase in intravascular fluid volume, as reflected by decreases in the hematocrit. Serial monitoring of the hematocrit is a useful method for evaluating the adequacy of intravascular fluid volume expansion, and satisfactory α-blockade is implied if the hematocrit decreases by about 5% (for example, from 45% to 40%). Normalization of intravascular fluid volume and systemic blood pressure produced by α-blockade before surgery also decreases the risk of intraoperative hypertension during manipulation of the tumor.

Persistence of tachycardia or cardiac dysrhythmias despite the presence of α-blockade is an indication for preoperative administration of drugs such as propranolol, 40 mg PO twice daily, to produce β-adrenergic blockade. The recommendation that β-blockade should not be instituted in the absence of α-blockade is based on the theoretical concern that a heart depressed by β-blockade might not be able to maintain an adequate cardiac output should unopposed α-mediated vasoconstriction from the release of catecholamines result in abrupt increases in systemic vascular resistance. In addition, administration of β-antagonists in the presence of a catecholamine-induced cardiomyopathy could precipitate congestive heart failure. Echocardiography may be useful for recognizing patients with suspected cardiomyopathy. Hyperglycemia is common preoperatively, although α-blockade facilitates the release of insulin and decreases the likelihood of hyperglycemia in patients with pheochromocytomas. The preoperative presence of hypercalcemia may indicate the presence of MEN that includes hyperparathyroidism (Table 22–22).[81, 83, 84]

Management of Anesthesia

Management of anesthesia for patients requiring excision of pheochromocytomas is based on administration of drugs that do not stimulate the sympathetic nervous system plus the use of invasive monitoring techniques to facilitate early and appropriate intervention when catecholamine-induced changes in cardiovascular function occur.[80, 81, 91–94] Continuation of α-antagonist therapy until the day of surgery is recommended. The argument that this treatment be discontinued preoperatively to unmask hypertensive responses during surgical palpation designed to locate the site of the tumor(s) is not necessary in view of the localizing accuracy of computed tomography. Furthermore, even with aggressive pharmacologically induced α-blockade, most patients show some degree of systemic blood pressure increase during surgical manipulation of the tumor. Concern that sustained α-blockade could contribute to refractory hypotension when vascular isolation of the tumor is accomplished has not been substantiated by clinical experience. β-Antagonist therapy should also be continued until the day of surgery. The times of significant intraoperative hazard to patients are (1) during tracheal intubation, (2) during manipulation of the tumor, and (3) after ligation of the tumor's venous drainage.

Clinical experience confirms that surgical excision of pheochromocytomas is often accompanied by varying degrees of intraoperative hemodynamic lability despite preoperative preparation with α- and β-adrenergic blocking drugs.[94] Nevertheless, there are few major perioperative complications, and mortality is rare. Identified risk factors for significant perioperative complications in these patients include large tumor size, prolonged surgery and anesthesia, and high preoperative levels of circulating catecholamines.[94]

Preoperative Medication

Preoperative medication is useful for decreasing the likelihood of anxiety-induced activation of the sympathetic nervous system. Administration of benzodiazepines, often with scopolamine, is a useful approach. Scopolamine is unlikely to produce an adverse heart rate change and greatly contributes to the sedative effect of preoperative medication. Morphine or other drugs that could release histamine and thus stimulate additional catecholamine release are avoided in these patients. If bilateral adrenalectomy is anticipated, supplemental cortisol treatment may be instituted at the same time as the preoperative medication.

Induction of Anesthesia

Placing a catheter in a peripheral artery to allow continuous monitoring of systemic blood pressure is useful before proceeding with induction of anesthesia. In the presence of adequate preoperative medication and local anesthesia, this invasive monitor can be placed without the risk of activating the sympathetic nervous system. Induction of anesthesia is most often accomplished with intravenous administration of a barbiturate, etomidate, or propofol. After the onset of unconsciousness, the depth of anesthesia should be increased by ventilating the lungs with nitrous oxide plus a volatile anesthetic. The choice of volatile anesthetics is based on the ability of these drugs to decrease sympathetic nervous system activity and their low likelihood of sensitizing the heart to the cardiac dysrhythmia effects of catecholamines. Although the most extensive clinical experience is with isoflurane, the ability to establish and change anesthetic concentrations rapidly with desflurane or sevoflurane is an attractive feature of these drugs for the management of anesthesia in patients with pheochromocytomas. The ability of rapid, large increases in the delivered concentration of desflurane to stimulate the sympathetic nervous system transiently should be considered when this drug is selected for management of anesthesia in these patients.

Mechanical ventilation of the patient's lungs is facilitated by producing skeletal muscle paralysis with nondepolarizing muscle relaxants deemed devoid of vagolytic or histamine-releasing effects. Pancuronium is an unlikely choice in view of its known cardiac effects, which could result in exaggerated systemic blood pressure increases in patients with pheochromocytomas. The use of succinylcholine has been questioned, as histamine release or compression of abdominal tumors by drug-induced skeletal muscle contractions (fasciculations) could provoke catecholamine release. Nevertheless, clinical experience has not supported a predictable adverse effect of this drug when administered to patients with pheochromocytomas.

Direct laryngoscopy for tracheal intubation is initiated only after establishing a surgical depth of anesthesia with volatile anesthetics (about 1.3 MAC). An adequate depth of anesthesia is necessary to minimize increases in systemic blood pressure associated with tracheal intubation. It may be helpful to administer lidocaine, 1 to 2 mg/kg IV, about 1 minute before initiating direct laryngoscopy, as this drug may attenuate the hypertensive response to tracheal intubation and decrease the likelihood of cardiac dysrhythmias. In addition, administration of short-acting opioids (fentanyl, sufentanil, remifentanil) just before initiating direct laryngoscopy may attenuate pressor responses. Nitroprusside or phentolamine must be readily available for administration should persistent hypertension accompany tracheal intubation. Nitroprusside, 1 to 2 μg/kg IV, as a rapid injection is effective for treating acute and persistent increases in systemic blood pressure. An alternative to nitroprusside is phentolamine, 1 to 5 mg IV, as intermittent injections.

Maintenance of Anesthesia

Anesthesia is often maintained with nitrous oxide plus volatile anesthetics such as isoflurane, desflurane, or sevoflurane. Delivered concentrations of volatile anesthetics are adjusted in response to changes in systemic blood pressure. Maintenance of anesthesia with nitrous oxide and opioids is an unlikely approach, as these drugs do not suppress hypertensive responses owing to catecholamine release. In addition, the ability to decrease the depth of anesthesia in the presence of persistent hypotension is not easily achieved when injected drugs are used for maintenance of anesthesia. Droperidol is not recommended in view of reports of systemic hypertension following its administration to patients with pheochromocytomas.[95] It is possible that droperidol may antagonize presynaptic dopaminergic receptors that normally inhibit the release of catecholamines, encouraging their release.

A continuous intravenous infusion of nitroprusside is necessary if systemic hypertension persists despite delivery of maximal concentrations of volatile anesthetic drugs (about 1.5 to 2.0 MAC). Reflex tachycardia accompanying nitroprusside-induced peripheral vasodilation is treated with continuous intravenous infusions of esmolol.[96,97] A β-adrenergic antagonist must be used cautiously in the presence of catecholamine-induced cardiomyopathy, as even minimal β-blockade can accentuate left ventricular dysfunction. Cardiac dysrhythmias are initially treated with lidocaine. Decreases in systemic blood pressure may accompany the prompt decreases in circulating concentrations of catecholamines that occur during ligation of the veins draining the pheochromocytoma. These decreases in systemic blood pressure are treated by decreasing the delivered concentration of volatile anesthetic as well as the

rapid intravenous infusion of crystalloids and/or colloids. Rarely, a continuous intravenous infusion of phenylephrine or norepinephrine is required until systemic vascular resistance can adapt to the decreased levels of endogenous α-adrenergic stimulation. Although experience is limited, there is no evidence to suggest avoidance of reversing the nondepolarizing neuromuscular blockade with anticholinesterase drugs plus anticholinergic drugs after excising a pheochromocytoma.

Monitoring

A pulmonary artery catheter is useful for monitoring the status of intravascular fluid volume in patients with pheochromocytomas, especially in the presence of catecholamine-induced cardiomyopathy.[98] In addition, the ability to measure cardiac output by thermodilution is helpful for evaluating cardiac function and the need for intervention with inotropic or vasodilator drugs. A central venous pressure catheter is an alternative to a pulmonary artery catheter, recognizing that left ventricular dysfunction might not be appreciated from this measurement, and thermodilution measurement of cardiac output is not possible. Transesophageal echocardiography provides much of the same information that is available from pulmonary artery catheter monitoring and may be viewed as a less invasive monitor. Monitoring arterial blood gases and pH, blood glucose concentrations, and electrolytes is recommended. Hyperglycemia is common before excising pheochromocytomas, whereas hypoglycemia may occur within minutes of the tumor removal as the α-adrenergic induced suppression of insulin release wanes.[99]

Postoperative Management

Invasive monitoring is continued during the postoperative period, as increases or decreases in systemic blood pressure are possible. Persistent hypotension that may be refractory to intravascular fluid volume replacement is the principal postoperative complication. It is tempting to ascribe postoperative hypotension to persistent effects of preoperative α-adrenergic blockade. However, it is more likely that hypotension reflects preoperative down-regulation of adrenergic receptors in the presence of excessive catecholamine secretion.[82] Conversely, a substantial number of patients remain hypertensive during the postoperative period despite removal of the pheochromocytoma. A high index of suspicion for hypoglycemia is maintained. Relief of postoperative pain (neuraxial opioids) may contribute to early tracheal extubation in these often young and otherwise healthy patients.

Regional Anesthesia

Regional anesthesia for excision of pheochromocytomas has been utilized successfully.[81] Despite the ability of this anesthetic technique to block the sympathetic nervous system, the postsynaptic α-adrenergic receptors can still respond to direct effects of sudden increases in the circulating concentrations of catecholamines. A specific disadvantage of a regional anesthetic is the absence of sympathetic nervous system activity if hypotension accompanies vascular isolation of the pheochromocytoma. In addition, the ability of awake or sedated patients to maintain adequate spontaneous alveolar ventilation may be impaired during intra-abdominal manipulation and retraction. Regional anesthesia is practical only if the surgical procedure is performed in the supine position.

▌ DYSFUNCTION OF THE TESTES OR OVARIES

The principal hormone secreted by the testes is testosterone, whereas the principal hormone secreted by the ovaries is progesterone. In adults, testosterone is responsible for spermatogenesis; and a metabolite, dihydrotestosterone, is responsible for external virilization. Ovulation and normal menses depend on the presence of ovarian hormones.

Klinefelter Syndrome

Klinefelter syndrome is the most common expression of testicular dysfunction, manifested as aspermatogenesis, decreased plasma testosterone concentrations, and testicular atrophy. The buccal smear for the Barr body (chromatin lumps) indicates an XXY chromosomal defect, which is diagnostic of the syndrome. Systemic effects of male hypogonadism include anemia, osteoporosis, fatigue, and skeletal muscle weakness.

Physiologic Menopause

Increases in human longevity means that many women live one-third or more of their lives without natural estrogen or progesterone. Menopause is almost complete cessation of estrogen production, accompanied by amenorrhea, which occurs at an average age of 51 years. The absence of estrogen has short-range (hot flashes), medium-range (vaginal atrophy), and long-range (osteoporosis) manifestations that can be relieved by exogenous estrogen replacement. The most significant medical consequence of menopause is osteoporosis and the risk of skeletal fractures, often involving the spine and hips. Normally, estrogen maintains the balance between bone formation and resorption; in the absence of estrogen, this balance is shifted toward bone resorption.

Premenstrual Syndrome

The abdominal discomfort (cramps) accompanying the ovulatory cycle probably reflects the effect of prostaglandins, accounting for the effectiveness of nonsteroidal antiinflammatory drugs in relieving pain. Premenstrual syndrome is a constellation of symptoms that appear the week before menstruation. There is no uniquely diagnostic physical finding or laboratory test, and treatment is symptomatic (analgesics, diuretics).

Ovarian Hyperstimulation Syndrome

Exogenous gonadotropin stimulation in association with ovulation induction for in vitro fertilization may be followed within 3 to 10 days by severe ovarian hyperstimulation, manifesting as ascites, pleural effusion, oliguria, hemoconcentration, electrolyte abnormalities, hypercoagulability, and hypotension. It is speculated that the production of prostaglandins by the ovarian follicle, as well as an alteration in the renin-angiotensin system, results in increased capillary permeability. This change allows edema formation (ascites) and fluid translocation (hypovolemia, oliguria). Hemoconcentration predisposes to increased blood viscosity and thromboembolic phenomena. Capillary leak has been associated with the development of acute respiratory distress syndrome; and liver dysfunction has been noted. The estimate that 0.4% to 4.0% of treatment cycles are associated with the development of severe ovarian hyperstimulation syndrome introduces the possibility that these patients could require anesthesia for termination of pregnancy or laparotomy.

The management of anesthesia in patients with severe ovarian hyperstimulation syndrome is influenced by the presence of hypovolemia and the impact of ascites on spontaneous ventilation.[100] The presence of ascites and the frequent presence of nausea and vomiting suggest the need to protect the patient's airway with a cuffed tracheal tube. Ketamine may be useful for induction and maintenance of anesthesia. Monitoring potentially rapid fluid fluxes may be facilitated by measuring cardiac filling pressures, especially if the planned surgery is extensive.

Turner Syndrome

Turner syndrome (gonadal dysgenesis) is due to the absence of a second X chromosome and is the most common sex chromosome abnormality in females, affecting an estimated 3% of all females conceived.[101] Manifestations of the syndrome include primary amenorrhea, genital immaturity, and short stature. Additional associated features that may influence the management of anesthesia include systemic hypertension, short neck, high palate, micrognathia, the occasional presence of aortic stenosis or coarctation of the aorta, pectus excavatum, and an absent kidney. Intelligence is usually normal.

Noonan Syndrome

Noonan syndrome (female pseudo-Turner syndrome) resembles Turner syndrome with respect to short stature, webbed neck, and facial characteristics. In contrast to Turner syndrome, Noonan syndrome is associated with mental retardation, right-sided cardiac lesions (pulmonic stenosis), and normal chromosomes. Noonan syndrome occurs in both genders. Males often have cryptorchidism and are rarely fertile, whereas females have normal fertility and anesthesia may be needed for delivery.

Potential anesthesia problems in patients with Noonan syndrome include difficult airway management and technical problems when performing regional anesthesia related to short stature and associated skeletal anomalies (lumbar lordosis, kyphoscoliosis, narrow spinal canal).[102–104] Clotting and platelet abnormalities may influence the selection of regional anesthetic techniques. Decreases in functional residual capacity produced by pregnancy are further exaggerated by the pectus deformity and kyphoscoliosis that are commonly present. Arterial hypoxemia may occur rapidly in view of the decreased functional residual capacity. Cardiac evaluation is indicated; and if echocardiography demonstrates pulmonic stenosis, it is important to consider the possible detrimental effects of excessive intravenous fluid administration, such as before regional anesthesia. Conversely, if patients are not adequately hydrated before spinal or epidural anesthesia, the hypotension that may result from sympathetic nervous system blockade can produce undesirable decreases in right ventricular stroke volume.

Many of the facial features of Noonan syndrome suggest the possibility of difficult airway management.[103] For example, the typical flattened mid-face and wide nasal base, high arched palate, micrognathia, and dental malocclusion combined with a webbed, sometimes fused neck may make conventional direct laryngoscopy difficult. These facial abnormalities usually become less marked with age and are not features of Turner syndrome. Other associated features with anesthetic implications include renal dysfunction and hepatosplenomegaly.

Stein-Leventhal Syndrome

Stein-Leventhal syndrome (polycystic ovary syndrome) accounts for up to 10% of the cases of primary amenorrhea. Ultrasonography is useful for recognizing ovarian enlargement. There is increased production of androgens, with hirsutism and increased muscularity. Height is usually normal, and congenital defects are unlikely. In the past, wedge resection of the ovary was used to improve the fertility of these patients. This disorder is currently treated with the antiestrogen drug clomiphene, which stimulates ovulation. Treatment of hirsutism includes suppression of androgen excess with prednisone. Long intervals of anovulation can be associated with the development of endometrial carcinoma, perhaps reflecting continuous exposure of the endometrium to estrogen unopposed by progesterone.

■ PITUITARY GLAND DYSFUNCTION

The pituitary gland, located in the sella turcica at the base of the brain, consists of the anterior pituitary and posterior pituitary. The anterior pituitary secretes six hormones under control of the hypothalamus (Table 22–23).[105] In this regard, the hypothalamus controls the function of the anterior pituitary by means of vascular connections (hormones travel via the hypophyseal portal veins to reach the anterior pituitary). The hypothalamic-anterior pituitary-target organ axis is comprised of tightly coordinated systems in which hormonal signals from the hypothalamus stimulate or inhibit secretion of anterior pituitary hormones, which in turn act on target organs and modulate hypothalamic and anterior pituitary activity ("closed loop or negative feedback system"). The posterior pituitary is composed of terminal neuron endings that originate in the hypothalamus. Vasopressin (antidiuretic hormone) and

Table 22–23 • Hypothalamic and Related Pituitary Hormones

Hypothalamic Hormone	Action	Pituitary Hormone or Organ Affected	Action
Corticotropin-releasing hormone	Stimulatory	Corticotropin	Stimulates secretion of cortisol Stimulates secretion of androgens
Thyrotropin-releasing hormone	Stimulatory	Thyrotropin	Stimulates secretion of thyroxine Stimulates secretion of triiodothyronine
Gonadotropin-releasing hormone	Stimulatory	Follicle-stimulating hormone Luteinizing hormone	Stimulates estradiol secretion* Stimulates progesterone secretion* Stimulates ovulation* Stimulates testosterone secretion† Stimulates spermatogenesis†
Growth hormone-releasing hormone	Stimulatory	Growth hormone	Stimulates production of insulin-like growth factor
Dopamine	Inhibitory	Prolactin	Stimulates lactation*
Somatostatin	Inhibitory	Growth hormone	
Vasopressin (antidiuretic hormone)	Stimulatory	Kidneys	Stimulates free-water reabsorption
Oxytocin	Stimulatory	Uterus	Stimulates uterine contractions*
		Breasts	Stimulates milk ejection*

* Actions in females.
† Actions in males.
Adapted from Vance ML. Hypopituitarism. N Engl J Med 1994;330:1651–62.

oxytocin are synthesized in the hypothalamus and are subsequently transported along the hypothalamic neuronal axons for storage in the posterior pituitary. Stimulus for the release of these hormones from the posterior pituitary arises from osmoreceptors in the hypothalamus that sense plasma osmolarity.

Overproduction of anterior pituitary hormones is most often reflected by hypersecretion of corticotropin (Cushing syndrome) by anterior pituitary adenomas (see "Hypercortisolism"). Hypersecretion of other tropic hormones rarely occurs. Underproduction of a single anterior pituitary hormone is less common than generalized pituitary hypofunction (panhypopituitarism).[105] The anterior pituitary gland is the only endocrine gland in which a tumor, most often a chromophobe adenoma, causes destruction by compressing the gland against the bony confines of the sella turcica. Metastatic tumor, most often from the breast or lung, also occasionally produces pituitary hypofunction. Endocrine features of panhypopituitarism are highly variable and depend on the rate at which the deficiency develops and the patient's age. For example, gonadotropin deficiency (amenorrhea, impotence) is typically the first manifestation of global pituitary dysfunction. Hypocortisolism occurs 4 to 14 days after hypophysectomy, whereas hypothyroidism is not likely to manifest before 4 weeks. Computed tomography and magnetic resonance imaging are useful for radiologic assessment of the pituitary gland.

Acromegaly

Acromegaly is due to excessive secretion of growth hormone in adults, most often by an adenoma in the anterior pituitary gland. Failure of plasma growth hormone concentrations to decrease 1 to 2 hours after ingestion of 75 to 100 g of glucose is presumptive evidence of acromegaly, as are growth hormone concentrations higher than 3 ng/ml. A skull radiograph and computed tomography are useful for detecting enlargement of the sella turcica, which is characteristic of anterior pituitary adenomas.

Signs and Symptoms

Manifestations of acromegaly reflect parasellar extension of the anterior pituitary adenomas and peripheral effects produced by the presence of excess growth hormone (Table 22–24). Headache and papilledema reflect increased intracranial pressure due to expansion of the anterior pituitary adenoma. Visual disturbances are due to compression of the optic chiasm by the expanding overgrowth of surrounding tissues. Overgrowth of soft tissues of the upper airway (enlargement of the tongue and epiglottis) and increased length of the mandible may make upper airway management difficult.[106–108] Polypoid masses reflect overgrowth of pharyngeal tissues, making the patient's upper airway susceptible to obstruction. Hoarseness and abnormal movement of the vocal cords or paralysis of a recurrent laryn-

Table 22–24 • Manifestations of Acromegaly

Parasellar
  Enlarged sella turcica
  Headache
  Visual field defects
  Rhinorrhea
Excess growth hormone
  Skeletal overgrowth (prognathism)
  Soft tissue overgrowth (lips, tongue, epiglottis, vocal cords)
  Connective tissue overgrowth (recurrent laryngeal nerve paralysis)
  Peripheral neuropathy (carpal tunnel syndrome)
  Visceromegaly
  Glucose intolerance
  Osteoarthritis
  Osteoporosis
  Hyperhydrosis
  Skeletal muscle weakness

geal nerve may be due to stretching by overgrowth of the cartilaginous structures. In addition, involvement of the cricoarytenoid joints can result in alterations in the patient's voice due to impaired movement of the vocal cords. The subglottic diameter may be decreased in acromegalic patients. Stridor or a history of dyspnea is suggestive of acromegalic involvement of the upper airway.

Peripheral neuropathy is common and likely reflects trapping of nerves by skeletal, connective, and soft tissue overgrowth. Flow through the ulnar artery may be compromised in patients exhibiting symptoms of carpal tunnel syndrome. Even in the absence of such symptoms, about one-half of patients with acromegaly have inadequate collateral blood flow through the ulnar artery in one or both hands. Glucose intolerance and, on occasion, diabetes mellitus requiring treatment with insulin reflects the effects of growth hormone on carbohydrate metabolism. The incidence of systemic hypertension, ischemic heart disease, osteoarthritis, and osteoporosis seems to be increased. Lung volumes are increased, and ventilation-to-perfusion mismatching may be increased. The patient's skin becomes thick and oily, skeletal muscle weakness may be prominent, and complaints of fatigue are common.

Treatment

Transsphenoidal surgical excision of pituitary adenomas is the preferred initial therapy.[109] When adenomas have extended beyond the sella turcica, surgery or radiation is no longer feasible; medical treatment with suppressant drugs (bromocriptine) may be an option.

Management of Anesthesia

Management of anesthesia for patients with acromegaly is complicated by changes induced by excessive secretion of growth hormone (Table 22–24). Particularly important are changes in the upper airway.[107–110] Distorted facial anatomy may interfere with placing an anesthesia face mask. Enlargement of the tongue and epiglottis predisposes to upper airway obstruction and interferes with visualization of the vocal cords by direct laryngoscopy. The distance between the lips and vocal cords is increased by overgrowth of the mandible. The glottic opening may be narrowed, owing to enlargement of the vocal cords, which combined with subglottic narrowing may necessitate use of a smaller internal diameter tracheal tube than would have been predicted on the basis of the patient's age and size. Nasal turbinate enlargement may preclude the passage of nasopharyngeal or nasotracheal airways. The preoperative history of dyspnea on exertion or the presence of hoarseness or stridor suggests involvement of the larynx by acromegaly. In this instance, indirect laryngoscopy may be indicated to quantitate the extent of vocal cord dysfunction. When difficulty placing a tracheal tube is anticipated, it may be prudent to consider an awake fiberoptic tracheal intubation. Indeed, the incidence of difficult laryngoscopy and tracheal intubation has been reported to be increased in acromegalic patients.[110, 111] Anticipation of the possible need to insert a smaller-diameter tracheal tube and minimizing the mechanical trauma to the upper airway and vocal cords are important considerations, as additional edema can result in airway obstruction after the tracheal tube is removed.

When placing a catheter in the radial artery it is important to consider the possibility of inadequate collateral circulation at the wrist.[112] Monitoring blood glucose concentrations is useful if diabetes mellitus or glucose intolerance accompanies acromegaly. Doses of nondepolarizing muscle relaxants are guided by the use of a peripheral nerve stimulator, particularly if skeletal muscle weakness exists before anesthesia induction. Skeletal changes that accompany acromegaly may make performance of regional anesthesia technically difficult or unreliable. There is no evidence that hemodynamic instability or alterations in pulmonary gas exchange accompany anesthesia in acromegalic patients.[110]

Diabetes Insipidus

Diabetes insipidus reflects the absence of vasopressin (antidiuretic hormone, ADH) owing to destruction of the posterior pituitary (neurogenic diabetes insipidus) or failure of renal tubules to respond to ADH (nephrogenic diabetes insipidus). Neurogenic and nephrogenic diabetes insipidus are differentiated on the basis of the response to desmopressin, which concentrates urine in the presence of neurogenic, but not nephrogenic, diabetes insipidus. Classic manifestations of diabetes insipidus are polydipsia and a high output of poorly concentrated urine despite increased serum osmolarity. Diabetes insipidus that develops during or immediately after pituitary gland surgery is generally due to reversible trauma to the posterior pituitary and is therefore transient.

Initial treatment of diabetes insipidus consists of intravenous infusion of electrolyte solutions if oral intake cannot offset polyuria. Chlorpropamide, an oral hypoglycemic drug, potentiates the effects of ADH on renal tubules and may be useful for treating nephrogenic diabetes insipidus. Treatment of neurogenic diabetes insipidus is with ADH administered intramuscularly every 2 to 4 days or by intranasal administration of DDAVP (desmopressin).

Management of anesthesia for patients with diabetes insipidus includes monitoring the urine output and serum electrolyte concentrations during the perioperative period.

Inappropriate Secretion of Antidiuretic Hormone

Inappropriate secretion of ADH can occur in the presence of diverse pathologic processes, including intracranial tumors, hypothyroidism, porphyria, and carcinoma of the lung, particularly undifferentiated small cell carcinoma. Inappropriate secretion of ADH is alleged to occur in most patients following major surgery. Inappropriately increased urinary sodium concentrations and osmolarity in the presence of hyponatremia and decreased serum osmolarity are highly suggestive of inappropriate ADH secretion. Hyponatremia is due to dilution, reflecting expansion of the intravascular fluid volume secondary to hormone-induced resorption of water by renal tubules. Abrupt decreases in serum sodium concentrations, especially less than 110 mEq/L, can result in cerebral edema and seizures.

Treatment of inappropriate secretion of ADH consists of restricted oral fluid intake (about 500 ml daily), antagonism of the effects of ADH on the renal tubules by administration of demeclocycline, and intravenous infusions of sodium chloride. Often restriction of oral fluid intake is sufficient treatment for inappropriate secretion of ADH not associated with symptoms secondary to hyponatremia. Restric-

tion of oral fluid intake and administration of demeclocycline, however, are not immediately effective in the management of patients manifesting acute neurologic symptoms due to hyponatremia. In these patients, intravenous infusions of hypertonic saline sufficient to increase serum sodium concentrations 0.5 mEq/L/hr are recommended. Overly rapid correction of chronic hyponatremia has been associated with a fatal neurologic disorder known as central pontine myelinolysis.[113]

References

1. Nathan DM. Diabetes mellitus. Sci Am Med 1997;1–24
2. Kjos SL, Buchanan TA. Gestational diabetes mellitus. N Engl J Med 1999;341:1749–56
3. Diabetes Control and Complications Trial Research Group. The effect of intensive treatment of diabetes in the development and progression of long-term complications in insulin-dependent diabetes mellitus. N Engl J Med 1993;329:977–86
4. Luzi L. Pancreas transplantation and diabetic complications. N Engl J Med 1998;339:115–7
5. Misbin RI, Green L, Stadel BV, et al. Lactic acidosis in patients with diabetes treated with metformin. N Engl J Med 1998;338:265–6
6. Mercker SK, Maier C, Doz P, et al. Lactic acidosis as a serious perioperative complication of antidiabetic biguanide medication with metformin. Anesthesiology 1997;87:1003–5
7. McAnulty GR, Robertshaw HJ, Hall GM. Anaesthetic management of patients with diabetes mellitus. Br J Anaesth 2000;85:80–90
8. Meigs JOB, Mittleman MA, Nathan DM, et al. Hyperinsulinemia, hyperglycemia, and impaired hemostasis: the Farmingham offspring study. JAMA 2000;283:221–8
9. Mordes D, Kreutner K, Metzger W, et al. Dangers of intravenous ritodrine in diabetic patients. JAMA 1982;248:973–5
10. Nathan DM. Hypoglycemia. Sci Am Med 1996;1–8
11. Ditser M, Camu F. Glucose homeostasis and insulin secretion during isoflurane anesthesia in humans. Anesthesiology 1988;68:860–8
12. Ferris FL, Davis MD, Aiello LM. Treatment of diabetic retinopathy. N Engl J Med 1999;341:667–78
13. Clark CM, Lee DA. Prevention and treatment of the complications of diabetes mellitus. N Engl J Med 1995;332:1210–7.
14. Partanen J, Niskanen L, Lehtinen J, et al. Natural history of peripheral neuropathy in patients with non-insulin dependent diabetes mellitus. N Engl J Med 1995;333:89–94
15. Warner MA, Warner ME, Martin JT. Ulnar neuropathy: incidence, outcome, and risk factors in sedated or anesthetized patients. Anesthesiology 1994;81:1332–40
16. Warner MA, Martin JT, Schroeder DR, et al. Lower extremity motor neuropathy associated with surgery performed on patients in a lithotomy position. Anesthesiology 1994;81:6–12
17. Watkins PJ. Diabetic autonomic neuropathy. N Engl J Med 1990;322:1078–9
18. Stoelting RK. Unique considerations in the anesthetic management of patients with diabetes mellitus. Curr Opin Anesth 1996;9:245–6
19. Kitamura A, Hoshino T, Kon T, et al. Patients with diabetic neuropathy are at risk of a greater intraoperative reduction in core temperature. Anesthesiology 2000;92:1311–8

20. Tsueda K, Huang KC, Diamond SW, et al. Cardiac sympathetic tone in anaesthetized diabetics. Can J Anaesth 1991; 38:20–3

21. O'Sullivan JJ, Conroy RM, Macdonald K, et al. Silent ischaemia in diabetic men with autonomic neuropathy. Br Heart J 1991;66:313–5

22. Ewing DJ, Campbell IW, Clarke BP. Assessment of cardiovascular effects of diabetic autonomic neuropathy and prognostic implications. Ann Intern Med 1980;92:308–11

23. Ciccarelli LO, Ford CM, Tsueda K. Autonomic neuropathy in a diabetic patient with renal failure. Anesthesiology 1986;64:283–7

24. Page MM, Watkins PJ. Cardiorespiratory arrest and diabetic autonomic neuropathy. Lancet 1978;1:14–6

25. Sampson MJ. Progression of diabetic autonomic neuropathy over a decade in insulin-dependent diabetics. Q J Med 1990;278:635–46

26. Lucas LF, Tsueda K. Cardiovascular depression after brachial plexus block in two diabetic patients with renal failure. Anesthesiology 1990;73:1032–5

27. Charlson ME, MacKanzie C, Gold JP. Preoperative autonomic function abnormalities in patients with diabetes mellitus and patients with hypertension. J Am Coll Surg 1994; 179:1–10

28. Wright RA, Clemente R, Wathen R. Diabetic gastroparesis: an abnormality of gastric emptying of solids. Am J Med Sci 1985;289:240–2

29. Reissell E, Orko R, Maunuksela E-L, et al. Predictability of difficult laryngoscopy in patients with long-term diabetes mellitus. Anaesthesia 1990;43:1024–7

30. Warner ME, Contreras MG, Warner MA, et al. Diabetes mellitus and difficult laryngoscopy in renal pancreatic transplant patients. Anesth Analg 1998;86:516–9

31. Eastwood DW. Anterior spinal artery syndrome after epidural anesthesia in a pregnant diabetic patient with scleredema. Anesth Analg 1991;73:90–1

32. Hirsch IB, Magill JOB, Cryer EG, et al. Perioperative management of surgical patients with diabetes mellitus. Anesthesiology 1991;74:346–59

33. Nathan DM. Long-term complications of diabetes mellitus. N Engl J Med 1993;328:1676–85

34. Burgos LUG, Bert TJ, Asiddao C, et al. Increased intraoperative cardiovascular morbidity in diabetics with autonomic neuropathy. Anesthesiology 1989;70:591–7

35. Alberti KG. Diabetes and surgery. Anesthesiology 1991;74:209–11

36. Milaskiewicz RM, Hall GM. Diabetes and anaesthesia: the past decade. Br J Anaesth 1992;68:198–206

37. Hall GM. Insulin administration in diabetic patients: return of the bolus? Br J Anaesth 1994;72:1–2

38. Kostopanagiotou G, Smyrniotis V, Arkadopoulos N, et al. Anesthetic and perioperative management of adult transplant recipients in nontransplant surgery. Anesth Analg 1999;89:613–22

39. Service JF. Hypoglycemic disorders. N Engl J Med 1995; 332:1144–52

40. Jacobs J, Vallejo R, DeSouza GO, et al. Severe hypoglycemia after labor epidural analgesia. Anesth Analg 2000;90:892–3

41. Muier JJ, Endres SM, Offord K, et al. Glucose management in patients undergoing operation for insulinoma removal. Anesthesiology 1983;59:371–5

42. Bennett-Guerrero E, Kramer DC, Schwinn DA. Effect of chronic and acute thyroid hormone reduction on perioperative outcome. Anesth Analg 1997;85:30–6

43. Farling PA. Thyroid disease. Br J Anaesth 2000;85:15–28

44. Franklyn JA. The management of hyperthyroidism. N Engl J Med 1994;330:1731–9

45. Weetman AP. Graves' disease. N Engl J Med 2000;343: 1236–48

46. Ikeda S, Schweiss FJ. Excessive blood loss during operation in the patient treated with propylthiouracil. Can Anaesth Soc J 1982;29:477–80

47. Hamilton WFD, Forrest AL, Gun A, et al. Beta-adrenoreceptor blockade and anesthesia for thyroidectomy. Anaesthesia 1984;39:335–42

48. Thorne AC, Bedford RF. Esmolol for perioperative management of thyrotoxic goiter. Anesthesiology 1989;71:291–4

49. Lee TC, Coffey BJ, Curvier BM, et al. Propranolol and thyroidectomy in the treatment of thyrotoxicosis. Ann Surg 1982;195:766–71

50. Peters KR, Nance P, Wingard DW. Malignant hyperthyroidism or malignant hyperthermia? Anesth Analg 1981;60: 613–5

51. Ambus T, Evans S, Smith NT. Thyrotoxicosis factitia in the anesthetized patient. Anesthesiology 1994;81:254–6

52. Redahan C, Karski JM. Thyrotoxicosis factitia in a post-aortocoronary bypass patient. Can J Anaesth 1994;41:969–72

53. Halpern SH. Anaesthesia for caesarean section in patients with uncontrolled hyperthyroidism. Can J Anaesth 1989; 36:454–9

54. Kaplan JA, Cooperman LH. Alarming reactions to ketamine in patients taking thyroid medication: treatment with propranolol. Anesthesiology 1971;35:229–30

55. Berman ML, Kuhnert L, Phythyon JM, et al. Isoflurane and enflurane-induced hepatic necrosis in triiodothyronine-pretreated rats. Anesthesiology 1983;58:1–5

56. Seino H, Dohi S, Aiyoshi Y, et al. Postoperative hepatic dysfunction after halothane or enflurane anesthesia in patients with hyperthyroidism. Anesthesiology 1986;64:122–5

57. Babad AA, Eger EI. The effects of hyperthyroidism and hypothyroidism on halothane and oxygen requirements in dogs. Anesthesiology 1969;29:1087–93

58. Cooper DS. Subclinical hypothyroidism. JAMA 1987;258: 246–7

59. Bennett-Guerrero E, Kramer DC, Schwinn DA. Effect of chronic and acute thyroid hormone reduction on perioperative outcome. Anesth Analg 1997;85:30–6

60. Murkin JM. Anesthesia and hypothyroidism: a review of thyroxine physiology, pharmacology, and anesthetic implications. Anesth Analg 1982;61:371–83

61. Levelle JP, Jopling MW, Sklar GS. Perioperative hypothyroidism: an unusual postanesthetic diagnosis. Anesthesiology 1985;63:195–7

62. Mogensen T, Hjortso N-C. Acute hypothyroidism in a severely ill surgical patient. Can J Anaesth 1988;35:74–5

63. Weinberg AD, Brennan MD, Gorman CA, et al. Outcome of anesthesia and surgery in hypothyroid patients. Arch Intern Med 1983;143:893–7

64. Mihai R, Farndon JR. Parathyroid disease and calcium metabolism. Br J Anaesth 2000;85:29–43

65. Heath DA. Hypercalcemia in malignancy: fluids and bisphosphonate are best when life is threatened. BMJ 1989;298: 1468–9

66. Al-Mohaya S, Naguib M, Abdelaif M, et al. Abnormal responses to muscle relaxants in a patient with primary hyperparathyroidism. Anesthesiology 1986;65:554–6

67. Roland EJL, Wierda JMKH, Turin BY, et al. Pharmacodynamic behavior of vecuronium in primary hyperparathyroidism. Can J Anaesth 1994;41:694–8

68. Drop LJ, Cullen DJ. Comparative effects of calcium chloride and calcium gluceptate. Br J Anaesth 1980;52:501–5

69. Orth DN. Cushing's syndrome. N Engl J Med 1995;332: 791–803

70. Weatherill D, Spence AA. Anaesthesia and disorders of the adrenal cortex. Br J Anaesth 1984;56:741–7

71. Aono J, Maniya K, Udea W. Abrupt onset of adrenal crisis during routine preoperative examination in a patient with unknown Addison's disease. Anesthesiology 1999;90: 313–4

72. Salem M, Tinsh RE, Bromberg J, et al. Perioperative glucocorticoid coverage: a reassessment 42 years after emergence of a problem. Ann Surg 1994;219:416–25

73. Kehlet H. A rational approach to dosage and preparation of parenteral glucocorticoid substitution therapy during surgical procedures. Acta Anaesthesiol Scand 1975;19:260–4

74. Knudsen L, Christiansen LA, Lorentzen JE. Hypotension during and after operation in glucocorticoid-treated patients. Br J Anaesth 1981;53:295–301

75. Udelsman R, Ramp J, Gallucci WT, et al. Adaptation during surgical stress: a reevaluation of the role of glucocorticoids. J Clin Invest 1986;77:1377–81

76. Symreng T, Karlberg BE, Kagedal B, et al. Physiological cortisol substitution of long-term steroid-treated patients undergoing major surgery. Br J Anaesth 1981;53:949–53

77. Ganguly A. Primary aldosteronism. N Engl J Med 1998; 339;1828–34

78. Gangat Y, Triner L, Baer L, et al. Primary aldosteronism with uncommon complications. Anesthesiology 1976;45: 542–4

79. Holland OB. Hypoaldosteronism: disease or normal response. N Engl J Med 1991;324:488–9

80. Hull CJ. Phaeochromocytoma: diagnosis, preoperative preparation and anaesthetic management. Br J Anaesth 1986;58:1453–8

81. Pullerits J, Ein S, Balfe JW. Anaesthesia for phaeochromocytoma. Can J Anaesth 1988;35:526–34

82. Prys-Roberts C. Phaeochromocytoma: recent progress in its management. Br J Anaesth 2000;85:44–57

83. Thomas JL, Bernardino ME. Pheochromocytoma in multiple endocrine adenomatosis. JAMA 1981;245:1467–9

84. Neumann HPH, Berger DP, Sigmund G, et al. Pheochromocytomas, multiple endocrine neoplasia type 2, and von Hippel-Lindau disease. N Engl J Med 1993;329:1531–8

85. Kirkendahl WM, Leighty RD, Culp DA. Diagnosis and treatment of patients with pheochromocytoma. Arch Intern Med 1965;115:529–36

86. Allen GC, Rosenberg H. Phaeochromocytoma presenting as acute malignant hyperthermia: a diagnostic challenge. Can J Anaesth 1990;37:593–5

87. Duncan MW, Compton P, Lazarus L, et al. Measurement of norepinephrine and 3,4-dihydroxyphenylglycol in urine and plasma for the diagnosis of pheochromocytoma. N Engl J Med 1988;319:136–42

88. Bravo EL, Giford RW. Pheochromocytoma: diagnosis, localization, and management. N Engl J Med 1984;311:1298–1303

89. Bravo E, Fouad-Tarazi R, Rossi G, et al. A reevaluation of the hemodynamics of pheochromocytoma. Hypertension 1990;15:128–31

90. Witteles RM, Kaplan EL, Roizen MF. Safe and cost-effective preoperative preparation of patients with pheochromocytoma. Anesth Analg 2000;91:302–4

91. Hamilton A, Sirrs S, Schmidt N, et al. Anaesthesia for phaeochromocytoma in pregnancy. Can J Anaesth 1997;44: 654–7

92. Mugawar M, Rajender Y, Purohit AK, et al. Anesthetic management of von Hippel-Lindau syndrome for excision of cerebellar hemangioblastoma and pheochromocytoma surgery. Anesth Analg 1998;86:673–4

93. Baillargeon J-P, Pek B, Teijeira J, et al. Combined surgery for coronary artery disease and pheochromocytoma. Can J Anesth 2000;47:647–52

94. Kinney MAO, Warner ME, vanHeerden JA, et al. Preanesthetic risks and outcomes of pheochromocytoma and paraganglioma resection. Anesth Analg 2000;91:1118–23

95. Bitter DA. Innovar-induced hypertensive crises in patients with pheochromocytoma. Anesthesiology 1979;50:366–9

96. Nicholas E, Deutschman CS, Allo M, et al. Use of esmolol in the intraoperative management of pheochromocytoma. Anesth Analg 1988;67:1114–7

97. Zakowski M, Kaufman B, Berguson P, et al. Esmolol use during resection of pheochromocytoma: report of three cases. Anesthesiology 1989;70:875–7

98. Mihm PG. Pulmonary artery pressure monitoring in patients with pheochromocytoma. Anesth Analg 1983;62: 1129–33

99. Levin H, Heefetz M. Phaeochromocytoma and severe protracted postoperative hypoglycaemia. Can J Anaesth 1990;37:477–8

100. Reed AP, Tausk H, Reynolds H. Anesthetic considerations for severe ovarian hyperstimulation syndrome. Anesthesiology 1990;73:1275–7

101. Saenger P. Turner's syndrome. N Engl J Med 1996;335: 1749–55

102. Dadabhoy ZP, Winnie AP. Regional anesthesia for cesarean section in a parturient with Noonan's syndrome. Anesthesiology 1988;68:636–8

103. McLure HA, Yentis SM. General anaesthesia for caesarean section in a parturient with Noonan's syndrome. Br J Anaesth 1996;77:665–8

104. Grange CS, Heid R, Lucas B, et al. Anaesthesia in a parturient with Noonan's syndrome. Can J Anaesth 1998;45:332–6

105. Vance ML. Hypopituitarism. N Engl J Med 1994;330:1651–62

106. Kitahata LM. Airway difficulties associated with anaesthesia in acromegaly. Br J Anaesth 1971;43:1187–90

107. Hassan SZ, Matz G, Lawrence AM, et al. Laryngeal stenosis in acromegaly. Anesth Analg 1976;55:57–60

108. Southwick JP, Katz J. Unusual airway difficulty in the acromegalic patient: indications for tracheostomy. Anesthesiology 1979;51:72–3

109. Melmed S. Acromegaly. N Engl J Med 1990;322:966–75

110. Seidman PA, Kofke WA, Policare R, et al. Anaesthetic complications of acromegaly. Br J Anaesth 2000;84:179–82

111. Schmitt H, Buchfelder M, Radespiel-Troger M, et al. Difficult intubation in acromegalic patients: incidence and predictability. Anesthesiology 2000;93:110–4

112. Compkin TV. Radial artery cannulation, potential hazard in patients with acromegaly. Anaesthesia 1980;35:1008–9

113. Sterns RH, Riggs JE, Schochet SS. Osmotic demyelination syndrome following correction of hyponatremia. N Engl J Med 1986;314:1535–42

23

Nutritional Diseases and Inborn Errors of Metabolism

The presence of nutritional disorders or inborn errors of metabolism may influence the management of anesthesia (Table 23–1).

▌ OBESITY

Obesity (body weight 20% or more above ideal weight) is a disorder of energy balance. It represents the most common and costly nutritional disorder in the United States, affecting an estimated one-third of the adult population.[1-3] Obesity is associated with increased morbidity and mortality and a wide spectrum of medical and surgical diseases (Table 23–2).[3] A measure of obesity is the body mass index (BMI), in which a value of 28 for men and 27 for women corresponds to 20% above ideal body weight (Table 23–3). A BMI higher than 28 is associated with increased morbidity due to stroke, ischemic heart disease, and diabetes that is three to four times the risk in the general population. A central distribution of body fat is associated with a higher risk of morbidity and mortality than a more peripheral distribution of body fat and may be a better indicator of the risk of morbidity than absolute body fat mass (see "Fat Storage").[1,2]

Pathogenesis

Obesity is a complex, multifactorial disease (mechanisms of fat storage, genetic, psychological); in simple terms, it occurs when net energy intake exceeds net energy expenditure over a prolonged period of time.[3] The primary form in which potential chemical energy is stored in the body is fat (triglyceride). Energy expenditure is determined by the energy costs of maintaining the integrated bodily functions

Table 23–1 • Nutritional Disorders and Inborn Errors of Metabolism

Nutritional
  Obesity
  Malnutrition
  Anorexia nervosa
  Bulimia nervosa
  Binge-eating disorder
  Vitamin imbalance disorders
Inborn errors of metabolism
  Porphyria
  Gout
  Pseudogout
  Hyperlipidemia
  Carbohydrate metabolism disorders
  Amino acid disorders
  Mucopolysaccharidoses
  Gangliosidoses

Table 23–3 • Calculation of Body Mass Index

$$\text{Body mass index (BMI)} = \frac{\text{weight (kg)}}{\text{height}^2 \text{ (m)}}$$

Example: A 150 kg, 1.8 m tall man has a BMI of 47 (more than 100% above ideal body weight). A similar patient weighing 80 kg has a BMI of 25.

(resting metabolic rate), thermic effect of activity, and heat produced by food digestion, absorption, and storage. The resting metabolic rate accounts for about 60% of total energy expenditure. The thermic effect of activity accounts for about 20% of total

energy expenditure in the average sedentary individual. This component can be increased by exercise. Exercise can increase the resting metabolic rate for as long as 18 hours after increased activity. It is likely that caloric restriction ("dieting") initiates a defense mechanism that decreases energy expenditure, which leads to slower weight loss during periods of caloric restriction and more rapid weight gain during periods of increased caloric intake.

The high caloric density and hydrophobic nature of triglycerides permits efficient energy storage without adverse osmotic effects. The amount of triglycerides in adipose tissues is the cumulative sum of the differences between energy (food) intake and energy expenditure (resting metabolism and physical activity) over time. The current availability of caloric dense foods and sedentary lifestyle promote weight gain. If daily energy intake exceeds energy expenditure by 2%, the cumulative effect after 365 days is about a 2.3 kg increase in body weight. Although there is great interest in dietary composition, it is unlikely that these factors play major roles in the pathogenesis of obesity. Protein and carbohydrate can be metabolically converted to fat, and there is no evidence that changing the relative proportion of protein, carbohydrate, and fat in the diet without reducing caloric intake promotes weight loss.[1] However, fat has a higher caloric density than proteins or carbohydrates, and its contribution to the palatability of foods promotes the ingestion of calories.

Table 23–2 • Medical and Surgical Conditions Associated with Obesity

Organ System	Side Effects
Respiratory system	Obstructive sleep apnea
	Obesity hypoventilation syndrome
	Restrictive lung disease
Cardiovascular system	Systemic hypertension
	Cardiomegaly
	Congestive heart failure
	Ischemic heart disease
	Cerebrovascular disease
	Peripheral vascular disease
	Pulmonary hypertension
	Deep vein thrombosis
	Pulmonary embolism
	Hypercholesterolemia
	Hypertriglyceridemia
	Sudden death
Endocrine system	Diabetes mellitus
	Cushing syndrome
	Hypothyroidism
Gastrointestinal system	Hiatal hernia
	Inguinal hernia
	Gallstones
	Fatty liver infiltration
Musculoskeletal system	Osteoarthritis of weight-bearing joints
	Back pain
Malignancy	Breast
	Prostate
	Cervical
	Uterine
	Colorectal

Adapted from: Adams JP, Murphy PG. Obesity in anaesthesia and intensive care. Br J Anaesth 2000;85:91–108.

Fat Storage

Surplus calories are converted to triglycerides and stored in adipocytes. This storage is regulated by the enzyme lipoprotein lipase. The activity of this enzyme varies in different parts of the body, being more active in abdominal fat and less active in hip fat. Increased morbidity and mortality associated with obesity depends on the amount of fat and its anatomic distribution. Central or android distribution of fat, which is more common in men, manifests as abdominal obesity. Abdominal fat deposits are metabolically more active than peripheral or gynecoid fat distribution (hips, buttocks, thighs) and are thus associated with a higher incidence of metabolic complications (dyslipidemias, glucose intolerance and diabetes mellitus, ischemic heart disease, congestive heart failure, stroke). For example, a waist-to-hip ratio higher than 1.0 in women and 0.8 in men increases the risk for ischemic heart disease, stroke, diabetes mellitus, and death independent of total body fat.[2, 3] Because men tend to accumulate abdominal fat, which is broken down by the more active form of lipoprotein lipase, they generally lose weight more readily than women, who accumulate hip fat. Stress and cigarette smoking stimulate cortisol production, which may facilitate deposition of excess calories as abdominal fat.

When triglycerides are deposited in fat cells, the cells initially increase in size until a maximum size is reached at which point the cells divide.[2] Moderate degrees of obesity (BMI less than 40) are likely to result in increased fat cell size, whereas extreme obesity (BMI higher than 40) is likely to result in adipocyte proliferation.

Metabolic Effects of Weight Change

The responses of both lean and obese individuals to experimental weight change support the notion that body fat content is regulated, meaning it is unlikely that behavior alone is the sole determinant of obesity.[1] The 24-hour energy expenditure per unit of lean body mass is similar in lean and obese individuals. Small decreases in body weight result in decreased energy expenditures that persist despite a caloric intake that is sufficiently decreased to maintain the lower weight. Thus a formerly obese person requires about 15% fewer calories to maintain "normal" body weight than persons of the same body composition who have never been obese. Should formerly obese patients return to the previous level of caloric intake, the resulting weight gain exceeds that previously lost because energy expenditures have been decreased, perhaps due to changes in the efficiency with which skeletal muscles convert chemical energy to mechanical work. Indeed, in both obese and lean subjects who lose weight there is an almost inevitable recidivism, with the lost weight rapidly regained. It is likely that obese patients who report failure to lose weight despite dieting in fact greatly underestimate their caloric intake and overestimate their physical activity.[4]

Genetic Factors

The importance of energy stores for survival and the ability to conserve energy in the form of adipose tissue at one time may have conferred a survival advantage. For this reason, humans are presumably enriched with genes that favor energy storage and diminish energy expenditure. However, the combination of easy access to calorically dense foods and a sedentary lifestyle have made the metabolic consequences of these genes maladaptive. Furthermore, the increasing prevalence of obesity and the inverse relation between obesity and social class confirm the co-existing importance of environmental factors in the development of obesity.

Treatment

The purpose of weight reduction should be to decrease morbidity rather than to meet a cosmetic standard of thinness.[1] A weight loss of only 5 to 20 kg may decrease systemic blood pressure and plasma lipid concentrations and enhance the control of diabetes mellitus. Lifestyle alterations in the form of increased physical activity and/or decreased caloric intake must be continued indefinitely. Serotonin-reuptake inhibitors (fenfluramine, phentermine) function as appetite suppressants but also produce unacceptable side effects (primary pulmonary hypertension) in some individuals. Sibutramine is an appetite suppressant that inhibits the reuptake of serotonin and norepinephrine, and orlistat is a lipase inhibitor that acts in the gastrointestinal tract and is not absorbed.

Surgery (vertical banded gastroplasty or gastric bypass) is usually recommended only for individuals with severe obesity (BMI higher than 40). Gastroplasty ("gastric reduction") is the most commonly performed procedure, and its efficacy is probably related to the increased sense of fullness (decreased gastric volume for food intake to about 50 ml) and symptoms of the "dumping syndrome" associated with passage of gastric contents into the intestines, which act as deterrents to eating. Patients who undergo gastroplasty are at risk for the development of intestinal obstruction and electrolyte disturbances.

Physiologic Disturbances Associated with Obesity

Obesity has potential detrimental effects on multiple organ systems including the patient's respiratory and cardiovascular systems (Table 23–2). Respiratory derangements associated with obesity include obesity hypoventilation syndrome and effects on lung volumes and gas exchange. Cardiovascular disease dominates the morbidity and mortality of obese individuals and manifests as ischemic heart disease, systemic hypertension, and congestive heart failure.

Morbidly obese individuals have limited mobility and may therefore appear to be asymptomatic even in the presence of significant respiratory and cardiovascular impairment. Exertional dyspnea and/or angina pectoris, although infrequent, may accompany periods of physical activity. Many obese individuals choose to sleep sitting up in a chair to avoid symptoms of orthopnea and paroxysmal nocturnal dyspnea.

Obstructive Sleep Apnea

Obstructive sleep apnea, characterized by frequent episodes of apnea or hypopnea during sleep, airway obstruction manifesting as snoring, daytime somnolence due to repeated episodes of fragmented sleep during the night, and physiologic changes that include arterial hypoxemia, arterial hypercarbia, polycythemia, systemic hypertension, pulmonary hypertension, and right ventricular failure, is present in 2% to 4% of middle-age adults, especially men (Table 23–4).[3, 5] An estimated 5% of obese subjects develop obstructive sleep apnea. In obese individuals, increased adipose tissue in the neck and pharyngeal tissues predisposes to airway narrowing.[5] Nonobese patients who develop obstructive sleep apnea often have tonsillar hypertrophy or craniofacial skeletal abnormalities (retrognathia) that predispose to airway narrowing or closure during sleep.

Table 23–4 • Manifestations and Risk Factors of Obstructive Sleep Apnea

---

Manifestations
    Frequent episodes of obstructive apnea (10 seconds or longer occurring five times or more per hour during sleep) or hypopnea (50% decrease in airflow or a decrease sufficient to decrease arterial oxygen saturation 4%)
    Snoring (characterized as ''heavy'')
    Daytime somnolence most likely reflecting sleep fragmentation (memory and concentration deficits, motor vehicle accidents)
    Physiologic changes
        Arterial hypoxemia
        Polycythemia
        Arterial hypercarbia
        Systemic hypertension (ischemic heart disease, cerebrovascular disease)
        Pulmonary hypertension (right ventricular failure)
Risk factors
    Male gender
    Middle age
    Obesity (body mass index > 30)
    Alcohol (evening ingestion)
    Drug-induced sleep

Pathogenesis

Apnea occurs when the pharyngeal airway collapses. Pharyngeal patency depends on the action of dilator muscles that prevent upper airway collapse. This pharyngeal muscle tone is decreased during sleep and in many individuals leads to significant narrowing of the airway with turbulent airflow and snoring. Increased inspiratory effort and the response to arterial hypoxemia and hypercarbia result in arousal, which in turn restores upper airway tone. The individual then falls asleep again, and the cycle repeats.

Risk Factors

The main predisposing factors for the development of obstructive sleep apnea are male gender, middle age, and obesity (BMI higher than 30), with other factors such as evening alcohol consumption or drug-induced sleep compounding the problem. For example, in addition to physiologic sleep, pharyngeal muscle tone may be decreased by drugs, especially alcohol. Obstructive sleep apnea is definitively diagnosed by polysonography in a sleep laboratory (observed episodes of apnea during sleep). An obstructive apneic episode is defined as 10 seconds or longer of total cessation of airflow despite continuous respiratory efforts against a closed airway. Sleep fragmentation is the most likely explanation for daytime somnolence, which is associated with impaired concentration, memory problems, and motor vehicle accidents.[6] Patients may complain of morning headaches due to nocturnal carbon dioxide retention and cerebral vasodilation.

Treatment

Positive airway pressure, delivered through a nasal mask, is the initial treatment of choice for clinically significant obstructive sleep apnea.[5] The level of positive pressure required to sustain patency of the patient's upper airway during sleep is determined in a sleep laboratory. Patients treated with positive airway pressure demonstrate improved neuropsychiatric function and a lessening of daytime somnolence. Patients with mild sleep apnea who do not tolerate positive airway pressure may benefit from nighttime application of oral appliances designed to enlarge the airway by keeping the tongue in an anterior position or by displacing the mandible forward. The use of drugs to treat obstructive sleep apnea (protriptyline, fluoxetine) has not been reliably effective in more severe cases of obstructive sleep apnea. Nocturnal oxygen therapy is a consideration for individuals who experience severe arterial oxygen desaturation.

Surgical treatment of obstructive sleep apnea includes tracheostomy (patients with severe apnea who do not tolerate positive airway pressure), palatal surgery (laser-assisted uvulopalatopharyngoplasty), and maxillofacial surgical procedures to enhance upper airway patency during sleep (genioglossal advancement). Patients with obstructive sleep apnea who have significant craniofacial abnormalities or who have had an unsuccessful genioglossal advancement, with or without uvulopalatopharyngoplasty, may benefit from maxillomandibular advancement.

Management of Anesthesia

Management of anesthesia in patients with a history of obstructive sleep apnea poses significant risks.[7-9] These patients may be exquisitely sensitive to all central nervous system depressant drugs, with a potential for upper airway obstruction or apnea with even minimal doses of these drugs. For these reasons, preoperative medication with sedatives including benzodiazepines or opioids is used sparingly if at all.

Induction and Maintenance. Upper airway abnormalities (decreased anatomic space to accommodate anterior displacement of the tongue) predisposing to difficult exposure of the glottic opening during direct laryngoscopy may also predispose to obstructive sleep apnea.[7] When awake these patients appear to compensate for compromising airway anatomy by increasing their craniocervical angulation, which increases the space between the mandible and cervical spine and elongates the tongue and soft tissues of the neck. This postural compensation is lost when these patients are rendered unconscious and paralyzed. Indeed, difficult tracheal intubation is a predictable problem in patients with a history of obstructive sleep apnea.[7]

All anesthetic drugs should be titrated to just the desired effect, preferably using short-acting inhaled (sevoflurane, desflurane, nitrous oxide) and/or injected (propofol) drugs. Nitrous oxide may be avoided in the presence of co-existing pulmonary hypertension. Neuromuscular blocking drugs characterized by rapid spontaneous recovery are most often selected. When feasible, regional anesthesia using a catheter to provide continuous anesthesia is useful. Perioperative monitoring for apnea, arterial oxygen desaturation, and the development of cardiac dysrhythmias is recommended.[8] Tracheal extubation is not considered until patients are fully conscious with intact upper airway reflexes and under controlled conditions in a monitored environment.

Postoperative Management. Patients with a history of obstructive sleep apnea are at increased risk for developing arterial hypoxemia during the postoperative period. Episodic arterial hypoxemia may occur early (first 24 hours) and later (2 to 5 days postoperatively). Early episodic arterial hypoxemia may be a reflection of opioid use either intraoperatively or to manage postoperative pain. Monitoring in an intensive care unit is indicated for some patients. The sitting position may be a useful postoperative posture to adopt to improve arterial oxygenation, especially in morbidly obese patients. Routine administration of oxygen during the postoperative period is controversial, as oxygen could increase the duration of apnea by delaying the arousal effect produced by arterial hypoxemia. Therefore it may be preferable to provide supplemental oxygen only when arterial oxygen desaturation is indicated by pulse oximetry.

Management of postoperative pain in patients with obstructive sleep apnea must consider the exquisite sensitivity of these patients to the ventilatory depressant effects of opioids. Even neuraxial opioids have been associated with unexpected degrees of ventilatory depression.[9] Regional analgesia is associated with a low incidence of apnea and periods of arterial hypoxemia, making this approach an attractive technique for providing postoperative analgesia. Nonsteroidal antiinflammatory drugs have considerable analgesic effects and are used frequently in these patients.

Specialized Surgical Procedures

Upper airway surgical procedures to treat patients with obstructive sleep apnea are often prolonged, especially when multiple procedures are needed concomitantly to address multiple levels of airway obstruction.[8] A general anesthetic with muscle relaxants is often selected for these patients. The arrangement of the anesthetic delivery system is influenced by the need for the surgeon to have complete access to the patient's head. A tracheostomy is mandatory before surgery that involves the base of the tongue. Tracheostomy may be exceedingly difficult in markedly obese patients with short necks. A cuffed armored nasotracheal tube is often utilized for mandibular and maxillomandibular surgery to permit occlusion of the teeth (intermaxillary fixation). Postoperatively, patients undergoing extensive corrective surgery are managed in an intensive care unit with oxygen supplementation, analgesics, and pulse oximetry monitoring.

Uvulopalatopharyngoplasty is performed with the patient supine and the head slightly elevated to enhance venous drainage. Local infiltration of an anesthetic solution containing epinephrine is likely to be utilized. Worsening of upper airway obstruction is possible during the early postoperative period due to the residual effects of anesthetic drugs or surgically induced upper airway edema. Acute upper airway obstruction may occur immediately following tracheal extubation.[8] A nasopharyngeal airway may be left in place to facilitate maintenance of airway patency following tracheal extubation. Continuous positive airway pressure and supplemental oxygen may be added following tracheal extubation. Postoperative analgesia with nonsteroidal antiinflammatory drugs is most often recommended. Monitoring of ventilation may be maintained for 24 to 48 hours postoperatively.

Obesity Hypoventilation Syndrome

Obesity hypoventilation syndrome is the long-term consequence of obstructive sleep apnea.[3] Obstructive sleep apnea is initially limited to nocturnal sleep with correction of respiratory acidosis during waking hours. As the obesity hypoventilation syndrome develops there is evidence of nocturnal alterations in the control of breathing manifesting as central apneic events (apnea without respiratory efforts). These nocturnal episodes of central apnea reflect progressive desensitization of the respiratory centers to nocturnal hypercarbia. At its extreme, obesity hypoventilation syndrome culminates in the *pickwickian syndrome,* which is characterized by obesity, daytime hypersomnolence, arterial hypoxemia, polycythemia, hypercarbia, respiratory acidosis, pulmonary hypertension, and right ventricular failure.

Lung Volumes

Obesity imposes a restrictive ventilation defect because of the weight added to the thoracic cage and the abdominal weight impeding motion of the diaphragm, especially with assumption of the supine position. The results of this added weight and associated splinting of the diaphragm are decreases in functional residual capacity (FRC), expiratory reserve volume (ERV), and total lung capacity, with the FRC declining exponentially with increasing BMI.[3] The FRC may be decreased to the point that small airway closure occurs with resulting ventilation-to-perfusion mismatching, right-to-left shunting, and arterial hypoxemia. Anesthesia accentuates these changes such that a 50% decrease in FRC occurs in obese anesthetized patients compared with a 20% decrease in nonobese individuals (Fig.

23–1).[3] The application of positive end-expiratory pressure (PEEP) improves the FRC and arterial oxygenation but at the expense of cardiac output and oxygen delivery.

The decrease in FRC impairs the ability of obese patients to tolerate periods of apnea, such as during direct laryngoscopy for tracheal intubation. Obese individuals are likely to experience arterial oxygen desaturation following induction of anesthesia despite preoxygenation. It reflects a decreased oxygen reservoir in their decreased FRC and an increase in oxygen consumption.

Gas Exchange

Morbidly obese individuals usually have only modest decreases in arterial oxygenation and increases in the alveolar-to-arterial oxygen difference, presumably reflecting ventilation-to-perfusion mismatching.[3] Nevertheless, arterial oxygenation may deteriorate markedly on induction of anesthesia, and increased concentrations of delivered oxygen are needed to maintain an acceptable PaO_2. In contrast to the likely decrease in PaO_2, the $PaCO_2$ and ventilatory response to carbon dioxide remain within a normal range in obese patients, reflecting the high diffusing capacity and favorable characteristics of the dissociation curve for carbon dioxide. As with oxygenation, however, the margin of reserve is small; administration of ventilatory depressant drugs, especially with the assumption of the supine position, may lead to carbon dioxide accumulation in obese patients.

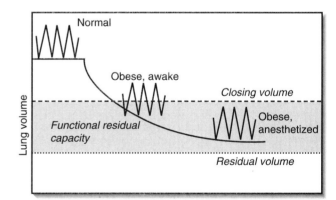

Figure 23–1 • Effects of severe obesity on functional residual capacity (FRC). Anesthesia and obesity are associated with decreases in FRC resulting in small airway closure, ventilation-to-perfusion mismatching, and impaired arterial oxygenation. (From Adams JP, Murphy PG. Obesity in anaesthesia and intensive care. Br J Anaesth 2000;85:91–108. © The Board of Management and Trustees of the British Journal of Anaesthesia. Reproduced by permission of Oxford University Press/British Journal of Anaesthesia.)

Lung Compliance and Resistance

Increasing BMI is associated with exponential decreases in respiratory compliance and resistance.[3] The decrease in lung compliance reflects accumulation of fat tissue in and around the chest wall and the effects of increased pulmonary blood volume. Decreased lung compliance is associated with decreases in FRC and impaired gas exchange. These changes in lung compliance and resistance result in rapid, shallow breathing patterns and increased work of breathing that is most marked when obese individuals assume the supine position.

Work of Breathing

Oxygen consumption and carbon dioxide production are increased in obese individuals as a result of the increased metabolic activity of the excess fat and the increased workload on supportive tissues. Normocapnia is maintained usually by increased minute ventilation, which results in increased oxygen cost (work) of breathing. Obese patients typically breathe rapidly and shallowly, as this pattern results in the least oxygen cost of breathing.

Systemic Hypertension

Mild to moderate systemic hypertension is present in 50% to 60% of obese patients.[3] Increased extracellular fluid volume resulting in hypervolemia and increased cardiac output is characteristic of obesity-induced hypertension. These changes are predictable, considering that each kilogram of fat contains 3000 meters of blood vessels. Cardiac output is estimated to increase 0.1 L/min for each kilogram of weight gain related to adipose tissue. Cardiomegaly and systemic hypertension most likely reflect increased cardiac output. Hyperinsulinemia, which is characteristic of obesity, can contribute to systemic hypertension by activating the sympathetic nervous system and causing sodium retention. Insulin resistance may be responsible for the enhancement of pressor activity of norepinephrine and angiotensin II.

Pulmonary hypertension is common in obese patients and most likely reflects the impact of chronic arterial hypoxemia or increased pulmonary blood volume (or both).

Ischemic Heart Disease

Obesity seems to be an independent risk factor for the development of ischemic heart disease and is more common in obese individuals with central distribution of fat. Other factors, such as systemic hypertension, diabetes mellitus, and hypercholesterolemia, which are common in obese individuals, compound the likely development of ischemic heart disease.

Congestive Heart Failure

Systemic hypertension leads to concentric left ventricular hypertrophy and a progressively noncompliant left ventricle, which when combined with hypervolemia increases the risk of congestive heart failure (Fig. 23–2).[3] Increases in epicardial fat are common in obese individuals, but fatty infiltration of the myocardium is uncommon and not responsible for congestive heart failure. Cardiac dysrhythmias in obese individuals may be precipitated by arterial hypoxemia, hypercarbia, ischemic heart disease, obese hypoventilation syndrome, and fatty infiltration of the cardiac conduction system. Left ventricular hypertrophy demonstrated by echocardiography is characteristic of obesity. Obesity-induced cardiomyopathy is associated with hypervolemia and increased cardiac output, and it reflects interactions with systemic hypertension and ischemic heart disease (Fig. 23–2).[3] Ventricular hypertrophy and dysfunction worsen with increasing duration of obesity. The increased demands placed on the cardiovascular system by obesity decrease the reserve of the cardiovascular system and limit exercise tolerance.

Morbidly obese patients tolerate exercise poorly, with any increase in cardiac output being achieved by increasing the heart rate without an increase in stroke volume or ejection fraction. Likewise, changing position from the sitting to the supine position is associated with increases in cardiac output, pulmonary capillary wedge pressure, and mean pulmonary artery pressure, together with decreases in heart rate and systemic vascular resistance.

Gastric Emptying

The notion that obese patients are at increased risk for aspiration and development of aspiration pneumonitis based on increased intra-abdominal pressure, delayed gastric emptying, and the increased incidence of hiatal hernia and gastroesophageal reflux is questionable.[3] In fact, obese patients without symptoms of gastroesophageal reflux have resistance gradients between the stomach and gastroesophageal junction similar to those in nonobese individuals in both the sitting and supine positions. Furthermore, although gastric volume is greater in obese individuals, gastric emptying may be more rapid in these subjects than in nonobese

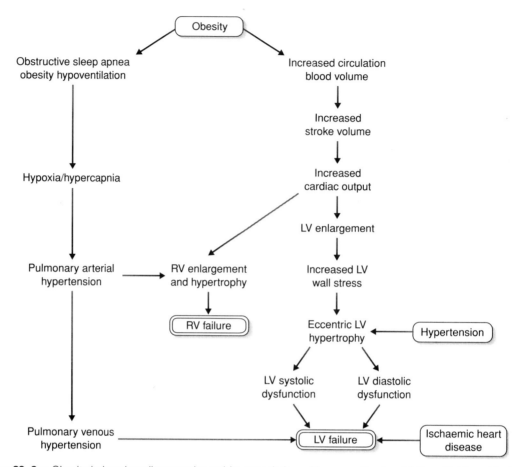

Figure 23–2 • Obesity-induced cardiomyopathy and its association with congestive heart failure [right ventricular (RV), left ventricular (LV)], systemic hypertension, and ischemic heart disease. (From Adams JP, Murphy PG. Obesity in anaesthesia and intensive care. Br J Anaesth 2000;85:91–108. © The Board of Management and Trustees of the British Journal of Anaesthesia. Reproduced by permission of Oxford University Press/British Journal of Anaesthesia.)

subjects. Nevertheless, because of the larger gastric capacity, the residual volume is larger in obese individuals.

Diabetes Mellitus

Glucose tolerance curves are often abnormal, and the incidence of diabetes mellitus is increased severalfold in obese patients. This finding is consistent with the resistance of peripheral tissues to the effects of insulin in the presence of increased adipose tissue. Indeed, obesity is an important risk factor for the development of non-insulin-dependent diabetes mellitus (NIDDM). In obese patients with NIDDM the catabolic response to surgery may necessitate the use of exogenous insulin during the perioperative period.

Hepatobiliary Disease

Abnormal liver function tests and fatty liver infiltration are frequent findings in obese patients. Despite evidence that volatile anesthetics are defluorinated to a greater extent in obese patients, there is no evidence of exaggerated anesthetic-induced hepatic dysfunction in obese patients. The risk of developing gallbladder and biliary tract disease is increased threefold in obese patients, perhaps reflecting abnormal cholesterol metabolism.

Thromboembolic Disease

The risk of deep vein thrombosis in obese patients undergoing surgery is approximately double that of nonobese individuals.[3] The increased risk of thromboembolic disease in obese patients presumably reflects the effects of polycythemia, increased abdominal pressure, and immobilization leading to venous stasis and increased abdominal pressure in deep veins.

Pharmacokinetics of Drugs

The physiological changes associated with obesity may lead to alterations in the distribution, binding, and elimination of many drugs.[3] The volume of distribution of drugs in obese individuals may be influenced by increased blood volume and cardiac output, decreased total body water (fat contains less water than other tissues), altered protein binding of drugs, and the lipid solubility of the drug being administered. The effect of obesity on protein binding of drugs, if any, is variable and not always predictable. Despite the occasional presence of liver dysfunction, hepatic clearance of drugs is not usually altered in obese individuals. Congestive heart failure and decreased hepatic blood flow could slow elimination of drugs that are highly dependent on liver clearance. Renal clearance of drugs may increase in obese individuals because of increased renal blood flow and glomerular filtration rate.

The impact of obesity on the appropriate dose of injected drugs is difficult to predict. Blood volume is likely to be increased, which would tend to decrease the plasma concentrations achieved following rapid intravenous injection of drugs. Conversely, fat has a low blood flow such that the increased doses calculated based on body weight could result in excessive plasma concentrations. The prudent approach is to calculate the initial dose of injected drug for administration to obese patients based on "ideal" body weight (reflects lean body mass) rather than actual body weight, which in obese patients overestimates the lean body mass. In this regard, drug doses can be initially determined based on ideal body weight, assuming it is 80 kg for females and 100 kg for males.[10] Subsequent doses are determined based on the pharmacologic response to the initial dose. Repeated injections of drugs, however, could result in cumulative drug effects and prolonged responses, reflecting storage of drugs in fat and subsequent release from this inactive depot into the systemic circulation as the plasma concentration of drug declines. Oral absorption of drugs is not influenced by obesity.

The notion that slow emergence of morbidly obese patients from the effects of general anesthesia reflects delayed release of the volatile anesthetic from fat stores is not accurate (see "Maintenance of Anesthesia").[3] Poor total fat blood flow limits the delivery of volatile anesthetics for storage such that slow emergence, if real, most likely reflects a central

nervous system effect. Overall, recovery times are often comparable in obese and lean individuals undergoing surgery that requires anesthesia lasting 2 to 4 hours.[3]

Management of Anesthesia

Management of anesthesia is influenced by obesity-induced alterations in physiologic function (Table 23–2).

Induction of Anesthesia

A detailed assessment of the obese patient's upper airway is performed before induction of anesthesia. Difficulties with mask ventilation and tracheal intubation may be considerable based on the presence of unique anatomic features (fat face and cheeks, short neck, large tongue, excessive palatal and pharyngeal soft tissue, restricted mouth opening, limited cervical and mandibular mobility, large breasts).[3] These anatomic features can present problems with airway maintenance, mask ventilation, and tracheal intubation in obese patients. Obese patients are traditionally presumed to be at increased risk for pulmonary aspiration during the induction of anesthesia, although there is no supporting evidence for this notion (see "Gastric Emptying"). Perhaps the greater risk of pulmonary aspiration is related to the potential for technically difficult tracheal intubation. In predetermined patients, awake tracheal intubation utilizing fiberoptic laryngoscopy may be selected.

The low FRC associated with obesity means that rapid decreases in arterial oxygenation may accompany direct laryngoscopy for tracheal intubation (Fig. 23–3).[11] The risk of arterial oxygen desaturation

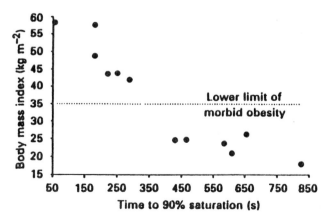

Figure 23–3 • Arterial oxygen saturation decreases to 90% more rapidly in morbidly obese patients, as quantitated by the body mass index. (From Berthoud MC, Peacock JE, Reilly CS. Effectiveness of preoxygenation in morbidly obese patients. Br J Anaesth 1991;67:464-6, with permission.)

emphasizes the importance of maximizing the oxygen content in the lungs before initiating direct laryngoscopy and monitoring arterial oxygen saturation continuously with pulse oximetry. Decreased FRC also leads to decreased mixing time for inhaled drugs, accelerating the rate of increase in the drug's alveolar concentration.

Maintenance of Anesthesia

The best choice of drugs or techniques for maintaining anesthesia in obese patients is not known. An increased incidence of fatty liver infiltration suggests caution when selecting drugs associated with postoperative liver dysfunction. Increased defluorination of volatile anesthetics in obese patients, however, has not been shown to result in hepatic or renal dysfunction. This increased defluorination observed after the administration of certain volatile anesthetics to obese patients does not seem to accompany the administration of sevoflurane to these patients. The possibility of prolonged responses to drugs stored in fat (volatile anesthetics, opioids, barbiturates) is not supported by delayed awakening from anesthesia in obese patients (see "Pharmacokinetics of Drugs").[3] Awakening of obese patients is prompter after exposure to desflurane or sevoflurane than after administration of isoflurane or propofol.[12] The rapid elimination of nitrous oxide is useful, but the frequent need for increased supplemental concentrations of oxygen may limit the usefulness of this inhaled drug in obese patients.

Spinal and Epidural Anesthesia

Spinal and epidural anesthesia may be technically difficult in obese patients, as bony landmarks are obscured. Local anesthetic requirements for spinal and epidural anesthesia in obese patients may be as much as 20% lower than in nonobese patients, presumably reflecting fatty infiltration and vascular engorgement caused by increased intra-abdominal pressure, which decreases the volume of the epidural space. As a result, it is difficult to predict reliably the sensory anesthesia level that will be achieved. It seems prudent to decrease the initial dose of local anesthetic administered for regional anesthesia when the body weight is greatly increased owing to excess adipose tissue.

Management of Ventilation

Controlled ventilation of the obese patient's lungs using large tidal volumes is often applied in an attempt to offset the decreased FRC and PaO_2 accompanying obesity. PEEP may improve ventilation-to-perfuson matching and arterial oxygenation in obese patients, but adverse effects on cardiac output and oxygen delivery may offset these benefits. The prone and head-down positions can further decrease chest wall compliance and the PaO_2 in obese patients. Assumption of the supine position by spontaneously breathing obese patients can decrease the PaO_2 and lead to cardiac arrest. Monitoring arterial oxygenation and ventilation is of increased importance in obese patients during the perioperative period.

Tracheal Extubation

Tracheal extubation is considered when obese patients are fully recovered from the depressant effects of anesthetics. Ideally, obese patients are allowed to recover in a head-up to sitting position. A history of obstructive sleep apnea or obesity hypoventilation syndrome mandates intense postoperative monitoring to ensure maintenance of a patient's upper airway and acceptable oxygenation and ventilation.

Postoperative Analgesia

Opioid depression of ventilation in obese patients is a concern, and the intramuscular route of administration may be unreliable owing to the unpredictable absorption of drugs. Patient-controlled analgesia is a commonly selected option for providing postoperative analgesia to obese patients. Doses of opioids used for patient-controlled analgesia are based on ideal body weight. Neuraxial opioids (continuous infusion of epidural solutions containing opioids and local anesthetics) comprise an effective method for producing postoperative analgesia in obese patients. Supplementation with oral analgesics such as nonsteroidal antiinflammatory drugs is useful. Supplemental oxygen administration and close observation, including pulse oximetry, are often utilized.

Postoperative Complications

Postoperative morbidity and mortality rates are higher in obese patients than in nonobese patients. Postoperative ventilation is more likely to be required in obese patients who have co-existing carbon dioxide retention and who have undergone prolonged surgery, especially abdominal operations. The semisitting position is often used during the postoperative period in attempts to decrease the likelihood of arterial hypoxemia. The hazards of obstructive sleep apnea and obesity hypoventilation syndrome may extend several days into the postoperative period. Arterial oxygenation should be closely monitored and supplemental oxygen provided as indicated by pulse oximetry and/or blood gas analysis of the PaO_2. The maximum decrease in PaO_2 typically occurs 2 to 3 days postoperatively. Weaning from mechanical ventilation may be difficult because of the increased work of breathing, decreased lung volumes, and ventilation-to-perfusion mismatching. Wound infection is twice as common. The likelihood of deep vein thrombosis and the risk of pulmonary embolism are increased, emphasizing the possible importance of early postoperative ambulation and the potential need for prophylactic subcutaneous heparin. Obese patients tend not to be able to mobilize their fat stores during critical illnesses and tend to rely on carbohydrates. The increased carbohydrate use increases the respiratory quotient and accelerates protein breakdown.

▌EATING DISORDERS

Eating disorders include anorexia nervosa, bulimia nervosa, and binge-eating disorders (Table 23–5).[13, 14] Bulimia nervosa and binge-eating disorder are encountered clinically more often than anorexia nervosa. All of these disorders are characterized by serious disturbances in eating (restriction or binging) and excessive concerns about body weight. Eating disorders typically occur in adolescent girls or young women, although 5% to 15% of cases of anorexia nervosa and bulimia nervosa and 40% of binge-eating disorders occur in boys and young men.[13]

Table 23–5 • Diagnostic Criteria for Eating Disorders

Anorexia nervosa
  Body mass index < 17.5
  Fear of weight gain
  Inaccurate perception of body shape and weight
  Amenorrhea
Bulimia nervosa
  Recurrent binge eating (twice a week for 3 months)
  Recurrent purging, excessive exercise, or fasting
  Excessive concern about body weight or shape
Binge-eating disorder
  Recurrent binge eating (2 days per week for 6 months)
  Eating rapidly
  Eating until uncomfortably full
  Eating when not hungry
  Eating alone
  Feeling guilty after a binge
  No purging or excessive exercise

Adapted from: Becker AE, Grinspoon SK, Klibanski A, et al. Eating disorders. N Engl J Med 1999;340:1092–8.

Anorexia Nervosa

Anorexia nervosa is a relatively rare disorder, having an incidence of 5 to 10 cases per 100,000 persons and a mortality of 5% to 10%.[14] About one-half the deaths result from medical complications associated with malnutrition, and the remainder are due to suicide associated with depression. The disease is characterized by striking decreases in food intake and excessive physical activity in the obsessive pursuit of thinness. Bulimic symptoms may be part of the syndrome. Females are most often affected, and weight loss exceeds 25% of normal body weight despite the patient's perception of being obese.

Signs and Symptoms

Marked, unexplained weight loss in adolescent girls is suggestive of anorexia nervosa. Among the more serious medical complications seen in patients with anorexia nervosa are those that affect the cardiovascular system. Cardiac changes include decreased cardiac muscle mass and myocardial contractility. Cardiomyopathy secondary to starvation and to the abuse of ipecac (used to induce vomiting) may be present. Sudden death has been attributed to ventricular cardiac dysrhythmias in these patients, presumably reflecting the effects of starvation and associated hypokalemia.

Amenorrhea is often seen soon after the onset of the disorder. Physical examination reveals marked emaciation, dry skin that may be covered with fine body hair, and cold, cyanotic extremities. Decreased body temperature, orthostatic hypotension, bradycardia, and cardiac dysrhythmias may reflect alterations in autonomic nervous system activity. Bone density is decreased as a result of poor nutrition and low estrogen concentrations, and long bones or vertebrae may fracture as a result of osteoporosis. Gastric emptying may be slowed, leading to complaints of gastric distress after eating. Starvation may impair cognitive function. Electrolyte abnormalities are unusual, although hypokalemia may occur in patients who induce self-vomiting or abuse diuretics and laxatives. Occasionally patients exhibit fatty liver infiltration and altered liver function tests. Renal complications may reflect long-term dehydration accompanied by hypokalemia resulting in irreversible damage to the renal tubules. Parturients are at increased risk of delivering low-birth-weight infants.

Treatment

Treatment of patients with anorexia nervosa is complicated by the patient's denial of the condition.

Psychopharmacologic treatment, including tricyclic antidepressants, fluoxetine, lithium, and antipsychotic drugs, has not been predictably successful. Selective serotonin reuptake inhibitors (fluoxetine) that are effective in obsessive-compulsive disorders may have some value for treating patients with anorexia nervosa.

Management of Anesthesia

There is a paucity of information relating to the management of anesthesia of patients with this eating disorder. Preoperative evaluation is based on the known pathophysiologic effects evoked by starvation. The electrocardiogram is useful for detecting evidence of cardiac dysfunction. Electrolyte abnormalities (hypokalemia), hypovolemia owing to dehydration, and delayed gastric emptying are preoperative considerations. Development of cardiac dysrhythmias in patients with anorexia nervosa have been attributed to the presence of hypokalemia, prolonged QT intervals, and possible imbalance of the autonomic nervous system.[15] Reversal of neuromuscular blockade and changes in $PaCO_2$ could contribute to the potential for the development of cardiac dysrhythmias in these patients. Experience is too limited to permit recommendations regarding specific anesthetic drugs, muscle relaxants, or anesthetic techniques in the presence of anorexia nervosa.

Bulimia Nervosa

Bulimia nervosa is characterized by episodes of binge-eating (a sense of loss of control over eating), purging, and dietary restriction.[14] Binges are most often triggered by a negative emotional experience. Purging usually consists of self-induced vomiting that may be facilitated by laxatives and/or diuretics. In most patients this disorder is chronic, with relapses and remissions. Depression, anxiety disorders, and substance abuse commonly accompany bulimia nervosa.

Signs and Symptoms

Findings on physical examination that suggest the presence of bulimia nervosa are dry skin, evidence of dehydration, and fluctuant hypertrophy of the salivary glands. Resting bradycardia is often present. The most common laboratory findings are increased serum amylase concentrations presumably of parotid gland origin. Metabolic alkalosis secondary to purging is frequently present with increased serum bicarbonate concentrations, hypochloremia,

and occasionally hypokalemia. Dental complications including periodontal disease are likely. Management of insulin-dependent diabetes mellitus is complicated in patients with co-existing bulimia nervosa.

Treatment

The most effective treatment of bulimia nervosa is cognitive-behavioral therapy. Pharmacotherapy with tricyclic antidepressants and selective serotonin reuptake inhibitors (fluoxetine) may be helpful. Potassium supplementation may be necessary in the presence of hypokalemia due to recurrent self-induced vomiting.

Binge-Eating Disorder

Binge-eating disorders resemble bulimia nervosa; but in contrast to patients with bulimia nervosa, these individuals do not purge and periods of dietary restriction are less striking.[14] The diagnosis of binge-eating disorders should be suspected in morbidly obese patients, particularly obese patients with continued weight gain or marked weight cycling. The disease is chronic and accompanied by weight gain. Like anorexia nervosa and bulimia nervosa, this disorder is frequently accompanied by depression, anxiety disorders, and personality disorders. The principal medical complication of binge-eating disorders is morbid obesity and associated systemic hypertension, NIDDM, hypercholesterolemia, and joint disorders. As in patients with bulimia nervosa, antidepressant medications are useful for treating those with binge-eating disorders.

MALNUTRITION AND VITAMIN DEFICIENCIES

Malnutrition is a medically distinct syndrome that is responsive to caloric support provided by enteral or total parenteral nutrition (hyperalimentation).[16, 17] Vitamin deficiencies are principally of historic interest but may still occur in severely malnourished patients.

Malnutrition

Signs and Symptoms

Malnourished patients are identified by the presence of serum albumin concentrations less than 3 g/dl and transferrin levels below 200 mg/dl. Skin test anergy (immunosuppression) also accompanies malnutrition. Critically ill patients often experience negative caloric intake complicated by hypermetabolic states due to increased caloric needs produced by trauma, fever, sepsis, and wound healing. It is estimated that a daily caloric intake of 1500 to 2000 calories is necessary to maintain basic energy requirements. An increase in body temperature of 1°C increases daily energy (caloric) requirements by about 15%. Multiple fractures increase energy needs by about 25% and major burns by about 100%. A large tumor, by virtue of its growth and metabolism, requires fuels that can exceed 100% of basic caloric requirements. Postoperatively, patients experience increased protein breakdown and decreased protein synthesis.[18]

Treatment

It is often recommended that patients who have lost more than 20% of their body weight be treated nutritionally before undergoing elective surgery. In this regard, provision of nutritional support for 7 days before surgery decreases postoperative complications, especially in patients with gastrointestinal cancer and elderly patients undergoing surgery for hip fractures.[17] Patients who are unable to eat or absorb food after 7 days postoperatively may require parenteral nutrition.

Enteral Nutrition

When the gastrointestinal tract is functioning, enteral nutrition can be provided by means of nasogastric or gastrostomy tube feedings. Continuous drip (100 to 120 ml/hr) is the method most frequently used for administering enteral feedings. Complications of enteral feedings are infrequent but may include hyperglycemia leading to osmotic diuresis and hypovolemia. Exogenous insulin administration is a consideration when blood glucose concentrations exceed 250 mg/dl. The high osmolarity of elemental diets (550 to 850 mOsm/L) is often the cause of diarrhea.

Total Parenteral Nutrition

Total parenteral nutrition (TPN) is indicated when the gastrointestinal tract is not functioning. TPN using an isotonic solution delivered through a peripheral vein is acceptable when patients require fewer than 2000 calories daily and the anticipated need for nutritional support is less than 14 days. When daily caloric requirements exceed 2000 calories or prolonged nutritional support is required, a catheter is placed in the subclavian vein to permit infusion of hypertonic parenteral solutions

(about 1900 mOsm/L) in a daily volume of about 40 ml/kg.

Potential complications of TPN are numerous (Table 23–6). Blood glucose concentrations are monitored, as hyperglycemia (higher than 250 mg/dl) may require treatment with exogenous insulin, whereas hypoglycemia may occur if the TPN infusion is abruptly discontinued (mechanical obstruction in the delivery tubing) and increased circulating endogenous concentrations of insulin persist. Hyperchloremic metabolic acidosis may occur because of the liberation of hydrochloric acid during the metabolism of amino acids present in most parenteral nutrition solutions. Parenteral feeding of patients with compromised cardiac function is associated with the risk of congestive heart failure owing to fluid overload. Increased production of carbon dioxide resulting from metabolism of large amounts of glucose may result in the need to initiate mechanical ventilation of the lungs or failure to wean patients from long-term ventilator support.[19] Parenteral nutrition solutions can support growth of bacteria and fungi, and catheter-related sepsis is a constant threat. In view of the risk of contamination, the use of hyperalimentation catheters for administering medications, obtaining blood samples, or monitoring central venous pressure, as during the perioperative period, is not recommended. Electrolyte abnormalities may include hypokalemia, hypomagnesemia, hypocalcemia, and hypophosphatemia. If intravenous hyperalimentation is continued during surgery, there should probably be a corresponding decrease in the infusion rates of other intravenous fluids to minimize the risk of fluid overload.

Vitamin Deficiencies

It is conceivable that administration of anesthesia for surgery will be required in patients with co-

---

Table 23–6 • Complications Associated with Total Parenteral Nutrition

Hyperglycemia
Nonketotic hyperosmolar hyperglycemic coma
Hypoglycemia
Hyperchloremic metabolic acidosis
Fluid overload
Increased carbon dioxide production
Catheter-related sepsis
Electrolyte abnormalities
Renal dysfunction
Hepatic dysfunction
Thrombosis of central veins

existing nutritional deficiencies of one or more of the essential vitamins. This situation is most likely to arise in chronic alcoholic patients. Although no specific anesthetic drugs or techniques can be recommended, it is important to appreciate the changes related to vitamin deficiencies to ensure proper medical judgment during the perioperative period.

Thiamine

Thiamine (vitamin B_1) deficiency (beriberi) is most likely to occur in chronic alcoholic patients who experience decreased dietary intake of thiamine. Decreased systemic vascular resistance and increased cardiac output may result in high-output cardiac failure in thiamine-deficient patients. This form of congestive heart failure is similar to the hyperdynamic heart failure that occurs in patients with large arteriovenous shunts. It may be difficult to differentiate congestive heart failure due to thiamine deficiency from the cardiomyopathy that accompanies chronic alcoholism. Memory loss (Korsakoff's psychosis) and skeletal muscle weakness may develop. Polyneuropathy with demyelination, paresthesias, and sensory deficits (glove and stocking distribution) are characteristic. Destruction of the peripheral sympathetic nervous system could impair compensatory vasomotor responses, manifesting as exaggerated decreases in systemic blood pressure in response to hemorrhage, positive-pressure ventilation of the lungs, or sudden changes in body position. Treatment of thiamine deficiency consists of administering intravenous preparations of this vitamin.

Ascorbic Acid

Deficiency of ascorbic acid (vitamin C) produces a clinical picture known as scurvy. Ascorbic acid is required for conversion of proline to hydroxyproline during the production of normal collagen. When ascorbic acid is deficient, manifestations of abnormal ground substance are present in all tissues. Capillary fragility, exhibited as petechial hemorrhages, is prominent in patients with ascorbic acid deficiency. Hemorrhage into joints and skeletal muscles can result. The failure of odontoblastic activity results in loosened teeth and gangrenous alveolar margins. Fibroblast activity is deficient, resulting in poor wound healing and decreased strength of new surgical incision sites. A catabolic state associated with negative nitrogen balance and potassium deficiency is also characteristic. Iron deficiency anemia is frequent, but the presence of macrocytic anemia suggests a concomitant folic acid deficiency. There are no special considerations for the management of anesthesia.

Nicotinic Acid

A deficiency of nicotinic acid (niacin) produces pellagra (black tongue). Nicotinic acid is part of nicotinamide adenine dinucleotide phosphate, an important component of cellular oxidation-reduction reactions. The body does not depend on exogenous nicotinic acid, as this vitamin can be manufactured from tryptophan. Patients with carcinoid tumors can develop pellagra, as available tryptophan is diverted to the formation of serotonin, rather than nicotinic acid. A diet with high maize content can lead to nicotinic acid deficiency, as corn contains large amounts of leucine, which interferes with the metabolism of tryptophan. Other causes of pellagra include malabsorption syndromes and chronic alcoholism.

Mental confusion, irritability, and peripheral neuropathy are characteristic of nicotinic acid deficiency. Administration of nicotinic acid usually reverses the central nervous system dysfunction in less than 24 hours. Gastrointestinal symptoms include achlorhydria and severe diarrhea, which can lead to hypovolemia and loss of electrolytes. Vesicular dermatitis involving the mucous membranes is also characteristic. Manifestations of dermatitis include stomatitis, glossitis, excessive salivation, and urethritis. There are no specific recommendations regarding the management of anesthesia.

Vitamin A

Vitamin A deficiency can result from dietary lack of foodstuffs that contain this vitamin (leafy vegetables, animal liver) or from malabsorption syndromes. Clinical manifestations of vitamin A deficiency include loss of night vision, conjunctival drying, and corneal destruction. Anemia from depressed hemoglobin synthesis is frequent. Management of anesthesia may include frequent application of artificial tears and keeping the patients' eyes closed during the intraoperative period.

An excess of vitamin A can produce irritability, hydrocephalus, hepatosplenomegaly, and anemia. Intracranial symptoms can be caused by intracranial hypertension secondary to cerebral sinus obstruction.

Vitamin D

Nutritional rickets is due to decreased availability of the active form of vitamin D. Gastrointestinal absorption of calcium is impaired when vitamin D is absent; there is also a tendency to develop hypocalcemia. This tendency is balanced by parathormone activity, which increases in response to low plasma calcium concentrations. The osteolytic activity of parathormone restores plasma calcium concentrations to near-normal levels at the expense of older bone, which becomes demineralized. New bone formation, which is dependent on plasma calcium concentrations, takes place in a normal manner. Therefore changes in the skeleton characteristic of rickets reflect unimpaired formation of new bone and breakdown of old bone. Thoracic kyphosis from this mechanism may be so severe it produces hypoventilation. Laboratory studies in the presence of vitamin D deficiency show normal to low plasma calcium concentrations, low plasma phosphate levels, increased plasma alkaline phosphatase concentrations, and low urinary excretion of calcium.

Vitamin K

Vitamin K is synthesized by bacteria residing in the gastrointestinal tract. Prolonged antibiotic therapy can eliminate these bacteria, leading to a prolonged prothrombin time. Because vitamin K is fat-soluble, a deficiency of this substance is likely whenever there is failure of fat absorption from the gastrointestinal tract. Decreased absorption of vitamin K from the gastrointestinal tract is most likely to occur when bile salts are excluded from the intestine.

▌ INBORN ERRORS OF METABOLISM

Inborn errors of metabolism manifest as a variety of metabolic defects that may complicate the management of anesthesia (Table 23–7). In some instances these defects are clinically asymptomatic and manifest only in response to specific triggering events, such as certain drugs or foodstuffs.

Porphyrias

Porphyrias are a group of inborn errors of metabolism characterized by the overproduction of porphyrins and their precursors. Porphyrins are essential for many vital physiologic functions including oxygen transport and storage. The synthetic pathway

Table 23–7 • Inborn Errors of Metabolism

- Porphyria
- Gout
- Pseudogout
- Hyperlipidemia
- Carbohydrate metabolism disorders
- Amino acid disorders
- Mucopolysaccharidoses
- Gangliosidoses

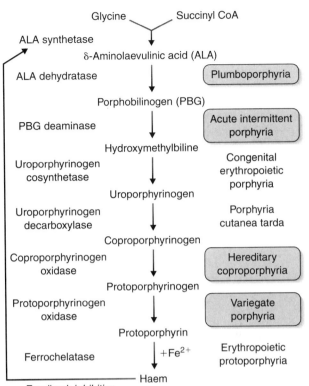

Figure 23–4 • Metabolic pathways for haem synthesis. Enzymes are noted on the feedback inhibition loop of the sequence, and the type of porphyria associated with the enzyme deficiency is designated on the right. Examples of acute porphyrias are indicated by the boxes. (From James MFM, Hift RJ. Porphyrias. Br J Anaesth 2000;85:143–53. © The Board of Management and Trustees of the British Journal of Anaesthesia. Reproduced by permission of Oxford University Press/British Journal of Anaesthesia.)

involved in the production of porphyrins is determined by a sequence of enzymes. A defect in any of these enzymes results in accumulation of the preceding intermediaries and produces a form of porphyria (Fig. 23–4).[20] In human physiology, heme is the most important porphyrin being bound to proteins to form hemoproteins that include hemoglobin and cytochromes (P_{450} isozymes, which are important for drug metabolism). Production of heme is controlled by the activity of the enzyme aminolevulinic acid (ALA) synthetase, which is present in mitochondria. The formation of ALA synthetase is controlled by the endogenous concentration of heme, ensuring that the level of heme production parallels requirements (Fig. 23–4).[20] ALA synthetase is readily inducible and can respond rapidly to increased heme requirements such as those resulting from the administration of drugs that require P_{450} for their metabolism. In the presence of porphyria, any increase in heme requirements results in accumulation of pathway intermediates immediately preceding the site of enzyme block (Fig. 23–4).[20]

Classification

Porphyrias are classified by the site of the enzyme defect (hepatic or erythropoietic, reflecting the major sites of heme production in the liver and bone marrow), the enzyme defect itself, or whether it causes acute symptoms (Table 23–8; Fig. 23–4).[20] Only acute forms of porphyria are relevant to the management of anesthesia, as they are the only forms of porphyria that may result in life-threatening reactions in response to certain drugs (Table 23–8).[20]

Acute Porphyrias

Acute porphyrias, with the exception of the rare plumboporphyria, are inherited as non-sex-linked autosomal dominant conditions with variable expression. The enzyme defects in porphyria are deficiencies rather than absolute deficits. Although there is no direct influence of gender on the pattern of inheritance, attacks occur more frequently in women and are most frequent during the third and fourth decades of life. Attacks are rare before puberty or following the onset of menopause. Acute attacks of porphyria are most commonly precipitated by events that decrease heme concentrations, thus increasing the activity of ALA synthetase and stimulating the production of porphyrinogens (Fig. 23–4).[20] Enzyme-inducing drugs are the most important triggering factors for the development of acute porphyrias. These acute attacks may also be precipitated by physiologic hormonal fluctuations such as those that accompany menstruation, fasting (such as before elective surgery), dehydration, stress (such as that associated with anesthesia and surgery), and infection. Pregnancy in these patients is often associated with spontaneous abortion. Furthermore,

pregnancy may be complicated by systemic hypertension and an increased incidence of low-birth-weight infants.

Signs and Symptoms

Acute attacks of porphyria are characterized by severe abdominal pain, autonomic nervous system instability, electrolyte disturbances, and neuropsychiatric manifestations ranging from mild disturbances to fulminating life-threatening events.[20] Skeletal muscle weakness that may progress to quadriparesis and respiratory failure is the most potentially lethal neurologic manifestation of acute attacks of porphyria. Central nervous system involvement with upper motor neuron lesions, cranial nerve palsies, and involvement of the cerebellum and basal ganglia is seen less frequently. Seizures may occur during an attack of acute porphyria. Psychiatric disturbances may develop, but it seems their incidence has been overemphasized.

Gastrointestinal symptoms accompanying abdominal pain include vomiting and diarrhea. Despite severe abdominal pain (may mimic acute appendicitis, acute cholecystitis, renal colic), clinical examination of the abdomen is typically normal. Abdominal pain is thought to relate directly to autonomic nervous system neuropathy. Dehydration and electrolyte disturbances involving sodium, potassium, and magnesium may be prominent in these patients. Tachycardia and systemic hypertension or less commonly hypotension are manifestations of cardiovascular instability.

Complete and prolonged remissions are likely between attacks, and many individuals with the genetic defect never develop symptoms. In this regard, patients at known risk for porphyria but previously asymptomatic ("silent or latent porphyria") may experience their first symptoms in response to inadvertent administration of triggering drugs during the perioperative period. ALA synthetase concentrations are increased during all acute attacks of porphyria.

Table 23–8 • Classification of Porphyrias

Acute
  Acute intermittent porphyria
  Variegate porphyria
  Hereditary coproporphyria
  Plumboporphyria
Nonacute
  Porphyria cutanea tarda
  Erythropoietic porphyrias
    Erythropoietic uroporphyria
    Erythropoietic protoporphyria

Adapted from: James MFM, Hift RJ. Porphyrias. Br J Anaesth 2000;85:143–53.

Triggering Drugs

Drugs may trigger an acute attack of porphyria by inducing the activity of ALA synthetase or interfering with the negative feedback control as the final common pathway (Fig. 23–4).[20] It is not possible to predict which drugs will be porphyrinogenic, although chemical groupings such as the allyl groups present on barbiturates and certain steroid structures have been incriminated in the production of porphyria. Only the acute forms of porphyria are affected by drug-induced enzyme induction. It is not clear why the manifestations of nonacute porphyria are not apparently affected by enzyme-inducing drugs. For example, potent enzyme inducers of ALA synthetase, including the anticonvulsants, do not exacerbate or precipitate porphyria cutanea tarda or the erythropoietic porphyrias. The labeling of drugs as safe or unsafe for patients with porphyria is often based on anecdotal experience with the use of the drugs in porphyric patients and reports of the induction of acute attacks.[20] Drugs may be tested in cell culture models for their ability to induce ALA synthetase activity or for their effects on porphyrin synthesis. Alternatively, the action of drugs on the porphyrin synthetic pathway can be investigated in animal models. Both cell culture and animal models tend to overestimate the porphyrino-genicity of drugs.

It is difficult to assess the porphyrinogenic potential of anesthetic drugs, as other factors such as sepsis or stress may precipitate a porphyric crisis coincidentally with administration of anesthesia. Any classification of anesthetic drugs with regard to their porphyrinogenicity is likely to be imperfect and arbitrary (Table 23–9).[20] Particular care is needed when selecting drugs for patients with acute intermittent porphyria or clinically active forms of porphyria and when prescribing drugs in combination, as exacerbation of porphyria is more likely under these circumstances.

Acute Intermittent Porphyria

Of all the acute porphyrias, acute intermittent porphyria affecting the central and peripheral nervous systems produces the most serious symptoms (systemic hypertension, renal dysfunction) and is the one most likely to be life-threatening. The defective enzyme is porphobilinogen deaminase, and the gene encoding this enzyme is located on chromosome 11 (Fig. 23–4).[20]

Variegate Porphyria

Variegate porphyria is characterized by neurotoxicity and cutaneous photosensitivity in which bullous skin eruptions occur on exposure to sunlight as a result of the conversion of porphyrinogens to porphyrins. The enzyme defect is at the level of protoporphyrinogen oxidase, and the gene encoding this enzyme is on chromosome 1 (Fig. 23–4).[20] The incidence of variegate porphyria is highest in South Africa.

Hereditary Coproporphyria

Acute attacks of hereditary coproporphyria are less common and severe than acute intermittent por-

Table 23–9 • Recommendations Regarding Use of Anesthetic Drugs in the Presence of Acute Porphyrias

Drug	Recommendation
Inhaled anesthetics	
Nitrous oxide	Safe
Isoflurane	Probably safe*
Sevoflurane	Probably safe*
Desflurane	Probably safe*
Intravenous anesthetics	
Propofol	Safe
Ketamine	Probably safe*
Thiopental	Avoid
Thiamylal	Avoid
Methohexital	Avoid
Etomidate	Avoid
Analgesics	
Acetaminophen	Safe
Aspirin	Safe
Codeine	Safe
Morphine	Safe
Fentanyl	Safe
Sufentanil	Safe
Ketorolac	Probably avoid†
Phenacetin	Probably avoid†
Pentazocine	Avoid
Opioid antagonists	
Naloxone	Safe
Neuromuscular blocking drugs	
Succinylcholine	Safe
Pancuronium	Safe
Atracurium	Probably safe*
Cisatracurium	Probably safe*
Vecuronium	Probably safe*
Rocuronium	Probably safe*
Mivacurium	Probably safe*
Anticholinergics	
Atropine	Safe
Glycopyrrolate	Safe
Anticholinesterases	
Neostigmine	Safe
Local anesthetics	
Lidocaine	Safe
Tetracaine	Safe
Bupivacaine	Safe
Mepivacaine	Safe
Ropivacaine	No data
Sedative and antiemetics	
Droperidol	Safe
Midazolam	Probably safe*
Lorazepam	Probably safe*
Cimetidine	Probably safe*
Ranitidine	Probably safe*
Metoclopramide	Probably safe*
Ondansetron	Probably safe*
Cardiovascular drugs	
Epinephrine	Safe
α-Agonists	Safe
β-Agonists	Safe
β-Antagonists	Safe
Diltiazem	Probably safe*
Nitroprusside	Probably safe*
Nifedipine	Probably avoid†

* Although safety is not conclusively established, the drug is unlikely to provoke acute porphyria.
† Use only if expected benefits outweigh the risks.
Adapted from: James MFM, Hift RJ. Porphyrias. Br J Anaesth 2000;85:143–53.

phyria or variegate porphyria. As in patients with variegate porphyria, neurotoxicity and cutaneous hypersensitivity are characteristic, though they tend to be less severe. The defective enzyme is coproporphyrinogen oxidase, encoded by a gene on chromosome 9 (Fig. 23–4).[20]

Porphyria Cutanea Tarda

Porphyria cutanea tarda is due to an enzymatic defect (decreased hepatic activity of uroporphyrinogen decarboxylase) transmitted as an autosomal dominant trait. ALA synthetase activity is not important, and drugs capable of precipitating attacks of other forms of porphyria do not provoke an attack of porphyria cutanea tarda. Likewise, neurotoxicity does not accompany this form of porphyria. Signs and symptoms of porphyria cutanea tarda most often appear as photosensitivity in men older than 35 years of age. Porphyrin accumulation in the liver is associated with hepatocellular necrosis. Anesthesia is not a hazard in affected patients, although the choice of drugs should take into consideration the likely presence of co-existing liver disease.

Erythropoietic Uroporphyria

Erythropoietic uroporphyria is a rare form of porphyria, transmitted as an autosomal recessive trait. In contrast to porphyrin synthesis in the liver, porphyrin synthesis in the erythropoietic system is responsive to changes in hematocrit and tissue oxygenation. Hemolytic anemia, bone marrow hyperplasia, and splenomegaly are often present. Repeated infections are common, and photosensitivity is severe. The urine of affected patients turns red when exposed to light. Neurotoxicity and abdominal pain do not occur, and administration of barbiturates does not adversely alter the course of the disease. Death usually occurs during early childhood.

Erythropoietic Protoporphyria

Erythropoietic protoporphyria is a more common, but less debilitating, form of erythropoietic porphyria. Signs and symptoms include photosensitivity, vesicular cutaneous eruptions, urticaria, and edema. In occasional patients cholelithiasis develops secondary to increased excretion of protoporphyrin. Administration of barbiturates does not adversely affect the course of the disease, and survival to adulthood is common.

Management of Anesthesia

Anesthesia has been implicated in the triggering of acute attacks of porphyria, although recent reports are rare.[20] Indeed, most patients with porphyria can be safely anesthetized assuming that appropriate precautions are taken. In this regard, patients with evidence of active porphyria or a history of past acute porphyric crises must be considered to be at increased risk. Short-acting drugs are presumed to be safe because their rapid elimination limits exposure time for enzyme induction to occur. Repeated or prolonged use (continuous intravenous infusions of propofol) could result in different responses. There is reason to believe that exposure to multiple potential enzyme-inducing drugs may be more dangerous than exposure to any one drug.

Preoperative Evaluation

The principles of safe anesthetic management of patients with porphyria depend on the identification of susceptible individuals and the determination of potential porphyrinogenic triggering drugs.[20] Laboratory identification of porphyric individuals is not easy, as many show only subtle or no biochemical abnormalities during asymptomatic phases. In the presence of a suggestive family history, determination of erythrocyte porphobilinogen activity is the most appropriate screening test for patients with suspected acute intermittent porphyria. In addition to a careful family history and thorough physical examination (often no clinical evidence or only subtle skin lesions), the presence or absence of peripheral neuropathy and autonomic nervous system instability is noted.

If an acute exacerbation of porphyria is suspected during the preoperative period, particular attention must be given to skeletal muscle strength and cranial nerve function, as symptoms related to these systems may predict impending respiratory failure and an increased risk of pulmonary aspiration. Cardiovascular examination may reveal systemic hypertension and tachycardia, which necessitate treatment before induction of anesthesia. Postoperative ventilation of the patient's lungs may be required during an acute porphyric crisis. During an acute exacerbation, severe abdominal pain may mimic a surgical abdomen. Preoperative preparation in patients experiencing an acute porphyric crisis should include careful assessment of fluid balance and electrolyte status.

Preoperative starvation should be minimized; but if a prolonged fast is unavoidable, administration of a glucose-saline infusion during the preoperative period may be considered, as caloric restriction has been linked to the precipitation of acute porphyria attacks. In view of the frequency with which hyponatremia is encountered during acute attacks of porphyria, intravenous fluids containing only glucose are not recommended.

Preoperative Premedication

Benzodiazepines are commonly selected for preoperative anxiolysis. Aspiration prophylaxis that includes antacids and/or H_2-receptor antagonists is acceptable. Cimetidine has been recommended for treatment of acute porphyric crises, as this drug may decrease heme consumption and inhibit ALA synthetase activity.[21] Cimetidine does not appear to be effective prophylactically.

Prophylactic Therapy

No specific prophylactic therapy is of proven benefit.[20] However, because carbohydrate administration can suppress porphyrin synthesis, administering oral carbohydrate supplements (20 g/hr) preoperatively may be recommended. If oral feedings are not acceptable, 10% glucose in saline is an option. Hematin has not been evaluated as prophylactic therapy.

Regional Anesthesia

There is no absolute contraindication to the use of regional anesthesia in patients with porphyria.[20] If a regional anesthetic is considered, it is essential to perform a neurologic examination before initiating the block to minimize the likelihood that worsening of any preexisting neuropathy would be erroneously attributed to the regional anesthetic. Autonomic nervous system blockade induced by the regional anesthetic could unmask cardiovascular instability, especially in the presence of autonomic nervous system neuropathy, hypovolemia, or both. There is no evidence that any local anesthetic has ever induced an acute attack of porphyria or neurologic damage in porphyric individuals.[20] Regional anesthesia has been safely administered to parturients with acute intermittent porphyria.[22] Regional anesthesia for patients experiencing acute intermittent porphyria, however, is not likely to be used because of concerns related to hemodynamic instability, mental confusion, and associated neuropathy.

General Anesthesia

The total dose of drugs administered and the length of exposure may influence the risk of triggering a porphyric crisis in vulnerable patients (Table 23–9).[20] In this regard, the availability of short-acting anesthetic drugs has likely contributed to the safety of anesthesia in the presence of porphyria. Perioper-

ative monitoring should consider the frequent presence of autonomic nervous system dysfunction and the possibility of labile systemic blood pressure.

Induction of Anesthesia. Propofol has been used safely for induction of anesthesia in patients with porphyria, although the use of prolonged continuous infusions of this drug are of unproven safety.[20] Ketamine has been used safely in the presence of quiescent acute intermittent porphyria. Use of etomidate is questionable, as it has been shown to be potentially porphyrinogenic in animal studies despite its safe use in this patient population. All barbiturates must be considered unsafe despite numerous reports of their safe administration to porphyric patients during the quiescent phase. Conversely, worsening of symptoms has been observed when thiopental is administered in the presence of a porphyric crisis.

Maintenance of Anesthesia. Nitrous oxide is well established as a safe inhaled anesthetic to administer to patients with porphyria. Safe use of isoflurane has been described.[20] The short duration of action of sevoflurane and desflurane are desirable characteristics for drugs to be administered to patients with porphyria, but experience is too limited to make recommendations.[20] Opioids have been administered safely to these patients. Neuromuscular blocking drugs, do not seem to introduce a predictable risk when administered to these patients.

Cardiopulmonary Bypass. Cardiopulmonary bypass is a potential risk for patients with porphyria, as the additional stress introduced by hypothermia, pump-induced hemolysis, blood loss and its consequent increase in heme demand by the bone marrow, and the large number of drugs administered could increase the risk of developing a porphyric crisis. Nevertheless, clinical experience does not support an increased incidence of porphyric crises in these patients when undergoing cardiopulmonary bypass.[20]

Treatment of a Porphyric Crisis

The first step in treating an acute porphyric crisis is removal of any known triggering factors. Adequate hydration and carbohydrates are necessary. Pain often necessitates treatment with opioids. Nausea and vomiting are treated with conventional antiemetics. β-Adrenergic blockers are administered to control tachycardia and systemic hypertension. Should seizures occur, traditional anticonvulsants are regarded as unsafe, necessitating use of a benzodiazepine. Electrolyte disturbances, including hypomagnesemia, are treated aggressively.

Hematin, 3 to 4 mg/kg IV over 20 minutes, is the only specific form of therapy for an acute porphyric crisis. It is presumed that hematin supplements the intracellular pool of heme and thus suppresses ALA synthetase activity. Heme arginate is more stable than hematin and lacks the potential adverse effects associated with hematin (renal failure, coagulopathy, thrombophlebitis). Somatostatin decreases the rate of formation of ALA synthetase and combined with plasmapheresis may effectively decrease pain and induce remission.

Gout

Gout is a disorder of purine metabolism that may be classified as primary or secondary. Primary gout is due to an inherited metabolic defect that leads to overproduction of uric acid. Secondary gout is hyperuricemia due to an identifiable cause, such as chemotherapeutic drugs used to treat leukemia, leading to the rapid lysis of purine-containing cells. Gout is characterized by hyperuricemia with recurrent episodes of acute arthritis owing to deposition of urate crystals in joints. Deposition of urate crystals typically initiates an inflammatory response that causes pain and limited motion of the joints. At least one-half of the initial attacks of gout are confined to the first metatarsophalangeal joint. Persistent hyperuricemia also results in deposition of urate crystals in extra-articular locations, manifested most often as nephrolithiasis. Urate crystal deposition can also occur in the myocardium, aortic valves, and extradural spinal regions. The incidence of systemic hypertension, ischemic heart disease, and diabetes mellitus are increased in patients with gout.

Treatment

Treatment of gout is designed to decrease the plasma concentrations of uric acid by administration of uricosuric drugs (probenecid) or inhibition of the conversion of purines to uric acid by xanthine oxidase (allopurinol). Colchicine, which lacks any effect on purine metabolism, is considered the drug of choice for management of acute gouty arthritis. It relieves joint pain presumably by modifying leukocyte migration and phagocytosis. The side effects of colchicine include vomiting and diarrhea. Large doses of colchicine can produce hepatorenal dysfunction and agranulocytosis.

Management of Anesthesia

Management of anesthesia in the presence of gout includes prehydration to facilitate continued renal elimination of uric acid. Sodium bicarbonate to alkalinize the urine also facilitates excretion of uric acid. As lactate can decrease the renal tubular secretion of uric acid, the use of lactated Ringer's solution may be questioned, although this is an unproven concern. Despite appropriate precautions, acute attacks of gout may follow surgical procedures for no apparent reason in patients with a history of gout.

Extra-articular manifestations of gout and side effects of drugs used to control the disease deserve consideration when formulating the plan for anesthesia management. Renal function is evaluated, as clinical manifestations of gout usually increase with deteriorating renal function. Abnormalities detected on the electrocardiogram could reflect urate deposits in the myocardium. The increased incidence of systemic hypertension, ischemic heart disease, and diabetes mellitus in patients with gout is considered. Although rare, adverse renal and hepatic effects may be associated with probenecid and colchicine. Limited temporomandibular joint motion from gouty arthritis, if present, can make direct laryngoscopy for tracheal intubation difficult.

Lesch-Nyhan Syndrome

Lesch-Nyhan syndrome is a genetically determined disorder of purine metabolism that occurs exclusively in males. Biochemically, the defect is characterized by decreased or absent activity of hypoxanthine-guanine phosphoribosyl transferase, leading to excess purine production and increased uric acid concentrations throughout the body. Clinically, patients are often mentally retarded and exhibit characteristic spasticity and self-mutilation patterns. Self-mutilation usually involves trauma to perioral tissues, and subsequnt scarification may present difficulties with direct laryngoscopy for tracheal intubation. Seizure disorders associated with this syndrome are often treated with benzodiazepines. Athetoid dysphagia may increase the likelihood of aspiration if vomiting occurs. Malnutrition is often present. Hyperuricemia is associated with nephropathy, urinary tract calculi, and arthritis. Death is often due to renal failure.

Management of anesthesia is influenced by co-existing renal dysfunction and possible impaired metabolism of drugs administered during anesthesia.[23] The presence of a spastic skeletal muscle disorder suggests caution about using succinylcholine. The sympathetic nervous system response to stress is enhanced, suggesting caution with administration of exogenous catecholamines to these patients.

Hyperlipoproteinemia

Abnormal increases in blood concentrations of lipids, cholesterol, or triglycerides is termed hyperlipoproteinemia. This term is more correct than hyperlipidemia because it emphasizes the importance of lipoproteins in the pathophysiology of atherosclerosis. The electrophoretic pattern produced by lipoproteins in the plasma is used to classify hyperlipoproteinemia into six categories (Table 23–10). Lipoproteins are classified as chylomicrons, very low density lipoproteins, intermediate density lipoproteins, low density lipoproteins, and high density lipoproteins. There is an inverse relation between high density lipoproteins and the development of ischemic heart disease. No absolute levels of cholesterol or triglycerides have been found to be diagnostic of hyperlipoproteinemia, but patients with blood cholesterol levels above the 90th percentile for gender and age are considered to be at increased risk for the development of atherosclerosis. The role of increased circulating concentrations of triglycerides in the development of ischemic heart disease is controversial.

Treatment of hyperlipoproteinemia includes diet (low fat, low cholesterol), smoking cessation, and drug therapy. Lowering the low density lipoprotein (LDL) cholesterol levels is associated with decreases in morbidity and mortality related to cardiac events. The 3-hydroxy-3-methylglutaryl coenzyme A (HMG-CoA) reductase inhibitors ("statin" drugs) comprise the class of drugs most effective for lowering LDL cholesterol concentrations. It has been demonstrated that postinfarction patients with LDL concentrations higher than 130 mg/dl benefit from drug therapy to lower these concentrations, ideally to less than 100 mg/dl. It is possible that beneficial effects of the statin drugs extend beyond their lipid-lowering effects, perhaps reflecting antiinflammatory effects that reduce the likelihood that atherosclerotic plaques will rupture.

Management of anesthesia in the presence of hyperlipoproteinemia is influenced by the possible presence of ischemic heart disease in these patients. Statin drugs used to lower serum cholesterol concentrations may be hepatotoxic, and laboratory evidence of this adverse effect may have implications for the management of anesthesia. Arterial insufficiency has been described following placement of an arterial catheter for intraoperative monitoring of systemic blood pressure.[24] Familial lipoprotein lipase deficiency is not associated with an increased risk of ischemic heart disease, but hepatosplenomegaly may be present.

Carnitine Deficiency

Carnitine deficiency is a rare condition associated with lipid storage disorders, manifesting as a systemic form and a myopathic form. Systemic carnitine deficiency is characterized by recurrent attacks of vomiting, diarrhea, and encephalopathy associated with metabolic acidosis, hypoglycemia, hyperammonemia, coagulation disorders, and increased serum aminotransferase concentrations reflecting hepatic dysfunction. Myopathic carnitine deficiency is characterized clinically by skeletal muscle weakness and cardiomyopathy. Carnitine is the essential cofactor in the enzymatic transport of long-chain

Table 23–10 • Characteristics of Hyperlipoproteinemia

Disorder	Cholesterol	Triglycerides	Xanthomas	Risk of Ischemic Heart Disease
Familial lipoprotein lipase deficiency (hyperchylomicronemia)	Normal	Increased	Eruptive	Very low
Familial dysbetalipoproteinemia	Increased	Increased	Palmar, plantar tendon	Very high
Familial hypercholesterolemia	Increased	Normal to increased	Tendon	Very high
Familial hypertriglyceridemia	Normal	Increased	Eruptive	Low
Familial combined hyperlipidemia	Markedly increased	Markedly increased	Palmar, plantar tendon	High
Polygenic hypercholesterolemia	Increased	Normal	Tendon	Moderate

fatty acids into the mitochondria in which they are oxidized.

Preoperative evaluation of patients with systemic carnitine deficiency includes assessment of the patient's neurologic status and blood glucose concentrations.[25] Cardiac evaluation is intended to determine the presence of cardiomyopathy. It is recommended that these patients receive their usual daily dose of carnitine on the morning of surgery. An intravenous infusion of glucose is initiated preoperatively and maintained throughout the perioperative period, guided by blood glucose concentrations. Administration of succinylcholine in the presence of skeletal muscle myopathy may be questioned.

Patients who require emergency surgery in the presence of a metabolic crisis are prepared with an intravenous infusion of glucose-containing solutions.[25] Electrolyte and acid-base derangements may require treatment. Carnitine should be administered intravenously if the patient's neurologic function does not improve with glucose. Hypoprothrombinemia may require treatment with fresh frozen plasma.

Tangier Disease

Tangier disease is characterized by an absence or marked deficiency of normal high density lipoproteins in plasma, resulting in the accumulation of cholesterol esters in numerous tissues (tonsils, spleen, lymph nodes, thymus, intestinal mucosa, nerves, cornea).[26] The principal clinical signs and symptoms are hyperplastic orange tonsils, splenomegaly, and relapsing peripheral neuropathies. Thrombocytopenia and platelet defects may occur and influence the selection of regional anesthesia. Tonsillar enlargement is a consideration during the preoperative evaluation of the patient's upper airway. In patients with peripheral neuropathies and skeletal muscle wasting, administration of succinylcholine may evoke hyperkalemia.

Propionic Acidemia

Propionic acidemia is a rare autosomal recessive inborn error of metabolism that results from deficient activity of the mitochondrial enzyme propionyl-CoA carboxylase. This disorder is characterized by repeated occurrences of severe metabolic ketoacidosis, usually precipitated by excessive protein intake or concurrent infections. Ketoacidosis develops because propionic acid inhibits citric acid cycle enzymes. Along with acidosis, manifestations

of propionic acidemia may include seizures, developmental retardation, hypotonia, episodic vomiting, pancreatitis, hyperammonemia, and cardiomyopathy. The acute management of acidosis and hyperammonemia focuses on hydration with fluids containing glucose and bicarbonate and treatment of the precipitating events.

Preoperative evaluation of patients with propionic acidemia is influenced by the acid-base balance, nutritional state, skeletal muscle tone, mental status, and gastrointestinal function.[27] Avoidance of events during the intraoperative period that precipitate metabolic acidosis (fasting, arterial hypoxemia, dehydration, hypotension) is important. When patients with propionic acidemia are fasting, they require glucose in their intravenous fluids to suppress protein catabolism and subsequent acidosis. Lactated Ringer's solutions are avoided, as lactate could contribute to acidemia. Muscle relaxants metabolized by ester hydrolysis are not recommended.

Disorders of Carbohydrate Metabolism

Disorders of carbohydrate metabolism usually reflect genetically determined enzyme defects (Table 23–11). The defect can result in a deficiency or an excess of precursors or end-products of metabolism that are normally involved in the formation of glycogen from glucose. In some instances an alternate metabolic pathway is utilized. Ultimately, signs and symptoms of specific disorders of carbohydrate metabolism reflect the effects produced by alterations in the amount of precursors or end-products of metabolism that result from the enzyme defects.

Glycogen Storage Disease Type 1a

Glycogen storage disease type 1a (von Gierke's disease) is due to the deficiency or lack of the enzyme glucose 6-phosphatase. As a result, glycogen cannot

---

Table 23–11 • Disorders of Carbohydrate Metabolism

Glycogen storage disease type 1a (von Gierke's disease)
Glycogen storage disease type 1b
Pompe's disease
McArdle's disease
Galactosemia
Fructose 1,6-diphosphate deficiency
Pyruvate dehydrogenase deficiency
Mucopolysaccharidoses
Gangliosidoses

be hydrolyzed in hepatocytes, neutrophils, and possibly other cells, leading to its intracellular accumulation.[28] Hypoglycemia can be severe, and oral feedings are required every 2 to 3 hours to maintain acceptable blood glucose concentrations. Chronic metabolic acidosis is present and may lead to osteoporosis. Mental retardation, growth retardation, and seizures due to hypoglycemia are likely. Hepatomegaly is due to accumulation of glycogen in the liver. Renal enlargement caused by accumulation of glycogen may manifest as chronic pyelonephritis. A hemorrhagic diathesis may be due to platelet dysfunction and manifest as recurrent epistaxis and bleeding after minor trauma and surgery. Facial and truncal obesity occur. Survival beyond 2 years of age is unusual, although surgical creation of a portocaval shunt may benefit occasional patients.

Management of anesthesia includes provision of exogenous glucose to prevent potentially unrecognized intraoperative hypoglycemia.[29] Monitoring the arterial pH and blood glucose concentration is helpful, as these patients often become acidotic owing to an inability to convert lactic acid to glycogen. In this regard, lactate-containing solutions for intravenous infusions are avoided to minimize the theoretic possibility of metabolic acidosis due to lactate administration during the perioperative period.

Glycogen Storage Disease Type 1b

Glycogen storage disease type 1b is a rare autosomal recessive disease in which glucose 6-phosphate, a product of metabolic cleavage of glycogen, cannot be transported to the inner surface of microsomes because of a deficiency in its transport system.[28] As such, this disease is a variant of glycogen storage disease type 1a. In glycogen storage disease type 1b, glycogen accumulates in the liver, kidneys, and intestinal mucosa; and glucose availability to tissues is impaired. Hypoglycemia and lactic acidosis ensue. Clinical signs and symptoms resemble those described for glycogen storage disease type 1a. In addition, type 1b patients may experience recurrent infections owing to impaired neutrophil activity.

Preoperative fasting is minimized, and glucose-containing infusions are administered intravenously throughout the perioperative period. Strict asepsis is important, and preoperative normalization of blood glucose concentrations may improve platelet function, thereby decreasing the likelihood of intraoperative bleeding. Intraoperative monitoring of blood glucose concentrations is recommended, as hypoglycemia may be profound and difficult to recognize during general anesthesia. Lactic acidosis develops as a result of the incomplete conversion of glycogen. For this reason monitoring

the arterial pH is helpful; administration of lactate-containing solutions is not recommended. Iatrogenic hyperventilation of the patient's lungs and associated respiratory alkalosis may stimulate release of lactate from skeletal muscles and aggravate metabolic acidosis. Treatment of metabolic acidosis includes administration of intravenous sodium bicarbonate.

Pompe's Disease

Pompe's disease is due to a specific glucosidase enzyme deficiency that results in glycogen deposits in smooth, striated, and cardiac muscle. Myocardial involvement is the most prominent feature, often manifesting clinically as congestive heart failure. Echocardiography may demonstrate cardiac hypertrophy and outflow tract obstruction (subaortic stenosis) owing to interventricular septal enlargement. A large, protruding, glycogen-infiltrated tongue and poor skeletal muscle tone predispose patients to upper airway obstruction. Impaired neurologic function manifests as a decreased cough and gag reflex and lack of coordination of swallowing. Aspiration and atelectasis are common.

Management of anesthesia considers the potential for upper airway obstruction when these patients are rendered unconscious. Volatile anesthetics may produce unexpected, exaggerated cardiac depression, especially if congestive heart failure is present. A decreased preload or afterload or an increased heart rate and/or myocardial contractility may precipitate subaortic stenosis. In view of skeletal muscle involvement, it may be prudent to avoid administering succinylcholine to these patients. A diagnostic skeletal muscle biopsy in the lower extremities has been performed using regional anesthesia.[30]

McArdle's Disease

McArdle's disease is caused by selective deficiency of myophosphorylase enzyme in skeletal muscles.[31] As a result of this enzyme deficiency, glycogen is not broken down to free glucose. Because glucose is not available as a source of adenosine triphosphate, the cells progressively lose adenosine triphosphate and become acidotic. Lactate production is impaired, and the characteristic increase in serum lactate concentrations that accompanies exercise is blunted. McArdle's disease manifests as skeletal muscle myalgias and myoglobinuria, sometimes progressing to rhabdomyolysis and renal failure.

During general anesthesia these patients are prone to the development of hypoglycemia, and rhabdomyolysis may develop if energy demands of skeletal muscles are increased. Intraoperative care includes supplying exogenous glucose to prevent adverse effects from unrecognized intraoperative hypoglycemia. Patients with McArdle's disease are presumed to be protected against developing malignant hyperthermia because skeletal muscles cannot undergo contracture. The occurrence of noncardiogenic pulmonary edema has been described, perhaps reflecting the triggering of an abnormal immune response to protamine in susceptible patients.[31] Myoglobinuria leading to renal failure can occur, emphasizing the potential value of hydration during the perioperative period. Mannitol may be considered if oliguria occurs despite volume replacement. The propensity for the development of myoglobinuria raises questions regarding the administration of succinylcholine, although this concern has not been substantiated by clinical experience. Because repeated episodes of skeletal muscle ischemia can lead to skeletal muscle atrophy, intraoperative use of a tourniquet on an extremity is not recommended.

Galactosemia

Galactosemia is due to a deficiency of galactokinase and an inability to convert galactose to glucose. As a result, galactose accumulates in various tissues, leading to the development of cataracts, cirrhosis of the liver, and mental retardation. Furthermore, increased plasma galactose concentrations can suppress release of glucose from the liver, causing hypoglycemia.

Galactosemia can be mild, with no symptoms until childhood; or it can result in hepatic failure and death during infancy. Treatment consists of avoiding foods with a high lactose content, such as milk. In the absence of hypoglycemia or hepatic dysfunction, there are no specific considerations for the management of anesthesia.

Fructose 1,6-Diphosphatase Deficiency

Fructose 1,6-diphosphatase deficiency means that the liver is unable to achieve efficient conversion of fructose, lactate, glycerol, and amino acids to glucose. When liver glycogen stores are depleted by starvation, hypoglycemia and metabolic acidosis are likely. Hepatomegaly, fatty liver infiltration, and skeletal muscle hypotonia are common.

Administration of sufficient glucose during the perioperative period is important.[32] The use of lactate-containing intravenous solutions is questionable, as these patients are unable to convert lactate

to glucose. As a result, metabolic acidosis could be produced by infusions of lactated Ringer's solution.

Pyruvate Dehydrogenase Deficiency

Pyruvate dehydrogenase deficiency results in an inability to convert pyruvate to acetyl coenzyme A, with the subsequent development of chronic metabolic (lactic) acidosis due to accumulation of pyruvate and lactate (Fig. 23–5).[33]

Management of anesthesia includes avoidance of events that could contribute to lactic acidosis, such as decreased cardiac output or hypothermia. The use of lactate-containing intravenous solutions is questionable, as their administration could increase plasma lactate concentrations. Lactic acidosis may be accentuated by carbohydrate loads, as delivered by glucose-containing solutions. Selection of drugs for induction and maintenance of anesthesia is influenced by possible drug-induced inhibitory effects on gluconeogenesis, which could enhance coexisting metabolic acidosis. Use of opioids has been recommended for these patients, but excessive depression of ventilation persisting into the postoperative period is possible. Overall, experience is too limited to justify recommendations about the selection of drugs for anesthesia.

Mucopolysaccharidoses

The mucopolysaccharidoses are a rare group of progressive familial diseases of connective tissue metabolism caused by absence or insufficiency of key enzymes catalyzing the metabolism of the three main components of connective tissue: dermatan sulfate, heparan sulfate, keratan sulfate.[34] As a result

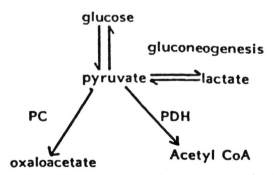

Figure 23–5 • Enzymatic reactions involving pyruvate, lactate, pyruvate dehydrogenase (PDH), and pyruvate carboxylase (PC). (From Dierdorf SF, McNiece WL. Anaesthesia and pyruvate dehydrogenase deficiency. Can Anaesth Soc J 1983;30:413–6, with permission.)

of these enzyme deficiencies, these substrates cannot be metabolized and so accumulate excessively in the skin, brain, heart, bone, liver, spleen, blood vessels, cornea, and tracheobronchial tree. Eight recognized syndromes are considered to represent the mucopolysaccharidoses (Table 23–12).[34, 35] All forms of mucopolysaccharidoses are characterized by progressive craniofacial, joint, and skeletal deformities and early death due to pulmonary infections or cardiac failure often before adulthood. Hurler syndrome is considered the prototypical defect, characterized by the most rapid progression, usually leading to death before 10 years of age. No definitive therapy is available for affected individuals. Indications for surgery are often to repair umbilical or inguinal hernias, for tonsillectomy, or to correct mandibular malformations.

Extensive preoperative evaluation of the upper airway, lungs, cervical spine, and heart and a thorough neurologic evaluation are recommended in patients with mucopolysaccharidoses scheduled for elective surgery.[34–36] Perioperative morbidity and mortality are common in these patients and are most often related to difficult airway management and tracheal intubation. Preoperative performance of magnetic resonance imaging to detect abnormalities of the spine (odontoid hypoplasia, thickening of the dura) may be helpful. Pulmonary infections are common and may necessitate treatment before surgery.

General anesthesia is most likely to be selected considering the young age of these patients and the predictable presence of mental retardation. Upper airway obstruction due to accumulation of glycosaminoglycans in the tongue and nasopharyngeal tissues suggests the possibility of technical difficulty when visualizing the glottic opening during direct laryngoscopy for tracheal intubation.[35–37] Micrognathia, a short neck, and restricted motion at the temporomandibular joint may further increase the technical difficulty associated with tracheal intubation. Hypoplasia of the odontoid and atlantoaxial subluxation, resulting in instability of the cervical spine, may be present.[38, 39] Spinal cord compression could follow direct laryngoscopy for tracheal intubation associated with hyperextension of the neck to facilitate glottic exposure. Compressive myelopathy due to thickening of the dura caused by accumulation of glycosaminoglycans has been described.[36] For all these reasons, awake fiberoptic laryngoscopy and tracheal intubation may be selected. It may be uniquely important to avoid extension and flexion movements of the patient's head during tracheal intubation or subsequent positioning for surgery. Intraoperative somatosensory evoked potential monitoring may be utilized especially if magnetic

resonance imaging confirms the preoperative presence of anatomic malformations of the spinal cord and vertebrae.

Co-existing cardiac valve disease, such as aortic regurgitation, or the presence of cardiomyopathy or ischemic heart disease reflecting infiltration of cardiac structures by glycosaminoglycans may influence the choice and dose of anesthetic drugs and muscle relaxants. Co-existing hepatic dysfunction is also a consideration when selecting drugs to be administered during anesthesia. Depressant effects of opioids are considerations if obstructive or restrictive ventilatory defects are reflected by copious airway secretions or skeletal deformities involving the vertebrae and thorax. Pulmonary hypertension may complicate chronic obstructive pulmonary disease in affected individuals. Delayed awakening from anesthesia has been described in a patient with Hunter syndrome.[40]

Gangliosidoses

Gangliosidoses (Gaucher's disease, Tay-Sachs disease, Niemann-Pick disease) are characterized by abnormalities of sphingolecithin metabolism resulting in damage to nerve membranes.

Gaucher's Disease

Gaucher's disease is an autosomal recessive disorder caused by an inherited deficiency of the enzyme glucocerebrosidase, which is necessary for the degradation of lipids containing sugars (glycolipids).[41] In the absence of this enzyme, extremely insoluble glucocerebrosidases accumulate in tissues, producing hepatosplenomegaly and bone lesions. This disease varies greatly in its severity; mild forms of the disease are encountered frequently, particularly among Ashkenazic Jews. Intravenous infusion of glucocerebroside is an effective but expensive treatment.

Fabry's Disease

Fabry's disease is an X-linked recessive lysosomal storage disorder caused by a deficiency of α-galactosidase A.[42] After Gaucher's disease, this is the second most prevalent metabolic storage disease. Intracellular accumulation of globotriaosylceramide, the glycolipid substrate of the deficient enzyme, leads to severe painful peripheral neuropathies (burning and aching pain in hands and feet) with progressive renal, cardiovascular, and cerebrovascular dysfunction and early death. The risk of stroke, uremia, and myocardial infarction is increased. Cardiac hyper-

Table 23–12 • Classification and Characteristics of Mucopolysaccharidoses

Eponym Type Prevalence	Enzyme Defect	Urinary Mucopolysaccharides	Progressive Craniofacial Deformities	Progressive Joint and Skeletal Deformities	Progressive Cardiac Involvement
Hurler I (H) 1:100,000	α-L-Iduronidase	Dermatan sulfate, heparan sulfate	Macrocephaly Coarse facies Macroglossia Hydrocephalus	Stiff joints Thoracolumbar kyphosis Odontoid hypoplasia Short neck Short stature	Coronary intimal and valvular thickening Mitral regurgitation Cardiomegaly
Scheie I (S) 1:500,000	α-L-Iduronidase	Dermatan sulfate	Coarse facies Macroglossia Prognathia	Short neck Normal stature	Aortic regurgitation
Hurler-Scheie I (HG) 1:100,000	α-L-Iduronidase	Dermatan sulfate, heparan sulfate	Macrocephaly Coarse facies Macroglossia Micrognathia	Diffuse joint limitation Short neck Short stature	Mitral and aortic valvular thickening and regurgitation
Hunter II 1:150,000	Iduronidate sulfatase	Dermatan sulfate	Macrocephaly Coarse facies Hydrocephalus	Diffuse joint limitation Short neck Short stature	Coronary intimal thickening Ischemic cardiomyopathy Minimal to none
San Filippo III (A to D)	Heparan sulfate	Heparan sulfate	Coarse facies	Stiff joints Lumbar vertebral dysplasia Short stature	
Morquio IV (A, B) 1:24,000 1:100,000	β-Galactosidase	Keratan sulfate	Coarse facies	Joint laxity Kyphoscoliosis Odontoid hypoplasia Short neck C1-2 and C2-3 subluxation Short stature	Aortic regurgitation
Maroteaux-Lamy VI 1:100,000	Arylsulfatase B	Dermatan sulfate	Macrocephaly Coarse facies Macroglossia	Joint stiffness Kyphoscoliosis Odontoid hypoplasia Short stature	Mitral and aortic valvular thickening and regurgitation
Sly VII Extremely rare	β-Glucuronidase	Dermatan sulfate, heparan sulfate	Macrocephaly Coarse facies	Joint flexion contractures Thoracolumbar gibbus Hip dysplasia	Mitral and aortic valvular thickening Aortic dissection Odontoid hypoplasia Short stature

Adapted from: Diaz JH, Belani KG. Perioperative management of children with mucopolysaccharidoses. Anesth Analg 1993;77:1261–70.

trophy, dysrhythmias, valvular insufficiency, and cardiac conduction abnormalities are common. The presence of angiokeratomas in skin and mucous membranes and characteristic benign corneal abnormalities facilitates the diagnosis, which is confirmed by documentation of decreased activity of α-galactosidase A in leukocytes.

Treatment is symptomatic, although intravenous infusions of α-galactosidase A may be helpful.[42] Alternatively, inhibitors of sphingoglycolipid synthesis may be useful. Neuropathic pain may respond to administration of carbamazepine, phenytoin, gabapentin, and lamotrigine.

Disorders of Amino Acid Metabolism

Although there are more than 70 known disorders of amino acid metabolism, most are rare. Classic manifestations include mental retardation, seizures, and aminoaciduria (Table 23–13). Metabolic acidosis, hyperammonemia, hepatic failure, and thromboembolism can also occur.

Management of anesthesia in patients with disorders of amino acid metabolism is directed toward maintenance of intravascular fluid volume and acid-base homeostasis. Use of anesthetics that could evoke seizures may be questionable in view of the likely presence of seizure disorders in these patients.

Phenylketonuria

Phenylketonuria is the prototype of disorders attributable to abnormal amino acid metabolism. Phenylalanine accumulates owing to an enzymatic deficiency of phenylalanine hydroxylase. Clinical features include mental retardation and seizures. The skin may be friable and vulnerable to damage from pressure or friction created by adhesive materials.

Homocystinuria

Homocystinuria is due to failure of transsulfuration of precursors of cystine, an important constituent of cross linkages in collagen. Manifestations of the disease reflect weakened collagen and include dislocation of the lens, osteoporosis, kyphoscoliosis, brittle light-colored hair, and malar flush.[43] Mental retardation may be prominent. The diagnosis of homocystinuria is confirmed by demonstrating homocystine in the urine as evidenced by the development of a characteristic magenta color upon exposure to nitroprusside. Thromboembolism can be life-threatening and is presumed to reflect activation of the Hageman factor by homocystine, resulting in

increased platelet adhesiveness. Attempts to minimize the likelihood of thromboembolism during the perioperative period should include administration of pyridoxine, which decreases platelet adhesiveness, preoperative hydration, infusion of dextran, and early ambulation.[43]

Maple Syrup Urine Disease

Maple syrup urine disease is a rare inborn error of metabolism that results from defective carboxylation of branched-chain amino acids. In the absence of adequate enzyme activity, consumption of foods containing branched-chain amino acids results in the accumulation of these amino acids and ketoacids in tissues and blood. Increased concentrations of leucine are usually greater than those of isoleucine or valine, as leucine is the predominant amino acid in most proteins. These amino acids result in a maple syrup odor in the urine.

Growth retardation and delayed psychomotor development are often a consequence of this chronic metabolic imbalance. Infection or fasting commonly results in acute metabolic decompensation, with increased plasma levels of branched-chain amino acids and ketoacids due to the breakdown of endogenous proteins. Increased plasma levels of ketoacids contributes to the production of metabolic acidosis. Hypoglycemia is a possibility, presumably reflecting the ability of increased plasma leucine concentrations to stimulate the release of insulin. A potentially fatal encephalopathy may accompany this disease.

Treatment is directed at decreasing the plasma levels of branched-chain amino acids and ketoacids with peritoneal dialysis or hemodialysis. Parenteral nutrition using preparations devoid of branched-chain amino acids may also be effective.[44]

Surgery and anesthesia introduce a number of hazards for the perioperative management of patients with maple syrup urine disease.[45] For example, catabolism of body proteins produced by surgery or infection could result in increased blood concentrations of branched-chain amino acids. Even blood in the gastrointestinal tract, as can occur following a tonsillectomy, produces an added metabolic load in patients with maple syrup urine disease. Accumulation of branched-chain amino acids in the circulation can produce neurologic deterioration during the perioperative period. The danger of hypoglycemia in affected patients is exacerbated by the period of fasting that precedes elective operations. Therefore it is useful to initiate intravenous infusions of glucose-containing solutions intraoperatively. Measurement of arterial pH is helpful for detecting metabolic acidosis due to accumulation

Table 23–13 • Disorders of Amino Acid Metabolism

Disorder	Mental Retardation	Seizures	Metabolic Acidosis	Hyperammonemia	Hepatic Failure	Thromboembolism	Other
Phenylketonuria	Yes	Yes	No	No	No	No	Friable skin
Homocystinuria	Yes/no	Yes	No	No	No	Yes	Hypoglycemia
Hypervalinemia	Yes	Yes	Yes	No	No	No	
Citrullinemia	Yes	Yes	No	Yes	Yes	No	Hypoglycemia
Branched-chain aciduria (maple syrup urine disease)	Yes	Yes	Yes	No	Yes	Yes	Neurologic deterioration during perioperative period
Methylmalonyl coenzyme A mutase deficiency			Yes	Yes			Acidosis intraoperatively Avoid nitrous oxide?
Isoleucinemia	Yes	Yes	Yes	Yes	Yes	No	Hypovolemia
Methioninemia	Yes	No	No	No	No	No	Thermal instability
Histidinuria	Yes	Yes/no	No	No	No	No	Erythrocyte fragility
Neutral aminoaciduria (Hartnup's disease)	Yes/no	Yes/no	Yes	No	No	No	Dermatitis
Arginemia	Yes		No	Yes	Yes	No	

of ketoacids in these patients. Significant metabolic acidosis during the perioperative period may necessitate treatment with intravenous administration of sodium bicarbonate.

Methylmalonyl-Coenzyme A Mutase Deficiency

Methylmalonyl-coenzyme A (MM-CoA) mutase deficiency is an inborn error of metabolism that can result in the formation of methylmalonic acidemia. Acute treatment includes intravenous administration of crystalloid solutions containing sodium bicarbonate. Events during the perioperative period that increase protein catabolism (fasting, bleeding into the gastrointestinal tract, stress responses, tissue destruction) may predispose to acidosis.

Experience with anesthesia is limited, and recommendations are based more on theory than on clinical experience.[46] For example, nitrous oxide may be avoided based on the theoretic concern that this inhaled anesthetic could predispose to methylmalonic acidemia in susceptible patients, reflecting nitrous oxide-induced inhibition of cobalamin coenzymes. The impact of preoperative fasting on amino acid metabolism and intravascular fluid volume is lessened by permitting clear fluid ingestion up to 2 hours before scheduled induction of anesthesia. Generous administration of intravenous fluids and glucose is also helpful for minimizing hypovolemia and protein catabolism.

References

1. Rosenbaum M, Leibel RL, Hirsch J. Obesity. N Engl J Med 1997;337:396–407
2. Agras WS. Obesity. Sci Am Med 1998;1–8
3. Adams JP, Murphy PG. Obesity in anaesthesia and intensive care. Br J Anaesth 2000;85:91–108
4. Lichtman SW, Pisarska K, Berman ER, et al. Discrepancy between self-reported and actual caloric intake and exercise in obese subjects. N Engl J Med 1992;327:1893–8
5. Strollo PJ, Rogers RM. Obstructive sleep apnea. N Engl J Med 1996;334:99–104
6. Suratt PM, Findley LJ. Driving with sleep apnea. N Engl J Med 1999;340:881–3
7. Hiremath AS, Hillman DR, James AL, et al. Relation between difficult tracheal intubation and obstructive sleep apnea. Br J Anaesth 1998;80:606–11
8. Boushra NN. Anaesthetic management of patients with sleep apnoea syndrome. Can J Anaesth 1996;43:599–616
9. Ostermeier AM, Roizen MF, Hautkappe M, et al. Three sudden postoperative respiratory arrests associated with epidural opioids in patients with sleep apnea. Anesth Analg 1997;85:452–60
10. Bouillon T, Shafer SL. Does size matter? Anesthesiology 1998;89:557–60
11. Berthoud MC, Peacock JE, Reilly CS. Effectiveness of preoxygenation in morbidly obese patients. Br J Anaesth 1991;67:464–6
12. Juvin P, Vadam C, Malek L, et al. Postoperative recovery after desflurane, propofol, or isoflurane anesthesia among morbidly obese patients: a prospective, randomized study. Anesth Analg 2000;91:714–9
13. Becker AE, Grinspoon SK, Klibanski A, et al. Eating disorders. N Engl J Med 1999;340:1092–8
14. Agras WS. The eating disorders. Sci Am Med 1998;1–7
15. Arnold DE, Rose RJ, Stoddard P. Intraoperative cardiac dysrhythmias in a patient with bulimic anorexia nervosa. Anesthesiology 1987;67:1003–5
16. Powell-Tuck J, Goode AW. Principles of enteral and parenteral nutrition. Br J Anaesth 1981;53:169–80
17. Rombeau JL, Rolandelli RH, Wilmore DW, et al. Enteral and parenteral nutritional support. Sci Am Med 1999;1–16
18. Carli F, Ramachandra V, Gandy J, et al. Effect of general anaesthesia on whole body protein turnover in patients undergoing elective surgery. Br J Anaesth 1990;65:373–9
19. Askanazi J, Nordenstrom J, Rosenbaum SH, et al. Nutrition for the patient with respiratory failure: glucose vs. fat. Anesthesiology 1981;54:373–7
20. James MFM, Hift RJ. Porphyrias. Br J Anaesth 2000;85:143–53
21. Jensen NF, Fiddler DS, Striepe V. Anesthetic considerations in porphyrias. Anesth Analg 1995;80:591–9
22. Kantor G, Rolbin SH. Acute intermittent porphyria and caesarean delivery. Can J Anaesth 1992;39:282–5
23. Larson LO, Wilkins RG. Anesthesia and the Lesch-Nyhan syndrome. Anesthesiology 1985;256:197–9
24. Cannon BW, Meshier WT. Extremity amputation following radial artery cannulation in a patient with hyperlipoproteinemia type V. Anesthesiology 1982;56:222–3
25. Rowe RW, Helander E. Anesthetic management of a patient with systemic carnitine deficiency. Anesth Analg 1990;71:295–7
26. Mentis SW. Tangier disease. Anesth Analg 1996;83:427–9
27. Harker HE, Emhardt JD, Hainline BE. Propionic acidemia in a four-month-old male: a case study and anesthetic implications. Anesth Analg 2000;91:309–11
28. Shenkman Z, Golub Y, Meretyk S, et al. Anaesthetic management of a patient with glycogen storage disease type 1b. Can J Anaesth 1996;43:467–70
29. Edelstine G, Hirshman CA. Hyperthermia and ketoacidosis during anesthesia in a child with glycogen-storage disease. Anesthesiology 1980;52:90–2
30. Rosen KR, Broadman LM. Anaesthesia for diagnostic muscle biopsy in an infant with Pompe's disease. Can Anaesth Soc J 1986;33:790–4
31. Lobato EB, Janelle GM, Urdaneta F, et al. Noncardiogenic pulmonary edema and rhabdomyolysis after protamine administration in a patient with unrecognized McArdle's disease. Anesthesiology 1999;91:303–5
32. Hashimoto Y, Watanabe H, Satou M. Anaesthetic management of a patient with heredity fructose-1,6-diphosphate deficiency. Anesth Analg 1978;57:503–6
33. Dierdorf SF, McNiece WL. Anaesthesia and pyruvate dehydrogenase deficiency. Can Anaesth Soc J 1983;30:413–6
34. Diaz JH, Belani KG. Perioperative management of children with mucopolysaccharidoses. Anesth Analg 1993;77:1261–70
35. Linstedt U, Maier C, Joehnk H, et al. Threatening spinal cord compression during anesthesia in a child with mucopolysaccharidosis VI. Anesthesiology 1994;80:227–9
36. Herrick IA, Rhine EJ. The mucopolysaccharidoses and anaesthesia: a report of clinical experience. Can J Anaesth 1988;35:67–73
37. Wilder RT, Belani KG. Fiberoptic intubation complicated by pulmonary edema in a 12 year old child with Hurler syndrome. Anesthesiology 1990;72:205–7

38. Birkinshaw K. Anaesthesia in a patient with an unstable neck: Morquio syndrome. Anaesthesia 1975;30:46–9

39. Jones AEP, Croley TF. Morquio syndrome and anesthesia. Anesthesiology 1979;51:261–2

40. Kreidstein A, Boorin MR, Crespi O, et al. Delayed awakening from general anaesthesia in a patient with Hunter syndrome. Can J Anaesth 1994;41:423–6

41. NIH Technology Assessment Panel on Gaucher Disease. Gaucher disease: current issues in diagnosis and treatment. JAMA 1996;275:548–53

42. Brady RO, Schiffmann R. Clinical features of and recent advances in therapy for Fabry disease. JAMA 2000;284:2771–5

43. Parris WCV, Quimby W. Anesthetic considerations for the patient with homocystinuria. Anesth Analg 1982;61:70–1

44. Berry GT, Heidenreich R, Kaplan P, et al. Branched-chain amino acid-free parenteral nutrition in the treatment of acute metabolic decompensation in patients with maple syrup urine disease. N Engl J Med 1991;324:175–8

45. Delaney A, Gal TJ. Hazards of anesthesia and operation in maple-syrup-urine disease. Anesthesiology 1976;44:83–6

46. Sharar SR, Haberkern CM, Jack R, et al. Anesthetic management of a child with methylmalonyl-coenzyme A mutase deficiency. Anesth Analg 1991;73:499–501

24

Diseases Due to Altered Hemoglobin Concentrations or Structures

Disease states may be related to abnormal concentrations (anemia, polycythemia) or structures (sickle cell disease) of hemoglobin. Oxygen-carrying capacity and adequacy of tissue oxygen delivery are often the most important clinical manifestations of these derangements.

ANEMIA

Anemia, like fever, is a sign of disease manifesting clinically as a numeric deficiency of erythrocytes (red blood cells, RBCs).[1] There is no single laboratory value that defines anemia. Indeed, the hematocrit may be unchanged despite acute blood loss, whereas in parturients decreased hematocrit values reflect increases in plasma volume and not anemia. Nevertheless, in adults anemia is usually defined as hemoglobin concentrations less than 11.5 g/dl (hematocrit 36%) for women and less than 12.5 g/dl (hematocrit 40%) for men. Decreases in hematocrit that exceed 1% every 24 hours can only be explained by acute blood loss or intravascular hemolysis.

The most important adverse effects of anemia are decreased tissue oxygen delivery owing to associated decreases in arterial content of oxygen (CaO_2). For example, decreases in hemoglobin concentrations from 15 g/dl to 10 g/dl result in a 33% decrease in CaO_2 (Table 24–1). Compensation for decreased CaO_2 is accomplished by a rightward shift of the oxyhemoglobin dissociation curve (facilitates release of oxygen from hemoglobin to tissues) and increased cardiac output as a reflection of decreased blood viscosity (Fig. 24–1). Furthermore, when oxygen delivery to tissues is inadequate, the kidneys release erythropoietin, which subsequently stimulates erythroid precursors in the bone marrow to

Table 24–1 • Calculation of Arterial Oxygen Content

$CaO_2 = (Hb \times 1.39)SaO_2 + PaO_2(0.003)$
where CaO_2 = arterial oxygen content (ml/dl); Hb = hemoglobin (g/dl); 1.39 = oxygen bound to hemoglobin (ml/g); SaO_2 = saturation of hemoglobin with oxygen; PaO_2 = arterial partial pressure of oxygen (mmHg); 0.003 = dissolved oxygen (ml/mmHg/dl)

Example: Hb = 15 g/dl, SaO_2 100%, PaO_2 100 mmHg

$CaO_2 = (15 \times 1.39)100 + 100(0.003) = 20.85 + 0.3 = 21.15$ ml/dl

Example: Hb = 10 g/dl, SaO_2 100%, PaO_2 100 mmHg

$CaO_2 = (10 \times 1.39)100 + 100(0.003) = 13.9 + 0.3 = 14.2$ ml/dl

Example: Hb = 10 g/dl, SaO_2 100%, PaO_2 500 mmHg

$CaO_2 = (10 \times 1.39)100 + 500(0.003) = 13.9 + 1.5 = 15.4$ ml/dl

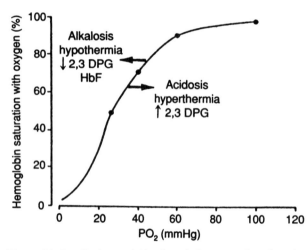

Figure 24–1 • Oxyhemoglobin dissociation curve describes the relation between SaO_2 and PaO_2. The PaO_2 at which SaO_2 is 50% is designated P_{50} (normal 26 mmHg). An increase in the P_{50} reflects a shift of the oxyhemoglobin dissociation curve to the right (increased 2,3-diphosphoglycerate level in red blood cells [RBCs], acidosis, increased body temperature); thus binding of oxygen to hemoglobin is less avid, facilitating its release to peripheral tissues. A decrease in the P_{50} reflects a shift in the oxyhemoglobin dissociation curve to the left (decreased 2,3-diphosphoglycerate level in RBCs, alkalosis, decreased body temperature); thus binding of oxygen to hemoglobin is more avid, impairing its release to peripheral tissues. Mixed venous blood has an SvO_2 of about 75% and a corresponding PvO_2 close to 40 mmHg. When the SaO_2 is about 90%, the corresponding PaO_2 is close to 60 mmHg.

produce additional RBCs. Fatigue and decreased exercise tolerance reflect the inability of the cardiac output to increase further and maintain tissue oxygenation, especially in anemic patients who become physically active. There are many causes and forms of anemia, with the most common causes of chronic anemia being iron deficiency, the presence of chronic diseases, thalassemia, and anemia due to acute blood loss (Table 24–2; Fig. 24–2).[1]

Iron Deficiency Anemia

Nutritional deficiency of iron is a cause of anemia only in infants and small children. In adults, iron deficiency anemia can only reflect depletion of iron stores owing to chronic blood loss, most likely from the gastrointestinal tract or from the female genital tract (menstruation). Parturients are susceptible to the development of iron deficiency anemia because of increased RBC mass during gestation and the needs of the fetus for iron. Symptoms of iron deficiency anemia depend on the actual hemoglobin concentrations.

Diagnosis

Patients experiencing chronic blood loss may not be able to absorb sufficient iron from the gastrointestinal tract to form hemoglobin as rapidly as RBCs are lost. As a result, RBCs are often produced with too little hemoglobin, resulting in microcytic hypochro-

Table 24–2 • Causes of Anemia

Iron deficiency anemia
Anemia of chronic disease
Thalassemia
    β-Thalassemia major
    β-Thalassemia minor
    α-Thalassemia
Acute blood loss
Aplastic anemia
    Fanconi syndrome
    Diamond-Blackfan syndrome
Megaloblastic anemia
    Vitamin B_{12} deficiency
    Folic acid deficiency
Hemolytic anemia
    Sickle cell disease
    Hereditary spherocytosis
    Paroxysmal nocturnal hemoglobinuria
    Glucose-6-phosphate dehydrogenase deficiency
    Pyruvate kinase deficiency
    Immune hemolytic anemia
Altered ability of hemoglobin to bind oxygen
    Methemoglobinemia
    Sulfhemoglobinemia

Anemia
Distribution of Causes

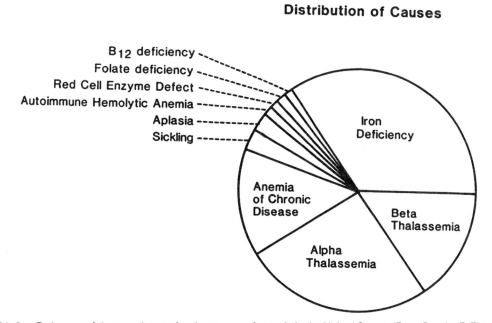

Figure 24–2 • Estimates of the prevalence of various types of anemia in the United States. (From Beutler E. The common anemias. JAMA 1988;259:2433–6, with permission.)

mic anemia. Nevertheless, most cases of iron deficiency anemia in the United States are mild, exhibiting hemoglobin concentrations of 9 to 12 g/dl. The absence of stainable iron in bone marrow aspirates is confirmatory for iron deficiency anemia. Demonstrations of decreased serum ferritin concentrations serve as cost-effective alternative tests to bone marrow examinations for the diagnosis of iron deficiency anemia.

Treatment

Treatment of iron deficiency anemia is with ferrous iron salts, such as ferrous sulfate administered orally. Iron stores are replenished slowly. Therapy should be continued for at least 1 year after the source of blood loss that caused the iron deficiency anemia is corrected. Favorable responses to iron therapy are characterized by increases in hemoglobin concentrations of about 2 g/dl in 3 weeks or return of hemoglobin concentrations to normal levels in 6 weeks. Continued bleeding is reflected by reticulocytosis and failure of hemoglobin concentrations to increase in response to iron therapy. Recombinant human erythropoietin may be used to treat drug-induced anemia or to improve hemoglobin concentrations before elective surgery.

Minimum acceptable hemoglobin concentrations that should be present before proceeding with elec-

tive surgery in patients with chronic anemia cannot be recommended. Although hemoglobin concentrations of 10 g/dl are commonly cited as a reference point, there is no evidence that hemoglobin values below this level mandates the need for perioperative RBC transfusions. Ultimately, the decision to administer RBCs during the perioperative period is influenced by the risks of anemia (decreased oxygen-carrying capacity) and the risks of transfusions (transmissible diseases, hemolytic and nonhemolytic transfusion reactions, immunosuppression).[2] The risks of anemia in addition to decreased tissue oxygen delivery vary among individuals, depending on co-existing medical diseases, age, and the magnitude of the blood loss. In this regard, decisions to transfuse patients to specific preoperative hemoglobin concentrations must be individualized, taking into consideration several factors (Table 24–3).

Although guidelines for perioperative management of anemia and the need for RBC transfusions have been developed (Table 24–3),[2,3] it is important to recognize that no controlled studies have documented the hemoglobin concentrations at which RBC transfusions prevent myocardial ischemia or infarction and improve clinical outcome. Furthermore, there is no evidence that postoperative morbidity (wound healing, infection) is adversely affected when surgery is performed in the presence

Table 24–3 • Guidelines for Blood Transfusions and Management of Blood Loss During the Perioperative Period

Hemoglobin concentrations >10 g/dl-transfusions rarely indicated

Hemoglobin concentrations < 6 g/dl-transfusions almost always indicated, especially when the anemia is acute

Hemoglobin concentrations 6–10 g/dl-decision to transfuse is determined by patient's risk for complications of decreased tissue oxygenation (patients with ischemic heart disease)

Transfusion trigger: not recommended for application to all patients as it ignores physiologic and surgical factors unique to individual patients

Preoperative autologous donation in selected patients

Intraoperative blood salvage when appropriate

Acute normovolemic hemodilution when appropriate

of mild to moderate anemia. Overall there is little evidence to support the efficacy of RBC transfusions, including transfusions in patients with cardiovascular disease.[2] The American College of Surgeons recommends RBC transfusions to normovolemic patients with anemia only if symptoms are present.[4] A hemoglobin level of 8 g/dl was suggested as a "transfusion trigger" by the Transfusion Practice Committee of the American Association of Blood Banks, whereas a threshold of 7 g/dl was suggested by the National Institutes of Health Consensus Conference on Perioperative Blood Transfusion.[5, 6] Nevertheless, there is some concern that liberalization of transfusion guidelines and increased acceptance of acute intraoperative decreases in hemoglobin concentrations may predispose certain patients to complications such as ischemic optic neuropathy (see Chapter 17).[7]

The ability of the cardiovascular system to compensate for decreases in CaO_2 by increasing the cardiac output is an important compensatory mechanism for maintaining tissue oxygen delivery, especially in acutely anemic patients. In resting adults undergoing normovolemic hemodilution, adequate tissue oxygen delivery is maintained at hemoglobin concentrations of 5 g/dl.[8] These data, however, may not be applicable to anesthetized patients undergoing surgery. Nevertheless, in anesthetized patients, acute normovolemic hemodilution to hemoglobin concentrations of 8 g/dl is associated with increases in cardiac output and decreases in systemic vascular resistance.[9]

Increased 2,3-diphosphoglycerate concentrations in RBCs are principally responsible for maintaining oxygen-carrying capacity in the presence of chronic anemia. In this regard, cardiac output does not increase in chronically anemic patients until hemoglo-

bin concentrations decrease to about 7 g/dl.[10] In vitro data suggest that peak oxygen-carrying capacity occurs at a hematocrit of 30%. Below this hematocrit level oxygen-carrying capacity decreases, whereas above this level the oxygen-carrying capacity may decrease as a result of decreased tissue blood flow owing to increased blood viscosity. Preoperative transfusions of packed RBCs can be administered to increase hemoglobin concentrations, recognizing that a period of about 24 hours is needed to restore intravascular fluid volume (Table 24–4). Compared with similar volumes of whole blood, packed RBCs produce about twice the increase in hemoglobin concentrations.

Management of Anesthesia

If elective surgery is performed in the presence of chronic anemia, it seems prudent to minimize the likelihood of significant changes that could further interfere with oxygen delivery to tissues. For example, drug-induced decreases in cardiac output or a leftward shift of the oxyhemoglobin dissociation curve owing to respiratory alkalosis from iatrogenic hyperventilation of the patient's lungs could interfere with tissue oxygen delivery. Decreased body temperature also shifts the oxyhemoglobin dissociation curves to the left. Decreased tissue oxygen requirements may accompany depressant effects of anesthetic drugs and hypothermia, offsetting the decreases in tissue oxygen delivery associated with anemia to unpredictable degrees. Nevertheless, signs and symptoms of inadequate tissue oxygen delivery due to anemia during anesthesia are difficult to appreciate. Efforts to offset the impact of surgical blood loss by such measures as normovolemic hemodilution and intraoperative blood salvage are considerations in selected patients. Monitoring cardiac function with transesophageal echocardiography may be useful for evaluating the

Table 24–4 • Basis for Decision to Administer Transfusions Preoperatively

Cause of anemia
Degree of anemia
Duration of anemia
Intravascular fluid volume
Urgency of surgery
Likelihood of intraoperative blood loss
Age of patient
Co-existing diseases
    Ischemic heart disease
    Cerebrovascular disease
    Peripheral vascular disease
    Lung disease

effects of anemia during the intraoperative course. Effects of anesthesia on the sympathetic nervous system and cardiovascular responses may blunt the usual increase in cardiac output associated with acute normovolemic anemia.[11]

Volatile anesthetics may be less soluble in the plasma of anemic patients, reflecting a decrease in the concentration of lipid-rich RBCs.[12] As a result, establishment of arterial partial pressures of volatile anesthetics in the plasma of anemic patients might be accelerated. Nevertheless, effects of decreased solubility of volatile anesthetics owing to anemia is probably offset by the impact of increased cardiac output. Therefore it seems unlikely that clinically detectable differences in the rate of induction of anesthesia or vulnerability to an anesthetic overdose would be present in anemic patients any more than in normal patients. Although supporting evidence is not available, it is likely that a decision to replace intraoperative blood loss with whole blood or packed RBCs will be made when hemoglobin concentrations decrease acutely to less than 7 g/dl, especially if there is co-existing anemia or cardiovascular or cerebrovascular disease. During the postoperative period it is important to minimize the occurrence of shivering or increases in body temperature, as these changes could increase total body oxygen requirements.

Anemia of Chronic Disease

Anemia of chronic disease is one of the most common forms of anemia (Table 24–5). There is nothing characteristic about the appearance of RBCs, and the underlying causes for the development of anemia in these patients is often unclear. The diagnosis of anemia of chronic disease remains largely one of exclusion. Iron accumulates in the reticuloendothelial system, and there appears to be a block in the release of iron from these cells to developing erythroblasts.

Attempts to treat anemia of chronic disease with iron replacement are not effective. In general, how-

ever, this form of chronic anemia is mild, only rarely requiring treatment with blood transfusions. Identifying and treating the underlying disease is the most effective therapy for the anemia.

Thalassemia

Thalassemia designates a number of inherited disorders characterized by decreased rates of synthesis or failure to synthesize structurally normal hemoglobin. Severe thalassemia (thalassemia major) is rare, whereas mild forms of this type of anemia (thalassemia minor) are common. No treatment is available for anemia due to thalassemia other than blood transfusions.

β-Thalassemia Major

β-Thalassemia major (Cooley's anemia) reflects an inability to form β-globin chains of hemoglobin. As a result, adult hemoglobin A is not formed, and anemia develops during the first year of life, as fetal hemoglobin (two α chains and two γ chains) disappears. Greek and Italian children are most often affected. Jaundice, hepatosplenomegaly, and susceptibility to infection are likely. Death due to cardiac hemochromatosis reflects the need for multiple transfusions to treat the chronic anemia. Indeed, supraventricular cardiac dysrhythmias and congestive heart failure are common. In this regard, it is important to appreciate that these patients are unusually sensitive to the effects of digitalis. Increased production of RBCs results in characteristic skeletal changes, including craniofacial deformities and thinning of cortical bone. Hemothorax and spinal cord compression may occur secondary to massive extramedullary hematopoiesis and destruction of vertebral bodies. Overgrowth of the maxillae can make visualization of the glottis difficult during direct laryngoscopy for tracheal intubation.

Treatment with hydroxyurea is helpful in some patients with sickle cell β-thalassemia (see "Sickle Cell Disease"). Bone marrow transplantation may be recommended in these patients, and splenectomy may be necessary if hypersplenism leads to pancytopenia.

β-Thalassemia Minor

β-Thalassemia minor reflects a heterozygote state (trait) that typically results in mild anemia. A relatively normal RBC count distinguishes anemia due to thalassemia minor from iron deficiency anemia. This form of anemia is encountered more frequently than previously realized.[1]

Table 24–5 • Chronic Diseases Associated with Anemia

Infections
Cancer
Connective tissue disorders
Acquired immunodeficiency syndrome
Alcoholic liver disease
Renal failure
Diabetes mellitus

α-Thalassemia

α-Thalassemia is due to the lack of production of α-chains of adult hemoglobin. A homozygous form of α-thalassemia is incompatible with life, resulting in intrauterine demise (fetal hydrops) or early neonatal death. Patients who are heterozygous for α-thalassemia (trait) characteristically acquire mild hypochromic and microcytic anemia. On occasion, blood transfusions to treat anemia or splenectomy to control hemolysis are necessary.

Acute Blood Loss

Orthostatic hypotension, tachycardia, and low central venous pressure suggest acute blood loss equivalent to at least 20% of the circulating blood volume (Table 24–6). The hematocrit may not reflect the anemia due to acute blood loss, as physiologic mechanisms for restoring plasma volume operate slowly. For example, the hematocrit does not decrease to a new plateau for as long as 3 days after acute blood loss.[13] The obvious treatment of anemia due to acute blood loss is correction of the cause leading to hemorrhage and prompt restoration of intravascular fluid volume with RBCs plus colloid or crystalloid solutions. Volume replacement with crystalloids or colloids is probably equally effective provided the crystalloids are administered at a dose of about 3 ml for every 1 ml of colloid.

Hemorrhagic shock (systolic blood pressure less than 90 mmHg, tachycardia, oliguria, metabolic acidosis, restlessness) is a potential complication of acute blood loss. The fundamental defect in hemorrhagic shock is decreased intravascular fluid volume leading to decreased venous return and cardiac output, with subsequent inadequate tissue perfusion. Increased sympathetic nervous system activity during acute hemorrhage is useful for redirecting blood flow to the brain and heart. Increased sympathetic nervous system activity for prolonged periods, however, with associated arteriolar vasoconstriction results in detrimental decreases in renal and splanchnic blood flow, one manifestation of which is oliguria. Furthermore, anaerobic metabolism is increased, manifesting as metabolic (lactic) acidosis.

Treatment of hemorrhagic shock is with infusion of whole blood. Crystalloid solutions are also indicated, as interstitial fluid shifts accompany acute hemorrhage. Administration of albumin to treat hypoalbuminemia or hypovolemia is controversial despite the fact that low serum albumin concentrations are independent predictors of morbidity.[14] Despite the theoretic advantages for using human albumin solutions as plasma substitutes, studies have shown that correcting hypoalbuminemia has no impact on the outcome in critically ill patients.[14]

Management of patients experiencing hemorrhagic shock often includes monitoring the systemic blood pressure, cardiac filling pressures, and urine output in attempts to optimize intravascular fluid volume replacement. Thermodilution measurements of cardiac output and calculation of systemic vascular resistance are helpful for determining the appropriate therapy. In this regard, dopamine or dobutamine may be useful in selected patients, especially when the goals of therapy include mild inotropic effects plus increased renal blood flow. Vasopressors are used sparingly to treat hemorrhagic shock, although it may be necessary to support cerebral and cardiac perfusion pressures with vasopressors until intravascular fluid volume can be replaced. Persistent metabolic acidosis probably reflects the continued presence of hypovolemia and inadequate oxygen delivery to tissues.

Induction and maintenance of anesthesia in the presence of hemorrhagic shock requires invasive monitoring of systemic blood pressure. Use of ketamine is supported by the known ability of this drug to stimulate the sympathetic nervous system and by the findings of a study in which survival was greater in acutely hemorrhaged rats when they were anesthetized with ketamine than when anesthetized with volatile anesthetics.[15] Nevertheless, other animal evidence suggests that ketamine, in contrast to volatile anesthetics, is associated with inadequate tissue perfusion, as reflected by the development of metabolic acidosis.[16] Clinically, adverse metabolic effects of ketamine may be offset by the benefit of maintaining perfusion pressures to vital organs until intravascular fluid volume can be restored.

Aplastic Anemia

Aplastic anemia refers to bone marrow failure characterized by destruction of rapidly growing cells normally present in the bone marrow.[17] Pancytope-

Table 24–6 • Clinical Signs Associated with Anemia Owing to Acute Blood Loss

Blood volume lost (%)	Signs
10	None
20–30	Orthostatic hypotension
	Tachycardia
	Central venous pressure
40	Hypotension
	Tachycardia
	Tachypnea
	Diaphoresis

nia is the most frequent presentation; in severely affected patients neutrophil counts are less than 200 cells/mm^3, and platelet counts are less than 20,000 cells/mm^3. The most common causes of destruction of bone marrow stem cells are cancer chemotherapeutic drugs and radiotherapy. Drug toxicity is mediated through intermediate metabolites that bind covalently to proteins and DNA. This form of bone marrow depression usually responds to removal of the offending drugs and to supportive treatment with RBC transfusions until surviving stem cells can repopulate the bone marrow. Other causes of aplastic anemia that are less responsive to treatment include solvents, irradiation, viral infections, and immunologic disorders. Severe pancytopenia occasionally occurs 1 to 2 months after an episode of apparent viral hepatitis.

Most patients with aplastic anemia respond favorably to immunosuppressive therapy with antilymphocyte globulin or corticosteroids.[17] An unexplained complication of aplastic anemia is the development of late clonal hematologic diseases (paroxysmal nocturnal hemoglobinuria, myelodysplasia, acute myelogenous leukemia) often 10 years after successful immunosuppressive therapy.

Fanconi Syndrome

Variations of aplastic anemia occur in pediatric patients. For example, Fanconi syndrome comprises congenital aplastic anemia plus numerous associated anomalies, including patchy hyperpigmentation, microcephaly, exaggerated tendon reflexes, strabismus, and short stature. Defects of the bones of the radial sides of the forearms and hands are frequent. Cleft palate may be present, and cardiac defects and abnormalities of the genitourinary tract have been observed. There is an increased incidence of malignancy in these patients. Treatment of Fanconi syndrome is with erythrocytes, corticosteroids, and androgens.

Diamond-Blackfan Syndrome

Diamond-Blackfan syndrome is a form of pure RBC aplasia, presenting as severe anemia during the first few months of life. Leukocyte and platelet production are normal. Anomalies associated with this syndrome include neck webbing and abnormalities of the first digits of the hands. These infants are treated with RBCs and corticosteroids. Splenectomy may be required for patients resistant to corticosteroids. An infantile form of RBC aplasia is associated with thymomas and myasthenia gravis. This association may reflect an immunologic mechanism or the presence of erythropoietic inhibitory factors. Thymec-

tomy cures about 30% of patients with this form of anemia.

Management of Anesthesia

Management of anesthesia for patients with aplastic anemia requires an understanding of the disease process and the drugs being used in its treatment.[18] For example, supplementation with corticosteroids may be necessary during the perioperative period. Anemia may be profound, requiring RBC transfusions before the induction of anesthesia. The vulnerability of these patients to infections in the presence of pancytopenia must be appreciated, and care must be taken to avoid iatrogenic infections from equipment used during the perioperative period. Thrombocytopenia introduces the risk of hemorrhage with even minor trauma. Tracheal intubation should be performed when indicated, but it must be recognized that trauma associated with this procedure could produce hemorrhage in the patient's airway. The choice of drugs used to produce anesthesia is not influenced by the presence of aplastic anemia, although the possible depressant effect of nitrous oxide on bone marrow is a consideration. Maintaining the PaO$_2$ near 100 mmHg and avoiding anesthetic-induced decreases in cardiac output are important goals during anesthesia to ensure optimal tissue oxygenation.

Megaloblastic Anemia

Megaloblastic anemia is most often due to deficiency of vitamin B$_{12}$ (cobalamin) and/or folic acid. Both vitamins must be supplied by the diet, as neither is produced in adequate amounts by intrinsic synthesis.

Vitamin B$_{12}$ Deficiency

Vitamin B$_{12}$ is released from ingested proteins in the stomach by enzymatic proteolysis. Absorption of released vitamin B$_{12}$ is dependent on a glycoprotein produced by the gastric parietal cells known as intrinsic factor. Malabsorption of vitamin B$_{12}$ from the small intestine due to disease or surgical resection is the usual cause of vitamin B$_{12}$ deficiency. In addition, atrophy of the gastric mucosa, presumably due to an autoimmune response, results in the absence of intrinsic factor and subsequent inability to absorb vitamin B$_{12}$. Pernicious anemia refers to megaloblastic anemia that reflects vitamin B$_{12}$ deficiency due to atrophy of the gastric mucosa and to a subsequent lack of intrinsic factor. The demonstration of decreased vitamin B$_{12}$ concentrations confirms the diagnosis of pernicious anemia. Thyroid disorders are more common in patients with pernicious anemia.

In addition to megaloblastic anemia, vitamin B_{12} deficiency is associated with bilateral peripheral neuropathy due to degeneration of the lateral and posterior columns of the spinal cord. There are symmetrical paresthesias with loss of proprioceptive and vibratory sensations, especially in the lower extremities. Gait is unsteady, and deep tendon reflexes are diminished. Memory impairment and mental depression may be prominent. These neurologic deficits are progressive unless parenteral vitamin B_{12} is provided. Nonmedical abuse of nitrous oxide may be associated with neurologic findings similar to those that accompany vitamin B_{12} deficiency and pernicious anemia.[19,20]

Management of anesthesia in patients with megaloblastic anemia due to vitamin B_{12} deficiency is influenced by the need to maintain delivery of oxygenated arterial blood to peripheral tissues. The presence of neurologic changes may detract from selection of regional anesthetic techniques or the use of peripheral nerve blocks. The use of nitrous oxide is questionable, as this drug has been shown to inhibit activity of methionine synthetase by oxidizing the cobalt atom of vitamin B_{12} from an active to an inactive state.[21] Even relatively short exposures to nitrous oxide may produce megaloblastic changes.[22]

Folic Acid Deficiency

Folic acid deficiency is the most common of the vitamin deficiencies. Because folic acid is essential for maturation of RBCs, it is not surprising that megaloblastic anemia develops when there is dietary deficiency of this vitamin. Manifestations of folic acid deficiency include a smooth tongue, hyperpigmentation, mental depression, and peripheral edema. Peripheral neuropathy may or may not accompany these changes. Liver dysfunction frequently occurs. Megaloblastic anemia is most likely to develop in severely ill patients, alcoholics, and parturients owing to deficiencies of folic acid in the diet. Phenytoin and other antiepileptic drugs, including barbiturates, are associated with megaloblastic anemia on rare occasions, presumably reflecting impaired gastrointestinal absorption of folate. Oral folic acid is effective in reversing megaloblastic anemia due to deficiencies of this vitamin.

Hemolytic Anemias

Anemia due to intravascular hemolysis is characterized by rapid decreases in the patient's hematocrit and increased serum concentrations of bilirubin.

Particles released from hemolyzed RBCs may lead to disseminated intravascular coagulation. Causes of hemolysis include abnormalities in the hemoglobin structure, abnormalities of RBC membranes, and RBC enzyme defects. These changes make RBCs so fragile they rupture easily as they pass through capillaries, especially in the spleen. Therefore even though the number of RBCs is normal, the life span (normally 90 to 120 days) is so shortened by the intravascular hemolysis that anemia results.

Sickle Cell Disease

Sickle cell disease represents an inherited disorder that ranges in severity from the usually benign sickle cell trait to the debilitating, often fatal sickle cell anemia.[23] The RBCs of African-Americans who are homozygous for hemoglobin S contain 70% to 98% hemoglobin S, and the development of sickle cell anemia (chronic hemolysis and acute episodic vaso-occlusive crises that may cause organ system failure) is a risk. Anemia is relatively well tolerated perhaps because of enhanced oxygen delivery to tissues by oxyhemoglobin S, as reflected by a rightward shift of the oxyhemoglobin dissociation curve ($P_{50} = 31$ mmHg). In contrast to anemia, sickle cell crises are life-threatening complications of sickle cell disease. About 8% of African-Americans are heterozygous carriers of the sickle cell trait (hemoglobin genotype AS), and about 40% of their hemoglobin is hemoglobin S. These individuals do not have anemia, nor do they need treatment. About 5% of those with sickle cell trait manifest hematuria at some time, and many cannot concentrate their urine; but these are clinically unimportant abnormalities. Confirmation of the presence of hemoglobin S depends on hemoglobin electrophoretic studies.

Pathophysiology

Sickle cell disease reflects the presence of a mutant hemoglobin (hemoglobin S) that is due to a valine substitution for glutamic acid on the β-globulin chain. Hemoglobin S has the singular property of forming insoluble globulin polymers when deoxygenated. Polymerization of hemoglobin S after deoxygenation is the fundamental molecular event that underlies the clinical manifestations of sickle cell disease. Sickle cell trait is benign because the cellular concentration of hemoglobin S is too low for polymerization to occur under most conditions, and it is hemoglobin S polymers that cause the cellular injury characteristic of sickle cell disease. Among hemolytic anemias, the vaso-occlusive features of sickle cell disease are unique.

The initiating event of a sickle cell crisis is unknown, nor is it clear why some patients have severe crises and others do not, although increased circulating concentrations of hemoglobin F may be protective. A low PO_2 is a recognized risk for sickling, and a PaO_2 less than 40 mmHg is likely to result in formation of sickle cells in patients who are homozygous for hemoglobin S. Sickling of RBCs in patients with sickle cell trait probably does not occur until the PaO_2 decreases to about 20 mmHg. The formation of sickle cells tends to be more extensive in veins than in arteries, emphasizing the importance of pH. The presence of acidosis favors the formation of sickle cells regardless of the prevailing PaO_2. A decrease in body temperature or exposure to a cold ambient environment promotes the formation of sickle cells by virtue of vasoconstriction. Likewise, increased blood viscosity, as may accompany dehydration, predisposes to sickling.

Signs and Symptoms

The signs and symptoms of sickle cell disease are due to chronic hemolysis and occlusion of blood vessels with sickle cells. These chronic events are periodically interrupted by acute exacerbations of the disease, which often include excruciating musculoskeletal and/or abdominal pain that may mimic surgical disease. An infarctive crisis may be triggered by trauma and infection, such as that associated with increased body temperature. In addition to infarctive events and hemolysis, patients with sickle cell anemia are susceptible to the development of aplastic and sequestration crises. Aplastic crises are characterized by bone marrow depression and a rapidly decreasing hematocrit, often in association with viral infections. Sequestration crises are due to depletion of circulating RBCs by virtue of pooling of these cells in the liver and spleen. Patients experiencing sequestration crises may become acutely hypovolemic.

Vaso-occlusion. Vaso-occlusion is the single most important pathophysiologic process that results in most of the acute complications of sickle cell disease (Table 24–7).[23, 24] Hemoglobin polymerization is the initial step in this process and significantly increases whole-blood viscosity. Once microvascular occlusion has occurred, the resultant hypoxia causes further sickling and the start of a vicious cycle that results in tissue infarction, release of inflammatory mediators, and pain. Multiple organ system dysfunction produced by infarctive events is the major reason prolonged survival is unlikely. Neurologic dysfunction is likely in patients with sickle cell anemia, manifesting most often as cere-

Table 24–7 • Signs and Symptoms of Sickle Cell Disease

Vaso-occlusive complications
  Painful episodes
  Stroke
  Acute chest syndrome
  Renal insufficiency
  Liver disease
  Splenic sequestration
  Proliferative retinopathy
  Priapism
  Spontaneous abortion
  Leg ulcers
  Osteonecrosis
Complications related to hemolysis
  Anemia (hematocrit 15–30%)
  Cholelithiasis
  Acute aplastic episodes
Infectious complications
  Streptococcus pneumoniae sepsis
  Escherichia coli sepsis
  Osteomyelitis

Adapted from: Steinberg MH. Management of sickle cell disease. N Engl J Med 1999;340:1021–30.

bral infarction in children and as intracranial hemorrhage in adults. Cardiomegaly most likely reflects cor pulmonale owing to repeated pulmonary emboli. Increased alveolar-to-arterial differences for oxygen most likely reflect pulmonary infarctive events. Infarctive events in the renal medulla lead to papillary necrosis with hematuria, impaired ability to concentrate urine, and ultimately renal failure. Hepatic damage may reflect impaired blood flow as a result of sickling in hepatic sinusoids where the PO_2 is low. Increased bilirubin loads from chronic hemolysis are associated with an increased incidence of chronic cholelithiasis. Autoinfarction of the spleen results in functional hyposplenism, which contributes to an increased risk of bacterial infections including osteomyelitis. Pneumococcal vaccine may be indicated as prophylaxis in adults, whereas children may require supplementary penicillin. Aseptic necrosis of the femoral head may necessitate total hip replacement. Chronic hemolysis is associated with poor skeletal growth and decreased fertility.

Acute episodes of severe pain (crises) lasting days or even weeks occur in the chest, abdomen, back, or extremities. Episodes of pain are sometimes triggered by infections, extreme temperatures, or physical or emotional stress; but more often these episodes are unprovoked and begin with little warning. Pain is more likely to start at night, perhaps because of nocturnal oxygen desaturation and relative dehydration. Acute pain crises are often accompanied by fever, but infection is rarely present. The occurrence of fever and leukocytosis in the absence of sepsis suggests that acute pain crises initiate an acute inflammatory syndrome.

Acute Chest Syndrome. The acute chest syndrome is a medical emergency, with mortality approaching 10%.[24] The pathogenesis of this syndrome is not well understood. Typically, patients present with an acute pain crisis, often affecting the lower chest wall. Fever, cough, pleuritic chest pain, arterial hypoxemia, pulmonary hypertension, and radiologic evidence of lung infiltrates especially in the lower bases of the lungs are likely. A substantial number of these patients have rib infarcts. Recurrent episodes of the acute chest syndrome are associated with progressive pulmonary fibrosis and chronic respiratory insufficiency.

Treatment of the acute chest syndrome includes delivery of supplemental oxygen and support of ventilation including continuous positive airway pressure and in some instances mechanical ventilation of the patient's lungs. Early intervention with exchange transfusions to achieve hemoglobin S concentrations less than 30% usually reverses respiratory failure. Inhaled nitric oxide may be beneficial in patients with the acute chest syndrome by dilating the pulmonary vasculature, decreasing the right ventricular afterload, and redistributing pulmonary blood flow to better ventilated areas of the patient's lungs.[25]

Treatment

Treatment for sickle cell disease can be characterized as general measures, treatment directed at the relief of symptoms (painful episodes, transfusions), and treatment directed at the prevention of complications (hydroxyurea, bone marrow transplantation).[23]

General Measures. Pneumococcal sepsis is a leading cause of death among infants with sickle cell anemia because a damaged spleen cannot clear pneumococci from the blood (pneumococcal vaccine is recommended). Antibiotics are often administered to patients with febrile episodes or the acute chest syndrome. Folic acid is prescribed to prevent megaloblastic anemia.

Painful Episodes. There is no standard method for treating pain associated with sickle cell disease, although opioids are often necessary, including patient-controlled analgesia (Table 24–8).[23] Extradural analgesia has been used in the management of acute sickle cell crises. Oral or intravenous fluids are necessary to prevent dehydration, which results in hemoconcentration and increased sickling. Nonsteroidal antiinflammatory drugs are effective for

Table 24–8 • Treatment of Pain in Patients with Sickle Cell Disease

Acute pain
  Fluid replacement (3–4 L daily in adults)
  Initiate analgesic treatment
    Administer opioids (morphine) at fixed intervals to relieve pain
    Administer opioids in smaller doses for breakthrough pain as needed
    Consider patient-controlled analgesia
    Consider use of adjunctive drugs (nonsteroidal antiinflammatory drugs)
    Follow responses with pain scales
Chronic pain
  Acetaminophen with codeine
  Fentanyl patches
  Nonsteroidal antiinflammatory drugs (osteonecrosis pain)

Adapted from: Steinberg MH. Management of sickle cell disease. N Engl J Med 1999;340:1021–30.

treating bone pain, although the presence of liver or renal insufficiency may limit the use of these drugs.

Transfusion. Transfusion of RBCs is not needed for the usual anemia or painful episodes associated with sickle cell disease. The goal of transfusions is to decrease hemoglobin S concentrations to less than 30%. Urgent transfusions are indicated for sudden, severe anemia in children when blood is sequestered in an enlarged spleen. Arterial hypoxemia accompanying the acute chest syndrome necessitates RBC transfusions and supplemental oxygen therapy. It is not clear if exchange transfusions are superior to conventional transfusions in patients with arterial hypoxemia.[23] Patients with renal failure and symptomatic anemia may benefit from transfusions and/or administration of erythropoietin.

Hydroxyurea. Hydroxyurea is effective in the treatment of sickle cell disease and associated anemia by virtue of its ability to stimulate production of hemoglobin F. Increased serum hemoglobin F concentrations decrease the severity of sickle cell disease by preventing the formation of hemoglobin S polymers. Long-term adverse effects of hydroxyurea therapy are unknown, although the incidence of leukemia is increased in patients with erythrocytosis (polycythemia) who are treated with this drug. The optimal dose of hydroxyurea is determined by the balance between hematologic toxicity as reflected by decreased circulating concentrations of granulocytes and platelets and increased serum concentrations of hemoglobin F.

Bone Marrow Transplantation. Bone marrow transplantation is used to treat sickle cell anemia in individuals less than 16 years of age who have experienced repeated serious complications (stroke, acute chest syndrome, refractory pain).

Management of Anesthesia

Anesthesia and surgery represent a special risk to patients with sickle cell disease.[23, 24] For patients undergoing general anesthesia, increasing the hematocrit to 30% with preoperative RBC transfusions is as effective for decreasing postoperative complications as more aggressive transfusion regimens designed to decrease hemoglobin S concentrations to less than 30% (Table 24–9).[23, 24] Therefore in patients undergoing elective procedures of intermediate to high risk, a relatively conservative transfusion program intended to increase the hematocrit to at least 30% (hemoglobin 10 g/dl or higher) is recommended. For minor surgical procedures there appears to be little benefit of preoperative RBC transfusions. In contrast, patients requiring emergency surgery are often at greatest risk for postoperative sickle cell disease-related complications, and optimal transfusion support of these patients often includes consultation with a hematologist. Patients with sickle cell trait do not require preoperative RBC transfusions, except possibly before open heart surgery or extensive thoracic surgery.[23]

Goals in the management of anesthesia include avoidance of circulatory stasis by maintaining hydration and proper patient positioning, maintaining arterial oxygenation, and avoiding acidosis, such as could accompany hypoventilation, as these events are known to trigger sickling in patients with sickle cell disease.[26] Likewise, maintenance of normal body temperature is desirable to minimize vasoconstriction and possible associated circulatory stasis.

Preoperative Period. Preoperative medication must not depress ventilation, which would lead to respiratory acidosis. Concentrations of inspired oxygen are increased to ensure maintenance of a normal to increased PaO_2. Monitoring the mixed venous oxygen partial pressures may be helpful for recognizing patients who are vulnerable to the onset of sickling and in whom therapeutic measures to increase oxygenation might be especially valuable. Administration of supplemental oxygen may be prudent if regional anesthetic techniques are selected. Prevention of circulatory stasis requires maintaining the intravascular fluid volume with intravenous infusion of crystalloid solutions and promptly correcting hypotension, which might interfere with optimal tissue perfusion. Although use of tourniquets on the extremities to provide a bloodless surgical field is generally discouraged in these patients, there is evidence that the use of tourniquets is not always contraindicated.[27] Theoretical hazards introduced by the use of extremity tourniquets include localized circulatory stasis, acidosis, and hypoxia, with the subsequent formation of sickle cells. Overzealous transfusion of RBCs can lead to undesirable increases in the viscosity of the blood, predisposing to circulatory stasis.

There is no evidence that specific anesthetic drugs are optimal for administration to patients with sickle cell disease. Indeed, there may be decreases in the number of circulating sickle cells during and immediately after general anesthesia.[28] Regional anesthetic techniques have been advocated in preference to general anesthesia, but the same precautions regarding ventilation, oxygenation, hypotension, and stasis of blood flow must be appreciated. Epidural or spinal anesthesia produces compensatory vasoconstriction and decreased PaO_2 in the nonblocked areas, making these areas theoretically vulnerable to infarction.[29] Cardiopulmonary bypass, with its attendant low peripheral blood flow plus hypothermia and acidosis, poses unique risks to patients with sickle cell disease. Patients with sickle cell trait seem to tolerate cardiopulmonary bypass with no increased risk.[30]

Postoperative Period. The postoperative period is a critical interval for patients with sickle cell disease. Incisional pain, use of analgesics, a high incidence of pulmonary infections, and expected decreases in arterial oxygenation predispose to sickling. Depending on the operative site, the PaO_2 may not return to preoperative levels for several

---

Table 24–9 • Perioperative Management of Patients with Sickle Cell Disease

Preoperative period
  Admit to hospital 12–24 hours before surgery to permit optimal hydration with intravenous fluids
  Treat obstructive lung disease with bronchodilators
  Transfuse to increase the hematocrit to 30% (not necessary before minor operations)
Intraoperative period
  Maintain arterial oxygenation
  Maintain hydration
  Maintain body temperature
  Replace blood loss when necessary
Postoperative period
  Maintain arterial oxygenation
  Continue intravenous fluids for hydration
  Consider incentive spirometry
  Consider overnight observation in the hospital

Adapted from: Steinberg MH. Management of sickle cell disease. N Engl J Med 1999;340:1021–30.

days. Supplemental oxygen and maintenance of intravascular fluid volume and body temperature are important considerations. The acute chest syndrome may occur as a postoperative complication, with a peak occurrence 48 hours after surgery.[23] Intraoperative arterial hypoxemia may cause postoperative acute chest syndrome. Postoperative analgesia; is often provided with patient-controlled analgesia; and in selected patients neuraxial opioids are useful.

Hemolytic Spherocytosis

Hereditary spherocytosis is characterized by abnormalities of RBC membranes that permit sodium to enter RBCs at an increased rate. Water enters the RBCs as well, resulting in swollen or spherocytic cells. These spherical cells, in contrast to normal biconcave RBCs, cannot be compressed and are vulnerable to rupture (hemolysis) with even slight compression as they pass through the spleen.

Anemia, reticulocytosis, and mild jaundice are characteristic expressions of hereditary spherocytosis. Infection or folic acid deficiency may trigger a hemolytic crisis with profound anemia, vomiting, and abdominal pain. Anemia and hyperbilirubinemia may be manifestations of this disease in neonates. Children with this defect may present with chronic mild anemia plus episodic decreases in hematocrit, particularly during bacterial infections. In elderly patients who have previously been able to compensate for these abnormalities, anemia may develop in response to the decreased ability to produce RBCs that accompanies aging. Cholelithiasis secondary to chronic hemolysis and increases in plasma bilirubin concentrations are common in patients with hereditary spherocytosis.

Treatment of patients with hereditary spherocytosis includes splenectomy if the anemia is severe. Splenectomy greatly decreases hemolysis, returning RBC survival to 80% of normal. Splenectomy, however, may be followed by an increased incidence of bacterial infections, especially with pneumococci, in these patients. Prophylactic pneumococcal vaccine may thus be indicated.

Paroxysmal Nocturnal Hemoglobinuria

Paroxysmal nocturnal hemoglobinuria is a rare acquired disorder characterized by acute episodes of thrombosis and complement-mediated hemolysis superimposed on a background of chronic hemolysis. The defect resulting in hemolysis is an abnormal sensitivity of RBC membranes to lytic actions of complement proteins.

Classically, patients are young adults who experience hemoglobinuria on first voiding after awakening. Nocturnal exacerbation of hemoglobinuria is presumed to reflect carbon dioxide retention and acidosis, leading to activation of complement proteins. There is a striking predisposition for venous thrombosis, especially involving the hepatic, splenic, portal, and cerebral veins reflecting a hypercoagulable state (see Table 25–3). Progressive diffuse hepatic vein thrombosis (Budd-Chiari syndrome) may be rapidly fatal. Thrombotic episodes have been attributed to direct activation of platelets by complement proteins.

Anesthesia may be a risk factor for hemoglobinuria in these patients should acidosis develop.[31] Surgery with associated trauma and venous stasis may accentuate the risk of thrombotic episodes. In this regard, preoperative hydration and treatment of precipitating factors such as sepsis are recommended.[32] Vigorous attempts to prevent infection are important for decreasing the likelihood of complement protein activation. There is no evidence that any specific anesthetic techniques or drugs are preferable, but maintenance of intraoperative hydration is important.[32] Because postoperative thrombosis is a risk, it has been suggested that anticoagulation with warfarin (Coumadin) be considered. Use of heparin for anticoagulation is controversial, as low doses may activate complement pathways. If RBC transfusions are needed, saline-washed RBCs may be selected to decrease the risk of leukocyte sensitization, antibody production against human leukocyte antigens, and reactions that may activate complement proteins.[31] Alternatively, administration of type-specific fresh RBCs is acceptable.

Glucose-6-Phosphate Dehydrogenase Deficiency

Glucose-6-phosphate dehydrogenase deficiency is the most common inherited RBC enzyme disorder.[33] This enzyme defect affects about 10% of African-American males in the United States. The gene for glucose-6-phosphate dehydrogenase enzyme is on the X chromosome, accounting for the predominance of this enzyme defect in males.

Chronic hemolytic anemia is the most common clinical manifestation of glucose-6-phosphate dehydrogenase deficiency. Drugs that form peroxides by interactions with oxyhemoglobin can trigger hemolysis in these patients (Table 24–10). Normally, these peroxides are inactivated by nicotinamide adenine dinucleotide phosphate (NADPH) and glutathione, produced by metabolic processes that depend on the enzymatic activity of glucose-6-phosphate dehydrogenase. The onset of disseminated intravascular coagulation may accompany drug-induced hemolysis. Although drugs used during anesthesia have not been incriminated as triggering agents, the onset

Table 24–10 • Drugs That May Induce Hemolysis in Patients with Glucose-6-Phosphate Dehydrogenase Deficiency

Nonopioid analgesics
    Phenacetin
    Acetaminophen
Antibiotics
    Nitrofurans
    Penicillin
    Streptomycin
    Chloramphenical
    Isoniazid
Sulfonamides
Antimalarial drugs
Miscellaneous
    Probenecid
    Quinidine
    Vitamin K analogues
    Methylene blue
    Nitroprusside (?)

of hemolysis and jaundice during the early postoperative period, especially in African-American males, suggest consideration of this diagnosis.[34] There is considerable variability in the hemolytic response to drugs; many drugs, such as aspirin, induce hemolysis only in large doses.

Pyruvate Kinase Deficiency

Pyruvate kinase deficiency is the most common of the enzyme defects in the anaerobic glycolytic pathway of RBCs. The results of this enzyme defect are RBC membranes that are highly permeable to potassium and vulnerable to rupture, as evidenced by the development of hemolytic anemia. Accumulation of 2,3-diphosphoglycerate in RBCs causes a shift of the oxyhemoglobin dissociation curve to the right to facilitate oxygen release from hemoglobin to the peripheral tissues. Splenectomy does not prevent hemolysis but does serve to decrease the rate of RBC destruction. Despite increased permeability of RBC membranes to potassium, the administration of succinylcholine has not been associated with hyperkalemia.

Immune Hemolytic Anemia

Immune hemolytic anemia is characterized by immunologic alterations in RBC membranes. An important aspect of evaluating patients with suspected immune hemolytic anemias is the Coombs' test. Coombs' antibody is an antibody to human immunoglobulin G. With the direct Coombs' test, antiserum is added to a sample of blood from the patient. The indirect Coombs' test consists of adding antiserum to a sample of plasma from the patient, to which have been added RBCs of known antigenicity. Clumping of RBCs in response to the added antiserum indicates the presence of antibodies to RBCs. This reaction is designated a positive direct or indirect Coombs' test. Immune hemolytic anemia may be due to drugs, diseases, or sensitization of RBCs.

Drug-Induced Hemolysis

α-Methyldopa causes time- and dose-dependent production of immunoglobulin G antibodies directed against Rh antigens on the surfaces of RBCs. Indeed, a positive direct Coombs' test is often present in patients being treated with α-methyldopa, but hemolysis occurs in fewer than 1% of patients receiving this drug. The mechanism for drug-induced stimulation of antibody production by α-methyldopa is unknown. Treatment consists of withdrawing the drug, which results in a rapid increase in the hemoglobin concentration, although the direct Coombs' test may remain positive for as long as 2 years.

High-dose penicillin therapy can also lead to hemolysis by attaching to RBCs to form haptens, which leads to the production of antibodies. Levodopa also occasionally produces an autoimmune hemolytic anemia.

Disease-Induced Hemolysis

Hypersplenism is a disease process that can be associated with hemolysis, anemia, leukopenia, and thrombocytopenia. It is presumed that an enlarged spleen has an increased blood flow and vascular surface area, exposing an unusually large proportion of RBCs and platelets to attack by phagocytes. For unknown reasons, hypersplenism produces marked increases in plasma volume, which results in dilutional anemia in addition to hemolytic anemia. Splenectomy may be necessary when anemia due to hemolysis is severe. If thrombocytopenia is present, it may be desirable to infuse platelets intraoperatively after the splenic pedicle has been surgically clamped.

Sensitization of RBCs

Sensitization of RBCs most often manifests as hemolytic disease of the newborn (erythroblastosis fetalis). Hemolysis of fetal RBCs occurs when maternal antibodies against fetal RBCs are produced and cross the placenta. Differences in the maternal and fetal ABO blood groups can cause this form of hemolysis. Severe anemia does not usually occur, however, because ABO antibodies are of the immunoglobulin M class and, as such, do not readily cross the placenta. More often, maternal development of antibodies to Rh antigens occurs after delivery of an Rh-positive infant. During subsequent pregnancies, RBCs of an Rh-positive fetus may undergo significant hemolysis from maternal antibodies directed against Rh antigens. The incidence of the development of maternal anti-Rh antibodies has decreased to less than 1% since the introduction of Rh-immune globulin (RhoGAM). This substance, when given to parturients within 72 hours of delivery, destroys fetal RBCs in the maternal circulation, preventing subsequent development of sensitization.

Clinical features of hemolytic disease of the newborn are related to anemia and hyperbilirubinemia. The fetus can be examined indirectly during gestation by periodic measurements of bilirubin concentrations in amniotic fluid samples. A fetus determined to be experiencing severe hemolysis may require intrauterine RBC transfusions or induced delivery. Hemolysis may continue after delivery, requiring fetal RBC transfusions. In addition, exchange transfusions of blood may be necessary to decrease serum concentrations of bilirubin in the newborn. Eventually maternal immunoglobulins against Rh antigens are excreted by the newborn, and hemolysis of RBCs ceases.

Hemoglobin Hammersmith

Hemoglobin Hammersmith is a rare unstable abnormal hemoglobin with low oxygen affinity. Hemolytic anemia is severe, requiring frequent RBC transfusions. These hemolytic episodes may be precipitated by systemic infections including tonsillitis. These patients are often chronically icteric. Monitoring during anesthesia may be complicated by hemoglobin Hammersmith interfering with the accurate functioning of conventional pulse oximetry (falsely low SpO_2, as hemoglobin Hammersmith is read as deoxyhemoglobin).[35]

Anemia Due to Temporary Formation of Abnormal Hemoglobins

There are more than 600 known hemoglobins with primary structural abnormalities (dyshemoglobins). Acute exposure to certain drugs may predispose genetically susceptible patients to the formation of hemoglobins that cannot optimally bind hemoglobin. Abnormal hemoglobins may be associated with altered absorption spectra resulting in erroneously low SpO_2 readings using pulse oximetry in the presence of methemoglobinemia and sulfhemoglobi-

nemia. In contrast, carboxyhemoglobin is read by conventional pulse oximetry as oxyhemoglobin.

Methemoglobinemia

Methemoglobin is hemoglobin A in which iron exists in the ferric rather than the normal ferrous state. The ferric form of iron is unable to bind oxygen. As a result, the oxygen-carrying capacity of arterial blood is decreased. In addition to an inability to combine reversibly with oxygen, methemoglobin shifts the oxyhemoglobin dissociation curve to the left, making it more difficult to release oxygen to tissues. Normally, methemoglobin concentrations are less than 1% owing to the effects of methemoglobin reductase enzyme. Congenital absence of this enzyme may predispose to the development of methemoglobinemia in patients receiving nitrate-containing compounds (nitroglycerin, benzocaine).[36, 37]

The diagnosis of methemoglobinemia is suggested by cyanosis in the presence of normal PaO_2 levels but low measured SaO_2 concentrations. Calculation of SaO_2 based on the measured PaO_2 using a nomogram does not detect the discrepancy between these two values, emphasizing the importance of measuring both PaO_2 and SaO_2 when methemoglobinemia is suspected. Decreased SpO_2 values, measured by pulse oximetry, associated with normal PaO_2 values may alert the anesthesiologist to the possible presence of methemoglobinemia. This occurs because the absorbance characteristics of methemoglobin are such that the pulse oximeter reads an SpO_2 of about 85% regardless of the PaO_2.[38] Cyanosis is usually present when plasma methemoglobin concentrations are about 15% (1.5 g/dl), although symptoms (lethargy, dizziness, headache) are unlikely to be present at methemoglobin levels of less than 20%.

Treatment of cyanosis caused by methemoglobinemia is with methylene blue, 1 mg/kg IV administered over 5 minutes, which transfers electrons from NADPH to methemoglobin. This dose may be repeated every 60 minutes if cyanosis persists, but it must be appreciated that methylene blue doses in excess of about 7 mg/kg may oxidize hemoglobin to methemoglobin. Recurrence of cyanosis after several hours presumably reflects release of nitrates from tissues into the peripheral blood. Methylene blue should not be administered to patients with glucose-6-phosphate dehydrogenase deficiency, as hemolysis may occur.

Sulfhemoglobinemia

Sulfhemoglobinemia, a rare cause of cyanosis, is usually drug-induced, reflecting oxidation of iron in hemoglobin by drugs.[39, 40] Drugs that stimulate the formation of methemoglobin are also capable of producing sulfhemoglobin. Sulfhemoglobinemia has been described in patients on both short-term and long-term metoclopramide therapy. The reason some patients develop sulfhemoglobinemia and others methemoglobinemia is not known. That sulfhemoglobinemia exists is suggested by the presence of decreased SpO_2 values, measured by pulse oximetry, despite normal PaO_2 levels.[40]

Sulfhemoglobin at a dose of 0.5 g/dl is needed to cause clinical cyanosis, compared with 1.5 g of methemoglobin per deciliter and 5 g of dexoxyhemoglobin per deciliter. Sulfhemoglobin cannot carry oxygen, but high concentrations of sulfhemoglobin are well tolerated because of a rightward shift of the oxyghemoglobin dissociation curve for normal hemoglobin, thus facilitating the release of oxygen to tissues. This is in contrast to methemoglobin, which causes a leftward shift of the oxyhemoglobin dissociation curve.

In contrast to methemoglobinemia, there is no pharmacologic treatment for sulfhemoglobinemia. The only means of removing sulfhemoglobin is by eventual destruction of the affected RBCs.

Myelodysplastic Syndrome

Myelodysplastic syndrome is a hematologic disorder characterized by cytopenia in the peripheral blood and normal to hypercellularity in the bone marrow with morphologic dysplastic changes.[41] Hemorrhage secondary to thrombocytopenia and infection secondary to leukopenia are the principal causes of morbidity in affected individuals. Uncontrolled bleeding may accompany surgery such as cesarean section. Regional anesthesia is avoided because of the risk of epidural bleeding associated with thrombocytopenia.

▮ POLYCYTHEMIA

Polycythemia (erythrocytosis) is defined as an increased number of circulating RBCs reflected as an increased hematocrit and elevated hemoglobin concentration. Major categories are relative polycythemia, secondary polycythemia, and primary polycythemia (polycythemia vera).[42]

Relative Polycythemia

Relative polycythemia most often occurs in middle-aged, obese, hypertensive men who have a chronic history of smoking ("smoker's polycythemia"). It is estimated that 0.5% to 0.7% of the normal male population in the United States manifests relative polycythemia. Increased production of RBCs most likely reflects a response to chronic decreases in the patient's PaO_2 to less than 60 mmHg. In addition, diuretics used to treat essential hypertension may accentuate plasma volume deficits and increases in hematocrit. Hematocrit values are usually less than 55%.

Smoker's polycythemia is another entity. Smoking generates carbon monoxide, leading to carboxyhemoglobin levels of 5% to 7% in those who smoke 30 cigarettes daily. In these patients, carboxyhemoglobin is unable to unload and transport oxygen, leading to the formation of hemoglobin that unloads oxygen poorly to peripheral tissues (P_{50} less than 26 mmHg). The end result is tissue hypoxia, which stimulates the production and release of erythropoietin. In addition, many cigarette smokers experience decreased plasma volume, contributing further to an increased hematocrit. The diagnosis of smoker's polycythemia is confirmed by measuring plasma carboxyhemoglobin concentrations at the end of the day. Because the carboxyhemoglobin half-time is about 4 hours, measurements obtained on arising in the morning following a period of cigarette abstinence, may give falsely low values. Cessation of smoking for about 5 days usually corrects the decreased plasma volume, and the hematocrit decreases.

Secondary Polycythemia

Polycythemia may occur when erythropoietin production is increased as a result of an appropriate compensatory response to chronic tissue hypoxia, as is seen at high altitude or with cardiopulmonary disease, obesity-hypoventilation syndrome, obstructive sleep apnea, or increased serum concentrations of carboxyhemoglobin. Increased erythropoietin production may accompany renal dysfunction and less often hepatic disorders. Because of the intricate regulation of erythropoietin production in the kidneys, distortion of renal anatomy (renal cysts, hydronephrosis, Bartter syndrome, renal cell carcinoma) can result in polycythemia. Androgens (testosterone) stimulate erythropoietin production by the kidneys and may lead to secondary polycythemia. Surreptitous injection of recombinant human erythropoietin to enhance athletic performance may be hazardous, as unmonitored increases in RBC production may cause significant polycythemia, which when combined with exercise-induced dehydration can be fatal.[42]

Primary Polycythemia (Polycythemia Vera)

Primary polycythemia is a neoplastic disorder that originates from a single neoplastic hematopoietic stem cell. This disease is slightly more common in men, and the incidence peaks at age 50 to 75 years. Polycythemia vera is considered one of a group of related stem cell disorders known as myeloproliferative disorders that include chronic myeloid leukemia, essential thrombocytopenia, and agnogenic myeloid metaplasia.

Signs and Symptoms

The natural history of polycythemia vera includes a latent, relatively asymptomatic prothrombotic phase followed by an overt proliferative phase during which the RBC mass expands and patients may manifest symptoms related to hyperviscosity (headache, cognitive dysfunction, weakness) and hypermetabolic changes (fever, weight loss, excessive diaphoresis). Erythromelalgia, episodic severe burning pain, and erythema in the fingers or toes are caused by digital ischemia and are highly suggestive of a myeloproliferative disorder. Physical examination usually reflects facial plethora, which is common to all patients with polycythemia. Diastolic hypertension is observed in about one-third of patients. Hepatosplenomegaly is likely to be present.

Laboratory Diagnosis

Hematocrit values higher than 60% in men or 57% in women are virtually diagnostic of primary or secondary polycythemia. There is a high prevalence of gastrointestinal bleeding in patients with polycythemia vera, which may result in a normal hematocrit. Leukocytosis and thrombocytosis are common. Serum uric acid concentrations are increased owing to the chronically increased production and destruction of RBCs. Bone marrow examination is not necessary for the diagnosis of polycythemia vera.

Treatment

The initial treatment of polycythemia vera includes phlebotomy with removal of 500 ml of blood one or two times a week until the target hematocrit value of less than 46% is achieved.[42] Iron deficiency anemia often develops and contributes to limiting the patient's ability to produce RBCs and the need for repeated phlebotomy. Myelosuppressive drugs such as hydroxyurea may be used in combination with phlebotomy, especially in patients considered to be at increased risk for thrombosis. Busulfan is an alternative to hydroxyurea. Administration of aspirin in an attempt to decrease the risk of thrombosis is not effective and increases the risk of gastrointestinal bleeding.

Complications

Bleeding and thrombosis (arterial and venous) are potential complications in patients with polycythemia vera who undergo surgery. These complications can be minimized by optimizing the patient's hematocrit prior to elective surgery. The hematocrit should be less than 46% to decrease the risk of thrombosis. Platelets are derived from the neoplastic clone cell and may not function normally, resulting in thrombosis or bleeding (bruising, epistaxis, gastrointestinal bleeding). Although platelets are often present in excess in patients with polycythemia vera, there is no clear relation between the absolute platelet count and the risk of thrombosis.

Clinical manifestations of thrombosis include myocardial infarction, ischemic stroke, transient ischemic attacks, peripheral arterial thrombosis, and deep vein thrombosis. Patients often note exacerbation of angina pectoris as their hematocrit increases. Hepatic vein thrombosis may occur, resulting in Budd-Chiari syndrome. A feared complication of polycythemia vera is its evolution to acute myeloid leukemia. Because of hyperuricemia, patients with polycythemia vera are at increased risk of developing gout or nephrolithiasis.

About 15% to 20% of patients with polycythemia vera progress to postpolycythemic myeloid metaplasia characterized by replacement of bone marrow with reticulin fibrosis. In these patients, hematopoiesis occurs in the liver and spleen, and hepatosplenomegaly may be massive. Splenic pain and infarction may accompany splenomegaly. Patients become progressively pancytopenic. Hypermetabolic symptoms (weight loss, chills, fever) and pruritus may respond to hydroxyurea.

■ DISORDERS OF LEUKOCYTES

Leukocytes are categorized as neutrophils, lymphocytes, eosinophils, basophils, and monocytes (Table 24–11). Certain clinical disorders alter the normal

Table 24–11 • Leukocyte Values in Peripheral Blood

Leukocyte	Range (cells/mm³)	Total (%)
Neutrophils	1800–7200	55
Lymphocytes	1500–4000	36
Eosinophils	0–700	2
Basophils	0–150	1
Monocytes	200–900	6

circulating concentrations of leukocytes (4,300–10,000 cells/mm³) in the peripheral blood.

Neutrophils

Neutrophils (polymorphonuclear leukocytes) are the first line of defense against bacterial infections, as they are attracted to sites of inflammation by chemotaxis. An important chemotaxic stimulus for migration of neutrophils to sites of inflammation is C5a, which is produced via activation of the complement system by combinations of bacterial antigens and antibodies. A variety of events may impair chemotaxis (diabetes mellitus, hemodialysis, alcohol ingestion, influenza, anesthetic drugs), predisposing patients for infections such as pneumonia. Despite the ability of anesthetic drugs to impair chemotaxis, there is no evidence that general anesthesia increases the risk of postoperative infections (see Chapter 27).

Neutrophilia most often reflects increased production of cells as a result of bacterial infection. Impaired egress of neutrophils from the systemic circulation is produced by exercise and corticosteroids. Neutropenia (neutrophil count less than 1800 cells/mm³) is common in patients with infectious mononucleosis and acquired immunodeficiency syndrome (AIDS). Chemotherapy may lead to neutropenia as a reflection of direct bone marrow suppression.

Administration of granulocyte colony-stimulating factors in efforts to increase granulocyte production are considerations in patients with neutropenia caused by chemotherapy, AIDS, thermal injury, or sepsis. Adverse effects of this treatment relevant to the management of anesthesia include pericardial and pleural effusions and generalized capillary leak syndromes, which may result in interstitial pulmonary edema and arterial hypoxemia.[43]

Lymphocytes

Lymphocytes are important in the production of immunoglobulins and recognition of foreign proteins. Lymphocytosis is typically associated with viral infections. Lymphocytopenia is a common finding in patients with AIDS.

Eosinophils

Eosinophils contain proteins that are toxic to parasites. Eosinophilia may accompany allergic reactions, fungal infections, and diseases such as polyar-

teritis nodosa and sarcoidosis.[44] Decreases in circulating serum eosinophil concentrations are not common signs of underlying disease.

Loffler Syndrome

Loffler syndrome is reflected in eosinophilia plus pulmonary infiltrates, cough, dyspnea, and increased body temperature. The syndrome is treated with corticosteroids.

Hypereosinophilic Syndrome

Hypereosinophilic syndrome is associated with cardiomyopathy, ataxia, peripheral neuropathy, and recurrent thromboembolism that may necessitate anticoagulation. Postoperative complications, including acute respiratory failure and coagulopathy, have been described in a patient with markedly increased eosinophil counts. In view of these complications, it may be useful to provide perioperative steroid coverage to patients presenting with eosinophilia prior to elective surgery.[45] Corticosteroids are effective by virtue of inhibiting eosinophil chemotaxis, adherence, and degranulation, thereby preventing the release of cytotoxic chemical mediators.

Basophils and Mast Cells

Basophils are circulating cells, whereas mast cells are predominantly present in tissues. These cells contain granules that release chemical mediators (histamine, leukotrienes, tryptase) during allergic reactions. Tryptase has no known physiologic function, and its presence in the circulation is confirmation that degranulation owing to an anaphylactic but not an anaphylactoid reaction has occurred.[46, 47]

Monocytes

Monocytes and their tissue counterparts macrophages are collectively referred to as the mononuclear phagocytic system (formerly known as the reticuloendothelial system). These cells are important in modifying immune function and may also act as phagocytes. Substances secreted by activated monocytes and macrophages include interleukin-1, tumor necrosis factor, interferon, and transforming growth factor.

References

1. Beutler E. The common anemias. JAMA 1988;259:2433–7
2. Chen AY, Carson JL. Perioperative management of anaemia. Br J Anaesth 1998;81:20–4

3. Practice guidelines for blood component therapy: a report by the American Society of Anesthesiologists Task Force on Blood Component Therapy. Anesthesiology 1996;84:732–47

4. American College of Physicians: Practice strategies for elective red blood cell transfusion. Ann Intern Med 1992;116:404–6

5. Grindon AJ, Tomasulo PS, Bergin JJ, et al. The hospital transfusion committee. JAMA 1985;253:540–3

6. Consensus Conference. Perioperative red blood cell transfusion. JAMA 1988;260:2700–3

7. Williams EL, Hart WM, Tempelhoff R. Postoperative ischemic optic neuropathy. Anesth Analg 1995;80:1018–29

8. Weiskopf RB, Viele MK, Feiner J, et al. Human cardiovascular and metabolic response to acute, severe, isovolemic anemia. JAMA 1988;279:217–21

9. Bak Z, Abildgard L, Lisander B, et al. Transesophageal echocardiographic hemodynamic monitoring during preoperative acute normovolemic hemodilution. Anesthesiology 2000;92:1250–6

10. Crosby ET. Perioperative haemotherapy. I. Indications for blood component transfusion. Can J Anaesth 1992;39:695–707

11. Ickx BE, Rigolet M, Van der Lingen P. Cardiovascular and metabolic response to acute normovolemic anemia: effects of anesthesia. Anesthesiology 2000;93:1011–6

12. Lerman J, Gregory GA, Eger EI. Hematocrit and the solubility of volatile anesthetics in blood. Anesth Analg 1984;63:911–4

13. Adamson J, Hillman RS. Blood volume and plasma protein replacement following acute blood loss in normal man. JAMA 1968;205:609–13

14. Nicholson JP, Wolmarans MR, Park GR. The role of albumin in critical illness. Br J Anaesth 2000;85:599–610

15. Longnecker DE, Sturgill BC. Influence of anesthetic agent on survival following hemorrhage. Anesthesiology 1976;45:516–21

16. Weiskopf RB, Townsley MI, Riordan KK, et al. Comparison of cardiopulmonary responses to graded hemorrhage during enflurane, halothane, isoflurane, and ketamine anesthesia. Anesth Analg 1981;160:481–91

17. Young NS, Maciejewski J. The pathophysiology of acquired aplastic anemia. N Engl J Med 1997;336:1365–72

18. Bruce DL, Koepke JA. Anesthetic management of patients with bone-marrow failure. Anesth Analg 1972;51:597–606

19. Kripke BJ, Talarico L, Shah NK, et al. Hematologic reaction to prolonged exposure to nitrous oxide. Anesthesiology 1977;47:342–8

20. Spence AA. Environmental pollution by inhalation anaesthetics. Br J Anaesth 1987;59:96–109

21. Koblin DD, Watson JE, Deady JE, et al. Inactivation of methionine synthetase by nitrous oxide in mice. Anesthesiology 1981;54:318–24

22. Berger JJ, Modell JH, Sypert GW. Megaloblastic anemia and brief exposure to nitrous oxide: a causal relationship? Anesth Analg 1988;67:197–8

23. Steinberg MH. Management of sickle cell disease. N Engl J Med 1999;340:1021–30

24. Vijay V, Cavenagh JD, Yate P. The anaesthetist's role in acute sickle cell crisis. Br J Anaesth 1998;80:820–8

25. Atz AM, Wessel DL. Inhaled nitric oxide in sickle cell disease with acute chest syndrome. Anesthesiology 1997;87:988–90

26. Esseltine DW, Baxter MRN, Bevan JC. Sickle cell states and the anaesthetist. Can J Anaesth 1988;35:385–403

27. Adu-Gyamfi Y, Sankarankutty M, Marwa S. Use of a tourniquet in patients with sickle-cell disease. Can J Anaesth 1993;40:24–7

28. Maduska AL, Guinee WS, Heaton JA, et al. Sickling dynamics of red blood cells and other physiologic studies during anesthesia. Anesth Analg 1975;54:361–5

29. Bridenbaugh PO, Moore DC, Bridenbaugh LD. Alterations in capillary and venous blood gases after regional-block anesthesia. Anesth Analg 1972;51:280–6

30. Djaiani GN, Cheng DCH, Carroll JA, et al. Fast-track cardiac anesthesia in patients with sickle cell abnormalities. Anesth Analg 1999;89:598–603

31. Kathirvel S, Prakash A, Lokesh BN, et al. The anesthetic management of a patient with paroxysmal nocturnal hemoglobinuria. Anesth Analg 2000;91:1029–31

32. Ogen GA. Cholecystectomy in a patient with paroxysmal nocturnal hemoglobinuria: anesthetic implications and management in the perioperative period. Anesthesiology 1990;72:761–4

33. Beutler E. Glucose-6-phosphate dehydrogenase deficiency. N Engl J Med 1991;324:169–75

34. Shapley JM, Wilson JR. Post-anaesthetic jaundice due to glucose-6-phosphate dehydrogenase deficiency. Can Anaesth Soc J 1973;20:390–2

35. Lang SA, Chang PC, Laxdal VA, et al. Haemoglobin Hammersmith precludes monitoring with conventional pulse oximetry. Can J Anaesth 1994;41:965–8

36. Gabel RA, Bunn HF. Hereditary methemoglobinemia as a cause of cyanosis during anesthesia. Anesthesiology 1974;40:516–8

37. Zurick AM, Wagner RH, Starr NJ, et al. Intravenous nitroglycerin, methemoglobinemia, and respiratory distress in a postoperative cardiac surgical patient. Anesthesiology 1984;61:464–6

38. Anderson ST, Hajduczek J, Barker SJ. Benzocaine-induced methemoglobinemia in an adult: accuracy of pulse oximetry with methemoglobinemia. Anesth Analg 1988;67:1099–1101

39. Schmitter CR. Sulfhemoglobinemia and methemoglobinemia: uncommon causes of cyanosis. Anesthesiology 1975;43:586–7

40. Aravindhan N, Chisholm DG. Sulfhemoglobinemia presenting as pulse oximetry desaturation. Anesthesiology 2000;93:883–4

41. Hara K, Saito Y, Morimoto N, et al. Anaesthetic management of caesarean section in a patient with myelodysplastic syndrome. Can J Anaesth 1998;45:157–63

42. Broudy VC. The polycythemias. Sci Am Med 1996;1–12

43. Tobias JD, Furman WL. Anesthetic considerations in patients receiving colony-stimulating factors (G-CSF and GM-SCF). Anesthesiology 1991;75:536–8

44. Rothenberg ME. Eosinophilia. N Engl J Med 1998;338:1592–1600

45. Samsoon G, Wood ME, Kinght-George AB, et al. General anaesthesia and the hypereosinophilia syndrome: severe postoperative complications in two patients. Br J Anaesth 1992;69:653–6

46. Laroche D, Vergnaud MC, Sillard B, et al. Biochemical markers of anaphylactoid reactions to drugs; comparison of plasma histamine and tryptase. Anesthesiology 1991;75:945–9

47. Renz CL, Laroche D, Thurn JD, et al. Tryptase levels are not increased during vancomycin-induced anaphylactoid reactions. Anesthesiology 1998;89:620–5

25

Coagulopathies

Coagulopathies may be hereditary or acquired (Table 25–1). Preoperative evaluation of patients for the presence of coagulation disorders includes the history, physical examination, and performance of appropriate laboratory tests. Careful exclusion of coagulation defects before the induction of anesthesia facilitates the differential diagnosis of intraoperative bleeding. One of the most important questions to ask preoperatively deals with hemostatic responses to prior operations (tonsillectomy, dental extractions). A history of drug ingestion (aspirin, oral anticoagulants) is confirmed. Physical examination may indicate the presence of petechiae, suggesting thrombocytopenia, abnormal platelet function, or defects in the integrity of the vascular walls.

Preoperative laboratory tests that constitute a screening coagulation profile are useful when the history or physical examination suggests the possibility of coagulation disorders, anticoagulant or antiplatelet drugs are being administered, coexisting diseases (hepatic, renal) are present that could alter coagulation, or the scheduled surgery may alter coagulation (cardiopulmonary bypass, liver transplantation). There is no evidence that preoperative performance of coagulation tests in asymptomatic patients is of any value.[1] When coagulation tests are indicated, the bleeding time, platelet count, prothrombin time (PT), activated partial thromboplastin time (PTT), and plasma fibrinogen concentration can provide information regarding all phases of coagulation (Table 25–2). To compensate for varying sensitivities of different thromboplastins utilized to determine the PT and thus permit comparison of values between laboratories, the international normalized ratio (INR) has been introduced.

Table 25–1 • Categorization of Coagulation Disorders

Hereditary
  Hemophilia A
  Hemophilia B
  Von Willebrand's disease
  Afibrinogenemia
  Factor V deficiency
  Factor VIII deficiency
  Hereditary hemorrhagic telangiectasia
  Protein C deficiency
  Antithrombin III deficiency
Acquired
  Disseminated intravascular coagulation
  Perioperative anticoagulation
  Intraoperative coagulopathies
    Dilutional thrombocytopenia
    Dilution of procoagulants
    Massive blood transfusions
    Type of surgery (cardiopulmonary bypass, brain trauma, orthopedic surgery, urologic surgery, obstetric delivery)
  Drug-induced hemorrhage
  Drug-induced platelet dysfunction
  Idiopathic thrombocytopenic purpura
  Thrombotic thrombocytopenic purpura
  Catheter-induced thrombocytopenia
  Vitamin K deficiency

Thromboelastography (TEG) may be considered in selected patients, especially if rapid perioperative evaluation of coagulation is desired. This test evaluates overall clot formation as a dynamic process, unlike standard coagulation tests, which measure isolated endpoints, permitting the diagnosis of procoagulant deficiencies (hemophilia), platelet dysfunction, fibrinolysis (disseminated intravascular coagulation, DIC), and hypercoagulation within 30 minutes of obtaining blood samples (Figs. 25–1, 25–2).[2, 3] TEG has been used extensively for coagulation monitoring during liver transplantation and may have applications in other clinical settings, including cardiovascular surgery, obstetric anesthesia, and trauma anesthesia (massive transfusion). Despite these potential applications, TEG has not achieved widespread use in the United States.[4]

HEREDITARY COAGULATION DISORDERS

Hereditary (congenital) coagulation disorders are usually due to the absence or decreased presence of a single procoagulant.[5] The three most common hereditary coagulating disorders are hemophilia A (factor VIII deficiency, classic hemophilia), hemophilia B (factor IX deficiency, Christmas disease), and von Willebrand's disease. Most often management of coagulation therapy for patients with hereditary coagulation disorders undergoing surgery is coordinated in consultation with a hematologist.

Hemophilia A

Hemophilia A is an X-linked recessive genetic disorder affecting approximately 2 per 10,000 male births, making it the most common hereditary coagulation disorder. The genetic defect results in the absence, severe deficiency, or defective functioning of plasma coagulation factor VIII (antihemophilia factor). Hemophilia A is the result of recent genetic mutations in approximately one-third of patients, such that no family history of bleeding disorders is present.

Signs and Symptoms

Hemophilia A is a clinically heterogeneous coagulation disorder reflecting the large number of molecular defects in the factor VIII gene. It is important to distinguish patients with severe hemophilia A, whose plasma has no detectable factor VIII, from those who have moderate hemophilia (1% to 4% of

Table 25–2 • Tests of Coagulation

Test	Normal Value	Measures
Bleeding time (Ivy)	3–10 minutes	Platelet function Vascular integrity
Platelet count	150,000–400,000 cells/mm^3	
Prothrombin time	10–12 seconds	Factors I, II, V, VII, X
Partial thromboplastin time	25–35 seconds	Factors I, II, V, VII, IX, X, XI, XII
Activated clotting time	90–120 seconds	Factors I, II, V, VII, IX, X, XI, XII
Thrombin time	9–11 seconds	Factors I, II
Fibrinogen	160–350 mg/dl	
Fibrin degradation products	< 4 μg/ml	
Thromboelastography	See Fig. 25–1	Procoagulants Platelets

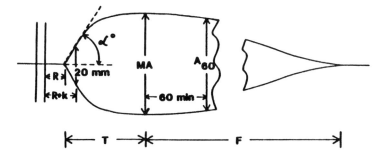

Figure 25–1 • Variables and normal values measured by thromboelastography. R, reaction time for initial fibrin formation, 6–8 minutes; R + K, coagulation time, 10–12 minutes; alpha°, clot formation rate, > 50 degrees; MA, maximum amplitude, 50–70 mm; A_{60}, amplitude 60 minutes after MA; F, whole-blood clot lysis time, > 300 minutes. (From Kang YG, Martin DJ, Marquez J, et al. Intraoperative changes in blood coagulation and thromboelastographic monitoring in liver transplantation. Anesth Analg 1985;64:888–96, with permission.)

the normal factor VIII level) or mild hemophilia (5% to 25% of the normal level). Mild or moderate hemophilia A is rarely complicated by episodes of unprovoked bleeding into joints. In fact, mild hemophilia A may be recognized in adults only after trauma or surgery, and there may be no history of bleeding.[6]

Clinical manifestations of hemophilia A are joint (knees, elbows, ankles, shoulders, hips) and skeletal muscle hemorrhages, easy bruising, and prolonged, potentially fatal hemorrhage after trauma or surgery, but no excessive bleeding after minor cuts or abrasions. Hemarthroses are often first noted when the affected child begins to walk. Bleeding into closed spaces can result in compression of peripheral nerves or vascular or airway obstruction. Intra-

cranial bleeding may be a cause of death in patients with hemophilia A.

Diagnosis

Hemophilia A is suspected when unusual bleeding is encountered in male patients. This suspicion is supported by screening laboratory tests that include a normal platelet count and PT but a prolonged activated PTT. Specific factor assays are then needed to determine the specific deficiency, as this is the only way to differentiate hemophilia A from hemophilia B (factor IX). Standardization of plasma reference values and assay methods make it possible to report factor VIII activity in international units, either as units per milliliter or units per deciliter.[6]

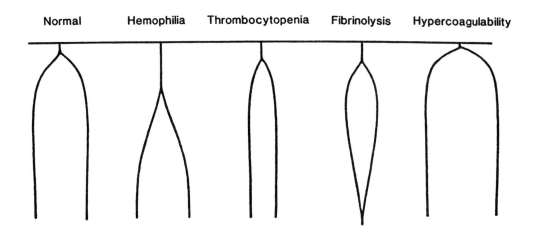

Figure 25–2 • Coagulopathy as reflected by the thromboelastograph. Compared with the normal thromboelastograph, an absence of coagulation factors (hemophilia) is characterized by a prolonged R and decreased α; thrombocytopenia or platelet dysfunction by a prolonged R and decreased MA and α; fibrinolysis by decreased MA, α, and F; and hypercoagulation by a shortened R and increased MA, α, and F. See Figure 25–1 for definition of abbreviations.

Treatment

Treatment of hemophilia A is with factor VIII concentrates. The amount of factor VIII required depends on the plasma level of factor VIII needed to treat the specific bleeding episode, and it must be sufficient to allow for the distribution of the factor throughout the body and its clearance from plasma.[6] In general, infusion of factor VIII 1 U/kg increases the plasma factor VIII level by 0.02 U/ml. Although minimal hemostatic levels of 0.3 U/ml are usually necessary to treat mild bleeding episodes, levels of 0.5 U/ml are generally considered the minimum for treating serious bleeding into joints or skeletal muscles. In cases of major surgery or life-threatening bleeding, normal circulating factor VIII levels must be maintained at all times. The short elimination half-time of factor VIII (about 8 hours) means that repeated doses are necessary unless factor VIII is administered by continuous intravenous infusion.

Pooled coagulation factor VIII concentrates that have not been heat-treated to inactivate viruses may transmit the human immunodeficiency virus (HIV) and hepatitis virus. Factor VIII produced by recombinant technology is comparable to plasma-derived factor VIII in its recovery and half-time characteristics and is effective for treating bleeding episodes. Because it is not derived from human plasma, recombinant factor VIII does not have the potential to transmit viral diseases. One of the most difficult problems in the clinical management of hemophilia is the development of antibodies to factor VIII in some patients. Factor VIII is a foreign protein that results in the formation of factor VIII inhibitors in 10% to 20% of patients.[6]

Desmopressin, 0.3 μg/kg IV, increases plasma levels of factor VIII and von Willebrand factor and can be administered to treat patients with mild or moderate hemophilia and von Willebrand's disease and to prepare patients for minor surgery. An obvious advantage of desmopressin therapy is the absence of the potential for disease transmission. Patients with severe hemophilia A do not respond to desmopressin.

Management of Anesthesia

Preoperative medication of patients with hemophilia A is ideally achieved with drugs administered orally. Although intramuscular injection of drugs is described as acceptable when factor VIII levels have been repleted, it seems prudent to avoid this route whenever possible.[7] Anticholinergic drugs can be administered intravenously before the induction of anesthesia if it is deemed a necessary part of the anesthesia. Maintenance of anesthesia is most often

with general anesthesia, as the risk of uncontrolled bleeding contraindicates the use of regional anesthesia techniques. Nevertheless, the uncomplicated use of an axillary block of the brachial plexus has been described in these patients.[7] Tracheal intubation need not be avoided, although hemorrhage into the tongue and neck could impair upper airway patency. When selecting anesthetic drugs, one should consider the likely presence of co-existing liver disease owing to hepatitis from prior blood or factor VIII transfusions. Likewise, the possible presence of acquired immunodeficiency syndrome (AIDS) must be considered. Superficial hemorrhage can be controlled by applying topical external pressure until treatment with factor VIII can be initiated.

Hemophilia B

Hemophilia B is an X-linked genetic coagulation disorder due to a defective or deficient factor IX molecule resulting in a hemorrhagic tendency. The inheritance pattern and clinical features are indistinguishable from those of hemophilia A.[6]

Diagnosis

The diagnosis of hemophilia B depends on demonstrating low or absent plasma factor IX concentrations in the presence of normal factor VIII activity. The activated PTT is prolonged in patients with hemophilia B.

Treatment

Treatment of hemophilia B is with factor IX concentrates, with the goal of maintaining plasma concentrations of this procoagulant higher than 30% of normal during the perioperative period. Dosing intervals of factor IX concentrates are based on elimination half-times of 24 hours. Preoperative preparation and management of anesthesia are as described for hemophilia A.

Von Willebrand's Disease

Von Willebrand's disease is inherited as an autosomal dominant trait affecting both genders, in contrast to X-linked hemophilia A and B. This coagulation disorder is caused by deficient or defective amounts of von Willebrand factor (vWF) in the patient's plasma. This factor is necessary for adherence of platelets to exposed endothelium. It is likely that factor VIII comprises two distinct molecules, with factor VIII:C and vWF present in the plasma as a complex. The incidence of von Willebrand's disease may be as high as 2% to 3% of the population, although severe (homozygous) von Willebrand's disease is much rarer, with an incidence similar to that of hemophilia A.[8]

Diagnosis

The diagnosis of von Willebrand's disease is suggested by the patient's history and the demonstration of prolonged bleeding times despite normal platelet counts. Affected patients have a lifelong history of bruising and mild bleeding usually from mucosal surfaces (epistaxis), but they are typically unaware of a bleeding disorder until they undergo surgery or experience trauma. Excessive bleeding, from surgery or trauma is localized to the site of surgery; hemarthroses and deep tissue bleeding, such as into skeletal muscles, are uncommon.

Treatment

Treatment of von Willebrand's disease consists of replacing vWF with cryoprecipitate.[8] Alternatively, desmopressin may stimulate the release of vWF, serving as an effective treatment in some patients. Because desmopressin seems to enhance fibrinolysis by causing the release of tissue plasminogen activator, concurrent administration of ε-aminocaproic acid may be recommended. Pregnancy stimulates increases in plasma vWF concentrations in parturients with mild to moderate forms of this coagulation disorder. Consequently, vaginal delivery usually occurs without adverse bleeding related to this disorder.

Afibrinogenemia

Congenital absence of fibrinogen activity may first present as persistent bleeding from the stump of the newborn's umbilical cord. Minor trauma can precipitate severe hemorrhage, but hemarthroses do not occur. Bleeding times, PT, PTT, and thrombin times are usually prolonged. Quantitative determination of serum fibrinogen concentrations demonstrates only trace amounts or the total absence of this procoagulant. Treatment is with fibrinogen or cryoprecipitate to increase serum fibrinogen concentrations to at least 50 mg/dl.

Factor V Deficiency

Factor V deficiency is inherited as an autosomal recessive trait affecting both genders. PT, PTT, and bleeding times are prolonged. Bleeding is most often from the mucous membranes, although hemorrhage from accidental trauma or surgery can be significant. Severe menorrhagia may be a manifestation of this disorder. Treatment of factor V deficiency is with fresh frozen plasma (FFP) to maintain serum factor V concentrations within the range of 5% to 20% of normal.[9]

Factor XII Deficiency

Factor XII (Hageman factor) deficiency is not associated with excessive bleeding after trauma or surgery despite prolonged in vitro clot formation. In fact, individuals with factor XII deficiency may be at risk for thromboembolic complications. Congenital deficiency of this factor is suggested when routine preoperative blood coagulation studies demonstrate a prolonged PTT despite a negative bleeding history. No substitution therapy is needed for these patients even during surgery.[10] Standard tests to monitor heparin activity depend on in vitro activation of factor XII, making it impossible to monitor heparin activity intraoperatively in these patients. Instead, heparin is administered according to weight-based protocols; a normal dose–response relation is assumed. Alternatively, measurement of serum heparin concentrations before and after cardiopulmonary bypass confirms maintenance of anticoagulation and its reversal in factor XII-deficient patients.[10]

Factor XIII Deficiency

Factor XIII deficiency results in an inability to form insoluble fibrin, manifesting at birth as persistent bleeding from the stump of the newborn's umbilical cord. During later life this procoagulant deficiency can result in delayed hemorrhage after accidental trauma or surgery. Central nervous system hemorrhage is common. The position of factor XIII in the coagulation pathway results in normal values for all the routine laboratory tests for coagulation. Treatment is with FFP or cryoprecipitate.[9]

Hereditary Hemorrhagic Telangiectasia

Hereditary hemorrhagic telangiectasia (Osler-Weber-Rendu syndrome) is an inherited non-sex-linked disorder characterized by an abnormal vascular ultrastructure resulting in telangiectasia, arteriovenous fistula formation (especially in the lungs), and the development of aneurysms throughout the cardiovascular system. High-output congestive heart failure may reflect the effect of systemic arteriovenous shunts, whereas arterial hypoxemia and paradoxical air embolism may reflect similar shunts in the patient's lungs. Epistaxis is a common event.

Management of anesthesia must take into consideration the possibility of hemorrhage from telangiectatic lesions that may be present in the oropharynx, trachea, and esophagus. Epidural anesthesia has been described for parturients in labor with Osler-Weber-Rendu syndrome; the risk of neurologic sequelae should be kept in mind in the event that the bleeding tendency leads to the formation of an epidural hematoma.[11]

Hereditary Thrombocytopenia

May-Hegglin anomaly, Fechtner syndrome, and the Sebastian platelet syndrome are rare forms of hereditary (autosomal dominant) thrombocytopenia.[12] All three of these conditions can cause bleeding in the absence of any apparent reason.

May-Hegglin Anomaly

May-Hegglin anomaly is a rare inherited disorder characterized by thrombocytopenia and a bleeding diathesis, manifesting commonly as purpura and epistaxis. Tests of platelet function are usually normal, but bleeding is due to a low platelet count, not platelet dysfunction. Because this anomaly is an autosomal dominant trait, a thrombocytopenic fetus would be expected in about one-half of afflicted parturients. Experience with the management of anesthesia in these patients is limited, although spinal anesthesia in a parturient has been described.[13]

Fechtner Syndrome

Fechtner syndrome is characterized by hematologic abnormalities similar to those in patients with May-Hegglin anomaly.[12] Although often asymptomatic and diagnosed accidentally, Fechtner syndrome can be associated with easy bruising, renal impairment, and hearing loss. Unexplained bleeding may occur despite normal platelet function. Management of anesthesia may include preoperative administration of platelets and desmopressin to improve platelet function.

Grey Platelet Syndrome

Grey platelet syndrome is a rare, inherited qualitative disorder of platelet function (deficiency of α granules) that presents clinically as a bleeding diathesis and thrombocytopenia. Patients may give a history of easy bruising, ecchymosis, recurrent epistaxis, and menorrhagia, but severe hemorrhage has most commonly been reported following surgical procedures including cesarean section.[14] The deficiency of α granules results in abnormalities of platelet secretion and secondary aggregation in response to various stimuli including collagen and thrombin.

α_2-Antiplasmin Deficiency

α_2-Antiplasmin deficiency is a rare congenital disease that results in activation of fibrinolysis and requires specific treatment with antifibrinolytic drugs.[15] Standard preoperative coagulation tests detect platelet and coagulation factor disorders but are unable to detect fibrinolysis disorders. Fibrinolysis should be suspected when a bleeding tendency is present but coagulation tests are normal. Bleeding as may occur in association with surgery is treated with ε-aminocaproic acid, which inhibits plasminogen activator and has direct antiplasmin activity that destroys excess plasmin.

Prekallikrein Deficiency

Prekallikrein deficiency (Fletcher factor deficiency) is a rare congenital defect that results in prolongation of the activated PTT and whole-blood clotting time.[16] Thrombin times, PT, and bleeding times are normal. Prekallikrein is a protein that is required for complete activation and optimal functioning of factor XII. In addition to congenital deficiency, prekallikrein deficiency has been associated with liver disease, septic shock, deep vein thrombosis, and DIC. Severe prekallikrein deficiency is not associated with clinically significant impairment of hemostasis or increased risks of central neuraxial bleeding should epidural or spinal anesthesia be utilized. Nevertheless, discovery of a prolonged PTT during the preoperative evaluation of patients necessitates the performance of several complex and time-consuming tests to elucidate the problem.[16]

Hypercoagulable States

Congenital and acquired hypercoagulable states occur when there is an imbalance between the anticoagulant and procoagulant activities of plasma in which the procoagulant activities predominate. A striking feature of these conditions is the focal nature of the thrombotic diathesis (Table 25–3).[17] For

Table 25–3 • Hypercoagulable States and Associated Vascular Bed-Specific Thrombosis Sites

Hypercoagulable State	Vascular Bed-Specific Thrombosis Site
Congenital	
Antithrombin III deficiency	
Heterozygous	Deep veins of legs
Homozygous	Deep veins and arteries
Protein C deficiency	Deep veins of legs
Protein S deficiency	Deep veins of legs
Factor V Leiden presence	Deep veins of legs and brain
	Coronary arteries (?)
Acquired	
Paroxysmal nocturnal hemoglobinuria	Portal and hepatic veins
Myeloproliferative diseases	Portal and hepatic veins
Antiphospholipid antibody syndrome	Arteries and veins
Warfarin-induced skin necrosis	Subcutaneous microvessels
Thrombotic thrombocytopenic purpura	All microvessels with exception of brain and lungs
Acute coronary artery syndrome	Coronary arteries presumed to reflect interplay of plaque rupture and alteration of a vascular bed-specific hemostatic circuit

Adapted from: Rosenberg RD, Aird WC. Vascular-bed-specific hemostasis and hypercoagulable states. N Engl J Med 1999;340: 1555–64.

example, congenital deficiencies of antithrombin III, protein C, and protein S are associated with an increased incidence of deep vein thrombosis of the lower but not the upper extremities. These hypercoagulable states do not predispose to arterial thrombosis as characterized by myocardial infarction (see Chapter 1). Acquired hypercoagulable states are also associated with vascular bed-specific thrombosis. Paroxysmal nocturnal hemoglobinuria and myeloproliferative diseases are characterized by an increased incidence of thrombosis of the hepatic, portal, and mesenteric veins.

Antithrombin III Deficiency

Antithrombin III (AT-III) inhibits activated clotting factors II and V. Deficiency of AT-III is associated with an increased incidence of thromboembolic disease and resistance to the anticoagulant effects of exogenously administered heparin. Acquired AT-III deficiency may occur in patients being treated with heparin and in those with DIC or severe liver disease. Women who take oral estrogen-containing contraceptives seem to be at increased risk of thromboembolism associated with decreased AT-III levels. The diagnosis of AT-III deficiency is confirmed by measuring plasma AT-III concentrations. Chronic treatment of AT-III deficiency is with oral anticoagulants, whereas acute correction is with administration of AT-III, as is present in specific concentrate preparations or FFP.

Protein C Deficiency

Protein C, a vitamin K-dependent anticoagulant protein synthesized in the liver, inhibits activated

clotting factors V and VIII and stimulates fibrinolysis.[18] Protein C deficiency may be inherited or acquired (liver disease, DIC, acute respiratory failure, after operation, after delivery, hemodialysis). Deficiency of protein C most often presents as a tendency for recurrent thromboembolic disease, including myocardial infarction, cerebral infarction, and pulmonary embolism. Thrombosis may be initiated by events associated with the perioperative period, including endothelial damage, immobility, and stasis of blood flow.[19] Because protein C deficiency does not cause abnormalities in routine screening coagulation tests (PT, PTT, bleeding times), it is important to maintain a high index of suspicion for patients who report a personal or family history of thromboembolic diseases at a young age. Oral anticoagulation is the treatment of choice to prevent thrombosis. Regional anesthetic techniques may be useful alternatives to general anesthesia in these patients.[20]

Protein S Deficiency

Protein S is a vitamin K-dependent anticoagulant protein that acts as a cofactor in the protein C-catalyzed inactivation of factors V and VIII. Protein S deficiency may be associated with an increased risk of venous thromboembolism.

Antiphospholipid Syndrome

Antiphospholipid syndrome, an autoimmune disorder, is characterized by venous or arterial thromboses, thrombocytopenia, and recurrent fetal losses reflecting the presence of autoantibodies directed against phospholipid–protein complexes. Antibodies present in patients with antiphospholipid syndrome may occur independently or in association with other autoimmune diseases, especially systemic lupus erythematosus. It is estimated that this syndrome occurs in 2% of the general population, and these patients may be at increased risk for developing ischemic heart disease and valvular heart disease, especially disease of the mitral valve. In addition, neurologic manifestations of antiphospholipid syndrome may include recurrent cerebral infarcts (strokes), headaches, and visual disturbances.

Patients with a history of antiphospholipid syndrome and at least one thrombotic episode are likely to present during the preoperative period while being treated with anticoagulants.[21] Regional anesthesia is not a likely choice in the presence of chronic anticoagulation. Prophylactic measures are taken to prevent thromboses, including the use of elastic stockings, avoidance of dehydration, and attempts to maintain normothermia. Monitoring anticoagulation in patients with antiphospholipid syndrome who require anticoagulation (cardiac surgery) is problematic.[22] Antiphospholipid antibodies inhibit phospholipid-dependent coagulation in vitro and interfere with laboratory testing of coagulation. Monitoring heparin anticoagulation in these patients can be accomplished by measuring activated clotting times.

■ ACQUIRED COAGULATION DISORDERS

Acquired coagulation disorders, in contrast to inherited disorders, are usually due to multiple abnormalities in the coagulation process (Table 25–1).

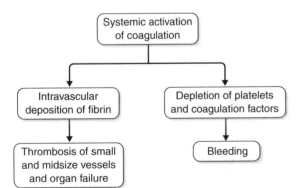

Figure 25–3 • Steps in disseminated intravascular coagulation. Systemic activation of coagulation leads to widespread intravascular deposition of fibrin and depletion of platelets and coagulation factors. As a result, thrombosis of small and mid-size vessels may occur, contributing to organ failure and possibly severe bleeding. (From Levi M, ten Cate H. Disseminated intravascular coagulation. N Engl J Med 1999;341:586–92. Copyright 1999 Massachusetts Medical Society, with permission.)

Table 25–4 • Clinical Conditions Associated with Disseminated Intravascular Coagulation

Sepsis
  Gram-negative sepsis
  Gram-positive sepsis
Trauma
  Head injury
  Fat embolism
Cancer
  Myeloproliferative disorders
  Solid tumors (pancreatic cancer, prostate cancer)
Obstetric complications
  Abruptio placentae
  Amniotic fluid embolism
Vascular disorders
  Aortic aneurysms
Immunologic disorders
  Allergic reactions
  Hemolytic transfusion reactions
  Transplant rejection

Adapted from: Levi M, ten Cate H. Disseminated intravascular coagulation. N Engl J Med 1999;341:586–92.

Disseminated Intravascular Coagulation

Disseminated intravascular coagulation (DIC) is characterized by widespread systemic activation of coagulation, which results in intravascular formation of fibrin and ultimately thrombotic occlusion of small and midsize vessels.[23] Intravascular coagulation can also compromise the blood supply to organs and, in conjunction with hemodynamic and metabolic derangements, may contribute to multiple organ system failure. At the same time, the consumption of platelets and coagulation factors may induce severe bleeding (Fig. 25–3).[23] Bleeding may be the presenting symptom in patients with DIC. Systemic formation of fibrin results from increased generation of thrombin, simultaneous suppression of physiologic anticoagulation mechanisms, and delayed removal of fibrin as a consequence of impaired fibrinolysis.

Causes

An acquired disorder, DIC occurs in a wide variety of clinical disorders (Table 25–4). Gram-negative sepsis and gram-positive sepsis are the most common clinical conditions associated with DIC. Cell-specific membrane components of the microorganisms (endotoxins, exotoxins) are responsible for triggering DIC. Another clinical condition frequently associated with DIC is severe trauma, particularly to the brain. Solid tumors and hematologic cancers may be complicated by DIC. DIC is a classic complication of obstetric conditions, such as abruptio placentae and amniotic fluid embolism.

Pregnancy-induced hypertension can be complicated by DIC. It may be difficult to differentiate between severe liver disease and DIC, as these two disorders produce similar laboratory abnormalities.

Diagnosis

There is no single laboratory test that can establish or rule out the diagnosis of DIC. A combination of tests in patients with clinical conditions known to be associated with DIC can be used to diagnose DIC in most cases.[23] In clinical practice, DIC can be diagnosed on the basis of the presence of a clinical condition known to be associated with this disorder, initial platelet counts of less than 100,000 cells/mm³, rapid decreases in platelet counts, prolongation of clotting times such as PT and the PTT, the presence of fibrin degradation products in the plasma, and low plasma concentrations of coagulation inhibitors such as antithrombin III.[23] Plasma fibrinogen levels may remain within the normal range despite considerable coagulation activity. Hypofibrinogenemia is useful diagnostically only in severe cases of DIC.

Treatment

The most important initial step in the treatment of DIC is management of the underlying clinical disorder responsible for triggering the coagulation process. Treating DIC without treating the underlying cause is destined to fail.[23] Supportive treatment may be necessary, but there is no consensus regarding the optimal treatment or supportive strategy. Patients with DIC and diffuse bleeding need supportive treatment different from that appropriate for patients with thrombotic obstruction of the vasculature and development of multiple organ system failure.

Anticoagulation

Theoretically, interrupting the coagulation process should be beneficial in patients with DIC. Treatment with heparin is probably helpful in those with DIC, particularly patients with clinically overt thromboembolism or extensive deposition of fibrin.[23] Relatively low doses of unfractionated heparin are administered continuously at hourly rates of 300 to 500 units IV. Low-molecular-weight heparin may be utilized as an alternative to unfractionated heparin.

Platelets and Plasma

Patients experiencing DIC characterized by low platelet counts and decreased circulating concentrations of procoagulant factors benefit from treatment with platelet concentrates and FFP. There is no evidence that this treatment is beneficial in patients with DIC not characterized by bleeding. The use of coagulation factor concentrates may not be recommended, as these concentrates are sometimes contaminated with activated coagulation factors, which could exacerbate the coagulation disorder. Furthermore, these concentrates contain only selected coagulation factors, whereas patients with DIC usually have deficiencies of all coagulation factors. Administration of supraphysiologic doses of antithrombin III may be helpful in patients with DIC and sepsis.

Antifibrinolytic Drugs

Antifibrinolytic drugs are effective in patients with bleeding, but administration of these drugs to patients with DIC is not generally recommended.[23] Because the deposition of fibrin in patients with DIC appears to be due in part to insufficient fibrinolysis, further inhibition of the fibrinolytic system does not seem desirable. Exceptions may include patients with DIC associated with cancer in whom antifibrinolytic drugs may control the bleeding.

Perioperative Anticoagulation

General Considerations

Long-term anticoagulation is usually reserved for patients with multiple episodes of venous thromboembolism, hereditary hypercoagulable states, cancer, mechanical heart valves, or atrial fibrillation (see Chapter 12). Anticoagulation decreases the risk of venous thromboembolism by about 80%, the risk of arterial thromboembolism in patients with mechanical heart valves by 75%, and the risk of arterial embolism in patients with nonvalvular atrial fibrillation by 66%.[24] Preoperative administration of warfarin poses problems when these patients need surgery. Interruption of warfarin treatment may increase the risk of venous thromboembolism, whereas continued treatment may increase the risk of postoperative bleeding. Nevertheless, postoperative bleeding due to preoperative administration of warfarin is rarely fatal or associated with major morbidity, whereas the consequences of venous or arterial thromboembolism (pulmonary embolus, stroke) may be fatal.

Independent of the intensity of preoperative anticoagulation, the perioperative risk of thromboembolism may be increased by other factors, in particular rebound hypercoagulable states caused by discontinuation of warfarin and the prothrombotic effect of surgery. There is evidence that surgery increases the risk of venous thromboembolism but not arterial

Table 25–5 • Impact of Anticoagulants on Tests of Coagulation

Anticoagulant	Factors Inhibited	Prothrombin Time	Partial Thromboplastin Time
Heparin			
Low dose	IX	Normal	Prolonged
High dose	II, IX, X	Prolonged	Prolonged
Warfarin			
Low dose	VII	Prolonged	Normal
High dose	II, VII, IX, X	Prolonged	Prolonged

thromboembolism in patients with atrial fibrillation or mechanical heart valves.[24]

Recommendations

Overall, there is no consensus on the appropriate perioperative management of anticoagulation for patients who have been receiving long-term warfarin therapy.[24] The effects of preoperative anticoagulant therapy on coagulation tests are influenced by the doses of drugs being administered (Table 25–5).

Warfarin

Perioperative management of patients being treated with warfarin preoperatively may include discontinuing the oral anticoagulant prior to elective surgery and instituting intravenous or subcutaneous heparin in selected patients (Table 25–6) (see Chapter 12).[24] If a patient's INR is between 2.0 and 3.0, four scheduled doses of warfarin are withheld to allow the INR to decrease spontaneously to 1.5 or less before surgery. The INR is measured a day before surgery to ensure adequate progress in the reversal of anticoagulation. If the INR remains higher than 1.8 at this time, an option is to administer 1 mg of vitamin K subcutaneously. Once the INR reaches 1.5, surgery can be safely performed.

After warfarin treatment is restarted, it takes about 3 days for the INR to reach 2.0. Therefore if warfarin is withheld for 4 days before surgery and treatment is restarted as soon as possible after surgery, patients can be expected to have a subtherapeutic INR for approximately 2 days before surgery and 2 days after surgery. However, because the INR is increased to some extent for much of this period, patients can still be expected to have partial protection against thromboembolism. The temporary discontinuation of warfarin thus exposes patients to a risk of thromboembolism equivalent to 1 day without anticoagulation before surgery and 1 day after surgery. Regardless of the approach to perioperative anticoagulation, patients must have a normal or nearly normal state of coagulation during surgery, so some increase in the risk of thromboembolism is unavoidable.

History of Venous Thromboembolism

Elective surgery should be avoided during the first 30 days after an acute episode of venous thromboembolism.[24] If this is not possible, intravenous heparin is administered before and after the surgical procedure while the INR is below 2.0. In these patients, if the PTT is in the therapeutic range, stopping continuous intravenous heparin therapy 6 hours before

Table 25–6 • Recommendations for Preoperative and Postoperative Anticoagulation in Patients Being Treated with Oral Anticoagulants

Indication	Before Surgery	After Surgery
Acute venous thromboembolism		
First 30 days	Heparin IV	Heparin IV
After 30 days	No change	Heparin IV
Recurrent venous thromboembolism	No change	Heparin SC
Acute arterial thromboembolism (first 30 days)	Heparin IV	Heparin IV
Mechanical heart valve	No change	Heparin SC
Nonvalvular atrial fibrillation	No change	Heparin SC

IV, intravenous; SC, subcutaneous.
Adapted from: Kearon C, Hirsh J. Management of anticoagulation before and after elective surgery. N Engl J Med 1997;336:1506–11.

surgery should be sufficient for heparin to be cleared before surgery. Heparin therapy is not restarted as a continuous intravenous infusion rate that is greater than the expected maintenance rate for about 12 hours after major surgery, and it should be delayed even longer if there is evidence of surgical bleeding.[24] The PTT is rechecked 12 hours after restarting heparin therapy to allow time for a stable anticoagulant response. Patients do not require preoperative intravenous heparin if the acute venous thromboembolism occurred more than 30 days previously, although postoperative heparin therapy may be recommended until warfarin therapy is resumed and the INR is above 2.0. Mechanical methods of prophylaxis, such as graduated compression stockings, or intermittent pneumatic compression stockings, are combined with pharmacologic therapy.

History of Arterial Thromboembolism

Elective surgery should be avoided during the first 30 days after an acute episode of arterial thromboembolism.[24] If this is not possible, preoperative intravenous heparin therapy is recommended. Postoperative heparin therapy is recommended for such patients only if the risk of postoperative bleeding is considered to be low. In all other patients who receive anticoagulants to prevent arterial embolism (mechanical heart valves, nonvalvular atrial fibrillation), the risk of arterial embolism is not high enough to justify preoperative or postoperative therapy with intravenous heparin. Intravenous heparin is avoided after major surgery because of the risk of bleeding. Subcutaneous low-dose heparin or low-molecular-weight heparin in doses used for prophylaxis against venous thromboembolism in high risk patients is recommended for hospitalized patients whose risk of arterial embolism does not justify intravenous heparin therapy. However, neither hospitalization to administer subcutaneous heparin nor the administration of subcutaneous heparin to outpatients seems justified.[24]

Regional Anesthesia or Neuraxial Analgesia

The prospect of administering spinal or epidural anesthetics or placing epidural catheters for postoperative neuraxial analgesia in patients who will receive heparin as prophylaxis against thromboembolic complications is a controversial clinical issue.[25] Even more controversial is the use of spinal or epidural anesthesia in patients who are already anticoagulated. If it is elected to administer a regional anesthetic to an anticoagulated patient, it is presumed that the benefits of the technique outweigh alternative approaches. The obvious concern is delayed hemorrhage from blood vessels that are damaged during performance of the regional anesthetic, leading to formation of an epidural or spinal hematoma and subsequent compression of the spinal cord and the onset of paraplegia. Even in the absence of regional anesthesia, there is a risk that epidural hematoma will occur spontaneously in anticoagulated patients.[26, 27]

Several large clinical studies have confirmed the safety of instituting heparin therapy in patients in whom the epidural catheter was previously placed and in whom clinically detectable bleeding was absent for at least 1 hour.[28-30] Postponement of surgery for 24 hours may be recommended if placement of the epidural catheter is associated with return of blood through the needle used for the placement or via the catheter. Timing of removal of the epidural catheter is also considered critical, as epidural bleeding could be initiated at this time. In this regard it is often recommended that the epidural catheter be removed 10 to 12 hours after the last dose of heparin and subsequent dosing with heparin be delayed for at least 1 hour after removing the catheter (Table 25–7).[29] Patients must be monitored closely during the perioperative period, including the time following catheter removal, for early signs of spinal cord compression (back pain, progression of numbness or weakness, bowel or bladder dysfunction) caused by an expanding epidural hematoma. Prompt recognition of an epidural hematoma as confirmed by computed tomography or magnetic resonance imaging is followed by decompressive laminectomy. Recovery of spinal cord function is unlikely if surgery is delayed more than 8 hours after the clinical onset of symptoms.[30]

In contrast to unfractionated heparin, low-molecular-weight heparin was intended to provide the potential advantage of distinguishing the antithrombotic effects from the bleeding effects of heparin. However, the incidence of epidural hematoma occurring spontaneously in treated patients and in association with regional anesthesia seems to be increased, resulting in concern about the safety of regional anesthesia and neuraxial analgesia in patients treated with low-molecular-weight heparin (Table 25–7).[29]

Intraoperative Coagulopathies

Intraoperative coagulopathies reflect alterations in the concentrations and function of circulating platelets and procoagulants. In addition, surgical stress may exert effects on coagulation.

Dilutional Thrombocytopenia

The most common cause of intraoperative coagulopathy is dilutional thrombocytopenia. Blood loss

Table 25-7 • Recommendations for Performance of Neuraxial Analgesia and Anesthesia in the Presence of Anticoagulants Administered for Thromboembolism Prophylaxis or Intraoperative Coagulation

Unfractionated (standard) minidose subcutaneous heparin
    No contraindication exists to neuraxial block.
    May consider delaying initiation of heparin therapy until after institution of the neuraxial block.
Unfractionated (standard) intravenous heparin for intraoperative coagulation
    Delay initiating heparin administration for 1 hour after needle placement for neuraxial block.
    Remove the epidural catheter 1 hour before any subsequent intravenous doses of heparin (assumes 12-hour dosing intervals) or 2–4 hours after the last dose of heparin.
    Consider the use of minimal concentrations of local anesthetics to permit early clinical detection of neurologic changes.
    Difficult neuraxial needle placement and/or appearance of blood in the needle or catheter does not mandate cancellation of the planned surgery; but if the operation proceeds, frequent postoperative monitoring of neurologic status is important.
Low-molecular-weight heparin
    Decision to perform neuraxial blocks is made on an individual basis.
    Difficult neuraxial needle placement and/or appearance of blood in the needle or catheter does not mandate cancellation of the planned surgery; but if the operation proceeds, it is important to delay initiation of low-molecular-weight heparin therapy for 24 hours.
    Delay epidural catheter removal for 10–12 hours after the last dose of low-molecular-weight heparin and do not administer any subsequent doses for 2 hours.
    Consider single-dose spinal anesthesia if regional anesthesia is required in patients being treated with low-molecular-weight heparin preoperatively.
    Perform frequent postoperative monitoring of neurologic status.
Oral anticoagulants
    Stop anticoagulant and allow normalization of prothrombin time (INR) before performing neuraxial block.
Antiplatelet drugs
    Treatment with these drugs does not interfere with performing neuraxial block.
Fibrinolytic and thrombolytic drugs
    Neuraxial block not recommended within 10 days of receiving these drugs.

Adapted from: Neuraxial Anesthesia and Anticoagulation, Consensus Statements. American Society of Regional Anesthesia, 1998.

that is replaced with crystalloids, colloids, packed red blood cells, or whole blood progressively dilutes platelet numbers. Massive blood transfusions are characterized as administration of 10 units or more of stored whole blood (equivalent to exchanging the patient's blood volume with transfused components). As much as 80% of the patient's estimated blood volume may have to be replaced before clinically significant thrombocytopenia occurs, assuming preoperative platelet counts were normal. Approximately 33% of the total platelet mass is contained in the patient's spleen and reticuloendothelial system. During surgical hemorrhage these platelets can be released into the systemic circulation. This is the reason that measured blood losses do not necessarily translate into similar decreases in circulating platelets. The presence of intraoperative dilutional thrombocytopenia is suggested by an abnormal TEG.[31] There is no justification for prophylactic administration of platelets to massively transfused patients. Each unit of platelets administered to adult patients can be expected to increase platelet counts by 5,000 to 10,000 cells/mm^3.

Dilution of Procoagulants

As with platelets, the dilutional effects of intraoperative fluid and blood administration on circulating plasma procoagulants may be somewhat offset by release of procoagulant proteins from the patient's liver. For example, surgical hemorrhage causes the release of fibrinogen from hepatic stores. Most plasma procoagulant concentrations are needed in only 30% of their normal concentrations for coagulation to continue. Nevertheless, fibrinogen concentrations below 150 mg/dl can contribute to coagulopathy. Factor V is also a consumable procoagulant, and decreases in its plasma concentrations may contribute to bleeding. Administration of platelets also contains 50 to 70 ml of plasma, resulting in delivery of procoagulants as well as platelets. There is no justification for prophylactic administration of fresh frozen plasma to massively transfused patients.[31]

Metabolic Changes

Metabolic changes that occur intraoperatively may contribute to the development of a coagulopathy. In this regard, metabolic acidosis, such as may accompany hypotension and poor tissue blood flow, can inhibit circulating procoagulants and platelet function. Rapid administration of large volumes of acidic blood products may contribute to metabolic acidosis. Citrate anticoagulant used in blood products may bind ionized calcium. Nevertheless, sufficient residual ionized calcium is usually present, and routine administration of ionized calcium during intraoperative blood administration is not likely to be necessary. In patients with normal liver function, the citrate present in stored blood is readily metabolized to bicarbonate.

Effects of Surgery

Surgery causes most patients to become hypercoagulable.[32] This response is nonspecific and seems to occur within the first hour of surgery and anesthesia. The dilutional effects associated with intraoperative fluid administration to offset surgical blood loss must overcome the effects of increased platelet and fibrinogen release before a coagulopathy develops. Intraoperative hypothermia has profound effects on enzyme systems, which may manifest as progressive prolongation of the PT and PTT and interference with normal platelet function.

Type of Surgery

Specific clinical surgical situations (cardiopulmonary bypass, brain trauma or surgery, orthopedic surgery, urologic surgery, obstetric delivery) may introduce risks for the development of intraoperative coagulopathies.

Cardiopulmonary Bypass

Cardiopulmonary bypass introduces the need for heparin anticoagulation and reversal with protamine plus the unavoidable presence of platelet destruction and plasmin activation. Excessive bleeding following cardiopulmonary bypass is most often due to acquired platelet dysfunction or heparin overdose.[33] This platelet dysfunction is most likely caused by contact between the platelets and the oxygenator. The degree of platelet dysfunction is directly proportional to the duration of cardiopulmonary bypass and is probably also related to the degree of hypothermia and the prophylactic use of semisynthetic penicillins and possibly to other drugs such as nitroglycerin and nitroprusside. In most patients platelet dysfunction is transient, lasting less than 1 hour. If bleeding persists, the treatment is infusion of platelet concentrates. Administration of hetastarch to increase the intravascular fluid volume in patients undergoing cardiac surgery may be avoided, as there is evidence that this synthetic colloid increases postoperative bleeding.[34]

Aprotinin administered in large doses before initiation of cardiopulmonary bypass decreases postoperative bleeding and transfusion requirements, especially in patients treated with aspirin and those undergoing repeated cardiac surgery.[35] The mechanism of this drug's beneficial effect may be inhibition of plasmin and kallikrein, resulting in inhibition of fibrinolytic activity. Aprotinin may also exert a protective effect on platelet function. These mechanisms are consistent with the notion that an acquired platelet defect is the most likely explanation when increased bleeding occurs after the conclusion of cardiopulmonary bypass.

Noncardiac Surgery and Obstetric Delivery

During orthopedic surgery trauma of the long bone marrow may cause extrusion of marrow fat and other debris into the circulation, resulting in a stimulus for coagulation and platelet deposition. One of the manifestations of this stimulation is the development of DIC. Lipids liberated during brain surgery and the tissue thromboplastins released during cerebral trauma or surgery create a high incidence of DIC or fibrinolysis. Surgical removal of the prostate can cause significant release of urokinase, thereby influencing plasmin activity. In the parturient, retained amniotic fluid or placental debris can trigger DIC if it enters the maternal circulation.

Drug-Induced Hemorrhage

Heparin overdose manifests as subcutaneous hemorrhage and deep tissue hematomas. This anticoagulant is inactivated in the liver and excreted by the kidneys, explaining the prolonged anticoagulant effects of heparin in patients with hepatorenal disease. Decreased body temperature is also associated with enhanced anticoagulant effects of heparin. The PT and PTT are prolonged; and the bleeding time is normal. Excessive heparin effect can be antagonized with the intravenous administration of protamine.

Overdoses of warfarin manifest as ecchymosis formation, mucosal hemorrhage, and subserosal bleeding into the walls of the gastrointestinal tract. The anticoagulant effect is due to the ability of warfarin to prevent carboxylation of vitamin K to its active form. The PT is markedly prolonged in the presence of warfarin overdose. Administration of FFP to provide vitamin K is necessary to treat acute hemorrhage owing to warfarin overdose.

Drug-Induced Platelet Dysfunction

Aspirin administered to patients irreversibly inhibits cyclooxygenase, which is responsible for platelet release of adenosine diphosphate (ADP), necessary for platelet aggregation. Indeed, prolongation of the bleeding time by 2 to 3 minutes is detectable within 3 hours of ingesting 300 mg of aspirin. Some apparently normal patients display marked sensitivity to the effects of aspirin; in these cases, bleeding times are greatly prolonged, and significant hemorrhage may occur during the perioperative period or following trauma. Uremic patients are especially sensitive to aspirin-induced bleeding. Phenylbutazone and indomethacin inhibit the platelet release reaction similar to aspirin; sodium salicylate has a lesser effect; and acetaminophen does not interfere with release of ADP from platelets.

Platelet dysfunction induced by aspirin persists for the life of the platelet, which may be for several days after discontinuation of aspirin. Therefore treatment of acute aspirin-induced hemorrhage consists of the transfusion of platelets that can release ADP. In response to this release reaction, platelets inhibited by aspirin can aggregate.

Drugs other than aspirin and related nonsteroidal antiinflammatory drugs may interfere with platelet release of ADP and with subsequent platelet aggregation. For example, alcohol, dextran, and certain antibiotics (carbenicillin, high doses of penicillin, many of the cephalosporins) interfere with platelet aggregation, manifesting as prolonged bleeding times. Volatile anesthetics and nitrous oxide studied using an in vitro model produce dose-related decreases in ADP-induced platelet aggregation.[36] It is possible that inhaled anesthetics change the surface characteristics of platelet cell membranes and thus interfere with platelet cohesion. The clinical importance of this effect on platelet aggregation, if any, is unknown.

A controversial question deals with performance of elective operations in the presence of known aspirin therapy (Table 25–7).[29] Although the bleeding time may return to normal within 72 hours after discontinuing aspirin, it may take 7 to 10 days for in vitro tests of platelet aggregation to normalize.[37] It has been suggested that the upper limit of bleeding times acceptable for performance of elective operations is 10 minutes.[38] Despite the concern that operative blood loss could be increased, there is evidence that perioperative blood loss is not increased in patients receiving daily aspirin doses of 1.2 to 3.6 g and undergoing hip replacement.[39] Likewise, there is no evidence that spinal or epidural anesthesia should be avoided in patients receiving antiplatelet drugs, although the incidence of blood-tinged cerebrospinal fluid or blood aspirated through the epidural or spinal needle may be increased in such patients.[40] Although the rarity of epidural hematomas is reassuring, there is a report of hematoma formation after regional anesthesia in the presence of aspirin-induced platelet dysfunction.[41] Postoperative neurologic monitoring is important in aspirin-treated patients receiving either epidural or spinal anesthetics for prompt detection of signs of spinal cord compression attributable to epidural hematoma formation.

Idiopathic Thrombocytopenic Purpura

Idiopathic thrombocytopenic purpura (ITP), or autoimmune thrombocytopenic purpura, is characterized by persistent thrombocytopenia caused by antiplatelet immunoglobulins that bind to platelet membranes, causing their premature rupture.[42] In addition to accelerated destruction, platelets in patients with ITP may not function normally, as reflected by prolonged bleeding times. The principal manifestations of thrombocytopenia are the formation of petechiae, characteristically at sites of increased internal or external pressure (oral mucosa, constricting clothing, legs). Intracranial hemorrhage is the principal cause of mortality in patients with ITP. Transplacental passage of anti-platelet antibodies may predispose neonates to spontaneous bleeding, including intracranial hemorrhage.

Causes

Otherwise healthy young females are most often afflicted with ITP, although many disease states and drugs may also be associated with thrombocytopenia that is indistinguishable from ITP (Table 25–8).

Heparin-induced thrombocytopenia may manifest as modest nonprogressive decreases in platelet counts that require no intervention or severe thrombocytopenia often to a level of less than 50,000 cells/mm^3 associated with thromboembolism, especially arterial thromboembolism. Heparin-dependent antibodies seem to be responsible for the severe form of heparin-induced thrombocytopenia, typically manifesting 4 to 6 days after initiation of anticoagu-

---

Table 25–8 • Factors Associated with Thrombocytopenia

Idiopathic
Heparin
Infectious mononucleosis
Acquired immunodeficiency syndrome
Hodgkin's disease
Systemic lupus erythematosus
Rheumatoid arthritis
Raynaud's phenomenon
Hyperthyroidism
Sepsis
Quinidine
Thiazide diuretics

lant therapy. Thrombocytopenia may occur 2 to 10 days after whole-blood transfusion, occurring most often in women exposed to alloantigens during a prior pregnancy.

Treatment

Treatment of ITP is initially with corticosteroids such as prednisone, which is presumed to interfere with macrophage attacks on platelets and eventually to decrease the amount of antiplatelet antibodies produced. Danazol and vincristine may serve as supplemental therapy or alternatives to corticosteroids. Immunosuppressive therapy must be used cautiously in parturients or patients with AIDS. If the platelet response to corticosteroids is inadequate or not sustained, splenectomy is indicated. The efficacy of splenectomy depends on eliminating the platelet-trapping role of the spleen and its function in producing antiplatelet antibodies. Cesarean section may be recommended when the fetus is affected by ITP to decrease the risk of cerebral trauma to the infant, which seems most likely if platelet counts are less than 50,000 cells/mm³.

Management of Anesthesia

It is recommended that corticosteroids be administered preoperatively to increase platelet counts to near 50,000 cells/mm³ at the induction of anesthesia. When surgery must be performed despite platelet counts less than 50,000 cells/mm³, administration of 6 units of platelet concentrate may be recommended at anesthetic induction and after ligation of the splenic pedicle. Management of anesthesia in these patients includes minimizing trauma to the upper airway, as during direct laryngoscopy for tracheal intubation. Regional anesthesia is rarely selected because of the potential for spontaneous hemorrhage. Corticosteroids are continued postoperatively until platelet counts increase.

Thrombotic Thrombocytopenic Purpura

Thrombotic thrombocytopenic purpura (TTP) is characterized by disseminated intravascular aggregation of platelets, presumably reflecting the presence of abnormal aggregating factors.[43] Clinical manifestations of TTP include thrombocytopenia, severe hemolytic anemia, central nervous system disturbances ranging from focal defects to seizures and coma, fever, mild renal dysfunction, and jaundice. Treatment of TTP is with antiplatelet drugs such as aspirin and with exchange plasmapheresis in an effort to provide the necessary absent factors or to remove toxic substances. Mortality from TTP may approach 60% to 80% during the first 10 days of the disease.

Catheter-Induced Thrombocytopenia

Thrombus formation on catheters placed in the systemic or pulmonary circulations is a predictable event.[44] Catheter-induced thrombogenicity is presumed to reflect the interaction of blood with the physicochemical and textural properties of the catheters. Catheters fabricated from polyvinyl chloride have been found to be particularly thrombogenic. For example, it has been demonstrated that a pulmonary artery catheter may induce thrombus formation within 1 to 2 hours after placement despite the use of a continuous infusion of heparinized saline through the catheter. By contrast, the use of a pulmonary artery catheter with heparin incorporated into the plastic material does not induce thrombus formation.[44] Although symptomatic pulmonary embolism is not a predictable event associated with the use of a thrombogenic pulmonary artery catheter, it seems logical to minimize the likelihood of thrombus formation if possible. Therefore the use of heparin-bonded pulmonary artery catheters may be a useful consideration.

Thrombocytopenia has also been associated with the use of pulmonary artery catheters.[45] Conceivably, increased platelet consumption owing to thrombus formation on pulmonary artery catheters is responsible for thrombocytopenia. In this regard, sequestration of platelets on pulmonary artery catheters becomes a possible explanation when thrombocytopenia occurs unexpectedly.

Vitamin K Deficiency

Vitamin K is necessary in the liver to facilitate the production of γ-carboxyglutamic acid required for the function of factors II, VII, IX, and X. Vitamin K deficiency occurs in the presence of malnutrition, gastrointestinal malabsorption, antibiotic-induced elimination of intestinal flora necessary for the synthesis of vitamin K, and obstructive jaundice. With obstructive jaundice, bile salts necessary for the absorption of vitamin K from the gastrointestinal tract cannot enter the intestine. The neonate lacks stores of vitamin K and can become deficient in this vitamin in the absence of supplemental therapy.

The diagnosis of vitamin K deficiency is based on documentation of a prolonged PT in the presence of a normal PTT. Treatment of a coagulation disorder owing to vitamin K deficiency is determined by the urgency of the situation. For example, treatment with a parenteral vitamin K analogue, such as phytonadione, requires 6 to 24 hours to exert beneficial effects. If active bleeding is present, administration of FFP is promptly effective.[46]

References

1. Rohrer MJ, Michelotti MC, Nahrwold DL. A prospective evaluation of the efficacy of preoperative coagulation testing. Am Surg 1988;208:554–62
2. Kang YG, Martin DJ, Marquez J, et al. Intraoperative changes in blood coagulation and thromboelastographic monitoring in liver transplantation. Anesth Analg 1985;64:888–96
3. Mallett SV, Cox DJA. Thrombelastography. Br J Anaesth 1992;69:307–13
4. Whitten CW, Greilich PE. Thromboelastography®: past, present, and future. Anesthesiology 2000;92:1223–5
5. Ellison N. Diagnosis and management of bleeding disorders. Anesthesiology 1977;47:171–80
6. Hoyer LW. Hemophilia A. N Engl J Med 1994;330:38–47
7. Sampson JF, Hamstra R, Aldrete JA. Management of hemophilic patients undergoing surgical procedures. Anesth Analg 1979;58:133–5
8. Cameron CB, Kobrinsky N. Perioperative management of patients with von Willebrand's disease. Can J Anaesth 1990;37:341–7
9. Consensus Conference. Fresh frozen plasma: indications and risks. JAMA 1985;253:551–3
10. Salmenpera M, Rasi V, Mattila S. Cardiopulmonary bypass in a patient with factor XII deficiency. Anesthesiology 1991;75:539–41
11. Waring PH, Shaw DB, Brumfield CG. Anesthetic management of a parturient with Osler-Weber-Rendu syndrome and rheumatic heart disease. Anesth Analg 1990;71:96–9
12. Mertzlufft F, Koster A, Steinhart H, et al. Fechtner's syndrome: considerations of anesthetic management. Anesth Analg 2000;90:1372–5
13. Kotelko DM. Anaesthesia for caesarean delivery in a patient with May-Hegglin anomaly. Can J Anaesth 1989;36:328–30
14. Laskey AL, Tobias JD. Anesthetic implications of the grey platelet syndrome. Can J Anesth 2000;47:1224–9
15. Paqueron X, Favier R, Richard P, et al. Severe postadenoidectomy bleeding revealing congenital alpha-2 antiplasmin deficiency in a child. Anesth Analg 1997;84:1147–9
16. Pasricha SK, Weiss H, Chen A. Spinal anesthesia in a patient with prekallikrein deficiency. Anesth Analg 1996;83:1325–6
17. Rosenberg RD, Aird WC. Vascular-bed-specific hemostasis and hypercoagulable states. N Engl J Med 1999;340:1555–64
18. Clouse LH, Comp PC. The regulation of hemostasis: the protein C system. N Engl J Med 1986;314:1298–1303
19. Sternberg TL, Bailey MK, Lazarchick J, et al. Protein C deficiency as a cause of pulmonary embolism in the perioperative period. Anesthesiology 1991;74:364–6
20. Wetzel RC, Marsh BR, Yaster M, et al. Anesthetic implications of protein C deficiency. Anesth Analg 1986;65:982–4
21. Menon G, Allt-Graham J. Anaesthetic implications of the anticardiolipin antibody syndrome. Br J Anaesth 1993;70:587–90
22. East CJ, Clements F, Mathew J, et al. Antiphospholipid syndrome and cardiac surgery: management of anticoagulation in two patients. Anesth Analg 2000;90:1098–1101
23. Levi M, Cate HT. Disseminated intravascular coagulation. N Engl J Med 1999;341:586–92
24. Kearon C, Hirsh J. Management of anticoagulation before and after elective surgery. N Engl J Med 1997;336:1506–11
25. Horlocker TT, Heit JA. Low molecular weight heparin: biochemistry, pharmacology, perioperative prophylaxis regimens and guidelines for regional anesthetic management. Anesth Analg 1997;85:874–85
26. Owens EL, Kasten GW, Hessel EA. Spinal subarachnoid hematoma after lumbar puncture and heparinization: a case report, review of the literature, and discussion of anesthetic implications. Anesth Analg 1986;65:1201–7
27. Wittebol MC, VanVeelen CWM. Spontaneous spinal epidural hematoma. Clin Neurol Neurosurg 1984;86:265–70
28. Rao TLK, El-Etr AA. Anticoagulation following placement of epidural and subarachnoid catheters: an evaluation of neurologic sequelae. Anesthesiology 1981;55:618–20
29. Neuraxial Anaesthesia and Anticoagulation, Consensus Statements. American Society of Regional Anesthesia, 1998
30. Vandeermeulen EP, Van Aken H, Vermylen J. Anticoagulants and spinal-epidural anesthesia. Anesth Analg 1994;79:1165–77
31. Murray DJ, Olson J, Strauss R, et al. Coagulation changes during packed red cell replacement of major blood loss. Anesthesiology 1988;69:839–46
32. Tuman KJ, McCarthy RJ, March RJ, et al. Effects of epidural anesthesia and analgesia on coagulation and outcome after major vascular surgery. Anesth Analg 1991;73:696–703
33. Harker LA. Bleeding after cardiopulmonary bypass. N Engl J Med 1986;314:1446–8
34. Knutson JE, Deering JA, Hall FW, et al. Does intraoperative hetastarch administration increase blood loss and transfusion requirements after cardiac surgery? Anesth Analg 2000;90:801–7
35. Levy JH, Bailey JM, Salmenpera M. Pharmacokinetics of aprotinin in preoperative surgical patients. Anesthesiology 1994;80:1013–8
36. Fauss BG, Meadows JC, Bruni CY, et al. The in-vitro and in-vivo effects of isoflurane and nitrous oxide in platelet aggregation. Anesth Analg 1986;65:1170–4
37. Hindman BJ, Koka BV. Usefulness of the post-aspirin bleeding time. Anesthesiology 1986;64:368–70
38. Macdonald R. Aspirin and extradural blocks. Br J Anaesth 1991;66:1–3
39. Amrein PC, Ellman L, Harris WH. Aspirin-induced prolongation of bleeding and perioperative blood loss. JAMA 1981;245:1825–8
40. Horlocker TT, Wedel DJ, Offord KP. Does preoperative antiplatelet therapy increase the risk of hemorrhagic complications associated with regional anesthesia? Anesth Analg 1990;70:631–4
41. Locke GE, Giorgio AJ, Biggers SL, et al. Acute spinal epidural hematoma secondary to aspirin-induced prolonged bleeding. Surg Neurol 1976;5:293–6
42. McMillan R. Chronic idiopathic thrombocytopenic purpura. N Engl J Med 1981;304:1135–7
43. Crain SM, Choudhury AM. Thrombotic thrombocytopenia: a reappraisal. JAMA 1981;246:1243–6
44. Hoar PF, Wilson RM, Mangano DT, et al. Heparin bonding reduces thrombogenicity of pulmonary-artery catheters. N Engl J Med 1981;305:993–5
45. Richman KA, Kim YL, Marshall BE. Thrombocytopenia and altered platelet kinetics associated with prolonged pulmonary-artery catheterization in the dog. Anesthesiology 1980;53:101–5
46. Consensus Conference. Fresh frozen plasma: indications and risks. JAMA 1985;253:551–3

Skin and Musculoskeletal Diseases

Diseases of the skin and musculoskeletal system manifest with obvious clinical signs, as both systems are readily visible. Occult systemic effects of many of these disorders may also be important.

■ EPIDERMOLYSIS BULLOSA

Epidermolysis bullosa is a group of hereditary diseases of the skin that may also involve mucous membranes, particularly those of the oropharynx and esophagus. This disease is categorized as simplex, junctional, and dystrophic (Fig. 26–1).[1] In the simplex type, epidermal cells are fragile, and mutations of genes encoding keratin intermediate filament proteins underlie the fragility. In the dystrophic types (incidence about 1 in every 300,000 births), the genetic mutation appears to be in the gene encoding the type of collagen that is the major component of anchoring fibrils.

Signs and Symptoms

Epidermolysis bullosa is characterized by bulla formation (blistering) due to separation within the epidermis followed by fluid accumulation. Bulla formation is typically initiated when lateral shearing forces are applied to the affected patient's skin. Pressure applied perpendicular to the skin is not as great a hazard. Bulla formation can occur with even minimal trauma or can occur spontaneously.

The simplex form of epidermolysis bullosa is characterized by a benign course and normal development. By contrast, patients with the junctional form of epidermolysis bullosa rarely survive beyond early childhood, with most dying from sepsis. Fea-

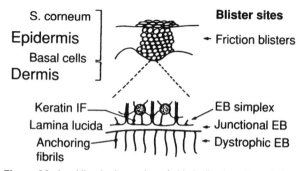

S. corneum

Epidermis

Basal cells

Dermis

Keratin IF

Lamina lucida

Anchoring fibrils

Blister sites

← Friction blisters

← EB simplex

← Junctional EB

← Dystrophic EB

Figure 26–1 • Histologic section of skin indicating sites of cleavage in friction blisters and for the three major types of epidermolysis bullosa (EB). (From Epstein EH. Molecular genetics of epidermolysis bullosa. Science 1992;256:799–803, with permission.)

tures that distinguish junctional epidermolysis bullosa from other forms are generalized blistering beginning at birth, absence of scar formation, and generalized mucosal involvement (skin, gastrointestinal, genitourinary, respiratory). In contrast to the junctional form, manifestations of epidermolysis bullosa dystrophica include severe scarring with fusion of the digits (pseudosyndactyly), constriction of the oral aperture (microstomia), and esophageal strictures. Teeth are often dysplastic. Malnutrition, anemia, electrolyte derangements, and hypoalbuminemia are common, most likely reflecting chronic infection, debilitation, and renal dysfunction. Survival beyond the second decade is unusual. Diseases associated with epidermolysis bullosa include porphyria, amyloidosis, multiple myeloma, diabetes mellitus, and hypercoagulable states. Mitral valve prolapse may accompany epidermolysis bullosa.

Treatment

Treatment of epidermolysis bullosa is symptomatic. Many of these patients are already receiving corticosteroids. Phenytoin has not been proved to be an effective treatment. Infection of bullae with *Staphylococcus aureus* or with β-hemolytic streptococci is common.

Management of Anesthesia

Management of anesthesia in patients with epidermolysis bullosa must include consideration of the drugs used to treat the disease.[2] For example, supplemental corticosteroids may be indicated during the perioperative period if patients have been chronically treated with these drugs. Avoidance of trauma to the skin and mucous membranes is crucial. Bulla

formation can be produced by trauma from tape, blood pressure cuffs, tourniquets, adhesive electrodes (as used to monitor the electrocardiogram or activity at the neuromuscular junction), and rubbing with alcohol wipes. If a systemic blood pressure cuff is used, it should be padded with loose cotton dressings. Intravenous and intra-arterial catheters should be sutured or held in place with gauze wraps rather than taped in place. Pulse oximetry using nonadhesive sensors is indicated.

Trauma from the anesthetic face mask must be minimized by gentle application against the patient's face. Lubrication of the patient's face and mask with cortisol ointment can be helpful. Upper airway instrumentation should be minimized, as the squamous epithelium lining the oropharynx and esophagus is more susceptible to trauma than is the columnar epithelium of the trachea. Frictional trauma to the oropharynx, as produced by oral airways, may result in large intraoral bulla formation and extensive hemorrhage from denuded mucosa. Nasal airways are equally hazardous. Esophageal stethoscopes should be avoided, as they can lead to the formation of intraoral or esophageal bullae. Hemorrhage from ruptured oral bullae has been treated successfully by epinephrine-soaked gauze applied to the bullae.

Tracheal intubation, despite theoretical hazards, has not been associated with laryngeal or tracheal complications in patients with epidermolysis bullosa dystrophica, and its more routine use in these patients has been recommended.[3] Indeed, laryngeal involvement with this form of the disease is rare, and tracheal bullae have not been reported. This finding is consistent with the greater resistance to disruption of the columnar epithelium that lines the trachea than the fragile squamous epithelium in the oral cavity. Generous lubrication of the laryngoscope blade with cortisol ointments and petroleum jelly (Vaseline) and selecting a smaller tracheal tube than usual is recommended. Chronic scarring of the oral cavity can result in a narrow oral aperture and immobility of the tongue, making tracheal intubation difficult. After tracheal intubation, the tube must be carefully immobilized with soft cloth bandages to prevent movement in the oropharynx. Tape is not used to hold the tracheal tube in place, and the tube must not exert lateral forces at the corners of the patient's mouth. At tracheal extubation it must be remembered that oropharyngeal suctioning can lead to life-threatening bulla formation. The risk of pulmonary aspiration may be increased by the presence of esophageal strictures. The safety of tracheal intubation in patients with junctional epidermolysis bullosa involving mucous membranes, including the respiratory epithelium, is unproven.[4]

Porphyria cutanea tarda has been reported to occur with increased frequency in patients with epidermolysis bullosa.[5] This type of porphyria does not have the same implications for management of anesthesia as does the presence of acute intermittent porphyria. Ketamine is a useful drug for avoiding airway manipulation when the operative procedure does not require controlled ventilation of the lungs or skeletal muscle relaxation. Despite the presence of dystrophic skeletal muscles, there is no evidence based on clinical experience that these patients are at increased risk of hyperkalemic responses when treated with succinylcholine.[6] There are no known contraindications to the use of inhaled anesthetic drugs in these patients. As alternatives to general anesthesia, regional anesthetic techniques (spinal, epidural, brachial plexus) have been recommended.[6]

▊ PEMPHIGUS

Pemphigus refers to a group of chronic autoimmune blistering (vesiculobullous) diseases that may involve extensive areas of the skin and mucous membranes. Cutaneous pemphigus is characterized by bullae in the skin and mucous membranes (mouth, upper airway, genitalia). Two histopathologically and clinically different types of pemphigus have been recognized: pemphigus vulgaris and pemphigus foliaceus. Cutaneous pemphigus closely resembles the oral manifestations of epidermolysis bullosa dystrophica. Involvement of the oropharynx is present in about 50% of patients with pemphigus. Extensive oropharyngeal involvement makes eating painful, and patients may decrease oral intake to the point that severe malnutrition develops. Skin denudation and bulla formation can result in significant fluid and protein loss. The risk of secondary infection is great.

Pemphigus is most likely an autoimmune disorder in which circulating antibodies attack antigenic sites on the epidermal cell surface, resulting in destruction of cells. In this regard, pemphigus may be associated with other autoimmune diseases including myasthenia gravis, systemic lupus erythematosus, Graves' disease, and immune thrombocytopenic purpura. As with epidermolysis bullosa, there may be an absence of intercellular bridges that normally prevent the separation of epidermal cells. Therefore frictional trauma may result in bulla formation. Occasionally, infection or drug sensitivity is the inciting event for bulla formation. Pemphigus vulgaris is the most common variant of pemphigus and is also the most significant because of the high incidence of oral lesions.

Treatment

Treatment of pemphigus with corticosteroids has decreased the mortality associated with this disease from 70% to 5%. Azathioprine, methotrexate, cyclophosphamide, and cyclosporine have also been used successfully for early treatment of pemphigus.

Management of Anesthesia

Management of anesthesia in patients with pemphigus and epidermolysis bullosa is similar.[2,7,8] Preoperative drug therapy must be considered. In this regard, supplementation of the usual corticosteroid doses may be necessary. Methotrexate produces immunosuppression, hepatorenal dysfunction, and depression of bone marrow activity but is unlikely to alter the activity of plasma cholinesterase enzyme. Azathioprine has been reported to antagonize nondepolarizing neuromuscular blockade, presumably reflecting inhibition of phosphodiesterase enzyme by this drug. Electrolyte derangements may reflect chronic fluid loss through bullous skin lesions that can result in dehydration and hypokalemia.

Airway management may be difficult because of co-existing bullae in the oropharynx.[9] Airway manipulations including direct laryngoscopy and tracheal intubation can result in acute bulla formation, severe upper airway obstruction, and bleeding. Nevertheless, numerous reports of uncomplicated elective tracheal intubation have been described. Likewise, regional anesthesia, although controversial, has been successfully administered to these patients.[8,10] Skin infection at the needle site selected for institution of regional anesthesia must be recognized and an alternative needle placement site selected. Infiltration with local anesthetic solutions is usually avoided because of the risk of skin sloughing and bulla formation at the injection site. Ketamine is useful for general anesthesia in selected patients.

▊ PSORIASIS

Psoriasis is a common chronic dermatologic disorder (affects 1% to 3% of the world's population) characterized by accelerated epidermal growth resulting in inflammatory erythematous papules covered with loosely adherent scales (chronic plaque psoriasis).[11] Skin lesions are remitting and relapsing, with one peak of onset being during adolescence and young adulthood (16 to 22 years of age) and the other during older age (57 to 60 years of age). Synthesis of deoxyribonucleic acid in the epidermis of these patients is four times that present in normal epidermis. Skin lesions, symmetrically distributed, typically involve the elbows, knees, hairlines, and presacral regions. An inflammatory asymmetrical arthropathy occurs in about 20% of patients with psoriasis. Uveitis and sacroiliitis associated with ascending vertebral body disease are common. High cardiac output congestive heart failure has also been observed. Generalized pustular psoriasis is a rare form of the disease that may be complicated by decreased plasma concentrations of albumin, sepsis, and renal failure.

Treatment

Treatment of psoriasis is directed at slowing the rapid proliferation of epidermal cells. Crude coal tar is effective because of its antimitotic actions and ability to inhibit enzymes. Although preparations containing coal tar cause clearance of plaques when used alone, they are usually used in combination with ultraviolet phototherapy. Their use is limited by their unpleasant odor and potential to irritate normal skin. Coal tar is frequently used in shampoo preparations to prevent psoriatic scaling of the scalp. In rare cases, skin cancer is associated with therapeutic use of coal tar. Ointments containing salicylic acid are the most widely used keratolytic agents, either alone or in combination with coal tar or topical corticosteroids. Topical corticosteroids are also effective, but the disease promptly recurs when treatment is discontinued. Application of corticosteroids under occlusive dressings can result in significant systemic absorption, with associated suppression of endogenous adrenal cortex activity. Systemic therapy with methotrexate, cyclosporine, and folate antagonists may be required for more severe cases. Toxic effects of these drugs include cirrhosis of the liver, renal failure, systemic hypertension, and pneumonitis.

Management of Anesthesia

Management of anesthesia must include consideration of the drugs being used for the treatment of psoriasis including topical corticosteroids and chemotherapeutic drugs. Skin trauma such as venipuncture and surgical incisions accentuates psoriasis in some patients. Patients with psoriasis can have marked increases in skin blood flow, which could contribute to altered thermoregulation.

▮ MASTOCYTOSIS

Mastocytosis is a rare disorder of mast cell proliferation that occurs in a cutaneous form (urticaria pigmentosa) and, in approximately 10% of cases, a systemic form.[12] Urticaria pigmentosa is usually benign and asymptomatic, with children being most often afflicted. In nearly one-half of these individuals the small red-brown macules most often present on the trunk and extremities disappear by adulthood. In the systemic form the mast cells proliferate in all organs, such as bone, liver, and spleen but not the central nervous system. Degranulation of mast cells with release of histamine, heparin, prostaglandins, and numerous enzymes (tryptases, hydrolases) may occur spontaneously or be triggered by nonimmune factors, including physical or psychological stimuli, alcohol, and drugs known to release histamine. A rare form of systemic mastocytosis, known as malignant aggressive systemic mastocytosis, is characterized by diffuse mast cell proliferation in parenchymal organs, thrombocytopenia, and hemorrhage. These patients often require splenectomy.

Signs and Symptoms

Classic symptoms of mastocytosis are thought to reflect massive degranulation of mast cells with anaphylactoid responses characterized by pruritus, urticaria, and cutaneous flushing. These changes may be accompanied by hypotension and tachycardia. Hypotension may be so severe as to be life-threatening. Although symptoms are commonly attributed to histamine release from mast cells, H_1- and H_2-receptor antagonists are not always protective and the incidence of bronchospasm is low, suggesting that vasoactive substances (prostaglandins) other than histamine may be involved.[13] Bleeding is unusual in these patients, even though mast cells contain heparin.

Management of Anesthesia

Management of anesthesia is influenced by the possibility of massive intraoperative degranulation and associated anaphylactoid symptoms.[12, 14] Although the intraoperative period for these patients is usually uneventful, there are reports of life-threatening anaphylactoid reactions with even minor surgical procedures, emphasizing the need to have resuscitation drugs such as epinephrine promptly available when anesthetizing these patients.[15, 16] Preoperative administration of H_1- and H_2-receptor antagonists is a consideration recognizing that these drugs do not interfere with the release of histamine from mast cells. Addition of prostaglandin inhibitors such as aspirin to the preoperative medication is a consideration, although aspirin may be questionable based on its alleged ability to initiate mast cell degranulation and its known effect on coagulation.[13] Paracetamol is a weak prostaglandin inhibitor that may be an alternative to aspirin.[12] Some recommend preoperative skin testing of drugs likely to be used during anesthesia in attempts to avoid anesthetics that might be likely to evoke degranulation.[12] Fentanyl, propofol, and vecuronium have been administered to these patients without evoking mast cell degranulation.[12] Even succinylcholine and meperidine have been administered without adverse effects.[15] Inhaled anesthetics are considered acceptable for administration to these patients. Monitoring serum tryptase concentrations during the perioperative period is useful for determining the occurrence of mast cell degranulation.[12]

ATOPIC DERMATITIS

Atopic dermatitis is the cutaneous manifestation of the atopic state. It is characterized by dry, scaly, eczematous, pruritic patches on the patient's face, neck, and flexor surfaces of the arms and legs. Pruritus is the primary symptom. Systemic antihistamines may be effective for decreasing pruritus, and corticosteroids may be indicated for short-term treatment of severe cases. Pulmonary manifestations of atopic states, such as asthma, hay fever, otitis media, and sinusitis, may influence management of anesthesia.

URTICARIA

Urticaria may be characterized as chronic urticaria and physical urticaria. Chronic urticaria (hives) and its associated angioedema affects 15% to 23% of the U.S. population, and in most cases the cause cannot be determined (Table 26–1).[17] With physical urticaria, physically stimulating the skin causes the formation of local wheals, itching, and in some cases angioedema (Table 26–1).[17] Cold urticaria accounts for 3% to 5% of all physical urticarias.[18] Urticarial vasculitis may be a presenting symptom of systemic lupus erythematosus and Sjögren syndrome.

Chronic Urticaria

Chronic urticaria is characterized by circumscribed wheals and localized areas of edema produced by extravasation of fluid through the blood vessel walls. The wheals are smooth, pink to red, and surrounded by a bright red flare; they usually are intensely pruritic, can be found anywhere on hairless or hairy skin, and last less than 24 hours. Wheals

Table 26–1 • Features of Common Types of Chronic Urticaria

Type of Urticaria	Age Range (years)	Clinical Features	Angioedema	Diagnostic Test
Chronic idiopathic	20–50	Pink or pale edematous papules or wheals Wheals often annular Pruritus	Yes	
Symptomatic dermatographism	20–50	Linear wheals with a surrounding bright-red flare at sites of stimulation Pruritus	No	Light stroking of skin causes wheal
Physical urticarias Cold	10–40	Pale or red swelling at sites of contact with cold surfaces or fluids Pruritus	Yes	Application of ice pack causes a wheal within 5 minutes of removing the ice (cold stimulation test)
Pressure	20–50	Swelling at sites of pressure (soles, palms, waist) lasting ≥ 24 hours Painful Pruritus	No	Application of pressure perpendicular to skin produces persistent red swelling after a latent period of 1–4 hours
Solar	20–50	Pale or red swelling at site of exposure to ultraviolet or visible light Pruritus	Yes	Radiation by a solar simulator for 30–120 seconds causes wheals in 30 minutes
Cholinergic	10–50	Monomorphic pale or pink wheals on trunk, neck, and limbs Pruritus	Yes	Exercise or hot shower elicits wheals

Adapted from: Greaves MW. Chronic urticaria. N Engl J Med 1995;332:1767–72.

lasting longer than 24 hours raise the possibility of other diagnoses including urticarial vasculitis. Chronic urticaria affects approximately twice as many women as men and often follows a remitting and relapsing course, with symptoms typically increasing at night. Angioedema describes urticaria involving the mucous membranes, particularly those of the mouth, pharynx, and larynx. Mast cells and basophils regulate urticarial reactions. When stimulated by certain immunologic factors (drugs, inhaled allergens) or nonimmunologic events, storage granules in these cells release histamine and other vasoactive substances such as bradykinins. These substances result in localized vasodilation and transudation of fluid characteristic of urticarial lesions.

Except for patients with chronic urticaria for whom avoidable causes can be identified (food additives), treatment is symptomatic. Antihistamines (H₁-receptor antagonists) are the principal treatment for mild cases, of recurring chronic urticaria. Terfenadine has a low potential for sedation and is adequate treatment for most mild cases, although high doses of this drug have been associated with cardiac dysrhythmias. Doxepin is a tricyclic antidepressant drug with significant H₁-antagonist actions that is particularly useful when severe urticaria is associated with mental depression. The combination of H₂-receptor antagonists and H₁-receptor antagonists produces some additional efficacy. When antihistamines do not control chronic urticaria, a course of systemic corticosteroids may be considered. The course of this treatment should be limited to 21 days, as prolonged use of corticosteroids is invariably associated with decreased efficacy and side effects. A 2% solution of ephedrine as a local spray is useful for treating oropharyngeal edema. Swelling involving the tongue may require urgent treatment with epinephrine.

All patients with chronic urticaria should be advised to avoid angiotensin-converting enzyme inhibitors, aspirin, and other nonsteroidal antiinflammatory drugs (NSAIDs).[17] A tepid shower temporarily alleviates the pruritus.

Cold Urticaria

Cold urticaria is characterized by development of urticaria and angioedema following exposure to local or environmental cold. The most common triggering factors are cold air currents, rain, aquatic activities, snow, cold foods and drinks, and contact with cold objects. Severe cold urticaria may be life-threatening, with laryngeal edema, bronchospasm, and hypotension.[19, 20] Diagnostic tests are based on skin stimulation with temperatures of 0°C to 4°C for 1 to 5 minutes (cold stimulation test). Immunologic mechanisms may be associated with the development of cold urticaria, and immunoglobulin E concentrations may be increased. Cutaneous mast cells rather than blood basophils are the target cells for degranulation, although basophil degranulation is possible with profound hypothermia. Tryptase is the most important marker of mast cell degranulation.

The primary objective of treatment is to prevent systemic reactions caused by known triggering mechanisms. Administration of antihistamines decreases the incidence of recurrence and prolongs the time to a positive cold stimulation test.

Management of anesthesia includes avoidance of drugs that are likely to evoke the release of histamine. Drugs requiring cold storage should be avoided or warmed before injection.[20] Other prophylactic measures include warming infusion fluids and increasing the ambient temperature of the operating room. Preoperative administration of H₁- and H₂-receptor antagonists and corticosteroids have been recommended for these patients especially when intraoperative decreases in body temperature are unavoidable as may be the case during operations requiring cardiopulmonary bypass.[19]

ERYTHEMA MULTIFORME

Erythema multiforme is an acute recurrent disorder of the skin and mucous membranes characterized by lesions ranging from edematous macules and papules to vesicular or bullous lesions that may ulcerate. Attacks are associated with viral diseases (especially herpes simplex), hemolytic streptococcal infections, neoplastic processes, collagen vascular diseases, and drug-induced hypersensitivity.

Stevens-Johnson syndrome is a severe manifestation of erythema multiforme associated with multisystem involvement. High fever, tachycardia, and tachypnea may occur. Drugs associated with the onset of this syndrome include antibiotics, analgesics, and over-the-counter medications. Corticosteroids are effective in the management of severe cases.

Hazards of administering anesthesia to patients with Stevens-Johnson syndrome are similar to those encountered in patients with epidermolysis bullosa.[21] For example, involvement of the respiratory tract can make management of the patient's upper airway and tracheal intubation difficult. The presence of pulmonary blebs can make these patients vulnerable to pneumothorax, particularly with positive intrathoracic pressure. In addition, the presence of pulmonary blebs might detract from the use of nitrous oxide. Ketamine has been utilized successfully for anesthesia in these patients.

SCLERODERMA

Scleroderma, or progressive systemic sclerosis, is characterized by inflammation, vascular sclerosis, and fibrosis of the skin and viscera. Microvascular changes produce tissue fibrosis and organ sclerosis. Injury to vascular endothelial cells results in vascular obliteration and leakage of serum proteins into interstitial spaces. These proteins produce tissue edema, lymphatic obstruction, and ultimately fibrosis. In some patients the disease evolves into the CREST syndrome (calcinoses, Raynaud's phenomenon, esophageal hypomotility, sclerodactyly, telangiectasias). The prognosis is poor and is related to the extent of visceral, rather than cutaneous, involvement. There is no known effective treatment for this disease. Corticosteroids should not be administered to patients with scleroderma.

The etiology of scleroderma is unknown, but the disease process has the characteristics of both a collagen disease and an autoimmune process. The typical onset is at 20 to 40 years of age, and women are most often afflicted. Pregnancy accelerates the progression of scleroderma in about half of patients. The incidence of spontaneous abortion, premature labor, and perinatal mortality is high.

Signs and Symptoms

Manifestations of scleroderma occur in the skin and musculoskeletal system, nervous system, cardiovascular system, lungs, kidneys, and gastrointestinal tract.

Skin and Musculoskeletal Systems

Skin exhibits mild thickening and diffuse nonpitting edema. As scleroderma progresses the skin becomes taut, leading to limited mobility and flexion contractures, especially of the fingers. Skeletal muscles may exhibit myopathy, manifesting as weakness of the proximal skeletal muscle groups. Plasma creatine kinase concentrations are typically increased. Mild inflammatory arthritis may occur, but most of the joint movement limitation is due to the thickened, taut overlying skin. Avascular necrosis of the femoral head may be present.

Nervous System

Peripheral or cranial nerve neuropathy in the presence of scleroderma has been ascribed to nerve compression by thickened connective tissues surrounding nerve sheaths. Facial pain suggestive of trigeminal neuralgia may also occur as a result of this thickening. Keratoconjunctivitis sicca exists in some patients and may predispose to corneal abrasions.

Cardiovascular System

Changes in the myocardium associated with scleroderma reflect sclerosis of small coronary arteries and the conduction system, replacement of cardiac muscle with fibrous tissue, and the indirect effects of systemic and pulmonary hypertension. These changes result in cardiac dysrhythmias, cardiac conduction abnormalities, and congestive heart failure. Intimal fibrosis of the pulmonary artery walls is associated with a high incidence of pulmonary hypertension, which may progress to cor pulmonale. Pulmonary hypertension is often present, even in asymptomatic patients. Pericarditis and pericardial effusion, with or without cardiac tamponade, are not infrequent occurrences. Changes in the peripheral vascular system are common and are characterized by intermittent vasospasm in small arteries of the digits. Oral or nasal telangiectasias may be present. Raynaud's phenomenon occurs in most cases and may be the initial manifestation of scleroderma.

Lungs

The effects of scleroderma on the lungs are a major cause of morbidity and mortality. Diffuse interstitial pulmonary fibrosis may occur independent of vascular changes that lead to pulmonary hypertension. Pulmonary fibrosis causes decreased inspiratory capacity and increased residual volume. Although dermal sclerosis does not decrease chest wall compliance, pulmonary compliance is diminished by fibrosis, and increased airway pressures may be required for adequate ventilation of the patient's lungs. Arterial hypoxemia resulting from decreased diffusion capacity is not unusual in these patients, even at rest.

Kidneys

Renal artery obstruction as a result of arteriolar intimal proliferation leads to decreased renal blood flow and systemic hypertension. Sudden development of accelerated systemic hypertension and irreversible renal failure is the most common cause of death in patients with scleroderma. Captopril may improve the impaired renal function that accompanies systemic hypertension in these patients.

Gastrointestinal Tract

Involvement of the gastrointestinal tract by scleroderma may manifest as dryness of the patient's oral mucosa (xerostomia). Progressive fibrosis of the gastrointestinal tract causes hypomotility of the lower esophagus and small intestine. Dysphagia is a common complaint and is due to hypomotility of the esophagus. Lower esophageal sphincter tone is decreased, with subsequent reflux of acidic gastric fluid into the esophagus. Symptoms from the resulting esophagitis can be treated with antacids. Bacterial overgrowth due to intestinal hypomotility can produce a malabsorption syndrome. Indeed, coagulation disorders may reflect malabsorption of vitamin K from the gastrointestinal tract. Broad-spectrum antibiotics are effective in the treatment of this type of malabsorption syndrome. Intestinal hypomotility may also manifest clinically as intestinal pseudo-obstruction. In this regard, prokinetic drugs are not effective motor stimulants, whereas somatostatin analogues, such as octreotide, may evoke intestinal contractions.

Management of Anesthesia

Preoperative evaluation of patients with scleroderma should focus attention on the multiple organ systems likely to be involved by the progressive changes associated with this disease.[22–24] Decreased mandibular motion and narrowing of the oral aperture due to taut skin must be appreciated before induction of anesthesia. Fiberoptic laryngoscopy may be necessary to facilitate tracheal intubation through a small oral opening. Oral or nasal telangiectasias may bleed profusely if traumatized during tracheal intubation. Intravenous access may be impeded by dermal thickening. Catheterization of peripheral arteries for monitoring systemic blood pressure introduces the same concerns present in patients with Raynaud's phenomenon. Cardiac evaluation, including auscultation of the chest and review of the electrocardiogram, may provide evidence of pulmonary hypertension. Because of chronic systemic hypertension and vasomotor instability, patients with scleroderma can have contracted intravascular fluid volumes, manifesting as hypotension, with vasodilation induced by drugs used to produce anesthesia. Relaxation of the lower esophageal sphincter makes these patients vulnerable to regurgitation and subsequent pulmonary aspiration should protective laryngeal reflexes be depressed. For this reason, efforts to increase gastric fluid pH with antacids or H_2-receptor antagonists before the induction of anesthesia may be recommended.

Intraoperatively, decreased pulmonary compliance may necessitate increased positive airway pressure to ensure adequate ventilation of the patient's lungs. Supplemental oxygen is indicated in view of impaired diffusion capacity and vulnerability for the development of arterial hypoxemia. Indeed, events known to increase pulmonary vascular resistance, such as respiratory acidosis and arterial hypoxemia, must be prevented. Acute increases in central venous pressure during administration of nitrous oxide could reflect pulmonary artery vasoconstriction due to effects of this inhaled anesthetic. The patient's eyes should remain protected at all times in view of the possibility of co-existing keratoconjunctivitis. The role of renal function is considered when selecting drugs dependent on this route for clearance from the plasma. Prolonged responses to local anesthetics have been observed, but the explanation or clinical significance is unclear. Furthermore, regional anesthesia may be technically difficult because of skin and joint changes that accompany scleroderma. Attractive features of regional anesthesia include postoperative analgesia and peripheral vasodilation, which might improve perfusion to the patient's lower extremities. Other measures to minimize peripheral vasoconstriction include maintenance of operating room ambient temperatures above 21°C and administration of warmed intravenous fluids. These patients may be sensitive to the ventilatory depressant effects of opioids, and postoperative support of ventilation may be required, especially in the presence of severe co-existing pulmonary disease.

■ PSEUDOXANTHOMA ELASTICUM

Pseudoxanthoma elasticum is a rare hereditary disorder of elastic tissues. Elastic fibers degenerate and calcify with time. The most striking feature of this condition, and often the basis for the diagnosis, is the appearance of angioid streaks in the patient's retinas. Substantial loss of visual acuity may result from these changes. Additional vision impairment may occur when vascular changes predispose to vitreous hemorrhage. Skin changes, consisting of yellowish, rectangular, elevated xanthoma-like lesions, primarily in the neck, axilla, and inguinal regions are often the earliest recognized clinical features. It is surprising that those tissues most rich in elastic fibers, such as the lungs, aorta, palms, and soles, are not affected by the disease process.

Gastrointestinal hemorrhage is a frequent occurrence in these patients. Degenerative changes in the walls of arteries supplying the gastrointestinal tract are thought to prevent constriction of these vessels in response even to minimal mucosal damage. The incidence of systemic hypertension and ischemic heart disease is increased in these patients. Endocardial calcification may involve the conduction system of the heart, predisposing these patients to cardiac dysrhythmias and sudden death. Involvement of cardiac valves with this disease process is frequent. Calcification of peripheral vessels, particularly of the radial or ulnar arteries, is common. Psychiatric disturbances often accompany the disease.

Management of anesthesia in the presence of pseudoxanthoma elasticum is based on an appreciation of the abnormalities associated with this disease.[25] The cardiovascular derangements that sometimes occur in these patients are probably the most important consideration. The increased incidence of ischemic heart disease is considered when establishing limits for acceptable changes in systemic blood pressure and heart rate. Monitoring the electrocardiogram is particularly important in view of the potential for cardiac dysrhythmias. The use of noninvasive blood pressure devices is an acceptable alternative to placing an intra-arterial catheter. Trauma to the mucosa of the upper gastrointestinal tract, as may be produced by instrumentation with a gastric tube or esophageal stethoscope, should be minimized. There are no specific recommendations regarding the choice of anesthetic drugs or techniques.

■ EHLERS-DANLOS SYNDROME

Ehlers-Danlos syndrome consists of a group of inherited connective tissue disorders (at least nine distinct types have been described) due to abnormalities of metabolism in type III collagen. Based on a definition of Ehlers-Danlos syndrome that includes, at a minimum, findings in both skin and joints, it is estimated that 1 in 5000 people are affected by this syndrome.[26] The only form of Ehlers-Danlos syndrome, associated with an increased risk of death is the form designated type IV (vascular) syndrome, which may be complicated by the sudden rupture of large blood vessels or disruption of the bowel.

Signs and Symptoms

All forms of Ehlers-Danlos syndrome cause clinical signs and symptoms including joint hypermobility, skin fragility, bruising and scarring, musculoskeletal discomfort, and susceptibility to osteoarthritis. The gastrointestinal tract, uterus, and blood vessels are particularly well endowed with type III collagen,

accounting for complications such as spontaneous rupture of the bowel, uterus, or major blood vessels. Premature labor and excessive bleeding with delivery are common obstetric problems. Dilation of the trachea is often present, and the incidence of pneumothorax is increased. Mitral regurgitation and cardiac conduction abnormalities are possible. Afflicted patients tend to exhibit extensive ecchymosis with even minimal trauma, but a specific coagulation defect has not been identified.

Management of Anesthesia

Management of anesthesia in patients with Ehlers-Danlos syndrome must consider the cardiorespiratory manifestations of this disease and the propensity for these patients to bleed excessively with interruption of vascular integrity.[27] Prophylactic antibiotics to protect against infective endocarditis may be indicated in the presence of cardiac murmurs suggestive of mitral regurgitation. Avoidance of intramuscular injections or instrumentation of the patient's nose or esophagus is important in view of the bleeding tendency. Trauma during direct laryngoscopy for tracheal intubation must be minimized. Likewise, placing an arterial or central venous catheter must be tempered with the realization that hematoma formation may be extensive. Extravasation of intravenous fluids due to a displaced venous cannula may go unnoticed because of the extreme distensibility of the skin. Maintenance of low airway pressures during assisted or controlled ventilation of the lungs seems prudent in view of the increased incidence of pneumothorax in these patients. Unsuspected coronary artery disease manifesting as intraoperative myocardial ischemia has been described.[28] There are no specific recommendations for drugs to provide anesthesia. Regional anesthesia is not recommended, however, because of the tendency of these patients to bleed and form extensive hematomas. Surgical complications include uncontrollable hemorrhage and postoperative wound dehiscence.

■ POLYMYOSITIS

Polymyositis (dermatomyositis) is a multisystem disease of unknown etiology, manifesting as nonsuppurative inflammation of skeletal muscles (inflammatory myopathy). Cutaneous changes include discoloration of the upper eyelids, periorbital edema, a scaly erythematous malar rash, and symmetrical erythematous atrophic changes over the extensor surfaces of joints. This characteristic rash has led to the alternate designation of this disease as dermatomyositis. It is speculated that abnormal immune system responses may be responsible for the slowly progressive skeletal muscle damage. The concept that altered cellular immunity causes polymyositis is supported by the fact that 10% to 20% of affected patients have occult neoplasms.

Signs and Symptoms

Weakness of skeletal muscles typically involves proximal skeletal muscle groups, including the flexors of the neck, shoulders, and hips. Patients may have difficulty climbing stairs. Dysphagia, pulmonary aspiration, and pneumonia may result from paresis of pharyngeal and respiratory muscles. Weakness of the intercostal muscles and diaphragm can contribute to ventilatory insufficiency. Necrosis of skeletal muscles results in increased serum creatine kinase concentrations that parallel the extent and rapidity of skeletal muscle destruction. There is no evidence that this disease affects the neuromuscular junction.

Heart block secondary to myocardial fibrosis or atrophy of the conduction system, left ventricular dysfunction, and myocarditis can occur. Polymyositis can also be associated with systemic lupus erythematosus, scleroderma, and rheumatoid arthritis. A widespread necrotizing vasculitis may be present with childhood forms of this disease.

Diagnosis

The diagnosis of polymyositis is confirmed by proximal skeletal muscle weakness, increased serum creatine kinase concentrations, and the presence of characteristic skin rashes. Electromyography may demonstrate a triad consisting of spontaneous fibrillation potentials, decreased amplitude of voluntary contraction potentials, and repetitive potentials on needle insertion. Skeletal muscle biopsy adds support to the clinical diagnosis. Muscular dystrophy or myasthenia gravis can mimic polymyositis.

Treatment

Corticosteroids are considered the treatment of choice for polymyositis, although their efficacy has not been proven in carefully controlled trials. Immunosuppressive therapy with methotrexate, azathioprine, or cyclosporine may be effective when the response to corticosteroids is inadequate. Inclusion body myositis mimics polymyositis, but involvement of distal muscles is characteristic, and these patients are often unresponsive to therapy.

Management of Anesthesia

Management of anesthesia must consider the vulnerability of patients with polymyositis to pulmonary aspiration.[29, 30] It has been recommended that drugs capable of triggering malignant hyperthermia be avoided in these patients if serum creatine kinase concentrations are increased.[30] In view of co-existing skeletal muscle weakness, there is a logical concern that these patients could display abnormal responses to muscle relaxants. Nevertheless, responses to nondepolarizing muscle relaxants (atracurium, vecuronium) and succinylcholine have been described as unchanged in the presence of polymyositis.[29, 30] Responses to succinylcholine may resemble those observed in patients with myotonic dystrophy. The possibility of postoperative skeletal muscle weakness, which can lead to ventilatory insufficiency, is a consideration.

■ SYSTEMIC LUPUS ERYTHEMATOSUS

Systemic lupus erythematosus (SLE) is a multisystem chronic inflammatory disease characterized by antinuclear antibody production, most often manifesting in young women (may affect as many as 1 in 1000 women).[31] Antinuclear antibodies have not been documented to be directly involved in the pathogenesis of the disease. Stress such as an infection, pregnancy, or surgery may exacerbate SLE. The onset of SLE may also be drug-induced. Drugs most frequently associated with SLE are procainamide, hydralazine, isoniazid, D-penicillamine, α-methyldopa, and occasionally nonbarbiturate anticonvulsants. Susceptibility to the development of SLE, as induced by hydralazine or procainamide, is related to the patient's acetylator phenotype. The disease is more likely to develop in patients who metabolize these drugs slowly (slow acetylators). The clinical picture of drug-induced SLE is similar to the spontaneous form of the disease, but progression is usually slower and symptoms are mild, consisting of arthralgia, a maculopapular rash, fever, anemia, and leukopenia. The natural history of SLE is highly variable, with the presence of nephritis and systemic hypertension being associated with a poorer prognosis. Pregnancy in patients with SLE, especially those who have nephritis or systemic hypertension, is associated with a substantial risk of exacerbating the disease and a poor prognosis for the fetus.

Diagnosis

Detection of antinuclear antibodies is a sensitive screening test for SLE. Because antinuclear antibodies occur in more than 95% of patients, it is difficult to be certain of the diagnosis in the absence of antibodies. The most common antibodies in patients with SLE are directed against nucleosomal DNA–histone complexes. A diagnosis of SLE is likely when patients have three of four typical manifestations: antinuclear antibodies, characteristic rash, thrombocytopenia, serositis or nephritis. Commonly, however, the presenting features consist of arthralgia or a nonspecific pattern of arthritis, vague central nervous system symptoms, a history of rash or Raynaud's phenomenon, and a weakly positive antinuclear antibody test.[31]

Signs and Symptoms

Clinical manifestations of SLE may be categorized as articular and systemic. Polyarthritis and dermatitis are the most common clinical manifestations of SLE. Many of the clinical manifestations of SLE are a consequence of tissue damage from vasculopathy mediated by immune complexes. Others, such as thrombocytopenia or the antiphospholipid syndrome, are the direct effects of antibodies to cell surface molecules or serum components.

Articular Manifestations

Symmetrical arthritis involving the hands, wrists, elbows, knees, and ankles is the most common manifestation of SLE, occurring in 90% of patients. Arthritis is characteristically episodic and migratory, with pain that is out of proportion to the signs of the synovitis present. Another form of skeletal involvement is avascular necrosis, which most often involves the head or condyle of the femur. Arthritis associated with SLE does not involve the spine.

Systemic Manifestations

Systemic manifestations appear in the central nervous system, heart, lungs, kidneys, liver, neuromuscular system, and skin.

Neurologic complications of SLE can affect any part of the *central nervous system*. Cognitive dysfunction, usually mild, occurs in about one-third of individuals with SLE. Psychological changes ranging from mood disturbances suggestive of schizophrenia to signs of organic psychosis with deterioration of intellectual capacity are seen in nearly one-half of patients with SLE. Most of the serious central nervous system manifestations appear to be the result of vascular abnormalities. Fluid and electrolyte disturbances, fever, systemic hypertension, uremia, infections, or drug-induced effects may contribute to central nervous system dysfunction. Atypical migraine headaches are common and may be accompanied by cortical visual disturbances. Aseptic meningitis related to drugs including NSAIDs is possible.

Pericarditis resulting in pericardial effusion, chest pain, and a friction rub is the most common *cardiac* manifestation of SLE. Myocarditis may result in abnormalities of cardiac conduction. Persistent tachycardia and congestive heart failure can develop, with extensive cardiac involvement. Valvular abnormalities may be identified by echocardiography. Left ventricular dysfunction has been demonstrated in young patients. Noninfectious endocarditis (Libman-Sacks endocarditis) may involve the aortic and mitral valves.

Pulmonary involvement by SLE may manifest as lupus pneumonia characterized by diffuse pulmonary infiltrates, pleural effusion, dry cough, dyspnea, and arterial hypoxemia. Pulmonary function studies in these patients commonly show a restrictive type of pulmonary disease. Recurrent atelectasis can result in the "shrinking lung syndrome" perhaps reflecting diaphragmatic dysfunction as a consequence of phrenic neuropathy. Pulmonary angiitis with lung hemorrhage may complicate severe SLE. Pulmonary vascular hypertension is present in some patients.

The most common *renal* abnormality in patients with SLE is glomerulonephritis with proteinuria, resulting in hypoalbuminemia. Hematuria is a frequent finding. Severe decreases in glomerular filtration rate can terminate in oliguric renal failure.

Liver function tests are abnormal in about 30% of patients with SLE. More severe liver disease is nearly always of infectious origin or due to misdiagnosed autoimmune hepatitis or primary biliary cirrhosis.

Neuromuscular manifestations also occur. Myopathy with weakness of proximal skeletal muscle groups and increased serum creatine kinase concentrations are often present. Tendinitis is common and can result in rupture of the tendons.

Hematologic abnormalities may also be present. Thromboembolism associated with antiphospholipid antibodies is an important cause of abnormalities in the central nervous system. Leukopenia, antibody granulocyte dysfunction, decreased complement levels, and functional asplenia have been implicated in the increased risk for development of infections. Thrombocytopenia and hemolytic anemia are present in some patients. The presence of circulating anticoagulants is reflected in a prolonged prothrombin time and activated partial thromboplastin time. Patients with circulating anticoagulants often manifest biologic false positive tests for syphilis.

Some patients have *cutaneous* manifestations. The classic butterfly nasal malar erythema rash occurs in only one-third of patients. This rash is usually transient and often accompanies exacerbations of the disease. A patchy maculopapular rash on the upper trunk and areas exposed to the sun is probably more common. Alopecia is another frequent manifestation of SLE exacerbation.

Treatment

Treatment is determined to a large extent by individual disease manifestations rather than the primary diagnosis.[31] There is no evidence that prophylactic treatment with low doses of corticosteroids is beneficial. Arthritis and serositis can often be controlled with aspirin or NSAIDs. Antimalarial drugs such as hydroxychloroquine and quinacrine are effective for many of the dermatologic manifestations of SLE. Patients should use sunscreens and avoid intense exposure to the sun. Thrombocytopenia and hemolytic anemia usually respond to moderate doses of corticosteroids. Danazol, intravenous low-dose vincristine, cyclophosphamide, or splenectomy is used when thrombocytopenia responds to glucocorticoid therapy. In view of the susceptibility to infections, the risk-to-benefit ratio of splenectomy is carefully considered. Corticosteroids effectively suppress glomerulonephritis and adverse changes in the cardiovascular system. Corticosteroid therapy is a major cause of morbidity in patients with SLE. A prominent cause of death during the course of SLE is coronary atherosclerosis, possibly related to treatment with corticosteroids. For many patients with severe manifestations of SLE, low-dose immunosuppressive treatment may be preferable to prolonged intensive treatment with corticosteroids.

Management of Anesthesia

Management of anesthesia is influenced by drugs used to treat SLE and by the magnitude of dysfunction of those organs damaged by the disease.[32] Laryngeal involvement, including mucosal ulceration, cricoarytenoid arthritis, and recurrent laryngeal nerve palsy, may be present in as many as 30% of patients.[33]

■ URBACH-WIETHE DISEASE

Urbach-Wiethe disease (lipoid proteinosis) is a rare recessively inherited multisystem disorder that affects primarily the skin and oral mucosa.[34] Deposition of hyaline material in the capillary walls and epithelial basement membranes leads to thickening of the skin or mucosa and a predisposition for minor trauma to result in widespread scarring. Laryngeal scarring manifests as hoarseness and may cause difficulty with tracheal intubation. Hyaline infiltration of the soft tissues and tongue may make direct laryngoscopy difficult, emphasizing the need to consider the use of a flexible fiberoptic laryngoscope. In view of the abnormal oral mucosa, the need for antisialagogues in the preoperative medication is doubtful. A decreased gag reflex may put these patients at risk for aspiration. Recommendations to avoid epileptogenic anesthetic drugs are based on the propensity of these patients to develop epilepsy.

■ CORNELIA de LANGE SYNDROME

Cornelia de Lange syndrome is a rare disorder believed to be due to hypoplasia of the mesenchyma. The maturation of most organ systems, including the central nervous system, is delayed. Mental retardation, hirsutism, and microbrachycephaly are likely to be present. Many of these patients die before 1 year of age, most often due to aspiration. Anesthetic experience is limited but may be characterized by increased sensitivity to depressant drugs, an increased risk of aspiration owing to the common presence of hiatal hernia, and difficult tracheal intubation due to a short neck, small mouth, and high arched palate.[35]

■ TUMORAL CALCINOSIS

Tumoral calcinosis usually presents as multiple soft tissue masses adjacent to large joints that appear radiologically as loculated calcifications. Joint motion is generally unaffected, but the masses may enlarge and interfere with skeletal muscle function. Treatment consists of early, complete excision of the mass. The principal anesthetic considerations are the rare involvement of the hyoid bone, hypothyroid ligament, and cervical intervertebral joints by the disease process, leading to difficult exposure of the glottic opening during direct laryngoscopy.[36]

■ MUSCULAR DYSTROPHY

Muscular dystrophy is a hereditary disease characterized by painless degeneration and atrophy of skeletal muscles.[37] There is progressive, symmetrical skeletal muscle weakness and wasting but no evidence of skeletal muscle denervation (intact sensation and reflexes). Mental retardation is often present. Increased permeability of skeletal muscle membranes precedes clinical evidence of muscular dystrophy. In order of decreasing frequency, muscular dystrophy can be categorized as pseudohypertrophic (Duchenne's muscular dystrophy), limb-girdle, facioscapulohumeral (Landouzy-Dejerine), nemaline rod myopathy, and oculopharyngeal dystrophy.

Pseudohypertrophic Muscular Dystrophy (Duchenne's Muscular Dystrophy)

Pseudohypertrophic muscular dystrophy is the most common (3 per 10,000 births) and most severe form of childhood progressive muscular dystrophy. The disease, caused by an X-linked recessive gene, becomes apparent in 2- to 5-year-old male children. Initial symptoms (waddling gait, frequent falling, difficulty climbing stairs) reflect involvement of the proximal skeletal muscle groups of the pelvis. Affected skeletal muscles may become larger as a result of fatty infiltration, accounting for the designation of this disorder as pseudohypertrophic. There is steady deterioration in skeletal muscle strength, resulting in confinement to a wheelchair by 8 to 11 years of age. Kyphoscoliosis may develop, reflecting the unopposed action of antagonists of the dystrophic muscles.[37] Skeletal muscle atrophy can predispose to long bone fractures. Serum creatine kinase concentrations are 30 to 300 times normal, even early in the disease, reflecting skeletal muscle necrosis and increased permeability of skeletal muscle membranes. Approximately 70% of female carriers of this disease also exhibit increased serum creatine kinase concentrations. Skeletal muscle biopsy early in the course of the disease may demonstrate necrosis and phagocytosis of muscle fibers. Death usually occurs at 15 to 25 years of age due to congestive heart failure and/or pneumonia.

Cardiopulmonary Dysfunction

Degeneration of cardiac muscle invariably accompanies muscular dystrophy. Characteristic changes on the electrocardiogram include tall R waves in V_1, deep Q waves in the limb leads, short PR intervals, and sinus tachycardia. Mitral regurgitation may be due to papillary muscle dysfunction and to decreased myocardial contractility.

Chronic weakness of inspiratory respiratory muscles and a decreased ability to cough can result in loss of pulmonary reserve and accumulation of secretions, which predispose to recurrent pneumonia. Respiratory insufficiency often remains covert because impaired skeletal muscle function prevents patients from exceeding their limited breathing capacity. As the disease progresses, kyphoscoliosis can contribute further to restrictive patterns of lung disease. Sleep apnea is possible and may contribute to the development of pulmonary hypertension. An estimated 30% of deaths among individuals with pseudohypertrophic muscular dystrophy are due to respiratory causes.[37]

Management of Anesthesia

Children with pseudohypertrophic muscular dystrophy often require anesthesia for skeletal muscle biopsy or correction of progressive orthopedic deformities.[38] Preparations for anesthesia in patients afflicted with pseudohypertrophic muscular dystrophy must take into consideration the implications of increased permeability of skeletal muscle membranes and decreased cardiopulmonary reserve.[37] Hypomotility of the gastrointestinal tract may delay gastric emptying, which in the presence of weak laryngeal reflexes increases the risk of pulmonary aspiration. Succinylcholine is contraindicated because of the risks of rhabdomyolysis, hyperkalemia, and cardiac arrest. Indeed, ventricular fibrillation that occurs during induction of anesthesia that included succinylcholine has been observed in patients later discovered to have pseudohypertrophic muscular dystrophy.[39] Succinylcholine-induced hyperkalemia during acute rhabdomyolysis is more likely to result in cardiac arrest and unsuccessful resuscitation than is the potassium efflux resulting from up-regulation of acetylcholine receptors.[40] Normal responses usually follow the administration of nondepolarizing muscle relaxants, although the possibility of prolonged responses should be considered when co-existing skeletal muscle weakness is prominent.[41]

Rhabdomyolysis, with or without cardiac arrest, has been observed in association with administration of volatile anesthetics to these patients even in the absence of neuromuscular blocking drugs.[42, 43] A malignant hyperthermia-like episode (rhabdomyolysis and cardiac arrest) has been reported in a patient with Becker muscular dystrophy undergoing surgery with anesthesia provided with isoflurane and skeletal muscle paralysis produced by rocuronium.[44] Dantrolene should be available, as there is an increased incidence of malignant hyperthermia in these patients.[45, 46] Malignant hyperthermia has been observed after only brief periods of halothane administration alone, although most cases have been triggered by succinylcholine or with prolonged inhalation of halothane. Regional anesthesia avoids many of the unique risks of general anesthesia in these patients; during the postoperative period it provides analgesia, which may facilitate chest physiotherapy.[47]

Monitoring is directed at early detection of malignant hyperthermia (capnography, body temperature) and cardiac depression. Postoperative pulmonary dysfunction must be anticipated and attempts made to facilitate clearance of secretions. Delayed pulmonary insufficiency may occur up to 36 hours postoperatively despite apparent recovery to the preoperative levels of skeletal muscle strength.

Limb-Girdle Muscular Dystrophy

Limb-girdle muscular dystrophies comprise a slowly progressive but relatively benign disease. The age of onset varies from the second to the fifth decades. The shoulder girdle or hip girdle may be the only skeletal muscle group involved.

Facioscapulohumeral Muscular Dystrophy

Facioscapulohumeral muscular dystrophy is characterized by slowly progressive wasting of facial, pectoral, and shoulder girdle skeletal muscles that begins during adolescence. Eventually the lower limbs are involved. Early symptoms include difficulty raising the arms above the head and difficulty smiling. The heart is not involved, and serum creatine kinase concentrations are seldom increased. Recovery from atracurium-induced neuromuscular blockade has been described as faster than normal.[48] The course of this muscular dystrophy is slow, and longevity is likely.

Nemaline Rod Muscular Dystrophy

Nemaline rod muscular dystrophy is an autosomal dominant disease characterized clinically by slowly progressive to nonprogressive symmetrical dystrophy of skeletal and smooth muscles. The diagnosis is confirmed by skeletal muscle biopsy and histologic examination for the presence of rods between normal myofibrils.

Affected individuals experience delayed motor development, generalized skeletal muscle weakness with decreased muscle mass, hypotonia, and loss of deep tendon reflexes. Bony abnormalities secondary to decreased skeletal muscle tone may manifest as micrognathia. These individuals develop typical dysmorphic features and abnormal gait but are generally of normal intelligence. Affected infants may present with hypotonia, dysphagia, respiratory distress, and cyanosis. Micrognathia and dental malocclusion are common. Other skeletal deformities include kyphoscoliosis and pectus excavatum. Restrictive lung disease may result from myopathy and scoliosis. Cardiac failure has been described perhaps reflecting involvement of the myocardium by the disease and associated progressive dilated cardiomyopathy.

Tracheal intubation may be difficult owing to associated anatomic abnormalities such as micrognathia and a high arched palate.[49] Consideration of awake fiberoptic tracheal intubation may be prudent.[50] Respiratory depressant effects of drugs may be exaggerated in these patients, reflecting respiratory muscle weakness (intercostal muscles, diaphragm) and chest wall abnormalities (scoliosis, kyphoscoliosis). Ventilation-to-perfusion mismatching is increased, and the ventilatory response to carbon dioxide may be blunted. Bulbar palsy and associated regurgitation and pulmonary aspiration may further complicate anesthetic management.

Responses to succinylcholine and nondepolarizing neuromuscular blocking drugs are unpredictable.[50] There is no conclusive evidence that administration of succinylcholine evokes excessive release of potassium. Resistance to the effects of succinylcholine has been described in patients who respond normally to pancuronium. Anesthetic complications typical of malignant hyperthermia have not been reported in patients with nemaline myopathy.[50] Unexpected myocardial depression could accompany administration of volatile anesthetics especially if the disease process involves the myocardium. Regional anesthesia must consider the possible respiratory compromise that could accompany high motor blocks. Exaggerated lumbar lordosis and kyphoscoliosis could make performance of regional anesthesia technically difficult.

Oculopharyngeal Dystrophy

Oculopharyngeal dystrophy is a rare variant of muscular dystrophy characterized by progressive dysphagia and ptosis. Although experience is limited, these patients may be at risk for aspiration during the perioperative period, and the sensitivity to muscle relaxants may be greatly enhanced.[51]

Emery-Dreifuss Muscular Dystrophy

Emery-Dreifuss muscular dystrophy is an X-linked recessive disorder characterized by the development of skeletal muscle contractures that precede the onset of skeletal muscle weakness in a humeroperoneal distribution.[52] Mental retardation is not present, and respiratory function is maintained. Cardiac involvement and associated cardiomyopathy may be life-threatening (congestive heart failure, thromboembolism). Atrial conduction defects with bradycardia are the principal manifestations of cardiomyopathy. In contrast to other muscular dystrophies, female carriers of this disorder may experience cardiac impairment.

MYOTONIC DYSTROPHY

Myotonic dystrophy designates a group of hereditary degenerative intrinsic diseases of skeletal muscles characterized by persistent contractures (myotonia) of skeletal muscles after voluntary contraction or following electrical stimulation (Table 26–2).[53] Peripheral nerves and the neuromuscular junctions are not affected. Electromyographic findings are diagnostic and characterized by prolonged discharges of repetitive muscle action potentials. The inability of skeletal muscles to relax after voluntary contraction or stimulation is diagnostic and results from abnormal calcium metabolism, as the cellular adenosine triphosphatase system fails to return calcium to the sarcoplasmic reticulum. Unsequestered calcium then remains available to produce sustained skeletal muscle contractions. This accounts for the failure of general anesthesia, regional anesthesia, or neuromuscular blocking drugs to prevent or relieve contraction of skeletal muscles. Infiltration of contracted skeletal muscles with solutions containing local anesthetics may induce relaxation. Quinine, 300 to 600 mg IV, has been reported to be effective in some cases. Increasing the ambient temperature in the operating room decreases the severity of myotonia and the incidence of postoperative shivering, which may precipitate contraction of skeletal muscles. Patients with myotonic disorders are susceptible to malignant hyperthermia. Most myotonic patients survive to adulthood with little impairment, and it is common for them to conceal their symptoms such

that they may present for unrelated surgery, with the underlying myotonia not being appreciated.

Myotonia Dystrophica

Myotonia dystrophica is the most common (2.4 to 5.5 per 100,000 population) and most serious form of myotonic dystrophy afflicting adults.[53, 54] It is inherited as an autosomal dominant trait, with the onset of symptoms during the second to third decades of life. Unlike other myotonic syndromes, myotonia dystrophica is a multisystem disease, although skeletal muscles are principally affected.

Treatment is symptomatic and may include the use of quinine, phenytoin, tocainide, or mexiletine. These drugs depress sodium influx into skeletal muscle cells and delay the return of membrane excitability. Death from pneumonia or congestive heart failure usually occurs by the sixth decade of life, reflecting the progressive involvement of skeletal, cardiac, and smooth muscles. High perioperative morbidity and mortality are caused principally by cardiopulmonary complications.

Signs and Symptoms

Myotonia dystrophica typically manifests as early facial weakness (expressionless facies), wasting and weakness of sternocleidomastoid muscles, ptosis, dysarthria, dysphagia, and inability to relax the handgrip (myotonia). The triad of characteristic features consists of mental retardation, frontal baldness, and cataract formation. Involvement of endocrine glands manifests as gonadal atrophy, diabetes mellitus, decreased thyroid function, and adrenal insufficiency. Slowed gastric emptying and intestinal pseudo-obstruction may be present. Occurrence of central sleep apnea in patients with myotonic dystrophy is recognized and probably accounts for the frequent presence of hypersomnolence. There is an increased incidence of cholelithiasis, especially in men. Exacerbation of symptoms during pregnancy is likely, and it is not unusual for uterine atony and retained placenta to complicate vaginal delivery.[54]

Cardiac dysrhythmias and conduction abnormalities presumably reflect myocardial involvement by the myotonic process. First-degree atrioventricular heart block is a common finding on the electrocardiogram before the clinical onset of symptoms. Up to 20% of these patients have evidence of mitral valve prolapse on echocardiography. Despite the relatively high incidence of mitral valve prolapse, systemic complications are rare. Reports of sudden death may reflect third-degree atrioventricular heart block. Weakness of pharyngeal and thoracic muscles

---

Table 26–2 • Classification of Myotonic Dystrophies

Myotonic dystrophy (myotonia atrophica, Steinert's disease)
Myotonia congenita (Thomsen's disease)
Paramyotonia congenita
Hyperkalemic periodic paralysis
Acid-maltase deficiency (Pompe's disease)
Schwartz-Jampel syndrome (chondrodystrophic myotonia)

renders these patients vulnerable to pulmonary aspiration of acidic gastric fluid.

Management of Anesthesia

Management of anesthesia in patients with myotonia dystrophica must consider the likely presence of cardiomyopathy, respiratory muscle weakness, and abnormal responses to the drugs used during anesthesia.[53, 55] It is presumed that even asymptomatic patients have some degree of cardiomyopathy and that myocardial depression produced by volatile anesthetics may be exaggerated. The need to treat cardiac dysrhythmias is anticipated. Anesthesia and surgery could theoretically aggravate co-existing cardiac conduction blockade by increasing vagal tone or causing transient hypoxia of the cardiac conduction system.

Administration of succinylcholine is not recommended, as prolonged skeletal muscle contractions occur. Conversely, the responses to nondepolarizing neuromuscular blocking drugs are normal.[56] Theoretically, reversal of neuromuscular blockade could precipitate skeletal muscle contractions by facilitating depolarization of the neuromuscular junction. Nevertheless, adverse responses do not predictably occur when neostigmine is used to reverse neuromuscular blockade in patients with myotonic dystrophy. Careful titration of neuromuscular blockade and administration of short-acting nondepolarizing muscle relaxants may obviate the need for pharmacologic reversal in selected patients.

Patients with myotonia dystrophica are sensitive to the ventilatory depressant effects of barbiturates, opioids, benzodiazepines, and propofol, most likely reflecting drug-induced central nervous system depression of ventilation superimposed on already weak and atrophic peripheral respiratory musculature. Furthermore, co-existing hypersomnolence and vulnerability to central sleep apnea may contribute to increased sensitivity to depressant drugs. There is a theoretical concern that these patients are susceptible to malignant hyperthermia. Myotonic contractions during surgical manipulation and use of electrocautery may interfere with surgical access. Drugs such as procainamide and phenytoin, which stabilize skeletal muscle membranes, may be helpful in this situation. Although high concentrations of volatile anesthetics may abolish myotonic contractions, it may be at the expense of cardiac depression. Postoperatively, local or regional anesthesia is useful for pain relief, and several hours of careful nursing surveillance is indicated. Intraoperative maintenance of body temperature and postoperative avoidance of shivering is important, as cold may induce myotonia.

Myotonia Congenita

Myotonia congenita is transmitted as a dominant characteristic and manifests at birth or during early childhood. Skeletal muscle involvement is widespread, but there is usually no involvement of other organ systems. The disease does not progress, nor does it result in decreased life expectancy. Patients with myotonia congenita respond to quinidine therapy. Myotonia congenita may be associated with susceptibility to malignant hyperthermia.[53]

Paramyotonia Congenita

Paramyotonia congenita is a rare autosomal dominant disorder characterized by generalized myotonia that is recognized during early childhood; and as with myotonia congenita, generalized muscular hypertrophy may occur.[53] This myotonia is viewed as paradoxical because, in contrast to other myotonias, the skeletal muscle stiffness is often exacerbated by exercise. Cold markedly aggravates the myotonia, and flaccid skeletal paralysis may be present after the muscles are warmed. Some patients with paramyotonia congenita develop skeletal muscle paralysis independent of myotonia, which may be related to serum potassium concentrations. For this reason there is some doubt that paramyotonia congenita and hyperkalemic periodic paralysis are separate entities.[53] The electromyogram may be normal at room temperature, but typical myotonic discharges become evident as skeletal muscles are cooled.

Hyperkalemic Periodic Paralysis

Hyperkalemic periodic paralysis is characterized by episodes of flaccid skeletal muscle paralysis associated with increased serum potassium concentrations. It is precipitated by cold, hunger, and emotional stress.[53] Most patients have clinical and electromyographic evidence of myotonia that is not present in patients manifesting familial hypokalemic periodic paralysis (see "Dyskalemic Familial Periodic Paralysis").

Preoperative depletion of total body potassium stimulated by the administration of furosemide or thiazide diuretics may be a consideration in patients with hyperkalemic periodic paralysis.[53] Potassium-containing fluids and drugs that evoke the release of potassium are avoided. Intravenous glucose infusions are administered to minimize carbohydrate depletion during fasting. Calcium gluconate administered intravenously is suggested for emergency treatment of hyperkalemia-induced skeletal muscle weakness. Intraoperative maintenance of body temperature is prudent.

Acid-Maltase Deficiency

Acid-maltase deficiency is a glycogen storage disease (Pompe's disease) presenting as pelvic girdle weakness and respiratory failure as a result of respiratory muscle weakness (see Chapter 23). Myotonic discharges are demonstrable, especially in the neck muscles; but they are rarely a predominant feature.

Schwartz-Jampel Syndrome

Schwartz-Jampel syndrome is a rare, progressive disorder of childhood comprising skeletal muscle stiffness, myotonia, and ocular, facial, and skeletal abnormalities including micrognathia.[53] Tracheal intubation is predictably difficult.[57] There is blepharospasm and tense puckering of the afflicted child's mouth. These children may be susceptible to malignant hyperthermia.

DYSKALEMIC FAMILIAL PERIODIC PARALYSIS

Dyskalemic familial periodic paralysis is a spectrum of diseases characterized by intermittent acute attacks of skeletal muscle weakness or paralysis (sparing only the bulbar musculature represented by muscles of respiration) associated with hypokalemia, hyperkalemia, or normokalemia (Table 26–3). The hyperkalemic form of periodic paralysis is much rarer than the hypokalemic form. It is speculated that paramyotonia congenita is a variant of the hyperkalemic form of hyperkalemic periodic paralysis (see "Hyperkalemic Periodic Paralysis").

Causes

The fundamental defect in patients with familial periodic paralysis is unknown, although mutations in calcium and sodium channels are associated with hypokalemic and hyperkalemic periodic paralysis, respectively. It is recognized that the mechanism of the disease is unrelated to any abnormality at the neuromuscular junctions. Skeletal muscle weakness provoked by glucose-insulin infusions confirms the presence of the hypokalemic form of familial periodic paralysis. Conversely, skeletal muscle weakness in response to oral administration of potassium confirms the presence of the hyperkalemic form of familial periodic paralysis. Acetazolamide has been recommended for the treatment of both forms of familial periodic paralysis; presumably this drug produces acidosis, which protects against hypokalemic paralysis. Protection in patients with hyperkalemic paralysis is provided by the ability of acetazolamide to promote renal excretion of potassium. The onset of unexpected postoperative skeletal muscle weakness may reflect familial periodic hypokalemic paralysis with or without additive effects being produced by lingering effects of nondepolarizing neuromuscular blocking drugs administered during surgery.

Management of Anesthesia

The nature of the potassium sensitivity in patients with dyskalemic familial periodic paralysis influ-

Table 26–3 • Clinical Features of Familial Periodic Paralysis

Type	Serum Potassium Concentration during Symptoms (mEq/L)	Precipitating Factors	Other Features
Hypokalemic	< 3.0	Large glucose meals Strenuous exercise Glucose-insulin infusions Stress Menstruation Pregnancy Anesthesia Hypothermia	Cardiac dysrhythmias ECG signs of hypokalemia
Hyperkalemic	> 5.5	Exercise Potassium infusions Metabolic acidosis Hypothermia	Skeletal muscle weakness may be localized to tongue and eyelids

ECG, electrocardiogram.

ences the management of anesthesia (Table 26–3). The goal of anesthesia is to avoid events that precipitate skeletal muscle weakness.[58–61] Hypothermia is avoided in patients with familial periodic paralysis, regardless of the nature of the potassium sensitivity. Increasing the ambient temperature of the operating room and warming the inhaled gases and intravenous fluids minimize intraoperative decreases in body temperature. In patients undergoing cardiopulmonary bypass, it may be necessary to maintain normothermia despite the common practice of using systemic hypothermia for many of these operations.[58] Nondepolarizing muscle relaxants are acceptable for administration to patients with familial periodic paralysis.[62, 63]

Hypokalemic Periodic Paralysis

Preoperative considerations include carbohydrate balance, correction of electrolyte abnormalities, and avoidance of events known to trigger hypokalemic attacks (psychological stress, cold, carbohydrate loads). Large carbohydrate meals are known to trigger hypokalemic episodes and should be avoided during the 24 hours preceding surgery in patients with the hypokalemic form of familial periodic paralysis. Glucose-containing intravenous solutions and drugs known to cause intracellular shifts of potassium (β-adrenergic agonists) are avoided. Mannitol is administered in place of potassium-losing diuretics should the operative procedure require drug-induced diuresis. Frequent perioperative monitoring (every 15 to 60 minutes) of serum potassium concentrations is useful, and aggressive interventions (potassium chloride up to 40 mEq/hr) are considerations. Hypokalemia may precede the onset of skeletal muscle weakness by several hours, allowing avoidance of these symptoms with potassium supplementation. Administration of short-acting neuromuscular blocking drugs is preferable to long-acting drugs when skeletal muscle relaxation is required for surgery. Succinylcholine, with its ability to increase serum potassium concentrations transiently, seems acceptable in these patients. Nevertheless, use of succinylcholine and other drugs known to trigger malignant hyperthermia is influenced by reports of this syndrome in patients with hypokalemic periodic paralysis.[64] Regional anesthesia has been safely utilized in these patients, although hypokalemia may be a consequence of epidural and other regional anesthetic techniques.[65]

Hyperkalemic Periodic Paralysis

Management of anesthesia in patients with hyperkalemic periodic paralysis includes preoperative potassium depletion with furosemide-induced diuresis, prevention of carbohydrate depletion during fasting with the administration of glucose-containing solutions, and avoidance of potassium containing solutions and potassium-releasing drugs such as succinylcholine.[62] As with the hypokalemic form of periodic paralysis, frequent monitoring of serum potassium concentrations is indicated, as is the availability of calcium for intravenous administration should signs of hyperkalemia appear on the electrocardiogram.

■ MYASTHENIA GRAVIS

Myasthenia gravis is an acquired chronic autoimmune disorder caused by a decrease in functioning acetylcholine receptors at the neuromuscular junctions owing to their destruction or inactivation by circulating antibodies (Fig. 26–2).[66] An estimated 70% to 80% of functional acetylcholine receptors are lost, explaining the easy exhaustion of these patients and the marked sensitivity to nondepolarizing muscle relaxants. Indeed, the hallmarks of the disease are weakness and rapid exhaustion of voluntary skeletal muscles with repetitive use followed by partial recovery with rest. Skeletal muscles innervated by cranial nerves (ocular, pharyngeal, and laryngeal muscles, representing bulbar muscles) are especially vulnerable, as reflected by the appearance of ptosis, diplopia, and dysphagia, which may be the initial symptoms of the disease. Myasthenia gravis is not a rare disease, with a prevalence of 50 to 125 cases per million population. Women 20 to 30 years of age are most often affected, whereas men are often older than 60 years of age when their disease manifests. Receptor-binding antibodies are present in the plasma of more than 80% of patients with myasthenia gravis. The origin of these antibodies is unknown, but a role of the thymus gland is suggested by the association of myasthenia gravis with thymus gland abnormalities. For example, hyperplasia of the thymus gland is present in more than 70% of patients with myasthenia gravis, and 10% to 15% of these patients have thymomas. Other conditions that cause weakness of the cranial and somatic musculature must be considered in the differential diagnosis of myasthenia gravis (Table 26–4).[66]

Classification

Myasthenia gravis may be classified on the basis of the skeletal muscles involved and the severity of the symptoms. Type I is limited to involvement of the extraocular muscles. About 10% of patients

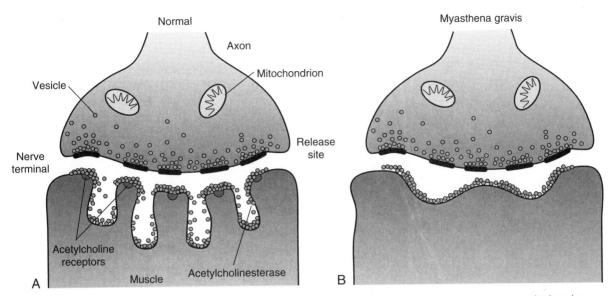

Figure 26–2 • Normal (*A*) and myasthenic (*B*) neuromuscular junctions. Compared with normal neuromuscular junctions, myasthenic neuromuscular junctions have fewer acetylcholine receptors, simplified synaptic folds, and widened synaptic spaces. (From Drachman DB. Myasthenia gravis. N Engl J Med 1994;330:1797–1810. Copyright 1994 Massachusetts Medical Society, with permission.)

Table 26–4 • Differential Diagnosis of Myasthenia Gravis

Condition	Symptoms and Characteristics	Comments
Congenital myasthenic syndromes	Rare Early onset Not autoimmune	Electrophysiologic and immunocytochemical tests required for diagnosis
Drug-induced myasthenia gravis Penicillamine	Triggers autoimmune myasthenia gravis	Recovery within weeks of discontinuing the drug

Nondepolarizing muscle relaxants
  Aminoglycosides
  Procainamide
	Increased sensitivity	Recovery after drug discontinuation

Lambert-Eaton syndrome	Oat cell cancer Fatigue	Incremental response on repetitive nerve stimulation Antibodies to calcium channels
Hyperthyroidism	Exacerbation of myasthenia gravis	Thyroid function abnormal
Graves' disease	Diplopia Exophthalmos	Thyroid-stimulating immunoglobulin present
Botulism	Generalized weakness Ophthalmoplegia	Incremental response on repetitive nerve stimulation Mydriasis
Progressive external ophthalmoplegia	Ptosis Diplopia Generalized weakness in some cases	Mitochondrial abnormalities
Intracranial mass compressing cranial nerves	Ophthalmoplegia Cranial nerve weakness	CT or MRI abnormalities

CT, computed tomography; MRI, magnetic resonance imaging.
Adapted from: Drachman DB. Myasthenia gravis. N Engl J Med 1994;330:1797–1810.

show signs and symptoms confined to the extraocular muscles and are considered to have ocular myasthenia gravis. Any extension beyond the ocular muscles is likely to involve the bulbar muscles. Patients in whom the disease has been confined to the ocular muscles for more than 3 years are unlikely to experience any progression in their disease. Type IIA is a slowly progressive, mild form of skeletal muscle weakness that spares the muscles of respiration. Responses to anticholinesterase drugs and occasionally corticosteroids are good in these patients. Type IIB is a more severe, rapidly progressive form of skeletal muscle weakness than that which occurs with type IIA. Responses to drug therapy are not as good, and muscles of respiration may be involved. Type III is characterized by an acute onset and rapid deterioration of skeletal muscle strength (within 6 months) and is associated with high mortality. Type IV is a severe form of skeletal muscle weakness that results from progression of type I or II.

Signs and Symptoms

The clinical course of myasthenia gravis is marked by periods of exacerbations and remissions. Electromyography demonstrates decreased voltage of skeletal muscle action potentials during repetitive stimulation. Ptosis and diplopia resulting from extraocular muscle weakness are the most common initial complaints. Weakness of pharyngeal and laryngeal muscles (bulbar muscles) results in dysphagia, dysarthria, and difficulty eliminating oral secretions. Skeletal muscle strength may be normal in well rested patients, but weakness occurs promptly with exercise. Arm, leg, or trunk weakness can occur in any combination and is usually asymmetrical in distribution. Skeletal muscle atrophy is unlikely. Patients with myasthenia gravis are at high risk for pulmonary aspiration of gastric contents. Myocarditis may result in atrial fibrillation and heart block. Myasthenia gravis may be associated with cardiomyopathy. Other diseases often considered autoimmune in origin can occur in association with myasthenia gravis. For example, decreased thyroid function is present in about 10% of patients with myasthenia gravis; rheumatoid arthritis, systemic lupus erythematosus, and pernicious anemia occur more commonly than in patients without myasthenia gravis. About 15% of infants born to mothers with myasthenia gravis demonstrate transient (2 to 4 weeks) skeletal muscle weakness. Infections, electrolyte abnormalities, pregnancy, emotional stress, and surgery may precipitate skeletal muscle weakness or exacerbate co-existing weakness. Antibiotics, particularly the aminoglycosides, can aggravate skeletal muscle weakness associated with myasthenia gravis. Isolated respiratory failure may be the presenting manifestation of myasthenia gravis.

Treatment

Treatment methods for myasthenia gravis include enhancing neuromuscular transmission with anticholinesterase drugs, surgical thymectomy, immunosuppression, and short-term immunotherapy, including plasma exchange and intravenous administration of immune globulins.[66]

Anticholinesterase Drugs

Anticholinesterase drugs are the first line of treatment for myasthenia gravis. Presumably, these drugs are effective because they inhibit the enzyme responsible for the hydrolysis of acetylcholine, which serves to increase the amount of neurotransmitter available at the neuromuscular junctions. Pyridostigmine is the most widely used anticholinesterase drug, producing an effect in 30 minutes and a peak effect in about 120 minutes. Oral pyridostigmine lasts longer (3 to 6 hours) and produces fewer side effects than occur with neostigmine. A 60 mg oral dose of pyridostigmine is equivalent to an intramuscular or intravenous dose of 2 mg. The pyridostigmine dose and schedule are tailored to the patient's responses, but the maximal useful dose of pyridostigmine rarely exceeds 120 mg every 3 hours. Higher doses may induce increased skeletal muscle weakness ("cholinergic crisis"). The presence of muscarinic side effects (salivation, miosis, bradycardia) plus accentuated skeletal muscle weakness after administration of edrophonium, 1 to 2 mg IV, confirms the diagnosis of cholinergic crisis. Although anticholinesterase drugs benefit most patients, improvements are usually incomplete and often wane after weeks or months of treatment.

Thymectomy

Surgical thymectomy as a treatment for myasthenia gravis is intended to induce remissions or at least permit improvement, allowing the doses of immunosuppressive medications to be decreased.[66] Generalized myasthenia gravis patients between the ages of puberty and about 60 years are candidates for surgical thymectomy. Preoperative preparation is intended to optimize the patient's strength (especially respiratory function), but immunosuppressive drugs should be avoided if possible because they increase the risk of infection. If the vital capacity is less than 2 L, plasmapheresis may be performed before surgery to improve the likelihood of spontaneous respiration during the postoperative period. Median sternotomy as an approach to the thymus gland optimizes removal of all thymic tissue. Alternatively, a cervical incision with mediastinoscopy has been advocated because it is associated with a smaller surgical incision and less postoperative pain. The use of neuraxial analgesia minimizes postoperative pain and thus enhances postoperative breathing. The need for anticholinesterase medications may be decreased for a few days postoperatively, and the benefits of thymectomy are often delayed until months after surgery. The mechanism by which thymectomy produces improvement is uncertain, although acetylcholine receptor antibody levels usually decrease following thymectomy.

Immunosuppressive Therapy

Immunosuppressive therapy (corticosteroids, azathioprine, cyclosporine) is indicated when skeletal muscle weakness is not adequately controlled by anticholinesterase drugs. Corticosteroids are the most commonly used and most consistently effective immunosuppressive drugs for the treatment of myasthenia gravis.[66] They are also associated with the greatest likelihood of adverse side effects.

Short-Term Immunotherapy

Plasmapheresis removes antibodies from the patient's circulation and produces short-term clinical improvements in patients with myasthenia gravis who are experiencing myasthenic crises or being prepared for thymectomy.[66] The beneficial effects of plasmapheresis are transient, and repeated treatments introduce risks of infection, hypotension, and pulmonary embolism. Indications for intravenous administration of immune globulins are the same as for plasmapheresis. The effect is temporary, and this treatment has no effect on the circulating concentrations of acetylcholine receptor antibodies.

Management of Anesthesia

Anesthesia for patients with myasthenia gravis is most often required for elective surgical procedures such as thymectomy.[67]

Preoperative Preparation

Drugs such as opioids should be used with caution, if at all, for preoperative medication. It is likely that patients with myasthenia gravis will require ventilatory support after surgery. For this reason it is useful to advise these patients during the preoperative interview that they will most likely have a tracheal tube in place when they awaken. Preoperatively, criteria that correlate with the likely need for controlled ventilation of the patient's lungs during the postoperative period following transsternal thymectomy include duration of the disease for longer than 6 years, the presence of chronic obstructive lung disease unrelated to myasthenia gravis, daily dose of pyridostigmine higher than 750 mg during the 48 hours preceding surgery, and a preoperative vital capacity less than 2.9 L.[68,69] These criteria are less predictive of the need for postoperative ventilatory support following transcervical thymectomy, suggesting that this less invasive surgical approach has a respiratory-sparing effect.

Muscle Relaxants

Antibodies decrease the number of functional acetylcholine receptors, which results in increased sensitivity to nondepolarizing muscle relaxants. The balance between active and nonfunctional acetylcholine receptors modulates the sensitivity to nondepolarizing muscle relaxants. Preoperative determination of train-of-four fade may be helpful for identifying the patients who will require less nondepolarizing muscle relaxants intraoperatively.[70] There is general agreement that initial muscle relaxant doses should be titrated against responses at the neuromuscular junction, as monitored with a peripheral nerve stimulator. Monitoring the neuromuscular blockade with a peripheral nerve stimulator and the responses evoked at the orbicularis oculi muscle may overestimate the degree of neuromuscular blockade in patients with myasthenia gravis.[71] For this reason it may be useful to monitor neuromuscular blockade at the orbicularis oculi muscle to avoid unrecognized persistent neuromuscular blockade in patients with myasthenia gravis.

It is possible that drugs used to treat myasthenia gravis influence the response to muscle relaxants independent of the disease process. For example, anticholinesterase drugs such as pyridostigmine not only inhibit true cholinesterase but also impair plasma cholinesterase activity, introducing the possibility of prolonged responses to succinylcholine. Conversely, anticholinesterase drugs theoretically antagonize the effects of nondepolarizing muscle relaxants. Nevertheless, this response does not seem to occur clinically. Corticosteroid therapy probably does not alter the dose requirements for succinylcholine. Conversely, corticosteroid therapy has been reported to produce resistance to the neuromuscular blocking effects of steroidal muscle relaxants such as vecuronium.[70]

Controlled measurements in patients with myasthenia gravis treated with pyridostigmine demonstrate resistance to the effects of succinylcholine (ED_{95} about 2.6 times normal) (Fig. 26–3).[72] Because the dose of succinylcholine commonly administered to normal patients (1.0 to 1.5 mg/kg) represents three to five times the ED_{95}, it is likely that adequate intubating conditions would be achieved in patients with myasthenia gravis using these doses. The mechanism by which patients with myasthenia gravis are resistant to succinylcholine is unknown, although the decreased number of acetylcholine receptors at the postsynaptic neuromuscular junctions may play a role.

In contrast to succinylcholine, patients with myasthenia gravis may exhibit exquisite sensitivity to nondepolarizing muscle relaxants. Nonparalyzing doses of nondepolarizing muscle relaxants intended to attenuate succinylcholine-induced fasciculations may produce profound skeletal muscle weakness if administered to patients with unrecognized myasthenia gravis. In patients with mild to moderate myasthenia gravis, the potency of atracurium is increased 1.7 to 1.9 times, compared with responses in normal patients (Fig. 26–4).[73] Patients with myasthenia gravis are also more sensitive to vecuronium.[74] Nevertheless, intermediate-acting muscle relaxants, as well as mivacurium, are eliminated rapidly and can be titrated to achieve the needed degree of skeletal muscle paralysis with confidence that drug effects can be predictably reversed at the conclusion of surgery.[67] When rapid onset of neuromuscular blockade is needed, it is important to recognize that resistance to succinylcholine may occur.

Induction of Anesthesia

Induction of anesthesia with short-acting intravenous anesthetics is acceptable for patients with myasthenia gravis. Logic suggests, however, that the respiratory depressant effects of these drugs could be accentuated. Tracheal intubation can be accomplished without muscle relaxants in many patients by taking advantage of co-existing skeletal muscle weakness and the relaxing effect of volatile anesthetics on skeletal muscles. Succinylcholine can be used to facilitate tracheal intubation, keeping in mind the need to decrease the initial dose of succinylcholine until responses at the neuromuscular junction can be documented with a peripheral nerve stimulator.

Maintenance of Anesthesia

Maintenance of anesthesia is often provided with nitrous oxide plus volatile anesthetics. Use of volatile anesthetics may decrease the dose of muscle relaxants needed or even eliminate the need for their intraoperative administration. Should administration of nondepolarizing muscle relaxants be necessary, the initial dose should be decreased at least one-half to two-thirds and the responses observed using a peripheral nerve stimulator. The inherent short duration of action of short- and intermediate-acting muscle relaxants are desirable characteristics when muscle relaxants are administered to these patients to facilitate tracheal intubation or provide maintenance of skeletal muscle relaxation.[74, 75] The ability to dissipate the effects of inhaled drugs at the conclusion of anesthesia is important for evaluating

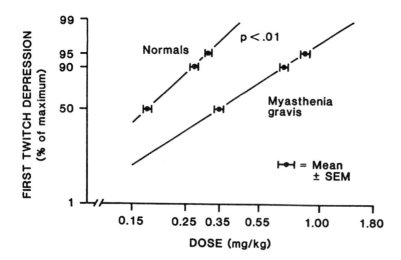

Figure 26–3 • Dose–response curves for succinylcholine in patients with myasthenia gravis are shifted to the right of curves for normal patients, indicating that myasthenic patients are resistant to the neuromuscular blocking effects of this muscle relaxant. (From Eisenkraft JB, Book WJ, Mann SM, et al. Resistance to succinylcholine in myasthenia gravis: a dose–response study. Anesthesiology 1988;69:760–3, with permission.)

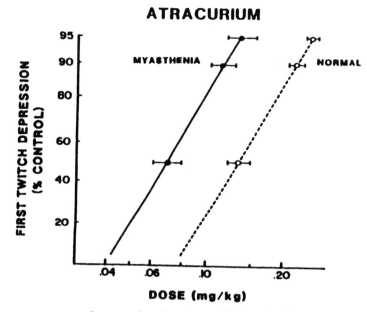

Figure 26–4 • Dose–response curves for atracurium in patients with myasthenia gravis. The curves are shifted to the left of the curves for normal patients, indicating that myasthenic patients are sensitive to the neuromuscular blocking effects of this muscle relaxant and presumably other nondepolarizing muscle relaxants as well. (From Smith CE, Donati F, Bevan DR. Cumulative dose-response curves for atracurium in patients with myasthenia gravis. Can J Anaesth 1989;36:402–6, with permission.)

skeletal muscle strength during the early postoperative period. Prolonged effects of opioids, especially on ventilation, detract from the use of these drugs for maintenance of anesthesia.

Postoperative Care

At the conclusion of surgery, it is wise to leave the tracheal tube in place until patients demonstrate an ability to maintain adequate levels of ventilation. Skeletal muscle strength often seems adequate during the early stages after anesthesia and surgery, only to deteriorate a few hours later. The need to

support ventilation of the lungs during the postoperative period should be anticipated for patients who demonstrate findings during the preoperative evaluation known to correlate with inadequate ventilation after surgery (see "Preoperative Preparation").

▮ MYASTHENIC SYNDROME

Myasthenic syndrome (Eaton-Lambert syndrome) is a rare disorder of neuromuscular transmission that resembles myasthenia gravis (Table 26–5).[76]

Table 26–5 • Comparison of Myasthenic Syndrome and Myasthenia Gravis

Parameter	Myasthenic Syndrome	Myasthenia Gravis
Manifestations	Proximal limb weakness (legs more than arms)	Extraocular, bulbar, and facial muscle weakness
	Exercise improves strength	Fatigue with exercise
	Muscle pain common	Muscle pain uncommon
	Reflexes absent or decreased	Reflexes normal
Gender	Males more often than females	Females more often than males
Co-existing pathology	Small cell lung cancer	Thymoma
Response to muscle relaxants	Sensitive to succinylcholine	Resistant to succinylcholine
	Sensitive to nondepolarizing muscle relaxants	Sensitive to nondepolarizing muscle relaxants
	Poor response to anticholinesterase	Good response to anticholinesterases

This syndrome of skeletal muscle weakness, originally described in patients with small cell carcinoma of the lung, has subsequently been described in patients with no evidence of cancer. Myasthenic syndrome is considered to be an autoimmune disease in which immunoglobulin G antibodies to presynaptic calcium channels are produced. The anticholinesterase drugs effective in the treatment of myasthenia gravis do not produce an improvement in patients with myasthenic syndrome.

Patients with myasthenic syndrome are sensitive to the effects of both succinylcholine and nondepolarizing muscle relaxants.[76] Antagonism of neuromuscular blockade with anticholinesterase drugs may be inadequate. The potential presence of myasthenic syndrome and the need to decrease the doses of muscle relaxants should be considered in patients with known cancer. Furthermore, this syndrome should be considered in patients undergoing such diagnostic procedures, as bronchoscopy, mediastinoscopy, or exploratory thoracotomy for suspected lung cancer.

▪ RHEUMATOID ARTHRITIS

Rheumatoid arthritis, the most common chronic inflammatory form of arthritis, affects about 1% of adults, with the incidence being two to three times higher in women than in men.[77, 78] The etiology of rheumatoid arthritis is unknown. The disease is characterized by symmetric polyarthropathy and significant systemic involvement (Table 26–6). Morning stiffness and involvement of the wrists and metacarpophalangeal joints helps distinguish rheumatoid arthritis from osteoarthritis, which typically affects weight-bearing joints and the distal interpha-langeal joints. The course of the disease is characterized by exacerbations and remissions. Rheumatoid nodules are typically present at pressure points, particularly below the elbow. Rheumatoid factor is an antiimmunoglobulin antibody that is present in up to 90% of patients with rheumatoid arthritis but not in those with osteoarthritis. The presence of rheumatoid factor, however, is not specific, being present in patients with SLE, pulmonary fibrosis, and viral hepatitis. Activation of cellular immune responses in genetically susceptible hosts may mark the beginning of rheumatoid arthritis. The cause of this response is unknown but may reflect virus-induced (Epstein-Barr) activation of B lymphocyte proliferation that culminates in proliferative synovitis.

Signs and Symptoms

The onset of rheumatoid arthritis in adults may be acute (involving single or multiple joints) or insidious (generating systemic manifestations that precede overt arthritis by months). In some patients the clinical course of rheumatoid arthritis coincides with trauma, a surgical procedure, childbirth, or exposure to extremes of ambient temperatures. Pregnancy often relieves the symptoms of rheumatoid arthritis, presumably owing to immunosuppression.

Joint Involvement

Morning stiffness is a hallmark of rheumatoid arthritis. Multiple joints, particularly in the hands, wrists, and knees, are affected at the same time in a symmetrical distribution. Fusiform swelling is typical of the involvement of the proximal interphalan-

Table 26–6 • Comparison of Rheumatoid Arthritis and Ankylosing Spondylitis

Parameter	Rheumatoid Arthritis	Ankylosing Spondylitis
Family history	Rare	Common
Gender	Female (30–50 years old)	Male (20–30 years old)
Joint involvement	Symmetrical polyarthropathy	Asymmetrical oligoarthropathy
Sacroiliac involvement	No	Yes
Vertebral involvement	Cervical	Total (ascending)
Cardiac changes	Pericardial effusion	Cardiomegaly
	Aortic regurgitation	Aortic regurgitation
	Cardiac conduction abnormalities	Cardiac conduction abnormalities
	Cardiac valve fibrosis	
	Coronary artery arteritis	
Pulmonary changes	Pulmonary fibrosis	Pulmonary fibrosis
	Pleural effusion	
Eyes	Keratoconjunctivitis sicca	Conjunctivitis
		Uveitis
Rheumatoid factor	Positive	Negative
HLA-B27	Negative	Positive

geal joints. Characteristically, these joints are painful and swollen and remain stiff for up to 3 hours after the start of daily activity. Synovitis of the temporo-mandibular joint may lead to marked limitation of mandibular motion. In patients whose disease is progressive and unremitting, nearly every joint is eventually affected, although joints of the thoracic, lumbar, and sacral spine are almost always spared.

In contrast to other sites of the spine, *cervical spine* involvement by rheumatoid arthritis is frequent and may result in pain and neurologic complications. The abnormality that has received the most attention is atlantoaxial subluxation and consequent separation of the atlanto-odontoid articulation. This deformity is best seen on lateral radiographs of the neck; with the patient's neck flexed, the separation of the anterior margin of the odontoid process from the posterior margin of the anterior arch of the atlas can exceed 3 mm. When this separation is severe, the odontoid process may protrude into the foramen magnum and exert pressure on the spinal cord or impair blood flow through the vertebral arteries. Often the odontoid process is eroded, minimizing complications on the spinal cord. Subluxation of the other cervical vertebrae may also occur. Magnetic resonance imaging has confirmed the frequency of cervical spine involvement by rheumatoid arthritis.

Cricoarytenoid arthritis is common in patients with generalized rheumatoid arthritis. With acute crico-arytenoid arthritis, hoarseness, pain on swallowing, dyspnea, and stridor may accompany tenderness over the larynx. Redness and swelling of the aryte-noids can be visualized by direct laryngoscopy. In the chronic state patients may be asymptomatic or may manifest variable degrees of hoarseness, dys-pnea, and upper airway obstruction manifesting as stridor. Cricoarytenoid arthritis may make it diffi-cult to manage these patients should tracheal intuba-tion be required.[79, 80]

Systemic Involvement

Many of the systemic manifestations of rheumatoid arthritis are most likely consequences of vasculitis due to deposition of immune complexes on the walls of small vessels with subsequent inflammatory reac-tions. Systemic involvement is usually most obvious in patients with severe articular disease.

In the *cardiovascular system*, pericardial thickening or effusion as determined by echocardiography is present in about one-third of patients with rheuma-toid arthritis. Pericardiectomy may be necessary to relieve cardiac tamponade. Cardiac involvement may also manifest as pericarditis, myocarditis, arte-ritis involving the coronary arteries, cardiac valve fibrosis, and formation of rheumatoid nodules in the cardiac conduction system. Aortitis with dilation of the aortic root may result in aortic regurgitation.

Vasculitis in small synovial blood vessels is an early finding in patients with rheumatoid arthritis, but more widespread vascular inflammation may also occur especially in older men. Clinically, pa-tients with rheumatoid vasculitis demonstrate poly-neuropathy (mononeuritis multiplex), skin ulcer-ations, and purpura. Neuropathy is presumed to be caused by deposition of immune complexes in the walls of blood vessels supplying the nerves. Mani-festations of visceral ischemia, including bowel per-foration, myocardial infarction, and cerebral infarc-tion, are possible.

The most common *pulmonary* manifestions of rheumatoid arthritis are pleural effusions. Rheuma-toid nodules occur in the pulmonary parenchyma and on pleural surfaces. On radiographic examina-tion these nodules may mimic tuberculosis or can-cer. Progressive pulmonary fibrosis, associated with cough, dyspnea, and diffuse changes on chest radio-graphs, are rare manifestations. Conversely, asymp-tomatic diffuse lung involvement characterized by interstitial inflammation and fibrosis may be com-mon.[81] Costochondral involvement may cause re-strictive changes with decreased lung volumes and vital capacity. The resulting ventilation-to-perfusion mismatch leads to decreased arterial oxygenation.

Neuromuscular involvement is seen, with loss of strength in skeletal muscles adjacent to joints with active synovitis being common. Peripheral neuropa-thies manifest as nerve compression, most often as-sociated with carpal tunnel involvement, although they may also be due to entrapment of the ulnar nerve at the elbow or branches of the sural nerve in the tarsal tunnel. Cervical nerve root compression is unlikely to accompany involvement of the cervical vertebrae by rheumatoid arthritis. Another type of neuropathy is a mild distal sensory neuropathy that affects the hands and feet.

The most common *hematologic* abnormality in pa-tients with rheumatoid arthritis is mild anemia, par-tially due to poor utilization of iron stores or chronic blood loss aggravated by drugs such as aspirin. Felty syndrome is rheumatoid arthritis with splenomeg-aly and leukopenia.

The *eyes* may also be affected. Keratoconjunctivitis sicca (Sjögren syndrome) occurs in about 10% of patients with rheumatoid arthritis. The cause is lack of tear formation due to impaired lacrimal gland function. As a result, patients experience sensations of grittiness with blinking. A similar process may involve the salivary glands, resulting in dryness of the mouth.

Mild abnormalities of *liver* function are common in patients with rheumatoid arthritis and may reflect the presence of Sjögren syndrome or use of salicylates. Rheumatoid arthritis is unlikely to evoke *renal* dysfunction other than that secondary to amyloidosis or use of drugs such as phenacetin, gold, or penicillamine.

Treatment

Treatment of rheumatoid arthritis includes efforts to relieve pain, preserve joint strength and function, and prevent deformities and attenuation of systemic complications. These objectives may be accomplished by the administration of drugs, utilization of physical therapy, and surgical intervention. Despite improved treatment regimens, there is little evidence that the outcome of rheumatoid arthritis has been significantly altered.[78]

Drug Therapy

Drug therapy is utilized to provide analgesia, control inflammation, and produce immunosuppression.[77]

Aspirin and Nonsteroidal Antiinflammatory Drugs

Aspirin remains an important drug for the initial treatment of rheumatoid arthritis, but its use has decreased because of the availability of newer NSAIDs. Aspirin decreases swelling in affected joints and relieves stiffness, but associated gastrointestinal blood loss and irreversible inhibition of platelet cyclooxygenase (COX) may necessitate discontinuation of aspirin. NSAIDs are probably no more effective than aspirin but produce fewer gastrointestinal side effects. The prostaglandin analogue misoprostol can suppress gastrointestinal toxicity of NSAIDs. Selective COX-2 inhibitors (rofecoxib) are as effective as analgesics and antiinflammatory drugs as COX-1 inhibitors (naproxen) but evoke fewer gastrointestinal side effects and do not interfere with platelet function. Nevertheless, both COX-1 and COX-2 drugs can adversely affect renal blood flow and glomerular filtration rate.[82]

Methotrexate

Methotrexate is the most effective second-line drug in the treatment of rheumatoid arthritis and has replaced treatment with gold salts in patients in whom NSAIDs do not adequately control symptoms.[83] Methotrexate is primarily antiinflammatory. Monitoring hematologic parameters (bone marrow suppression) and liver function (cirrhosis) is necessary in individuals being treated with methotrexate.

Anticytokine Therapy

Interference with the function of tumor necrosis factor (TNF), either by drug-induced receptor blockade or by giving monoclonal antibodies, is effective in treating rheumatoid arthritis.[84] TNF is a proinflammatory cytokine that is overproduced in joints of patients with rheumatoid arthritis. There is evidence that drugs (infliximab, etanercept) acting as TNF inhibitors are more effective than methotrexate and are associated with a lower risk of joint damage.[84] Because TNF is important in host defense and possibly tumor surveillance, impairment of these functions could theoretically be undesirable. For these reasons, these drugs may not be acceptable for administration to individuals with active infections. Development of SLE may also be a risk of this therapy.

Corticosteroids

Corticosteroids are potent antiinflammatory drugs that decrease joint swelling, pain, and morning stiffness in patients with rheumatoid arthritis. However, the doses of systemic corticosteroids necessary to maintain desirable effects are often associated with long-term side effects (osteoporosis, osteonecrosis, increased susceptibility to infection, myopathy, poor wound healing). It is believed that corticosteroids neither alter the course of rheumatoid arthritis nor affect the ultimate degree of damage to the joints. Intra-articular corticosteroids may produce beneficial effects lasting, on average, about 3 months; but repeated injections may result in increased cartilage destruction and osteonecrosis.

Immunosuppressive Drugs

Alkylating drugs (particularly cyclophosphamide) and antimetabolites such as azathioprine may be considered in patients with severely symptomatic disease who are unresponsive to more conventional drug therapy. Cyclophosphamide also effectively controls rheumatoid vasculitis in some patients. Hematologic toxicity, gastrointestinal toxicity, and hemorrhagic cystitis are possible complications in patients treated with cyclophosphamide. Azathioprine is less toxic but has only modest efficacy.

Surgery

Indications for surgery in patients with rheumatoid arthritis include intractable pain and impaired function.[77] Eroded cartilage, ruptured ligaments, and progressive destruction of bone can lead to functional impairment that is amenable only to surgical treatment. Arthroscopic surgery is utilized to remove cartilaginous fragments and to perform a partial synovectomy. Stabilization of certain joints such as the wrist and ankle may be needed to improve overall patient function. When joints are destroyed by the disease process, total joint replacement (hip, knee, shoulder, elbow) is often considered.

Management of Anesthesia

Multiple organ system involvement and side effects of drugs used to treat rheumatoid arthritis must be appreciated when planning the management of anesthesia. Preoperatively, patients should be evaluated for airway problems due to the disease process. Compromise of the patient's airway may occur at the cervical spine, temporomandibular joints, and cricoarytenoid joints. For example, flexion deformity of the cervical spine may make it impossible to straighten the neck, and upper airway obstruction is likely when these patients are rendered unconscious. Atlantoaxial subluxation may be present, particularly in those with severe hand deformities and rheumatoid nodules. Radiologic demonstration that the distance from the anterior arch of the atlas to the odontoid process exceeds 3 mm confirms the presence of atlantoaxial subluxation. The importance of atlantoaxial subluxation lies in the fact that the displaced odontoid process can compress the cervical spinal cord or medulla in addition to occluding the vertebral arteries. In its presence, care must be taken during direct laryngoscopy for tracheal intubation to avoid excessive movement of the patient's head and neck, thereby minimizing the likelihood of further displacement of the odontoid process and damage to the underlying spinal cord. It may be prudent to evaluate patients preoperatively to determine if there is interference with vertebral artery blood flow during flexion, extension, or rotation of the head and cervical spine. This may be accomplished by asking awake patients to demonstrate head movements or positions that can be tolerated without discomfort.

Limitation of movement at the temporomandibular joints must be recognized before the induction of anesthesia. The combination of limited mobility of these joints and the cervical spine may make visualizing the glottic opening by direct laryngoscopy difficult or impossible. Tracheal intubation before induction of anesthesia using fiberoptic laryngoscopy may be indicated when preoperative evaluation suggests that direct visualization of the glottic opening will be difficult. Involvement of the cricoarytenoid joints by arthritic changes is suggested by the preoperative presence of hoarseness or stridor and by the observation of erythema and edema of the vocal cords during direct laryngoscopy, making identification of the glottic opening difficult or impossible (Fig. 26–5).[79, 80] Diminished or even absent movement of these joints may result in narrowing of the glottic opening and subsequent interference with translaryngeal passage of the tracheal tube or an increased risk of cricoarytenoid joint dislocation.[79, 80]

Preoperative pulmonary function studies plus measurement of arterial blood gases and pH may be indicated if severe lung disease due to rheumatoid arthritis is suspected. The effect of aspirin on clotting

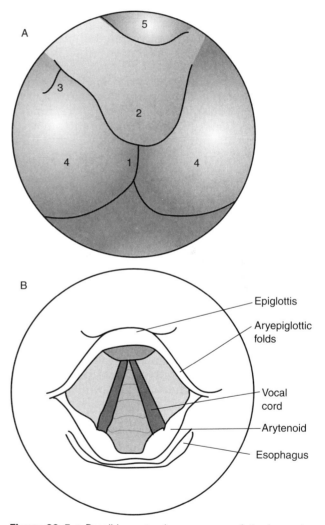

Figure 26–5 • Possible anatomic appearance of the larynx in patients with rheumatoid arthritis involving the upper airway (A) compared with normal anatomy (B). 1, glottic opening; 2, epiglottis; 3, aryepiglottic fold; 4, arytenoid; 5, vallecula. (From Vetter TR. Acute airway obstruction due to arytenoiditis in a child with juvenile rheumatoid arthritis. Anesth Analg 1994;79:1198–200. © 1994, Lippincott Williams & Wilkins, with permission.)

must be considered. Exogenous corticosteroid supplementation may be indicated in patients being treated chronically with these drugs. The presence of anemia and its implications should be appreciated. The need for postoperative ventilatory support should be anticipated if severe restrictive lung disease is present preoperatively. Postextubation laryngeal obstruction may occur in patients with cricoarytenoid arthritis.[79]

SPONDYLARTHROPATHIES

Spondylarthropathies are a group of nonrheumatic arthropathies, that include ankylosing spondylitis (Marie-Strumpell disease), Reiter's disease, juvenile chronic polyarthropathy, and enteropathic arthropathies. These diseases are characterized by involvement of the sacroiliac joints, peripheral inflammatory arthropathy, and the absence of rheumatic nodules or detectable circulating rheumatoid factor (Table 26–6). Causes of these seronegative spondylarthropathies are unknown, but there is often an association with human leukocyte antigen (HLA) designated B27.

Ankylosing Spondylitis

Ankylosing spondylitis is a chronic, usually progressive inflammatory disease involving the articulations of the spine and adjacent soft tissues (Table 26–6). Spinal disease begins in the sacroiliac joints and moves cranially. The degree of spinal disease ranges from only sacroiliac involvement alone to complete ankylosis of the spine. Hip involvement occurs in about one-third of patients. Back pain characterized by morning stiffness that improves with activity and exercise plus radiographic evidence of sacroiliitis is highly suggestive of this diagnosis. The disease occurs predominantly in men 20 to 30 years of age. The strong familial incidence is supported by the finding that 90% of patients with this diagnosis are HLA-B27-positive compared with only 6% of the general population. Ankylosing spondylitis is often erroneously diagnosed as back pain due to lumbar disc degeneration. Examination of the patient's spine may demonstrate skeletal muscle spasms, loss of lordosis, and decreased mobility involving the entire vertebral column.

Systemic involvement manifests as weight loss, fatigue, and low grade fever. Conjunctivitis and uveitis occur in about 25% of patients. Distinctive pulmonary abnormalities associated with ankylosing spondylitis include apical cavitary lesions with fibrosis and pleural thickening that mimics tuberculosis. Arthritic involvement of the thoracic vertebral and costovertebral articulations may result in decreased compliance of the chest wall, with associated decreases in vital capacity.

Treatment

Treatment of ankylosing spondylitis is with exercises designed to maintain joint mobility plus antiinflammatory drugs. Indomethacin or phenylbutazone are commonly used. Bone marrow depression is a potential adverse effect of these drugs. The prognosis is good with early detection and treatment.

Management of Anesthesia

Management of anesthesia in patients with ankylosing spondylitis is influenced by the magnitude of upper airway involvement by the disease, the presence of restrictive patterns of breathing due to costochondral rigidity and flexion deformity of the thoracic spine, and the degree of cardiac involvement. Awake fiberoptic tracheal intubation is performed if the spinal column deformity is extensive.[85] Excessive manipulation of the cervical spine could injure the spinal cord. Intraoperatively, ventilation of the lungs should be supported, as the chest wall is stiff and breathing is diaphragmatic. Neurologic monitoring is a consideration for patients undergoing corrective spinal deformity surgery. Epidural or spinal anesthesia is an acceptable alternative to general anesthesia in the presence of ankylosing spondylitis and perineal or lower limb surgery.[85] Regional anesthesia may be technically difficult owing to limited joint mobility and closed interspinous spaces, although ossification of the ligamentum flavum is uncommon in these patients. Sudden or excessive decreases in systemic vascular resistance are poorly tolerated when aortic regurgitation is present.

Reiter's Disease

Reiter's disease occurs in young men and consists of nonspecific urethritis, uveitis, and arthritis. Predisposing factors are a unique genetic makeup (HLA-B27-positive) plus bacterial infections with *Shigella* or *Chlamydia* organisms. Most of the signs of this disease persist for only a few days, but arthritis progresses to sacroiliitis and spondylitis in about 20% of patients. Cricoarytenoid arthritis can also occur. Hyperkeratotic skin lesions cannot be distinguished from psoriasis, and the two diseases frequently appear to overlap. No cure has been found for Reiter's disease. Symptomatic management is with indomethacin or phenylbutazone.

Juvenile Chronic Polyarthropathy

The pathology of chronic juvenile polyarthropathy is similar to that of adult rheumatoid arthritis. Growth abnormalities may occur if arthritis appears before puberty. Hepatic dysfunction may be present, but cardiac involvement is unusual. An acute form of polyarthritis, which presents as fever, rash, lymphadenopathy, and splenomegaly in young children who are negative for rheumatoid factor and HLA-B27, is designated Still's disease. Aspirin is a common, useful therapy. Corticosteroids effectively control this disease but have limited usefulness, as they may induce growth retardation when administered to young patients.

Enteropathic Arthropathies

Approximately 20% of patients with granulomatous ileocolitis or ulcerative colitis exhibit acute migratory inflammatory polyarthritis, most often involving the large joints of the lower extremities. Remissions occur spontaneously, although subsequent recurrence may parallel exacerbations of the underlying disease. Treatment is directed at controlling the underlying gastrointestinal disorder.

Inflammatory bowel disease may also be associated with sacroiliitis and occasionally with severe ankylosing spondylitis. There is no correlation between the severity of the bowel disorder and spondylitis. Treatment is as described for ankylosing spondylitis.

A postintestinal bypass syndrome consisting of arthropathy and dermatitis is well documented. The cause is unknown, although immune mechanisms have been implicated.

▌ OSTEOARTHRITIS

Osteoarthritis is a degenerative process that affects the articular cartilage (see Chapter 33). This process differs from rheumatoid arthritis in that there is minimal inflammatory reaction. The pathogenesis is unclear but may be related to joint trauma. Advancing age and a genetic predisposition are important associated factors. Pain that is usually present on motion, is relieved by rest. Stiffness tends to disappear rapidly with joint motion, in contrast to the morning stiffness associated with rheumatoid arthritis, which may last several hours.

Characteristically, one to several joints are affected by osteoarthritis. The knees and hips are common sites of involvement. Bony enlargements, referred to as Heberden's nodes, are seen at the distal interphalangeal joints. There may be degenerative disease of the vertebral bodies and intervertebral discs, which may be complicated by protrusion of the nucleus pulposus and compression of nerve roots. Degenerative changes are most significant in the middle to lower cervical spine and in the lower lumbar areas. Spinal fusion is unusual, in contrast to its common occurrence in ankylosing spondylitis. Radiographic findings may show narrowing of the intervertebral disc spaces and osteophyte formation.

Treatment of osteoarthritis is symptomatic and includes application of heat, mild analgesics, and antiinflammatory drugs including aspirin and specific NSAIDs. Symptomatic improvement with application of heat may be due to an increased pain threshold in warm tissues compared to that in cold tissues. Corticosteroids are not recommended, as they may contribute to degenerative joint changes. Reconstructive joint surgery (total hip or knee replacement) may be recommended when pain due to osteoarthritis is persistent and disabling.

▌ PAGET'S DISEASE

Paget's disease of bone is characterized by excessive osteoblastic and osteoclastic activity, resulting in abnormally thickened but weak bones.[86] The cause is unknown but may reflect an excess of parathyroid hormone or a deficiency of calcitonin. A familial tendency is present, with white men over 40 years of age affected most often. Bone pain is the most common symptom. Complications of Paget's disease involve bones (fractures and neoplastic degeneration), joints (arthritis), and the nervous system (nerve compression, paraplegia). Hypercalcemia and renal calculi may occur. The most characteristic radiographic feature of Paget's disease is localized enlargement of bone. Lytic and sclerotic bone changes may involve the skull. If the skull is affected, it may be grossly enlarged, and irreversible hearing loss may occur. Radionuclide bone scanning is the most reliable means to identify lesions due to Paget's disease. Serum alkaline phosphatase concentrations (reflects bone formation) and urinary hydroxyproline excretion (reflects bone resorption) are usually increased.

Treatment of Paget's disease is designed to alleviate bone pain and to minimize or prevent progression of the disease. Calcitonin is a hormone secreted by the thyroid gland that inhibits osteoclast activity and rapidly decreases bone resorption. Treatment with calcitonin decreases pain, biochemical abnormalities, and radiographic abnormalities associated with Paget's disease; and it may stabilize the hearing loss due to Paget's disease. Intravenous administration of plicamycin decreases the pain and bone turnover in these patients but is associated with bone marrow, liver, and renal toxicity. Bisphosphonates (etidronate, pamidronate, alendronate) induce marked and prolonged inhibition of bone resorption by decreasing osteoclastic activity. In contrast to the short-lived effects of calcitonin, disease activity remains low for many months, sometimes years, after treatment with bisphosphonates is stopped. Radiographically confirmed repair of osteolytic lesions may occur in response to treatment with bisphosphanates.

Conservative treatment of fractures in patients with Paget's disease is associated with a high risk of delayed union. Patients with Paget's disease who have severe osteoarthritis of the hips or knees often benefit from elective joint replacement. Rarely, osteotomy must be performed to correct bowing deformities of long bones. Patients with evidence of peripheral nerve compression, radiculopathy, or spinal cord compression require decompressive surgery.

■ MARFAN SYNDROME

Marfan syndrome, a disorder of connective tissue, is inherited as an autosomal dominant trait.[87] The incidence is 4 to 6 per 100,000 live births, and the mean age of survival is 32 years. Characteristically, these patients have long tubular bones, giving them a tall stature and an "Abe Lincoln" appearance. Additional skeletal abnormalities include a high arched palate, pectus excavatum, kyphoscoliosis, and hyperextensibility of the joints. Early development of pulmonary emphysema is characteristic and may further accentuate the impact of restrictive lung disease related to kyphoscoliosis. There is a high incidence of spontaneous pneumothorax in these patients. Ocular changes characterized by lens dislocation, myopia, and detachment of the retina occur at some time in more than one-half of patients with Marfan syndrome.

Cardiovascular System

Abnormalities that involve the cardiovascular system are responsible for nearly all premature fatalities in patients with Marfan syndrome. Defective tensile strength in the connective tissues of the aorta and heart valves leads to dilation, dissection, and rupture of the aorta and to prolapse of the cardiac valves, especially of the mitral valve. Mitral regurgitation is a common abnormality, reflecting mitral valve prolapse. The risk of bacterial endocarditis is increased in the presence of valvular heart disease. Cardiac conduction abnormalities, especially bundle branch block, are common. Echocardiography is particularly useful for detecting cardiac abnormalities in otherwise asymptomatic individuals. Prophylactic β-adrenergic blocker therapy may be recommended for patients in whom the thoracic aorta becomes dilated. By contrast, prophylactic surgical replacement of the aortic valve and ascending aorta is indicated for patients in whom the diameter of the proximal thoracic aorta exceeds 6 cm and in whom substantial aortic regurgitation is present. Extension of an aortic dissection through the sinus of Valsalva into the pericardium can lead to sudden cardiac tamponade. Pregnancy poses a unique risk of rupture or dissection of the aorta in parturients with Marfan syndrome.

Management of Anesthesia

Preoperative evaluation of patients with Marfan syndrome should concentrate on cardiopulmonary abnormalities.[88] Prophylactic antibiotics are appropriate if valvular heart disease is present. In most patients, skeletal abnormalities have little impact on the patient's upper airway. Care should be exercised, however, to avoid extreme movements of the mandible, as these patients are susceptible to temporomandibular joint dislocation. In view of the possibility of weakened walls of the thoracic aorta, it is prudent to avoid sustained increases in systemic blood pressure, as can occur during direct laryngoscopy for tracheal intubation or in response to painful surgical stimulation. Invasive monitoring including transesophageal echocardiography may be a consideration. A high index of suspicion must be maintained for the development of pneumothorax.

■ KYPHOSCOLIOSIS

Kyphoscoliosis is a deformity of the costovertebral skeletal structures characterized by an anterior flexion (kyphosis) and lateral curvature (scoliosis) of the patient's vertebral column. Idiopathic kyphoscoliosis, which accounts for 80% of cases, commonly begins during late childhood and may progress in severity during periods of rapid skeletal growth. The incidence of idiopathic kyphoscoliosis is about 4 per 1000 population. Diseases of the neuromuscular system, such as poliomyelitis, cerebral palsy, and muscular dystrophy, may be associated with kyphoscoliosis. There seems to be a familial predisposition of this disease, with females affected about four times more often than males.

Signs and Symptoms

Curves of more than 40 degrees are considered severe and are most likely to be associated with physiologic derangements in cardiac and pulmonary function. Restrictive lung disease and pulmonary hypertension progressing to cor pulmonale are the principal causes of death in patients with kyphoscoliosis. As the scoliosis curve worsens, more lung tissue is compressed, resulting in decreased vital capacity and dyspnea with mild exertion. The work of breathing is increased by abnormal mechanical properties of the thorax and, to a lesser degree, by increased airway resistance resulting from small lung volumes. The alveolar-to-arterial difference for oxygen is increased. The $PaCO_2$ is usually normal, but relatively minor insults such as bacterial or viral upper respiratory tract infections may result in acute respiratory failure. A poor cough reflex contributes to frequent pulmonary infections. Pulmonary hypertension reflects increased pulmonary vascular resistance due to compression of lung vasculature by the spinal curvature and pulmonary vascular responses to arterial hypoxemia.

Management of Anesthesia

Preoperatively, it is important to assess the severity of the physiologic derangements produced by the skeletal deformity. Pulmonary function tests, with special attention to the vital capacity and forced expiratory volume in 1 second (FEV_1), reflect the magnitude of restrictive lung disease. Arterial blood gases and pH are helpful for detecting unrecognized arterial hypoxemia or acidosis that could be contributing to pulmonary hypertension. These patients may enter the preoperative period with pneumonia due to chronic aspiration. Certainly, any reversible component of pulmonary dysfunction, such as bacterial infection or bronchospasm, should be corrected before an elective operation is performed. Preoperative depressant drugs must be administered with caution, if at all, in view of the narrow margin of ventilatory reserve in these patients and the adverse effects on pulmonary vascular resistance that would occur with respiratory acidosis due to hypoventilation.

Intraoperatively, ventilation of the lungs should be controlled to facilitate adequate arterial oxygenation and elimination of carbon dioxide. Adequacy of oxygenation is confirmed by pulse oximetry. Although no specific drug or drug combinations can be recommended as optimal, it should be remembered that nitrous oxide may increase pulmonary vascular resistance, presumably by direct vasoconstrictive effects on the pulmonary vasculature. Monitoring the central venous pressure may provide an early warning of increased pulmonary vascular resistance produced by nitrous oxide. Signs of malignant hyperthermia (hypercapnia, acidosis, tachycardia, increased body temperature) must be appreciated, as it has been suggested that there is an increased incidence of this syndrome in patients with scoliosis.[89]

If surgery is undertaken to *correct the spinal curvature*, special anesthetic considerations are given to intraoperative blood loss and recognition of surgically induced spinal cord damage. Controlled hypotension with combinations of volatile anesthetics and vasodilators such as nitroprusside may be selected in attempts to minimize intraoperative blood loss. As the spinal curvature is straightened, excess traction on the spinal cord may result in ischemia manifesting as paralysis during the postoperative period. Intraoperative maneuvers designed to detect spinal cord ischemia include pharmacologic reversal of neuromuscular blockade and discontinuation of the volatile anesthetic until the patient is sufficiently awake to move both legs on request, confirming that the spinal cord is intact ("wake-up test"). Inhalation anesthesia is then reestablished and the operation completed. Monitoring the somatosensory cortical evoked potentials is also useful to confirm an intact spinal cord. The advantage of monitoring somatosensory evoked potentials is that patients need not be awakened intraoperatively. If this approach is selected, it must be appreciated that many drugs, including volatile anesthetics, interfere with the interpretation of the evoked potentials. Therefore a nitrous oxide-opioid technique is often recommended, and a continuous intravenous infusion of propofol is also acceptable. Continuous infusion of opioids and/or propofol maintains any drug-induced changes in the evoked potentials at constant levels, making it easier to interpret changes due to spinal cord damage.[90] Unfortunately, postoperative paralysis may still occur despite the absence of any intraoperative abnormality in the somatosensory evoked potentials, emphasizing that this monitor reflects only the sensory (dorsal column function) and not the motor (ventral column function), integrity of the spinal cord. For these reasons a wake-up test is still recommended. In this regard, the test can often be done by utilizing short-acting opioids such as remifentanil or propofol from which prompt awakening occurs when the drug infusion is discontinued. Postoperatively, the principal concern is restoration of adequate ventilation. Slow weaning from the ventilator is often necessary in patients with severe kyphoscoliosis, regardless of the operative procedure.

ACHONDROPLASIA

Achondroplasia is the most common cause of disproportionate dwarfism, occurring predominantly in females, with an incidence of 1.5 per 10,000 births.[91] Transmission is by an autosomal dominant gene, although an estimated 80% of cases represent spontaneous mutations. Indeed, fertility among achondroplastic dwarfs is low. The basic defect is thought to be a decrease in the rate of endochondral ossification, that, when coupled with normal periosteal bone formation, leads to short tubular bones. The predicted height for achondroplastic males is 132 cm and for females 122 cm. Kyphoscoliosis and genu varum are common. Premature fusion of the bones at the base of the skull occurs in achondroplasia, resulting in a shortened skull base and a small stenotic foramen magnum. This change may result in infantile hydrocephalus or damage to the cervical spinal cord. For example, central sleep apnea experienced by achondroplastic dwarfs may be a function of brain stem compression due to foramen magnum stenosis. Pulmonary hypertension, leading to cor pulmonale, is probably the most common cardiovascular disturbance that develops in dwarfs. Mental and skeletal muscle development are normal, as is life expectancy for those who survive the first year of life.

Management of Anesthesia

Management of anesthesia in achondroplastic dwarfs may be influenced by difficulties with airway management, cervical spine instability, and the potential for spinal cord trauma with neck extension (Table 26–7).[92] Pituitary dwarfism is more likely to be associated with proportionately smaller airways

without anatomic abnormalities. A short laryngoscope handle, a range of blades, and oral or nasal airways appropriate for pediatric patients should be available for those with pituitary dwarfism. The anatomy of adult patients with pituitary dwarfism, including the size of the tracheal tubes, is more similar to that of pediatric patients than of normal-size adult patients.[92]

Achondroplastic dwarfs characteristically undergo a number of specific procedures, including suboccipital craniectomy for foramen magnum stenosis, laminectomy for spinal column stenosis or nerve root compression, and ventricular peritoneal shunts.[91] Abnormal bone growth is responsible for several potential anesthesia-related problems.[93, 94] A preoperative history of obstructive sleep apnea may predispose to the development of upper airway obstruction after sedation or induction of anesthesia. Facial features characterized by a large protruding forehead, short maxilla, large mandible, flat nose, and large tongue suggest difficulty attaining a suitable fit with an anesthesia face mask and maintenance of a patent upper airway. Despite these characteristics, clinical experience has not confirmed any difficulty with maintaining an upper airway or achieving tracheal intubation in most of these patients.[93]

In dwarfs with cervical kyphosis, tracheal intubation may be difficult because of an inability to align the axes of the airway. In achondroplastic dwarfs the size of the base of the skull may be decreased secondary to premature fusion of the cranium, a narrow foramen magnum, functional fusion of the atlanto-occipital joint with odontoid hypoplasia, atlantoaxial instability, bulging discs, and severe cervical kyphosis. Hyperextension of the patient's neck during direct laryngoscopy for tracheal intubation should be avoided, if possible, considering the likely presence of foramen magnum stenosis. The clinical impression of an anatomically abnormal upper airway or cervical spine may be confirmed by computed tomography or magnetic resonance imaging. Fiberoptic-guided tracheal intubation may be a consideration in selected patients. Weight rather than age is the best guide for predicting the proper-size endotracheal tube for these patients.[93]

Excess skin and subcutaneous tissues may make establishment of peripheral intravenous lines technically difficult. Achondroplastic dwarfs undergoing suboccipital craniectomy, especially in the sitting position, are at high risk for venous air embolism, emphasizing the potential value of a right atrial catheter.[95] Placing such catheters is technically difficult, however, because of the patient's short neck and the difficulty of identifying landmarks that may be obscured by excess soft tissues. Monitoring

Table 26–7 • Characteristics of Achondroplastic Dwarfs that May Influence Management of Anesthesia

Upper airway obstruction
Difficult exposure of the glottic opening
Restrictive lung disease
Obstructive sleep apnea
Central sleep apnea
Pulmonary hypertension
Cor pulmonale
Hydrocephalus
Compressive spinal cord and nerve root syndromes
   Foramen magnum stenosis
   Odontoid hypoplasia with cervical instability
   Kyphoscoliosis
Thermal regulation dysfunction (hyperthermia)

somatosensory evoked potentials is useful during operations that may be associated with brain stem or spinal cord injury. As with surgery to correct kyphoscoliosis, it is important to remember that somatosensory evoked potentials reflect the integrity of the dorsal, not the ventral, columns of the spinal cord. Achondroplastic dwarfs seem to respond normally to drugs used for anesthesia and skeletal muscle relaxation. Anesthetic techniques that permit rapid awakening may be desirable for prompt evaluation of neurologic function.

Regional anesthesia in achondroplastic dwarfs may be considered for cesarean section, which is mandated by the small, contracted pelvis in these patients combined with near-normal infant birth weights.[96] Technical difficulties may occur because of kyphoscoliosis and a narrow epidural space and spinal canal. Indeed, the small epidural space may make it difficult to introduce a catheter or obtain free flow of cerebrospinal fluid. Neurologic changes may occur during later life because of compression of the spinal cord by osteophytes, prolapsed intervertebral discs, or deformed vertebral bodies. There are no data confirming appropriate doses of local anesthetics for epidural or spinal anesthesia in these patients. For this reason, epidural anesthesia may be preferable to spinal anesthesia, as it permits titration of local anesthetic doses to achieve desired sensory levels of blockade.

Russell-Silver Syndrome

Russell-Silver syndrome is a form of dwarfism characterized by intrauterine growth retardation with subsequent severe postnatal growth impairment, dysmorphic facial features including mandibular and facial hypoplasia, limb asymmetry, congenital heart defects, and a constellation of endocrine abnormalities including hypoglycemia, hypoadrenocortical insufficiency, and hypogonadism.[97] Pseudohydrocephalus has been used to describe the facial features characteristic of this syndrome. Developmental and hormonal abnormalities tend to normalize with age, and individuals with this syndrome are likely to achieve adult heights near 150 cm. Hypoglycemia may be responsible for diaphoresis, tachycardia, and seizures. Rapid depletion of limited hepatic glycogen stores, especially in small-for-gestational-age neonates may predispose to hypoglycemia. The risk of hypoglycemia diminishes as the child grows and is usually not present after about 4 years of age.

Preoperative evaluation considers the glucose status, especially in neonates most at risk for hypoglycemia.[97] Intravenous infusions containing glucose may be indicated preoperatively. Unexplained tachycardia, diaphoresis, or excessive somnolence after anesthetic emergence may reflect hypoglycemia. Infants with Russell-Silver syndrome may be especially prone to intraoperative hypothermia because of their large surface-to-volume ratio. Facial manifestations of this syndrome (similar to those in Goldenhar and Treacher Collins syndromes) may make direct laryngoscopy and exposure of the glottic opening difficult. A tracheal tube smaller than the predicted size may be needed. Obtaining a good mask fit may be difficult owing to facial asymmetry. Administration of drugs, such as muscle relaxants, on the basis of body weight rather than body surface area may result in relative underdosing.

■ BACK PAIN

Low back pain is the most common musculoskeletal complaint requiring medical attention and the fifth most common reason for physician visits (Table 26–8).[98] An increased risk for back pain is associated with the male gender, frequent lifting of heavy objects, and smoking. In most patients the cause of pain cannot be determined with certainty and is usually attributed to muscular or ligamentous strain, facet joint arthritis, or disc pressure on the annulus fibrosus, vertebral end-plate, or nerve roots.[98]

Acute Back Pain

Back pain improves within 30 days in 90% of patients. Among patients with acute low back pain, continuing ordinary activities within the limits permitted by the pain leads to more rapid recovery than bed rest or back-mobilizing exercises.[99] Pain arising from inflammation initiated by mechanical or chemical insult to the surrounding nerve root may be responsive to epidural administration of corticosteroids. Few patients experience symptomatic relief from epidural corticosteroids if the first injection was of no help, if radicular pain has been present for more than 6 months, or if laminectomy has been previously performed. Patients with persistent pain after 30 days of conservative treatment (NSAIDs) may be evaluated for systemic illnesses. A herniated lumbar disc should be considered in patients with symptoms of radiculopathy, as suggested by pain radiating down the leg with symptoms reproduced by straight leg raising. Magnetic resonance imaging may be necessary to confirm a herniated disc, but findings should be interpreted with caution because many asymptomatic persons

Table 26–8 • Differential Diagnosis of Low Back Pain

Mechanical low back or leg pain (97%)
  Idiopathic low back pain (lumbar sprain or strain)
    (70%)
  Degenerative processes of discs and facets (age-
    related) (10%)
  Herniated disc (4%)
  Spinal stenosis (3%)
  Osteoporotic compression fractures (4%)
  Spondylolisthesis (2%)
  Traumatic fracture (< 1%)
  Congenital disease (< 1%)
    Severe kyphosis
    Severe scoliosis
  Spondylolysis
Nonmechanical spinal conditions (1%)
  Cancer (0.7%)
    Multiple myeloma
    Metastatic cancer
    Lymphoma and leukemia
    Spinal cord tumors
    Retroperitoneal tumors
    Primary vertebral tumors
  Infection (0.01%)
    Osteomyelitis
    Paraspinal abscess
    Epidural abscess
  Inflammatory arthritis
    Ankylosing spondylitis
    Psoriatic spondylitis
    Reiter syndrome
    Inflammatory bowel disease
Visceral disease (2%)
  Disease of pelvic organs
    Prostatitis
    Endometriosis
    Pelvic inflammatory disease
  Renal disease
    Nephrolithiasis
    Pyelonephritis
    Perinephric abscess
  Aortic aneurysm
  Gastrointestinal disease
    Pancreatitis
    Cholecystitis
    Penetrating ulcer

Percentages indicate the estimated incidence of these conditions in adult patients.
Adapted from: Deyo RO, Weinstein JN. Low back pain. N Engl J Med 2001;344:363–70.

have disc abnormalities. Most lumbar disc herniations producing sciatica occur at the L4-5 and L5-S1 vertebral interspaces. Surgical intervention is indicated in patients with persistent sciatica and evidence of a herniated disc on magnetic resonance imaging or myelogram computed tomographic scanning.

Lumbar Spinal Stenosis

Lumbar spinal stenosis is narrowing of the central spinal canal or its lateral recesses typically from hypertrophic degenerative changes in spinal structures (extensive degenerative disc disease and osteophyte formation) occurring most often in elderly patients with chronic back pain associated with sciatica (see Chapter 33). Patients typically complain of pain, numbness, and weakness in the buttocks that extends to one or both legs. Symptoms are usually exacerbated by standing or walking and improve when patients assume the flexed or supine position ("neurogenic claudication").[98] The diagnosis of lumbar spinal stenosis is confirmed by magnetic resonance imaging or myelogram computed tomography. Although conservative measures are helpful in some patients, surgical decompression by multilevel laminectomy and fusion is considered for those with progressive functional deterioration.

OTHER MUSCULOSKELETAL SYNDROMES

Rotator Cuff Tear

Rotator cuff tear is the most common pathologic entity involving the shoulders.[100] The prevalence of partial- to full-thickness rotator cuff tears is 5% to 40% as determined at postmortem examinations of adults older than 40 years of age. The incidence of rotator cuff tears increases with age, with approximately 50% of individuals older than 55 years of age demonstrating arthrographically detectable rotator cuff tears. Other shoulder diagnoses are less common. Adhesive capsulitis (frozen shoulder) occurs in approximately 2% of the adult population and in 11% of the adult diabetic population. The prevalence of calcific tendinitis ranges from 3% to 7%. Shoulder pain, largely related to rotator cuff tears, ranks second only to back and neck pain as a cause of dysfunction in the working population (see Chapter 17).[100]

Corticosteroid injections into the subacromial space may provide symptomatic relief in patients with impingement syndromes with or without rotator cuff tears, adhesive capsulitis, or supraspinatus tendinitis. Arthroscopic release or manipulation under anesthesia may be utilized in an attempt to restore shoulder motion. Arthroscopic acromioplasty has been utilized for impingement syndromes. Arthroscopic rotator cuff repairs are possible, but most often this repair is performed as an open procedure.[100] Total shoulder replacement (replacement of humeral and glenoid articular surfaces) reduces shoulder pain in most patients.

Brachial plexus anesthesia utilizing the interscalene approach and continuous infusion of local anesthetic solutions provides anesthesia for shoulder procedures as well as postoperative analgesia.[101, 102] Ipsilateral hemidiaphragmatic paresis is an unavoidable side effect of the interscalene approach utilized for anesthesia in patients undergoing shoulder surgery. For this reason, interscalene block may be avoided in patients with severe chronic obstructive pulmonary disease or neuromuscular diseases in which decreases in the forced vital capacity would not be acceptable. Continuous infusion devices utilizing a roller pump mechanism have been observed to produce electrocardiographic artifacts that can mimic atrial flutter or atrial fibrillation.[103] Venous air embolism has been described during shoulder arthroscopy in which air was used as a joint-distending agent.[104] Wound infiltration and lavage with solutions containing a long-acting local anesthetic such as ropivacaine also provide postoperative analgesia following major shoulder surgery.[105]

Floppy Infant Syndrome

Floppy infant syndrome is a term used to describe infants who have weak, hypotonic skeletal muscles owing to neuromuscular or nonneuromuscular causes. Diminished cough reflex, aspiration, and recurrent pneumonia are common. Weakness of the bulbar musculature may cause difficulty swallowing and breathing. Progressive weakness and atrophy of skeletal muscles leads to contractures and kyphoscoliosis.

Management of anesthesia, as for skeletal muscle biopsies to confirm the diagnosis, may be associated with increased sensitivity to nondepolarizing muscle relaxants, hyperkalemia, and cardiac arrest after administration of succinylcholine. Susceptibility to malignant hyperthermia, which may be present in patients with skeletal muscle myopathies, limits the use of certain inhaled anesthetics and muscle relaxants. Ketamine is useful for providing surgical anesthesia without depressing ventilation while avoiding muscle relaxants and other potential triggering drugs for malignant hyperthermia.[106]

Hyperekplexia

Hyperekplexia ("stiff baby syndrome") is a rare genetic syndrome characterized by intense skeletal muscle rigidity manifesting immediately after birth.

Similarities between this syndrome and hyperexplexia (exaggerated startle response to sudden noises or movement) are remarkable; they may even be the same disease. Electromyography demonstrates continuous skeletal muscle activity with only rare periods of quiescence. Choking, vomiting, and difficulty with swallowing are common; motor development is delayed, but intelligence is normal. Skeletal muscle stiffness disappears gradually during the first years of life.

Experience with this syndrome is too limited to make recommendations regarding anesthesia. In a single affected infant resistance to succinylcholine was observed, whereas the response to pancuronium and neostigmine were considered normal.[107] In this same patient substantial increases in the resting tension of skeletal muscles were observed during the onset of action of succinylcholine. Release of potassium was not enhanced after administration of succinylcholine. Responses to volatile anesthetics and nitrous oxide seem predictable in these patients.

Tracheomegaly

Tracheomegaly is characterized by marked dilation of the trachea and bronchi, due to congenital defects of elastic and smooth muscle fibers of the tracheobronchial tree or their destruction after radiotherapy, especially to the head and neck.[108] The diagnosis is confirmed by a tracheal diameter of more than 30 mm on chest radiographs. Symptoms include chronic productive cough and frequent pulmonary infections, most likely reflecting chronic aspiration. Tracheal and bronchial walls are abnormally flaccid and may collapse, especially during vigorous coughing. Aspiration is a possibility during general anesthesia, especially if maximal inflation of the tracheal tube cuff fails to provide an airtight seal.

Alcoholic Myopathy

Acute and chronic forms of proximal skeletal muscle weakness occur frequently in alcoholic patients. Distinction of alcohol myopathy from alcoholic neuropathy is based on proximal, rather than distal, skeletal muscle involvement, increased serum creatine kinase concentrations, myoglobinuria in acute cases, and rapid recovery after cessation of alcohol consumption.

Freeman-Sheldon Syndrome

Freeman-Sheldon syndrome ("whistling face syndrome") is a rare congenital disorder characterized by facial and skeletal abnormalities.[109] The three basic abnormalities are microstomia with pouting lips reflecting hypoplasia of facial muscles, camptodactyly with ulnar deviation of the fingers, and talipes equinovarus. Many of the features of this syndrome are due to an underlying myopathy. Skeletal muscle contractures lead to a short neck and cephalad positioning of the larynx, restrictive lung disease, and kyphoscoliosis. Chronic upper airway obstruction reflects involvement of oral and nasal pharyngeal muscles. Difficulty swallowing may lead to malnourishment. Patients with this syndrome frequently present for surgical correction of musculoskeletal or facial abnormalities.

Anesthetic challenges include difficult airway management, a risk of malignant hyperthermia, and postoperative pulmonary complications. Intravenous cannulation may be difficult in patients with this syndrome owing to thickened subcutaneous tissues and frequent extremity surgery. Difficult airway management may result from microstomia, micrognathia, small nasal passages, kyphoscoliosis, and upper airway obstruction. The rami of the mandible may be hypoplastic and the malar bones small. Diffuse fibrosis of the orbicularis oris muscle and dermal fibrous bands along the vermilion border of the lower lip may be responsible for the contracted oral aperture. Neuromuscular blockade may have limited effect on these fibrous changes. In view of the possible susceptibility to malignant hyperthermia, nontriggering anesthetics (propofol, fentanyl, midazolam, regional nerve blocks) are recommended. Postoperative pulmonary complications (pneumonia, recurrent respiratory infections, respiratory insufficiency) may result from intercostal myopathy and loss of lung volumes.

Prader-Willi Syndrome

Prader-Willi syndrome manifests at birth as skeletal muscle hypotonia, which may be associated with weak swallowing and cough reflexes and upper airway obstruction. Nasogastric feeding may be necessary during infancy. The syndrome progresses during childhood and is characterized by hyperphagia leading to obesity plus endocrine abnormalities including hypogonadism and diabetes mellitus. The pickwickian syndrome develops in some patients. There is little growth in height, and patients remain short. Mental retardation is often severe. There is a high frequency of chromosome 15 deletion in patients with this syndrome, and an autosomal-recessive mode of inheritance has been proposed. It has been suggested that the incidence of Prader-

Willi syndrome is little different from that of the trisomy 21 defect.

The principal concerns for management of anesthesia in these patients are skeletal muscle hypotonia and altered metabolism of carbohydrates and fat.[110] Weak skeletal musculature is associated with an ineffective cough and an increased incidence of pneumonia. Intraoperative monitoring of blood glucose concentrations and provision of exogenous glucose is necessary, as these patients continue to use circulating glucose to manufacture fat rather than to meet basal energy needs. When calculating doses of drugs, one should consider the decreased skeletal muscle mass and increased fat content in these patients. Although not substantiated, it is predictable that muscle relaxant requirements could be decreased in the presence of skeletal muscle hypotonia. Succinylcholine has been administered without incident to these patients.[110]

Micrognathia, high arched palate, strabismus, a straight ulnar border, and congenital dislocation of the hip may be present. Dental caries associated with enamel defects are common. Chronic regurgitation of gastric contents (rumination) occurs frequently in these patients and may contribute to the development of dental caries and to an increased incidence of perioperative aspiration pneumonitis.[111] Disturbances in thermoregulation, often characterized as intraoperative rises in body temperature and metabolic acidosis, have been observed, although a relation to malignant hyperthermia has not been established.[110] Seizures are associated with this syndrome, suggesting caution when using drugs known to stimulate the central nervous system. Cardiac dysfunction does not seem to accompany this syndrome.

Prune-Belly Syndrome

Prune-belly syndrome is characterized by congenital agenesis of the lower central abdominal musculature and the presence of urinary tract anomalies.[112] Recurrent respiratory tract infections reflect an impaired ability to cough effectively. It is unlikely that muscle relaxants are necessary during the management of anesthesia.

Hallermann-Streiff Syndrome

Hallermann-Streiff syndrome is characterized by oculomandibulodyscephaly and dwarfism. The nose and mandible are hypoplastic, the teeth brittle, and the temporomandibular joints weak and easily dislocated. These airway abnormalities make direct laryngoscopy for tracheal intubation difficult and hazardous. Awake fiberoptic nasotracheal intubation can be difficult if the nares are hypoplastic.[113]

Dutch-Kentucky Syndrome

Dutch-Kentucky syndrome is a rare inherited disorder characterized by decreased ability to open the mouth owing to trismus and flexion deformity of the fingers, which occurs with wrist extension (pseudocamptodactyly). Enlarged coronoid processes may be the cause of trismus. Foot deformities and shorter-than-normal stature are frequently present. When these patients require surgery, management of the airway may be facilitated by fiberoptic laryngoscopy.[114]

Coffin-Siris Syndrome

Coffin-Siris syndrome ("fifth digit syndrome") is a rare genetic disorder characterized by absent fifth digit fingernails or a hypoplastic fifth finger terminal phalanx, mental retardation, severe growth retardation, infant feeding difficulties, hypotonia, and coarse facies.[115] Management of anesthesia is complicated by the need to communicate with mentally retarded and uncooperative patients plus facial malformations that make direct laryngoscopy for tracheal intubation difficult.

Williams-Beuren Syndrome

Williams-Beuren syndrome is a rare entity characterized by mental retardation, hypercalcemia with associated kidney dysfunction and corneal opacities, kyphoscoliosis, and skeletal muscle hypotonia. Characteristic facies include broad forehead, pointed chin, flattened nasal bridge, large upper lip, and prognathism. Aortic regurgitation is present in more than 50% of these patients. The presence of stenosis of the left subclavian artery can result in unequal systemic blood pressure measurements in the upper extremities.

Arthrogryposis Multiplex Congenita

Arthrogryposis multiplex congenita is a rare syndrome characterized by joint contractures and multiple organ system congenital abnormalities.[116] Cardiac abnormalities include aortic stenosis, coarctation of the aorta, and cyanotic heart disease. Airway problems are introduced by micrognathia, high arched palate, and cervical spine abnormalities. Decreased skeletal muscle mass may be associated with increased sensitivity to muscle relaxants. In view of the myopathy associated with this disease, there is an unsubstantiated concern about possible susceptibility to malignant hyperthermia. Regional anesthesia has been successfully conducted, but deformities of the vertebral column may make the technique technically difficult.

Smith-Lemli-Opitz Syndrome

Smith-Lemli-Opitz syndrome is characterized by mental, motor, and growth retardation, microcephalus, hypoplasia of the external genitalia, and syndactyly of the toes. The prognosis is poor, with death frequently occurring in infancy due to pulmonary infections or congenital heart defects. Sudden skeletal muscle rigidity in response to the administration of halothane has been described, suggesting that these patients may be susceptible to malignant hyperthermia.[117]

Multiple Pterygium Syndrome

Multiple pterygium syndrome is a rare, autosomal recessive disorder that involves webbing of the skin across joints, cleft palate, syngnathia (congenital bands of tissue between the maxilla and mandible), ankyloglossia (extensive adhesions of the tongue to the palate), micrognathia, and webbing of the neck.[118] These anomalies limit mouth opening, displace the tongue posteriorly, obscure visualization of the pharynx, and prevent neck extension. Patients have pterygia (contracture bands) across many of their joints that significantly limit mobility. They may require operations for repair of cleft palate, syndactyly, scoliosis, congenital hip dislocation, and inguinal and umbilical hernias.

Airway management is the principal concern in these patients.[118] As children grow older, airway management is likely to become more difficult as a result of increased airway deformity by pterygia. This syndrome differs from many other congenital syndromes in which airway management becomes easier as children grow older and larger. Although evidence is lacking, there is concern that patients with multiple pterygium syndrome could be susceptible to malignant hyperthermia. Nevertheless, volatile anesthetics and the ability to maintain spontaneous breathing are viewed as being more important than the theoretical risk of malignant hyperthermia.

Holt-Oram Syndrome (Heart-Hand Syndrome)

Holt-Oram syndrome is an inherited disorder characterized by anomalies of the upper limbs (often hypoplastic thumbs) and heart.[119] Cardiac abnormalities include atrial septal defects, ventricular septal defects, tetralogy of Fallot, endocardial cushion defects, total anomalous pulmonary venous return, and disturbances in cardiac rhythm (bradycardia, atrioventricular heart block). Sudden death may occur. Survival of individuals with this syndrome depends on the severity of the associated cardiac anomalies.

Poland Syndrome

Poland syndrome is a rare anomaly characterized by congenital absence of the pectoralis minor muscle and its nerve supply.[120] Defects in the chest wall are variable, with the absence or rudimentary development of anterior portions of the second through fifth ribs and their costal cartilages. As the thoracic cage grows, the defect enlarges. Lung herniation can occur during Valsalva maneuvers or crying. The presence of chest wall defects with no underlying skeletal structures makes this condition similar to an open chest. Negative pressure generated during inspiration leads to retraction of the chest wall in the region of the defect during inspiration and expansion during exhalation. The ipsilateral arm, forearm, and hand are hypoplastic. Associated anomalies include dextrocardia, scoliosis, hemivertebrae, inguinal hernias, renal aplasia, and displacement of the liver into the chest. Möbius syndrome is an extreme expression of this syndrome with associated facial musculature paralysis and cranial nerve palsies.

Mitochondrial Myopathies

Mitochondrial myopathies are a heterogeneous group of disorders of skeletal muscle energy metabolism.[121] Mitochondria produce the energy requirements of skeletal muscle cells through the redox reactions of the electron transfer chain and oxidative phosphorylation, thereby producing adenosine triphosphate. Defects in this process result in exercise intolerance, fatigue, skeletal muscle pain, and progressive weakness. The morphologic hallmark is large subsarcolemmal accumulations of abnormal mitochondria that appear as red-staining granules ("red-flagged fibers"). Disorders of mitochondrial metabolism may also involve other organ systems with high energy demands (brain, heart, liver, kidneys).

Kearns-Sayre Syndrome

Kearns-Sayre syndrome is a rare mitochondrial myopathy accompanied by progressive external ophthalmoplegia, pigmented degeneration of the retina, and heart block due to involvement of the cardiac conduction system.[122] Dilated cardiomyopathy and associated congestive heart failure may be present.

General anesthesia may be administered to these patients, keeping in mind the risk of drug-induced myocardial depression and the development of cardiac conduction defects.[122] Even though skeletal muscle weakness is not present, it is prudent to monitor respiratory status, especially during the early postoperative period, to ensure complete recovery from lingering effects of anesthetic drugs or muscle relaxants.

MELAS Syndrome

MELAS syndrome is a multisystem disorder characterized clinically by stroke-like episodes, seizures, dementia, recurrent headaches, vomiting, and evidence of mitochondrial dysfunction in the form of lactic acidosis.[123] Lactic acidosis most likely results from defects in the respiratory chain necessitating anaerobic metabolism of glucose. Cardiac abnormalities include conduction defects and cardiomyopathy. Death is usually attributed to respiratory failure.

Limb weakness indicative of skeletal muscle wasting suggests caution when administering succinylcholine to these patients. There may also be an association between skeletal muscle abnormalities and susceptibility to malignant hyperthermia. For this reason it may be prudent to consider patients with mitochondrial myopathies to be susceptible to malignant hyperthermia.[121] The presence of increased serum lactate concentrations emphasizes the need to maintain normal blood glucose concentrations. The direct myocardial depressant effects of anesthetic drugs, especially volatile anesthetics, must be minimized. Careful titration of sedatives and opioids is important, as these patients may manifest decreased ventilatory responses to arterial hypoxemia and hypercarbia. The preoperative presence of seizures, peripheral neuropathies, and renal disease have potential importance when selecting anesthetic drugs and anesthetic techniques.[123]

Multicore Myopathy

Multicore myopathy is a heterogeneous group of diseases characterized by proximal skeletal muscle weakness with decreases in muscle mass and musculoskeletal abnormalities (scoliosis, high arched palate).[124] Recurrent chest infections are common and often reflect the severity of associated kyphoscoliosis. Unlike other myopathies, serum creatine kinase concentrations are generally normal in these individuals. Intelligence is usually normal, and the myopathy typically has a benign course.

Cardiomyopathy may accompany this myopathy, suggesting the value of preoperative assessment with echocardiography.[124] Respiratory function is evaluated especially in the presence of kyphoscoliosis and recurrent chest infections. Difficulty swallowing and an inability to clear secretions detected during the preoperative period may reflect pharyngeal and laryngeal (bulbar) muscle involvement. Careful assessment of swallowing and cough preoperatively and titration of opioid and sedative doses are prudent measures. Postoperative aspiration may be associated with impaired protective upper airway reflexes and lingering effects of drugs administered during anesthesia. Although an anesthetic designed to avoid all known triggering drugs for malignant hyperthermia is not considered necessary, it is important to recognize the potential relation between multicore myopathy and malignant hyperthermia.[124]

Centronuclear Myopathy

Centronuclear myopathy is a rare congenital myopathy characterized by progressive skeletal muscle weakness of the extraocular, facial, neck, and limb muscles.[125] Development of scoliosis with restrictive lung disease is the most important physiologic manifestation of the disease's progress. Congenital heart disease and cardiomyopathy have been described. Serum creatine kinase concentrations are usually normal. The association of ptosis and strabismus with this myopathy increases the likelihood that these children must undergo surgery.

Management of anesthesia is influenced by the known potential for muscle relaxants to potentiate co-existing skeletal muscle weakness and the possibility of triggering malignant hyperthermia. In this regard, muscle relaxants may be avoided and a nontriggering general anesthetic technique utilized.[125] The preoperative presence of micrognathia, restrictive lung disease, and gastroesophageal reflux have important anesthetic implications.

Meige Syndrome

Meige syndrome is an idiopathic dystonic disorder that manifests as blepharospasm and oromandibular dystonia; it most often affects middle-age to elderly women. Median facial muscle spasms are characterized by symmetrical dystonic contractions of the facial muscles. Dystonia is aggravated by stress and disappears during sleep. The pathophysiologic cause of this disease is unknown but may be related to dopamine hyperreactivity or dysfunction of basal ganglia. Drug therapy (antidopaminergics, anticholinergics, acetylcholine agonists, γ-aminobutyric acid agonists) may be somewhat effective, and facial nerve block has been reported to provide sustained relief (up to 9 months).[126]

Spasmodic Dysphonia

Spasmodic dysphonia is a laryngeal disorder characterized by adductor or abductor dystonic spasms of the vocal cords.[127] This syndrome typically manifests as abnormal phonation but on rare occasions is associated with respiratory distress. Stress can exacerbate it, and associated neurologic symptoms (tremors, weakness, dystonia of other skeletal muscle groups) are present in most afflicted patients. Botulinum toxin, which blocks neuromuscular transmission, may be effective for treating the spasms of torticollis, blepharospasm, and spasmodic dysphonia.

Preoperative fiberoptic or direct laryngoscopy may be necessary to define anatomic abnormalities and to estimate airway dimensions.[127] The presence of laryngeal stenosis may necessitate the use of smaller-than-usual tracheal tubes. The risk of pulmonary aspiration may be increased by vocal cord dysfunction caused by therapeutic interventions such as botulinum toxin injection or recurrent laryngeal nerve interruption. Continued monitoring during the postoperative period is important, as these patients may experience respiratory difficulties.

Juvenile Hyaline Fibromatosis

Juvenile hyaline fibromatosis is a rare syndrome characterized by the presence of numerous dermal and subcutaneous nodules. Patients may have hypertrophic gingivae, osteolytic bone lesions, and stunted growth with normal mental development. Resistance to the effects of succinylcholine has been described in patients with juvenile hyaline fibromatosis.[128]

Chondrodysplasia Calcificans Punctata

Chondrodysplasia calcificans punctata is a rare congenital syndrome caused by peroxisomal dysfunction; it manifests as erratic cartilage calcification resulting in bone and skin lesions, cataracts, and cardiac malformations.[129] In surviving children, abnormal growth leads to dwarfism, kyphoscoliosis, limb shortness, and subluxation of the hips. There is no available treatment, but orthopedic procedures are often necessary to offset functional limitations of the disease and to stabilize spinal and limb malformations. Tracheal cartilage may be involved by the disease process resulting in tracheal stenosis, which may complicate perioperative airway management.[129]

Erythromelalgia

Erythromelalgia manifests as painful, swollen, erythematous extremities.[130] Intense, burning pain and increased temperature of the involved extremities are hallmarks of the disease. The lower extremities are most often involved, and males are affected twice as often as females. Primary or idiopathic erythromelalgia occurs more frequently than secondary erythromelalgia, which is most commonly associated with myeloproliferative disorders such as thromboembolism or polycythemia vera. Intravascular platelet aggregation may be prominent. Aspirin may be effective treatment in patients in whom erythromelalgia is associated with thrombocytopenia. The only effective treatment of the severe pain associated with erythromelalgia is immersion of the afflicted extremity in ice water. Neuraxial opioids and local anesthetics may provide some, but not total, pain relief.[130]

Farber's Lipogranulomatosis

Farber's lipogranulomatosis is an inherited disorder due to a deficiency of ceramidase that results in accumulation of ceramide in tissues (pleura, pericardium, synovial lining of joints, liver, spleen, lymph nodes).[131] Progressive arthropathy, psychomotor retardation, and nutritional failure are present, and most afflicted individuals die by 2 years of age owing to airway (oral cavity granulomas) and ventilation problems. Acute renal and hepatic failure may reflect accumulation of ceramide in these organs. Difficult airway management is a predictable problem in patients in whom the disease process involves granuloma formation in the pharynx or on the larynx.[131] Tracheal intubation may be avoided in patients with upper airway involvement because postoperative laryngeal edema or bleeding from laryngeal granulomas is possible.

McCune-Albright Syndrome

McCune-Albright syndrome consists of a triad of physical signs characterized as osseous lesions (polyostotic fibrous dysplasia), melanotic cutaneous macules (café au lait spots), and sexual precocity (autonomous ovarian steroid secretion). Conductive and neural deafness occurs when osseous lesions involve the temporal bone, with resultant ocular or cochlear impingement. Osseous fractures are likely during childhood. In addition to the classic triad, some patients show endocrine dysfunction, especially hyperthyroidism, growth hormone excess, and hypophosphatemia.

Important anesthetic implications are identification of associated endocrine abnormalities, especially hyperthyroidism (see Chapter 23).[132] Perioperative steroid supplementation is a consideration when adrenal hyperactivity is present because these patients may exhibit altered cortisol responses to stress. Vascular fragility may make venous access difficult. These patients have increased bone fragility, and care is indicated during intraoperative positioning and padding. Tracheal intubation may be difficult because of airway distortion associated with acromegaly or hypertrophy of soft tissues in the upper airway.[132]

Klippel-Feil Syndrome

Klippel-Feil syndrome is characterized by a short neck resulting from a reduced number of cervical vertebrae or fusion of several vertebrae into an osseous mass. Movement of the neck is limited, and associated skeletal abnormalities include spinal canal stenosis or kyphoscoliosis. Mandibular malformations and micrognathia may be present. There is an increased incidence of cardiac and genitourinary anomalies in these patients. Management of anesthesia must consider the risk of neurologic damage during direct laryngoscopy in the presence of cervical spine instability.[133] Preoperative lateral neck radiographs help evaluate the stability of the cervical spine.

Osteogenesis Imperfecta

Osteogenesis imperfecta is a rare, autosomal dominant, inherited disease of connective tissues that affects bones, sclera, and the inner ear.[134] Bones are extremely brittle because of defective collagen production. The incidence is higher in females. Clinically, osteogenesis imperfecta manifests as one of two forms: osteogenesis imperfecta congenita and osteogenesis imperfecta tarda. With the congenita form fractures occur in utero, and death is usually during the perinatal period. The tarda form typically manifests during childhood or early adolescence with the presence of blue sclera (due to defective collagen production), fractures with trivial trauma, kyphoscoliosis as a reflection of collapsed vertebral bodies, bowing of the femur and tibia, and gradual onset of otosclerosis and deafness. Impaired platelet function in these patients may manifest as mild bleeding tendencies. Increased body temperature with hyperhydrosis may occur in patients with osteogenesis imperfecta. Increased serum thyroxine concentrations associated with increased oxygen consumption occur in at least 50% of patients with this disease.

Management of anesthesia is influenced by co-existing orthopedic deformities and vulnerability for additional fractures during the perioperative period.[135] Patients with osteogenesis imperfecta often have decreased range of motion of the cervical spine owing to remodeled bone formation. Tracheal intubation must be accomplished with minimal manipulation and trauma, as cervical and mandibular fractures may occur. Awake fiberoptic tracheal intubation is prudent if co-existing orthopedic deformities make it difficult to visualize the glottic opening using direct laryngoscopy. Succinylcholine-induced fasciculations may produce fractures. Dentition is often defective, and teeth may be vulnerable to damage, as during direct laryngoscopy. Associated kyphoscoliosis and pectus excavatum may decrease vital capacity and chest wall compliance with resulting arterial hypoxemia due to ventilation-to-perfusion mismatching. Automated blood pressure cuffs may be hazardous, as overinflation may result in fractures. Regional anesthesia is acceptable in selected patients, as it avoids the need for tracheal intubation; but it may be technically difficult because of kyphoscoliosis. The coagulation status is often evaluated before selecting regional anesthetic techniques in view of the association of osteogenesis imperfecta with prolonged bleeding times despite normal platelet counts. Desmopressin may be effective in restoring normal platelet function. In view of the potential for increased body temperature, it is probably important to monitor the temperature continuously. The increase in body temperature is usually mild and not a forerunner of malignant hyperthermia.

Fibrodysplasia Ossificans

Fibrodysplasia ossificans is a rare inherited autosomal dominant disease, usually manifesting before 6 years of age and characterized clinically by interstitial myositis and proliferation of connective tissue. The term myositis ossificans is also applied to this disease, but fibrodysplasia ossificans is more correct, because it is principally a disease of connective tissue rather than skeletal muscles. Connective tissues undergo cartilaginous and osteoid transformation, eventually leading to displacement of skeletal muscle mass by ectopic bone formation. Ectopic bone formation typically affects skeletal muscles of the elbows, hips, and knees, leading to serious limitations of joint movement. Cervical spine involvement is common, with varying degrees of cervical fusion and the possibility of atlantoaxial subluxation. There may be temporomandibular joint involvement with obvious implications for tracheal intubation. Skeletal muscles of the face, larynx, eyes, anterior abdominal wall, diaphragm, and heart usually escape involvement.

During the early stages of the disease fever may occur at the same time localized lumps appear in affected skeletal muscles. Alkaline phosphatase activity is increased during active phases of the disease. Restrictive patterns of breathing reflect limitation of rib movement. Progression to respiratory failure is rare, although pneumonia is a common complication. Abnormalities on the electrocardiogram may include ST segment changes and right bundle branch block. Deafness may occur, but mental retardation is unlikely.

Treatment directed at halting the progression of this disease is unsuccessful, principally because the pathogenesis remains unknown.[136] Corticosteroids, which decrease bone formation by inhibiting periosteal cell proliferation, provide relief in a few patients, but it is unlikely they can affect the eventual outcome. Warfarin has been used because of anecdotal reports of subjective improvement in the mobility of patients with ectopic calcifications.

Deformities of the Sternum

Pectus carinatum (outward protuberance of the sternum) and pectus excavatum (inward concavity of the sternum) produce psychological problems, but functional consequences are rare. In general, narrowing of the distance between the posterior sternum and the anterior border of the vertebral bodies to as little as 2 cm (normal is 8 cm in adults) can be tolerated with respect to cardiopulmonary function. Nevertheless, pectus excavatum may rarely be associated with increased cardiac ventricular filing pressures and atrial dysrhythmias, especially during exercise. Obstructive sleep apnea may be more common in young children with pectus excavatum, perhaps reflecting inward movement of a pliable costochondral apparatus due to the effect of negative intrathoracic pressure generated by airway obstruction.

Macroglossia

Macroglossia is an infrequent but potentially lethal postoperative complication that is most often associated with posterior fossa craniotomies performed in the sitting position, presumably reflecting extremes of neck flexion or head rotation.[137] Speculated causes of macroglossia include arterial compression, venous compression (excessive neck flexion, head-down position), or mechanical compression (teeth, oral airways, tracheal tubes); or it may have a neurogenic origin. Venous obstruction leading to arterial insufficiency and resulting in reperfusion injury may be the primary etiology in many of these cases. When the onset of macroglossia is immediate it is easily recognized, and airway obstruction does not occur as tracheal extubation is delayed. In some patients, however, initial obstruction to venous outflow from the tongue may lead to the development of regional ischemia because of compression of the lingual arteries, followed by reperfusion injury that does not occur until venous outflow obstruction is relieved. As a result, the onset of macroglossia may be delayed (30 minutes or longer) with the risk of complete airway obstruction occurring at an unexpected time during the postoperative period.[137]

References

1. Epstein EH. Molecular genetics of epidermolysis bullosa. Science 1992;256:799–803
2. Smith GB, Shribman AJ. Anaesthesia and severe skin disease. Anaesthesia 1984;39:443–55
3. James I, Wark H. Airway management during anesthesia in patients with epidermolysis bullosa dystrophica. Anesthesiology 1982;56:323–6
4. Holzman RS, Worthen HM, Johnson K. Anaesthesia for children with junctional epidermolysis bullosa (lethalis). Can J Anaesth 1987;34:395–9
5. Spargo PM, Smith GB. Epidermolysis bullosa and porphyria. Anaesthesia 1989;44:79–83
6. Kelly RE, Koff HD, Rothaus KO, et al. Brachial plexus anesthesia in eight patients with recessive dystrophic epidermolysis bullosa. Anesth Analg 1987;66:1318–20.
7. Jeyaram C, Torda TA. Anesthetic management of cholecystectomy in a patient with buccal pemphigus. Anesthesiology 1974;40:600–1
8. Abouleish EI, Elias MA, Lopez M, et al. Spinal anesthesia for cesarean section in a case of pemphigus foliaceus. Anesth Analg 1997;84:449–50
9. Drenger B, Zidenbaum M, Reifen E, et al. Severe upper airway obstruction and difficult intubation in cicatricial pemphigoid. Anaesthesia 1986;41:1029–31
10. Prasad KK, Chen L. Anesthetic management of a patient with bullous pemphigoid. Anesth Analg 1989;69:437–40
11. Greaves MW, Weinstein GD. Treatment of psoriasis. N Engl J Med 1995;332:581–8
12. Borgeat A, Ruetsch YA. Anesthesia in a patient with malignant systemic mastocytosis using a total intravenous anesthetic technique. Anesth Analg 1998;86:442–4
13. Roberts LJ, Sweetman BJ, Lewis RA, et al. Increased production of prostaglandin D_2 in patients with systemic mastocytosis. N Engl J Med 1980;303:1400–4
14. Lerno G, Slaats G, Coenen E, et al. Anaesthetic management of systemic mastocytosis. Br J Anaesth 1990;65:254–7
15. Coleman MA, Liberthson RR, Crone RK, et al. General anesthesia in a child with urticaria pigmentosa. Anesth Analg 1980;59:704–6
16. Hosking MP, Warner MA. Sudden intraoperative hypotension in a patient with asymptomatic urticaria pigmentosa. Anesth Analg 1987;66:344–6
17. Greaves MW. Chronic urticaria. N Engl J Med 1995;332:1767–72
18. Kotou-Fili K, Borici-Mazi R, Kapp A, et al. Physical urticaria: classification and diagnosis guidelines. Allergy 1997;52:504–13
19. Johnston WE, Moss J, Philbin DM, et al. Management of cold urticaria during hypothermic cardiopulmonary bypass. N Engl J Med 1982;306:219–21
20. Arino P, Aguado L, Cortada V, et al. Cold urticaria associated with intraoperative hypotension and facial edema. Anesthesiology 1999;90:907–9
21. Cucchira RF, Dawson B. Anesthesia in Steven-Johnson syndrome: report of a case. Anesthesiology 1971;35:537–9
22. Younker D, Harrison B. Scleroderma and pregnancy: anaesthetic considerations. Br J Anaesth 1985;57:1136–9
23. Thompson J, Conklin KA. Anesthetic management of a pregnant patient with scleroderma. Anesthesiology 1983;59:69–71
24. D'Angelo R, Miller R. Pregnancy complicated by severe preeclampsia and thrombocytopenia in a patient with selceroderma. Anesth Analg 1997;85:839–41
25. Krechel SLW, Ramirez-Inawant RC, Fabian LW. Anesthetic considerations in pseudoxanthoma elasticum. Anesth Analg 1981;60:344–7
26. Pyeritz RE. Ehlers-Danlos syndrome. N Engl J Med 2000;342:730–2
27. Brighouse D, Guard B. Anaesthesia for caesarean section in a patient with Ehlers-Danlos syndrome type IV. Br J Anaesth 1992;69:517–9
28. Price CM, Ford S, Jones S, et al. Myocardial ischaemia associated with Ehlers-Danlos syndrome. Br J Anaesth 1996;76:464–6
29. Saarnivaara LHM. Anesthesia for a patient with polymyositis undergoing myectomy of the cricopharyngeal muscle. Anesth Analg 1988;67:701–2
30. Brown S, Shupak RC, Patel C, et al. Neuromuscular blockade in a patient with active dermatomyositis. Anesthesiology 1992;77:1031–3
31. Mills JA. Systemic lupus erythematosus. N Engl J Med 1994;330:1871–9
32. Davies SR. Systemic lupus erythematosus and the obstetrical patient: implications for the anaesthetist. Can J Anaesth 1991;38:790–5
33. Espana A, Gutierrez JM, Soria C, et al. Recurrent laryngeal nerve palsy in systemic lupus erythematosus. Neurology 1990;40:1143–6
34. Kelly JE, Simpson MT, Jonathan D, et al. Lipoid proteinosis: Urbach-Wiethe disease. Br J Anaesth 1989;63:609–11
35. Sargent WW. Anesthetic management of a patient with Cornelia de Lange syndrome. Anesthesiology 1991;74:1162–3
36. Kasuda H, Akazawa S, Shimizu R, et al. Difficult endotracheal intubation in a patient with tumoral calcinosis. Anesth Analg 1992;74:159–61

37. Smith CL, Bush GH. Anaesthesia and progressive muscular dystrophy. Br J Anaesth 1985;57:1113–8

38. Sethna NF, Rockoff MA, Worthen HM, et al. Anesthesia-related complications in children with Duchenne muscular dystrophy. Anesthesiology 1988;68:462–5

39. Sullivan M, Thompson WK, Hill GD. Succinylcholine-induced cardiac arrest in children with undiagnosed myopathy. Can J Anaesth 1994;41:497–501

40. Gronert GA. Cardiac arrest after succinylcholine: mortality greater with rhabdomyolysis than receptor upregulation. Anesthesiology 2001;94:523–9

41. Wiesel S, Bevan JC, Samuel J, et al. Vecuronium neuromuscular blockade in a child with mitochondrial myopathy. Anesth Analg 1991;72:696–9

42. Goresky GV, Fox RG. Inhalation anesthetics and Duchenne's muscular dystrophy. Can J Anaesth 1999;46:525–8

43. Chalkiadis GA, Branch KG. Cardiac arrest after isoflurane anaesthesia in a patient with Duchenne's muscular dystrophy. Anaesthesia 1990;45:22–6

44. Kleopa K, Rosenberg H, Heiman-Patterson T. Malignant hyperthermia-like episode in Becker muscular dystrophy. Anesthesiology 2000;93:1535–7

45. Rosenberg H, Heiman-Patterson T. Duchenne's muscular dystrophy and malignant hyperthermia: another warning. Anesthesiology 1983;59:362

46. Wang JM, Stanley TH. Duchenne muscular dystrophy and malignant hyperthermia: two case reports. Can Anaesth Soc J 1986;33:492–7

47. Murat I, Esteve C, Montay G, et al. Pharmacokinetics and cardiovascular effects of bupivacaine during epidural anesthesia in children with Duchenne muscular dystrophy. Anesthesiology 1987;67:249–52

48. Dresner DL, Ali HH. Anaesthetic management of a patient with facioscapulohumeral muscular dystrophy. Br J Anaesth 1989;62:331–4

49. Cunliffe M, Burrows FA. Anaesthetic implications of nemaline rod myopathy. Can Anaesth Soc J 1985;32:543–7

50. Stackhouse R, Chelmow D, Dattel BJ. Anesthetic complications in a pregnant patient with nemaline myopathy. Anesth Analg 1994;79:1195–7

51. Landrum AL, Eggers GWN. Oculopharyngeal dystrophy: an approach to anesthetic management. Anesth Analg 1992;75:1043–5

52. Jensen V. The anaesthetic management of a patient with Emery-Dreifuss muscular dystrophy. Can J Anaesth 1996;43:968–71

53. Russell SH, Hirsch NP. Anaesthesia and myotonia. Br J Anaesth 1994;72:210–6

54. Aldredge LM. Anaesthetic problems in myotonic dystrophy: a case report and review of the Aberdeen experience comprising 48 general anaesthetics in a further 16 patients. Br J Anaesth 1985;57:1119–30

55. Cope KD, Miller JN. Local and spinal anesthesia for cesarean section in a patient with myotonic dystrophy. Anesth Analg 1986;65:687–90

56. Nightingale P, Healy TEJ, McGuinness K. Dystophica myotonica and atracurium. Br J Anaesth 1985;57:1131–5

57. Theroux MC, Kettrick RG, Khine HH. Laryngeal mask airway and fiberoptic endoscopy in an infant with Schwartz-Jampel syndrome. Anesthesiology 1995;82:605

58. Lema G, Urzua J, Moran S, et al. Successful anesthetic management of a patient with hypokalemic familial periodic paralysis undergoing cardiac surgery. Anesthesiology 1991;74:373–5

59. Viscomi CM, Ptacek LJ, Dudley D. Anesthetic management of familial hypokalemic periodic paralysis during parturition. Anesth Analg 1999;88:1081–2

60. Walsh F, Kelly D. Anaesthetic management of a patient with familial normokalemic periodic paralysis. Can J Anaesth 1996;43:684–6

61. Hecht ML, Valtysson B, Hogan K. Spinal anesthesia for a patient with calcium channel mutation causing hypokalemic periodic paralysis. Anesth Analg 1997;84:461–4

62. Ashwood EM, Russell WJ, Burrow DD. Hyperkalemic periodic paralysis. Anaesthesia 1992;47:579–84

63. Rodney RT, Shannon EC, Sun T, et al. Atracurium and hypokalemic familial periodic paralysis. Anesth Analg 1988;67:782–3

64. Lambert C, Blanloeil Y, Horber RK, et al. Malignant hyperthermia in a patient with hypokalemic periodic paralysis. Anesth Analg 1994;79:1012–4

65. Lofgren A, Hahn RG. Hypokalemia from intercostal nerve block. Reg Anesth 1994;19:247–54

66. Drachman DB. Myasthenia gravis. N Engl J Med 1994;330:1797–1810

67. Baraka A. Anaesthesia and myasthenia gravis. Can J Anaesth 1992;39:476–86

68. Leventhal SR, Orkin FK, Hirsh RA. Prediction of the need for postoperative mechanical ventilation in myasthenia gravis. Anesthesiology 1980;53:26–30

69. Eisenkraft JB, Papatestas AE, Kahn CH, et al. Predicting the need for postoperative mechanical ventilation and myasthenia gravis. Anesthesiology 1986;65:79–82

70. Parr SM, Robinson BJ, Rees D, et al. Interaction between betamethasone and vecuronium. Br J Anaesth 1991;67:447–51

71. Itoh H, Shibata K, Yoshida M, et al. Neuromuscular monitoring at the orbicularis oculi may overestimate the blockade in myasthenic patients. Anesthesiology 2000;93:1194–7

72. Eisenkraft JB, Book WJ, Mann SM, et al. Resistance to succinylcholine in myasthenia gravis: a dose-response study. Anesthesiology 1988;69:760–3

73. Smith CE, Donati F, Bevan DR. Cumulative dose-response curves for atracurium in patients with myasthenia gravis. Can J Anaesth 1989;36:402–6

74. Nilsson E, Meretoja OA. Vecuronium dose-response and requirements in patients with myasthenia gravis. Anesthesiology 1990;73:28–32

75. Baraka A, Tabboush Z. Neuromuscular response to succinylcholine-vecuronium sequence in three myasthenic patients undergoing thymectomy. Anesth Analg 1991;72:827–30

76. Small S, Ali HH, Lennon VA, et al. Anesthesia for unsuspected Lambert-Eaton myasthenic syndrome with autoantibodies and occult small cell lung carcinoma. Anesthesiology 1992;76:142–5

77. Firestein GS. Rheumatoid arthritis. Sci Am Med 2000;1–15

78. Harris ED. Rheumatoid arthritis: pathophysiology and implications for therapy. N Engl J Med 1990;322:1277–88

79. Funk D, Raymon F. Rheumatoid arthritis of the cricoarytenoid joints: an airway hazard. Anesth Analg 1975;54:742–5

80. Vetter TR. Acute airway obstruction due to arytenoiditis in a child with juvenile rheumatoid arthritis. Anesth Analg 1994;79:1198–200

81. Cervantes-Perez P, Toro-Perez AH, Rodreguez-Jurado P. Pulmonary involvement in rheumatoid arthritis. JAMA 1980;243:1715–9

82. Bombardier C, Laikne L, Reicin A, et al. Comparison of upper gastrointestinal toxicity of rofecoxib and naproxen in patients with rheumatoid arthritis. N Engl J Med 2000;343:1520–8

83. Weinblatt ME, Coblyn JS, Fox DA, et al. Efficacy of low-dose methotrexate in rheumatoid arthritis. N Engl J Med 1985;312:818–23

84. Bathon JM, Martin RW, Fleischmann RM, et al. A comparison of etanercept and methotrexate in patients with early rheumatoid arthritis. N Engl J Med 2000;343:1586–93

85. Schelew BL, Vaghadia H. Ankylosing spondylitis and neuraxial anaesthesia: a 10 year review. Can J Anaesth 1996; 43:65–8

86. Delmas PD, Meunier PJ. The management of Paget's disease of bone. N Engl J Med 1997;336:558–66

87. Pyeritz RE, McKusick VA. The Marfan syndrome: diagnosis and management. N Engl J Med 1979;300:772–7

88. Tritapepe L, Voci P, Pinto G, et al. Anaesthesia for caesarean section in a Marfan patient with recurrent aortic dissection. Can J Anaesth 1996;43:1153–5

89. Kafer ER. Respiratory and cardiovascular functions in scoliosis and the principles of anesthetic management. Anesthesiology 1980;52:339–51

90. Pathak KS, Brown RH, Nash CL, et al. Continuous opioid infusion for scoliosis fusion surgery. Anesth Analg 1983;62:841–5

91. Berkowitz ID, Raja SN, Bender KS, et al. Dwarfs: pathophysiology and anesthetic implications. Anesthesiology 1990;73: 739–59

92. Ratner EF, Hamilton CL. Anesthesia for cesarean section in a pituitary dwarf. Anesthesiology 1998;89:253–4

93. Mayhew JF, Katz J, Miner M, et al. Anaesthesia for the achondroplastic dwarf. Can Anaesth Soc J 1986;33:216–21

94. Kallman GN, Fening E, Obiaya MD. Anaesthetic management of achondroplasia. Br J Anaesth 1986;58:117–9

95. Katz J, Mayhew JF. Air embolism in the achondroplastic dwarf. Anesthesiology 1985;63:205–7

96. Cohen SE. Anesthesia for cesarean section in achondroplastic dwarfs. Anesthesiology 1980;52:264–6

97. Dinner M, Goldin EZ, Ward R, et al. Russell-Silver syndrome: anesthetic implications. Anesth Analg 1994;78: 1197–9

98. Deyo RA, Weinstein JN. Low back pain. N Engl J Med 2001;344:363–70

99. Malmivaara A, Hakkinen U, Aro T, et al. The treatment of acute low back pain-bed rest, exercises, or ordinary activity? N Engl J Med 1995;332:351–5

100. Burkhart SS. A 26-year-old woman with shoulder pain. JAMA 2000;284:1559–67

101. Klein SM, Grant SA, Greengrass RA, et al. Interscalene brachial plexus block with continuous catheter insertion system and a disposable infusion pump. Anesth Analg 2000;91: 1473–8

102. Singelyln FJ, Seguy S, Gouverneur JM. Interscalene brachial plexus analgesia after open shoulder surgery: continuous versus patient-controlled infusion. Anesth Analg 1999;89: 1216–20

103. Toyoyama H, Kariya N, Toyoda Y. Electrocardiographic artifacts during shoulder arthroscopy using a pressure-controlled irrigation pump. Anesth Analg 2000;90:856–7

104. Hegde RT, Avatgere RN. Air embolism during anaesthesia for shoulder arthroscopy. Br J Anaesth 2000;85:925–7

105. Horn E-P, Schroeder F, Wilhelm S, et al. Wound infiltration and drain lavage with ropivacaine after major shoulder surgery. Anesth Analg 1999;89:1461–6

106. Ramchandra DS, Anisya V, Gourie-Deve M. Ketamine monoanaesthesia for diagnostic muscle biopsy in neuromuscular disorders in infancy and childhood: floppy infant syndrome. Can J Anaesth 1990;37:474–6

107. Cook WP, Kaplan RF. Neuromuscular blockade in a patient with stiff-baby syndrome. Anesthesiology 1986;65:525–8

108. Parris WSCV, Johnson AC. Tracheomegaly. Anesthesiology 1982;56:141–3

109. Cruickshanks GF, Brown S, Chitayat D. Anesthesia for Freeman-Sheldon syndrome using a laryngeal mask airway. Can J Anesth 1999;46:783–7

110. Yamashita M, Koishi K, Yamaya R, et al. Anaesthetic considerations in the Prader-Willi syndrome: report of four cases. Can Anaesth Soc J 1983;30:179–84

111. Sloan TB, Kaye CI. Rumination risk of aspiration of gastric contents in the Prader-Willi syndrome. Anesth Analg 1991;73:492–5

112. Hannington-Kiff JG. Prune-belly syndrome and general anaesthesia: case report. Br J Anaesth 1970;42:649–52

113. Ravindran R, Stoops CM. Anesthetic management of a patient with Hallermann-Streiff syndrome. Anesth Analg 1979;58:254–5

114. Vaghadia H, Blackstock D. Anaesthetic implications of the trismus pseudocamptodactyly (Dutch-Kentucky or Hech Beals) syndrome. Can J Anaesth 1988;35:80–5

115. Dimaculangan DP, Lokhandwala BS, Wlody DJ, et al. Difficult airway in a patient with Coffin-Siris syndrome. Anesth Analg 2001;92:554–5

116. Quance DR. Anaesthetic management of an obstetrical patient with arthrogryposis multiplex congenita. Can J Anaesth 1988;35:612–14

117. Petersen WC, Crouch ER. Anesthesia-induced rigidity, unrelated to succinylcholine, associated with Smith-Lemli-Opitz syndrome and malignant hyperthermia. Anesth Analg 1995;80:606–8

118. Kuzma PJ, Calkins MD, Kline MD, et al. The anesthetic management of patients with multiple pterygium syndrome. Anesth Analg 1996;83:430–2

119. Shono S, Higa K, Kumano K, et al. Holt-Oram syndrome. Br J Anaesth 1998;80:856–7

120. Sethuraman R, Kannan S, Bala I, et al. Anaesthesia in Poland syndrome. Can J Anaesth 1998;45:277–9

121. Rosaeg OP, Morrison S, MacLeod JP. Anaesthetic management of labour and delivery in the parturient with mitochondrial myopathy. Can J Anaesth 1996;43:403–7

122. Kitoh T, Mizuno K, Otagiri T, et al. Anesthetic management for a patient with Kearns-Sayre syndrome. Anesth Analg 1995;80:1240–2

123. Thompson VA, Wahr JA. Anesthetic considerations in patients presenting with mitochondrial myopathy, encephalopathy, lactic acidosis, and stroke-like episodes (MELAS) syndrome. Anesth Analg 1997;85:1404–6

124. Gordon CP, Litz S. Multicore myopathy in a patient with anhidrotic ectodermal dysplasia. Can J Anaesth 1992;39: 966–8

125. Gottschalk A, Heiman-Patterson T, deQuevedo R 2nd, et al. General anesthesia for a patient with centronuclear (myotubular) myopathy. Anesthesiology 1998;89:1018–20

126. Kobayashi A, Lee M, Tanaka Y. Successful treatment of Meige's syndrome with facial nerve block. Anesthesiology 1994;80:1396–8

127. Manoub M, Rao U, Motta P, et al. Recurrent postoperative stridor requiring tracheosotomy in a patient with spasmodic dysphonia. Anesthesiology 2000;92:893–5

128. Baraka A. Succinylcholine resistance in a patient with juvenile hyaline fibromatosis. Anesthesiology 1997;87:1250–2

129. Karoutsos S, Lansade A, Terrier G, et al. Chondrodysplasia punctata and subglottic stenosis. Anesth Analg 1999;89: 1322–3

130. Rauck RL, Naveira F, Speight KL, et al. Refractory idiopathic erythromelalgia. Anesth Analg 1996;82:1097–1101

131. Asada A, Tatekasa S, Terai T, et al. The anesthetic implications of a patient with Farber's lipogranulomatosis. Anesthesiology 1994;80:206–9

132. Langer RA, Yook I, Capan LM. Anesthetic considerations in McCune-Albright syndrome: case report with literature review. Anesth Analg 1995;80:1236–9

133. Naguib M, Farag H, Ibfrahim AED. Anaesthetic considerations in Klippel-Feil syndrome. Can Anaesth Soc J 1986;33: 66–70

134. Marini JC, Gerber NL. Osteogenesis imperfecta: rehabilitation and prospects for gene therapy. JAMA 1997;277: 746–50

135. Cho E, Dayan SS, Marx GF. Anaesthesia in a parturient with osteogenesis imperfecta. Br J Anaesth 1992;68:422–3

136. Newton MC, Allen PW, Ryan DC. Fibrodysplasia ossificans progressive. Br J Anaesth 1990;64:246–50

137. Lam RM, Vavilala MS. Macroglossia: compartment syndrome of the tongue? Anesthesiology 2000;92:1832–5

27

Infectious Diseases

Infectious diseases, although rarely an indication for surgery, may influence the management of anesthesia.[1] Patients with known transmissible diseases receive special attention with respect to use of disposable equipment. When handling blood and body fluids one must consider the possible presence of undiagnosed infectious diseases in all patients. Infection is the most common cause of fever, reflecting the effect of endogenous pyrogens (cytokines) on the hypothalamic setpoint. There is no direct evidence that fever is beneficial to the host, whereas high fever may cause seizures in children (0.5 to 6.0 years of age) and altered sensorium in adults. In elderly patients or those with cardiopulmonary disease, fever can precipitate cardiac dysrhythmias, myocardial ischemia, and congestive heart failure, reflecting increased oxygen consumption that cannot be met by increasing the cardiac output. Significant increases in body temperature should be treated in young children, elderly or debilitated individuals, and those with cardiopulmonary disease. Aspirin-like drugs are used to lower body temperature owing to increased hypothalamic setpoints. If physical cooling methods are utilized without antipyretic drugs, homeostatic mechanisms continue to attempt to increase body temperature, resulting in intense vasoconstriction and shivering.

■ PROPHYLACTIC ANTIBIOTICS

Prophylactic antibiotics are used for many of the commonly performed surgical procedures. Because of their broad antimicrobial spectrum and low toxicity, cephalosporins are likely choices for preoperative prophylaxis when the most common pathogens are normal skin, gastrointestinal, and genitourinary flora. Timing of antibiotic administration should coincide with bacterial inoculation, emphasizing that prophylactic drugs need not be routinely administered before the induction of anesthesia. Prolongation of prophylactic antibiotic therapy beyond the first postoperative day probably affords no additional protection.

The incidence of allergic reactions to cephalosporins is low, and administration of these antibiotics to patients with a history of allergy to penicillin is controversial. Similarity in chemical structure between the two classes of drugs suggests the possibility of cross-sensitivity, although it seems to be a remote possibility.[2] Nevertheless, it is common to avoid cephalosporins in patients who have a history of life-threatening allergic reactions to penicillin.

Vancomycin, when utilized prophylactically, is likely to be administered as a continuous intravenous infusion often over 15 to 30 minutes to minimize the risk of drug-induced histamine release and associated hypotension. Allergic reactions to vancomycin have been associated with cardiovascular collapse.[3, 4] The frequent dependence of antibiotics on renal clearance must be considered when determining the dose being administered to patients with renal insufficiency.

INFECTIONS DUE TO GRAM-POSITIVE BACTERIA

Organisms categorized as gram-positive bacteria include pneumococci, streptococci, and staphylococci. These organisms are frequently implicated as causes of infections that may contribute to significant morbidity in hospitalized patients.

Pneumococci

There are more than 80 distinct serotypes of the *Pneumococcus* genus (*Streptococcus pneumoniae*).[5] These serotypes differ by virtue of the polysaccharide polymers that form their outer capsules. These capsules are crucial to the virulence of pneumococci, as they allow these bacteria to resist phagocytosis. Capsular polysaccharides from the 14 most prevalent serotypes of pneumococci have been incorporated into a pneumococcal vaccine.[6] Pneumococci remain the most important cause of bacterial pneumonias, accounting for about 60% of these infections. Acute otitis media, due to spread of pneumococci from the nasopharynx, is one of the most frequent bacterial infections in children. The nasopharynx is the natural habitat of pneumococci. In rare instances, meningitis reflects the spread of pneumococcal organisms from the middle ear or nasal sinuses. An uncommon pneumococcal syndrome is overwhelming infection after surgical splenectomy.

Penicillin (or other antibiotics with similar antimicrobial spectrums) remains the drug of choice to treat infections due to pneumococci. Pneumococcal vaccine is indicated in patients at risk of infection, including those with chronic cardiopulmonary disease, sickle cell disease, cirrhosis of the liver, or nephrosis and patients who are immunosuppressed.[6] The vaccine may be useful in the management of patients with Hodgkin's disease, who are at risk for pneumococcal sepsis following staging laparotomy and splenectomy. It should be appreciated that responses to this vaccine are often inadequate following chemotherapy and radiotherapy.

Streptococci

Streptococci are diverse groups of gram-positive bacteria that reside in humans as part of the normal bacterial flora. Based on comparisons of their carbohydrate cell walls, streptococci are divided into 18 groups designated A through H and K through T.

Group A Streptococci

Group A streptococci (*Streptococcus pyogenes*) comprise one of the most common and ubiquitous groups of human pathogens. They are responsible for a wide array of infections, the most frequent of which are acute pharyngitis and superficial skin infections (Table 27–1).[7]

Mechanism of Transmission

The most important mode of transmission of group A streptococci is droplets originating from asymptomatic nasopharyngeal carriers or from patients

---

Table 27–1 • Infections Due to Group A Streptococci

Pharyngitis ("strep throat") and tonsillitis
Superficial skin infections (impetigo, pyoderma)
Deep skin infections (cellulitis, erysipelas)
Sinusitis
Otitis
Pneumonia
Bacteremia (endocarditis, meningitis, osteomyelitis)
Scarlet fever
Peritonsillar and retropharyngeal abscess
Pueperal sepsis
Nonsuppurative sequelae (acute rheumatic fever, acute glomerulonephritis)

with pharyngitis. Group A streptococci elaborate enzymes that account for the ability of these organisms to produce inflammation and to spread rapidly to adjacent tissues. Among these enzymes are streptolysin O and streptolysin S, which are responsible for hemolysis (the reason for their designation as β-hemolytic streptococci) and inactivation of leukocytes. Streptokinase enzyme elaborated by certain streptococci is responsible for promoting fibrinolysis. Elaboration of hyaluronidase enzyme by streptococci facilitates spread of infection to adjacent tissues owing to the ability of this enzyme to digest hyaluronic acid present in connective tissues.

Manifestations

Group A streptococci are the most common causes of bacterial pharyngitis and tonsillitis. Elaboration of erythrogenic toxin is responsible for scarlet fever. Acute rheumatic fever occurs only after pharyngitis caused by group A streptococci. Rheumatic fever is most likely to develop in patients 5 to 15 years old. Typically, symptoms of rheumatic fever manifest 1 to 3 weeks following streptococcal infections. Antibodies formed against streptococcal antigens are the most likely mechanism by which prior infections with group A streptococci produce delayed tissue damage. This tissue damage may manifest as pericarditis, myocarditis, or endocarditis. The mitral and aortic valves are often involved in the disease process. An acute migratory arthritis occurs in more than half of the patients in whom rheumatic fever develops. Early treatment of pharyngitis due to infections with group A streptococci prevent subsequent attacks of rheumatic fever. Aspirin can control the fever and articular manifestations associated with acute rheumatic fever.

Superficial infections of the epidermis due to group A streptococci are known as impetigo. Impetigo is highly contagious and predisposes to the poststreptococcal infection syndrome known as glomerulonephritis. Surgical wound infections due to streptococci often manifest as acute increases in body temperature despite a relatively benign-appearing incision site.

Deep skin infections due to group A streptococci are known as erysipelas and cellulitis. Osteomyelitis, meningitis, and endocarditis are potential complications of group A streptococcal bacteremia. Group A streptococci are the classic cause of postpartum infections.

Treatment

Penicillin is the drug of choice to treat infections due to group A streptococci. Alternatives to penicillin include erythromycin and clindamycin. One should not rely on tetracyclines, as many strains of group A streptococci are resistant to this antibiotic.

Streptococcal Toxic Shock Syndrome

Septic shock and multiorgan failure in children and adults may be associated with severe, invasive (less often noninvasive) group A streptococcal infections.[8] This syndrome is believed to be mediated by streptococcal exotoxins and is most commonly associated with necrotizing fasciitis or myositis and pneumonia. Necrotizing fasciitis or myositis requires extensive soft tissue débridement and/or amputation on an emergency basis. Organ dysfunction (increased serum creatinine concentrations) may precede the onset of hypotension that reflects myocardial depression, peripheral vasodilation, and hypovolemia. Hyperkalemia may require urgent hemodialysis. Rhabdomyolysis may occur with necrotizing fasciitis or myositis. Coagulopathy with disseminated intravascular coagulation is frequently present. Acute respiratory failure and fulminant pneumonia may manifest, and bacteremia is often present.

Recommended antibiotic treatment includes high doses of penicillin plus clindamycin. Vasopressors are usually required, and optimization of the intravascular fluid volume status may be monitored using measurements from a pulmonary artery catheter. Correction of coagulation abnormalities with blood products is needed to permit surgical débridement of infected tissues. Ketamine may be useful for induction and maintenance of anesthesia in severely hypotensive patients. The need for continued inotropic and ventilatory support is anticipated into the postoperative period.

Group B Streptococci

Group B streptococci are the most common cause of bacterial sepsis in neonates. Infections due to these organisms are most often associated with prematurity and prolonged rupture of the membranes. Pneumonia or meningitis is present in about one-half of neonates who have an infection due to these organisms. Mortality ranges from 20% to 75% despite aggressive treatment with antibiotics. Neurologic sequelae are often present in neonates who survive. Despite demonstrations of a decreased incidence of necrotizing enterocolitis in high risk infants treated with antibiotics, routine use of antibiotics is limited by the concern about the development of resistant organisms.

Group D Streptococci

Group D streptococci reside in the gastrointestinal and genitourinary tracts. These enterococci are relatively common causes of superficial wound infections, urinary tract infections, peritonitis, endocarditis, and bacteremia. Infections with group D streptococci are most likely to be seen in patients with co-existing diseases of the genitourinary or gastrointestinal tract. Treatment of infections due to group D streptococci are difficult, as these organisms are unique among streptococci in that they are resistant to penicillin.

Staphylococci

The two important species of staphylococci are *Staphylococcus aureus* and *Staphylococcus epidermidis*. Unlike pneumococci and streptococci, there is no satisfactory serologic classification of staphylococci.

Staphylococcus aureus

Staphylococcus aureus is a widely distributed organism; and asymptomatic carriers or persons with staphylococcal lesions act as reservoirs of infection. The incidence of nasal carriage is 15% to 50% in hospital populations. The incidence is even higher among intravenous drug users and patients with insulin-dependent diabetes mellitus. Contamination of the hands with nasal secretions is the primary mode of transmission.

The most frequent manifestations of *S. aureus* infections are superficial infections (conjunctivitis, furuncle, paronychia) and soft tissue infections (cellulitis, mastitis, surgical incision). These organisms are among the principal causes of septic arthritis and osteomyelitis. Staphylococcal bacteremia may result in endocarditis and meningitis. Staphylococci do not cause pharyngitis and are responsible for fewer than 10% of all bacterial pneumonias.

Staphylococcal invasion of the gastrointestinal tract may take two forms. With one form, ingestion of staphylococcal enterotoxin results in vomiting and diarrhea within 3 to 6 hours after consumption of food contaminated with *S. aureus*. Characteristically, these symptoms are not accompanied by fever. With the second form, staphylococcal enterocolitis is caused by the intestinal overgrowth of *S. aureus* in patients receiving broad-spectrum oral antibiotics.

Staphylococcus aureus is usually resistant to penicillin. Effective antibiotics include aminoglycoside and cephalosporin antibiotics, oxacillin, and nafcillin. In addition to therapy with antibiotics, other measures may be necessary, such as removing such portals of entry as indwelling venous catheters and surgical drainage.

Staphylococcal toxic shock syndrome is a potentially fatal multisystem illness due to *S. aureus* infection and production of toxins. This syndrome is associated with tampon use during menstruation and with the use of vaginal contraceptive sponges. Toxic shock syndrome may be a complication of staphylococcal pneumonia that follows an influenza-like illness (postinfluenza toxic shock syndrome).[9] Other nonmenstrual causes of toxic shock syndrome have been related to nasal packing, childbirth and abortion, surgical wound infections, and vaginal infections.

Criteria for the diagnosis of toxic shock syndrome include fever, diffuse macular erythroderma, and hypotension. Desquamation is a characteristic feature of this syndrome but is not an early finding. Evidence of multisystem involvement may include diarrhea, skeletal muscle myalgia (increased serum creatine kinase concentrations), renal dysfunction (increased serum creatinine concentrations), hepatic dysfunction (increased serum aminotransaminase and bilirubin concentrations), disseminated intravascular coagulation, and thrombocytopenia. Isolation of toxin-producing *S. aureus* from secretions of affected patients further supports the diagnosis of toxic shock syndrome.

Staphylococcus epidermidis

Staphylococcus epidermidis is an organism of low pathogenic potential that is universally present as part of the normal skin flora. Because of its ubiquity, *S. epidermidis* is frequently isolated from clinical specimens, including blood cultures. Nevertheless, these organisms are most often skin contaminants rather than true pathogens, producing infections only in patients with severe underlying medical problems.

A frequent manifestation of infection with *S. epidermidis* is bacteremia resulting from an infected intravenous catheter. Many affected patients have associated persistent low grade fevers, with periodic marked increases in body temperature. Signs of thrombophlebitis may or may not be present. Removal of contaminated intravenous catheters is the most important aspect of therapy. In this regard, use of antiseptic-impregnated central venous catheters decreases the risk of catheter-related bacteremia.[10]

The most difficult therapeutic problem caused by *S. epidermidis* is infection of prosthetic heart valves. This infection typically has a subacute course, but eradication of organisms is difficult owing to their resistance to many of the available antibiotics.

INFECTIONS DUE TO GRAM-NEGATIVE BACTERIA

Clinically important diseases caused by infections with gram-positive bacteria include *Escherichia coli*-induced diarrhea, salmonellosis, shigellosis, and cholera. Manifestations of these diseases are seen primarily in the gastrointestinal tract.

Escherichia coli-Induced Diarrhea

Escherichia coli is an important constituent of the normal gastrointestinal flora. Some strains of *E. coli*, however, are not part of the normal flora and produce diarrhea ("traveler's disease") when introduced into the gastrointestinal tract by contaminated food or water. Clinical manifestations include abrupt onset of abdominal cramps and watery diarrhea. Absence of fever is consistent with the failure of these organisms to invade other tissues or to produce inflammation. This form of diarrhea cannot be distinguished clinically from shigellosis. The most important aspect of treatment is fluid and electrolyte replacement.

Salmonellosis

Gastroenteritis accounts for about two-thirds of all infections with *Salmonella*. Ingestion of these organisms is followed in 8 to 48 hours by abdominal cramps, vomiting, and diarrhea. Abdominal pain is typically periumbilical or is localized to the right lower quadrant. As such, this pain can mimic acute appendicitis, cholecystitis, or a ruptured viscus. Antibiotics are not effective.

Enteric fever (thyroid fever) is characterized by sustained gram-negative bacteremia and by persistent fever. There may be associated dysfunction of multiple organ systems. Chloramphenical is the recommended treatment.

Shigellosis

Shigellosis is an acute inflammatory disease of the gastrointestinal tract that ranges in severity from mild nonspecific diarrhea to classic dysentery. Initial manifestations of infection with these gram-negative organisms include fever, abdominal cramps, and watery diarrhea. Treatment is with tetracycline antibiotics.

Cholera

Cholera is an acute diarrheal disease produced by enterotoxin secreted by *Vibrio cholerae* organisms. Humans are the only known hosts, so transmission can occur only through infected human excrement. These organisms are exquisitely sensitive to gastric acid; thus persons who are achlorhydric or who are taking antacids are more susceptible to cholera.

Diarrhea is massive and watery. Hourly fluid loss may be equivalent to 1000 ml of isotonic fluid at the peak of the disease. Hypotension, tachycardia, and metabolic acidosis reflect large fluid and electrolyte losses. Fever is characteristically absent. Treatment is with fluid and electrolyte replacement and eradication of gram-negative organisms with tetracycline antibiotics.

INFECTIONS DUE TO SPORE-FORMING ANAEROBES

Spore-forming gram-positive anaerobes that cause invasive infections are normally found in the lower gastrointestinal tract of humans and animals and in soil contaminated with their excrement. These organisms are strict anaerobes and are protected from the lethal effects of oxygen by forming spores. Introduction of spores into wounds (puncture wounds, burns, uterine instrumentation, subcutaneous injections by intravenous drug abusers) sets the stage for the conversion of spores into exotoxin-producing vegetative forms. The species most often responsible for disease in humans are *Clostridium perfringens*, *Clostridium tetani*, and *Clostridium botulinum*. Exotoxins elaborated by vegetative forms of these organisms cause clostridial myonecrosis, tetanus, and botulism, respectively.

Clostridial Myonecrosis

Clostridial myonecrosis ("gas gangrene") is due to infection with *C. perfringens*. The incubation period is 8 to 72 hours, after which there is a sudden onset of localized skeletal muscle pain and swelling.

Signs and Symptoms

Necrosis of skeletal muscles and alterations in the integrity of the capillary membranes are caused by elaboration of an exotoxin (lecithinase) by these organisms. A brownish discharge with a foul odor is characteristic. In addition to the exotoxin, these organisms liberate hydrogen and carbon dioxide, which is responsible for crepitus over involved skeletal muscles, and the associated swelling can cause compression of surrounding blood vessels.

Systemic effects of infection with *C. perfringens* are prominent. Tachycardia and fever are followed by hypotension and oliguria. Presumably, these responses reflect decreased intravascular fluid volume due to massive tissue edema. Anemia, jaundice, and hemoglobinuria are due to intravascular hemolysis in association with *Clostridium* bacteremia. Renal failure may be a consequence of hemoglobinuria.

Treatment

Treatment of clostridial myonecrosis is immediate surgical débridement of infected tissues. Penicillin or an equivalent antibiotic is administered to eradicate organisms not removed by débridement and to control bacteremia.

Management of Anesthesia

Management of anesthesia for surgical débridement must take into consideration the multiple physiologic derangements that accompany infection with these organisms.[11] Preoperatively, important considerations include the status of the intravascular fluid volume, oxygen-carrying capacity of the blood, and renal function. Ketamine is useful for the induction and maintenance of anesthesia. Use of nitrous oxide may be avoided based on the theoretical concern that it would cause expansion of gas pockets produced by clostridial infection. This seems unlikely, however, as these gas pockets are relatively avascular. Likewise, the release of potassium from necrotic skeletal muscles following administration of succinylcholine seems unlikely, as the involved skeletal muscles are avascular and thus effectively isolated from the systemic circulation.

In vitro oxygen exposure to less than 2.5 atmospheres of pressure does not inhibit release of the clostridial exotoxin. Therefore delivery of oxygen concentrations higher than those needed to maintain adequate arterial oxygenation during surgery seems to offer no advantages. Renal function must be considered when selecting nondepolarizing muscle relaxants that may depend on renal clearance mechanisms. Use of electrocautery may be questioned in view of the production of hydrogen gas by clostridial organisms. Regional anesthesia is not recommended because clostridial organisms could theoretically be introduced into other sites by needles used to place the local anesthetic. Furthermore, blockade of the peripheral sympathetic nervous system might be undesirable in the presence of an unstable cardiovascular system.

Postoperatively, these patients are not likely to be sources of cross-infections to other patients as *C. perfringens* organisms are neutralized when exposed to air. Therefore strict isolation of these patients is not mandatory.

Tetanus

Tetanus is caused by the gram-negative bacillus *Clostridium tetani*. Elaboration of the neurotoxin tetanospasmin by vegetative forms of these organisms is responsible for the clinical manifestations of tetanus. With the exception of botulinum toxin, tetanospasmin is the most powerful poison known to humans. Tetanospasmin, when elaborated into wounds, spreads centrally along motor nerves to the spinal cord or enters the systemic circulation to reach the central nervous system. This toxin affects the nervous system in several areas. In the spinal cord tetanospasmin suppresses inhibitory internuncial neurons, resulting in generalized skeletal muscle contractions ("spasms"). In the brain there is fixation of toxin by gangliosides. The fourth cerebral ventricle is believed to have selective permeability for tetanospasmin, resulting in early manifestations of trismus and neck rigidity. Sympathetic nervous system hyperactivity may manifest as the disease progresses.[12]

Signs and Symptoms

Trismus is the presenting symptom of tetanus in 75% of patients. The greater strength of the masseter muscles, compared with the opposing digastric and mylohyoid muscles, results in "lockjaw." Indeed, these patients may initially seek dental attention. Rigidity of the facial muscles results in the characteristic appearance described as the "sardonic smile" (risus sardonicus). Spasm of laryngeal muscles can occur at any time. Intractable pharyngeal spasms following tracheal extubation has been described in patients with unrecognized tetanus.[13] Dysphagia may be due to spasm of the pharyngeal muscles. Spasm of the intercostal muscles and the diaphragm interferes with adequate ventilation. The rigidity of abdominal and lumbar muscles accounts for the opisthotonic posture. Skeletal muscle spasms are tonic and clonic in nature, and are excruciatingly painful. Furthermore, the increased skeletal muscle work is associated with dramatic increases in oxygen consumption, and peripheral vasoconstriction can contribute to increased body temperature.

External stimulation, including sudden exposure to bright light, unexpected noise, or tracheal suction, can precipitate generalized skeletal muscle spasms, leading to inadequate ventilation and then death. Hypotension has been attributed to myocarditis. Isolated and unexplained tachycardia may be early manifestations of hyperactivity of the sympathetic nervous system. More often this hyperactivity manifests as transient systemic hypertension. Sympathetic nervous system responses to external stimuli are exaggerated, as demonstrated by cardiac tachydysrhythmias and labile systemic blood pressure. In addition, excessive sympathetic nervous system activity is associated with intense peripheral vasoconstriction, diaphoresis, and increased urinary excretion of catecholamines. Inappropriate secretion of antidiuretic hormone manifesting as hyponatremia as well as decreased plasma osmolarity may occur.

Treatment

Treatment of patients with tetanus is directed toward controlling the skeletal muscle spasms, preventing sympathetic nervous system hyperactivity, supporting ventilation, neutralizing circulating exotoxin, and surgically débriding the affected area to eliminate the source of the exotoxin. Diazepam, 40 to 100 mg IV daily, is useful for controlling skeletal muscle spasms. If skeletal muscle spasms are not controlled by diazepam, administration of nondepolarizing muscle relaxants and mechanical ventilation of the patient's lungs via a tracheal tube are necessary. Indeed early, aggressive protection of the patient's upper airway is important, as laryngospasm may accompany generalized skeletal muscle spasms. Overactivity of the sympathetic nervous system is best managed with intravenous administration of β-antagonists such as propranolol or esmolol. Continuous epidural anesthesia has also been utilized to control tetanus-induced sympathetic nervous system hyperactivity.[14] The circulating exotoxin is neutralized with intramuscular human hyperimmune globulin. This neutralization does not alter the symptoms already present but does prevent additional exotoxin from reaching the central nervous system. Penicillin destroys the exotoxin-producing vegetative forms of C. tetani.

Management of Anesthesia

General anesthesia including tracheal intubation is a useful approach for surgical débridement. Such débridement is delayed until several hours after the patient has received antitoxin because tetanospasmin is mobilized into the systemic circulation during surgical resection. Monitoring often includes continuous recording of systemic blood pressure via an intra-arterial catheter and measuring the central venous pressure. Volatile anesthetics are useful for maintenance of anesthesia if excessive sympathetic nervous system activity is present. Cardiac irritability is unlikely to be accentuated by volatile anesthetics other than halothane. Drugs such as lidocaine, esmolol, and nitroprusside are kept readily available to treat excessive sympathetic nervous system activity during the perioperative period.

Botulism

Botulism is due to effects of a neurotoxin elaborated by Clostridium botulinum. This neurotoxin interferes with presynaptic release of acetylcholine from preganglionic nerve endings and at the neuromuscular junctions. The diagnosis of botulism is a consideration in any patient with acute symmetrical skeletal muscle weakness or paralysis leading to acute respiratory failure. The incubation period is 18 to 36 hours after ingestion of food contaminated with these organisms.

◼ INFECTIONS DUE TO SPIROCHETES

Infections due to spirochetes are represented by syphilis and Lyme disease.

Syphilis

Syphilis is a sexually transmitted infection caused by the spirochete Treponema pallidum. Humans are the only known hosts. Disease of more than 4 years' duration is rarely transmissible. An untreated parturient, however, can transmit syphilis to her fetus, regardless of the stage of the disease.

Clinical manifestations of syphilis depend on the chronologic stage of the disease. The first clinical sign is the chancre, which develops at the inoculation site after 3 to 4 weeks of incubation. Secondary syphilis (characterized by widespread mucocutaneous lesions, lymphadenopathy, and splenomegaly) develops about 6 weeks after the chancre has healed. During the latent stage of the disease there are no clinical or cerebrospinal fluid abnormalities, but serologic tests are positive.

The tertiary stage of syphilis is characterized by destructive lesions in the central nervous system, peripheral nervous system, and cardiovascular system. Tabes dorsalis (locomotor ataxia) develops 15 to 20 years after the initial infection with syphilis. Posterior nerve root dysfunction and posterior column degeneration result in ataxia with a broad-based gait, hypotonic bladder, and jabbing pains that typically occur in the legs. Sudden attacks of abdominal pain may mimic a surgical abdomen.

Cardiovascular syphilis most often manifests as aortitis with dilation of the aortic ring and subsequent aortic regurgitation. An aneurysm due to syphilis almost always involves the ascending thoracic aorta and only rarely the abdominal aorta. Diagnosis of aortitis due to syphilis is a consideration whenever an adult presents with isolated aortic regurgitation and positive serology. Linear calcifications in the wall of the ascending aorta that are visible on chest radiographs and positive serology suggest that the aneurysm is due to syphilis.

Lyme Disease

Lyme disease (Lyme borreliosis) is caused by the spirochete *Borrelia burgdorferi,* which is transmitted to humans by tick bites.[15] Certain species of mice are critical to the life cycle of this spirochete, and deer appear to be important to the tick. Although distribution of the disease is worldwide, its name, Lyme disease, reflects its initial description in a clustering of Lyme, Connecticut children who were thought to have juvenile rheumatoid arthritis.

Lyme disease, like other spirochetal infections, is characterized by multisystem involvement in clinically distinct stages with manifestations that undergo remissions and exacerbations. Erythema chronicum migrans is the initial unique clinical marker for Lyme disease. This classic cutaneous manifestation begins as an area of redness that expands to a diameter ranging from 3 to 6 cm. Malaise and fatigue, headache, fever, and chills often accompany the skin involvement. Some patients have evidence of meningeal irritation, encephalopathy, lymphadenopathy, and hepatitis. Cranial neuritis, including bilateral facial nerve palsy, may occur. Neurologic abnormalities typically last for months but usually resolve completely. Within several weeks after the onset of illness, in about 8% of patients cardiac involvement develops, most often manifesting as fluctuating degrees of atrioventricular heart block lasting 7 to 10 days. Rarely, mild left ventricular dysfunction occurs. The duration of the cardiac involvement is usually brief (3 days to 6 weeks), but it may recur. Arthritis develops in 60% of infected individuals, manifesting a few weeks to as long as 2 years after the onset of the illness. Typically, arthritis consists of migratory musculoskeletal pain, which may recur for years. In about 10% of patients with arthritis, involvement of large joints becomes chronic, with erosion of cartilage and bone.

Laboratory abnormalities early during the course of Lyme disease include increased erythrocyte sedimentation rates, serum concentrations of hepatic transaminase enzymes, and serum concentrations of immunoglobulin M proteins. These changes typically return to normal within several weeks. Mild anemia may be present. Renal function tests are not altered.

Treatment of Lyme disease is initially with tetracycline antibiotics followed by penicillin and erythromycin. Despite antibiotic treatment, nearly one-half of patients continue to experience minor symptoms such as headache, fatigue, and musculoskeletal pains.

▪ INFECTIONS DUE TO MYCOBACTERIA

Infections with mycobacteria manifest clinically as tuberculosis and leprosy.

Tuberculosis

Myobacterium tuberculosis is an obligate aerobe responsible for tuberculosis.[16] These organisms survive most successfully in tissues with high oxygen concentrations, which is consistent with the increased incidence of tuberculosis in the apices of the lungs.

Epidemiology

In the past, most cases of tuberculosis in the United States were due to reactivation of an infection, especially in elderly individuals.[16] At present, most cases of tuberculosis occur in racial and ethnic minorities, foreign-born individuals from areas where tuberculosis is endemic (Asia), intravenous drug abusers, and those with acquired immunodeficiency syndrome (AIDS). The appearance of multidrug-resistant strains of *Myocobacterium tuberculosis* has been the reason for the resurgence of tuberculosis worldwide.

Transmission

Almost all *M. tuberculosis* infections result from aerosol (droplet) inhalation. It has been estimated that up to 600,000 droplet nuclei are expelled with each cough and remain viable for several days. Although a single infectious unit is capable of causing infection in susceptible individuals, prolonged exposure in closed environments is optimal for transmission of infection. It is estimated that 90% of patients infected with *M. tuberculosis* never become symptomatic and are identified only by conversion of the tuberculin skin test. Often patients who acquire the infection early in life do not become symptomatic until much later. Patients who are human immunodeficiency virus (HIV)-positive, however, tend to acquire active tuberculosis soon after infection.

Diagnosis

The diagnosis of tuberculosis is based on the presence of clinical symptoms, the epidemiologic likelihood of infection, and the results of diagnostic tests.[16] Symptoms of pulmonary tuberculosis often include persistent nonproductive cough, anorexia, weight loss, chest pain, hemoptysis, and night sweats. The most common test for tuberculosis is the tuberculin skin (Mantoux) test. The skin reaction is read in 48 to 72 hours, and a positive reading is generally defined as an induration of more than 10 mm. For patients with AIDS, a reaction of 5 mm or more is considered positive.

Chest radiographs are important for the diagnosis of tuberculosis. Apical or subapical infiltrates are highly suggestive of infection. Bilateral upper lobe infiltration with the presence of cavitation is also common. Patients with AIDS may demonstrate a less classic picture on chest radiography, which may be further confounded by the presence of *Pneumocystis carinii* pneumonia. Tuberculous vertebral osteomyelitis (Pott's disease) is a common manifestation of extrapulmonary tuberculosis.[17]

Sputum smears and cultures are also used to diagnose tuberculosis. Smears are examined for the presence of acid-fast bacilli. This test is based on the ability of mycobacteria to take up and retain neutral red stains after an acid wash. It is estimated that 50% to 80% of individuals with active tuberculosis have positive sputum smears. Although the absence of acid-fast bacilli does not rule out tuberculosis, a positive sputum culture containing *M. tuberculosis* provides a definitive diagnosis.

Risk to Health Care Workers

Health care workers are at increased risk for occupational acquisition of tuberculosis.[16] For example, tuberculosis is twice as prevalent in physicians as in the general population. Persons involved with autopsies are uniquely at risk. Nosocomial outbreaks of tuberculosis have occurred especially among AIDS patients. The Centers for Disease Control and Prevention (CDC) has issued guidelines for the prevention of occupationally acquired tuberculosis among health care workers (Table 27–2).[16, 18]

Table 27–2 • Centers for Disease Control Guidelines for Prevention of Occupationally Acquired Tuberculosis

Early diagnosis
    Availability and access to diagnostic tests
    Improved tests and reporting of results
Source controls
    Contain infectious nuclei from coughs and sneezes
    Patient isolation
    Personal respirators
Engineering controls
    Negative-pressure patient environment
    Minimum of six environmental air changes every hour
    Ultraviolet light sources
    High efficiency particulate filters
    Personal respirators
Decontamination
    Sterilization and disinfection of equipment
Screening/treatment
    Annual tuberculin testing
    Availability and compliance with chemoprophylaxis
    Bacille Calmette Guérin (BCG) vaccination

Anesthesiologists are at increased risk for nosocomial tuberculosis by virtue of events surrounding the induction and maintenance of anesthesia that may induce coughing (tracheal intubation, tracheal suctioning, mechanical ventilation).[16] Bronchoscopy is a high risk procedure associated with conversion of the tuberculin skin test in anesthesiologists. As a first step in preventing occupational acquisition of tuberculosis, anesthesia personnel should participate in annual tuberculin screening such that any conversion can be promptly treated with chemotherapy. A baseline chest radiograph is indicated when a positive tuberculin test first manifests.

Treatment

Antituberculosis chemotherapy has decreased mortality from tuberculosis by more than 90%.[16] With adequate treatment, more than 90% of patients who have susceptible strains of tuberculosis have bacteriologically negative sputum smears within 3 months. In the United States vaccination with BCG (bacille Calmette Guérin) is not recommended, as regular tuberculin testing coupled with preventive therapy is more cost-effective.

Patients who have positive skin tests should receive chemotherapy with isoniazid. The toxicity of isoniazid manifests in the peripheral nervous system, liver, and possibly the kidneys. Neurotoxicity can be prevented by daily administration of pyridoxine. Hepatotoxicity is most likely to be related to metabolism of isoniazid by hepatic acetylation. Depending on the genetically determined traits, patients may be characterized as slow or rapid acetylators. Hepatitis appears to be more common in rapid acetylators, consistent with the greater production of hydrazine, a potentially hepatotoxic metabolite of isoniazid. Persistent elevations of serum transaminase concentrations mandate that isoniazid be discontinued, but mild, transient increases do not. In addition to toxic effects in the liver, metabolites of isoniazid, which contain a hydrazine moiety, may also increase defluorination of volatile anesthetics.[19]

Other drugs used to treat tuberculosis include streptomycin and rifampin. Adverse effects of rifampin include thrombocytopenia, leukopenia, anemia, and renal failure. Hepatitis associated with increases in serum aminotransaminase concentrations occur in about 10% of patients being treated with rifampin.

Management of Anesthesia

The preoperative assessment of patients considered to be at risk for tuberculosis includes a detailed history, including the presence of a persistent cough and the tuberculin status.[16] Universal precautions are indicated, as these patients may have AIDS or hepatitis B. Elective surgical procedures should be postponed until patients are no longer considered infectious. Patients are considered noninfectious if they have received antituberculous chemotherapy, are improving clinically, and have had three consecutive negative sputum smears. If surgery cannot be delayed, it is important to limit the number of involved personnel; and high risk procedures (bronchoscopy, tracheal intubation and suctioning) should be performed in a negative-pressure environment whenever possible. Patients should be transported to the operating room wearing a tight-fitting face mask to prevent casual exposure of others to airborne bacilli.

A high efficiency particulate air filter is placed in the anesthesia delivery circuit between the Y-connector and the mask, laryngeal mask airway, or tracheal tube. Bacterial filters are placed on the exhalation limb of the anesthesia delivery circuit to decrease the discharge of tubercle bacilli into the ambient air. Sterilization of anesthesia equipment (laryngoscope blades) is with standard methods utilizing a disinfectant that destroys tubercle bacilli. Use of a dedicated respirator is recommended.[16] Positive-pressure ventilation has been associated with massive hemoptysis in a patient with old pulmonary tuberculosis leading to the recommendation that maintenance of spontaneous breathing may be indicated in selected patients.[20] Postoperative care should, if possible, take place in an isolation room, preferably with negative pressure.

Leprosy

Leprosy is a chronic granulomatous infection caused by *Mycobacterium leprae*.[21] The disease has a worldwide distribution, with the highest incidence in India. Pregnancy may unmask the disease or aggravate existing symptoms.

Signs and Symptoms

Lepromatous leprosy is primarily a disease of the skin, mucosa of the upper respiratory tract, and peripheral nerves. Nerve involvement results in motor paralysis and sensory loss that is attributable to the affinity of *M. leprae* for Schwann cells. Leprosy is also a systemic disease affecting multiple organs during the bacillemic phase. Involvement of the cardiovascular system may manifest as prolongation of the QT interval, ST-T wave changes, and cardiac dysrhythmias on the electrocardiogram. Orthostatic hypotension may be due to altered autonomic nervous system function. Anatomic involvement of the respiratory tract includes the nose, pharynx (uvula), and larynx. Impaired ventilatory responses ("respiratory dysautonomia") are presumed to reflect altered function of chemoreceptors. Granulomatous changes in the liver and renal involvement manifesting as interstitial nephritis and rapidly progressive glomerulonephritis are possible. Secondary amyloidosis is a recognized complication of lepromatous leprosy. The anterior chamber of the eye is affected eventually in almost all infected individuals. Chronic osteomyelitis is a feature of the late stages of leprosy. Skeletal muscle myositis and neuropathic disuse atrophy of skeletal muscles are likely.

Treatment

Leprosy is treated with the folate antagonist dapsone (diphenylsulfone). Adverse effects of this treatment include hemolytic anemia, methemoglobinemia, agranulocytosis, hepatitis, peripheral neuropathy, and psychosis. Other than increased serum liver aminotransaminase concentrations, rifampin produces fewer side effects than dapsone and may be an alternative treatment.

Management of Anesthesia

Leprosy affects many organ systems relevant to the management of anesthesia. Nevertheless, reported experience with anesthesia in these patients is limited.[21] Hematologic side effects of drugs used to treat leprosy are important considerations during the preoperative evaluation. Evidence of hepatic and renal dysfunction is sought. The presence of peripheral neuropathy may influence the choice of regional anesthesia. Indirect laryngoscopy may be useful prior to induction of anesthesia to determine the presence of upper airway involvement by leprosy. Autonomic nervous system dysfunction may influence cardiovascular responses to general and regional anesthesia. Leprosy is a highly infectious disease, with the nasal mucosa harboring organisms that are discharged during sneezing. Bacilli can also exit through ulcerated cutaneous lesions. Local application of rifampin drops or spray destroys most of the bacilli.

■ SYSTEMIC MYCOTIC INFECTIONS

The three most common mycotic infections are blastomycosis, coccidioidomycosis, and histoplasmosis. All three diseases are caused by specific fungi that gain entry into the host by inhalation. Clinical manifestations resemble tuberculosis and include pulmonary cavitary lesions. Sporotrichosis differs from other systemic fungal infections because of its wide geographic distribution. Furthermore, the portal of entry and major site of infection is the skin. Pulmonary cavitary disease is rarely present.

Treatment

Amphotericin B administered intravenously is the drug of choice to eradicate invading organisms that cause these three fungal diseases. Amphotericin B can produce adverse renal and hematologic reactions, however. For example, a decreased glomerular filtration rate is unavoidable during therapy with this drug. It may be necessary to discontinue amphotericin temporarily to maintain serum creatinine concentrations below 3 mg/dl. Renal tubular acidosis, hypokalemia, and hypomagnesemia occur frequently; and exogenous electrolyte replacement is often necessary. Adverse hematologic effects typically manifest as anemia. Fever, chills, and hypotension may occur within the first few hours following intravenous administration of amphotericin B; and ventricular fibrillation has been observed after its rapid intravenous infusion. Hepatotoxicity is not produced by this drug.

Blastomycosis

Blastomycosis is caused by the fungus *Blastomyces dermatitidis*, which is endemic in the southeastern and south central portions of the United States. Pulmonary involvement manifests as cavitary disease of the upper lung lobes. Fever, productive cough, hemoptysis, and simultaneous involvement of other organ systems, particularly skin and skeleton, are present in many patients. Surgery may be necessary to treat persistent pulmonary cavities or to correct deforming orthopedic lesions.

Coccidioidomycosis

Coccidioidomycosis is caused by the fungus *Coccidioides immitis*, which is endemic in the southwestern United States. Positive skin tests may be the only evidence of systemic infection with this fungus. Pulmonary cavitary disease is often discovered on routine chest radiographs. The most serious extrapulmonary manifestation of coccidioidomycosis is meningitis. Meningitis due to this organism is an indication for intrathecal administration of amphotericin B. Surgical intervention may be necessary to treat hydrocephalus resulting from the meningitis. Arthralgia develops in 10% to 20% of patients with coccidioidomycosis.

Histoplasmosis

Histoplasmosis is an infection of phagocytic cells of the reticuloendothelial system caused by the fungus *Histoplasma capsulatum*. This fungus is endemic in the eastern and central portions of the United States and grows particularly well in soil contaminated with fecal material from birds. Most individuals infected with this fungus are asymptomatic or manifest symptoms indistinguishable from those of the common cold. The presence of positive skin tests confirms infection with this fungus.

Chronic cavitary histoplasmosis is predominantly a disease of middle-age and elderly men who also have chronic obstructive pulmonary disease. Surgical ablation of pulmonary cavities combined with intravenous administration of amphotericin B may be necessary in the presence of cavitary lung disease. Disseminated histoplasmosis is most likely to occur in elderly or immunosuppressed patients.

■ INFECTIONS DUE TO *MYCOPLASMA*

Mycoplasma pneumoniae, formerly designated a pleuropneumonia-like organism, is the smallest known living organism. Infections with *M. pneumoniae* produce pneumonia, also known as primary atypical pneumonia. Pneumonia in urban populations is often due to these organisms. Erythromycin and tetracyclines are the antibiotics of choice for treating primary atypical pneumonia.

Mycoplasma pneumoniae pneumonia manifests with subacute onset of a nonproductive cough and pharyngitis. Headache, chills, and fever up to 40°C are present in most patients. Congested tympanic membranes are present in 10% to 20% of patients. Peripheral leukocyte counts are normal in most patients, which helps exclude bacterial pneumonia. About 50% of patients show a fourfold or more increase in the cold agglutinin titer (1 : 128 or higher). By contrast, low titers (less than 1 : 32) may occur with infectious mononucleosis and pneumonias caused by adenovirus or influenza viruses. Infection characteristically spreads slowly throughout a family household.

INFECTIONS DUE TO RICKETTSIAL ORGANISMS

Rocky mountain spotted fever and Q fever are caused by rickettsial organisms. Antibiotics of choice to eradicate these organisms are chloramphenicol and tetracyclines.

Rocky Mountain Spotted Fever

Rocky mountain spotted fever is an acute tick-borne illness caused by *Rickettsia rickettsii*. The disease manifests as a sudden onset of fever, headache, and rash that begins on the extremities and spreads to the individual's chest and abdomen. The rash is the most useful diagnostic sign. Abdominal pain may be prominent, suggesting the need for surgical exploration. Thrombocytopenia occurs in nearly one-half of infected individuals. Involvement of the myocardium may manifest as nonspecific ST segment and T wave changes on the electrocardiogram.

Q Fever

Q fever is an acute systemic infection caused by a rickettsial organism known as *Coxiella burnetii*. Infection with this organism produces a clinical picture similar to that of *Mycoplasma pneumoniae* pneumonia. Q fever differs from other diseases caused by rickettsial organisms in that there is no rash. Furthermore, the infection is by airborne organisms in infected feces, not by injection from tick bites. Hepatosplenomegaly, jaundice, abnormal liver function tests, and endocarditis may occur.

VIRAL INFECTIONS OF THE UPPER RESPIRATORY TRACT

Influenza viruses, rhinoviruses, and adenoviruses are responsible for infections of the respiratory tract. These infections occur in all age groups but are most frequent in adults. Virus transmission is a common event in hospitals.[22]

Influenza Virus

Infection with influenza virus produces an acute febrile illness associated with myalgia, malaise, and headache. The syndrome is commonly referred to as influenza. The most important reservoirs for viral particles are the nasopharyngeal secretions of infected persons. Thus anesthesia personnel are likely to experience frequent contact with the virus and contribute to its spread. Influenza is usually self-limited unless it is complicated by bacterial infection or the presence of co-existing chronic pulmonary disease. Indeed, pneumonia due to secondary bacterial infections is the most common complication following influenza. In this regard, it seems likely that influenza causes damage to mucosal surfaces of the tracheobronchial tree, which together with impaired mucociliary transport promotes colonization with bacteria such as *Pseudomonas aeruginosa*. Severe myositis can be associated with myocarditis. Rarely, Guillain-Barré syndrome follows infection with influenza A.

Influenza immunization must be repeated annually because antigenic shifts in the virus necessitate production of new vaccines to protect against new epidemic strains.[23] A polyvalent vaccine is often produced that contains antigens from the influenza A and B strains that are expected to predominate. It is estimated that the vaccine is about 60% effective for decreasing the mortality rate due to influenza in high risk patients, including the elderly and those with chronic cardiovascular or pulmonary disease (children with asthma). Pneumococcal and influenza vaccines may be administered concurrently. Neurologic complications, including Guillain-Barré syndrome, are not associated with the influenza vaccine.

Amantadine and rimantadine are antiviral drugs that specifically inhibit influenza A virus. Administered prophylactically, amantadine and rimantadine are highly effective in preventing influenza A and providing postexposure prophylaxis to household contacts. These drugs also ameliorate symptoms when administered within the first 48 hours of infection. Side effects, which occur in 5% to 10% of patients, include insomnia; and seizures are a possibility when excessive drug levels accumulate in patients in renal failure. Inhaled zanamivir is a potent inhibitor of influenza A and B virus neuraminidases and is effective in treating acute influenza in adults.[23, 24]

Rhinovirus

Rhinovirus is responsible for one-third or more of adult common colds (viral rhinosinusitis). Transmission is most likely by inoculation from contaminated environmental surfaces or from the skin of infected individuals. Airborne transmission by cough or sneeze is unlikely. The classic syndrome includes acute coryza, malaise, and slight fever. Infection occurs most often in the winter, but reasons for this seasonal incidence are not known. Postexposure prophylaxis with intranasal interferon may prevent respiratory symptoms in those exposed to infected individuals.

It may be difficult to distinguish viral rhinosinusitis from bacterial sinusitis (maxillary toothache, purulent nasal discharge). Viral infections of the upper respiratory tract are the most common causes of acute cough. Chronic cough most likely reflects postnasal drip syndrome, gastroesophageal reflux disease, chronic bronchitis due to cigarette smoking, or treatment with angiotensin enzyme-converting inhibitors.

Adenovirus

Adenovirus produces an acute febrile illness associated with pharyngitis and cough, which most commonly affects children or semiclosed populations, such as military recruits. Another illness caused by adenovirus is highly contagious pharyngoconjunctival fever, which manifests as pharyngitis, conjunctivitis, and fever and usually affects children and young adults. Epidemic keratoconjunctivitis is easily transmitted by contaminated fingers. When caring for patients known to have adenoviral illnesses, handwashing and use of gloves should decrease the risk of iatrogenic spread of the virus.

Respiratory Syncytial Virus

Respiratory syncytial virus is the most frequent cause of infant pneumonia and bronchiolitis. Hospital personnel act as transmitters of infections to children by carrying contaminated secretions on their hands and clothes. The antiviral drug ribavirin may be effective in the treatment of respiratory syncytial virus bronchiolitis or pneumonia.

Parainfluenza Virus

Parainfluenza virus is the principal cause of laryngotracheobronchitis in children. Transmission occurs by person-to-person contact or by large droplet spread.

Human Papilloma Virus

Recurrent respiratory papillomatosis is an increasingly common viral infection in children caused by the human papilloma virus. Progressive formation of multiple papillomas in the respiratory tract requires surgical removal to prevent speech difficulties and upper airway obstruction. The initial presentation of this disease is variable, and it is often mistaken for asthma, bronchitis, croup, or laryngomalacia. The most common symptoms are changes in the voice, hoarseness, or stridor that usually precedes respiratory difficulty. Papillomas are typically located near the vocal cords. The clinical course is characterized by multiple recurrences, and the disease may persist into adulthood. Laser ablation, although not curative, is the accepted treatment for these papillomas. Unexpected complete airway obstruction during the induction of anesthesia has been described.[25]

Management of Anesthesia

Decisions to proceed with or delay elective operations that require general anesthesia in patients with concurrent viral upper respiratory tract infections or a recent history of such infections is a controversial clinical issue.[26–30] Despite some disagreement in the literature, it appears prudent to avoid anesthesia that requires tracheal intubation in patients with or recovering from viral upper respiratory tract infections.[26] This is particularly applicable in children; data supporting an increased likelihood of complications in adults with viral upper respiratory tract infections are less convincing.[27] Evidence for an increased incidence of complications when anesthesia is administered to at-risk patients includes a threefold increase in the incidence of intraoperative bronchospasm and laryngospasm in asymptomatic patients with a recent history of viral upper respiratory tract infections.[28] Reports of perioperative arterial hypoxemia in patients with asymptomatic viral upper respiratory tract infections are supported by data from virus-infected animals demonstrating increased intrapulmonary shunting and perhaps increased oxygen consumption by inflamed pulmonary tissues.[29] Viral infections are associated with exacerbations of asthma and chronic obstructive pulmonary disease. Even in patients without co-existing lung disease, viral infections of the upper respiratory tract can cause temporary airway hyperresponsiveness, emphasizing the importance of considering the possible adverse effects of tracheal intubation in these patients.

Concern about the potential increased risk of administering anesthesia to children with viral upper respiratory tract infections has resulted in recommendations for delaying elective operations for 2 to 6 weeks.[30] If this recommendation is accepted, the potential safe time for administering a general anesthetic is limited, considering that children, especially those younger than 2 years of age, experience five to ten viral upper respiratory tract infections annually. The greatest risk of airway complications when anesthesia is administered in the presence of viral upper respiratory tract infections seems to be in children less than 1 year of age, whereas the risk is much less in children older than 5 years of age, presumably because of the presence of anatomically larger airways.

When anesthesia cannot be delayed in patients with viral upper respiratory tract infections, it is helpful to consider potential problems (airway hyperreactivity, arterial hypoxemia, postoperative laryngeal edema).[27-30] In this regard, administration of supplemental oxygen and extension of monitoring with pulse oximetry into the postoperative period are reasonable considerations. Increased airway responsiveness suggests the need to establish suppressant concentrations of volatile anesthetics before tracheal intubation and during the surgery. Because vagally mediated reflex bronchoconstriction is an almost universal occurrence, the use of atropine to interrupt this reflex arc before tracheal intubation is a consideration. General anesthesia does not increase the incidence of pulmonary complications in patients with uncomplicated viral upper respiratory tract infections who are undergoing minor operations (myringotomy) without tracheal intubation.[26]

■ INFECTIONS DUE TO HERPES VIRUSES

Herpes viruses include seven human viruses and multiple animal viruses (Table 27–3). All human herpes viruses replicate primarily in cell nuclei and share the properties of latency and reactivation. Sites of reactivation vary and include neural ganglion cells and B lymphocytes.

Table 27–3 • Human Herpes Viruses

Herpes simplex virus type 1 (HSV-1)
Herpes simplex virus type 2 (HSV-2)
Varicella zoster
Cytomegalovirus
Epstein-Barr
Human herpesvirus type 6 (HHV-6)
Human herpesvirus type 7 (HHV-7)

Herpes Simplex Virus

Herpes simplex virus type 1 (HSV-1) and type 2 (HSV-2) are characterized by unique routes of transmission and different clinical manifestations (Table 27–4). Although viral titers are increased and transmission is more likely when lesions are present, asymptomatic excretion of virus particles is common. The spread of infection through contact with oral secretions may be an occupational hazard for health care workers, emphasizing the importance of wearing gloves. After initial infection, the HSV travels along sensory nerve pathways to ganglion cells, where viral DNA remains dormant only to be reactivated by certain events such as immunosuppression. After activation, the virus reverses its course and spreads peripherally by sensory nerve pathways.

The most common and significant infection caused by HSV-1 is keratitis, which may lead to destruction of the cornea. Herpetic infection of the digits (whitlow) is possible in personnel who experience sustained direct contact with oral, pharyngeal, or tracheal secretions from infected individuals. Despite pain that occurs with paronychial involvement, it is stressed that treatment should not include surgical drainage, as this may cause entrance of HSV-1 into the deep pulp space and secondary bacterial infection. Infected health care personnel should refrain from dealing with chronically ill, debilitated, or immunosuppressed patients until their viral lesions resolve.

Table 27–4 • Comparison of Herpes Simplex Viruses

Parameter	HSV-1	HSV-2
Route of transmission	Oral	Genital
Manifestations	Oral-labial Ocular Whitlow Encephalitis	Genital Perianal and anal Whitlow

Acyclovir is the drug of choice for treating HSV infections; it is effective topically, orally, and intravenously. Clearance of acyclovir is dependent on renal excretion, but the overall toxicity of this drug is minimal. Rapid intravenous administration, however, has been associated with renal dysfunction and transient increases in serum liver aminotransaminase concentrations. The carrier solution for acyclovir is alkaline, and thrombophlebitis is possible following intravenous administration.

Varicella-Zoster Virus

Herpes zoster follows endogenous reactivation of the virus, which is believed to persist in sensory ganglia in quiescent states after initial episodes of varicella. The incidence of herpes zoster is dramatically increased in immunosuppressed patients. Indeed, the development of herpes zoster in an asymptomatic carrier of HIV is often a forerunner of impending AIDS. An attack of herpes zoster is often preceded by pain that may persist for several days before the unilateral vesicular lesions appear. Individual attacks of herpes zoster are usually limited to one to three dermatomes. The most common complication of herpes zoster is postherpetic neuralgia, which may be severe and resistant to treatment, particularly in elderly patients (see Chapter 17). Encephalitis occurs as a complication of herpes zoster, primarily in immunosuppressed individuals.

Cytomegalovirus

Cytomegalovirus (CMV) is a ubiquitous virus that has a significant role in many diseases, including a heterophile-negative mononucleosis syndrome and disseminated disease in immunosuppressed hosts. Transmission occurs by contact with infected secretions or leukocyte-containing blood products. Infections of parturients may result in damage to the immature fetal central nervous system. Blood transfusions and organ transplantation may also transmit CMV from asymptomatic donors to previously uninfected recipients. There is no evidence of a risk of transmission of CMV from infected patients to hospital personnel.[31] Dormant CMV infections may be reactivated in patients with compromised T lymphocyte function, as in transplant patients or individuals with AIDS. Matching of seronegative transplant or transfusion recipients with seronegative organs or blood donors may decrease the frequency of CMV transmission. Mononucleosis due to CMV manifests as fever, adenopathy, splenomegaly, hepatitis, and atypical lymphocytes in the patient's blood. Hepatitis is mild and only rarely progresses to chronic liver disease.

Epstein-Barr Virus

Epstein-Barr virus (EBV) is a member of the herpesvirus family and infects more than 90% of humans, persisting for the lifetime of the host.[32] Infection of humans with EBV usually occurs by contact with oral secretions. The virus replicates in cells in the oropharynx, and nearly all seropositive persons actively shed virus in the saliva. Resting memory B cells are thought to be the site of persistent EBV presence in the body. Infection of humans with EBV results in humoral and cellular immunity to the virus. The finding of antibodies directed against the viral structural proteins is important for the diagnosis of EBV infection, whereas the cellular immune response is more important for the control of EBV infection.

Epstein-Barr viral infections are responsible for or associated with several clinical syndromes including several forms of cancer (Table 27–5).[32] In the future, vaccination against EBV may become available for patients who remain seronegative for the virus. A relation between EBV infection and chronic fatigue syndrome is not documented, as antibody titers for EBV may be only slightly increased.

Infectious mononucleosis is the result of EBV infection in adolescents and adults, most often manifesting as the triad of fever, lymphadenopathy, and splenomegaly. Most patients with infectious mononucleosis develop leukocytosis with an absolute increase in circulating mononuclear cells, heterophile antibodies, increased serum aminotransferase concentrations as evidence of mild hepatitis, and atypical lymphocytes. Jaundice develops in 10% to 20% of patients. Autoimmune hemolytic anemia may be

Table 27–5 • Clinical Syndromes and Epstein-Barr Virus Infection

Infectious mononucleosis
Chronic active Epstein-Barr virus infection
X-linked lymphoproliferative disease
Cancer
   Nasopharyngeal cancer
   Burkitt's lymphoma
   Hodgkin's disease
   Lymphoproliferative disease
Acquired immunodeficiency syndrome
   Oral hairy leukoplakia
   Lymphoid interstitial pneumonitis
   Non-Hodgkin's lymphoma

Adapted from: Cohen JI. Epstein-Barr virus infection. N Engl J Med 2000;343:481–92.

present. Encephalitis, meningitis, or Guillain-Barré syndrome develops in fewer than 1% of patients with infectious mononucleosis. Splenic rupture is rare but is a consideration when abdominal pain occurs. Hyperplasia of the tonsils and adenoids or edema of the uvula or epiglottis can compromise the patency of the upper airway.[33] EBV myocarditis has been associated with intraoperative cardiac arrest.[34] Most of the manifestations of mononucleosis can be attributed to the proliferation and activation of T cells in response to infection. Transmission is by oral-to-oral contact, and the incubation period is about 28 days. The diagnosis of infectious hepatitis is confirmed by the presence of heterophile antibodies.

Treatment of infectious mononucleosis is symptomatic. Acyclovir inhibits EBV replication and decreases viral shedding, but it has no effect on the symptoms, which are primarily due to the immune response to the virus. Corticosteroids shorten the duration of fever and oropharyngeal symptoms associated with infectious mononucleosis. Severe complications of the disease, such as impending upper airway obstruction, acute hemolytic anemia, cardiac involvement, and neurologic changes, are likely to be treated with corticosteroids.

X-linked lymphoproliferative disease is inherited, affecting males who are resistant to EBV infection. These individuals may die from infectious mononucleosis or malignant lymphomas.

Nasopharyngeal cancer nearly always contains EBV genomes. Increases in EBV-specific antibody titers are often present in these patients.

Burkitt's lymphoma is a malignant lymphoma that may be associated with malaria and tumors that develop in the patient's mandible. Infection with malaria is thought to diminish the T cell control of proliferating EBV-infected B cells and enhance their proliferation.

Epstein-Barr virus DNA is often detected in tumors of patients with Hodgkin's disease. Patients with Hodgkin's disease may have increased titers of antibodies to EBV structural proteins before the onset of lymphoma or with the development of lymphoma.

Epstein-Barr virus is associated with lymphoproliferative disease in patients with AIDS. These patients have impaired T cell immunity and are unable to control the proliferation of EBV-infected cells. They present with symptoms of infectious mononucleosis or with fever and localized or disseminated lymphoproliferation involving lymph nodes, liver, lungs, kidneys, bone marrow, and the central nervous system.

Patients with acquired immunodeficiency syndrome have 10 to 20 times as many circulating EBV-infected B cells as do healthy individuals. T cells from patients with AIDS suppress EBV-infected B cells less effectively than do cells from normal individuals.

ACQUIRED IMMUNODEFICIENCY SYNDROME

Acquired immunodeficiency syndrome describes the occurrence of life-threatening opportunistic infections, Kaposi's sarcoma, or both in patients who manifest profound immunodepression unrelated to drug therapy or known co-existing diseases. The syndrome is initiated by a human T lymphotropic retrovirus known as human immunodeficiency virus type 1 (HIV-1). A related retrovirus, HIV-2, may also cause AIDS, though it is generally less pathogenic than HIV-1. As the virus replicates, T lymphocytes are damaged or destroyed, leading to cell-mediated immunodeficiency and leaving the host unable to cope with a variety of infectious diseases and cancers. Despite the immunosuppression caused by HIV-1, the infected host is able to mount an immune response to the virus after infection. These antibodies form the basis for most of the diagnostic tests for AIDS but offer little protection against development of the disease.

Transmission

Transmitted by intimate sexual contact and blood-borne contamination, HIV-1 initially presented in homosexual men, but the epidemic in the United States has gradually shifted to involve a larger proportion of individuals who acquire AIDS through intravenous drug abuse or intimate heterosexual contact. Sexual contact is a relatively inefficient mode of HIV-1 transmission; blood-borne contact and transfusion of infected blood products are more efficient routes. Transmission of AIDS through blood product transfusions and organ transplantation has been almost eliminated in the United States, with the risk of acquiring HIV-1 after receiving one unit of blood estimated to be 1 in 500,000 units transfused.[35]

Administration of zidovudine (AZT) during the perinatal period greatly decreases maternal transmission of HIV-1 to the newborn. Postexposure prophylaxis with AZT after needlestick injuries decreases the risk of acquiring HIV-1 by about 80% (see "Prevention of Nosocomial Transmission of HIV-1"). AIDS is not transmitted by casual contact in the workplace, schools, or nosocomial environments. There is no evidence of airborne transmission of HIV-1. HIV-1 may survive for prolonged periods (3 to 7 days) outside the host, yet the virus is highly susceptible to destruction by mycobacterial disinfectants or sodium hypochlorite (bleach) as well as low levels of heat (10 minutes at 50°C). Common hospital sterilization techniques using ethylene oxide, steam, and boiling water kill HIV-1.

Natural History

The last stage of a disease process, AIDS has an average course of 10 years.[35] The initial stages of HIV-1 infection may be subclinical or associated with a mononucleosis-like syndrome characterized by symptoms including fever, maculopapular eruption, aseptic meningitis, and lymphadenopathy. This constellation of symptoms occurs in 40% to 60% of patients with primary HIV-1 infection. Other clinical signs include oral or vaginal thrush, herpes zoster, new or worsening eczema, and unexplained weight loss. The primary infection syndrome typically follows inoculation with the virus by 2 to 8 weeks and resolves spontaneously over 2 to 4 weeks. Most patients experience no overt clinical manifestations of illness for 6 to 10 years after the primary infection. Patients who experience symptomatic primary infection have a significantly poorer prognosis than those who undergo asymptomatic seroconversion. As HIV infection progresses, patients are at increased risk for clinical manifestations directly associated with the disease, including encephalopathy, dementia, anemia, and HIV-1-associated wasting. Death is usually the result of wasting, opportunistic infections, or cancer.

Diagnosis

A formal diagnosis of AIDS is made when the CD4$^+$ T cell count decreases to fewer than 200 cells/mm^3 or when patients experience the first AIDS-defining opportunistic infections (*Pneumocystis carinii* pneumonia most common, cryptococcosis, CMV infection, mycobacterium infection) or cancer (Kaposi's sarcoma, B cell lymphoma) reflecting progressive immunodeficiency. Laboratory abnormalities that should prompt testing for HIV-1 are unexplained leukopenia and thrombocytopenia. The CD4$^+$ T cell count (50 to 100 cells/mm^3) is the most useful indicator of immunologic dysfunction and the immediate risk for opportunistic infections with specific viral, bacterial, fungal, and mycobacterial organisms. In most patients the clinical syndromes produced by opportunistic pathogens represent reactivation of latent infections acquired earlier in life that become symptomatic as cellular immunity declines.

Serologic tests, which are most often based on enzyme-linked immunsorbent assay (ELISA) technology, are highly sensitive and specific for HIV-1. Positive results by ELISA are confirmed by a second test, such as the Western blot assay, which detects antibodies to specific HIV-1 antigens. Serologic testing is repeated at 6, 12, and 24 weeks after an initial potential exposure to allow sufficient time for possible seroconversion. HIV-1 testing is a consideration for any individual expected to be at increased risk because of lifestyle and is strongly recommended for parturients.[35]

Treatment

The initial medical management of HIV-1 infection involves antiretroviral chemotherapy and prophylaxis against opportunistic infections through vaccination (pneumococcal vaccine, hepatitis B, influenza) and chemoprophylaxis (tuberculosis, *Pneumocystis carinii* pneumonia).

Antiretroviral Chemotherapy

Antiretroviral chemotherapy to achieve suppression of viral replication often includes combination drug therapy with two nucleoside analogue reverse transcriptase inhibitors (AZT, didanosine, zalcitabine, stavudine, lamivudine) and a potent protease inhibitor (saquinavir, ritonavir, indinavir, nelfinavir). Failure to achieve near-complete suppression of viral replication results in the emergence of drug resistance. In fact, development of resistance to antiretroviral drugs has been an inevitable consequence of drug treatment.

Antiretroviral drugs must be taken according to rigid oral drug administration schedules to achieve maximal benefits. Although the maximum effects of antiretroviral chemotherapeutic drug combinations may not be evident for as long as 20 weeks, a decrease in plasma HIV-1 RNA concentrations should be detectable by the second week of treatment. Once the initial drug regimen adequately suppresses viral replication, patients are followed for drug-induced toxicity and loss of antiretroviral effect, reflected in the plasma HIV-1 RNA concentrations. When suppression of viral replication is lost, the drug combination regimen is altered by substituting new drugs.

The major dose-limiting toxicity of AZT is suppression of myelopoiesis and erythropoiesis. The development of anemia and granulocytopenia is related to drug dosage and stage of the disease. Bone marrow suppression produced by AZT is exacerbated by concurrent use of other myelosuppressive drugs. Hepatic failure has been associated with AZT treatment, especially in obese patients and those with co-existing liver disease.

Didanosine is associated with pancreatitis and peripheral neuropathy. Didanosine-associated peripheral neuropathy is generally reversible by stopping the drug or decreasing its dosage. Pancreatitis is seen more often in patients with advanced stages of AIDS and may occur with such rapidity that monitoring the serum amylase or lipase concentrations is not helpful for preventing this complication. Peripheral neuropathy is the major dose-limiting toxicity associated with zalcitabine and stavudine. Lamivudine is occasionally associated with suppression of the erythroid and myeloid elements of the bone marrow, although this complication is less likely than with AZT.

Indinavir is often associated with transient hyperbilirubinemia, which is reversible and not dose-limiting. The principal dose-limiting toxicity of indinavir is formation of renal stones. Attention to hydration may decrease the risk of this drug-induced nephrolithiasis. Ritonavir is difficult to administer because of its side effects, which include circumoral paresthesias, gastrointestinal toxicity, and effects on hepatic metabolism of a variety of other chemotherapeutic drugs. In addition, its unpalatability limits the clinical utility of this drug. Nelfinavir is well absorbed and has few adverse effects other than diarrhea.

Prophylaxis Against Opportunistic Infections

Vaccinations produce better immunologic responses in persons with high $CD4^+$ T cell counts. Certain live attenuated vaccines, such as oral polio vaccines, should not be administered to HIV-1 infected individuals. Antiretroviral chemotherapy is associated with improved cell-mediated immune responsiveness, including responsiveness to vaccines. Patients with positive tuberculin skin tests may be treated with isoniazid. Trimethoprim-sulfamethoxazole, dapsone, or atovaquone provide prophylaxis for *Pneumocystis carinii* pneumonia and *Toxoplasma gondii* encephalitis (see "Infections of Immunosuppressed Hosts").

Prevention of Nosocomial Transmission of HIV-1

Transmission of HIV-1 to health care providers caring for AIDS patients is a concern. For this reason, it is important for health care workers to implement universal blood and body fluid precautions when contact with blood and body fluids is unavoidable

(Table 27–6).[36] The overall risk of acquiring HIV-1 after a percutaneous exposure with a sharp instrument contaminated with HIV-1-infected body fluids is approximately 1 in 300.[37] The risk of HIV-1 transmission is increased when the injury involves a sharp instrument that has been in a blood vessel and when the exposure is more severe than a simple needlestick. The administration of AZT after percutaneous exposures is associated with an 80% decrease in the risk of HIV-1 transmission.[37] Based on this observation, the CDC recommends that the risk of acquiring HIV-1 should be stratified on the basis of the nature of the injury; moreover, for all significant exposures, the CDC recommends prompt chemoprophylaxis consisting of at least two drugs to which the virus is unlikely to be resistant (Table 27–7).[35, 38]

Management of Anesthesia

Management of anesthesia assumes that all patients are potentially HIV-positive or infected with other blood-borne pathogens. In this regard, appropriate universal ("barrier") precautions are necessary, which include wearing gloves, masks, and protective eyewear during invasive procedures including placement of intravascular catheters and tracheal intubation (Table 27–6).[36] Universal precautions are particularly important in emergency situations in which the risk of blood exposure is increased and the infection status of the patient is unknown. Attempts to cap needles after use are not recommended, as accidental needlesticks are a potential risk of this practice. Health care workers with breaks in normal skin integrity (cuts, dermatitis, acne)

Table 27–6 • Universal Precautions to Prevent Transmission of Human Immunodeficiency Virus

Blood and body fluid precautions should be used for all patients, recognizing that it is not possible to identify infected patients reliably

Use barrier precautions to prevent skin and mucous membrane exposure to blood or body fluids that may contain blood
    Wear gloves
    Wear protective eye shields if droplets likely
    Take care to prevent injury when handling sharp devices—do not recap needles

Health care workers with exudative skin lesions should refrain from direct patient care

Use equipment for cardiopulmonary resuscitation that obviates the need for mouth-to-mouth resuscitation

Adapted from: Recommendations for prevention of HIV transmission in health-care setting. MMWR Morb Mortal Wkly Rep 1987;36:629–33.

Table 27–7 • Antiretroviral Chemoprophylaxis of Percutaneous Exposures to HIV-1-Infected Materials

Source Material	Antiretroviral Prophylaxis	Antiretroviral Regimen
Percutaneous exposure		
Blood		
Highest risk	Recommended	AZT plus lamivudine plus indinavir
Increased risk	Recommended	AZT plus lamivudine with or without indinavir
No increased risk	Offer	AZT plus lamivudine
Fluid containing visible blood or other potentially infectious fluid (semen, vaginal secretions, CSF, amniotic fluid) or tissue	Offer	AZT plus lamivudine
Other body fluids (urine)	Do not offer	
Mucous membrane exposure		
Blood	Offer	AZT plus lamivudine with or without indinavir
Fluid containing visible blood or other potentially infectious fluid (semen, vaginal secretions, CSF, amniotic fluid) or tissue	Offer	AZT with or without lamivudine
Other body fluids (urine)	Do not offer	
Skin exposure (increased risk)*		
Blood	Offer	AZT plus lamivudine with or without indinavir
Fluid containing visible blood or other potentially infectious fluid (semen, vaginal secretions, CSF, amniotic fluid) or tissue	Offer	AZT with or without lamivudine
Other body fluids (urine)	Do not offer	

AZT, zidovudine; CSF, cerebrospinal fluid.
* Risk is considered to be increased with exposure to high titers of HIV-1, prolonged contact, an extensive area, or an area in which skin integrity is visibly compromised. For skin exposures without increased risk, the risk of drug toxicity exceeds the possible benefits.
Adapted from: Schooley RT. Acquired immunodeficiency syndrome. Sci Am Med 1998;1–14.

should be particularly careful to cover these sites when dealing with AIDS patients. Hands and other contaminated surfaces should be promptly washed if accidental contamination with blood or other body fluids occurs. There is no evidence that gowns, hoods, or strict patient isolation are of value; patients with AIDS may be transported to the operating room by the usual routes and personnel. Patients with AIDS wear masks only if it is believed that transmission of opportunistic infections is decreased by the mask.

Lack of evidence for spread of HIV-1 by airborne routes does not eliminate the concern regarding anesthesia equipment, as airway secretions can be mixed with blood, which is a medium for transmission.[39] Use of disposable anesthetic circuits, soda lime canisters, and ventilator bellows may be recommended, although routine sterilization destroys HIV-1. Laryngoscopes and other nondisposable items that have touched mucosal membranes or contacted blood or secretions from an AIDS patient should remain separated from clean equipment; the contaminated equipment should be thoroughly washed with detergent and water and either gas- or steam-sterilized or subjected to appropriate disinfection.[40] Surgeons use disposable gowns and drapes

that are discarded in the usual manner for contaminated materials. Surgical specimens are labeled to indicate the presence of infection in the patient. Instruments are sterilized in the usual manner, and operating rooms are cleaned with dilute (1 : 10) solutions of sodium hypochlorite, which destroys HIV-1. Care is taken to avoid spilling undiluted sodium hypochlorite, which generates fumes when it contacts proteins, such as those present in dried blood.

The choice of anesthetic drugs, techniques, and monitors is influenced by accompanying systemic manifestations of AIDS and any associated opportunistic infections. For example, oxygenation may be impaired by pneumonia due to *Pneumocystitis carinii*. Nutrition may be inadequate and blood volume decreased. Anemia from chronic infection is predictable. Care should be taken when placing vascular catheters and tracheal tubes to avoid introducing bacteria into the patient. An increased index of suspicion for the development of perioperative adrenal insufficiency may be reasonable based on the common involvement of the adrenal glands in AIDS patients. Upper airway obstruction and difficulty placing a tracheal tube may accompany supraglottic Kaposi's sarcoma.[41] Postoperatively, these patients are managed in the postanesthesia care unit according to criteria reserved for management of patients with communicable diseases. Nurses assigned to the care of AIDS patients should not take care of other patients concurrently.

■ MYOCARDITIS

Myocarditis is an insidious disease that is defined clinically as inflammation of the heart muscle.[42] Patients are often asymptomatic, and the diagnosis may not be suspected until postmortem studies are performed. Such studies suggest that myocarditis is a major cause of sudden death (accounting for approximately 20% of cases) in adults less than 40 years of age.[42]

The cause of myocarditis often remains unknown, although a large variety of infections (viral, bacterial, protozoa), systemic diseases, drugs, and toxins have been implicated. Enterovirus has been identified in patients with myocarditis and idiopathic dilated cardiomyopathy. Adenoviruses may also be responsible for myocarditis. The most common myocarditis worldwide is Chagas' disease caused by the parasitic protozoan *Trypanosoma cruzi*. A relatively common form of drug-induced myocarditis is due to doxorubicin. Drug-induced allergic myocarditis is a consideration in the presence of eosinophilic infiltrates in the myocardium. Cocaine may be associated with the acute onset of cardiac dysfunction, presumably reflecting its profound vasoconstrictive effects.

The clinical spectrum of myocarditis is varied, ranging from asymptomatic patients who may have abnormalities on the electrocardiogram to patients with fulminant congestive heart failure.[42] Patients may present with a history of a recent flu-like syndrome accompanied by fever, arthralgias, and malaise. Laboratory tests may show leukocytosis, increased erythrocyte sedimentation rates, eosinophilia, or increases in the cardiac fractions of creatine kinase. The electrocardiogram may show ventricular cardiac dysrhythmias or heart block, or it may mimic the findings of acute myocardial infarction or pericarditis. Endomyocardial biopsy remains the best method for definitively diagnosing myocarditis.

Supportive care is the first line of treatment for patients with myocarditis.[42] In the presence of congestive heart failure, administration of diuretics, angiotensin-converting enzyme inhibitors, and peripheral vasodilators (nitroglycerin, nitroprusside) may be required. Digoxin has been associated with increased mortality in an animal model and should be used with caution and only at low doses. In the presence of fulminant congestive heart failure, intra-venous administration of inotropes or implantation of ventricular assist devices (or both) may be considered.

■ NOSOCOMIAL INFECTIONS

Nosocomial infections are those that occur during the course of hospitalization. Common sites and causes include the urinary tract (*Escherichia coli*), respiratory tract (*Klebsiella pneumoniae*, *Pseudomonas aeruginosa*), and surgical incision sites. Risk factors for nosocomial infections include aspiration of gastric fluids, chronic obstructive pulmonary disease, and thoracic and upper abdominal surgery. Patients who require mechanical ventilation are at increased risk for developing pneumonia. Nosocomial pneumonia is an important cause of morbidity and mortality in hospitalized patients, accounting for about 18% of all hospital-acquired infections. In adults, acute bacterial meningitis is often nosocomial and due generally to gram-negative bacteria. Nosocomial infections are often resistant to treatment with antibiotics. Transmission of viruses is common in hospitals, and most of these infections involve the respiratory tract. Thorough handwashing by staff between patients is an effective way to decrease the role of hospital personnel in transmitting bacterial and viral infections. Use of gloves likewise protects both patients and hospital personnel.

Anesthesia Equipment

The role of bacterial contamination of the anesthesia machine and equipment and the subsequent development of pulmonary infections and cross-infections among patients is controversial.[22, 43] It is assumed that equipment used to deliver anesthesia is a potential source of bacterial contamination for patients. On the basis of this assumption, use of disposable anesthetic delivery circuits containing built-in bacterial filters has been advocated. Nevertheless, routine use of these filters has not been shown to alter the incidence of postoperative pneumonia or other types of infection compared with similar surgical patients receiving anesthesia through circuits without bacterial filters. Furthermore, anesthesia administered to patients with known colonization of gram-negative bacteria does not produce contamination of the anesthesia machine with significant levels of bacteria.[44] These observations suggest that basic hygienic management of equipment used to deliver anesthetic gases can provide safety from the standpoint of cross-infections among patients and prevents the development of nosocomial infections from these sources. Bacteria placed in vaporizers containing liquid volatile anesthetics do not survive. The role of anesthesia equipment in transmitting viral illnesses has not been determined, but airborne transmission of intracellular viruses seems less likely than that of extracellular bacteria.[22] High humidity in the anesthesia circuit speeds inactivation of viruses. Furthermore, anesthetic concentrations of liquid volatile anesthetics may inhibit viral replication.[45]

Gram-Negative Bacteremia

About one-half of primary nosocomial bacteremias are associated with gram-negative bacteria. The most frequent presentation of gram-negative bacteremia is fever, chills, and leukocytosis, without systemic hypotension. Chills and fever may not be apparent in elderly, debilitated, or immunosuppressed patients.

Regional Anesthesia and Bacteremia

Selection of epidural or spinal anesthesia in the presence of bacteremia is influenced by the concern that the needle might introduce infected blood into the subarachnoid or epidural space, leading to the development of meningitis or an epidural abscess.[46] Nevertheless, performance of diagnostic lumbar puncture in patients with fever or bacteremia of unknown origin is not associated with evidence that dural puncture leads to meningitis in these patients. Available data support the conclusion that spinal anesthesia need not be avoided in patients at risk for transient, low grade, intraoperative bacteremia (urologic and obstetric patients) after dural puncture.[46] Performance of epidural or spinal anesthesia in patients with evidence of systemic infections is an acceptable consideration, provided appropriate antibiotic therapy has been initiated and the patient has shown a positive response to therapy, as evidenced by a decrease in fever.[46] In those rare patients in whom central nervous system infections follow regional anesthesia, it is not appropriate to assume a cause-and-effect relation between the anesthetic and the infection. Indeed, most cases of meningitis and epidural abscess occur spontaneously.

■ SEPSIS AND SEPTIC SHOCK

Sepsis is an infection-induced syndrome defined as the presence of two or more manifestations of a systemic inflammatory response (systemic inflammatory response syndrome) (Table 27–8).[47, 48] Sepsis is considered severe when it is associated with organ dysfunction, hypoperfusion (lactic acidosis, oliguria, altered mentation), or hypotension (septic shock).[49] Each year sepsis develops in more than 500,000 patients in the United States, with the resulting mortality about 50%.[47]

Pathogenesis

The host response is probably as important a cause of sepsis as the site of infection or the type of microorganism. Normally, an immunologic cascade ensures a prompt protective response to microbial invasion in humans.[47] An impaired immunologic response may permit infections to become established, whereas poorly regulated immunologic responses may harm patients by releasing endogenously generated inflammatory substances. The complexity of these immunologic responses makes the development of pharmacologic interventions difficult. Conceptually, one approach is to prevent infection in high risk patients with antibiotics and immune stimulants and then provide brief, targeted immunosuppressive therapy (antitoxins, coagulation inhibitors, antiinflammatory cytokines) if sepsis ensues.[47]

Biochemical events in sepsis include the involvement of cytokines (tumor necrosis factor, interleukin-1, interleukin-8), which are immunoregulatory peptides. A trigger such as a microbial toxin stimulates the production of tumor necrosis factor and interleukin-1, which in turn promote endothelial cell leukocyte adhesion, release of proteases and arachidonate metabolites, and activation of clotting. Interleukin-8, a neutrophil chemotaxis, may have an especially important role in perpetuating tissue inflammation.

Arachidonic acid metabolites of thromboxane A_2 (vasoconstrictor), prostacyclin (vasodilator), and prostaglandin E_2 participate in the generation of fever, tachycardia, tachypnea, ventilation-perfusion abnormalities, and lactic acidosis.[47] A cyclooxygenase inhibitor, ibuprofen, suppresses production of

---

Table 27–8 • Identification of Systemic Inflammatory Response Syndrome

Body temperature >38°C or <36°C
Heart rate >90 beats/min
Respiratory rate >32 breaths/min or $PaCO_2$ <32 mmHg
Leukocytosis or leukopenia

these metabolites and the associated symptoms but does not seem to alter outcome.

The lungs are the most common sites of infection followed by the abdomen and urinary tract. In 20% to 30% of patients, a definite site of infection is not determined.[47] Pleural, peritoneal, and paranasal sinus infections may be overlooked even with the use of computed tomography. Positive blood cultures are the accepted proof of infection, but blood cultures are positive in only approximately 30% of patients. Patients with negative blood cultures but presumed to be infected and patients with serious inflammatory conditions not caused by infections (pancreatitis) have clinical signs and symptoms and physiologic changes similar to those with documented infections. In patients with confirmed infections, no single pathogen predominates, suggesting that the host response is more important for the outcome of sepsis.

Organ Failure

Effective treatment of organ failure is critically important, as the cumulative burden of organ failure is responsible for the mortality associated with sepsis. The average risk of death increases by 15% to 20% for each additional organ system that fails.[47] A median of two organ systems fail during severe sepsis with an associated mortality of 30% to 40%. Pulmonary dysfunction occurs often and early and persists, whereas shock, which also occurs early, resolves rapidly or is fatal. Serious abnormalities of liver function, coagulation, and central nervous system function tend to occur hours to days after the onset of sepsis and persist for intermediate periods. In addition to the number of organ systems that fail, the severity of the failure (level of arterial oxygenation, serum creatinine concentrations) parallels the prognosis. Most organ failures resolve within 30 days in survivors of sepsis.

Pulmonary Dysfunction

Sepsis places extreme demands on the lungs, requiring increased minute ventilation at the same time the compliance of the lungs is decreased, airway resistance is increased, and skeletal muscle efficiency is impaired.[47] Detection of sepsis is facilitated by the nearly universal presence of tachypnea and arterial hypoxemia. Acute respiratory failure may develop rapidly (a sustained respiratory rate of more than 30 breaths/min signals impending failure) even when arterial oxygenation is maintained.[50] Timely tracheal intubation and institution of mechanical ventilation of the patient's lungs decreases respiratory muscle oxygen requirements and the

risk of aspiration. Nearly 85% of patients require mechanical ventilatory support for 7 to 14 days.[47] There is no compelling evidence that any one ventilation strategy is preferable (see Chapter 16). The use of positive end-expiratory pressure and supplemental oxygen to maintain arterial oxygen saturations between 88% and 92% is acceptable, as higher oxygen saturations accomplish little additional oxygen delivery.

Cardiovascular Dysfunction

Shock is considered to be present when the systolic blood pressure is less than 90 mmHg and is unresponsive to intravenous fluids or requires support with vasoactive drugs. Circulatory adequacy is reflected by mentation, urinary output, and skin perfusion. Septic shock is initially characterized by low cardiac filling pressures (pulmonary capillary wedge pressures less than 8 mmHg), low cardiac output, and normal to increased systemic vascular resistance, especially before intravascular fluid volume repletion (often a 4- to 6-L deficit) is accomplished. Volume depletion reflects decreased oral fluid intake, increased fluid losses (bleeding, vomiting, tachypnea, fever, increased vascular permeability), and increased venous capacitance. A high cardiac output and decreased systemic vascular resistance typically follow intravascular fluid volume repletion. Fluid administration is guided by responses to therapy (systemic blood pressure, urinary output, cardiac filling pressures, cardiac output, mixed venous oxygen saturations), and colloid has no proven value over crystalloid solutions.

Systemic hypotension that persists after intravascular fluid volume repletion is often the result of low systemic vascular resistance, occasionally combined with impaired myocardial contractility and low cardiac output.[47, 51] Decreases in myocardial contractility are the result of myocardial depressant factors. Left ventricular dysfunction in patients with sepsis can be demonstrated by transesophageal echocardiography. β-Adrenergic agonists (dopamine) can often improve myocardial contractility, and α-adrenergic agonists (phenylephrine) can often increase systemic vascular resistance.

Lactic acidosis may reflect global tissue ischemia due to inadequate oxygen delivery or regional (organ-specific) ischemia.[47] Because regional ischemia usually results from disordered local autoregulation or cellular dysfunction, it is unlikely to respond to increases in oxygen delivery. Although it is difficult to demonstrate that administration of bicarbonate improves cardiovascular performance, it is common practice to treat systemic acidosis (pH less than 7.2) with intravenous sodium bicarbonate. Correction of the derangement causing anaerobic metabolism is more beneficial that normalizing arterial pH in the presence of continued anaerobic metabolism.

Central Nervous System Dysfunction

Central nervous system dysfunction (septic encephalitis) is often an early symptom of sepsis, particularly in elderly patients.[51] Cumulative effects of hypotension, arterial hypoxemia, and treatment with sedatives and analgesics are responsible for changes in mentation. Polyneuropathy associated with sepsis and multiple organ system dysfunction may occur for unknown reasons. Decreased Glasgow Coma Scale scores that are not due to medications are usually the result of arterial hypoxemia or intracranial hemorrhage.[47]

Renal Dysfunction

Transient oliguria is common and temporally related to hypotension, whereas anuria is rare. Correcting any intravascular fluid deficits usually reverses oliguria. Renal failure requiring dialysis occurs in fewer than 5% of septic patients.[47]

Gastrointestinal Dysfunction

The liver is a mechanical and immunologic filter for portal blood and may be a major source of cytokines that cause lung injury.[47] Abnormalities in serum liver aminotransaminase and bilirubin concentrations are common; but like renal failure, hepatic failure is uncommon in septic patients. Nevertheless, ischemic hepatitis ("shock liver") may occur, characterized by sudden massive increases in serum concentrations of aminotransferase enzymes. Septic shock usually causes ileus, which typically persists for 24 to 48 hours after hypotension is corrected. Protein and caloric requirements are increased, and malnutrition is prevalent in patients with sepsis. Hemodynamically stable patients who have not recently undergone abdominal surgery can usually be fed enterally.

Coagulation Dysfunction

Coagulation abnormalities are common in patients with sepsis presenting for surgery, presumably reflecting vitamin K deficiency (poor dietary intake, liver dysfunction, impaired absorption, antibiotic-induced inhibition of gastrointestinal flora) and effects on factors II, VII, IX, and X.[51] This change is accompanied by prolongation of the prothrombin times and, if severe, prolongation of the plasma thromboplastin times. Thrombocytopenia due to increased platelet destruction is a common finding in patients with sepsis and septic shock, even in the absence of disseminated intravascular coagulation. Sepsis and septic shock often result in direct activation of the coagulation cascade and simultaneous fibrinolysis. Disseminated intravascular coagulation may occur in the setting of sepsis and septic shock.

Treatment

Treatment of patients with sepsis, especially those manifesting evidence of septic shock, includes identification and eradication of the infection utilizing appropriate antibiotics and/or surgical drainage (Table 27–9).[51] The hemodynamic goals of therapy for patients with sepsis and septic shock are maintenance of perfusion pressures that provide adequate blood flow and optimal oxygen delivery. The key to managing hypotension and optimizing oxygen delivery is aggressive intravascular volume repletion with intravenous fluids. Treatment of severe sepsis with recombinant human activated protein C decreases mortality but may be associated with an increased risk of bleeding.

Antibiotic Therapy

Antibiotic therapy is necessary but not sufficient for the treatment of sepsis and paradoxically may precipitate septic changes by liberating microbial products.[47] A common approach is to initiate broad-spectrum antibiotic coverage when the pathogens are uncertain and then narrow the therapeutic spectrum when the pathogens are identified.

Supportive Therapy

Considered important to the overall outcome of patients who develop sepsis are timely provision of enteral nutrition; prevention of nosocomial infections, gastric stress ulcers, skin breakdown, and deep vein thrombosis; and judicious use of sedation.[47] Prophylaxis against stress ulcers includes administration of histamine antagonists, proton pump inhibitors, or sucralfate especially to high risk patients undergoing mechanical ventilation. In selected patients, administration of heparin (unfractionated or low molecular weight) and/or utilization of venous compression devices are recommended to decrease the risk of deep vein thrombosis.

Management of Anesthesia

Management of anesthesia for patients with sepsis is influenced by the status of the intravascular fluid

Table 27-9 • Guidelines for Treatment of Patients with Septic Shock

Abnormality	Intervention	Therapeutic Goals
Infection	Antibiotics Surgical drainage	Eradication of infection
Cardiovascular dysfunction		
Hypotension	Intravascular volume repletion Vasopressors	Mean arterial pressure at least 60 mmHg Pulmonary capillary wedge pressure at least 14–18 mmHg
Tissue hypoperfusion	Intravascular volume repletion Vasopressors Inotropes	Hemoglobin at least 10 g/dl Oxygen saturation above 88% Cardiac index above 4 L/min/m² Normalize blood lactate concentrations
Pulmonary dysfunction	Mechanical ventilation Supplemental oxygen	Oxygen saturation above 88% Minimize alveolar-arterial oxygen gradient
Renal dysfunction	Intravascular volume repletion Vasopressors Inotropes	Normalize serum creatinine concentrations Adequate urine output
Liver dysfunction	Intravascular volume repletion Vasopressors	Normalize serum aminotransferase concentrations

Adapted from: Parrillo JE. Pathogenic mechanisms of septic shock. N Engl J Med 1993;328:1471–7.

volume and cardiovascular function.[51] Normal preoperative systemic blood pressure may not ensure adequate intravascular fluid volume. Assessment of heart rate, urine output, and mentation may facilitate evaluation of intravascular fluid volume during the preoperative period. The hemodynamic status is stabilized with intravenous fluids and drugs (vasopressors, inotropes) prior to the induction of anesthesia.

Sepsis is often associated with ileus, and these patients are considered to be at risk for aspiration during the perioperative period. Consideration of preoperative ventilatory status (arterial blood gases) may allow predictions as to the likely need for postoperative mechanical ventilation. Typically, drug infusions are continued until the patient arrives in the operating room. Patients receiving total parenteral nutrition may develop hypoglycemia if the infusion is abruptly discontinued.

Plans for monitoring often include an intra-arterial catheter placed before induction of anesthesia. Adequate venous access is obtained with large-bore intravenous catheters. Placing a central venous or pulmonary artery catheter may be useful. Transesophageal echocardiography is an alternative monitor for assessing the intravascular fluid volume status and myocardial contractility.

There are no specific anesthetic induction or maintenance techniques for patients with sepsis or septic shock. Avoidance of sudden decreases in systemic vascular resistance makes induction of anesthesia with ketamine an attractive consideration. The potential for succinylcholine to evoke the release of excessive amounts of potassium is a theoretical risk

in the presence of prolonged intra-abdominal sepsis.[51] In animals, sepsis is associated with decreased anesthetic requirements.[50] Blood product availability is ensured before induction of anesthesia. Inotropic and vasopressor infusions are often prepared in anticipation of their need during surgery.

Postoperative management is provided in an intensive care unit with continued monitoring of the patient's vital signs. Mechanical control of ventilation is often continued into the postoperative period especially if hemodynamic instability persists or if inotropic support of the circulation is needed.

INFECTIVE ENDOCARDITIS

Infective endocarditis is a microbial infection that implants on heart valves or on the walls of the endocardium. Streptococcal organisms account for nearly one-half of cases. Gram-negative bacteria and fungi are rare causes of infective endocarditis. Morbidity and mortality remain significant despite improvements in antibiotic therapy.

Predisposing Factors

Infective endocarditis cannot occur without preceding bacteremia (Table 27–10).[52] Operative procedures that are predictably associated with transient bacteremia include dental treatments resulting in bleeding of the gingiva and surgical procedures or instrumentation of the upper airway, gallbladder, lower gastrointestinal tract, and genitourinary tract.

Table 27–10 • Estimated Risk of Infective Endocarditis Associated with Co-Existing Cardiac Disorders

High risk
  Prosthetic heart valves
  Previous infective endocarditis
  Cyanotic congenital heart disease
  Patent ductus arteriosus
  Aortic regurgitation
  Aortic stenosis
  Mitral regurgitation
  Mitral stenosis and regurgitation
  Ventricular septal defect
  Coarctation of the aorta
  Surgically repaired intracardiac lesions with residual
    hemodynamic abnormalities
Intermediate risk
  Mitral valve prolapse with regurgitation
  Pure mitral stenosis
  Tricuspid valve disease
  Pulmonic stenosis
  Asymmetrical septal hypertrophy
  Bicuspid aortic valve or calcific aortic stenosis with
    minimal hemodynamic abnormality
  Degenerative valvular disease in elderly patients
  Surgically repaired intracardiac lesions with minimal to
    no hemodynamic abnormality, less than 6 months
    after operation
Low risk
  Mitral valve prolapse without regurgitation
  Trivial valvular regurgitation on echocardiography
    without structural abnormality
  Isolated atrial septal defect
  Arteriosclerotic plaques
  Coronary artery disease
  Cardiac pacemaker
  Surgically repaired intracardiac lesions with minimal to
    no hemodynamic abnormality, more than 6 months
    after operation

Adapted from: Durack DT. Prevention of infective endocarditis. N Engl J Med 1995;332:38–44.

Parenteral drug injections, as by intravenous drug abusers, or prolonged placement of indwelling venous catheters, as used for hyperalimentation, can also lead to bacteremia. Patients with prosthetic heart valves are at the greatest risk for infective endocarditis when transient bacteremia occurs. The incidence of infective endocarditis is also increased in patients with congenital or acquired heart defects that result in turbulent blood flow. For example, mitral regurgitation, aortic regurgitation, bicuspid aortic valves, and ventricular septal defects (as present in patients with tetralogy of Fallot) produce turbulent blood flow and are associated with an increased incidence of infective endocarditis. Patients with aortic or pulmonic stenosis have a lower probability of infection; infective endocarditis rarely develops in patients with mitral stenosis or an atrial septal defect.

Antibiotic Prophylaxis

Prophylactic use of antibiotics is recommended in susceptible patients when surgical procedures associated with bacteremia are planned (Table 27–11).[52] Even in the absence of known heart disease, the presence of diastolic heart murmurs must be assumed to represent organic heart disease that requires prophylactic antibiotic therapy during the perioperative period. Patients who are receiving chronic antibiotic therapy because of prior rheumatic fever should also receive additional antibiotics, as doses of antibiotics used for rheumatic fever prophylaxis are likely to be inadequate to protect against the development of infective endocarditis.

Bactericidal antibiotics are typically selected to provide prophylaxis against infective endocarditis. Prophylactic antibiotic therapy must be initiated before surgery, as the drug must be present in tissues, as well as in blood, to provide protection. Further-

Table 27–11 • Recommendations for Prophylaxis During Various Surgical Procedures That May Cause Bacteremia

Prophylaxis recommended
  Dental operations associated with gingival or mucosal
    bleeding (includes professional cleaning)
  Tonsillectomy or adenoidectomy
  Surgery involving the gastrointestinal or respiratory
    tract mucous membranes
  Bronchoscopy with a rigid bronchoscope
  Sclerotherapy for esophageal varices
  Esophageal dilation
  Gallbladder surgery
  Cystoscopy and urethral dilation
  Uretheral catheterization if urinary infection is present
  Urinary tract surgery (prostate surgery)
  Incision and drainage of infected tissues
  Vaginal hysterectomy
  Vaginal delivery complicated by infection
Prophylaxis not recommended
  Dental procedures not likely to cause bleeding
    (adjustment of orthodontic appliances, fillings above
    the gum line)
  Intraoral injection of local anesthetic
  Shedding of primary teeth
  Tympanoplasty tube insertion
  Tracheal intubation
  Bronchoscopy with flexible fiberoptic bronchoscope
    (with or without biopsy)
  Cardiac catheterization
  Gastrointestinal endoscopy (with or without biopsy)
  Cesarean section
  Procedures performed in the absence of infection
    (urethral catheterization, dilatation and curettage,
    uncomplicated vaginal delivery, therapeutic
    abortion, insertion or removal of intrauterine
    devices, sterilization procedures, laparoscopy)

Adapted from: Durack DT. Prevention of infective endocarditis. N Engl J Med 1995;332:38–44.

Table 27–12 • Infective Endocarditis Prophylaxis

Procedure	Organism	Antibiotic Selection		
		Routine	Allergic to Penicillin	Prosthetic Heart Valve
Dental treatment	α-Hemolytic streptococcus	Penicillin	Vancomycin or erythromycin	Penicillin plus streptomycin
Tonsillectomy Adenoidectomy Nasotracheal intubation Bronchoscopy		Amoxicillin		
Hepatobiliary tract	Enterococcus	Penicillin or ampicillin plus gentamicin or streptomycin	Vancomycin	As for routine
Cardiac surgery	Staphylococcus	Penicillinase-resistant penicillins or cephalosporins	As for routine	As for routine

more, antibiotic therapy must be continued for 48 to 72 hours after surgery. The antibiotic regimen selected should consider the type of bacteria likely to enter the systemic circulation during the operative procedure (Table 27–12).

α-Hemolytic streptococci are most likely to enter the circulation during dental procedures or surgical manipulation of the upper respiratory tract. Amoxicillin, 3 g administered orally 1 hour before the procedure followed by 1.5 g 6 hours later, is highly effective against these organisms (Table 27–12).[52] Vancomycin, clindamycin, or erythromycin is selected for patients with a history of allergy to penicillin. Combined use of penicillin and streptomycin is recommended for patients with prosthetic heart valves, as these patients are at increased risk for infective endocarditis.

Bacteremia due to *enterococci* is most likely to follow instrumentation or surgery on the gallbladder, lower gastrointestinal tract, or genitourinary tract. For patients at high risk undergoing surgical procedures involving these systems, parenteral ampicillin plus gentamicin or vancomycin plus gentamicin are recommended.[52] Gram-negative bacteremia may also occur after surgical procedures in these areas, but such organisms rarely produce infective endocarditis.

Staphylococci are the organisms most likely to invade the systemic circulation during surgery that requires cardiopulmonary bypass. Antibiotics effective against staphylococci include penicillinase-resistant penicillins and cephalosporins (Table 27–12).

Signs and Symptoms

Infective endocarditis is considered in patients with heart murmurs, anemia, and fever, particularly if there is a history of co-existing cardiac disease or of recent surgical procedures. Evidence of systemic embolization, including cerebrovascular occlusion and hematuria, may reflect dissemination of emboli from vegetations present on cardiac valves. Congestive heart failure is the most frequent cardiac complication. Acute aortic or mitral regurgitation can reflect destruction or perforation of cardiac valve leaflets. Mitral regurgitation can also be due to rupture of chordae tendineae. Cardiac conduction abnormalities may indicate extension of valvular infection into the ventricular septum. Cardiac rhythm disturbances, such as ventricular premature beats, may reflect myocarditis.

Operative intervention for valve replacement must be performed in patients with infective endocarditis in whom intractable congestive heart failure develops. Ideally, surgery is delayed until high doses of appropriate antibiotics can be administered to reduce the likelihood of infection of the new valve.

CENTRAL NERVOUS SYSTEM INFECTIONS

Central nervous system infections are life-threatening emergencies that require prompt, accurate diagnosis and treatment. Computed tomography and magnetic resonance imaging are useful for evaluating the possible presence of space-occupying lesions that result from central nervous system infections. Examination of the cerebrospinal fluid (CSF) is important in the differential diagnosis of central nervous system infections. Imaging studies, however, may be needed to exclude intracranial lesions before a diagnostic lumbar puncture is performed. Third-generation cephalosporins have improved the treatment of central nervous system infections.

Meningitis

Meningitis manifests as fever, headache, vomiting, nuchal rigidity, and obtundation. Cranial nerve dysfunction involving primarily the third, fourth, sixth, or seventh cranial nerves appears in up to 20% of patients with bacterial meningitis. Seizures may occur, and occasionally cerebral edema with associated increases in intracranial pressure (ICP) is present. Coagulopathies ranging from thrombocytopenia to disseminated intravascular coagulation may accompany bacteremia and hypotension in the presence of meningitis. Characteristic CSF findings in the presence of bacterial meningitis include increased numbers of neutrophils, glucose concentration less than 50% of the blood glucose concentration, and increased protein concentrations.

A definitive diagnosis of meningitis requires isolation of the causative organisms from the CSF. *Haemophilus influenzae* is the most commonly identified pathogen followed by *Streptococcus pneumoniae*, and *Neisseria meningitidis*.[53] Meningococcal meningitis is the only form of bacterial meningitis that occurs in epidemic form. Recurrent episodes of bacterial meningitis are most often the result of anatomic defects (traumatic or surgical) that permit access of bacteria to the CSF.

Optimal antibiotic treatment of meningitis requires that the drugs used for treatment have bactericidal effects in CSF.[53] The presence of meningitis enhances penetration of antibiotics into the CSF, and achieving a rapid bactericidal effect at this site is a primary goal of therapy. In the absence of a documented causative organism, the recommended approach is administration of broad-spectrum cephalosporins supplemented in young infants and older adults with ampicillin. In patients with recent head trauma or neurosurgery and those with CSF shunts, broad-spectrum antibiotics effective against gramnegative and gram-positive organisms should be administered in combination (ceftazidime and vancomycin). Empirical corticosteroid therapy (dexamethasone) may be administered on the basis that inflammatory cytokines contribute to CSF inflammation and cerebral edema.[53] Vaccinations against *Haemophilus influenzae*, *Streptococcus pneumoniae*, and *Neisseria meningitidis* may decrease the risk of meningitis due to these organisms. When cerebral edema occurs, conventional methods (diuretics, corticosteroids) to decrease ICP are indicated. Fluid restriction is indicated initially to minimize the occurrence of cerebral edema. Acute control of seizures is often achieved with intravenous administration of diazepam, whereas maintenance therapy may be with phenytoin.

Brain Abscess

Brain abscess can result from direct extension of contiguous infections (paranasal sinuses), retrograde venous spread (otitis media), or hematogenous spread (lung abscesses, right-to-left intracardiac shunts), typically in the distribution of the middle cerebral artery. Manifestations of brain abscesses are most often those of an expanding intracranial mass with obtundation, headache, focal neurologic findings, and seizures. Evidence of increased ICP is somnolence, vomiting, and cranial nerve palsies. Lumbar puncture is not recommended when brain abscesses are thought to be present because of the risk of brain herniation. Computed tomography is highly sensitive for detecting brain abscesses larger than 1 cm in diameter and for subsequent resolution of the abscess. Magnetic resonance imaging has greater sensitivity than computed tomography for soft tissue lesions and does not require injection of contrast dyes.

Prompt antibiotic therapy and often surgical aspiration or excision are necessary in the management of brain abscesses. Emergency surgical decompression is indicated whenever increased ICP leads to evidence of brain herniation. Cerebral edema is managed with diuretics and corticosteroids during the perioperative period. Seizures are common sequelae of brain abscesses.

Epidural Abscess

Lumbar epidural abscesses associated with epidural anesthesia usually present 24 to 72 hours after performance of the block with severe backache, local tenderness, paraspinal muscle spasm, and fever associated with leukocytosis.[54] Sensory findings are absent or reflected only by paresthesias, whereas motor deficits manifest as flaccid skeletal muscle paralysis. Meningismus may be present, and the erythrocyte sedimentation rate is likely to be increased. In the absence of needle or catheter placement in the epidural or subarachnoid space, infection is most often derived from bloodstream transmission, vertebral osteomyelitis, or contiguous infections. A history of back trauma is present in about 30% of afflicted patients. Introduction of needles into the lumbar area in the presence of an epidural abscess can lead to bacterial meningitis.

Magnetic resonance imaging is the most sensitive modality for evaluating the spine when infection is suspected. Computed tomography is also useful for determining the presence of extradural compression of the spinal cord. Laminectomy should be performed promptly when epidural abscess is diagnosed to minimize the likelihood of permanent neurologic deficits.

BACTERIAL INFECTIONS OF THE UPPER RESPIRATORY TRACT

Bacterial infections of the upper respiratory tract frequently follow processes that impair normal host defense mechanisms. For example, clearance of pulmonary secretions may be impaired owing to the decreased activity of cilia or impaired cough reflexes. Viral respiratory tract infections are often the cause of impaired respiratory defense mechanisms. No infection of the respiratory tract is more rapidly progressive or potentially lethal than acute epiglottitis (see Chapter 32).

Acute Sinusitis

Acute sinusitis (inflammation of the sinus epithelium) is a common consequence of upper respiratory tract infections and manifests as nasal discharge, fever, leukocytosis, and facial pain that typically increases when the patient leans forward. Nasopharyngeal instrumentation (nasotracheal tubes, nasogastric tubes, nasal packing) in traumatized patients may predispose to sinusitis. Sinusitis should be considered when fever occurs without a known focus in patients with nasotracheal tubes in place.[55, 56] Nasal polyps or deviation of the nasal septum may also predispose to sinusitis by obstructing sinus drainage. Maxillary and frontal sinusitis are more common in adults, whereas infection of the ethmoid sinus predominates in children. Maxillary sinusitis is characterized by pain and tenderness over the patient's suborbital areas. Pain is often referred to the teeth. Frontal sinusitis produces pain and tenderness over the patient's forehead. Patients with ethmoid sinusitis typically complain of retroorbital pain.

Acute sinusitis responds well to decongestants and analgesics. Although most patients do not require antibiotics, administration of ampicillin or amoxicillin is often recommended in patients who fail to respond to decongestants. Sinusitis that leads to intracranial infections by bony spread or through venous channels requires treatment with high doses of antibiotics and surgical drainage.

Administration of anesthesia that includes nitrous oxide to patients with sinusitis introduces the consideration of increased pressures in the sinuses in the event that nitrous oxide enters any aircontaining portion of the sinuses more rapidly than nitrogen is absorbed. Clinical experience does not support the validity of this theoretical concern.

Chronic Sinusitis

Chronic sinusitis is a prevalent disease that affects an estimated 14% of the U.S. population and accounts for millions of physician office visits.[57] Of interest is the observation that chronic rhinosinusitis is an almost invariable feature of cystic fibrosis. Mutations in the gene responsible for cystic fibrosis may be associated with the development of chronic rhinosinusitis in the general population.[57]

Acute Otitis Media

Otitis media results when bacteria spread from the nasopharynx to the normally sterile middle ear. Abnormal eustachian tube reflux or obstruction caused by viral or allergic nasopharyngitis may lead to infection. Pain, fever, and hearing loss are the classic presenting symptoms. The diagnosis is based on the presence of bulging tympanic membranes and obscured landmarks. The differential diagnosis of acute otitis media includes serous otitis media. Serous otitis media differs from the purulent form in that fever and pain are absent. In contrast to purulent otitis media, tympanic membranes are usually retracted despite the presence of fluid in the middle ear, and the bony landmarks are usually preserved.

Treatment of acute otitis media includes decongestants, analgesics, and antibiotics, most often amoxicillin. Myringotomy does not hasten recovery but is indicated for patients with intractable pain. Tympanoplasty tubes may be helpful in children with repeated recurrences of otitis media. Acute mastoiditis was once a common sequela of acute otitis media but is now, with the routine use of antibiotics, an unusual complication. Nevertheless, the benefits of antibiotics in the treatment of acute otitis media appear to be modest. Otitis media is often the surgical diagnosis in children undergoing adenoidectomy and tonsillectomy, which is the most commonly performed major surgical operation among children in the United States. The value of this operation is limited and transient and should not be considered a first surgical intervention in children whose only indication is recurrent acute otitis media.[58] Chronic otitis media is characterized by hearing loss and perforation of the tympanic membranes. Peripheral perforations of the tympanic membranes may be associated with invasive cholesteatomas.

Administration of nitrous oxide in the presence of known inflammation or edema of the eustachian tubes must consider the blood gas solubility of this inhaled anesthetic relative to air. For example, the middle ear is an air-filled cavity that vents passively by way of the eustachian tube when pressures exceed about 20 cmH$_2$O. Nitrous oxide diffuses into the middle ear more rapidly than nitrogen leaves, and middle ear pressures may become excessive if decompression through the eustachian tubes is not possible. Rupture of the tympanic membrane following anesthesia that included nitrous oxide has been attributed to this mechanism.[59] Conversely, negative middle ear pressures may develop after discontinuation of nitrous oxide, leading to serous otitis.

Pharyngitis

Viruses are the most common cause of pharyngitis, and treatment is symptomatic. Group A streptococci are more likely to cause tonsillitis than pharyngitis. As it is impossible to distinguish clinically between streptococcal and viral pharyngitis, throat cultures are necessary. Antibiotics, most often oral penicillin V or erythromycin, are important for eradication of bacterial infections and prevention of rheumatic fever and local suppurative complications. Because rheumatic fever can be prevented, even if therapy is delayed up to 9 days after the onset of symptoms treatment need not be initiated until the results of throat cultures are available. Tonsillectomy was once commonly performed in children to prevent recurrent pharyngitis, but this practice has been largely abandoned.

Peritonsillar Abscess

Peritonsillar abscess ("quinsy") is a complication of streptococcal tonsillitis. Dysphagia impairs swallowing of saliva, leading to drooling; and pain and edema result in a muffled voice. The affected tonsil is visibly displaced toward the midline, and the soft palate may be edematous. Trismus occurs in some patients. Traditional treatment consists of parenteral administration of penicillin and surgical drainage. Alternatively, oral administration of antibiotics and needle aspiration have produced acceptable results, avoiding the need for hospitalization.

Retropharyngeal Infections

Retropharyngeal infections are most common during childhood because lymph nodes in this region atrophy during adulthood. Fever, dysphagia, respiratory stridor, and bulging of the posterior wall of the pharynx are present. Lateral radiographs of the neck may demonstrate soft tissue swelling and forward displacement of the larynx. Penicillin is the antibiotic of choice, and surgical drainage is necessary to prevent upper airway obstruction and extension of infection to the mediastinum. Strategies for airway management in patients with retropharyngeal infections in the presence of airway compromise include fiberoptic laryngoscopy and obtaining a surgical airway as the first-line approach.[17]

Parapharyngeal infections are characterized by severe trismus, externally visible inflammation behind the angle of the jaw, and medial displacement of the tonsils. Treatment consists of the intravenous administration of penicillin and drainage from behind the angle of the mandible.

Ludwig's Angina

Ludwig's angina is cellulitis of the submandibular, sublingual, and submental regions. It is most frequently caused by streptococci and is characterized by fever and rapidly progressive edema of the anterior neck and floor of the mouth. Elevation of the tongue impedes swallowing, and upper airway obstruction is a potentially fatal complication. Tracheal intubation may not be possible, necessitating a tracheostomy to preserve the airway. Broad-spectrum antibiotics are indicated, and surgical decompression may be required.

Acute Epiglottitis (Supraglottitis)

Acute epiglottitis is becoming a rare disease in children and is being encountered predominantly among adults, especially those with co-existing diseases associated with immunosuppression (see Chapter 32).[60] The reason for the decline in acute epiglottitis in children is presumed to reflect vaccination against Haemophilus influenzae, the most common bacterial pathogen implicated in epiglottitis. There is no consensus on the optimal management of adult patients with acute epiglottitis.[60] In adults sore throat and dysphagia are the most common presenting symptoms; and the classic "muffled voice" is observed infrequently.[60] It is agreed that patients presenting with imminent or actual airway obstruction should have an artificial airway (tracheal intubation, tracheostomy) established promptly; management of patients with mild symptoms is controversial, with opinions ranging from vigilant monitoring to elective tracheal intubation.

The rationale for elective tracheal intubation before signs of airway obstruction occur is the lack of reliable criteria for distinguishing patients who may sustain sudden airway obstruction from those whose course may be benign. Nevertheless, for adult patients with acute epiglottitis without severe respiratory distress on presentation, routine prophylactic tracheal intubation appears unnecessary if observation facilities and personnel skilled in airway management are available.[60]

PULMONARY PARENCHYMAL INFECTIONS

Pulmonary parenchymal infections typically develop after events that impair normal host defense mechanisms, such as viral infections that alter the physical and chemical characteristics of the normally protective mucus secreted in the airways. Indeed, the seasonal increase in viral infections during winter months is typically associated with an increased incidence of bacterial pneumonia. Immunosuppressed patients, especially those with AIDS, are vulnerable to a broad range of pulmonary pathogens. Patients with chronic obstructive pulmonary disease are vulnerable to bacterial infections in the lungs because of impaired mucociliary transport and inefficient cough mechanisms. Cigarette smoke may contribute to an increased incidence of pulmonary infections by virtue of the inhibition of ciliary activity by smoke.

Bacterial Pneumonia

Pneumococci remain the most frequent cause of bacterial pneumonia in adults, with streptococci also a common cause. Inhalation of oropharyngeal secretions containing these bacteria, rather than droplet spread from person to person, is responsible for most pneumococcal pneumonias. Oropharyngeal secretions are often inhaled during normal sleep. Nevertheless, bacterial pneumonia is uncommon in healthy patients because of efficient host defense mechanisms. By contrast, alcoholism, drug abuse, and neurologic disorders can impair consciousness and predispose to the inhalation of bacteria-containing secretions and subsequent development of pneumonia. Pneumonia due to gram-negative bacteria occurs most often in chronically ill and debilitated patients who are confined to bed.

Diagnosis and Treatment

Bacterial pneumonia is characterized by an initial chill, followed by abrupt onset of fever and copious sputum production. Segmental distribution of the infective process results in bronchopneumonia. Lobar pneumonia is present when infection includes more than one segment of a pulmonary lobe or multiple lobes are involved. Nevertheless, classic physical and radiographic findings of lobar consolidation may be absent. Dehydration can minimize abnormalities seen on chest radiographs in the presence of bacterial pneumonia. Polymorphonuclear leukocytosis is typical, and arterial hypoxemia may occur in severe cases of bacterial pneumonia. Arterial hypoxemia reflects right-to-left shunting of blood due to perfusion of alveoli filled with inflammatory exudates. Microscopic examination of sputum plus cultures and sensitivity testing are necessary for the etiologic diagnosis of pneumonia and selection of appropriate antibiotic treatment. In addition to antibiotic therapy, adequate hydration through administration of fluids or humidification of inhaled gases is important for optimizing clearance of secretions.

Acute Bronchitis versus Pneumonia

The distinction between acute bronchitis and bacterial pneumonia is anatomic, rather than etiologic, as the same organisms can cause both diseases. Patients with bacterial pneumonia are more likely to develop high fevers, bacteremia, and arterial hypoxemia. Chest radiographs typically show infiltrates in patients with pneumonia. Changes associated with chronic lung disease and bronchitis, however, can mimic pulmonary infiltrates.

Legionnaires' Disease

Legionnaires' disease is caused by the gram-negative bacillus *Legionella pneumophila.* This disease manifests with a prodromal phase of myalgia, malaise, and headache followed by high fever, shaking chills, nonproductive cough, tachypnea, and often pleuritic pain. Obtundation is common; and abdominal pain, vomiting, and diarrhea may be present. Extrapulmonary manifestations include peritonitis, pericardial involvement, and acute renal failure. Mild cases of legionnaires' disease may resemble *Mycoplasma pneumoniae* pneumonia. Erythromycin is the antibiotic of choice for treating this disease.

Aspiration Pneumonia

Aspiration is probably the mechanism responsible for most bacterial (mixed flora) pneumonias. Most patients with depressed consciousness experience pharyngeal aspiration, which in the presence of underlying diseases that impair host defense mechanisms and alterations in oropharyngeal flora, may manifest as aspiration pneumonia. Alcohol abuse, drug abuse, head trauma, seizures and other neurologic disorders, and administration of sedatives are most often responsible for the development of aspiration pneumonia. Patients with abnormalities of deglutition or esophageal motility resulting from placement of nasogastric tubes, esophageal cancer, bowel obstruction, or repeated vomiting are prone to aspiration of gastric contents. Poor oral hygiene and periodontal disease predispose to aspiration pneumonia because of the presence of increased bacterial flora. Induction and recovery from anesthesia may place patients at increased risk for aspiration of gastric contents.

Clinical manifestations of pulmonary aspiration depend in large part on the nature and volume of aspirated material. Aspiration of large volumes of acidic gastric fluid (Mendelson's syndrome) produces fulminating pneumonia and arterial hypoxemia. Aspiration of particulate material may result in airway obstruction, and smaller particles may produce atelectasis. Radiographically, infiltrates are most common in dependent areas of the patient's lungs.

Penicillin-sensitive anaerobes are the most likely cause of aspiration pneumonia. Clindamycin is an alternative to penicillin and may be superior for treating necrotizing aspiration pneumonia and lung abscess. Hospitalization or antibiotic therapy alters the usual oropharyngeal flora such that aspiration pneumonia in hospitalized patients often involves pathogens that are uncommon in community-acquired pneumonias.

It is important to distinguish between bacterial and nonbacterial pneumonia. Nonbacterial pneumonia, such as *Mycoplasma pneumoniae* pneumonia, most frequently occurs in previously healthy and young patients. In contrast to bacterial pneumonia, the presence of nonbacterial pulmonary infections is suggested by a nonproductive cough and an absence of leukocytosis. Interstitial infiltrates on the chest radiograph also suggest a nonbacterial etiology.

Lung Abscess

Lung abscess is most likely to develop after bacterial pneumonia. Alcohol abuse and poor dental hygiene are frequently present in patients in whom a lung abscess develops. Septic pulmonary embolization, which is most common in intravenous drug abusers, may also result in formation of a lung abscess. Chest radiography is needed to establish the presence of a lung abscess. Findings of an air-fluid level signifies rupture of the abscess into the bronchial tree, and

foul-smelling sputum is characteristic. Antibiotics are the mainstay of treatment of a lung abscess. Surgery is indicated only when complications such as empyema occur. Thoracentesis is necessary to establish the diagnosis of empyema, and treatment requires chest tube drainage and antibiotics. Surgical drainage is necessary to treat chronic empyema.

▮ INTRA-ABDOMINAL INFECTIONS

Peritonitis and subphrenic abscess are intra-abdominal infections that can present during the perioperative period. Both of these processes can be confused with pneumonia.

Peritonitis

Peritonitis is a localized to diffuse inflammatory process involving the peritoneum. Diffuse inflammation of the peritoneum typically follows breakdown of the integrity of the gastrointestinal tract, as may occur with appendicitis, diverticulitis, or trauma. Multiple organisms most likely contribute to the disease process when peritonitis is due to these events. Acute pancreatitis can also mimic bacterial peritonitis. Likewise, abdominal pain associated with an acute peptic ulcer, cholecystitis, mesenteric artery occlusion, acute porphyria, and diabetic acidosis suggest peritonitis. Occasionally, bacterial peritonitis develops in patients with systemic lupus erythematosus.

Peritonitis has also been observed in patients with alcoholic cirrhosis of the liver. The most common causative organism in these patients is *Escherichia coli*. For this reason, examination of ascitic fluid is useful in patients with cirrhosis of the liver who develop abdominal pain or unexplained fever. Gentamicin is a useful antibiotic for treating peritonitis due to *E. coli*.

Subphrenic Abscess

Subphrenic abscess should be suspected in patients who have undergone abdominal surgery and subsequently exhibit unexplained fever. The frequent presence of pleural effusions in association with subphrenic abscess can be attributed erroneously to bacterial pneumonia. A wide separation between the upper margin of the gastric air bubble and diaphragm, as demonstrated on chest radiography, suggests a subphrenic abscess. Leukocytosis is almost always present. Treatment of subphrenic abscess is with surgical drainage plus antibiotics. The antibiotic can be changed, if indicated, when results of cultures of the abscess fluid are available.

URINARY TRACT INFECTIONS

Urinary tract infection is the most common of all bacterial infections affecting humans. During the first 50 years of life it predominates in females. Symptoms range from asymptomatic bacteriuria to acute pyelonephritis. Most patients complain of dysuria and frequency. Urinalysis indicates hematuria and the presence of protein. The most common etiologic organisms are gram-negative bacteria such as *Escherichia coli*. Ampicillin is usually effective in the treatment of otherwise uncomplicated urinary tract infections.

Acute bacterial prostatitis is a febrile illness associated with fever, chills, pelvic pain, dysuria, and urinary frequency. The most common causative organism is *E. coli*. Chronic bacterial prostatitis may require surgical removal of the gland.

OSTEOMYELITIS

Osteomyelitis is a difficult to treat infection characterized by progressive inflammatory destruction of bone.[61] Normal bone is highly resistant to infection, which can occur only as a result of a large inoculum, trauma, or the presence of foreign bodies (prostheses). Certain major causes of infection, such as *Staphylococcus aureus*, adhere to bone by expressing receptors (adhesions) for components of bone matrix. Identification of the causative microorganism(s) is necessary for diagnosis and treatment. Surgical sampling or a needle biopsy of infected tissues provides important information. Computed tomography and magnetic resonance imaging are useful for detection and assessment of osteomyelitis.

In patients undergoing bone surgery antibiotics should be administered intravenously 30 minutes before skin incision and for no longer than 24 hours after surgery.[61] For orthopedic surgery on closed fractures, antistaphylococcal penicillins and cephalosporins decrease the incidence of postoperative infections. Patients receiving prosthetic devices have a high susceptibility to infection when only a few microorganisms of low pathogenicity, such as *Staphylococcus epidermidis*, are present. For such procedures the use of surgical rooms with laminar airflow and prophylactic antibiotic treatment have decreased the rate of infection from prosthetic devices to less than 2%.

FEVER OF UNDETERMINED ORIGIN

Fever of undetermined origin is characterized by temperature increases exceeding 38.3°C on several occasions during at least a 21-day period. Most patients with fever of undetermined origin are subsequently shown to have infections, cancer, or connective tissue disorders. Two major systemic infections to consider are tuberculosis and infective endocarditis. Localized infections to consider include hepatic abscess, subphrenic abscess, and urinary tract infection. Viral infections usually do not produce fevers lasting 21 days or longer, the one important exception being infections due to CMV. Ultrasonography and computed tomography are useful for detecting hidden sites of infection, significantly decreasing the number of biopsies required to make the diagnosis.

INFECTIONS IN IMMUNOSUPPRESSED HOSTS

The principal causes of morbidity and mortality in immunosuppressed hosts are often infections, rather than the primary illness. In this regard, therapeutic regimens that can adversely influence the ability of patients to withstand infections include antibiotics, radiation therapy, corticosteroids, and cancer chemotherapeutic drugs (see Chapter 28). Development of resistant organisms is a major adverse side effect of antibiotic treatment. Radiation therapy and treatment with corticosteroids or cancer chemotherapeutic drugs may adversely affect host immune mechanisms by impairing the function of numbers of neutrophils. The absolute level of circulating neutrophils required to prevent infection is not known, although the risk of sepsis is increased when concentrations are less than 1000 cells/mm³. Neutropenia is the most important factor predisposing to bacterial infections in the presence of cancer or after organ transplantation. Other conditions that predispose to infections in immunosuppressed hosts include malnutrition, diabetes mellitus, uremia, splenectomy, and breaks in the mucocutaneous lining that separates patients from microbes. In this regard, radiation therapy may damage mucocutaneous surfaces, providing portals of entry for microorganisms. An indirect effect of immunosuppressive therapy, especially in patients receiving organ transplants, is the activation of latent CMV or EBV infections.

A common presenting symptom of infections in immunosuppressed patients is fever without localized findings. In this regard, special care must be taken to maintain asepsis during percutaneous introduction of intravascular catheters or performance of regional anesthesia. Use of indwelling Hickman-Broviac catheters for venous access, especially in neutropenic patients, may become sources of bacteremia. Most of these catheter infections can be successfully treated with antibiotics, leaving the catheters in place. Prevention of infections in immunosuppressed patients is improved by avoiding hospitalization for procedures that can be performed in outpatient environments and by utilizing indwelling vascular and urinary catheters only when necessary.

Pneumonia is the most common infectious cause of death in immunosuppressed hosts. A potentially fatal bacteremia may be associated with trivial-appearing pulmonary infiltrates on chest radiographs. Fungal infections are problems in immunosuppressed hosts, as reflected by the common presence of candidiasis. Aspergillosis is an airborne fungal infection that rarely occurs in immunocompetent patients, but in immunocompromised patients it is likely to result in bronchopneumonia and bronchitis. The initial manifestations of aspergillosis pneumonia include fever, dyspnea, nonproductive cough, and hemoptysis, with an occasional life-threatening hemorrhage. Rapid, extensive invasion of blood vessels provides access of *Aspergillus* to the systemic circulation, causing a high incidence of spread, particularly to the patient's brain and heart. Cryptococcosis (torulosis) is a systemic fungal disease that may cause pneumonia and meningitis. Treatment of disseminated fungal infections is with intravenous administration of amphotericin B.

Pneumocystitis carinii is a protozoan organism that is a common opportunistic cause of interstitial pneumonia in immunosuppressed patients, especially those with AIDS. These organisms may be present in the lungs of healthy persons, suggesting that immunosuppression reactivates latent infections causing pneumonitis. *P. carinii* pneumonia typically manifests as sudden onset of fever, nonproductive cough, tachypnea, and progressive dyspnea. The degree of arterial hypoxemia and extent of the infiltrates on chest radiographs correlates best with the breathing rate. The classic radiographic presentation is diffuse, bilateral symmetrical interstitial and alveolar infiltrative patterns that are predominantly perihilar in distribution. Arterial blood gases are sensitive measurements of pulmonary involvement. The definitive diagnosis entails the demonstration of *P. carinii* organisms in airway secretions or lung tissue specimens. A lung biopsy may be necessary to establish the diagnosis. During anesthesia these patients may require high inspired concentrations of oxygen with or without positive end-expiratory pressure. Trimethoprim-sulfamethoxazole, dap-sone, or atovaquone provide treatment for *P. carinii* pneumonia.

References

1. Browne RA, Chernesky MA. Infectious diseases and the anaesthetist. Can J Anaesth 1988;35:655–65
2. Kelkar PS, Li JTC. Cephalosporin allergy. N Engl J Med 2001;345:804–9
3. Mayhew JF, Deutsch S. Cardiac arrest following administration of vancomycin. Can Anaesth Soc J 1985;32:178–81
4. Symons NLP, Hobbes AFT, Leaver HK. Anaphylactoid reactions to vancomycin during anaesthesia: two clinical reports. Can Anaesth Soc J 1985;32:178–81
5. Mufson MA. Pneumococcal infections. JAMA 1981;246:1942–8
6. Shapiro ED, Berg AT, Austrian R, et al. The protective efficacy of polyvalent pneumococcal polysaccharide vaccine. N Engl J Med 1991;325:1453–60
7. Bisno AL. Group A streptococcal infections and acute rheumatic fever. N Engl J Med 1991;325:783–93
8. Baxter F, McChesney J. Severe group A streptococcal infection and streptococcal toxic shock syndrome. Can J Anesth 2000;47:1129–40
9. MacDonald KL, Osterholm MT, Hedberg CW, et al. Toxic shock syndrome: a newly recognized complication of influenza and influenza like illness. JAMA 1987;157:1053–8
10. Veenstra DL, Saint S, Sullivan S. Cost-effectiveness of antiseptic-impregnated central venous catheters for the prevention of catheter-related bloodstream infection. JAMA 1999;282:554–60
11. Laflin MJ, Tobey RE, Reves JG. Anesthetic considerations in patients with gas gangrene. Anesth Analg 1976;55:247–51
12. Tsueda K, Oliver OB, Richter RW. Cardiovascular manifestations of tetanus. Anesthesiology 1974;40:588–92
13. Baronia AK, Singh PK, Dhiman RK. Intractable pharyngeal spasm following tracheal extubation in a patient with undiagnosed tetanus. Anesthesiology 1991;75:1111–2
14. Southorn PA, Blaise GA. Treatment of tetanus-induced autonomic nervous system dysfunction with continuous epidural blockade. Crit Care Med 1986;14:251–2
15. Steere AC. Lyme disease. N Engl J Med 1989;321:586–96
16. Tait AR. Occupational transmission of tuberculosis: implications for anesthesiologists. Anesth Analg 1997;85:444–51
17. Pollard BA, El-Beheiry H. Pott's disease with unstable cervical spine, retropharyngeal cold abscess and progressive airway obstruction. Can J Anesth 1999;46:772–5
18. Centers for Disease Control. Guidelines for preventing the transmission of Myobacterium tuberculosis in health care facilities. MMWR Morb Mortal Wkly Rep 1994;43:1–13
19. Rich SA, Sbordone L, Mazze RI. Metabolism by rat hepatic microsomes of fluorinated ether anesthetics following isoniazid administration. Anesthesiology 1980;53:489–93
20. Wang Y-L, Hong C-L, Chung HS, et al. Massive hemoptysis after the initiation of positive pressure ventilation in a patient with pulmonary tuberculosis. Anesthesiology 2000;92:1480–2
21. Mitra S, Gombar KK. Leprosy and the anesthesiologist. Can J Anesth 2000;47:1001–7
22. DuMoulin GC, Hedley-Whyte J. Hospital-associated viral infection and the anesthesiologist. Anesthesiology 1983;59:51–65
23. Couch RB. Prevention and treatment of influenza. N Engl J Med 2000;343:1778–88

24. Hayden FG, Gubareva LV, Monto AS, et al. Inhaled zanamivir for the prevention of influenza in families. N Engl J Med 2000;343:1282–9

25. Dalmeida RE, Mayhew JF, Driscoll B, et al. Total airway obstruction by papillomas during induction of anesthesia. Anesth Analg 1996;83:1332–4

26. Jacoby DB, Hirshman CA. General anesthesia in patients with viral respiratory infections: an unsound sleep. Anesthesiology 1991;74:969–72

27. Fennelly ME, Hall GM. Anaesthesia and upper respiratory tract infections: a non-existent hazard? Br J Anaesth 1990;64:535–6

28. Tait AR, Knight PR. Intraoperative respiratory complications in patients with upper respiratory tract infections. Can J Anaesth 1987;34:300–3

29. Kinouchi K, Tanigami H, Tashiro C, et al. Duration of apnea in anesthetized infants and children required for desaturation of hemoglobin to 95%: the influence of upper respiratory infection. Anesthesiology 1992;77:1105–7

30. Cohen MM, Cameron CB. Should you cancel the operation when a child has an upper respiratory tract infection? Anesth Analg 1991;72:282–8

31. Balfour CL, Balfour HH. Cytomegalovirus is not an occupational risk for nurses in renal transplant and neonatal units: results of prospective surveillance study. JAMA 1986;256:1909–14

32. Cohen JI. Epstein-Barr virus infection. N Engl J Med 2000;343:481–92

33. Meyers EF, Krupin B. Anesthetic management of emergency tonsillectomy and adenoidectomy in infectious mononucleosis. Anesthesiology 1975;42:490–1

34. Fayon M, Gauthier M, Blanc VF, et al. Intraoperative cardiac arrest due to the oculocardiac reflex and subsequent death in a child with occult Epstein-Barr virus myocarditis. Anesthesiology 1995;83:622–4

35. Schooley RT. Acquired immunodeficiency syndrome. Sci Am Med 1998;1–14

36. Recommendations for prevention of HIV transmission in health care settings. MMWR Morb Mortal Wkly Rep 1987;36:629–33

37. Cardo DM, Culver DH, Ciesielski CA, et al. A case-control study of HIV seroconversion in health-care workers after percutaneous exposure: Centers for Disease Control and Prevention Needlestick Surveillance Group. N Engl J Med 1997;337:1485–93

38. Public health service guidelines for the management of health-care worker exposures to HIV and recommendations for postexposure prophylaxis. MMWR Morb Mortal Wkly Rep 1998;47:1–5

39. Schwartz D, Schwartz T, Cooper E, et al. Anaesthesia and the child with HIV infection. Can J Anaesth 1991;38:626–33

40. Kunkel SE, Warner MA. Human T-cell lymphotropic virus type III (HTLV-III) infection: how it can affect you, your patients, and your anesthetic practice. Anesthesiology 1987;66:195–207

41. Miner JE, Egan TD. An AIDS-associated cause of the difficult airway: supraglottic Kaposi's sarcoma. Anesth Analg 2000;90:1223–6

42. Feldman AM, McNamara D. Myocarditis. N Engl J Med 2000;343:1388–98

43. Feeley TW, Hamilton WK, Xavier B, et al. Sterile anesthetic breathing circuits do not prevent postoperative pulmonary infection. Anesthesiology 1981;54:369–72

44. DuMoulin GC, Saubermann AJ. The anesthesia machine and circle system are not likely to be sources of bacterial contamination. Anesthesiology 1977;47:353–8

45. Knight PR, Bedows E, Nahrwold ML, et al. Alterations in influenza virus pulmonary pathology induced by diethyl ether, halothane, enflurane, and pentobarbital anesthesia in mice. Anesthesiology 1983;58:209–15

46. Chestnut DH. Spinal anesthesia in the febrile patient. Anesthesiology 1992;76:667–9

47. Wheeler AP, Bernard GR. Treating patients with severe sepsis. N Engl J Med 1999;340:207–14

48. Bone RC. Sepsis, sepsis syndrome, and the systemic inflammatory response syndrome (SIRS). JAMA 1995;273:155–6

49. Parrillo JE. Pathogenetic mechanisms of septic shock. N Engl J Med 1993;328:1471–7

50. Gill R, Martin C, McKinnon T, et al. Sepsis reduces isoflurane MAC in a normotensive animal model of sepsis. Can J Anaesth 1995;42:631–5

51. Baxter F. Septic shock. Can J Anaesth 1997;44:59–72

52. Durack DT. Prevention of infective endocarditis. N Engl J Med 1995;332:38–44

53. Quagliarello VJ, Scheld WM. Treatment of bacterial meningitis. N Engl J Med 1997;336:708–16

54. Manourian AC, Dickman CA, Drayer BP, et al. Spinal epidural abscess: three cases following spinal epidural injection demonstrated with magnetic resonance imaging. Anesthesiology 1993;78:204–7

55. Hansen M, Paulsen MR, Bendixen DK, et al. Incidence of sinusitis in patients with nasotracheal intubation. Br J Anaesth 1988;61:231–2

56. Souweine B, Mom T, Traore O, et al. Ventilator-associated sinusitis: microbiological results of sinus aspirates in patients on antibiotics. Anesthesiology 2000;93:1255–60

57. Wang X-J, Moylan B, Leopold DA, et al. Mutation in the gene responsible for cystic fibrosis and predisposition to chronic rhinosinusitis in the general population. JAMA 2000;284:1814–9

58. Paradise JL, Bluestone CD, Colborn DK, et al. Adenoidectomy and adenotonsillectomy for recurrent acute otitis media: parallel randomized clinical trials in children not previously treated with tympanoplasty tubes. JAMA 1999;282:945–53

59. Perreault L, Normandin N, Plamondon L, et al. Tympanic membrane rupture after anesthesia with nitrous oxide. Anesthesiology 1982;57:325–6

60. Park KW, Darvish A, Lowenstein E. Airway management for adult patients with acute epiglottitis: a 12 year experience at an academic medical center (1984–1995). Anesthesiology 1998;88:254–61

61. Lew DP, Waldvogel FA. Osteomyelitis. N Engl J Med 1997;336:999–1007

28

Cancer

Cancer is the second most frequent cause of death in the United States, exceeded only by heart disease. Cancer develops in one of every three Americans, and one of every five cancer victims die from the effects of their disease. The number of deaths is increasing as a reflection of the growing elderly population and a decrease in the number of deaths from heart disease.

▎MECHANISM

Cancer results from accumulation of mutations in genes that regulate cellular proliferation.[1] Genes are involved in carcinogenesis by virtue of inherited traits that predispose to cancer (altered metabolism of potentially carcinogenic components, decreased level of immune system function) or mutation of normal genes into oncogenes. The inheritance of a mutated allele is commonly followed by the loss of the second allele from a somatic cell, leading to inactivation of a tumor suppressor gene and triggering of malignant transformations. A critical gene related to cancer in humans is the tumor suppressor *p53*.[1] This gene is not only essential for cell viability, it is critical for monitoring damage to deoxyribonucleic acid (DNA). Inactivation of *p53* is an early step in the development of many types of cancer.

Stimulation of oncogene formation by carcinogens (tobacco, alcohol, sunlight) is estimated to be responsible for 80% of cancers in the United States. Tobacco use accounts for more cases of cancer than all other known carcinogens combined. The fundamental events that cause cells to become malignant are alterations in the structure of DNA. The responsible mutations occur in cells of target tissues, with these cells becoming the ancestors of the entire future tumor cell population. Clonal evolution to even more undifferentiated cells reflects high mutation rates and contributes to the development of tumors that are resistant to drugs, hormones, and antibody therapies. Mutations have no effect on germ cells and are not transmitted genetically.

Cancer cells must evade the host's immune surveillance systems, which are designed to seek out and destroy tumor cells. Most mutant cells stimulate the host's immune system to form antibodies (see "Immunology of Cancer Cells"). Some cancer cells may also become metastatic. It seems likely that many cancers reflect activation of genes that promote production of tumor cells. In support of a protective role of the immune system is the increased incidence of cancer in immunosuppressed patients, such as those with acquired immunodeficiency syndrome (AIDS) and those receiving organ transplants.

▮ DIAGNOSIS

Cancer often becomes clinically evident when tumor bulk compromises the function of vital organs. The initial diagnosis of cancer is often by aspiration cytology or biopsy (needle, incisional, excisional). Monoclonal antibodies that recognize antigens for specific cancers (prostate, lung, breast, ovary) may aid in the diagnosis of cancer (see "Immunology of Cancer Cells"). A commonly used staging system for solid tumors is the TNM system based on tumor size (T), lymph node involvement (N), and distant metastasis (M). This system further groups patients into stages ranging from the best prognosis (stage 1) to the poorest prognosis (stage 3 or 4). Tumor invasiveness is related to the release of various tumor mediators that modify the surrounding microenvironment in such a way as to permit cancer cells to spread along the lines of least resistance. Lymphatics lack a basement membrane such that local spread of cancer is influenced by the anatomy of the regional lymphatics. For example, regional lymph node involvement occurs late in squamous cell cancer of the vocal cords because these structures have few lymphatics, whereas regional lymph node involvement is an early manifestation of supraglottic cancer because this region is rich in lymphatics. Imaging techniques including computed tomography and magnetic resonance imaging are used for further delineation of tumor presence and its spread.

▮ TREATMENT

Treatment of cancer includes chemotherapy, radiation, and surgery. Surgery is often necessary for the initial diagnosis of cancer (biopsy) and subsequent definitive treatment to remove the entire tumor or distant metastases or to decrease the tumor mass. Palliative and rehabilitative therapy may require surgery. Adequate relief of acute and chronic pain associated with cancer is a mandatory part of the patient's treatment.

Chemotherapy

Drugs administered for cancer chemotherapy may produce significant side effects (Table 28–1).[2,3] These side effects may have important implications for the management of anesthesia during surgical procedures for treatment of cancer and operations unrelated to the presence of cancer (see "Management of Anesthesia").

Angiogenesis Inhibitors

Cancer cells secrete proteins that facilitate angiogenesis (creation of new blood vessels) and tissue invasion, such as vascular endothelial growth factor, fibroblast growth factors, and matrix metalloproteinases. Signaling proteins have been identified, such as Flk-1 kinase, that are activated in endothelial cells after binding of angiogenic growth factors. Drugs that prevent angiogenesis, such as endostatin, may be useful in the treatment of cancer.[4]

Acute and Chronic Pain

Cancer patients may experience acute pain associated with pathologic fractures, tumor invasion, surgery, radiation, and chemotherapy.[5] A frequent source of pain is related to metastatic spread of the cancer, especially to bones. Nerve compression or infiltration may be causes of pain. Patients with cancer who experience pain frequently exhibit signs of depression and increased anxiety.

Pathophysiology

Organic causes of cancer pain may be subdivided into nociceptive or neuropathic pain.[5] Nociceptive pain includes somatic and visceral pain and refers to pain due to the peripheral stimulation of nociceptors in somatic or visceral structures. Somatic pain is related to tumor involvement of somatic structures such as bones or skeletal muscles and is often described as "aching," "stabbing," or "throbbing."[5] Visceral pain is related to lesions in a hollow or solid viscus and is described as "diffuse," "gnawing," or "crampy" if a hollow viscus is involved. It is more commonly described as "aching" or "sharp" if a solid viscus is involved. Nociceptive pain is usually responsive to nonopioids and opioids. Neuropathic pain involves peripheral or central afferent neural pathways and is commonly described as "burning" or lancinating pain. Patients experiencing neuropathic pain often respond poorly to opioids.

Drug Therapy

Drug therapy is the cornerstone of cancer pain management because of its efficacy, rapid onset of action, and relatively low cost.[5] Mild to moderate cancer pain is initially treated with nonsteroidal antiinflammatory drugs (NSAIDs) and acetaminophen. NSAIDs are especially effective for managing bone pain, which is the most common cause of cancer pain. The next step in management of moderate to severe pain includes addition of codeine or one of its analogues. When cancer pain is severe, opioids are the major drugs used. Morphine is the most commonly selected opioid and can be administered orally. When the oral route of administration is inadequate, alternative routes (intravenous, subcutaneous, epidural, intrathecal, transmucosal, transdermal) are considered. Fentanyl is available in transdermal and transmucosal delivery systems. There is no maximum safe dose of morphine and other mu agonist opioids. Only titration of opioids to the desired patient response is useful for determining the optimal dose for specific patients. Tolerance to opioids does occur but need not be a clinical problem. Unnecessary fear of addiction is a major reason opioids are underused despite the fact that addiction is rare when these drugs are correctly used to treat pain in cancer patients.

Tricyclic antidepressant drugs are recommended for those who remain depressed despite improved pain control. These drugs are also effective in the absence of depression and appear to have direct analgesic effects and cause potentiation of opioids. Anticonvulsants are useful for management of chronic neuropathic pain. Corticosteroids can lower pain perception, have a sparing effect on opioid requirements, improve mood, increase appetite, and lead to weight gain.

Neuraxial Administration

Morphine may be administered intrathecally or epidurally for management of acute and chronic cancer pain.[5] Spinal opioids may be delivered for weeks to months by placing a long-term, subcutaneously tunneled, exteriorized catheter or by using implantable drug delivery systems. The implantable systems can be intrathecal or epidural and feature a drug reservoir or an implanted infusion device often with external reprogramming. Patients are typically considered for neuraxial opioid administration only when systemic opioid administration has failed as a result of the onset of intolerable adverse (systemic) side effects or adequate analgesia has not been achieved. Neuraxial administration of opioids is usually successful, although some patients require a low concentration of local anesthetic to achieve adequate pain control.

Neurolytic Procedures

Neurolytic procedures intended to destroy sensory components of nerves cannot be used without also destroying motor and autonomic nervous system fibers. Important aspects of determining the suitability of destructive nerve blocks are the location and quality of the pain, the effectiveness of less destructive treatment modalities, the patient's life expectancy, the inherent risks associated with the block, and the availability of experienced anesthesiologists to perform the procedures.[5] In general, constant pain is more amenable to destructive nerve blocks than is intermittent pain.

Neurolytic celiac plexus blocks (alcohol, phenol) have been utilized to treat pain originating from abdominal viscera (pancreatic cancer). The blocks are associated with serious side effects. Analgesia usually lasts 6 months or longer. Neurosurgical procedures (neuroablative or neurostimulatory) for managing cancer pain are reserved for patients unresponsive to other, less invasive procedures. Cordotomy involves interruption of the spinothalamic tract in the spinal cord and is considered for treatment of unilateral pain involving the lower extremity, thorax, or upper extremity. Dorsal rhizotomy involves interruption of sensory nerve roots and is utilized when pain is localized to specific dermatomal levels. Dorsal column stimulators or deep brain stimulators may be utilized in selected patients.

■ IMMUNOLOGY OF CANCER CELLS

Tumor cells are antigenically different from normal cells and may therefore elicit immune reactions similar to those that cause rejection of histoincompatible allografts. Antigens present in cancer cells but not in normal cells are designated tumor-specific antigens. Conversely, tumor-associated antigens (α-fetoprotein, prostate-specific antigen, carcinoembryonic antigen) are present in cancer cells and normal cells, but concentrations are higher in tumor cells. Because tumor-associated antigens may be

Table 28–1 • Adverse Side Effects Associated with Cancer Chemotherapeutic Drugs

	Immunosuppression	Thrombocytopenia	Leukopenia	Anemia	Cardiac Toxicity	Pulmonary Toxicity
Alkylating agents						
Busulfan (Myleran)	+	+++	+++	+++		++
Chlorambucil (Leukeran)	+	++	++	++		+
Cyclophosphamide (Cytoxan)	++++	+	++	+		+
Melphalan (Alkeran)	+	++	++	++		+
Thiotepa (Thiotcpa)	+	+++	+++	+++		+
Antimetabolites						
Methotrexate (Methotrexate)	+++	+++	+++	+++		+
6-Merceptopurine (Purinethol)	+++	++	++	++		
Thioguanine (Thioguanine)	+++	+	++	++		
5-Fluorouracil (Fluorouracil)	++++	+++	+++	+++		
Plant alkaloids						
Vinblastine (Velban)	++	+	+++	+		
Vincristine (Oncovin)	++	+	++	+		
Antibiotics						
Doxorubicin (Adriamycin)		+	+++	++	+++	
Daunorubicin (Daunomycin)	+	++	+++	++	+++	
Bleomycin (Blenoxane)		+	+	+		+++
Mithramycin (Mithracin)	+	++++	++++	+++		
Nitrosoureas						
Carmustine (BiCNU)		++	++	++		+
Lomustine (CeeNU)		+++	+++	++		
Enzymes						
L-Asparaginase (Elspar)	++	+	+	+		

+, minimal; ++, mild; +++, moderate; ++++, marked.
ADH, antidiuretic hormone.
Adapted from: Selvin BL. Cancer chemotherapy: Implications for tha anesthesiologist. Anesth Analg 1981;60:425–34, with permission.

present in normal tissues, measurements of these antigens may be less useful for the diagnosis of cancer than for monitoring patients with known malignant disorders.

Antibodies to tumor-associated antigens can be used for the immunodiagnosis of cancer. In this regard, the use of monoclonal antibodies to detect proteins encoded by oncogenes or other types of tumor-associated antigens is a commonly used method for identifying cancer. Monoclonal antibod-ies to various tumor-associated antigens can be la-beled with radioisotopes and injected to monitor the spread of cancer or be used as carriers of immu-notoxins or drugs. The enormous antigenic diversity of many forms of cancer makes the development of an effective vaccine a formidable task. Alternatively, attempts may be made to enhance a patient's overall level of immunity with nonspecific immunopotenti-ators such as bacillus Calmette Guérin (BCG) and interferons. Most spontaneously occurring tumors

Renal Toxicity	Hepatic Toxicity	CNS Toxicity	Peripheral Nervous System Toxicity	Autonomic Nervous System Toxicity	Stomatitis	Plasma Cholinesterase Inhibition	Other
++					+	+	Adrenocortical-like effect (+) Hemolytic anemia (++)
	+	+				+	Hemolytic anemia (++)
+	+				+	++	Hemolytic anemia (++) Hemorrhagic cystitis (+++)
						+	Inappropriate ADH secretion (+)
						++	Hemolytic anemia (++)
							Hemolytic anemia (++)
++	+				+++		
++	+++				+		
	+++				+		
		+			+++		
			+	+	+		Inappropriate ADH secretion (+)
+		+	++	++			
	+				++		Red urine (+)
					++		Red urine (+)
					+++		
++	++	+			+++		Coagulation defects (+++) Hypocalcemia (+) Hypokalemia (+)
+					+		
	+				+		
+	+++	+			+		Hemorrhagic pancreatitis (+) Coagulation defects (+)

appear to be weakly antigenic, whereas others can activate suppressor T cells to dampen the intensity of immune responses to tumor antigens.

▪ PARANEOPLASTIC SYNDROMES

Paraneoplastic syndromes manifest as pathophysiologic disturbances that may accompany cancer (Table 28–2). Certain of these pathophysiologic disturbances [superior vena cava obstruction, increased intracranial pressure (ICP), pericardial tamponade, renal failure, hypercalcemia] may manifest as acute life-threatening medical emergencies.

Fever and Weight Loss

Fever may accompany any type of cancer but is particularly likely with metastases to the liver. Increased body temperature and perhaps lactic acidosis may accompany rapidly proliferating tumors, such as leukemias and lymphomas. Fever may reflect tumor necrosis, inflammation, the release of

Table 28–2 • Pathophysiologic Manifestations of Paraneoplastic Syndromes

Fever
Anorexia
Weight loss
Anemia
Thrombocytopenia
Coagulopathies
Neuromuscular abnormalities
Ectopic hormone production
Hypercalcemia
Hyperuricemia
Tumor lysis syndrome
Adrenal insufficiency
Nephrotic syndrome
Ureteral obstruction
Pulmonary hypertrophic osteoarthropathy and clubbing
Pericardial effusion
Pericardial tamponade
Superior vena cava obstruction
Spinal cord compression
Brain metastasis

toxic products by cancer cells, and the production of endogenous pyrogens. Acidosis results from increased anaerobic glycolysis of the hypoxic proliferating tumor cells, especially when hepatic function is concomitantly impaired.

Anorexia and weight loss are frequent occurrences in patients with cancer, especially lung cancer. In addition to the psychological effects of cancer on appetite, cancer cells compete with normal tissues for nutrients and may eventually cause nutritive death of normal cells. Hyperalimentation is indicated for nutritional support when malnutrition is severe, especially before elective surgery.

Hematologic Abnormalities

Anemia most likely reflects the direct effects of cancer, such as gastrointestinal ulceration with bleeding or tumor replacement of bone marrow. Cancer chemotherapy is another common cause of bone marrow depression and anemia. Acute hemolytic anemia may accompany lymphoproliferative diseases. Solid tumors, especially metastatic breast cancer, can lead to pancytopenia. In contrast to anemia, an increased amount of erythropoietin, as produced by a hypernephroma or hepatoma, can result in polycythemia. Thrombocytopenia may be due to chemotherapy or the presence of an unrecognized cancer. Disseminated intravascular coagulation may occur in patients with advanced cancer, especially in the presence of hepatic metastases. There is an association between venous thromboembolism and a subsequent diagnosis of cancer. Cancer diagnosed at the same time as,

or within 1 year after, an episode of venous thromboembolism is often associated with an advanced stage of cancer and a poor prognosis.[6] Recurrent venous thrombosis due to unknown mechanisms may be associated with pancreatic cancer.

Neuromuscular Abnormalities

Neuromuscular abnormalities occur in 5% to 10% of patients with cancer. The most common manifestations are skeletal muscle weakness (myasthenic syndrome) associated with lung cancer. Prolonged responses to depolarizing and nondepolarizing muscle relaxants have been observed in patients with co-existing skeletal muscle weakness, particularly when weakness is associated with undifferentiated small cell lung cancers.

Ectopic Hormone Production

Active hormones are produced by a number of tumors, resulting in predictable physiologic effects (Table 28–3).

Hypercalcemia

Cancer is the most common cause of hypercalcemia is hospitalized patients, reflecting local osteolytic activity from bone metastases (especially breast cancer) or the ectopic hormonal activity associated with tumors that arise from the kidneys, lungs, pancreas, or ovaries. The rapid onset of hypercalcemia that occurs in patients with cancer may manifest as lethargy and coma. Polyuria and dehydration may accompany hypercalcemia, which is further exaggerated by bone pain and resulting immobility. Opioids administered to relieve pain can result in further immobility, vomiting, or dehydration.

Tumor Lysis Syndrome

Tumor lysis syndrome is caused by sudden therapeutic destruction of tumor cells, leading to the release of precursors of uric acid, potassium, and phosphate. This syndrome occurs most often after treatment of hematologic neoplasms, such as acute lymphoblastic leukemia. Acute renal failure can accompany hyperuricemia. Likewise, hyperkalemia and resulting cardiac dysrhythmia are more likely in the presence of renal dysfunction. Conversely, hyperphosphatemia can lead to secondary hypocalcemia, which increases the risk of cardiac dysrhyth-

Table 28–3 • Ectopic Hormone Production

Hormone	Associated Cancer	Manifestations
Corticotropin	Lung (small cell) Thyroid (medullary) Thymoma Carcinoid Non-beta islet cell of pancreas	Cushing syndrome
Antidiuretic hormone	Lung (small cell) Pancreas Lymphomas	Water intoxication
Gonadotropin	Lung (large cell) Ovary Adrenal	Gynecomastia Precocious puberty
Melanocyte-stimulating hormone	Lung (small cell)	Hyperpigmentation
Parathyroid hormone	Renal Lung (squamous) Pancreas Ovary	Hyperparathyroidism
Thyrotropin	Choriocarcinoma Testicular (embryonal)	Hyperthyroidism
Thyrocalcitonin	Thyroid (medullary)	Hypocalcemia
Insulin	Retroperitoneal tumors	Hypoglycemia

mias from hypokalemia and can cause neuromuscular symptoms such as tetany.

Adrenal Insufficiency

Adrenal insufficiency caused by complete replacement of the adrenal glands by metastatic tumor is rare. More often there is relative adrenal insufficiency owing to partial replacement of the adrenal cortex by tumor or suppression of adrenal cortex function by prolonged treatment with corticosteroids. Adrenal insufficiency is most often seen in patients with metastatic disease due to melanoma, retroperitoneal tumors, lung cancer, or breast cancer. The stress of the perioperative period may unmask adrenal insufficiency. Clinical manifestations include fatigue, dehydration, oliguria, and cardiovascular collapse. Treatment of acute adrenal insufficiency consists of rapid intravenous administration of cortisol followed by continuous infusion of cortisol until oral replacement can be initiated.

Renal Dysfunction

Renal complications of cancer may reflect invasion of the kidneys by tumor, damage from tumor products, or chemotherapy. Deposition of tumor antigen-antibody complexes on the glomerular membrane may result in changes considered characteristic of the nephrotic syndrome. Extensive retroperitoneal cancer can lead to bilateral ureteral obstruction and fatal uremia, especially in patients with cancer of the cervix, bladder, or prostate. Percutaneous nephrostomy is indicated if a ureter is totally obstructed. Chemotherapy can destroy large numbers of cells; acute hyperuricemic nephropathy due to precipitation of uric acid crystals in the renal tubules is prevented by administration of allopurinol in combination with hydration and urinary alkalinization. Methotrexate and cisplatin are the chemotherapeutic drugs most often associated with nephrotoxicity. Acute hemorrhagic cystitis is a rare complication of cyclophosphamide therapy.

Acute Respiratory Complications

The acute onset of dyspnea may reflect extension of the tumor or the effects of chemotherapy. Bleomycin-induced interstitial pneumonitis and fibrosis is the most commonly encountered pulmonary complication of chemotherapy. Elderly patients and those with co-existing lung disease, prior use of radiotherapy, or currently receiving high doses of bleomycin are at greatest risk of pulmonary toxicity. Pulmonary toxicity rarely occurs when the total doses of bleomycin are less than 150 mg/m^2. The most common symptoms of interstitial pneumonitis are the insidious onset of nonproductive cough, dyspnea, tachypnea, and occasionally fever 4 to 10 weeks after initiation of bleomycin therapy. These symptoms appear in 3% to 6% of patients treated with bleomycin. Incipient toxicity can be detected by measuring the diffusion capacity of the lungs for carbon monoxide. The alveolar-to-arterial difference for oxygen is often increased in affected patients. The appearance of radiographic changes, such as bilateral diffuse pulmonary infiltrates, probably portends irreversible pulmonary fibrosis. In the absence of a biopsy, the clinical and radiographic features of bleomycin-induced pneumonitis may be difficult to distinguish from pneumonia due to *Pneumocystis carinii*. Corticosteroids are the only treatment for the acute effects of drug-induced pneumonitis, but interstitial and alveolar fibrosis are irreversible.

Acute Cardiac Complications

Pericardial effusion caused by metastatic invasion of the pericardium can lead to the sudden onset of cardiac tamponade. Lung cancer seems to be the most common cause of pericardial tamponade. Malignant pericardial effusion is the most common cause of electrical alternans on the electrocardiogram (ECG). Paroxysmal atrial fibrillation or flutter may be an early manifestation of malignant involvement of the pericardium or myocardium. Optimal treatment of malignant pericardial effusion consists of prompt removal of the fluid followed by surgical creation of a pericardial window (see Chapter 9).

Cardiac toxicity manifesting as life-threatening cardiomyopathy occurs in 1% to 5% of patients treated with doxorubicin or daunorubicin. Cardiotoxicity may manifest initially as symptoms suggestive of an upper respiratory tract infection (nonproductive cough) followed by rapidly progressive congestive heart failure (CHF) that is often refractory to cardiac inotropic drugs or mechanical cardiac assistance. Cardiomegaly and/or pleural effusion may be evident on chest radiographs. QRS voltages on the ECG may be decreased. Patients who have undergone radiation therapy, particularly to the mediastinum, or patients who are on concurrent cyclophosphamide therapy seem to be more susceptible to the development of cardiomyopathy.[7] Impairment of left ventricular function for as long as 3 years after discontinuing the doxorubicin has been observed.[8] In contrast to life-threatening cardiomyopathy, about 10% of treated patients show nonspecific, usually benign changes on the ECG (nonspecific ST-T wave changes, low QRS voltages, atrial or ventricular premature beats) that do not necessarily reflect an underlying cardiomyopathy.

Superior Vena Cava Obstruction

Obstruction of the superior vena cava is caused by spread of cancer into the mediastinum or direct invasion of vessel walls by disease, most often lung cancer. Engorgement of veins above the waist occurs, particularly the jugular veins and those in the extremities. Dyspnea and airway obstruction may be present. Edema of the arms and face is usually prominent. Hoarseness may reflect edema of the vocal cords. Increased ICP manifests as nausea, seizures, and decreased levels of consciousness and is most likely due to increased cerebral venous pressures. Treatment consists of prompt radiation or chemotherapy, as determined by the histopathology of the cancer, to decrease the size of the tumor and thus relieve venous and airway obstruction. In this regard, bronchoscopy and mediastinoscopy to obtain a tissue diagnosis can be hazardous, especially in the presence of co-existing airway obstruction and increased pressure in the mediastinal veins.

Spinal Cord Compression

Spinal cord compression results from the presence of metastatic lesions in the epidural space, most often reflecting breast, lung, or prostate cancer or lymphoma. Symptoms incude pain, skeletal muscle weakness, sensory loss, and autonomic nervous system dysfunction. Myelography may be necessary to visualize the limits of compression, but the associated lumbar puncture may exacerbate the symptoms and necessitate prompt surgical intervention. Computed tomography is an alternative to myelography. Radiation therapy is a useful treatment when neurologic deficits are partial. In this regard, corticosteroids are often administered to minimize any inflammatory reaction and edema that can result from radiation directed to tumors in the epidural space. Once total paralysis has developed, the results of surgical laminectomy or of radiation to decompress the patient's spinal cord are equally poor.

Increased Intracranial Pressure

Metastatic brain tumors, most often from the lung and breast, present initially as mental deterioration, focal neurologic defects, and seizures. Computed tomography is the most useful diagnostic test. Treatment of acute increases in ICP caused by metastatic lesions includes corticosteroids, diuretics, and mannitol (see Chapter 17). Radiation is the usual palliative treatment, whereas surgery may be considered for patients with single metastatic lesions. Intrathecal administration of chemotherapeutic drugs is necessary when the meninges are involved.

■ MANAGEMENT OF ANESTHESIA

Preoperative evaluation of patients with cancer includes consideration of possible pathophysiologic side effects of the disease and recognition of the potential adverse side effects associated with cancer chemotherapeutic drugs (Tables 28–1, 28–2, 28–3).[2,3]

Side Effects of Chemotherapy

Clinical tests to detect preoperatively side effects related to treatment with chemotherapeutic drugs may be useful (Table 28–4).

Pulmonary and Cardiac Toxicity

The possible presence of pulmonary and cardiac toxicity is a consideration for patients being treated with chemotherapeutic drugs known to be associated with this complication. In this regard, the preoperative history of drug-induced pulmonary fibrosis (dyspnea, nonproductive cough) or CHF may influence the subsequent conduct of anesthesia. For example, in patients treated with bleomycin, it may be helpful to monitor arterial blood gases and arterial oxygenation (SpO_2) and to titrate intravascular fluid replacement, keeping in mind that these patients may be at risk for the development of interstitial pulmonary edema presumably caused by impaired lymphatic drainage owing to drug-induced pulmonary fibrosis. Suggestions that bleomycin increases the likelihood of oxygen toxicity in the presence of high inspired concentrations of oxygen are not supported by animal and patient data.[9,10] Nevertheless, it may be prudent to consider administration of colloid solutions to these patients and to adjust the delivered oxygen concentrations to those values that provide the desired SpO_2. Depressant effects of anesthetic drugs on myocardial contractility may be

---

Table 28–4 • Preoperative Tests in Patients with Cancer

Hematocrit
Platelet count
White blood cell count
Prothrombin time
Electrolytes
Liver function tests
Renal function tests
Blood glucose concentrations
Arterial blood gases
Chest radiography
Electrocardiography

---

enhanced in patients with drug-induced cardiac toxicity.

Neurotoxicity

Anticancer chemotherapy can cause a number of neurotoxic side effects including peripheral neuropathy and encephalopathy.[11]

Peripheral Neuropathy

Vinca alkaloids, particularly vincristine, affect the microtubules, causing sensorimotor peripheral neuropathy. Virtually all patients treated with vincristine develop paresthesias in their digits. Autonomic nervous system neuropathy may accompany these drug-induced changes, which are reversible. Cisplatin causes dose-dependent large-fiber neuropathy by damaging dorsal root ganglia. Loss of proprioceptive sensation in these patients may be sufficiently severe to interfere with ambulation. Performance of regional anesthesia in patients being treated with cisplatin chemotherapy may be influenced by the realization that cisplatin neurotoxicity is possibly present though unrecognized in a large percentage of patients receiving this drug.[12] Furthermore, cisplatin neurotoxicity may extend several months beyond discontinuation of treatment. Severe diffuse brachial plexopathy has been described following interscalene blockade in a patient receiving cisplatin chemotherapy ("pharmacologic double crush syndrome").[12] Paclitaxel causes dose-dependent sensory ataxia that may be accompanied by paresthesias in the hands and feet and proximal skeletal muscle weakness. Corticosteroids (prednisone or its equivalent at 60 to 100 mg daily) may cause a myopathy characterized by weakness of the neck flexors and proximal weakness of the extremities. The first sign of corticosteroid-induced neurotoxicity is difficulty assuming the standing position from the sitting position. Respiratory muscles may be affected. Corticosteroid-induced peripheral neuropathy usually resolves when the drugs are discontinued.

Encephalopathy

Many cancer chemotherapeutic drugs can cause encephalopathy. High-dose cyclophosphamide may be associated with acute delirium. High-dose cytarabine may cause acute delirium or cerebellar degeneration, which are usually reversible. Reversible acute encephalopathy may accompany the intravenous or intrathecal administration of methotrexate. Prolonged administration of methotrexate, especially in conjunction with radiation therapy, can lead to progressive dementia.

Preoperative Preparation

Preoperatively, correction of nutrient deficiencies, anemia, coagulopathy, and electrolyte abnormalities may be needed. Nausea and vomiting are the most common and distressing side effects of chemotherapy and, to some extent, of radiation treatment. Metoclopramide, droperidol, and serotonin antagonist drugs such as ondansetron may help control nausea in these patients during the preoperative period. Tricyclic antidepressants may be useful for potentiating the analgesic effects of opioids and producing some inherent analgesia. Opioids used for management of cancer-induced pain may be responsible for preoperative sedation.

The presence of hepatic or renal dysfunction may influence the choice of anesthetic drugs and muscle relaxants. Although not a consistent observation, the possibility of prolonged responses to succinylcholine is a consideration in patients being treated with alkylating chemotherapeutic drugs.[8] Attention to aseptic technique is important, as immunosuppression occurs with most chemotherapeutic drugs. Immunosuppression produced by anesthesia, surgical stimulation, or even blood transfusions during the perioperative period may exert undefined effects on the patient's subsequent responses to cancer.

Postoperative Considerations

Postoperative mechanical support of the patient's ventilation is often required, particularly following invasive or prolonged operations and in patients with preoperative drug-induced pulmonary fibrosis. Patients with drug-induced cardiac toxicity are more likely to experience postoperative cardiac complications.[8]

COMMON CANCERS ENCOUNTERED IN CLINICAL PRACTICE

The most commonly encountered cancers in adults are lung cancer, breast cancer, colon cancer, and prostate cancer. Lung cancer is the second most common malignancy in men surpassed only by prostate cancer, whereas in women the incidence of lung cancer is increasing and is exceeded only by breast cancer.

Lung Cancer

Lung cancer is the leading cause of cancer deaths among men and women and accounts for nearly one-third of all cancer deaths in the United States.[13–17] It is largely a preventable disease, as more than 90% of lung cancer deaths are related to cigarette smoking. The high mortality resulting from lung cancer (15% survival after 5 years) reflects, in part, its aggressive biology and advanced state when the diagnosis is confirmed. On the basis of present trends, the probability at birth of eventual death from lung cancer is 8% for males and 4% for females.[13]

Etiology

The strong association of cigarette smoking with lung cancer is established. Smoking marijuana produces a substantially greater respiratory burden of carbon monoxide and tar than smoking a similar quantity of tobacco and thus may pose an additional risk factor for lung cancer in cigarette smokers. The mutagens of carcinogens present in cigarette smoke may cause chromosomal damage and eventual malignant events. Other carcinogens that cause lung cancer include ionizing radiation (by-product of coal and iron mining), asbestos (increases the incidence of lung cancer in nonsmokers and acts as a synergistic co-carcinogen with tobacco smoke), and naturally occurring radon gas. Adjuvant radiotherapy for breast cancer following mastectomy is associated with an increased risk of lung cancer.

Cessation of cigarette smoking decreases the incidence of lung cancer to that of nonsmokers after about 10 to 15 years have elapsed. There is a familial risk of lung cancer that is related to genetic and ecogenetic factors and to exposure to passive smoking. Inhalation of secondhand smoke increases the risk of lung cancer and contributes to the development of childhood respiratory infections and asthma. Cigarette smokers who develop emphysema are at increased risk for the development of lung cancer. AIDS may be associated with an increased incidence of lung cancer.

Signs and Symptoms

Patients with lung cancer present with features related to the extent of the disease, including local and regional manifestations, signs and symptoms of metastatic disease, and various paraneoplastic syndromes related indirectly to the cancer (Table 28–2).[13] Cough, hemoptysis, wheezing, stridor, dyspnea, or pneumonitis from obstruction of airways with fever and sputum production may be presenting clinical symptoms. Mediastinal metastases may cause hoarseness (recurrent laryngeal nerve compression), superior vena cava syndrome, cardiac dysrhythmias, or CHF from pericardial effusion and tamponade. Pleural effusion results in increasing dyspnea and often chest pain. Generalized weakness, fatigue, anorexia, and weight loss are common.

Histologic Subtypes

Clinical manifestations of lung cancer vary with the histologic subtype (Table 28–5).[13] Non-small-cell lung cancer, which includes squamous cell, adenocarcinoma, and large cell carcinoma, accounts for 75% to 80% of all new cases of lung cancer.[16]

Squamous cell cancers arise in major bronchi or their primary divisions (central origin) and are usually detected by sputum cytology. These tumors tend to grow slowly and may reach a large size before they are detected based on hemoptysis and bronchial obstruction with associated atelectasis, dyspnea, and fever from pneumonia. Cavitation may be evident on chest radiographs.

Adenocarcinomas most often originate in the lung periphery. These tumors commonly present as subpleural nodules and have a tendency to invade the pleura and induce pleural effusions that contain malignant cells. Lung adenocarcinomas may be difficult to differentiate morphologically from malignant mesothelioma or adenocarcinoma that has metastasized from other sites (breast, gastrointestinal tract, pancreas).

Large cell carcinomas are usually peripheral in origin and present as a large, bulky tumor. Like adenocarcinomas, these tumors metastasize early, preferentially to the central nervous system.

Small cell carcinomas are usually a central bronchial origin with a high frequency of early lymphatic invasion especially to lymph nodes in the mediasti-num and metastases to liver, bone, central nervous system, adrenal glands, and pancreas. Prominent mediastinal lymphadenopathy may lead to the erroneous diagnosis of malignant lymphoma. Superior vena cava syndrome may result from mediastinal compression, and atelectasis (but not hemoptysis) is possible. Small tumor cells have a marked propensity to produce polypeptides resulting in metabolic abnormalities. These patients do not usually present before the disease process is extensive as reflected by distant metastases (especially bone).

Diagnosis

Cytologic analysis of sputum is often sufficient for diagnosis of lung cancer, especially when the cancer arises in proximal endobronchial locations where shedding of cells is likely to occur. Peripheral lesions as small as 3.0 mm can be detected by high resolution computed tomography. Lung cancer screening has been recommended for patients who are at highest risk, such as cigarette smokers with airflow obstruction, as measured by spirometry.[14, 17] Despite new diagnostic techniques, the overall 5-year survival rates remain about 14%, and most patients still present with advanced disease.

Flexible fiberoptic bronchoscopy, in combination with a biopsy, brushings, or washings is a standard procedure for initial evaluation of lung cancer. Peripheral lung lesions can be diagnosed by percutaneous fine-needle aspiration guided by fluoroscopy, ultrasonography, or computed tomography scanning. Video-assisted thoracoscopic surgery is useful for diagnosing peripheral lung lesions and pleura-based tumors. Computed tomography scanning is sensitive for detecting pulmonary metastases. Brain magnetic resonance imaging and head computed tomography scans are useful for detecting metastases even in patients without neurologic abnormalities. Mediastinal computed tomography scanning

Table 28–5 • Clinical and Pathologic Features of Lung Cancer

Histologic Subtype	Incidence (%)	5-Year Survival (%)		Associated Symptoms
		All Cases	Resectable Cases	
Squamous cell	25–40	11	40	Hypercalcemia
Adenocarcinoma	30–50	5	30	Hypercoagulability
				Osteoarthropathy
Large cell	10	4	30	Gynecomastia
				Galactorrhea
Small cell	15–24	2	5–10	Inappropriate ADH secretion
				Ectopic corticotropin secretion
				Eaton-Lambert syndrome

ADH, antidiuretic hormone.
Adapted from: Skarin AT. Lung cancer. Sci Am Med 1997;1–20.

is important for staging lung cancer, and cervical mediastinoscopy is indicated in patients with enlarged central nodes detected by computed tomography scanning. Anterior mediastinoscopy is used for examining lymph nodes that cannot be visualized with the cervical mediastinoscope. This approach requires a small incision in the left second intercostal space. Alternatively, video-assisted thoracoscopy may provide similar information to anterior mediastinoscopy.

Treatment

Surgical resection (lobectomy, pneumonectomy) is the most effective treatment for lung cancer. In patients with impaired pulmonary function, wedge resection may be selected. Resectability refers to the extent of the disease and whether the tumor can be entirely removed, as determined by staging procedures. Operability refers to the medical status of the patient and includes an assessment of the patient's tolerance to surgery and the amount of functional lung tissue. It is estimated that about 30% of patients with newly diagnosed non-small cell lung cancers have locally advanced inoperable disease at the time of diagnosis, whereas another 40% have confirmed metastatic disease.[16] Even among the 30% considered surgically curable, recurrent metastatic disease develops in about half within 5 years. For these reasons, many patients with non-small cell lung cancers are candidates for chemotherapy alone or in combination with surgery or radiation therapy. Standard thoractomy is the preferred surgical approach except in patients with cardiopulmonary impairment, in whom video-assisted thoracoscopy is often preferred, especially for limited wedge resection or even lobectomy.

The 5-year survival is unaffected by traditional adjuvant treatments, including radiation, chemotherapy (cyclophosphamide, doxorubicin, cisplatin), immunotherapy, or combinations of these treatments. Surgery has little effect on survival when the disease has spread to unilateral mediastinal lymph nodes but without distant metastases. Radiotherapy is effective in palliating symptoms from tumor invasion in most patients.

Management of Anesthesia

Management of anesthesia in patients with lung cancer includes preoperative consideration of tumor-induced effects that may manifest as malnutrition, pneumonia, pain, and ectopic endocrine effects such as hyponatremia (Table 28–3). The propensity of lung cancer to metastasize to the brain and bones is of possible significance when evaluating patients. When resection of lung tissue is planned, it is important to evaluate underlying pulmonary and cardiac function, especially for the presence of pulmonary hypertension.

Hemorrhage and pneumothorax are the most frequently encountered complications of mediastinoscopy. Positive-pressure ventilation of the lungs during mediastinoscopy is recommended to minimize the risk of venous air embolism. The mediastinoscope can also exert pressure against the right subclavian artery, causing loss of a pulse distal to the site of compression and an erroneous diagnosis of cardiac arrest. Likewise, unrecognized compression of the right carotid artery may manifest as a postoperative neurologic deficit. Bradycardia during mediastinoscopy may be due to stretching of the vagus nerve or trachea by the mediastinoscope.

Colorectal Cancer

Colon cancer is second only to lung cancer as a cause of cancer death in the United States.[18, 19] The incidence and mortality from this cancer has not changed appreciably during the past five decades. More than 99% of colorectal cancers are adenocarcinomas, and the disease generally occurs in adults older than 50 years.

Etiology

Most colorectal cancers arise from premalignant adenomatous polyps. Large polyps, especially those larger than 1.5 cm in diameter, are more likely to contain invasive cancer. Although adenomatous polyps are common (present in more than 30% of patients older than 50 years), fewer than 1% of adenomatous polyps ever become malignant. It is thought that adenomatous polyps require more than 5 years of growth before they become clinically significant. The evolution of normal colonic mucosa first to a benign adenomatous polyp that contains cancer and then to life-threatening invasive cancer is associated with a series of genetic events that involve the mutational activation of a proto-oncogene and the loss of several genes that normally suppress tumor genesis.

Most colorectal cancers appear to be related to diet, with the disease occurring in the greatest incidence among individuals in upper socioeconomic classes living in urban areas. There is a direct correlation between calories consumed, dietary fat and oil, and meat protein. Available data indicate that a high intake of animal fat is the dietary element that is most strongly associated with the risk of colon cancer. As many as 25% of patients with colorectal cancer have a family history of the disease, which suggests involvement of a genetic factor. Inflammatory bowel disease is associated with an increased incidence of colorectal cancer. Cigarette smoking for more than 35 years appears to increase the risk of colorectal cancer.

Diagnosis

The rationale for colorectal cancer screening is that earlier detection of localized superficial tumors and precancerous lesions in asymptomatic individuals increases the surgical cure rate.[18-20] Screening programs (digital rectal examination, examination of the stool for occult blood, colonoscopy) appear to be particularly useful for persons who have first-degree relatives with a history of the disease, especially if these relatives experience the disease before 55 years of age. There is evidence that either annual or biennial fecal occult blood testing decreases the incidence of colorectal cancer.[21]

Signs and Symptoms

The presenting signs and symptoms of colorectal cancer reflect the anatomic location of the cancer.[18] Because stool is relatively liquid as it passes into the right colon through the ileocecal valve, tumors in the cecum and ascending colon can become large and markedly narrow the bowel lumen without causing obstructive symptoms. Ascending colon cancers frequently ulcerate, leading to chronic blood loss in the stool. These patients experience symptoms related to chronic iron deficiency anemia, including fatigue and in some patients angina pectoris.

Stool becomes more concentrated as it passes into the transverse colon. Transverse colon cancers cause abdominal cramping, occasional bowel obstruction, and even perforation. Abdominal radiographs reveals characteristic abnormalities in the colonic gas pattern, reflecting narrowing of the lumen ("napkin ring lesion"). Colon cancers developing in the rectosigmoid portion of the large intestine result in tenesmus and narrowing of the stool. Anemia is unusual despite the passage of bright red blood from the rectum (often attributed to hemorrhoids).

Colorectal cancers initially spread to regional lymph nodes and then through the portal venous circulation to the liver, which represents the most common visceral site of metastases. Colorectal cancers rarely spread to the lungs, bones, or brain in the absence of liver metastases. Preoperative increases in the serum concentrations of carcinoembryonic antigen (CEA) suggest that the tumor will recur following surgical resection. CEA is a glycoprotein that is also increased in the presence of other cancers (stomach, pancreas, breast, lung) and non-

malignant conditions (alcoholic liver disease, inflammatory bowel disease, cigarette smoking, pancreatitis).

Treatment

The prognosis for patients with adenocarcinoma of the colorectum depends on the depth of tumor penetration into the bowel wall and the presence or absence of regional lymph node involvement and distant metastases (liver, lung, bone). Radical surgical resection (lymph nodes draining the involved bowel and blood vessels) offers the best potential for cure of patients with invasive colorectal cancer. Surgical management of cancers that arise in the distal rectum may necessitate a permanent sigmoid colostomy (abdominoperineal resection). Because most recurrences after resection occur within 3 to 4 years, the cure rate for colorectal cancer is often estimated by 5-year survival rates.

Radiation therapy is a consideration in patients with rectal tumors, as the risk of recurrence following surgery is significant. Postoperative radiation therapy causes transient diarrhea and cystitis, although chronic damage to the small intestine and bladder is uncommon. Use of chemotherapy in patients with advanced colorectal cancers (5-fluorouracil) rarely is associated with a satisfactory response.

Management of Anesthesia

Management of anesthesia for surgical resection of colorectal cancers may be influenced by disease-induced anemia and the effects of metastases, as may be present in the liver, lungs, bones, or brain. Chronic large bowel obstruction probably does not increase the risk of aspiration during induction of anesthesia, although abdominal distension could interfere with adequate ventilation and oxygenation. Blood transfusion during surgical resection of colorectal cancers has been alleged to be associated with decreased patient survival time.[22] Presumably this effect, if real, could reflect immunosuppression produced by transfused blood. For this reason, careful review of the risks and benefits of blood transfusions in these patients may be prudent.

Prostate Cancer

Prostate cancer is the second leading cause of death among men who die because of cancer.[23] The reported number of cases of prostate cancer has increased dramatically, presumably reflecting the widespread use of prostate-specific antigen (PSA) testing. The incidence of prostate cancer is highest in African-Americans, and the lowest incidence is in Asians. Prostate cancer is often not detected during the patient's lifetime, being discovered during autopsy as asymptomatic, occult foci of well differentiated prostate cancer. The presence of the hereditary prostate cancer (HPC-1) gene mutation greatly increases the risk of developing prostate cancer. The possibility that previous vasectomy may be associated with an increased risk of prostate cancer is not substantiated. Prostate cancer is almost always an adenocarcinoma.

Diagnosis

The use of PSA-based screening has changed the way prostate cancer is diagnosed. Increased serum PSA concentrations (normal concentrations increase with aging) may indicate the presence of prostate cancer in asymptomatic men and thus prompt a digital rectal examination (Table 28-6).[23] Detection of a discrete nodule or diffuse induration on digital rectal examination leads to suspicion of prostate cancer, especially in the presence of impotence or symptoms of urinary obstruction (frequency, nocturia, hesitancy, urgency). However, the rectal examination can evaluate only the posterior and lateral aspects of the patient's prostate. If the rectal examination indicates the possible presence of cancer, transrectal ultrasonography is utilized regardless of the PSA concentration. There is a much greater likelihood of detecting cancer if the PSA level is higher than 10 ng/ml, regardless of the findings on rectal examination. Abnormal results on ultrasonography (cancer is hypoechoic) can help direct the biopsy. Infrequently, patients present with symptoms of metastatic disease, such as diffuse bone pain and weight loss.

Treatment

Focal, well differentiated prostate cancers are usually cured by transurethral resection. Nevertheless, progressive disease may develop in up to 16% of

these patients within 8 years.[23] For this reason, more aggressive treatment such as radical prostatectomy or radiation may be indicated in subsets of these patients, especially those less than 65 years of age. If lymph nodes are involved, radical prostatectomy or definitive radiation therapy is often recommended. Radical prostatectomy may be performed via a retropubic or perineal approach. The retropubic approach permits the surgeon to take lymph node samples from frozen sections before beginning the prostatectomy. Radiation therapy can be delivered either by an external beam using a linear accelerator or by implantation of iodine-125 or radioactive gold into the prostate. The decision to select surgery or radiation is based on the side effects of each treatment. Impotence and urinary incontinence are risks of radical prostatectomy. Radiation therapy produces impotence less often but debilitating cystitis or proctitis may develop. Attempts to preserve the neurovascular bundles on each side of the prostate may decrease the risk of impotence following surgery. Brachytherapy is implantation of radioactive seeds of iodine or palladium into precise sites in the prostate gland. Cryosurgery involves inserting probes containing liquid nitrogen into the prostate causing cellular necrosis and sloughing.

Hormonal ablative therapy is indicated for management of metastatic prostate cancer, as these cancers are under the tropic influence of androgens. The goals of androgen deprivation is to produce regression of the disease and to produce castrate levels of testosterone and dihydrotestosterone. Such goals can be obtained by surgical castration, administration of exogenous estrogens such as diethylstilbestrol, use of analogues of luteinizing hormone-releasing hormone (LHRH) that inhibit the release of pituitary gonadotropins, use of antiandrogens such as flutamide that block the action of androgens at target tissues, and use of combination therapy, such as an antiandrogen in combination with an LHRH agonist or bilateral orchiectomy.

When advanced prostate cancers become resistant to hormone therapy, incapacitating bone pain often develops. Systemic chemotherapy with cyclophosphamide, 5-fluorouracil, cisplatin, and doxorubicin (each alone or in combinations) is often effective in palliating pain. In the terminal phases of the disease, high doses of prednisone for short periods often produce subjective improvement.

Breast Cancer

Women in the United States have a 12.6% lifetime risk of developing breast cancer, and the risk of death from breast cancer is 3.6%.[24] Most women in

Table 28-6 • Age-Specific Prostate-Specific Antigen Concentrations

Age (years)	Normal (ng/ml)
40–49	0–2.5
50–59	0–3.5
60–69	0–4.5
70–79	0–6.5

Adapted from: Garnick MB. Prostate cancer. Sci Am Med 1997;1–10.

whom breast cancer is diagnosed do not die from the disease, with the cure rate estimated to be 70%. It is estimated that more than 2 million women in the United States are living with a history of breast cancer. Because of increased awareness and use of screening mammography, in situ cancers now account for about 20% of newly diagnosed cases of breast cancer.

Risk Factors

The principal risk factors for development of breast cancer are increasing age (75% of cases occur in patients older than 50 years of age) and family history (a first-degree relative diagnosed when younger than 50 years of age increases the risk three- to fourfold). An estimated 5% to 8% of breast cancers occur in high risk families. Reproductive risk factors that increase the risk of breast cancer include early menarche, late menopause, late first pregnancy, and nulliparity, which all are presumed to prolong exposure of the breasts to estrogen. Two breast cancer susceptibility genes (BRCA1, BRCA2) are mutations that are inherited as autosomal dominant traits.

Screening

Recommended screening strategies for breast cancer include the triad of breast self-examination, clinical breast examination by a professional, and screening mammography. Clinical breast examination by a professional and regular mammography appear to decrease mortality from breast cancer by 25% to 30% in women older than 50 years. Annual screening mammography is recommended for women older than 40 years who are at standard risk for breast cancer. An estimated 10% to 15% of breast cancers are not detected by mammography suggesting that alternative screening methods (ultrasonography, magnetic resonance imaging) may be of value in selected patients.

Prognosis

Axillary node status and tumor size are the two most important determinants of outcome in patients with early breast cancer. Other established prognostic factors include estrogen receptor and progesterone receptor content of the primary tumor and its histologic grade. An absence of estrogen receptor and progesterone receptor expression is associated with a poorer prognosis. Most tumors that express receptors are responsive to endocrine therapy.

Treatment

Although radical mastectomy (removal of the involved breast, axillary contents, and underlying chest wall musculature) was the principal treatment for invasive breast cancer in the past, it is seldom utilized in current practice.[25] Breast conservation therapy, involving lumpectomy with radiation therapy, and modified radical mastectomy, involving removal of the breast and axillary nodes, provide similar survival rates. Because the likelihood of distant micrometastatic spread is highly correlated with the number of lymph nodes involved, axillary dissection provides useful prognostic information. Therapeutic benefit from axillary node dissection is minimal. The morbidity associated with breast cancer surgery is largely related to side effects of lymph node dissection (lymphedema and restricted arm motion). Obesity, weight gain, and infection in the arm are additional risk factors for the development of lymphedema. To minimize the chance of lymphedema, it is reasonable to protect the ipsilateral arm from venipuncture, compression, infection, and exposure to heat. Alternatively, sentinel lymph node mapping involves injection of a radioactive tracer or isosulfan blue dye into the area around the primary breast tumor. The injected substance tracks rapidly to the dominant axillary lymph node ("sentinel node"). If the sentinel node is tumor-free, the remaining lymph nodes are likely to be tumor-free and further axillary surgery can be avoided. Administration of isosulfan blue dye causes transient decreases in SpO_2, as measured by pulse oximetry.[26] In typical patients, maximal SpO_2 decreases of 3% occur 25 minutes after injection of isosulfan blue.

Radiation is an important component of breast conservation therapy, as lumpectomy alone is associated with a high incidence of recurrence. The value of postmastectomy radiation is not confirmed, and cardiac toxicity is a risk. As a result, postmastectomy radiation is often reserved for women with extensive local disease, such as skin and chest wall invasion, or extensive lymph node involvement.

Systemic Treatment

The recognition that many women with early-stage breast cancer already have distant micrometastases at the time of diagnosis is the rationale for systemic therapy. Systemic therapy is intended to prevent or delay recurrence of the disease. Ovarian ablation, tamoxifen therapy, and chemotherapy are the most commonly utilized modes of systemic therapy.

Tamoxifen. Tamoxifen is a mixed estrogen agonist-antagonist that has become the most commonly prescribed antineoplastic drug.[25] The principal beneficial effect of tamoxifen is related to its interactions with estrogen receptors. In patients with minimal or no estrogen receptor expression in their tumors, tamoxifen does not alter outcome. Conversely, tamoxifen therapy for 5 years in patients with estrogen receptor, positive tumors was associated with significant decreases in the incidence of recurrence and mortality 10 years after the initial diagnosis. Benefits of tamoxifen therapy are similar for node-positive and node-negative patients.

Tamoxifen can cause body temperature disturbances, vaginal discharge, and increases the risk of developing uterine endometrial cancer. Megestrol (progestin) may be administered to decrease the severity of body temperature disturbances associated with tamoxifen treatment. Tamoxifen lowers the serum concentrations of cholesterol and low density lipoproteins, but the importance of these effects on lowering the risk of ischemic heart disease is unclear.[24] Tamoxifen preserves bone density in postmenopausal women by its proestrogenic effects and may decrease the incidence of osteoporotic fractures of the hip, spine, and radius. There is an increased risk of thromboembolic events, including deep venous thrombosis, pulmonary embolism, and stroke. Raloxifene, like tamoxifen, is a selective estrogen-receptor modulator.

Chemotherapy. Combination chemotherapy decreases the rate of recurrence and mortality from breast cancer, and the effects are present in node-positive and node-negative patients. The absolute benefit seems to be in node-positive women less than 50 years of age. A commonly utilized combination chemotherapy regimen includes cyclophosphamide, methotrexate, and 5-fluorouracil. Regimens including doxorubicin, paclitaxel, and docetaxel are also being utilized. The chemotherapy dose is an important determinant of cell kill. Conventional adjuvant chemotherapy usually begins within a few months after surgery. Use of primary chemotherapy preceding surgery or radiation is a consideration in selected patients in attempts to decrease tumor size and improve breast conservation. In high risk women with multiple positive lymph nodes, high-dose chemotherapy with alkylating drugs combined with autologous bone marrow transplantation is a consideration.

Chemotherapy for breast cancer can have adverse effects that typically resolve following treatment (nausea and vomiting, hair loss, bone marrow suppression). Induction of menopause is a common concern in young patients. The most serious late sequelae of chemotherapy are leukemia and doxorubicin-induced cardiac impairment. Clinically significant CHF develops in 0.5% to 1.0% of women treated with standard anthracycline-based chemotherapy regimens. Patients with symptoms of cardiac disease or CHF should be evaluated with an ECG and echocardiography. Myelodysplastic syndromes or acute myeloid leukemia can arise after chemotherapy, but the incidence is low (0.2% to 1.0%). The development of cytopenia in breast cancer patients following chemotherapy may be evidence of these chemotherapy-related side effects. High-dose radiation may be associated with plexopathy or nerve damage, pneumonitis, pulmonary fibrosis, and cardiac damage.

Supportive Treatment

Palliation of symptoms and prevention of complications are primary goals when treating advanced breast cancer. Bone is the most common site of breast cancer metastases. Regular administration of bisphosphonates (pamidronate, clodronate) in addition to hormone therapy or chemotherapy can decrease bone pain and lower the incidence of bone complications by virtue of inhibiting osteoclast activity. Erythropoietin may be useful for diminishing symptoms of chemotherapy-related bone marrow suppression. The cardiotoxicity of doxorubicin may be decreased through the use of the cardioprotective drug dexrazoxane or liposomal preparations.[25] Adequate pain control is usually achieved with sustained-release oral and transdermal opioid preparations.

Management of Anesthesia

Preoperative evaluation of patients for side effects related to chemotherapy is recommended. Placement of intravenous catheters in the ipsilateral arm is avoided, as exacerbation of lymphedema and the susceptibility to infection are considerations. It is also useful to protect the ipsilateral arm from compression and exposure to heat. The presence of bone pain and pathologic fractures is considered when selecting regional anesthesia and when positioning patients during surgery. Preoperative administration of opioids is helpful for patients experiencing pain prior to arriving in the operating room. Selection of anesthetic drugs, techniques, and special monitoring is influenced more by the planned surgical procedure than the presence of breast cancer. If isosulfan blue dye is injected during the surgical procedure, it is likely that pulse oximetry will demonstrate a transient and spurious decrease in the measured SpO_2 value (about a 3% decrease occurring approximately 25 minutes after injection of the dye).[26]

LESS COMMON CANCERS ENCOUNTERED IN CLINICAL PRACTICE

Less common cancers encountered clinically include cardiac tumors, head and neck cancer, cancers involving the endocrine glands, liver, gallbladder, genitourinary tract, and reproductive organs. Lymphomas and leukemias are examples of cancers involving the lymph glands and blood-forming elements.

Cardiac Tumors

Cardiac tumors may be primary or secondary and benign or malignant. Metastatic cardiac involvement occurs 20 to 40 times more often than do primary tumors.

Cardiac Myxomas

Cardiac myxomas account for more than one-half of all benign cardiac tumors that occur in adults.[27] Myxomas often show considerable movement within the cardiac chamber during the cardiac cycle. About 70% of cardiac myxomas occur in the left atrium, and the remaining 30% are in the right atrium.

Signs and Symptoms

Signs and symptoms of cardiac myxomas reflect interference with filling and emptying of the involved cardiac chamber and release of emboli composed of myxomatous material or thrombi that have formed in the tumor (Table 28–7). Left atrial myxomas may mimic mitral valve disease with the development of pulmonary edema. Conversely, right atrial myxomas mimic tricuspid disease and are associated with impaired venous return and evidence of right heart failure. Right atrial myxomas may manifest as isolated tricuspid stenosis (mimics constrictive pericarditis), dyspnea, and arterial hypoxemia. Embolism occurs in 30% to 40% of patients

---

Table 28–7 • Signs and Symptoms of Cardiac Myxomas

Refractory congestive heart failure
Unexplained cardiac rhythm disturbances
Syncope related to body position changes
Unexplained systemic or pulmonary emboli
Pulmonary hypertension of unknown cause

---

with cardiac myxomas.[27] Because most myxomas are located in the left atrium, systemic embolism is particularly frequent. In most patients the cerebral arteries including the retinal arteries, are involved. Cardiac myxomas may occur as part of a syndrome that includes cutaneous myxomas, myxoid fibroadenomas of the breast, pituitary adenomas, and adrenocortical hyperplasia with Cushing syndrome.

Diagnosis

Echocardiography can be utilized to determine the location, size, shape, attachment, and mobility of cardiac myxomas. There are reports of the incidental discovery of cardiac myxomas during intraoperative transesophageal echocardiography monitoring of patients undergoing emergency surgery for embolectomy of a peripheral artery.[28, 29] In this regard, any surgically removed emboli should be examined microscopically for myxomatous material. Cardiac myxomas at least 0.5 to 1.0 cm in diameter can be identified by computed tomography and magnetic resonance imaging.

Treatment

Surgical resection of cardiac myxomas is usually curative. After the diagnosis has been established, prompt surgery is indicated because of the possibility of sudden death and embolic complications. In most cases cardiac myxomas can be removed easily because they are pedunculated. Intraoperative fragmentation of the tumor and embolism are carefully avoided. All chambers of the heart are examined to eliminate the presence of multifocal tumors. Mechanical damage to the heart valve or adhesion of the tumor to valve leaflets may necessitate valve replacement.

Management of Anesthesia

Anesthetic considerations in patients with cardiac myxomas include the possible presence of low cardiac output and arterial hypoxemia owing to obstruction at the tricuspid valve.[30, 31] Symptoms of obstruction to blood flow may be exacerbated by changes in body position. The presence of a right atrial myxoma prohibits placement of right atrial or pulmonary artery catheters. Supraventricular cardiac dysrhythmias may follow surgical removal of atrial myxomas. In some patients, permanent cardiac pacing is needed because of atrioventricular conduction disturbances.

Metastatic Cardiac Tumors

Metastatic cardiac tumors are present in about 10% of all patients who die from cancer, but only 5% to

10% of these patients are symptomatic. Tumors most likely to metastasize to the heart include lung and breast cancer, Kaposi's sarcoma, and leukemia. Manifestations of metastatic cardiac tumors most often reflect pericardial metastases. Malignant pericardial perfusions are often hemorrhagic, and cardiac tamponade is possible. The pericardium is sometimes encased in tumor, producing a disorder resembling cardiomyopathy or constrictive pericarditis. Atrial fibrillation may be an early manifestation of malignant involvement of the pericardium. Malignant pericardial effusions are the most common cause of electrical alternans on the ECG. Echocardiography, computed tomography, and magnetic resonance imaging are all useful in the diagnosis of pericardial and cardiac metastases. Treatment is most often related to management of pericardial effusions that may produce cardiac tamponade.

Primary Malignant Tumors

Primary malignant tumors involving the heart are most often a form of sarcoma and are more likely to occur in the right heart than the left heart. Signs and symptoms reflect intracavitary growth of the tumor, including pulmonary artery outflow tract obstruction. Sudden onset and rapid progression of refractory CHF, especially right ventricular failure, is common, as is syncope. Tumor invasion of the myocardium and compromise of the coronary circulation may resemble myocardial ischemia and infarction.

Head and Neck Cancers

Head and neck cancers account for about 5% of all cancers in the United States, with a predominance in men older than 50 years of age. Most patients have a history of excessive cigarette smoking and alcohol abuse. The most common sites of metastases are lungs, liver, and bone. Hypercalcemia may be associated with bone metastases, whereas altered liver function tests presumably reflect alcohol-induced disease. Preoperative nutritional therapy may be indicated before surgical resection of the tumor, which often uses laser technology. The goals of chemotherapy, if selected, are to decrease the bulk of the primary tumors or known metastases, thereby enhancing the efficacy of subsequent surgery or radiation. A secondary goal is eradication of subclinical occult micrometastases.

Thyroid Cancer

Clinically detectable thyroid cancers constitute fewer than 1% of all human cancers.[32] Papillary and follicular (differentiated) thyroid cancers are among the most curable cancers. Thyroid cancers are more frequent in women. External radiation to the neck during childhood increases the risk of papillary thyroid cancers. Nuclear accidents that result in exposure to radioactive isotopes of iodine have direct carcinogenic effects on the thyroid. Medullary thyroid cancers may be associated with pheochromocytomas in an autosomal dominant disorder known as multiple endocrine neoplasia type 2 (MEN 2). This type of thyroid cancer typically produces large amounts of thyrocalcitonin, providing a sensitive measure of the presence of the disease as well as its cure.

Surgical resection of all tumor tissue in the neck (leaving no more than 2 to 3 g of thyroid tissue) results in lower recurrence rates than a more limited thyroidectomy. Risks of total thyroidectomy include recurrent laryngeal nerve injuries and hypoparathyroidism. Even with total thyroidectomy, often some thyroid tissue remains, as detected by postoperative scanning with iodine-131. In patients with papillary thyroid cancers, paratracheal and tracheoesophageal lymph nodes are dissected. The growth of thyroid tumor cells is controlled by thyrotropin, and inhibition of thyrotropin secretion with thyroxine improves survival rates.

Esophageal Cancer

Excessive alcohol consumption and chronic cigarette smoking are thought to be independent risk factors responsible for 80% or more of the esophageal cancers in the United States. Dysphagia and weight loss are the initial symptoms of esophageal cancer in 90% of patients. The disease is usually incurable by the time these clinical symptoms are present. The lack of a serosal layer around the esophagus and the presence of an extensive lymphatic system result in rapid spread of the tumor, especially to the liver and lungs. Difficulty swallowing may result in regurgitation and the risk of aspiration.

The results of primary radiation therapy resemble those of radical surgery, with a 5-year survival rate of about 5%. Chemotherapy and radiation may be instituted prior to attempting surgical resection. Palliation may include surgical placement of a feeding tube or a polyvinyl esophageal prosthesis.

The likelihood of underlying alcohol-induced liver disease, chronic obstructive pulmonary disease from cigarette smoking, and cross-tolerance with other anesthetic drugs is a consideration during anesthetic management of affected patients. Furthermore, extensive weight loss often parallels decreases in intravascular fluid volume, manifesting as hypotension during induction and maintenance of anesthesia.

Gastric Cancer

The incidence of gastric cancer has decreased dramatically since 1930, when it was the leading cause of cancer-related death among men in the United States.[33] Loss of gastric acidity and the appearance of pernicious anemia contributes to the development of gastric cancer. The presenting features of gastric cancer (indigestion, epigastric distress, anorexia) are indistinguishable from those of benign peptic ulcers. About 90% of gastric cancers are adenocarcinomas, and about 50% of them occur in the distal portion of the stomach. Gastric cancer is usually far advanced when symptoms such as weight loss and ascites appear.

Complete surgical eradication of gastric tumors with resection of adjacent lymph nodes is the only treatment that may be curative.[33] Resection of the primary lesion can also offer the most effective means of symptomatic palliation. Gastric cancer is relatively resistant to radiation therapy. Chemotherapy is not greatly effective for managing patients with gastric cancer.

Liver Cancer

Liver cancer occurs most often in men with cirrhosis of the liver caused by hepatitis B. Initial manifestations are often a painful mass in the right upper quadrant accompanied by weight loss. There is often compression of the inferior vena cava and/or portal vein and synthesis of abnormal prothrombin molecules, resulting in impaired coagulation. Liver function tests are likely to be abnormal. Computed tomography of the liver can determine the anatomic location of the tumor, although angiography is more useful for distinguishing hepatocellular cancer (hypervascular) from hepatic metastases (hypovascular) and for determining if the tumor is resectable. Radical surgical resection or liver transplantation offers the only hope for survival. Most patients with liver cancer are not surgical candidates because of extensive cirrhosis and impaired liver function. Chemotherapy is of limited value, whereas radiation is principally useful for pain relief.

Gallbladder Cancer

Gallbladder cancer is uncommon in the United States, occurring more often in females and being discovered unexpectedly during performance of cholecystectomy to treat cholelithiasis. The risk of gallbladder cancer in patients with asymptomatic cholelithiasis is no greater than the operative mortality for cholecystectomy. Therefore cholecystectomy is not recommended as a prophylactic measure for gallbladder cancer. When gallbladder cancer is invasive at discovery, the 5-year survival rate is less than 5% despite radical surgery, postoperative irradiation, and chemotherapy.

Pancreatic Cancer

Pancreatic cancer, despite its low incidence, is the fourth most common cause of cancer-related mortality. There is no evidence linking this cancer to alcohol abuse, caffeine ingestion, cholelithiasis, or diabetes mellitus, but cigarette smoking shows a positive correlation. About 95% of pancreatic cancers are ductal adenocarcinomas, with most occurring in the head of the pancreas. Abdominal pain, anorexia, and weight loss are often insidious initial symptoms. Pain suggests retroperitoneal invasion and infiltration of splanchnic nerves. Jaundice reflects biliary obstruction in patients with tumor in the head of the pancreas. Diabetes mellitus is rare in patients who develop pancreatic cancer.

Pancreatic cancer may appear as a localized mass or as diffuse enlargement of the gland on computed tomography of the abdomen. Biopsy of the lesion is needed to confirm the diagnosis.

Complete surgical resection is the only effective treatment of ductal pancreatic cancer. Patients most likely to have resectable lesions are those with tumors in the head of the pancreas that cause painless jaundice. Extrapancreatic spread eliminates the possibility of surgical cure. The two most commonly employed surgical resection techniques are total pancreatectomy and pancreatoduodenectomy (Whipple procedure). Total pancreatectomy is technically easier but has the disadvantage of producing diabetes mellitus and malabsorption. Only 10% of patients who undergo complete resection survive 5 years, whereas the median survival for patients with unresectable tumors is 5 months. Palliative procedures include surgical diversion of the biliary system, radiation, and chemotherapy. Celiac plexus block with alcohol or phenol is the most effective intervention for treating the pain associated with pancreatic cancer (see "Acute and Chronic Pain").[5] Complications of celiac plexus block include hypotension due to sympathetic nervous system denervation, especially in chronically ill hypovolemic patients. Computed tomography may be used to confirm proper needle placement before injecting any solution intended to act on the celiac plexus.

Renal Cell Cancer

Renal cell cancer most often manifests in men as hematuria, flank pain, and a palpable mass. Risk factors include a family history and cigarette smoking. Renal ultrasonography helps identify renal cysts, and computed tomography and magnetic resonance imaging are useful for determining the presence and extent of renal cancers. Evaluation for distant metastases includes chest radiographs, bone scan, and liver function tests. Altered laboratory values may include eosinophilia and liver function abnormalities. High-output CHF, when it occurs, is presumed to reflect the development of a renal arteriovenous fistula. The only curative treatment for renal adenocarcinoma limited to the kidneys is radical nephrectomy with regional lymphadenectomy. Radical nephrectomy is not helpful in patients with distant metastases, whereas chemotherapy may show some efficacy, although the 5-year survival is less than 5%.

Bladder Cancer

Bladder cancer occurs most often in men and is associated with cigarette smoking and chronic exposure to chemicals, as used in the textile and rubber industries. The most common presenting feature is gross, painless hematuria. The urine survivin assay appears to provide a practical and noninvasive test to identify patients with new or recurrent bladder cancer.[34] Metastatic disease is characterized by involvement of adjacent lymph nodes and spread to the lungs, liver, and bones.

Treatment of noninvasive bladder cancer includes endoscopic resection and intravesical chemotherapy. Carcinoma in situ of the bladder, unlike that of the uterine cervix, often behaves virulently and may require cystectomy to help prevent muscle invasion and metastatic spread. Traditional treatment for metastatic disease often includes preoperative radiation followed by cystectomy and chemotherapy. The most common urinary diversion is ureteroileostomy. Alternatively, creation of an artificial bladder from segments of the patient's colon may obviate the need for external diversion.

Testicular Cancer

Although testicular cancer is rare, it is the most common cancer in young males and represents a tumor that can be cured even when distant metastases are present. Orchipexy before 2 years of age is recommended for cryptorchidism to decrease the risk of testicular cancer. Initial manifestations of testicular cancer are usually the appearance of a painless mass. When the diagnosis is suspected, an inguinal orchiectomy is performed and the diagnosis histologically confirmed. A transcrotal biopsy is not performed, as disruption of the scrotum may predispose to local recurrences and metastatic spread to inguinal lymphatics. Germ cell cancers, which account for 95% of testicular cancers, can be subdivided into seminomas and nonseminomas. Seminomas often metastasize through regional lymphatics to the retroperitoneum and mediastinum, and nonseminomas spread hematogenously to viscera, especially the liver and lungs. Abdominal and pelvic computed tomography are useful for assessing metastatic disease.

Patients with seminomas that do not extend beyond the retroperitoneal lymph nodes are treated with radiation. Chemotherapy is recommended when seminomas are advanced. Nonseminomas are not radiation sensitive and are treated with retroperitoneal lymph node dissection, often with adjuvant chemotherapy. Side effects of chemotherapy in these patients may include anemia, cardiac toxicity, pulmonary toxicity, nephrotoxicity, and peripheral neuropathy (see "Management of Anesthesia," "Side Effects of Chemotherapy").

Uterine Cervix Cancer

Uterine cervix cancer is the most common gynecologic cancer in females aged 15 to 34 years. Viruses such as herpes simplex and human papillomavirus may predispose to uterine cervix cancer. Carcinoma in situ as detected by a Papanicolaou (Pap) smear is treated with a cone biopsy, whereas disease that has metastasized is treated with radiation therapy, surgery, and chemotherapy.

Uterine Cancer

Cancer involving the uterine endometrium occurs most frequently in women 50 to 70 years of age and may be associated with obesity, systemic hypertension, and diabetes mellitus. Women who smoke heavily may be at decreased risk for uterine endometrial cancer, presumably reflecting decreased estrogen levels caused by cigarette smoking.[35] Common manifestations of uterine cancer are vaginal bleeding in menopausal or perimenopausal women. The initial evaluation of these patients often includes fractional dilation and curettage. In the absence of metastatic disease, a total abdominal hysterectomy and bilateral salpingo-oophorectomy with or without radiation is the treatment. Hormonal therapy, usually with progesterone, is useful for treating patients with metastatic disease. Chemotherapy has not been widely utilized for endometrial cancer.

Ovarian Cancer

Ovarian cancer is most likely to develop in women who experience early menopause or who have family histories of ovarian cancer. Advanced disease is usually present when the disease is discovered, often including omental metastases, reflecting lymphatic drainage of the ovaries through retroperitoneal lymph nodes. Surgery is the treatment of early-stage ovarian cancer, often followed by chemotherapy or radiation. The efficacy of chemotherapy is increased when the tumor mass has been decreased by surgery. Intraperitoneal chemotherapy is indicated in selected patients.

Cutaneous Melanoma

The incidence of cutaneous melanoma is increasing more rapidly than that of any other cancer, affecting as many as 1 in every 90 Americans.[36] There is evidence that sunlight (ultraviolet light) is an important environmental factor in the pathogenesis of melanoma. Melanoma is suspected when there is a change in color, size, shape, or surface of a mole. The initial treatment of a suspected lesion is excisional biopsy. Evidence of metastatic disease is most likely in the lymph nodes, brain, liver, lungs, and bones. Metastatic melanomas are usually incurable, with palliation provided by regional lymph node dissection, radiation, and chemotherapy.

Bone Cancer

Bone cancer manifests as multiple myeloma, osteosarcoma, Ewing's tumor, and chondrosarcoma.

Multiple Myeloma

Multiple myeloma (plasma cell myeloma, myelomatosis) is a malignant neoplasm characterized by poorly controlled growth of a single clone of plasma cells, which are immunoglobulin-secreting cells. Multiple myeloma accounts for 10% to 15% of hematologic cancers and 1% of all cancers.[37, 38] The disease is more common in elderly patients, and it occurs twice as often in African-Americans as in Caucasians. The cause of multiple myeloma is unknown;

and its extent, complications, sensitivity to drugs, and clinical course vary greatly among patients.

Signs and Symptoms

The most frequent manifestations of multiple myeloma are painful pathologic fractures (often vertebral collapse), anemia, thrombocytopenia, neutropenia, hypercalcemia, renal failure, and recurrent bacterial infections reflecting bone marrow invasion by tumor cells.[37] Extension into the spinal cord can produce extramedullary compression. Other extramedullary sites of tumor invasion include the liver, spleen, nasopharynx, and paranasal sinuses. Peripheral neuropathy may reflect segmental demyelination. Inactivation of plasma procoagulants by myeloma proteins may interfere with coagulation. These proteins may also prolong the bleeding time by interfering with platelet function. The presence of hypercalcemia from excessive bone destruction should be suspected in patients with myeloma who develop nausea, fatigue, confusion, or polyuria. Renal insufficiency occurs in about 25% of patients with multiple myeloma due to deposition of an abnormal protein (Bence Jones protein) in renal tubules. Dehydration must be avoided, especially in patients with Bence Jones proteinuria, as they are at risk for the development of nephropathy. Amyloidosis or immunoglobulin deposition disease, which causes or contributes to renal failure in some patients, should be suspected if albuminuria is present. Unexplained high-output CHF has been observed in patients with multiple myeloma.[39] Recurrent bacterial infections are a major cause of morbidity in patients with multiple myeloma and are most common in those with bone marrow depression and impaired immune responses due to advanced disease or those with granulocytopenia caused by chemotherapy. The combination of hypogammaglobulinemia, granulocytopenia, and low cell-mediated immunity increases the risk of infection. Development of fever in patients with multiple myeloma is an indication for antibiotic therapy. In an estimated 20% of patients, multiple myeloma is diagnosed by chance in the absence of symptoms when screening laboratory studies reveal increased serum protein concentrations.

Treatment

Treatment of symptomatic multiple myeloma most often includes chemotherapy with intermittent courses of melphalan and prednisone. Mild granulocytopenia and/or thrombocytopenia may accompany treatment with melphalan. Drug-induced remission is characterized by at least a 75% decrease in production of serum myeloma proteins and a 95% decrease in Bence Jones proteinuria. The median duration of remission is about 2 years and the median survival approximately 3 years. Fewer than 10% of patients live longer than 10 years, and there is no evidence that this disease is ever cured.[37] Other chemotherapeutic combinations have included vincristine, doxorubicin, and dexamethasone.

The pain of vertebral compression fractures may be relieved by chemotherapy, but local radiation combined with high-dose corticosteroid therapy is necessary if pain is severe. Signs of spinal cord compression due to an extramedullary plasmacytoma require early confirmation with magnetic resonance imaging and prompt radiation. Urgent decompressive laminectomy may be needed if radiation is not effective to avoid permanent paralysis. Chemotherapy reverses mild renal failure in many patients with multiple myeloma, whereas temporary hemodialysis may be necessary in the presence of severe renal failure to permit time for chemotherapy to become effective. Erythropoietin therapy may be indicated to treat anemia. Prevention of dehydration is important if hypercalcemia is present. Hypercalcemia requires prompt treatment with intravenous infusions of saline and administration of furosemide (see Chapter 21). Bed rest is avoided, as inactivity leads to mobilization of calcium and the formation of venous thrombi due to venous stasis.

Management of Anesthesia

The presence of compression fractures emphasizes the need for caution when positioning these patients during anesthesia and surgery. Postoperatively, pathologic fractures of the ribs may impair ventilation and predispose to the development of pneumonia. Altered responses to drugs owing to abnormal circulating immunoglobulins plus hypoalbuminemia are theoretical but undocumented concerns.

Osteosarcoma

Osteosarcoma occurs most often in adolescents and typically involves the long bones. A genetic predisposition is suggested by the association of this tumor with retinoblastoma. Computed tomography is used to assess the extent of the primary lesion and the existence of metastatic disease, especially in the lungs. Serum alkaline phosphatase concentrations are likely to be increased in the presence of metastatic disease. Treatment consists of chemotherapy followed by surgical excision. Success of chemotherapy may permit limb salvage procedures in selected patients. Pulmonary resection may be indicated in patients with isolated metastatic lung lesions.

Ewing's Tumor

Ewing's tumor or sarcoma usually occurs in patients less than 30 years of age and most often involves the pelvis, femur, and tibia. Metastatic disease is usually present at diagnosis. Treatment consists of surgery, local radiation, and chemotherapy.

Chondrosarcoma

Chondrosarcoma usually involves the pelvis, ribs, or upper end of the femur or humerus in young adults. This tumor grows slowly and is treated by radical surgical excision.

■ LYMPHOMAS AND LEUKEMIAS

Hodgkin's Disease

Hodgkin's disease is a lymphoma that has both an infective (Epstein-Barr virus) and genetic association. Another factor that appears to predispose to the development of lymphoma is impaired immunity as present in patients with an organ transplant or AIDS. The most useful diagnostic test in patients with suspected lymphomas is lymph node biopsy.

A typical onset of Hodgkin's disease is a painless enlarging mass that classically appears in the patient's neck. Pruritus can be generalized and severe. Cyclic increases in body temperature and unexplained weight loss may occur. Superior vena cava obstruction reflects invasion of the mediastinum by tumor. Moderately severe anemia is often present. Chest radiographs often reflect involvement of the lungs that also often invades the liver and spleen. Peripheral neuropathies and spinal cord compression may occur as a direct result of tumor growth. Bone marrow and central nervous system involvement is unusual in Hodgkin's disease but not in other lymphomas.

Surgical exploration of the patient's abdomen permits evaluation of the spread of Hodgkin's disease and is the basis for classifying lymphomas in preparation for selecting appropriate therapy. Radiation therapy is curative for localized Hodgkin's disease, and there is general agreement that advanced Hodgkin's disease can be cured by combination chemotherapy.[40] Autologous bone marrow or peripheral blood stem cell transplantation are considerations for patients who experience relapses despite prior successful chemotherapy.

Leukemia

Leukemia is the uncontrolled production of leukocytes owing to cancerous mutation of lymphogenous cells or myelogenous cells. Lymphocytic leukemias begin in lymph nodes and are named according to the type of hematopoietic cells that are primarily involved. Myeloid leukemias begin as cancerous production of myelogenous cells in bone marrow with spread to extramedullary organs. The principal difference between normal cells and leukemia cells is the ability of the latter to continue to divide. The result is an expanding mass of cells that infiltrate the bone marrow, rendering patients functionally aplastic. Anemia may be profound. Eventually, bone marrow failure is the cause of fatal infections or hemorrhage due to thrombocytopenia. In addition to bone marrow, leukemia cells may infiltrate the liver, spleen, lymph nodes, and meninges, producing signs of dysfunction at these sites. Extensive use of nutrients by rapidly proliferating cancerous cells depletes amino acids, leading to patient fatigue and metabolic starvation of normal tissues.

Acute Lymphoblastic Leukemia

Acute lymphoblastic leukemia accounts for about 15% of all leukemias in adults. Central nervous system dysfunction is common. Affected patients are highly susceptible to life-threatening opportunistic infections, including those due to *Pneumocystis carinii* and cytomegalovirus. Chemotherapy may cure as many as 70% of children with acute lymphoblastic leukemia and often produces remissions in adults.[41]

Chronic Lymphocytic Leukemia

Chronic lymphocytic leukemia is one of the most common leukemias in adults, accounting for about 25% of all leukemias, especially in elderly patients. This form of leukemia rarely occurs in children.[41] The diagnosis of chronic lymphocytic leukemia is confirmed by the presence of lymphocytosis and lymphocytic infiltrates in bone marrow. Signs and symptoms are highly variable, with the extent of bone marrow infiltration often determining the clinical course. Autoimmune hemolytic anemia and hypersplenism that results in pancytopenia and thrombocytopenia may be prominent. Lymph node enlargement may obstruct the ureters. Recurrent infections may require repeated antibiotic therapy or intravenous infusion of immunoglobulins. Chemotherapy with alkylating drugs is the indicated therapy, as corticosteroids do not destroy leukemic lymphocytes. Splenectomy occasionally is necessary.

Adult T Cell Leukemia

Adult T cell leukemia, a rapidly fatal disease, is characterized by leukocytosis, hepatosplenomegaly,

cutaneous lesions, and hypercalcemia. Lytic bone lesions are the likely explanation for hypercalcemia. A human retrovirus termed human T cell lymphotropic virus type 1 (HTLV-1) has been isolated from affected patients. Opportunistic infections caused by *Pneumocystis carinii* and cytomegalovirus are common, as is central nervous system involvement.

Acute Myeloid Leukemia

Acute myeloid leukemia is characterized by increases in the number of myeloid cells in the affected individual's bone marrow and arrest of their maturation, frequently resulting in hematopoietic insufficiency (granulocytopenia, thrombocytopenia, anemia) with or without leukocytosis.[42] In the United States the annual incidence of acute myeloid leukemia is approximately 2.4 per 100,000 adults, and this incidence increases to 12.6 per 100,000 adults 65 years of age or older.

Clinical signs and symptoms of acute myeloid leukemia are diverse and nonspecific, but they are usually attributable to the leukemic infiltration of the bone marrow, with resulting cytopenia.[42] Typically, patients present with complaints of fatigue, hemorrhage, infections, and fever due to decreases in erythrocytes, platelets, or leukocytes. Dyspnea on exertion is common. Leukemic infiltration of various organs (hepatomegaly, splenomegaly, lymphadenopathy), bones, gingiva, and the central nervous system can produce a variety of symptoms. Hyperleukocytosis (more than 100,000 cells/mm^3) can result in symptoms of leukostasis (ocular and cerebrovascular dysfunction or bleeding). Metabolic abnormalities may include hyperuricemia and hypocalcemia.

The primary objective when treating acute myeloid leukemia is to induce remission and thereafter prevent relapse.[42] Chemotherapy with daunorubicin and cytarabine is administered to induce remission. Complete remission can be achieved in 70% to 80% of patients who are 60 years of age or younger and in about 50% of older patients. Bone marrow transplantation may be a consideration in selected patients.

Chronic Myeloid Leukemia

Chronic myeloid leukemia manifests as massive hepatosplenomegaly, often in the presence of leukocyte counts that exceed 50,000 cells/mm^3. High leukocyte counts may predispose to vascular occlusion. Anemia and thrombocytopenia may be profound in affected patients. Hyperuricemia is likely and is treated with allopurinol. Leukopheresis, splenectomy, and chemotherapy are often employed. Traditional treatment of chronic myeloid leukemia is with busulfan, although bone marrow transplantation may be the most effective treatment in selected patients.

Chemotherapy for Treatment of Leukemia

A kilogram of leukemia cells (about 10^{12} cells) appears to be a lethal mass. Symptoms leading to the diagnosis of leukemia are unlikely until the tumor load is about 10^9 cells. Chemotherapy is intended to decrease the number of tumor cells so organomegaly regresses and function of the bone marrow improves. Drugs used for chemotherapy are principally those that depress the activity of bone marrow, such that hemorrhage and infection become the determinants of maximum acceptable doses. Destruction of tumor cells by chemotherapy produces a uric acid load that may result in urate nephropathy and gouty arthritis. Nutritional support of patients undergoing chemotherapy may be necessary to prevent hypoalbuminemia and loss of immunocompetence.

Bone Marrow Transplantation for Treatment of Leukemia

Bone marrow transplantation offers an opportunity for cure of otherwise fatal nonmalignant and malignant diseases (Table 28–8).[43, 44] Autologous bone marrow transplantation entails donation of the patient's own bone marrow for subsequent reinfusion, whereas allogeneic transplantation uses bone mar-

row from immunocompatible donors. Regardless of the type of bone marrow transplantation, recipients must undergo a preoperative regimen designed to achieve functional bone marrow ablation produced by combinations of total body radiation and chemotherapy. Bone marrow is usually harvested by repeated aspirations from the donor's posterior iliac crest. For allogeneic bone marrow transplantation with major AB incompatibility between donor and recipient, it is necessary to remove mature erythrocytes from the graft to avoid hemolytic transfusion reactions. Removal of T cells from the allograft can decrease the risk of graft-versus-host disease.

Processing of the harvested bone marrow (eradicating malignant cells, removing incompatible erythrocytes) may take 2 to 12 hours. The condensed bone marrow volume (about 200 ml) is then infused into the recipient through an indwelling central venous catheter. From the systemic circulation, the bone marrow cells pass into the recipient's bone marrow, providing the microenvironment necessary for maturation and differentiation of the cells. The time of bone marrow engraftment is usually 10 to 28 days, during which time protective isolation of the patient is often utilized. While awaiting engraftment, it may be necessary to administer platelets to maintain the count above 20,000 cells/mm^3 and erythrocytes to maintain the hematocrit above 25%.

Anesthesia for Bone Marrow Transplantation

General anesthesia or regional anesthesia is needed to aspirate bone marrow from the donor's iliac crests. Nitrous oxide may be avoided in the donor because of potential bone marrow depression associated with the use of this drug. Nevertheless, there is no evidence that nitrous oxide administered during bone marrow harvesting adversely affects marrow engraftment and subsequent function. Brief heparinization before removal of bone marrow may influence the selection of spinal or epidural anesthesia. The volume of peripheral blood loss parallels the quantity of marrow harvested, emphasizing the substantial fluid loss that may accompany this procedure. Blood replacement may be necessary, either with autologous blood transfusions or by reinfusion of separated erythrocytes obtained during the harvest. The decision to place a Foley catheter is individualized and is influenced by the donor's general health, anticipated duration of the procedure, and estimated blood volume of bone marrow to be harvested. Postoperative complications are rare, although discomfort at bone puncture sites is predictable.

Table 28–8 • Diseases Treated by Bone Marrow Transplantation

Nonmalignant diseases
  Aplastic anemia
  Thalassemia
  Sickle cell disease
  Immunodeficiency disorders
    Wiskott-Aldrich syndrome
    Chediak-Higashi syndrome
  Genetic disorders
Malignant diseases
  Acute myeloid leukemia
  Myelodysplastic syndrome
  Acute lymphoblastic leukemia
  Chronic myelogenous leukemia
  Chronic lymphocytic leukemia
  Multiple myeloma
  Non-Hodgkin's lymphoma
  Hodgkin's disease
  Neuroblastoma
  Breast cancer
  Testicular cancer
  Malignant melanomas

Complications of Bone Marrow Transplantation

In addition to prolonged myelosuppression, bone marrow transplantation is associated with several unusual complications.[44]

Graft-versus-Host Disease. Graft-versus-host disease is a life-threatening complication of bone marrow transplantation manifesting as organ system dysfunction most often involving the skin, liver, and gastrointestinal tract (Table 28–9). It is unclear why the kidneys are usually spared. The most life-threatening complication is often the profound immunosuppression that accompanies this disease. This response occurs when immunologically competent cells in the graft target antigens on the recipient's cells.

Graft-verus-host disease can be divided into two somewhat distinct clinical entities: acute disease, which occurs during the first 30 to 60 days after bone marrow transplantation, and chronic disease, which develops at least 60 to 90 days after transplantation.[44] Patients undergoing allogeneic bone marrow transplantation typically undergo prophylactic treatment (cyclosporine, methotrexate, corticosteroids, removal of T cells from the graft) for acute graft-versus-host disease. Even with prophylaxis, however, most adult patients experience some degree of graft-versus-host disease after allogeneic bone marrow transplantation. The chronic form of graft-versus-host disease shares certain clinical characteristics with other immunologic disorders, such as scleroderma.

Graft Rejection. Rejection of a bone marrow graft in most patients represents destruction of the graft by immunologically active cells in the host.[44] The approach to prevention of graft rejection is use of preparative regimens that are maximally immunosuppressive.

Pulmonary Complications. A common cause of death following allogeneic bone marrow transplantation is interstitial pneumonitis manifesting as fever, pulmonary infiltrates, arterial hypoxemia, and acute respiratory failure.[44] When interstitial pneumonitis occurs 60 days or more after bone marrow transplantation, it is most often due to cytomegalovirus. Patients at greatest risk for pulmonary complications are those with severe graft-versus-host disease. Diffuse alveolar hemorrhage may occur following autologous bone marrow transplantation for unknown reasons. Treatment with high doses of corticosteroids is often effective in these patients.

Veno-Occlusive Disease of the Liver. Veno-occlusive disease of the liver may occur following allogeneic and autologous bone marrow transplantation.[44] Primary symptoms of veno-occlusive disease include jaundice, hepatomegaly, ascites, and unexpected weight gain. Progressive hepatic failure and often renal failure develop in severely affected patients, and the mortality is high.

References

1. Haber D. Roads leading to breast cancer. N Engl J Med 2000;343:1566–8
2. Selvin BL. Cancer chemotherapy: implications for the anesthesiologist. Anesth Analg 1981;60:425–34
3. Klein DS, Wilds PR. Pulmonary toxicity of antineoplastic agents: anaesthetic and postoperative implications. Can Anaesth Soc J 1983;30:399–405
4. Folkman J. Clinical applications of research on angiogenesis. N Engl J Med 1995;333:1757–63
5. Ashburn MA, Lipman AG. Management of pain in the cancer patient. Anesth Analg 1993;76:402–16
6. Sorensen HT, Mellemkjaer L, Olsen JH, et al. Prognosis of cancers associated with venous thromboembolism. N Engl J Med 2000;343:1846–50
7. Dillman JB. Safe use of succinylcholine during repeated anesthetics in a patient treated with cyclophosphamide. Anesth Analg 1987;66:351–3
8. Burrows FA, Hickey PR, Colan S. Perioperative complications in patients with anthracycline chemotherapeutic agents. Can Anaesth Soc J 1985;32:149–57
9. LaMantia KR, Glick JH, Marshall BE. Supplemental oxygen does not cause respiratory failure in bleomycin-treated surgical patients. Anesthesiology 1984;60:65–7
10. Matalon S, Harper WV, Nickerson PA, et al. Intravenous bleomycin does not alter the toxic effects of hyperoxia in rabbits. Anesthesiology 1986;64:614–9
11. Posner JB. Neoplastic disorders. Sci Am Med 1998;1–12
12. Hebl JR, Horlocker TT, Pritchard DJ. Diffuse brachial plexopathy after interscalene blockade in a patient receiving cisplatin chemotherapy: the pharmacologic double crush syndrome. Anesth Analg 2001;92:249–51
13. Skarin AT. Lung cancer. Sci Am Med 1997;1–20
14. Petty TL. Screening strategies for early detection of lung cancer: the time is now. JAMA 2000;284:1977–80
15. Frame PS. Routine screening for lung cancer? Maybe someday, but not yet. JAMA 2000;284:1980–3
16. Carney DN, Hansen HH. Non-small-cell lung cancer-stalemate or progress? N Engl J Med 2000;343:1261–2

Table 28–9 • Manifestations of Graft-Versus-Host Disease

Pancytopenia and immunodeficiency
Oral ulceration and mucositis
Esophageal ulceration
Diarrhea with fluid and electrolyte loss
Hepatitis with coagulopathy
Bronchiolitis obliterans
Interstitial pneumonitis
Pulmonary fibrosis
Renal failure

17. Patz EF, Goodman PC, Bepler G. Screening for lung cancer. N Engl J Med 2000;343:1627–33
18. Mayer RJ. Gastrointestinal cancer. Sci Am Med 1996;1–22
19. Frazier AL, Colditz GA, Fuchs CS, et al. Cost-effectiveness of screening for colorectal cancer in the general population. JAMA 2000;284:1954–61
20. Ranshoff DF, Lang CA. Screening for colorectal cancer. N Engl J Med 1991;325:37–41
21. Mandel JS, Church TR, Bond JH, et al. The effect of fecal occult-blood screening on the incidence of colorectal cancer. N Engl J Med 2000;343:1603–7
22. Fielding LP. Red for danger: blood transfusion and colorectal cancer. BMJ 1985;291:841–3
23. Kantoff PW. Prostate cancer. Sci Am Med 2000;1–9
24. Burstein HJ, Winer EP. Primary care for survivors of breast cancer. N Engl J Med 2000;343:1086–94
25. Davidson NE. Breast cancer. Sci Am Med 1999;1–13
26. Vokach-Brodsky L, Jeffrey SS, Lemmens HJM, et al. Isosulfan blue affects pulse oximetry. Anesthesiology 2000;93:1002–3
27. Reynen K. Cardiac myxomas. N Engl J Med 1995;333:1610–7
28. Swenson JD, Bailey PL. The intraoperative diagnosis of atrial myxoma by transesophageal echocardiogram. Anesth Analg 1995;80:180–2
29. Brooker RF, Butterworth JF, Klopfenstein HS. Intraoperative diagnosis of left atrial myxoma. Anesth Analg 1995;80:183–4
30. Lebovic S, Koorn R, Reich DL. Role of two dimensional trans-oesophageal echocardiography in the management of a right ventricular tumor. Can J Anaesth 1991;38:1050–4
31. Moritz HA, Azad SS. Right atrial myxoma: case report and anesthetic considerations. Can J Anaesth 1989;36:212–4
32. Schulmberger MJ. Papillary and follicular thyroid carcinoma. N Engl J Med 1998;338:297–306
33. Fuchs CS, Mayer RJ. Gastric carcinoma. N Engl J Med 1995;333:32–41
34. Smith SD, Wheeler MA, Plescia J, et al. Urine detection of survivin and diagnosis of bladder cancer. JAMA 2001;285:324–8
35. Lesko SM, Rosenberg L, Kaufman DW, et al. Cigarette smoking and the risk of endometrial cancer. N Engl J Med 1985;313:593–7
36. Koh KH. Cutaneous melanoma. N Engl J Med 1991;325:171–82
37. Alexanian R, Dimopoulos M. The treatment of multiple myeloma. N Engl J Med 1994;330:484–9
38. Dunbar CE, Nienhuis AW. Multiple myeloma: new approaches to therapy. JAMA 1993;269:2412–6
39. McBridge W, Jackman JD, Gammon RS, et al. High-output cardiac failure in patients with multiple myeloma. N Engl J Med 1988;319:1651–6
40. DeVita V, Hubbard SM. Hodgkin's disease. N Engl J Med 1993;328:560–5
41. Pui C-H. Childhood leukemias. N Engl J Med 1995;332:1618–29
42. Lowenberg B, Downing JR, Burnett A. Acute myeloid leukemia. N Engl J Med 1999;341:1051–62
43. Stein RA, Messino MJ, Hessel EA. Anaesthetic implications for bone marrow transplant recipients. Can J Anaesth 1990;37:571–8
44. Armitage JO. Bone marrow transplantation. N Engl J Med 1994;330:827–37

29

Diseases Related to Immune System Dysfunction

The immune system, which consists of a number of lymphoid organs (thymus, lymph nodes, tonsils, spleen) is responsible for protecting the host against infection and recognizing foreign substances. Immunologically active cells of the immune system are lymphocytes, characterized as B lymphocytes and T lymphocytes (Fig. 29–1). Humoral immunity is mediated by B lymphocytes that differentiate into antibody-producing plasma cells when stimulated by antigens. Antibodies are secreted by plasma cells as a heterogeneous group of plasma proteins designated immunoglobulins (Ig), classified as IgG, IgA, IgM, IgD, and IgE on the basis of electrophoretic and serologic properties (Table 29–1). Most antibodies are IgGs, and antigens that preferentially induce IgE antibodies are designated allergens. Cellular immunity that may result in rejection of transplanted foreign tissues is mediated by T lymphocytes. The complement system, composed of 18 plasma proteins, serves as the principal humoral effector of immunologically induced inflammation. Complement activation can be initiated by the classic pathway (antigen-antibody interaction) or the alternative pathway (bacterial polysaccharides) (Fig. 29–2).[1] Although both pathways result in formation of the same critical component, C3, each pathway appears to have a distinct role in protecting the body against autoimmune diseases (classic pathway) or against infections (alternative pathway). A deficiency of the protein that normally regulates progression of the complement cascade (C1 inhibitor protein) is associated with uncontrolled accumulation of the components of the complement system (see "Hereditary Angioedema").

◼ ALLERGIC REACTIONS

Allergic reactions may be due to an antigen-antibody interaction (anaphylaxis, immune-mediated hyper-

611

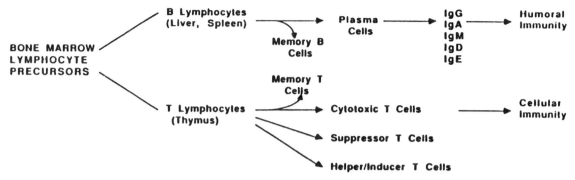

Figure 29–1 • Immune system.

sensitivity), release of chemical mediators in the absence of antigen-antibody interactions (anaphylactoid, chemical), or activation of the complement pathway.[2] An anaphylactoid reaction reflects massive release of histamine from basophils in response to administration of certain drugs (muscle relaxants, opioids, protamine) that have the inherent ability to displace this vasoactive mediator from cells (see "Drug Allergy"). This histamine release is independent of antigen-antibody interactions, emphasizing that such responses may occur in susceptible patients exposed to drugs for the first time.

Anaphylaxis

Anaphylaxis is a life-threatening manifestation of antigen-antibody interactions.[2] This type of allergic reaction is possible whenever prior exposure to antigens (drugs, foods, venoms) have evoked production of antigen-specific IgE antibodies, thereby sensitizing the host.[2] Subsequent exposure of the host to the same or chemically similar antigens results in antigen-antibody interactions that initiate explosive degranulation of mast cells and basophils. Initial manifestations usually occur within 10 minutes of exposure to antigens. Vasoactive mediators released

by degranulation of mast cells and basophils are responsible for the clinical manifestations of anaphylaxis (Table 29–2). Urticarial rash and pruritus are likely in patients who experience anaphylaxis. Primary vascular collapse occurs in about 25% of cases of fatal anaphylaxis and is frequently associated with myocardial ischemia and cardiac dysrhythmias. Extravasation of up to 50% of the intravascular fluid volume into extracellular fluid spaces reflects marked increases in capillary permeability that accompany anaphylaxis. Indeed, hypovolemia is a likely cause of hypotension in these patients, although negative inotropic actions of leukotrienes could also play a role (Table 29–2). Laryngeal edema, bronchospasm, and arterial hypoxemia may accompany anaphylaxis.

Diagnosis

Diagnosis of anaphylaxis is suggested by the dramatic nature of the clinical manifestations in close temporal relation to exposure to antigens. When only a few symptoms are present, however, the response may mimic pulmonary embolism, acute myocardial infarction, aspiration, or a vasovagal reaction. Anesthetic drugs may alter vasoactive mediator release, possibly delaying early recognition of

Table 29–1 • Properties of Human Immunoglobulins

Parameter	IgG	IgA	IgM	IgD	IgE
Location	Plasma Amniotic fluid	Plasma Saliva Tears	Plasma	Plasma	Plasma
Plasma concentration (mg/dl)	550–1900	60–333	45–145	0.3–30.0	Trace
Half-time (days) Function	23 Immunity Defense against infections	6 Topical defense against infections	5 Lysis of bacterial cell walls	3 Not known	2.5 Anaphylaxis

CLASSICAL PATHWAY

ALTERNATIVE PATHWAY

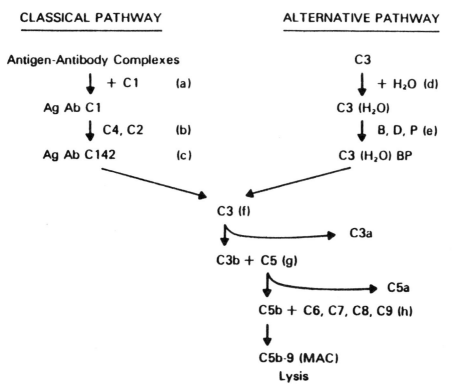

Figure 29–2 • Complement system consists of the classic pathway and the alternative pathway. (From Frank MM. Complement in the pathophysiology of human disease. N Engl J Med 1987;316:1525–30, with permission.)

anaphylaxis.[3] Conversely, it is conceivable that blockade of the innervation of the adrenal glands could accentuate the symptoms of anaphylaxis by preventing endogenous release of catecholamines. Importantly, hypotension and cardiovascular col-lapse may be the only manifestations of anaphylaxis in patients rendered unconscious by general anesthesia.

The initial in vivo response of plasma IgE concentrations during anaphylaxis is a decrease reflecting the complexing of antibodies with newly injected antigens (Fig. 29–3).[4] After this initial decrease, there is often an overshoot of the plasma IgE concentrations. The absence of changes in the plasma concentrations of complement proteins supports the occurrence of allergic reactions due to anaphylaxis. Further immunologic and biochemical proof of anaphylaxis is provided by increases in plasma tryptase concentrations in blood samples collected within 1 to 2 hours after the suspected allergic drug reaction and a sample collected 5 to 6 hours later.[5,6] Tryptase, a neutral protease stored in mast cells, is liberated into the systemic circulation during anaphylactic but not anaphylactoid reactions, thereby verifying that mast cell activation with mediator release has occurred and serving to distinguish immunologic from chemical reactions.[7] Tryptase samples remain stable for several days, and the amount of increase in the patient's serum generally reflects the severity of the reaction. Plasma histamine concentrations return to baseline within 30 to 60 minutes of the reac-

Table 29–2 • Vasoactive Mediators Released During Antigen/Antibody-Induced Degranulation

Vasoactive Mediator	Physiologic Effect
Histamine	Increased capillary permeability Peripheral vasodilation Bronchoconstriction
Leukotrienes	Increased capillary permeability Intense bronchoconstriction Negative inotropy Coronary artery vasoconstriction
Prostaglandins	Bronchoconstriction
Eosinophil chemotactic factor	Attraction of eosinophils
Neutrophil chemotactic factor	Attraction of neutrophils
Platelet-activating factor	Platelet aggregation and release of vasoactive amines

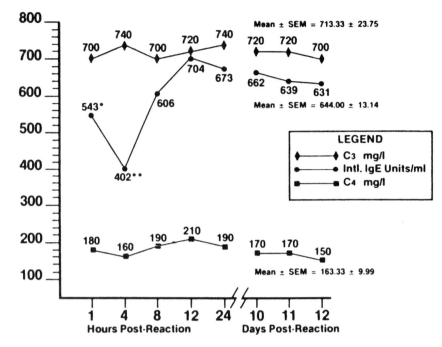

Figure 29–3 • A patient experiencing an anaphylactic reaction to thiopental manifested a decrease followed by an overshoot in the plasma concentrations of immunoglobulin E (IgE). Concentrations of complement proteins C3 and C4 were unchanged. (From Lilly JK, Hoy RH. Thiopental anaphylaxis and reagin involvement. Anesthesiology 1980;53:335–7, with permission.)

tion, so the test sample must be obtained immediately. Urinary methylhistamine levels remain elevated for a longer time.

Identification of the offending antigens is provided by a positive intradermal test (wheal and flare more than 4 mm in diameter), which confirms the presence of specific IgE antibodies. This test, however, has inherent risks, emphasizing the need to begin with injections of dilute preservative-free solutions of suspected antigens (10 to 20 μl). The radioallergosorbent test (RAST) and enzyme-linked immunosorbent assay (ELISA) are commercially available antigen preparations that combine with antibodies in the patient's plasma that are specific for the test antigens.[8]

Treatment

The three immediate goals when treating anaphylaxis are reversal of arterial hypoxemia, replacement of intravascular fluid volume, and inhibition of further cellular degranulation with release of vasoactive mediators (Table 29–3).[9] Often 1 to 4 L of balanced salt and/or colloid solutions must be infused rapidly to restore intravascular fluid volume and systemic blood pressure.

When anaphylaxis is life-threatening, *epinephrine* is indicated in doses of 10 to 100 μg IV.[10] Early intervention with intravenous administration of epinephrine is critical for reversing the life-threatening events characteristic of anaphylaxis. Epinephrine, by increasing intracellular concentrations of cyclic adenosine monophosphate (cAMP), restores membrane permeability and thus decreases the release of vasoactive mediators. The β-agonist effects of epinephrine also relax bronchial smooth muscles. The dose of epinephrine should be doubled and repeated every 1 to 3 minutes until satisfactory systemic blood pressure responses are obtained. This titration approach decreases the likelihood of undesirable overshoots of the systemic blood pressure produced by epinephrine. When anaphylaxis is not life-threatening, subcutaneous epinephrine 0.3 to 0.5 mg in a 1 : 1000 dilution is the standard adult dose.

Table 29–3 • Treatment of Anaphylactic Reactions
Supplemental oxygen
Balanced salt solutions or colloids
Epinephrine
Diphenhydramine
β_2-Agonists
Corticosteroids

Administration of *antihistamines* such as diphenydramine, 50 to 100 mg IV, to adults competes with membrane receptor sites normally occupied by histamine and perhaps decreases the manifestations of anaphylaxis such as hypotension, pruritus, and bronchospasm. There is no evidence, however, that administration of antihistamines is effective in treating anaphylaxis once vasoactive mediators have been released. Furthermore, bronchospasm and the negative inotropic effects due to leukotrienes are not influenced by antihistamines.

β₂-Agonists such as albuterol delivered by metered-dose inhalers have replaced aminophylline in the treatment of bronchospasm associated with anaphylaxis.

Corticosteroids (cortisol or methylprednisolone) are often administered intravenously to patients experiencing life-threatening anaphylaxis. Although these drugs have no known effect on degranulation or antigen-antibody interactions, the favorable effects of corticosteroids may reflect enhancement of the β-agonist effects of other drugs and inhibition of the release of arachidonic acid responsible for the production of leukotrienes and prostaglandins. Corticosteroids may be uniquely helpful in patients experiencing life-threatening allergic reactions due to activation of the complement system.

Allergic Rhinitis

Allergic rhinitis is an IgE-mediated inflammatory disease involving the nasal mucous membranes. Symptoms usually begin during childhood and are often seasonal when pollens (antigens) come into direct contact with respiratory tract mucosa, leading to the release of vasoactive mediators from submucosal mast cells.[2] Nasal pruritus, rhinorrhea, lacrimation, and sneezing are common symptoms. These symptoms may be aggravated by nonspecific irritants such as cigarette smoke. Inflammatory or infectious sinusitis may result in maxillofrontal headaches, postnasal discharge, and persistent nasal stuffiness. Increased numbers of eosinophils in nasal secretions are often present, whereas increased numbers of eosinophils may be present in the peripheral blood of patients with allergic or nonallergic rhinitis. Atopic dermatitis is often associated with allergic rhinitis. Viral upper respiratory tract infections and hormone-related rhinitis (premenstrual or during pregnancy) may mimic allergic rhinitis, presenting a dilemma during the preoperative evaluation of patients scheduled for elective surgery. In contrast to allergic rhinitis, symptoms of viral respiratory tract infections are usually short-lived (less than 7 days) and include fever and the presence of neutrophils in nasal secretions.

Treatment of allergic rhinitis includes avoidance of offending allergens, the use of antihistamines, and administration of allergen-specific immunotherapy. Terfenadine is an H_1-receptor antagonist that has minimal sedative effects and is effective in the treatment of seasonal allergic rhinitis. In addition, a sympathomimetic drug (pseudoephedrine, phenylpropanolamine) may be useful for symptomatic relief. Increased systemic blood pressure and heart rate may accompany the use of sympathomimetics for this purpose. Nasal inhalation of cromolyn and/or corticosteroids may be useful for resistant cases. Nasal corticosteroids do not seem to suppress the patient's adrenal glands.

Allergic Conjunctivitis

Allergic conjunctivitis is the ocular equivalent of allergic rhinitis and reflects local mediator release as a result of antigen-antibody interactions. Pruritus is usually a prominent symptom, and a history of allergic rhinitis is almost always present. Many topical preparations used to treat allergic conjunctivitis contain combinations of antihistamines and vasoconstrictors.

Allergic Asthma

Allergic asthma manifests as reversible airway obstruction and bronchospasm accompanied by inflammation of the airways and increased bronchial smooth muscle reactivity (see Chapter 14). This response is triggered by specific allergens and may be aggravated by viral infections, smoke, air pollution (sulfur dioxide), and food or drug preservatives (sodium metabisulfite). Sodium metabisulfite is sometimes utilized as a preservative for anesthetic drugs, including a generic formulation of propofol,[11] and in susceptible patients it may evoke bronchospasm. Symptoms are highly variable but usually include wheezing, cough, and dyspnea. Treatment includes administration of β_2-agonists, corticosteroids, and cromolyn.

Food Allergy

Food allergy results from antibody-mediated degranulation of gastrointestinal tract mast cells when exposed to specific antigens. Abdominal pain and diarrhea are likely. Systemic anaphylaxis may occur within minutes or hours. Intraoperative anaphylactic reactions after administration of protamine to neutralize heparin is more likely in patients allergic to seafood, emphasizing the derivation of this drug from salmon sperm.[12]

Drug Allergy

Epidemiology

In the general population, penicillin accounts for most fatal anaphylactic drug reactions. Drug sensitivity has been implicated in 4.3% of anesthesia-related deaths reported in the United Kingdom.[13] In Australia such reactions occur once in every 5000 to 25,000 anesthesias, for 3.4% mortality.[14] The incidence of allergic drug reactions during anesthesia seems to be increasing, presumably reflecting the frequent administration of several drugs to the same patient and cross-sensitivity among drugs. Allergic reactions to drugs may reflect anaphylaxis, drug-induced release of histamine (anaphylactoid reactions), or activation of the complement system. More than one mechanism may be involved in the production of allergic drug reactions in the same patient. Regardless of the mechanism responsible for life-threatening allergic drug reactions, the manifestations and treatment are identical (Table 29–3).

It is not possible to predict reliably which patients are likely to experience anaphylaxis after administration of drugs that are usually innocuous. Nevertheless, patients with a history of allergy (asthma, food, drugs) have an increased incidence of anaphylaxis, primarily as a reflection of genetic predisposition to form increased amounts of IgE antibodies. Patients allergic to penicillin have three- to fourfold greater risks of experiencing allergic reactions to any drug. A history of allergy to specific drugs elicited during the preoperative evaluation is helpful, but it must be appreciated that prior uneventful exposure to drugs such as thiopental does not eliminate the possibility of anaphylaxis on subsequent exposures.[13, 15-17] Initial injections of small test doses of drugs are more likely to unmask idiosyncratic reac-

tions than to prevent anaphylaxis. For example, 5 mg of protamine is equivalent to 60×10^{15} molecules. Although the severity of anaphylaxis is likely to be related to the total dose of antigens injected, the rarity of allergic drug reactions does not support the routine use of test doses of drugs during the perioperative period.[18] Conversely, the magnitude of histamine release produced on reexposure to drugs that previously resulted in anaphylactoid reactions can be decreased by reducing the dose of drug and slowing its rate of infusion.[16] Because histamine is the principal vasoactive mediator released during anaphylactoid reactions, it may be useful to provide prophylaxis during the preoperative period to patients who, on the basis of history, are deemed likely to display such reactions. Prophylaxis may include corticosteroids and H_1- and H_2-receptor antagonists, although severe allergic reactions can still occur.[19]

Allergic drug reactions must be distinguished from drug intolerance, idiosyncratic reactions, and drug toxicity (Table 29–4). The occurrence of undesirable pharmacologic effects at low doses of the drugs reflects intolerance, whereas idiosyncratic reactions are undesirable responses to drugs independent of the doses administered. Evidence of histamine release along veins into which drugs are injected reflects localized and nonimmunologic release of histamine insufficient to evoke anaphylactoid reactions. Patients manifesting this localized response should not be diagnosed as allergic to the drug. It is estimated that plasma histamine concentrations must double before hypotension occurs. Pretreatment with H_1- and H_2-receptor antagonists is more effective for controlling symptoms associated with local drug-induced histamine release than those accompanying anaphylactoid reactions. Presumably, fewer vasoactive mediators are involved in localized drug-induced responses, with histamine being the most important mediator.

Perioperative Period

Allergic drug reactions have been reported with virtually all drugs that may be injected during the

Table 29–4 • Differential Diagnosis of Drug Allergy versus Drug Toxicity

Parameter	Drug Allergy	Drug Toxicity
Mechanism	Antigen-antibody interactions	Dependent on chemical properties of drug
Manifestations	Hypotension	Variable for each drug
	Bronchospasm	
	Urticaria	
Predictability	Poor	Good based on animal and human studies
Prior exposure	Required	Not required
Dose-related	No	Yes
Onset	Usually within 10 minutes	Usually delayed
Incidence	Low	High, especially if dose is sufficient

administration of anesthesia (Table 29–5).[16, 17, 20] The exception to this generalization may be ketamine and benzodiazepines. Cardiovascular collapse is the predominant manifestation of life-threatening allergic drug reactions in anesthetized patients, whereas bronchospasm is present in fewer patients.[20] It is important to consider the possible role of latex sensitivity when presumed allergic reactions to drugs occur. In fact, many allergic reactions previously attributed to drugs may, in fact, represent latex allergy.[21, 22] It is estimated that as many as 15% of allergic reactions during anesthesia are due to latex.

Most drug-induced allergic reactions manifest within 10 minutes of an intravenous injection of the offending drug. The important exception is the allergic response to latex, which is typically delayed for as long as 30 minutes. An allergic reaction should be considered whenever there are abrupt decreases in systemic blood pressure and increases in heart rate that exceed 30% of the control value. In about 10% of patients the only manifestation of an intraoperative allergic reaction is systemic hypotension. Extravasation of fluid into the extracellular fluid space reflects marked increases in capillary permeability, and the resulting hypovolemia is the most likely cause of hypotension during drug-induced allergic reactions. Bronchospasm may be particularly severe and difficult to treat in patients with chronic obstructive pulmonary disease.

Muscle Relaxants

Muscle relaxants are responsible for more than 60% of drug-induced allergic reactions during the perioperative period.[23, 24] It is estimated that 50% of patients who experience allergic reactions to muscle relaxants are also allergic to other muscle relaxants. Cross-sensitivity among muscle relaxants emphasizes the structural similarities of these drugs, especially the presence of one or more antigenic quaternary ammonium groups. Indeed, IgE antibodies to

choline are likely to be present in patients who have experienced allergic reactions to succinylcholine and other muscle relaxants. Drug-induced histamine release from mast cells and basophils is also a possibility with any of the muscle relaxants, especially when they are rapidly administered intravenously in large doses.

Induction Drugs

Allergic reactions after the administration of *barbiturates* for the induction of anesthesia are rare (1 in about 30,000 anesthesias) but are often life-threatening. Most reported cases are in patients with a history of allergies (food allergies, rhinitis, asthma) and prior uneventful exposure to barbiturates during anesthesia.[15] As little as 10 μg of thiopental administered intravenously may induce evidence of anaphylaxis in highly sensitized patients. Allergic reactions may occur after administration of thiobarbiturates or oxybarbiturates, although in vitro data suggest that methohexital is less likely to evoke the release of histamine.[25]

Life-threatening allergic reactions have occurred after the first or subsequent exposure to *propofol*.[20] Patients with a history of allergy to other drugs seem to be more vulnerable to propofol allergy, perhaps reflecting the presence of common antigenic groups (phenyl nucleus, isopropyl side chain) in propofol and other chemicals (muscle relaxants, local anesthetics, antibiotics, dermatologic preparations). Bronchospasm occurs more often in patients experiencing allergic reactions to propofol than with other anesthetic drugs.

Local Anesthetics

Local anesthetic-induced allergic reactions are rare despite the frequent use of these drugs and the common labeling of patients as allergic to drugs in this class. It is estimated that only 1% of all local anesthetic reactions are allergic reactions. The mechanism of adverse responses to local anesthetics can often be determined by careful questioning of patients and review of past medical records describing the events. For example, the occurrence of hypotension and seizures is characteristic of systemic reactions due to excessive blood levels of local anesthetics, as is most likely to occur with accidental intravascular injections during performance of regional anesthesia (epidural, brachial plexus, intercostal). These responses to excessive blood levels of local anesthetics are often erroneously attributed to allergic reactions. Tachycardia and systemic hypertension associated with injection of a local anesthetic most likely reflect systemic absorption of epinephrine that was present in the local anesthetic solution. The rare patient who

---

Table 29–5 • Causes of Allergic Reactions During the Perioperative Period

Muscle relaxants
Barbiturates
Propofol
Local anesthetics (especially ester derivatives)
Opioids
Volatile anesthetics (especially halothane)
Protamine
Antibiotics
Blood and plasma volume expanders
Intravascular contrast media
Vascular graft material
Latex-containing medical equipment

exhibits urticaria, laryngeal edema, and broncho-constriction may well be experiencing a local anesthetic-induced allergic reaction.

Ester-based local anesthetics that are metabolized to the highly antigenic compound paraaminobenzoic acid (PABA) are more likely than amide-based local anesthetics that are not metabolized to PABA to evoke allergic reactions.[26] Local anesthetic solutions may also contain methylparaben or propylparaben as preservatives with bacteriostatic and fungistatic properties. The structural similarity of these preservatives to PABA may render them antigenic. As a result, anaphylaxis may be due to prior stimulation of antibody production by the preservatives and not the local anesthetic.

A common clinical problem deals with the safety of administering local anesthetics to patients with a history of allergy to this class of drugs. It is generally agreed that cross-sensitivity does not exist between ester- and amide-based local anesthetics. Therefore it should be acceptable to administer amide-based local anesthetics to patients with a history of being allergic to ester-based local anesthetics. The reverse of this recommendation would also be true. It must be remembered, however, that use of preservative-free local anesthetic solutions is important, as preservatives may be responsible for allergic reactions erroneously attributed to local anesthetics. All factors considered, it seems reasonable to recommend intradermal testing with preservative-free alternative local anesthetics in occasional patients who describe convincing allergic histories and in whom failure to document a safe local anesthetic drug would prevent the use of local or regional anesthesia.

Opioids

Anaphylaxis after administration of opioids is rare, perhaps reflecting the similarity of these drugs to naturally occurring substances known as endorphins.[27] Fentanyl has been associated with allergic reactions following systemic and neuraxial administration.[28] Morphine, but not fentanyl or its related derivatives, may directly evoke the release of histamine from mast cells and basophils, producing anaphylactoid reactions in susceptible patients.

Volatile Anesthetics

Clinical manifestations of halothane-induced hepatitis that suggest a drug-induced allergic reaction include eosinophilia, fever, rash, and prior exposure to halothane (see Chapter 18). The plasma of patients with a clinical diagnosis of halothane hepatitis may contain antibodies that react with halothane-induced liver antigens (neoantigens). These neoantigens are formed by the covalent interaction of reactive oxidative trifluoroacetyl halide metabolites of halothane with hepatic microsomal proteins. Acetylation of liver proteins, in effect, changes these proteins from self to nonself (neoantigens), resulting in the formation of antibodies against this now foreign protein. It is presumed that subsequent antigen-antibody interactions are responsible for the liver injury associated with halothane-induced hepatitis. Similar oxidative halide metabolites are also produced after exposure to enflurane, isoflurane, and desflurane, but not sevoflurane, emphasizing the possibility of cross-sensitivity among certain volatile anesthetics in susceptible patients. Considering the magnitude of the metabolism of these volatile drugs, it is predictable that the incidence of anesthetic-induced allergic hepatitis would be greatest after halothane, intermediate with enflurane, minimal with isoflurane, and remote with desflurane (metabolism 10-fold less than with isoflurane).

Protamine

Anaphylactic reactions following administration of protamine are more likely to occur in patients who are allergic to seafoods (protamine is derived from salmon sperm) and in patients with diabetes mellitus who are being treated with protamine-containing insulin preparations.[12, 13, 29–31] Presumably, small amounts of protamine in certain insulin preparations stimulates the production of antibodies such that anaphylaxis occurs when large doses of protamine (antigen) are administered to neutralize the effects of heparin. Nevertheless, there are also data suggesting that the incidence of reactions to protamine is no higher in patients treated with NPH insulin than in nondiabetics. Vasectomized or infertile men may develop circulating antibodies to spermatozoa, but any increased risk of allergic reactions to protamine is undocumented and seems unlikely, as antibody titers are low. Protamine is also capable of directly evoking histamine release from cells; in susceptible patients protamine may activate the complement pathway and evoke the release of thromboxane, leading to bronchoconstriction and pulmonary hypertension.[32] Patients known to be allergic to protamine present a therapeutic dilemma when neutralization of heparin is required because no alternative anticoagulant drug to reverse the effects of protamine is available. Spontaneous dissipation of the anticoagulant effects of heparin is prolonged and may be associated with excessive perioperative blood loss, especially after successful weaning from cardiopulmonary bypass.

Antibiotics

The structural similarity between penicillin and cephalosporins (both contain β-lactam rings) suggests the possibility of cross-sensitivity. Nevertheless, the incidence of life-threatening allergic reactions following administration of cephalosporins is low (0.02%), and the incidence of allergic reactions to cephalosporins is minimally (if at all) increased in patients with a history of penicillin allergy.[33] Vancomycin may produce life-threatening allergic reactions in susceptible patients even when its intravenous administration rate is greatly slowed.[34-36]

Blood and Plasma Volume Expanders

Allergic reactions to properly crossmatched blood occur in about 3% of patients, with manifestations ranging from pruritus, urticaria, and fever to noncardiogenic pulmonary edema. Synthetic plasma protein solutions (dextran, hydroxyethyl starch solutions) have been implicated in anaphylaxis and anaphylactoid reactions, with manifestations ranging from a cutaneous rash and modest hypotension to shock and bronchospasm. Low-molecular-weight dextran cannot induce antibody formation, but this material may react with antibodies formed previously in response to exposure to polysaccharides of viral or bacterial origin. Dextran may also activate the complement system, producing signs of allergic reactions.

Intravascular Contrast Media

Iodine in intravascular contrast media injected intravenously for radiologic studies evokes allergic reactions in about 5% of patients. The risk of allergic reactions is probably increased in patients with a history of allergies to other drugs or foods. Many of the allergic reactions to contrast media seem to be anaphylactoid and can be modified by pretreatment with corticosteroids or diphenhydramine and limitation of the iodine dose.

Vascular Graft Material

Profound vasodilation and hypotension accompanied by evidence of disseminated intravascular coagulation has been observed in association with the placement of vascular graft materials.[37] Presumably, plasticizers used to bind and combine the inert graft material together are responsible for the release of vasoactive mediators in rare but susceptible patients. Because transient hypotension is frequent following restoration of blood flow after aortic reconstruction grafting, it is possible that an allergic reaction is not a possible explanation, even if hypotension is more severe or persistent than usual. Treatment consists of replacing the graft with material from a different manufacturer.

Latex-Containing Medical Devices

Cardiovascular collapse during anesthesia and surgery has been attributed to anaphylaxis triggered by latex (natural rubber).[38-42] A feature that appears to distinguish latex-induced allergic reactions from drug-induced allergic reactions is the delayed onset (typically longer than 30 minutes) after the start of surgery. By contrast, most drug-induced allergic reactions occur within 10 minutes following intravenous administration of the drug. It is presumed that it takes time for the responsible antigens to be eluted from rubber gloves and absorbed across mucous membranes into the systemic circulation in amounts sufficient to cause allergic reactions. Contact with latex at mucosal surfaces is probably the most significant route of latex exposure. In addition, inhalation of latex antigens is a common route of exposure and sensitization in health care workers. Corn starch powder in gloves is not likely to be immunogenic but, rather, acts as an airborne vehicle because the powder absorbs latex antigens, which are then inhaled when gloves are placed on the hands.

Diagnosis. Sensitized patients develop IgE antibodies directed specifically against latex antigens. Skin-prick testing can confirm latex hypersensitivity, but standardization of latex antigen extracts is important. A nonammoniated latex extract has been reported to have 95% sensitivity and 100% specificity.[43] Anaphylaxis has occurred during skin prick testing. In vitro tests to detect latex-specific IgE antibodies include RASTs (use radioactivity to detect antibodies) and ELISAs. These tests are equally sensitive and specific and avoid the risk of anaphylaxis associated with skin testing. The principal disadvantage is the time required to obtain results (often several days), which limits their value as part of the preoperative evaluation and preparation of patients. Patients with confirmed latex allergy should wear "identification bracelets."

Questions about itching, conjunctivitis, rhinitis, rash, or wheezing after wearing latex gloves, following dental or gynecologic examinations involving latex gloves, or inflating toy balloons may be helpful for identifying sensitized patients. Operating room personnel and patients with spina bifida have an increased incidence of latex allergy that is presumed to reflect frequent exposure to latex devices (bladder catheters, gloves). Latex sensitivity is recognized as an occupational hazard for operating room personnel. In these individuals, latex sensitivity most often manifests as cutaneous sensitivity from direct contact with latex gloves or airway changes due to inhalation of latex antigens. The incidence of latex sensitivity in anesthesiologists may exceed 15%.[44] Health care workers are at increased risk for developing severe latex allergic reactions should they become patients and undergo a surgical procedure.

Management of Anesthesia. Patients who are in high risk categories for latex sensitivity (spina bifida, multiple prior operations, health care workers, atopic individuals, history of fruit allergies) should be questioned for symptoms related to exposure to natural rubber during their daily routine or prior surgical procedure. If necessary, an allergy consult is obtained to discuss perioperative management. Because latex allergy is IgE-mediated, administration of H_1- and H_2-receptor antagonists and corticosteroids is a consideration but not routine practice. Intraoperative management is characterized by a "latex-free environment."[45] Nonlatex gloves (styrene, neoprene) are used by all personnel who may be in contact with patients, especially their mucous membranes. Medications should not be withdrawn from multidose bottles with latex caps or injected through latex ports on intravenous delivery tubing. Adhesive tape, intravenous and bladder catheters, drains, anesthesia delivery tubing, ventilator bellows, endotracheal tubes, laryngeal mask airways, nasogastric tubes, blood pressure cuffs, pulse oximeter probes, electrocardiogram pads, and syringes are selected on the basis of being latex-free (polyvinyl, synthetic rubber, plastics). Despite these precautions, it can never be guaranteed that allergic reactions to latex will not occur.[46]

ANESTHESIA AND IMMUNOCOMPETENCE

Exposure to anesthesia and performance of surgery may alter immunocompetence manifesting as alterations in the incidence of infections and responses to cancer.[47–49]

Resistance to Infection

It is conceivable that anesthesia-induced depression of the immune system can increase the development of postoperative infections or augment co-existing infections. For example, local and inhaled anesthetics (nitrous oxide) may produce dose-dependent inhibition of mobilization and migration of polymorphonuclear leukocytes.[47, 48] Nevertheless, the effects produced by these drugs are probably clini-

cally insignificant, considering the usual duration of anesthesia and the doses of drugs administered. Indeed, the incidence of postoperative infections seems more likely related to surgical trauma and to an associated release of cortisol and catecholamines, which are known to inhibit phagocytosis. In the absence of surgical stimulation, anesthetic drugs are not predictably associated with increased circulating concentrations of cortisol or catecholamines. The consensus, based on available information, is that the effects of anesthetics on resistance to infections are transient, reversible, and of minor importance compared with the prolonged immunosuppressive effects of cortisol and catecholamines released as part of the hormonal response to surgery.[47] Mild perioperative hypothermia (less than 36°C) has also been described as being associated with an increased risk of postoperative infection.[50]

If hormonal responses to surgical stimulation are undesirable with respect to infection risk, it could be reasoned that light anesthesia, which does not reliably attenuate sympathetic nervous system activity, is less desirable than deeper levels of anesthesia. It is likely that 1.5 MAC of volatile anesthetics or more than 1 mg/kg of morphine is necessary to prevent sympathetic nervous system responses to surgical skin incisions in 50% of patients.[51] Sternal incisions that require cutting bone seem to require higher concentrations of anesthesia to block sympathetic nervous system responses. Regional anesthesia may also decrease the hormonal responses to surgical stimulation.[48] Despite these observations, there is no evidence that the incidence of postoperative infections can be altered by the depth of anesthesia or the techniques selected to produce anesthesia.

Possible bacteriostatic effects of anesthetic drugs must also be considered. Local anesthetics have been shown to have such effects on a wide variety of organisms at concentrations achievable with topical applications.[48] Clinical applications of this observation are that topical anesthesia, used for bronchoscopy, could influence the incidence of positive cultures. Conversely, concentrations of local anesthetics in the circulation, in association with regional anesthesia or after intravenous administration, do not alter bacterial growth. Likewise, volatile anesthetics do not have bacteriostatic effects.[48] Liquid volatile anesthetics, however, may be bactericidal. Volatile anesthetics in doses as low as 0.2 MAC produce dose-dependent inhibition of measles virus replication and decrease mortality in mice receiving intranasal influenza virus.[52]

Resistance to Cancer

Immunocompetence is essential for host resistance to cancer. It is a clinical impression that some patients with a preoperative diagnosis of cancer experience rapid growth of their tumors after anesthesia and surgery. Conceivably, drugs administered to produce anesthesia could enhance tumor cell replication and spread by decreasing host resistance. Despite these concerns, there is no evidence that short-term effects of anesthetic drugs are of any significance in the resistance of hosts to cancer.[49] As with infections, the more important concern is immunosuppression produced by hormonal responses to surgical stimulation. If hormonal responses are indeed undesirable with respect to host resistance to cancer, it seems logical to suppress these responses with either regional or deep general anesthesia. It should be emphasized, however, that there is no evidence to support the validity of this speculation.

In contrast to concerns in patients with cancer, immunosuppression secondary to hormonal responses produced by surgical stimulation could be beneficial for patients undergoing organ transplant. Nevertheless, if such benefits do occur, they are probably too small or transient to be of any significance during the early transplant period.

DISORDERS OF IMMUNOGLOBULINS

X-Linked Agammaglobulineima

X-linked agammaglobulinemia (congenital agammaglobulinemia) is a genetically transmitted disorder characterized by recurrent bacterial infections, decreased to absent plasma concentrations of all immunoglobulin classes, and an inability to produce antibodies even in response to intense antigenic stimulations (Table 29–1).[53] Infants are born with maternal IgG, so manifestations of the disease are not seen before about 9 months of age. As the name implies, only males are affected, although rare cases with similar clinical features have been described in females. The principal defect appears to be the absence of mature B lymphocytes, such that antibodies cannot be produced (Fig. 29–1). By contrast, T lymphocytes are normal, and cell-mediated immunity (graft rejection) is intact (Fig. 29–1). *Pneumocystitis carinii* pneumonia may be the presenting manifestation of this disorder. Recurrent infections may lead to chronic sinusitis and bronchiectasis.

Treatment of X-linked agammaglobulinemia consists of intravenous or intramuscular administration of gamma globulin to maintain plasma IgG concentrations close to 400 to 500 mg/dl.[54] The half-time of IgGs used for this purpose is about 30 days, which is longer than normal, emphasizing the relation of the catabolism of IgG to the amount of IgG (Table 29–1). The presence of infection results in more rapid catabolism of IgG. Antibiotics are indicated when bacterial infections occur.

Acquired Hypoimmunoglobulinemia

Acquired hypoimmunoglobulinemia does not appear to be genetically determined and usually does not manifest until after puberty. Symptoms and treatment are the same as for X-linked agammaglobulinemia. This syndrome is associated with autoimmune diseases and malabsorption syndromes.

Selective Immunoglobulin A Deficiency

Selective IgA deficiency occurs in 1 of every 600 to 800 adults. With this condition plasma IgA concentrations are less than 5 mg/dl, but the concentrations of other immunoglobulins are normal (Table 29–1). Recurrent sinus and pulmonary infections are the most common symptoms, although many patients are asymptomatic, and their disorder remains undetected until they are screened as potential blood donors. About 40% of these patients produce anti-IgA antibodies and may experience life-threatening anaphylaxis when transfused with blood containing IgA. Therefore these patients should receive blood or blood components obtained only from IgA-deficient donors.

Cold Autoimmune Diseases

Cold autoimmune diseases are characterized by the presence of abnormal circulating proteins that may agglutinate in response to decreased body temperature (Table 29–6).[55]

Cryoglobulinemia

Cryoglobulinemia is a disorder in which circulating abnormal proteins (cold agglutinins or cryoglobulins) precipitate on exposure to cold, leading to activation of complement pathways, platelet aggregation, and consumption of clotting factors. Hyperviscosity of the plasma is prominent, and acute renal failure may accompany microvascular thrombosis. Indeed, renal dysfunction eventually occurs in more than 20% of patients. Normally, symptoms occur only when blood temperature falls below 33°C.

Management of anesthesia in patients with cryoglobulinemia includes maintenance of body temperature above the thermal reactivity of the cryoglobulins during the perioperative period.[56] This goal is

Table 29–6 • Cold Autoimmune Diseases

Disease	Thermal Reactivity (°C)	Associated Conditions	Response to Cold Exposure
Cryoglobulins	17–33	Macroglobulinemia	Hyperviscosity Platelet aggregation Renal failure
Cold hemagglutinin disease	15–32	None	Acrocyanosis Hemolysis Raynaud's phenomenon
Paroxysmal cold hemoglobinuria	10–15	Syphilis	Hemolysis Jaundice Renal failure
Acquired cold autoimmune disease	4–25	Mycoplasma Mononucleosis Leukemia	Acrocyanosis Hyperviscosity Hemolysis

facilitated by increasing the ambient temperature of the operating rooms, using warming blankets, and ventilating the patient's lungs with humidified and warmed gases. Passing intravenous fluids through a blood warmer before delivery to patients also decreases loss of body heat during anesthesia.

Patients scheduled for operations requiring cardiopulmonary bypass present significant challenges.[55] Use of systemic hypothermia may be contraindicated, and cold cardioplegia solutions may cause intracoronary hemagglutination with inadequate distribution of cardioplegia solutions, thrombosis, ischemia, or infarction. Alternatives to cold cardioplegia are ischemic arrest for brief periods of time. Plasmapheresis may be helpful for decreasing plasma concentrations of immunoglobulins. Efforts to maintain body temperature above the thermal reactivity of the cryoglobulins must also be extended into the postoperative period.

Cold Hemagglutinin Disease

Cold hemagglutinin disease is characterized by the presence of IgM autoantibodies in the plasma that react with antigens on the patient's erythrocytes in the presence of decreased body temperature. This reaction may activate the complement system, leading to severe intravascular hemolysis. Cold hemagglutinins may predispose to vascular occlusion in exposed and therefore chilled areas of the patient's body. Symptoms such as acrocyanosis of the extremities and Raynaud's phenomenon occur when the blood has cooled below a critical temperature ("thermal threshold"). Severe intravascular hemolysis due to perioperative hypothermia has been described. The diagnosis of cold hemagglutinin disease is suggested by the presence of hemolytic anemia and signs of vascular occlusion. Cold agglutinin disease may be caused by lymphomas or other ma-

lignancies or infections such as *Mycoplasma* pneumonia, or it may be idiopathic.

The principal method for protecting patients with cold hemagglutinin disease is avoidance of cold environments. Cyclophosphamide is often used to suppress the IgM-producing cells. Plasmapheresis reduces symptoms and lowers IgM levels in patients with cold hemagglutinin disease, but the effect is transient and treatment must be repeated to maintain depressed antibody titers. Splenectomy may be necessary when anemia is severe, which indicates sequestration of erythrocytes in the spleen. Treatment may also include infusion of packed erythrocytes that are warmed to decrease the likelihood of cold hemagglutination. Exchange transfusions and plasmapheresis may be useful when acute hemolysis is occurring. Occasionally, high doses of corticosteroids are useful for decreasing the degree of hemolysis.

Patients with severe cold hemagglutinin disease undergoing surgical procedures (often splenectomy), when exposed to cold operating room environments, are at risk of developing agglutination, causing acrocyanosis, Raynaud's phenomenon, purpura, gangrene, or immune complex nephritis. Hemolysis may also occur in cold operating rooms, resulting in severe anemia, hemoglobinuria, and renal failure. The use of preoperative plasmapheresis and intraoperative forced air convective warming to minimize hemolysis in patients with severe cold agglutinin hemolytic anemia has been utilized for perioperative management of these patients.[57]

Multiple Myeloma

Multiple myeloma is due to neoplastic proliferation of single-clone immunoglobulin-secreting cells (see Chapter 28).

Waldenström's Macroglobulinemia

Waldenström's macroglobulinemia is due to proliferation of a malignant plasma cell clone that secretes IgM, resulting in marked increases in plasma viscosity. The bone marrow is infiltrated with malignant lymphocytes, as are the liver, spleen, and lungs. Anemia and an increased incidence of spontaneous hemorrhage are common findings in these patients. In contrast to multiple myeloma, Waldenström's macroglobulinemia rarely involves the skeletal system. As a result, renal dysfunction due to hypercalcemia is unlikely.

Treatment of Waldenström's macroglobulinemia consists of plasmapheresis to remove the abnormal proteins and diminish the viscosity of plasma. This is especially important before transfusion of blood, which may abruptly increase the patient's hematocrit and plasma viscosity. Chemotherapy is also instituted in attempts to decrease the proliferation of cells responsible for production of abnormal immunoglobulins.

Amyloidosis

Amyloidosis encompasses several disorders characterized by the accumulation of insoluble fibrillar proteins (amyloid) in various tissues, including the heart, vascular smooth muscle, kidneys, adrenal glands, gastrointestinal tract, peripheral nerves, and skin.[58, 59] The natural history of primary amyloidosis is poorly understood, and the disease is not clinically diagnosed until it is far advanced. The development of amyloidosis is frequently associated with multiple myeloma, rheumatoid arthritis, and prolonged antigenic challenges, as may be produced by chronic infections. Sudden death is common, occurring in one-third of patients.[60]

Signs and Symptoms

Macroglossia is a classic feature of amyloidosis that occurs in about 20% of patients. The enlarged, stiff tongue may cause problems with swallowing and speaking and could interfere with visualizing the glottic opening by direct laryngoscopy. Salivary gland involvement with extension into adjacent skeletal muscles can produce upper airway obstruction and mimic angioneurotic edema. Cardiac involvement is common and may manifest as disturbed conduction of cardiac impulses and the appearance of life-threatening heart block. With cardiac amyloidosis acute-onset right heart failure is the predominant sign, whereas left heart function is preserved until late in the disease.[61] Pulmonary amyloidosis rarely causes symptoms, and dyspnea is most likely due to congestive heart failure. Renal involvement with amyloid results in the nephrotic syndrome. Amyloid deposition in joints causes pain and limitation of motion. In contrast to the absence of central nervous system involvement, sensory and motor disturbances may reflect peripheral nerve involvement. Carpal tunnel syndrome may occur as a result of median nerve compression. Infiltration of the autonomic nervous system manifests as delayed gastric emptying and postural hypotension. Amyloidosis of the gastrointestinal tract may produce malabsorption, ileus, hemorrhage, and intestinal obstruction. Hepatomegaly is a common finding, but hepatic dysfunction is uncommon. Amyloid deposits may trap factor X or evoke fibrinolysis, leading to an increased likelihood of bleeding.

Diagnosis

The diagnosis of amyloidosis is based on clinical suspicion and tissue biopsy.[58] The prognosis of amyloidosis varies, but it is generally poor especially if symptomatic cardiac involvement is present. The frequent presence of amyloid deposits in the wall of the rectum makes rectal biopsy the common initial diagnostic approach.

Treatment

Treatment of amyloidosis is generally ineffective and is directed toward symptomatic support of the affected organs. Chemotherapy with intermittent oral melphalan and prednisone may be efficacious. The nephrotic syndrome requires general supportive and diuretic therapy, and renal failure can be successfully treated by dialysis. Renal transplantation may be considered in selected patients. Congestive heart failure may initially respond to diuretics but is often resistant to any treatment. Calcium channel blockers and β-blockers are not utilized to treat cardiac amyloidosis. An external cardiac pacemaker may be indicated in patients with symptomatic bradycardia. Gastric motility drugs may be of some benefit. Liver transplantation is indicated in selected patients.

Management of Anesthesia

Macroglossia may interfere with maintenance of a patent upper airway and subsequent direct laryngoscopy for tracheal intubation. Delayed gastric emptying may accompany amyloidosis that affects the gastrointestinal tract. The depressant effects of anesthetic drugs could theoretically enhance cardiac amyloidosis effects. Fatal perioperative myocardial infarction and postoperative ventricular fibrillation have been described in patients with cardiac amyloidosis.[60, 61] Impaired renal function may influence the selection of drugs dependent on renal clearance mechanisms. Peripheral nerve involvement is considered when selecting regional anesthesia and positioning patients during surgery.

Hyperimmunoglobulinemia E Syndrome

Hyperimmunoglobulinemia E (Job) syndrome is a rare disorder characterized by recurrent bacterial infections of the skin, sinuses, and lungs, with IgE plasma concentrations at least 10 times normal and neutrophils having a variable chemotactic defect. Most infections are due to *Staphylococcus aureus*. Bacteremia may occur, and mucocutaneous candidiasis is likely. Despite antibiotic therapy, these patients are likely to present repeatedly for surgical drainage of abscesses. Management of anesthesia must consider the risk of epidural abscesses if an epidural or spinal anesthetic is considered.[62] A prolonged response to succinylcholine in the absence of an obvious explanation has been described in a patient with this disorder.[63]

Wiskott-Aldrich Syndrome

Wiskott-Aldrich syndrome is inherited as an X-linked recessive disease, thus affecting only males. The syndrome is characterized by thrombocytopenia, eczema, and increased susceptibility to infections. Thrombocytopenia is the result of rapid platelet destruction caused by intrinsic defects in platelets. Presenting features are usually related to thrombocytopenia and associated hemorrhage. Plasma IgM concentrations are often decreased. Treatment consists of platelet transfusions, as the thrombocytopenia is resistant to corticosteroids and is not improved by splenectomy.

Ataxia Telangiectasia

Ataxia telangiectasia is characterized by progressive cerebellar ataxia beginning during childhood, recurrent sinus and pulmonary infections, and the subsequent development of telangiectasia of the bulbar conjunctivae. Most patients are found to have absent or decreased plasma concentrations of IgA and IgE. The function of T lymphocytes may also be impaired, and there is a high incidence of lymphoma in these patients. Skin manifestations may include café au lait spots and sclerodermoid changes. Disor-

ders of glucose metabolism may be present. A familial incidence suggests that this disease is inherited as an autosomal recessive disorder.

DISORDERS OF THE COMPLEMENT SYSTEM

Disorders of the complement system are uncommon, and most manifest as hereditary angioedema. Deficiencies of complement proteins 2 and 3 may also occur.

Hereditary Angioedema

Hereditary angioedema is a rare autosomal dominant disorder. It is due to decreased functional activity of the plasma complement protein known as "C1 esterase inhibitor," manifesting as episodic and sometimes life-threatening airway edema (Fig. 29–2).[1, 64, 65] In the absence of C1 esterase inhibitor activity, the initial activation of the complement pathway is not regulated, leading to the release of vasoactive mediators (possibly bradykinin) that increase vascular permeability. Attacks may occur spontaneously but are more often initiated by trauma, particularly a dental procedure or conceivably direct laryngoscopy and tracheal intubation. Emotional stress is responsible for triggering attacks in 30% to 40% of patients.[64]

Diagnosis

Hereditary angioedema is diagnosed on the basis of family history, prior attacks of angioedema, and documentation of low or absent levels of C1 esterase inhibitor. Functional levels of C1 inhibitor activity in the blood are approximately 30% of normal values. About 15% of patients, however, have normal levels of C1 inhibitor, but most of it is nonfunctional.

Signs and Symptoms

Hereditary angioedema is characterized by episodic and painless edema (increased vascular permeability) of the skin (face and extremities) and mucous membranes (respiratory and gastrointestinal tract). Laryngeal edema is the most dangerous manifestation and can lead to complete upper airway obstruction and asphyxiation. Abdominal cramps may reflect edema in the small intestine and, on occasion, falsely suggest the need for exploratory laparotomy. Attacks typically last 48 to 96 hours.

Treatment

Treatment of hereditary angioedema includes long-term prophylaxis, short-term prophylaxis, and treatment of acute attacks.[65]

Long-Term Prophylaxis

Long-term prophylaxis is not necessary in every patient, being reserved for those with a history of repeated debilitating attacks associated with facial and laryngeal edema. The two classes of drugs utilized for long-term prophylaxis are anabolic steroids (stanozolol 2 mg daily, danazol 600 mg daily) and antifibrinolytics (aminocaproic acid, tranexamic acid). Anabolic steroids are believed to increase hepatic synthesis of C1 esterase inhibitor, whereas antifibrinolytics are believed to act by inhibiting plasmin activation. Several days of treatment are needed with each of these classes of drugs to achieve a therapeutic effect. Children and parturients are rarely treated because of the harmful side effects (masculinization, hepatic dysfunction) that may accompany administration of anabolic steroids.

Short-Term Prophylaxis

Short-term prophylaxis is indicated for patients with hereditary angioedema who are not receiving long-term prophylaxis but who are scheduled for dental procedures or surgical procedures that require tracheal intubation.[65] Such therapy can be provided by a 5- to 7-day course of anabolic steroids (stanozolol) before surgery or by intravenous administration of C1 esterase inhibitor concentrates or fresh frozen plasma immediately before surgery. Purified preparations of C1 esterase inhibitor concentrate administered intravenously prevent attacks of hereditary angioedema and can be used to treat acute attacks.[64] Fresh frozen plasma is a source of C1 esterase inhibitor; 2 to 4 units administered 24 hours before surgery can prevent airway swelling during the intraoperative and postoperative periods.

Acute Attack

Intravenous infusions of C1 esterase inhibitor concentrates, 25 units/kg, during acute attacks of hereditary angioedema are likely to evoke therapeutic responses within 60 minutes of beginning the infusions.[64, 65] Fresh frozen plasma may also be administered to provide C1 esterase inhibitor. Acute attacks do not respond to treatment with anabolic steroids, corticosteroids, antihistamines, catecholamines, or antifibrinolytics. Should upper airway obstruction develop during acute attacks of hereditary angi-

oedema, tracheal intubation is life-saving until the edema subsides.

Management of Anesthesia

Pretreatment of patients with hereditary angioedema prior to elective surgery may include administration of an anabolic steroid (stanozolol) and intravenous administration of C1 esterase inhibitor concentrates or fresh frozen plasma during the 24 hours preceding surgery especially to patients in whom airway trauma (including placement of a laryngeal mask airway or tracheal tube) is anticipated.[65–67] It seems prudent to ensure the ready availability of C1 esterase inhibitor concentrates for intravenous infusion should an acute attack occur. If patients are receiving prophylaxis therapy, these drugs are continued throughout the perioperative period. Incidental trauma to the patient's oropharynx, such as that produced by suctioning, should be minimized. Intramuscular injections do not seem to cause problems in these patients. Regional anesthetic techniques are reasonable considerations if their selection negates the predictable need to use a laryngeal mask airway or tracheal intubation. Nevertheless, tracheal intubation should not be avoided in these patients if this intervention can contribute to safe conduct of the anesthesia, recognizing that airway trauma may worsen laryngeal edema and necessitate emergency tracheostomy. The potential for laryngeal distortion secondary to edema may render laryngeal mask airways ineffective. The choice of drugs to produce general or regional anesthesia is not influenced by the presence of hereditary angioedema.

Emergency Airway Management

Emergency management of the patient's airway during an acute attack of laryngeal edema includes administration of supplemental oxygen and consideration of tracheal intubation. The presence of airway edema limits the usefulness of fiberoptic laryngoscopy. When performing emergency laryngoscopy, it is important to have personnel and equipment available to perform an urgent tracheostomy. Airway swelling may become so severe that even tracheostomy may be ineffective in providing a patent airway. Swelling may extend into the airway to such an extent that death is inevitable in the absence of specific replacement therapy.[65]

Complement Protein C2 Deficiency

Complement protein C2 deficiency occurs in about 1 of every 10,000 individuals. About half of these patients have a history of systemic lupus erythematosus or a related disorder such as Schönlein-Henoch purpura. This association may reflect viral origins for these diseases and complement participation in viral neutralization.

Complement Protein C3 Deficiency

Complement protein C3 deficiency is associated with increased susceptibility to life-threatening bacterial infections. Complement-mediated functions, such as bactericidal activity, chemotaxis, and opsonization, are absent in C3-deficient plasma. Patients who are homozygous for C5-C8 complement protein deficiency may also display increased susceptibility to infections.

▌ AUTOIMMUNE DISEASES

Autoimmune diseases occur when the host's own tissues act as self-antigens to evoke the production of autoantibodies (Table 29–7) (see Chapter 26).[68] The resulting antigen-antibody interactions produce tissue injury. Normally, T lymphocytes are responsi-

Table 29–7 • Examples of Autoimmune Diseases

Organ-specific diseases
  Insulin-dependent diabetes mellitus
  Myasthenia gravis
  Graves' disease
  Thyroiditis
  Addison's disease
  Pernicious anemia
  Male infertility
  Primary biliary cirrhosis
  Chronic active hepatitis
  Crohn's disease
  Autoimmune hemolytic anemia
  Psoriasis
Systemic diseases
  Rheumatic fever
  Rheumatoid arthritis
  Ankylosing spondylitis
  Systemic lupus erythematosus
  Scleroderma
  Polymyositis
  Goodpasture syndrome
  Chronic graft-versus-host disease
  Hypereosinophilic syndrome
  Lyme disease
  Kawasaki disease
  Immunoglobulin A deficiency
  Hereditary complement deficiency
  Vasculitis
  Sarcoidosis

ble for blocking antibody production to host antigens. Failure of suppressor T lymphocytes to prevent antibody production by B lymphocytes may result in autoimmune diseases. Cyclosporine suppresses immune responses by inhibiting helper T lymphocytes but does not inhibit antigen-induced activation of suppressor T lymphocytes. It is possible that self-antigens are modified by combining with drugs (hydralazine, procainamide) or viruses that then stimulate antibody production. Similar mechanisms may be at work when streptococcal antigens induce formation of antibodies to heart valves (rheumatic fever) or neuronal tissues (Sydenham's chorea) in genetically susceptible patients. Myasthenia gravis is characterized by the development of autoantibodies to acetylcholine receptors at the neuromuscular junctions. Patients with Graves' disease may produce autoantibodies that act on receptors, leading to increased synthesis of cAMP. Vasculitis is often part of autoimmune diseases, being limited to a single organ such as the kidneys or becoming generalized.

References

1. Walport MJ, Complement, N Engl J Med 2001;344:1058–66, 1140–51
2. Kay AB. Allergy and allergic diseases. N Engl J Med 2001;344:30–7, 109–13
3. Kettelkamp NS, Austin DR, Cheek DBC, et al. Inhibition of d-tubocurarine-induced histamine release by halothane. Anesthesiology 1987;66:666–9
4. Lilly JK, Hoy RH. Thiopental anaphylaxis and reagin involvement. Anesthesiology 1980;53:335–7
5. Laroche D, Vergnaud M-C, Sillard B, et al. Biochemical markers of anaphylactoid reactions to drugs. Anesthesiology 1991;75:945–9
6. Matthey P, Wang P, Finegan BA, et al. Rocuronium anaphylaxis and multiple neuromuscular blocking drug sensitivities. Can J Anaesth 2000;47:890–3
7. Renz CL, Laroche D, Thurn JD, et al. Tryptase levels are not increased during vancomycin-induced anaphylactoid reactions. Anesthesiology 1998;89:620–5
8. Fisher MM, Baldo BA, Silbert BS. Anaphylaxis during anesthesia: use of radioimmunoassays to determine etiology and drugs responsible in fatal cases. Anesthesiology 1991;75:1112–5
9. Sage DJ. Management of acute anaphylactoid reactions. Int Anesthesiol Clin 1985;23:175–86
10. Barach EM, Nowak RM, Lee TG, et al. Epinephrine for treatment of anaphylactic shock. JAMA 1984;251:2118–22
11. Generic propofol debate evolves. Anesth Patient Safety Found Newslett 1999;14:13–7
12. Knape JTA, Schuller JL, deHaan P, et al. An anaphylactic reaction to protamine in a patient allergic to fish. Anesthesiology 1981;55:324–5
13. Weiss ME, Adkinson NF, Hirshman CA. Evaluation of allergic drug reactions in the perioperative period. Anesthesiology 1989;71:483–6
14. Fisher MM, More DG. The epidemiology and clinical features of anaphylactic reactions in anaesthesia. Anaesth Intensive Care 1981;9:226–34

15. Etter MS, Helrich M, Mackenzie CF. Immunoglobulin E fluctuation in thiopental anaphylaxis. Anesthesiology 1980;52:181–3

16. Beaven MA. Anaphylactoid reactions to anesthetic drugs. Anesthesiology 1981;55:3–5

17. Moudgil GC. Anaesthesia and allergic drug reactions. Can Anaesth Soc J 1986;33:400–14

18. Bochner BS, Lichtenstein LM. Current concepts: anaphylaxis. N Engl J Med 1991;324:1785–91

19. Bruno LA, Smith DS, Bloom MJ, et al. Sudden hypotension with a test dose of chymopapain. Anesth Analg 1984;63:533–5

20. Laxenaire M-C, Mata-Bermejo E, Moneret-Vautrin DA, et al. Life-threatening anaphylactoid reactions to propofol. Anesthesiology 1992;77:275–80

21. Sethna NF, Brown RH, Christie JM, et al. Latex anaphylaxis in a child with a history of multiple anesthetic drug allergies. Anesthesiology 1992;77:372–5

22. Zucker-Pinchoff B, Chandler MJ. Latex anaphylaxis masquerading as fentanyl anaphylaxis: retraction of a case report. Anesthesiology 1993;79:1153–4

23. Harle DG, Baldo BA, Fisher MM. Cross-reactivity of metocurine, atracurium, vecuronium and fazadinium with IgE antibodies from patients unexposed to these drugs but allergic to other myoneural blocking drugs. Br J Anaesth 1985;57:1073–6

24. Laxenaire MC. Epidemiology of anesthetic anaphylactoid reactions: fourth multicenter survey (July 1994–December 1996). Ann Fr Anesth Reanim 1999;18:796–809

25. Hirshman CA, Edelstein RA, Ebertz JM, et al. Thiobarbiturate-induced histamine release in human skin mast cells. Anesthesiology 1985;63:353–6

26. Brown DT, Beamish D, Wiedsmith JAW. Allergic reaction to an amide local anaesthetic. Br J Anaesth 1981;53:435–7

27. Levy JH, Rockoff MA. Anaphylaxis to meperidine. Anesth Analg 1982;61:301–3

28. Bennett MJ, Anderson LK, McMillan JC, et al. Anaphylactic reaction during anaesthesia associated with positive intradermal skin test to fentanyl. Can Anaesth Soc J 1986;33:75–8

29. Moorthy SS, Pond W, Rowland RG. Severe circulatory shock following protamine (an anaphylactic reaction). Anesth Analg 1980;59:77–8

30. Weiss ME, Nyhan D, Peng Z, et al. Association of protamine IgE and IgG antibodies with life-threatening reactions to intravenous protamine. N Engl J Med 1989;320:886–92

31. Levy JH, Schwieger IM, Zaidan JR, et al. Evaluation of patients at risk for protamine reactions. J Thorac Cardiovasc Surg 1989;98:200–4

32. Morel DR, Zapol WM, Thomas ST, et al. C5a and thromboxane generation associated with pulmonary vaso- and bronchoconstriction during protamine reversal of heparin. Anesthesiology 1987;66:597–604

33. Anne S, Reisman RE. Risk of administering cephalosporin antibiotics to patients with histories of penicillin allergy. Ann Allergy Asthma Immunol 1995;74:167–70

34. Symons NLP, Hobbes AFT, Leaver HK. Anaphylactoid reactions to vancomycin during anaesthesia: two clinical reports. Can Anaesth Soc J 1985;32:178–81

35. Mayhew JF, Duetsch S. Cardiac arrest following administration of vancomycin. Can Anaesth Soc J 1985;32:65–6

36. Lyon GD, Bruce DL. Diphenhydramine reversal of vancomycin-induced hypotension. Anesth Analg 1988;67:1109–10

37. Roizen MF, Rodgers GM, Valone FH, et al. Anaphylactoid reactions to vascular graft material presenting with vasodilation and subsequent disseminated intravascular coagulation. Anesthesiology 1989;71:331–8

38. Hirshman CA. Latex anaphylaxis. Anesthesiology 1992;77:223–5

39. Calenda E, Durand JP, Petit J, et al. Anaphylactic shock produced by latex. JAMA 1991;265:2844–7

40. Holzman RS. Latex allergy: an emerging operating room problem. Anesth Analg 1993;76:635–41

41. Moneret-Vautrin DA, Laxenaire MC, Bavoux F. Allergic shock to latex and ethylene oxide during surgery for spina bifida. Anesthesiology 1990;73:556–8

42. Slater JE. Rubber anaphylaxis. N Engl J Med 1989;320:1126–30

43. Hamilton RG, Adkinson NF. Multi-center Latex Skin Testing Study Task Force: diagnosis of natural rubber latex allergy: multicenter latex skin testing efficacy study. J Allergy Clin Immunol 1998;102:482–90

44. Konrad C, Fieber T, Gerber H, et al. The prevalence of latex sensitivity among anesthesiology staff. Anesth Analg 1997;84:629–33

45. Holzman RS. Clinical management of latex-allergic children. Anesth Analg 1997;85:529–33

46. Setlock MA, Cotter TP, Rosner D. Latex allergy: failure of prophylaxis to prevent severe reaction. Anesth Analg 1993;76:650–2

47. Walton B. Effects of anaesthesia and surgery on immune status. Br J Anaesth 1979;51:37–43

48. Duncan PG, Cullen BF. Anesthesia and immunology. Anesthesiology 1976;45:522–38

49. Lewis RE, Cruse JM, Hazelwood J. Halothane-induced suppression of cell-mediated immunity in normal and tumor bearing C3Hf/He mice. Anesth Analg 1980;59:666–71

50. Sessler DI. Mild perioperative hypothermia. N Engl J Med 1997;336:1630–7

51. Roizen MF, Horrigan RW, Frazer BM. Anesthetic doses blocking adrenergic (stress) and cardiovascular responses to incision-MAC BAR. Anesthesiology 1981;54:390–8

52. Knight PR, Bedows E, Nahrwold ML, et al. Alterations in influenza virus pulmonary pathology induced by diethyl ether, halothane, enflurane, and pentobarbital anesthesia in mice. Anesthesiology 1983;58:209–15

53. Fosen FS, Cooper MD, Wedgwood RJP. The primary immunodeficiencies. N Engl J Med 1984;311:235–42

54. Buckley RH, Schiff RI. The use of intravenous immune globulin in immunodeficiency diseases. N Engl J Med 1991;325:110–7

55. Park JV, Weiss CI. Cardiopulmonary bypass and myocardial protection: management problems in cardiac surgical patients with cold autoimmune disease. Anesth Analg 1988;67:75–8

56. Diaz JH, Cooper ES, Oschner JL. Cardiac surgery in patients with cold autoimmune diseases. Anesth Analg 1984;63:349–52

57. Beebe DS, Bergen L, Palahniu RJ. Anesthetic management of a patient with severe cold agglutinin hemolytic anemia utilizing forced air warming. Anesth Analg 1993;76:1144–6

58. Falk RH, Comenzo RL, Skinner M. The systemic amyloidoses. N Engl J Med 1997;337:898–909

59. Mizutani AR, Ward CF. Amyloidosis associated bleeding diatheses in the surgical patient. Can J Anaesth 1990;37:910–2

60. Wang MMJ, Pollard JB. Postoperative ventricular fibrillation and undiagnosed primary amyloidosis. Anesthesiology 2000;92:871–2

61. Kotani N, Hashimoto H, Muraoka M, et al. Fatal perioperative myocardial infarction in four patients with cardiac amyloidosis. Anesthesiology 2000;92:873–5

62. Miller FL, Mann DL. Anesthetic management of a pregnant patient with the hyperimmunoglobulin E (Job's) syndrome. Anesth Analg 1990;70:454–6

63. Guzzi LM, Stamatos JM. Job's syndrome: an unusual response to a common drug. Anesth Analg 1992;75:139–40

64. Waytes AT, Rosen FS, Frank MM. Treatment of hereditary angioedema with a vapor-heated C1 inhibitor concentrate. N Engl J Med 1996;334:1630–4

65. Jensen NF, Weiler JM. C1 esterase inhibitor deficiency, airway compromise, and anesthesia. Anesth Analg 1998;87:480–8

66. Wall RT, Frank M, Hahn M. A review of 25 patients with hereditary angioedema requiring surgery. Anesthesiology 1989;71:309–11

67. Sarantopoulos CD, Bratanow NC, Stowe DF, et al. Uneventful propofol anesthesia in a patient with coexisting hereditary coproporphyria and hereditary angioneurotic edema. Anesthesiology 2000;92:607–9

68. Dalakas MC. Polymyositis, dermatomyositis, and inclusion-body myositis. N Engl J Med 1991;325:1487–98

Psychiatric Diseases and Substance Abuse

The prevalence of psychiatric diseases increases the likelihood that these diseases will co-exist in patients undergoing anesthesia and surgery. Important considerations are the potential drug interactions introduced by medications used to treat psychiatric illness. Substance abuse and drug dependence may also be viewed as types of psychiatric diseases. Substance abuse and suicide represent significant occupational hazards for anesthesiologists compared with other nonoperating room physicians.[1]

MENTAL DEPRESSION

Mental depression is the most common psychiatric disorder (affects 2% to 4% of the population) and is distinguished from normal sadness and grief by the severity and duration of the mood disturbances and the presence of fatigue, loss of appetite, and insomnia. Patients with mental depression who have had a manic episode are classified as having bipolar disease, or manic-depressive disorder. There is a familial pattern of major mental depression, and females are affected more often than males. About 15% of patients with major depression commit suicide. Pathophysiologic causes of major mental depression are unknown, although abnormalities of amine neurotransmitter pathways are the most likely etiologic factors. Cortisol hypersecretion is present in many of these patients.

Diagnosis

The diagnosis of major mental depression is based on the persistent presence of at least five characteristics and the exclusion of organic causes or a normal

Depressed mood
Decreased interest in daily activities and physical
 appearance
Fluctuations in body weight
Insomnia or hypersomnia
Fatigue
Decreased ability to concentrate
Recurrent thoughts of suicide

reaction to the death of a loved one (Table 30–1). Alcoholism and major depression often occur together; and it is presumed that toxic effects of alcohol on the brain are responsible. Mental depression and dementia may be difficult to distinguish in elderly patients. All patients with depression should be evaluated for the potential to commit suicide. Suicide is the tenth leading cause of death in the United States, and for physicians younger than 40 years of age it ranks first. More than 90% of overdose suicide victims have been under the care of a physician shortly before their death, emphasizing the importance of recognizing at risk patients. Hopelessness is the most important aspect of depression associated with suicide.

Treatment

Treatment of mental depression is with antidepressant drugs and/or electroconvulsive therapy (ECT).[2] An estimated 70% to 80% of patients respond to pharmacologic therapy, and at least 50% who do not respond to antidepressants do respond favorably to ECT. ECT is usually reserved for patients resistant to antidepressant drugs or those with medical contraindications to treatment with these drugs. Patients with mental depression plus psychotic symptoms (delusions, hallucinations, catatonia) require both antidepressant and antipsychotic drugs. The concept that antidepressant drugs work by increasing the availability of norepinephrine and serotonin is not supported by the observation that these drugs require 14 to 28 days to effect symptomatic improvement, whereas the effects on neurotransmitter uptake are prompt. Instead, the effects of these drugs on the regulation of neurotransmitter receptor function over several days is a more likely explanation for the therapeutic effects.

Selective Serotonin Reuptake Inhibitors

Selective serotonin reuptake inhibitors (SSRIs) comprise the most broadly prescribed class of antide-

pressants and are the drugs of choice to treat mild to moderate mental depression. These drugs are also effective for treating panic disorders and at high doses for obsessive-compulsive disorders. Compared with tricyclic antidepressants, the SSRIs have little effect on norepinephrine reuptake. Although their mechanism of action is unknown, it is presumed that effects on serotonin receptors are necessary for a therapeutic effect. Unlike tricyclic antidepressant drugs, SSRIs lack anticholinergic effects and do not cause postural hypotension or delayed conduction of cardiac impulses; they also do not appear to have an effect on seizure thresholds (Table 30–2). Common side effects of SSRIs are insomnia, agitation, headache, nausea, diarrhea, and sexual dysfunction. Appetite suppression is associated with fluoxetine therapy.

Among SSRIs, fluoxetine is a potent inhibitor of certain hepatic cytochrome P_{450} enzymes.[3] As a result, this drug may increase plasma concentrations of drugs that depend on hepatic metabolism for clearance. For example, addition of fluoxetine to treatment with tricyclic antidepressant drugs may result in two- to fivefold increases in the plasma concentrations of tricyclic drugs. Cardiac antidysrhythmia drugs and some β-adrenergic antagonists may be metabolized by the same enzyme systems that are inhibited by fluoxetine, resulting in potentiation of these drug's effects. Monoamine oxidase inhibitors (MAOIs) combined with fluoxetine may cause the development of a serotonin syndrome characterized by anxiety, restlessness, chills, ataxia, and insomnia. The combination of fluoxetine and lithium or carbamazepine may also provoke this potentially fatal syndrome.

Other Second-Generation Antidepressants

Other second generation antidepressants include drugs (bupropion, venlafaxine, trazodone) unrelated to SSRIs, tricyclic antidepressants, or MAOIs (Table 30–2). These drugs may serve as alternative therapies for patients who do not respond to SSRIs. Bupropion, like the SSRIs, has no anticholinergic effects, does not produce postural hypotension, and lacks significant effects on conduction of cardiac impulses. Unlike SSRIs, bupropion is not associated with significant drug interactions. Venlafaxine, like tricyclic antidepressants, inhibits norepinephrine reuptake but does not produce anticholinergic effects or postural hypotension. Trazodone inhibits serotonin uptake and may also act as a serotonin agonist via an active metabolite. Although effective in the management of mental depression, it greatest efficacy is in the treatment of insomnia. Combination

Table 30–2 • Antidepressant Drugs Used to Treat Psychiatric Diseases

Drug	Sedative Potency	Anticholinergic Potency	Orthostatic Hypotension	Cardiac Dysrhythmia Potential
Selective serotonin uptake inhibitors				
Fluoxetine	+	+	+	0
Paroxetine	+	+	+	0
Sertaline	+	+	+	0
Fluvoxamine	+	+	+	0
Other second-generation antidepressants				
Bupropion	+	+	+	0
Venlafaxine	+	+	*	0
Trazodone	+++	+	+++	0
Nefazodone	++	+	++	0
Tricyclic antidepressants				
Amitriptyline	+++	++++	+++	++
Amoxapine	+	+	++	++
Clomipramine	+++	+++	+++	++
Desipramine	+	+	+++	++
Doxepin	+++	++	++	++
Imipramine	++	++	+++	++
Nortriptyline	+	+	+	++
Protriptyline	+	+++	+	++
Trimipramine	+++	++	++	++
Related polycyclics				
Anixaoube	+	+	++	++
Malprotiline	++	+	++	++

0, none; +, mild; ++, moderate; +++, marked; ++++, greatest.
* May cause systemic hypertension.

therapy with these drugs and MAOIs is not recommended.

Tricyclic Antidepressants

Before the availability of SSRIs, tricyclic antidepressants were the most commonly prescribed drugs for treating mental depression. Side effects of antidepressant drugs influence drug choice because all of these drugs are equally effective if administered in equivalent doses (Table 30–2). Generally, tricyclic antidepressants producing sedation are selected for patients describing insomnia. It is useful to minimize drug-induced anticholinergic effects (tachycardia, blurred vision, dry mouth, delayed gastric emptying, urinary retention), especially in elderly patients or in individuals with glaucoma or prostatic hypertrophy. All tricyclic antidepressants exert some anticholinergic effects, with the most pronounced effects accompanying the use of amitriptyline and protriptyline. In addition to causing sedative and anticholinergic effects, tricyclic antidepressants can cause cardiovascular abnormalities, including orthostatic hypotension and cardiac dysrhythmias. Tricyclic antidepressants tend to slow both atrial and ventricular depolarization, manifesting as increased PR and QT intervals and widened QRS complexes on the patient's electrocardiogram

(ECG). These changes on the ECG, in the absence of excessive plasma concentrations of the drug, are probably benign and gradually disappear with continued therapy (see "Tricyclic Antidepressant Overdose").[4] Previous suggestions that tricyclic antidepressants increased the risk of cardiac dysrhythmias and sudden death have not been substantiated in the absence of drug overdoses. Even in the presence of co-existing cardiac dysfunction, tricyclic antidepressants have no adverse effects on left ventricular function and may even have cardiac antidysrhythmia properties.[5, 6] Nevertheless, it is possible that patients with co-existing heart block or prolonged QT intervals on the ECG may be at increased risk of cardiac toxicity. Decreased cardiac toxicity for doxepin has not been confirmed. The polycyclic drug maprotiline has a tendency to cause seizures at upper therapeutic dose ranges.

It is usually possible to taper the dose of antidepressant drugs in patients with primary depressive illnesses who have been symptom-free for about 6 months. A few patients require long-term treatment, whereas patients whose mental depression is secondary to treatable medical illnesses may require only short courses of antidepressant therapy. If tricyclic antidepressant therapy is contraindicated because of the patient's cardiac status, ECT may be recommended.

Treatment with tricyclic antidepressants need not be discontinued before administration of anesthesia for elective operations. Alterations in responses to drugs administered during the perioperative period, however, should be anticipated in treated patients. For example, increased availability of neurotransmitters in the patient's central nervous system can result in increased anesthetic requirements.[7] Likewise, increased availability of norepinephrine at postsynaptic receptors in the peripheral sympathetic nervous system can be responsible for exaggerated systemic blood pressure responses following administration of indirect-acting vasopressors, such as ephedrine. If vasopressors are needed during the perioperative period, a direct-acting drug such as phenylephrine may be useful. If systemic hypertension requires treatment, peripheral vasodilating drugs such as nitroprusside are effective. The potential for hypertensive crises is greatest during acute treatment (first 14 to 21 days) with tricyclic antidepressants, whereas chronic treatment is associated with down-regulation of receptors and a decreased likelihood of exaggerated systemic blood pressure responses following administration of sympathomimetic drugs.[8]

Chronic treatment with tricyclic antidepressants may alter the responses to pancuronium. For example, tachydysrhythmias have been observed following administration of pancuronium to patients anesthetized who were also receiving imipramine.[9] Presumably there is an interaction between tricyclic antidepressants and the anticholinergic and sympathetic nervous stimulating effects of pancuronium. Theoretically, ketamine might produce adverse responses similar to those seen with pancuronium when administered to patients being treated with tricyclic antidepressants. The dose of exogenous epinephrine necessary to produce ventricular cardiac dysrhythmias during anesthesia provided with volatile anesthetics may be decreased by prior acute treatment with imipramine. It is conceivable that treatment with tricyclic antidepressants could also accentuate the cardiac dysrhythmogenic potential of systemically absorbed exogenous epinephrine, as could occur when epinephrine-containing local anesthetic solutions are utilized for peripheral nerve blocks or epidural anesthesia. Conversely, chronic imipramine therapy does not alter the incidence of cardiac dysrhythmias, presumably because of compensatory mechanisms at sympathetic nerve endings. Theoretically, drugs that produce seizure activity on the electroencephalogram (EEG) should be avoided in patients being treated with antidepressant drugs that are also associated with seizure activity. In animals, tricyclic antidepressants augment the analgesic and ventilatory depressant effects of opioids and the sedative effects of barbiturates. If these effects also occur in patients, it is possible that drug doses should be decreased to avoid exaggerated or prolonged effects.[10] Postoperatively, the likelihood of delirium and confusion might be increased by additive anticholinergic effects of the tricyclic antidepressants and centrally active anticholinergic drugs used for preoperative medication.

Monoamine Oxidase Inhibitors

Patients who do not respond to antidepressants may benefit from treatment with MAOIs (phenelzine, isocarboxazid, tranylcypromine). In contrast to tricyclic antidepressants, MAOIs have negligible anticholinergic effects and do not sensitize the heart to the cardiac dysrhythmogenic effects of epinephrine. The principal clinical problem associated with use of these drugs is the possible occurrence of severe systemic hypertension if treated patients ingest foods that contain tyramine (cheeses, wines) or receive drugs characterized as sympathomimetics (Table 30–3). Systemic hypertension reflects inhibition of the enzyme activity of monoamine oxidase, which results in increased availability of norepinephrine. Therefore sympathomimetic drugs such as ephedrine, which act by stimulating the release of norepinephrine, can precipitate hypertension. Likewise, tyramine in foods acts as a potent stimulus for the release of norepinephrine, explaining the resulting systemic hypertension if susceptible patients ingest tyramine-containing foods. Orthostatic hypotension is the most common side effect observed in patients being treated with MAOIs. The mechanism for this hypotension is unknown, but it may reflect accumulation of false neurotransmitters such as octopamine, which are less potent than norepinephrine. This mechanism may also explain the antihypertensive effects observed with chronic use of MAOIs.

Although uncommon, adverse interactions between MAOIs and opioids have been observed.[11, 12] Systemic hypertension, hypotension, hyperthermia, depression of ventilation, seizures, and coma may follow administration of opioids to patients being

---

Table 30–3 • Side Effects of Monoamine Oxidase Inhibitors

Sedation
Blurred vision
Orthostatic hypotension
Peripheral neuropathy
Systemic hypertension in response to ingestion of tyramine-containing foods
Hyperthermia in response to opioid administration

treated with MAOIs. Meperidine has been the opioid most often incriminated, but the same syndrome can occur with other opioids. Explanations for these adverse responses include decreased or slowed metabolism of the opioid, mass sympathetic nervous system discharge caused by the opioid, formation of toxic metabolites of the opioid, and increased central nervous system concentrations of serotonin.

Management of Anesthesia

Anesthesia can be safely conducted in patients being chronically treated with MAOIs despite earlier recommendations that these drugs be discontinued 14 to 21 days before elective operations to permit time for regeneration of new enzyme.[11-13] Furthermore, it is not a realistic recommendation to discontinue MAOIs before elective procedures that require anesthesia, such as ECT, as patients may be placed at increased risk for suicide.

Proceeding with anesthesia and surgery in patients being treated with MAOIs may influence the selection of drugs and the doses administered. For example, opioids should probably be avoided in the preoperative medication of patients being treated with MAOIs. Likewise, in the absence of specific indications, inclusion of anticholinergic drugs in the preoperative medication is probably not necessary. Benzodiazepines are acceptable for pharmacologic treatment of preoperative anxiety in these patients. Induction of anesthesia can be safely accomplished with drugs administered intravenously, keeping in mind that central nervous system effects and depression of ventilation may be exaggerated. The exception to this generalization is ketamine in view of the ability of this drug to stimulate the sympathetic nervous system. Serum cholinesterase activity may decrease in patients treated with phenelzine, suggesting the need to adjust the succinylcholine dose.[12] Nitrous oxide combined with volatile anesthetics is acceptable for maintenance of anesthesia. Selection of specific volatile anesthetics may be influenced by the ability of drugs such as halothane to evoke cardiac dysrhythmias in the presence of catecholamines and by the possibility of MAOI-induced hepatic dysfunction, as reflected in liver function tests. It is conceivable, but unproven, that anesthetic requirements are increased owing to increased concentrations of norepinephrine present in the central nervous system. Fentanyl has been administered intraoperatively to patients being treated with MAOIs without apparent adverse effects.[11, 12] The choice of nondepolarizing muscle relaxants is not influenced by treatment with MAOIs, with the possible exception of pancuronium. Spinal or epidural anesthesia is acceptable, although the potential for these anes-thetic techniques to produce hypotension and the consequent need for vasopressors may mitigate in favor of general anesthesia.[14] Epinephrine added to local anesthetic solutions should probably be avoided when regional anesthetic techniques are selected.

During anesthesia and surgery it is important to avoid stimulating the sympathetic nervous system (as produced by arterial hypoxemia, hypercarbia, hypotension, topical cocaine spray, or injection of indirect-acting vasopressors) to decrease the incidence of systemic hypertension and cardiac dysrhythmias.[15] If vasopressors are needed, direct-acting drugs such as phenylephrine are recommended. Even with this drug, the dose should probably be decreased to minimize the likelihood of an exaggerated hypertensive response. Nevertheless, ephedrine has also been administered with no apparent adverse effects.[12] In this regard, the potential for hypertensive crisis is greatest during acute treatment with MAOIs (first 14 to 21 days), whereas chronic treatment is associated with down-regulation of receptors and a decreased likelihood of exaggerated systemic blood pressure responses following administration of sympathomimetics.[8]

Postoperative Care

Provision of analgesia during the postoperative period is influenced by the potential adverse interactions between opioids and MAOIs. If opioids are needed for postoperative pain management, morphine or fentanyl is the preferred drug, but the dose should be the least amount necessary to achieve analgesia. Alternatives to opioids for providing postoperative analgesia includes administration of nonopioid analgesics, peripheral nerve blocks with local anesthetics, and the use of transcutaneous electrical nerve stimulation. Neuraxial opioids provide effective analgesia, but experience is too limited to permit recommendations regarding use of this approach in patients being treated with MAOIs.

Electroconvulsive Therapy

Electroconvulsive therapy is indicated for treating severe mental depression in patients who are unresponsive to drugs or who become acutely suicidal.[16-18] Increased intracranial pressure is a contraindication to ECT. To minimize memory impairment, ECT is often administered only to the nondominant hemisphere. When administered in brief-pulse waveforms it uses only one-third to one-fourth the voltage used when administered in sine waveforms. Although the mechanism of action of ECT is unknown, it is likely that therapeutic efficacy is related to the amount of current passed through the brain. The previous concept that the therapeutic benefit of ECT depended on the duration of the electrically induced seizure is not substantiated. The electrical stimulus produces a grand mal seizure consisting of a brief tonic phase followed by a more prolonged clonic phase. The EEG shows changes similar to those present during spontaneous grand mal seizures. Typically, about eight treatments are necessary, with more than 75% of treated patients showing a favorable response.

Side Effects

Side effects of ECT manifest principally in the cardiovascular and central nervous systems (Table 30–4).[18] An initial vagal discharge may lead to bradycardia, with decreased systemic blood pressure followed by sympathetic nervous system activation and increased heart rate and systemic blood pressure. These changes may be undesirable in patients with ischemic heart disease. Indeed, the most common causes of death following ECT are myocardial infarction and cardiac dysrhythmias.[19] Ventricular premature beats presumably reflect excess sympathetic nervous system activity. Increased T wave amplitude on the ECG simulating hyperkalemia may accompany ECT, presumably reflecting an imbalance of autonomic nervous system activity, as electrically induced seizure activity is not known to cause potassium release.[20] Venous return to the heart is decreased by the increased intrathoracic pressure that accompanies the seizure and/or positive-pressure ventilation of the lungs.

Cerebral blood flow increases up to sevenfold, reflecting increased cerebral oxygen consumption in the presence of the electrically induced seizure. The resulting increase in intracranial pressure is transient but may prohibit the use of ECT in patients with known space-occupying lesions or head injury.

■ **Table 30–4** • Side Effects of
■ Electroconvulsive Therapy

■ Parasympathetic nervous system stimulation
    Bradycardia
    Hypotension
■ Sympathetic nervous system stimulation
    Tachycardia
    Systemic hypertension
    Cardiac dysrhythmias
Increased cerebral blood flow
Increased intracranial pressure
Increased intraocular pressure
Increased intragastric pressure
Hypoventilation

Increased intraocular pressure is an inevitable side effect of electrically induced seizures and may detract from the use of ECT in patients with glaucoma. Increased intragastric pressure also occurs during seizure activity. Transient apnea plus postictal confusion may follow the seizure. The common long-term effect of ECT is memory impairment.

Management of Anesthesia

Anesthesia is usually administered to ensure patient comfort during ECT.[16] Patients are fasted, but preanesthetic medication is not recommended, as drug-produced sedation could prolong the period of recovery following ECT. Administration of atropine or glycopyrrolate intravenously 1 to 2 minutes before induction of anesthesia and delivery of the electrical current may be useful for decreasing the likelihood of bradycardia that may accompany ECT. Centrally acting anticholinergic drugs such as atropine may have additive effects with the central and peripheral anticholinergic effects of tricyclic antidepressants, manifesting as delirium and confusion during the postanesthetic period. For this reason, glycopyrrolate may be recommended when ECT is administered to patients being treated with tricyclic antidepressants, although many patients have undergone ECT safely without prior administration of anticholinergic drugs.[18] Nitroglycerin ointment applied 45 minutes before ECT decreases the magnitude of treatment-induced hypertension and thus may be useful in patients considered to be at risk for myocardial ischemia.[21, 22] Likewise, esmolol, 100 to 200 mg IV administered 1 minute before induction of anesthesia and 2 minutes before ECT, attenuates increases in systemic blood pressure and heart rate following ECT.[23] The duration of seizure activity is shortened by the higher dose of esmolol. Monitoring the ECG is useful for recognizing ECT-induced cardiac dysrhythmias.

Methohexital, 0.5 to 1.0 mg/kg IV, is a frequent choice for induction of anesthesia prior to ECT. Thiopental has no advantage over methohexital and might be associated with longer recovery times. Prior treatment of patients with tricyclic antidepressants or MAOIs could enhance the sedative effects of barbiturates. Propofol, 1.5 mg/kg IV, is an alternative to methohexital, being associated with a lower systemic blood pressure and heart rate in response to ECT compared with barbiturates.[24] Recovery time is similar following administration of methohexital or propofol, but an anticonvulsant effect of propofol is suggested by a shortened duration of electrically induced seizures in patients receiving this drug (Fig. 30–1).[24]

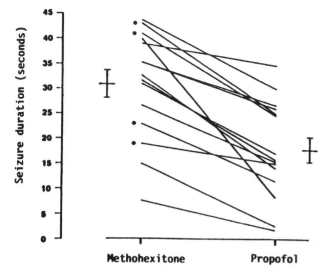

Figure 30–1 • Mean duration of an electrically induced seizure in the same patient was longer in the presence of methohexitone (methohexital) than in the presence of propofol. The lines labeled with an asterisk (*) represent patients receiving treatment with a benzodiazepine. Bars represent mean ± SE for each drug. (From Rampton AJ, Griffin RM, Stuart CS, et al. Comparison of methohexital and propofol for electroconvulsive therapy: effects of hemodynamic responses and seizure duration. Anesthesiology 1989;70:412–7, with permission.)

Intravenous injection of succinylcholine promptly after the induction of anesthesia for ECT is intended to attenuate the potentially dangerous skeletal muscle contractions and bone fractures that can be produced by seizure activity. Although the amount of succinylcholine administered varies, doses of 0.3 to 0.5 mg/kg IV are usually sufficient to attenuate contraction of skeletal muscles adequately and still permit visual confirmation of seizure activity. The most reliable method to confirm electrically induced seizure activity is the EEG. Alternatively, spontaneous movement of the patient's arm that has been isolated from the circulation by applying a tourniquet before administering succinylcholine is evidence that a seizure has occurred. Pretreatment with nonparalyzing doses of nondepolarizing muscle relaxants before administration of succinylcholine has not been evaluated in these patients. Ventilation support and delivery of supplemental oxygen is recommended both before production of the seizure and until the effects of succinylcholine have dissipated. Denitrogenation of the patient's lungs with oxygen before production of seizures decreases the likelihood of arterial hypoxemia if it becomes difficult to support ventilation in the presence of seizure-induced skeletal muscle contractions. Furthermore, it is important to recognize that apnea lasting up to 2 minutes can

follow ECT in the absence of succinylcholine. Monitoring arterial hemoglobin oxygen saturations with pulse oximetry is useful when guiding the need for supplemental oxygen and mechanical support of ventilation in patients undergoing ECT. Use of a peripheral nerve stimulator confirms the degree of neuromuscular blockade produced by succinylcholine and identifies patients with previously unrecognized atypical cholinesterase enzyme. Because repeated anesthesia is necessary, it is possible to establish the dose of the anesthetic induction drug and succinylcholine that produces the most predictable and desirable effects in each patient. Succinylcholine-induced myalgia is remarkably uncommon, occurring in only about 2% of patients undergoing ECT. There is no evidence that succinylcholine-induced release of potassium is increased by ECT.[20]

Occasionally, ECT is necessary in a patient with a permanently implanted artificial cardiac pacemaker. Fortunately, most artificial cardiac pacemakers are shielded and are not adversely affected by the electrical currents necessary to produce seizures. Nevertheless, it seems prudent to have an appropriate external magnet available to ensure the capability of converting pacemakers to asynchronous modes should malfunction occur in response to the externally delivered electrical current. In addition, continuous monitoring of the ECG, use of a Doppler sensor, and palpation of peripheral arterial pulses document the uninterrupted function of artificial cardiac pacemakers.

Safe and successful use of ECT has been described in patients following cardiac transplantation.[25] In such patients the lack of vagal innervation to the heart eliminates the risk of bradydysrhythmias. Increased systemic blood pressure and heart rate can still occur as a reflection of catecholamine release in response to electrically induced seizures.

▌ MANIA

Mania is an autosomal dominant disease with variable penetrance. It manifests clinically as sustained periods of mood elevation and, in severe cases, delusions and hallucinations (Table 30–5). Presumably,

Table 30–5 • Manifestations of Mania

Inflated self-esteem
Decreased need for sleep
Flight of ideas
Short attention span
Increased verbalization

there are abnormalities in neuroendocrine pathways that result in aberrant regulation of one or more amine neurotransmitter systems. This hypothesis is consistent with the observation that therapeutic effects occur over a period of 14 to 28 days rather than immediately, which would be the explanation if mania were caused by an excess or deficiency of specific neurotransmitters.

Treatment

Mania necessitates prompt treatment with lithium, which requires about 14 days before improvement is noted. When manic symptoms are severe, lithium is usually administered in combination with an antipsychotic (haloperidol) until the acute symptoms abate, allowing tapering and discontinuation of the antipsychotic.

Lithium

Lithium is efficiently absorbed after oral administration; its therapeutic serum concentration for acute mania is 1.0 to 1.2 mEq/L and for prophylaxis 0.6 to 0.8 mEq/L. Monitoring serum lithium concentrations by flame photometry about 12 hours after the last oral dose may be recommended to decrease the likelihood of toxicity. The therapeutic effects of lithium are most likely related to actions on second messenger systems based on phosphatidylinositol turnover. Lithium also affects transmembrane ion pumps and has inhibitory effects on adenylate cyclase.

Toxicity is likely when serum concentrations of lithium exceed 2 mEq/L, with symptoms of skeletal muscle weakness, ataxia, sedation, and widening of the QRS complexes on the ECG. Atrioventricular heart block, hypotension, and seizures may accompany severe lithium toxicity. Lithium inhibits release of thyroid hormones and results in hypothyroidism in about 5% of patients. Long-term administration of lithium occasionally results in a vasopressin-resistant diabetes insipidus-like syndrome (polyuria, polydipsia) that resolves when the drug is discontinued. T wave flattening or inversion on the ECG may occur, but these changes are considered benign. Cardiac conduction disturbances are rare, although patients with co-existing sinus node dysfunction should probably have artificial cardiac pacemakers in place before initiating treatment with lithium. Leukocytosis in the range of 10,000 to 14,000 cells/mm^3 is possible in lithium-treated patients.

Lithium is excreted almost entirely by the kidneys Resorption of lithium occurs at proximal convoluted renal tubules and is inversely related to the concentrations of sodium in the glomerular filtrate. For this reason, administration of loop diuretics or thiazide diuretics, which enhance the renal excretion of sodium, increases the resorption of lithium and thus increases serum lithium concentrations by as much as 50%. Administration of sodium-containing solutions or osmotic diuretics favors renal excretion of lithium in patients who show evidence of lithium toxicity.

Carbamazepine

Carbamazepine, an anticonvulsant, is particularly useful for treating patients who are unresponsive to lithium. Side effects of this drug include leukopenia, aplastic anemia, and hepatotoxicity, emphasizing the importance of performing periodic blood counts and liver function tests.

Management of Anesthesia

Evidence of lithium toxicity is important to consider during the preoperative evaluation of treated patients.[26] Review of the most recent serum lithium concentration measurements may be useful. In view of the potential resorption of lithium in the presence of decreased sodium concentrations, it is reasonable to administer sodium-containing intravenous solutions during the perioperative period. Likewise, stimulation of urine output with loop or thiazide diuretics could adversely increase serum lithium concentrations. Inclusion of lithium in the measurements of the patient's serum electrolytes during the perioperative period is a consideration. Monitoring the ECG for evidence of lithium-induced changes is useful for recognizing the effect of excessive serum lithium concentrations on the conduction of cardiac impulses. Association of sedation with lithium therapy suggests that anesthetic requirements for injected and inhaled anesthetic drugs may be decreased in these patients. Monitoring neuromuscular blockade is indicated, as the duration of succinylcholine and nondepolarizing muscle relaxants may be prolonged in the presence of lithium.[27]

■ SCHIZOPHRENIA

Schizophrenia is the most common psychotic disorder, accounting for about 20% of all patients treated for mental illness. The essential features of the illness include an array of symptoms, such as delusions, hallucinations, flattened affect, social or occupational dysfunction including withdrawal, and changes in appearance and hygiene. In some patients the disorder is persistent, whereas in others there are exacerbations and remissions. Although the pathophysiology of schizophrenia has not been delineated, therapeutic drug development has been influenced by the hypothesis that certain dopamine pathways are overactive in affected individuals.[28]

Treatment

Treatment of schizophrenia is with antipsychotic drugs, which most likely exert their effects by inhibiting dopamine binding at postsynaptic dopamine receptors (Table 30–6). Although antipsychotic drugs have an array of adverse effects (autonomic, neuroendocrine, cardiac, ophthalmic, hematologic), their therapeutic index is high and side effects are rarely serious or irreversible (Table 30–7).[28] The most troublesome side effects are neurologic and include acute dystonia, akathisia (restlessness), parkinsonism, and tardive dyskinesia or tardive dystonia. Among patients receiving short-term treatment with antipsychotic drugs, 50% to 70% manifest some clinically important extrapyramidal side effects. These effects may diminish after 2 to 3 months, but they often persist to some degree for as long as the antipsychotic drug is taken. Antipsychotic drugs are not known to have teratogenic effects.

Acute dystonia (contraction of skeletal muscles of the neck, mouth, and tongue; tremor) responds to

---

Table 30–6 • Drugs Used to Treat Schizophrenia

Phenothiazines
  Chlorpromazine
  Thioridazine
  Prochlorperazine
  Perphenazine
  Triflupromazine
  Fluphenazine
Thioxanthenes
  Chlorprothixene
  Thiothixene
Butyrophenones
  Haloperidol
Dibenzoxazepines
  Loxapine
Dihydroindolones
  Molindone
Dibenzodiazepines
  Clozapine
Benzisoxazoles
  Risperidone
Long-acting injectable preparations
  Fluphenazine
  Haloperidol

Adapted from: Kane JM. Schizophrenia. N Engl J Med 1996;334:34–41.

Table 30–7 • Side Effects of Antipsychotic Drugs

Central nervous system
  Extrapyramidal symptoms
    Acute dystonia
    Akathisia
    Parkinsonism
    Tardive dyskinesia
  Sedation
  Cognitive impairment
  Dysregulation of body temperature control
  Seizures
  Toxic psychosis
  Autonomic nervous system dysfunction
    Hypotension
    Tachycardia
    Dry mouth
    Blurred vision
    Urinary retention
  Neuroleptic malignant syndrome
Cardiovascular system
  Prolonged QT intervals
  Torsades de pointes
Respiratory
  Pharyngeal and laryngeal dysfunction
  Respiratory dyskinesia
Endocrine
  Amenorrhea
  Galactorrhea
  Weight gain
Hematologic
  Leukopenia
  Agranulocytosis
Gastrointestinal
  Decreased bowel motility
  Cholestatic jaundice
Ophthalmic
  Increased intraocular pressure
  Opacities of lens and cornea

Adapted from: Kane JM. Schizophrenia. N Engl J Med 1996;334:34–41.

---

administration of diphenhydramine, 25 to 50 mg IV. Tardive dyskinesia is characterized by choreoathetoid movements, which usually develop after several months of treatment with antipsychotic drugs and may be irreversible, especially in elderly patients. Orthostatic hypotension is more likely to occur when high doses of antipsychotic drugs produce α-adrenergic blockade. This may be an important consideration during the management of anesthesia, as intraoperative decreases in systemic blood pressure could be exaggerated. This is particularly true with acute blood loss or institution of positive pressure ventilation of the patient's lungs, as compensatory sympathetic nervous system-mediated vasoconstriction is attenuated by drug-induced α-adrenergic blockade. Rarely, antipsychotic drugs prolong the QT interval on the ECG and predispose to ventricular fibrillation. Agranulocytosis is the most important adverse effect of clozapine. The period of maximal risk is 4 to 18 weeks after initiation of therapy especially in older women. Seizures may occur more often with clozapine than with other antipsychotic drugs. Clozapine is the only antipsychotic for which the risk of tardive dyskinesia is low or nonexistent. The presence of drug-induced sedation preoperatively may parallel decreased anesthetic requirements.

Neuroleptic Malignant Syndrome

Neuroleptic malignant syndrome is a rare, potentially fatal complication of antipsychotic drug therapy that is presumed to reflect drug-induced interference with dopamine's role in central thermoregulation, perhaps in patients with predisposed skeletal muscles.[28-30] This syndrome usually manifests during the first few weeks of treatment or following an increase in drug dose. Clinical manifestations of neuroleptic malignant syndrome usually develop over a 24- to 72-hour period and include high fever, severe skeletal muscle rigidity, autonomic nervous system instability (tachycardia, labile systemic blood pressure, cardiac dysrhythmias, diaphoresis), altered consciousness, and increased serum creatine kinase concentrations reflecting skeletal muscle damage. Skeletal muscle spasm may be so severe that mechanical support of ventilation becomes necessary. Renal failure may occur owing to myoglobinuria and dehydration. For unknown reasons, liver function tests are often abnormal.

Treatment of neuroleptic malignant syndrome is immediate cessation of antipsychotic drug therapy, administration of bromocriptine (5 mg PO every 6 hours) or dantrolene (up to 6 mg/kg daily as a continuous intravenous infusion) in attempts to decrease skeletal muscle rigidity, and supportive therapy (ventilation, hydration).[28-30] Bromocriptine, a dopamine agonist, may be associated with hypotension. ECT has alleviated some of the syndrome's components including fever and diaphoresis and has improved the level of consciousness. Benzodiazepines may provide a transient decrease in symptoms. Anticholinergic drugs are not effective in decreasing skeletal muscle rigidity. Mortality approaches 20% in untreated patients, with causes of death being cardiac dysrhythmias, congestive heart failure, hypoventilation, renal failure, and thromboembolism. Patients who have this syndrome are likely to experience recurrences when treatment with antipsychotic drugs is resumed. Starting with low doses of antipsychotic drugs or considering of alternative therapies (lithium, ECT) are possible approaches in these patients.

Because a common pathophysiology has been suggested for neuroleptic malignant syndrome and malignant hyperthermia, the possibility that patients with a history of neuroleptic malignant syndrome are vulnerable to developing malignant hyperthermia is an important factor when considering general anesthesia, especially when administering succinylcholine to these patients for ECT.[28] Nevertheless, there is no evidence of a pathophysiologic link between the two syndromes, and succinylcholine can be safely administered to patients receiving ECT for treatment of neuroleptic malignant syndrome.[28, 31, 32] However, until any association between neuroleptic malignant syndrome and malignant hyperthermia is disproved, careful metabolic monitoring of general anesthesia is recommended.

ANXIETY DISORDERS

Anxiety disorders can be responses to exogenous stimuli (situational anxiety, pain, angina pectoris) or endogenous stimuli (Table 30–8). Anxiety resulting from identifiable stresses is usually self-limited and rarely requires pharmacologic treatment. Nevertheless, for patients whose anxiety is unusually severe, a short course of low-dose benzodiazepine therapy (diazepam 5 mg PO three times daily) is often helpful. A single dose of benzodiazepine may be useful for treating specific phobias such as fear of flying. Performance anxiety ("stage fright") is a special type of situational anxiety that is better treated with β-antagonists (propranolol 20 to 40 mg PO) that do not produce sedation. Endogenous ligands that have effects opposite to those of the benzodiazepines (anxiogenic) have been identified and support the hypothesis that abnormalities of the endogenous benzodiazepine system are responsible for many anxiety states.

Panic disorders appear to be inherited and are characterized as discrete periods of intense fear that are not triggered by a severe anxiogenic stimulus. This

Table 30–8 • Manifestations of Anxiety Disorders

Tremor
Dyspnea
Tachycardia
Diaphoresis
Insomnia
Irritability
Polyuria
Fatigue
Diarrhea
Skeletal muscle tension

disorder is often accompanied by dyspnea, tachycardia, diaphoresis, paresthesias, nausea, chest pain, and fear of dying. An unexplained observation is that infusion of lactate may provoke panic attacks in susceptible individuals. Tricyclic antidepressants or MAOIs are effective for treating panic attacks. Delayed recovery from anesthesia has been attributed to co-existing hysteria.[33]

AUTISM

Autism is a developmental disorder characterized by disturbances in the rate of development of physical, social, and language skills, although specific cognitive abilities may be present. Abnormal responses to sensory inputs manifest as hyperreactivity that alternates with hyporeactivity. The prevalence of this syndrome is estimated as 4.7 per 10,000 live births, with males affected five times more often than females. Enlarged cerebral ventricles may be present, and seizures frequently begin during late childhood. The cause of this syndrome is unknown, but proposed etiologic factors include viral encephalitis and metabolic disorders. Congenital or familial factors are suggested by the occurrence of autism in twins or siblings. No treatment alters the natural history of this disorder, and life expectancy is normal. The long-range prognosis is poor, and many patients are classified as mentally retarded. Drug therapy is symptomatic and works best when aimed at controlling specific behaviors.

SUBSTANCE ABUSE AND DRUG OVERDOSE

Substance abuse may be defined as self-administration of drug(s) that deviate(s) from accepted medical or social use, which if sustained can lead to physical and psychological dependence. The incidence of substance abuse and drug-related deaths is high among physicians, especially during the first 5 years after medical school graduation.[1] Dependence is diagnosed when patients manifest at least three of nine characteristic symptoms, with some of the symptoms having persisted for at least 1 month or occurred repeatedly (Table 30–9).[34] Physical dependence has developed when the presence of a drug in the body is necessary for normal physiologic function and prevention of withdrawal symptoms. Typically, the withdrawal syndrome consists of a rebound in the physiologic systems modified by the drug. Tolerance is a state in which tissues become accustomed to the presence of a drug such that increased doses of that drug become necessary to pro-

Table 30–9 • Characteristic Symptoms for Psychoactive Drug Dependence

Drug taken in higher doses or for longer periods than intended
Unsuccessful attempts to decrease use of drug
Increased time spent obtaining the drug
Frequent intoxication or withdrawal symptoms
Restricted social or work activities because of drug use
Continued drug use despite social or physical problems related to drug use
Evidence of tolerance to effects of the drug
Characteristic withdrawal symptoms
Drug use to avoid withdrawal symptoms

duce effects similar to those observed initially with smaller doses. Substance abuse patients can manifest cross-tolerance to drugs, making it difficult to predict analgesic or anesthetic requirements.[35] Most often, chronic substance abuse results in increased analgesic and anesthetic requirements, whereas additive or even synergistic effects may occur in the presence of acute substance abuse. It is important to recognize the signs of drug withdrawal during the preoperative period. Certainly, acute drug withdrawal should not be attempted during the preoperative period.

Diagnosis

Substance abuse is often first suspected or recognized during the medical management of another disorder [hepatitis, acquired immunodeficiency syndrome (AIDS), pregnancy]. Patients almost always have a concomitant personality disorder and display antisocial traits. Sociopathic characteristics (school dropouts, criminal records, multiple drug abuse) seem to predispose to, rather than result from, drug addiction. About 50% of patients admitted to hospitals with factitious disorders are drug abusers, as are some chronic pain patients. Psychiatric consultation is recommended in all cases of substance abuse.

Drug overdose is the leading cause of unconsciousness observed in patients admitted to emergency departments; often more than one class of drugs as well as alcohol have been ingested. Conditions other than drug overdose may result in unconsciousness, emphasizing the importance of laboratory tests (electrolytes, blood glucose concentrations, arterial blood gases, renal and liver function tests) for confirming the diagnosis. The depth of central nervous system depression can be estimated on the basis of responses to painful stimulation, activity of the gag reflex, presence or absence of hypotension, breathing rate, and size and responsiveness of the patient's pupils.

Treatment

Regardless of the drug or drugs ingested, the manifestations are similar; assessment and treatment proceed simultaneously. The first step is to secure the patient's airway and support ventilation and circulation. Absence of a gag reflex is confirmatory evidence that protective laryngeal reflexes are dangerously depressed. In this situation, a cuffed tracheal tube should be placed to protect the patient's lungs from aspiration. Body temperature is monitored, as hypothermia frequently accompanies unconsciousness due to a drug overdose. Decisions to attempt removal of ingested substances (gastric lavage, forced diuresis, hemodialysis) depend on the drug ingested, the time since ingestion, and the degree of central nervous system depression. Gastric lavage may be beneficial if less than 4 hours has elapsed since ingestion. Gastric lavage or pharmacologic stimulation is not recommended when the ingested substances are hydrocarbons or corrosive materials or when protective laryngeal reflexes are not intact. After gastric lavage or emesis, activated charcoal can be administered to absorb any drug remaining in the patient's gastrointestinal tract. Hemodialysis may be considered when potentially fatal doses of drugs have been ingested, when there is progressive deterioration of cardiovascular function, or when normal routes of metabolism and renal excretion are impaired. Treatment with hemodialysis is of little value when the ingested drugs are highly bound to proteins or avidly stored in tissues because of their lipid solubility.

Alcoholism

Alcoholism is defined as a primary chronic disease with genetic, psychosocial, and environmental factors that influence its development and manifestations.[36] Alcoholism affects at least 10 million Americans and is responsible for 200,000 deaths annually. Up to one-third of adult patients have medical problems related to alcohol (Table 30-10). A diagnosis of alcoholism requires a high index of suspicion combined with nonspecific but suggestive symptoms (gastritis, tremor, history of falling, unexplained episodes of amnesia). The possibility of alcoholism is often overlooked in the elderly.

Male gender and family history of alcohol abuse are the two major risk factors for alcoholism. Adoption studies indicate that male children of alcoholic

Table 30–10 • Medical Problems Related to Alcoholism

Central nervous system effects
  Psychiatric disorders (depression, antisocial behavior)
  Nutritional disorders (Wernicke-Korsakoff)
  Withdrawal syndrome
  Cerebellar degeneration
  Cerebral atrophy
Cardiovascular effects
  Dilated cardiomyopathy
  Cardiac dysrhythmias
  Systemic hypertension
Gastrointestinal and hepatobiliary effects
  Esophagitis
  Gastritis
  Pancreatitis
  Hepatic cirrhosis (portal hypertension manifesting as esophageal varices or hemorrhoids)
Skin and musculoskeletal effects
  Spider angiomas
  Myopathy
  Osteoporosis
Endocrine and metabolic effects
  Decreased serum testosterone concentrations (impotence)
  Decreased gluconeogenesis (hypoglycemia)
  Ketoacidosis
  Hypoalbuminemia
  Hypomagnesemia
Hematologic effects
  Thrombocytopenia
  Leukopenia
  Anemia

parents are more likely to become alcoholic, even when raised by nonalcoholic adoptive parents. Other forms of psychiatric disease such as mental depression or sociopathy are not increased in the children of alcoholic parents. Inherited differences in the activity of alcohol dehydrogenase among ethnic groups has not been documented.

Although alcohol appears to produce widespread nonspecific effects on cell membranes, there is evidence that many of its neurologic effects are mediated by actions on receptors for the inhibitory neurotransmitter, γ-aminobutyric acid (GABA).[36] When GABA binds to receptors, it causes chloride channels in the receptors to open, thereby hyperpolarizing the neurons and making the occurrence of depolarization less likely. Alcohol appears to increase GABA-mediated chloride ion conductance. A shared site of action for alcohol, benzodiazepines, and barbiturates would be consistent with the ability of these different classes of drugs to produce cross-tolerance and cross-dependence.

Treatment

Treatment of alcoholism mandates total abstinence from alcohol ingestion. Disulfiram may be administered as an adjunctive drug along with psychiatric counseling. The unpleasantness of symptoms (flushing, vertigo, diaphoresis, nausea, vomiting) that accompanies alcohol ingestion in the presence of disulfiram is intended to serve as a deterrent to the patient's urge to deviate from alcohol abstinence. These symptoms reflect the accumulation of acetaldehyde from oxidation of alcohol, which cannot be further oxidized because of disulfiram-induced inhibition of aldehyde dehydrogenase activity. Compliance with long-term disulfiram therapy is often poor, and this drug has not been documented to have advantages over placebo for achieving total alcohol abstinence.[37] Medical contraindications to disulfiram include pregnancy, cardiac dysfunction, hepatic dysfunction, renal dysfunction, and peripheral neuropathies. Emergency treatment of an alcohol–disulfiram interaction includes intravenous infusions of crystalloid solutions and occasionally transient maintenance of systemic blood pressure with vasopressors.

Overdose

Intoxicating effects of alcohol parallel its blood concentrations. In patients who are not alcoholics, blood alcohol levels of 25 mg/dl are associated with impaired cognition and incoordination. At blood alcohol concentrations higher than 100 mg/dl, signs of vestibular and cerebellar dysfunction (nystagmus, dysarthria, ataxia) increase. Autonomic nervous system dysfunction may result in hypotension, hypothermia, stupor, and ultimately coma. Intoxication with alcohol is often defined as blood alcohol concentrations higher than 80 to 100 mg/dl, and levels higher than 500 mg/dl are usually fatal owing to depressed ventilation. Chronic tolerance from prolonged excessive alcohol ingestion may cause alcoholic patients to remain sober despite potentially fatal blood alcohol concentrations. The critical aspect of treating life-threatening alcohol overdoses is maintenance of ventilation. Hypoglycemia may be profound if excessive alcohol consumption is associated with food deprivation. It must be appreciated that other central nervous system depressant drugs are often ingested simultaneously with alcohol.

Withdrawal Syndrome

Physiologic dependence on alcohol manifests as a withdrawal syndrome when the drug is discontinued or when there is decreased intake.[36]

Early Manifestations

The earliest and most common withdrawal syndrome is characterized by generalized tremors that may be accompanied by perceptual disturbances (nightmares, hallucinations), autonomic nervous system hyperactivity (tachycardia, hypertension, cardiac dysrhythmias), nausea, vomiting, insomnia, and mild confusional states with agitation. These symptoms usually begin within 6 to 8 hours after substantial decreases in blood alcohol concentrations and are typically most pronounced at 24 to 36 hours. These withdrawal symptoms can be suppressed by the resumption of alcohol ingestion or by administration of benzodiazepines, β-antagonists, or α2-agonists. In clinical situations, diazepam is usually administered to produce sedation; a β-antagonist is included if tachycardia is present. The ability of sympatholytic drugs to attenuate these symptoms suggests a role of autonomic nervous system hyperactivity in the etiology of alcohol withdrawal syndrome.

Delirium Tremens

About 5% of patients experiencing alcohol withdrawal syndrome exhibit delirium tremens, a life-threatening medical emergency. Delirium tremens occurs 2 to 4 days after the cessation of alcohol ingestion, manifesting as hallucinations, combativeness, hyperthermia, tachycardia, hypertension, hypotension, and grand mal seizures.

Treatment of delirium tremens must be aggressive, with administration of diazepam, 5 to 10 mg IV every 5 minutes, until the patient becomes sedated but remains awake. Administration of β-adrenergic antagonists such as propranolol or esmolol is useful to suppress manifestions of sympathetic nervous system hyperactivity. The goal of β-antagonist therapy is to decrease the patient's heart rate to less than 100 beats/min. Protection of the upper airway with a cuffed tracheal tube is necessary in some patients. Correction of fluid, electrolyte (magnesium, potassium), and metabolic (thiamine) derangements is important. Lidocaine is usually effective when cardiac dysrhythmias occur despite correction of electrolyte abnormalities. Physical restraint may be necessary to decrease the risk of self-injury or injury to others. Despite aggressive treatment, mortality from delirium tremens is about 10%, principally due to hypotension, cardiac dysrhythmias, or seizures.

Wernicke-Korsakoff Syndrome

Wernicke-Korsakoff syndrome reflects a loss of neurons in the cerebellum (Wernicke's encephalopathy) and loss of memory (Korsakoff's psychoses) due to the lack of thiamine (vitamin B1), which is required for the intermediary metabolism of carbohydrates (see Chapter 24). This syndrome is not an alcohol withdrawal syndrome, but its occurrence establishes that these patients are, or have been, physically dependent on alcohol. In addition to ataxia and memory loss, many of the patients exhibit global confusion states, drowsiness, nystagmus, and orthostatic hypotension. An associated peripheral polyneuropathy is almost always present.

Treatment of Wernicke-Korsakoff syndrome consists of intravenous administration of thiamine, with normal dietary intake if possible. Because carbohydrate loads may precipitate this syndrome in thiamine-depleted patients, it may be useful to administer thiamine before initiation of glucose infusions to malnourished or alcoholic patients.

Alcohol and Pregnancy

Alcohol crosses the placenta and may result in decreased birth weight. High blood concentrations of alcohol (more than 150 mg/dl) may result in the fetal alcohol syndrome, characterized by craniofacial dysmorphology, growth retardation, and mental retardation. There is an increased incidence of cardiac malformations, including patent ductus arteriosus and septal defects.

Management of Anesthesia

Management of anesthesia in patients being treated with disulfiram should consider the potential presence of disulfiram-induced sedation and hepatotoxicity. Decreased drug requirements could reflect additive effects with co-existing sedation or the ability of disulfiram to inhibit metabolism of drugs other than alcohol. For example, disulfiram may potentiate the effects of benzodiazepines. Acute, unexplained hypotension during general anesthesia could reflect inadequate stores of norepinephrine due to disulfiram-induced inhibition of dopamine β-hydroxylase.[38] This hypotension may respond to ephedrine, but direct-acting sympathomimetics such as phenylephrine may produce more predictable responses in the presence of norepinephrine depletion. Use of regional anesthesia may be influenced by occasional patients who are treated with disulfiram and in whom polyneuropathy develops. Alcohol-containing solutions, as used for skin cleansing, probably should be avoided in disulfiram-treated patients.

Cocaine

Cocaine use for nonmedical purposes is a public health problem with important economic and social consequences.[39, 40] Myths associated with cocaine abuse are that it is sexually stimulating, nonaddictive, and physiologically benign. In fact, cocaine is highly addictive; casual use is not possible once addiction occurs, and life-threatening side effects accompany its use. Cocaine produces sympathetic nervous system stimulation by blocking the presynaptic uptake of norepinephrine and dopamine, thereby increasing the postsynaptic concentrations of these neurotransmitters. Because of this blocking effect, dopamine remains in high concentrations in synapses, producing the characteristic "cocaine high."

Side Effects

Acute cocaine administration is known to cause coronary vasospasm, myocardial ischemia, myocardial infarction, and ventricular cardiac dysrhythmias, including ventricular fibrillation. Associated systemic hypertension and tachycardia further increase the myocardial oxygen requirement at a time when coronary oxygen delivery is decreased by the effects of cocaine on coronary blood flow. Cocaine use can cause myocardial ischemia and hypotension that lasts as long as 6 weeks after discontinuing cocaine use.[41] Excessive sensitivity of the coronary vasculature to catecholamines after chronic exposure to cocaine may be due in part to cocaine-induced depletion of dopamine stores. Lung damage and pulmonary edema have been observed in patients who smoke cocaine. Cocaine-abusing parturients are at higher risk for spontaneous abortions, abruptio placentae, and fetal malformations. Cocaine causes dose-dependent decreases in uterine blood flow, and it may produce hyperpyrexia, which can contribute to seizures. There is a temporal relation between the recreational use of cocaine and cerebrovascular accidents.[42] Chronic cocaine abuse is associated with nasal septal atrophy, agitated behavior, paranoid thinking, and heightened reflexes. Symptoms associated with cocaine withdrawal include fatigue, mental depression, and increased appetite. Death due to cocaine use has occurred with all routes of administration (intranasal, oral, intravenous, inhalation by smoking) and is usually due to apnea, seizures, or cardiac dysrhythmias. Persons with decreased plasma cholinesterase activity (elderly patients, parturients, those with severe liver disease) may be at risk for sudden death when using cocaine because this enzyme is essential for metabolizing the drug.

Cocaine overdose evokes overwhelming sympathetic nervous system stimulation of the cardiovascular system. Uncontrolled systemic hypertension may result in pulmonary and cerebral edema, whereas the effects of increased circulating catecholamine concentrations may include coronary artery vasoconstriction, spasm, and platelet aggregation.

Treatment

Treatment of cocaine overdose includes administration of nitroglycerin to manage myocardial ischemia.[43] Although esmolol has been recommended for treating tachycardia due to cocaine overdose, there is evidence that β-adrenergic blockade accentuates cocaine-induced coronary artery vasospasm.[44] α-Adrenergic blockade may be effective in the treatment of coronary vasoconstriction due to cocaine, but in the presence of hypotension this intervention is questionable. Administration of intravenous benzodiazepines such as diazepam is effective for controlling seizures associated with cocaine toxicity. Active cooling procedures may be necessary if hyperthermia accompanies cocaine overdose.

Management of Anesthesia

Management of anesthesia in patients acutely intoxicated with cocaine must consider the vulnerability of these patients to myocardial ischemia and cardiac dysrhythmias. Any event or drug likely to increase already enhanced sympathetic nervous system activity must be carefully considered before its selection. It seems prudent to have nitroglycerin readily available to treat signs of myocardial ischemia associated with tachycardia or systemic hypertension. Unexpected patient agitation during the perioperative period may reflect the effects of cocaine ingestion.[45] Increased anesthetic requirements may be present in acutely intoxicated patients, presumably reflecting increased concentrations of catecholamines in the central nervous system.[46] Thrombocytopenia associated with cocaine abuse may influence the selection of regional anesthesia in these patients.

In the absence of acute intoxication, chronic abuse of cocaine has not been shown to be predictably associated with adverse anesthetic interactions, although the possibility of cardiac dysrhythmias remains a constant concern. Rapid metabolism of cocaine probably decreases the likelihood that acutely intoxicated patients will present in the operating room. Administration of topical cocaine plus epinephrine for medically indicated purposes followed by the administration of volatile anesthetics that sensitize the myocardium may exaggerate the cardiac-stimulating effects of cocaine. Cocaine utilization for medically indicated uses should be avoided in patients with systemic hypertension or coronary artery disease and in patients receiving drugs that potentiate the effects of catecholamines, such as MAOIs.

Opioids

Contrary to common speculation, opioid dependence rarely develops from the use of these drugs to treat acute postoperative pain. It is possible to become addicted to opioids in less than 14 days, however, if the drug is administered daily in ever-increasing doses. Opioids are abused orally, subcutaneously, or intravenously for their euphoric and analgesic effects. Numerous medical problems are encountered in opioid addicts, especially intravenous abusers (Table 30–11). Evidence for the presence of these medical problems in opioid addicts should be sought during the preoperative evaluation. Tolerance may develop to some of the effects of opioids (analgesia, sedation, emesis, euphoria, hypoventilation) but not to others (miosis, constipation). Fortunately, as tolerance increases, so does the lethal dose of the opioid. In general, there is a high degree of cross-tolerance between drugs with morphine-like actions, although tolerance wanes rapidly when addicts are withdrawn from opioids.

Overdose

The most obvious manifestations of opioid overdose (usually heroin) are slow breathing rates with a normal to increased tidal volume. Pupils are usually miotic, although mydriasis may occur if hypoventilation results in severe arterial hypoxemia. Central nervous system manifestations range from dysphoria to unconsciousness; seizures are unlikely. Pulmonary edema occurs in a large proportion of patients experiencing heroin overdose. The etiology of pulmonary edema is poorly understood; but arterial hypoxemia, hypotension, neurogenic mechanisms, and drug-related pulmonary endothelial damage are considerations. Gastric atony is a predictable

---

Table 30–11 • Medical Problems Associated with Chronic Opioid Abuse

Acquired immunodeficiency syndrome (AIDS)
Hepatitis
Cellulitis
Superficial skin abscesses
Septic thrombophlebitis
Tetanus
Endocarditis with or without pulmonary emboli
Systemic septic emboli and infarctions
Aspiration pneumonitis
Adrenal gland dysfunction
Malaria
Malnutrition
Positive and false-positive serologies
Transverse myelitis

accompaniment of acute opioid overdose. Fatal opioid overdose is most often an outcome of fluctuation in the purity of street products or the combination of opioids with other central nervous system depressants. Naloxone is the specific opioid antagonist administered to maintain acceptable breathing rates, usually more than 12 breaths/min.

Withdrawal Syndrome

Although withdrawal from opioids is rarely life-threatening, it is unpleasant and may complicate management during the perioperative period. In this regard it is useful to consider the time to onset, peak intensity, and duration of withdrawal after abrupt withdrawal of opioids (Table 30–12). Opioid withdrawal symptoms develop within seconds after intravenous administration of naloxone. Conversely, it is usually possible to abort the withdrawal syndrome by reinstituting administration of the abused opioid or by substituting methadone (2.5 mg equivalent to 10 mg of morphine). Clonidine may also attenuate opioid withdrawal symptoms presumably by replacing opioid-mediated inhibition (absent during withdrawal) with α_2-agonist-mediated inhibition of the sympathetic nervous system in the brain.[47]

Opioid withdrawal symptoms often include manifestations of excess sympathetic nervous system activity (diaphoresis, mydriasis, systemic hypertension, tachycardia). Craving for the drug and anxiety are followed by yawning, lacrimation, rhinorrhea, piloerection (origin of the term "cold turkey"), tremors, skeletal muscle and bone discomfort, and anorexia. Insomnia, abdominal cramps, diarrhea, and hyperthermia may develop. Skeletal muscle spasms and jerking of the legs (origin of the term "kicking the habit") follow, and cardiovascular collapse is possible. Seizures are rare, and their occurrence should introduce a consideration of other etiologies, such as unrecognized barbiturate withdrawal or underlying epilepsy.

Rapid Opioid Detoxification

Rapid opioid detoxification utilizing high doses of opioid antagonists (nalmefene) administered to patients during general anesthesia followed by naltrexone maintenance has been proposed as a cost-effective alternative to conventional detoxification approaches.[48] There is evidence that opioid withdrawal, primarily involving the nucleus locus coeruleus, peaks and then recovers to near baseline within 4 to 6 hours after administering high doses of opioid antagonists. Subsequent administration of naloxone to patients who have undergone rapid detoxification under general anesthesia should produce no evidence of opioid withdrawal, confirming rapid achievement of opioid detoxification. In contrast to conventional detoxification achieved by gradual tapering of opioid doses, the unpleasant aspects of opioid withdrawal are passed through in a few hours during which time patients are anesthetized, which contributes to an increased success rate.

Profound increases in serum catecholamine concentrations during anesthesia-assisted opioid detoxification have been described manifesting as changes in systolic blood pressure or tachycardia.[48] Prior administration of clonidine may blunt these changes. During anesthesia, manifestations of sympathetic nervous system hyperreactivity may be treated with pharmacologic interventions such as administration of β-adrenergic antagonists. Deep general anesthesia with skeletal muscle paralysis and controlled ventilation of the patient's lungs may be recommended. Although general anesthesia seems to be safely tolerated during rapid opioid detoxification, there is some concern regarding the occurrence of cardiac dysrhythmias (prolonged QT intervals) and postoperative mortality.[49] Naltrexone is often administered in the postanesthesia care unit, with adjunct medications (midazolam, ketorolac, clonidine) being administered as needed. The occurrence of mild to moderate withdrawal symptoms for 3 to 4 days after rapid opioid detoxification is expected.

Management of Anesthesia

Opioid addicts should have opioids or methadone maintained during the perioperative period. Preoperative medication may also include opioids.[50] Opi-

| Table 30–12 • Time Course of Opioid Withdrawal Syndrome |
Drug	Onset	Peak Intensity	Duration
Meperidine Dihydromorphine	2–6 hours	8–12 hours	4–5 days
Codeine Morphine Heroin	6–18 hours	36–72 hours	7–10 days
Methadone	24–48 hours	3–21 days	6–7 weeks

oid agonist-antagonists are not recommended, as these drugs could precipitate acute withdrawal reactions. There is no advantage in trying to maintain anesthesia with opioids, as doses greatly in excess of normal are likely to be required. Furthermore, chronic opioid use leads to cross-tolerance to other central nervous system depressants that may manifest as decreased analgesic responses to inhaled anesthetics such as nitrous oxide (Fig. 30–2).[51] Conversely, acute opioid administration decreases anesthetic requirements. Maintenance of anesthesia is most often with volatile anesthetics, remembering that these patients are likely to have underlying liver disease. There is a tendency for perioperative hypotension to occur, which may reflect inadequate intravascular fluid volume secondary to chronic infections, fever, malnutrition, adrenocortical insufficiency, or inadequate opioid concentrations in the brain.[52]

Management of anesthesia for rehabilitated opioid addicts and patients on antagonist therapy often includes volatile anesthetics. Regional anesthesia may have a role in some patients, but it is important to remember the tendency for hypotension to occur, the increased incidence of positive serology, the occasional presence of peripheral neuritis, and the rare occurrence of transverse myelitis.

Opioid addicts often seem to experience exaggerated degrees of postoperative pain. For reasons that are not clear, satisfactory postoperative analgesia may be achieved when average doses of meperidine are administered in addition to the usual daily maintenance dose of methadone or other opioids. Methadone has minimal analgesic activity with respect to management of postoperative pain. Levomethadyl, like methadone, is a mu opioid agonist that has a long half-life owing to its active metabolites. As a result, an advantage of levomethadyl over methadone is the option for less than daily doses.[53] Alternative methods of postoperative pain relief in these patients include continuous regional anesthesia with local anesthetics, neuraxial opioids, and transcutaneous electrical nerve stimulation.

Barbiturates

Chronic barbiturate abuse is not associated with major pathophysiologic changes. These drugs are most commonly abused orally for their euphoric effects to counter insomnia and to antagonize the stimulant effects of other drugs. There is tolerance to most of the actions of these drugs and cross-tolerance to other central nervous system depressants. Although the barbiturate doses required to produce sedative or euphoric effects increase rapidly, lethal doses do not increase at the same rate or to the same magnitude. Thus a barbiturate abuser's margin of error, in contrast to that of opioid addicts, decreases as barbiturate doses are increased to achieve the desired effect.

Overdose

Central nervous system depression is the principal manifestation of barbiturate overdose. Barbiturate blood levels correspond with the degree of central nervous system depression (slurred speech, ataxia, irritability), with excessively high blood levels resulting in loss of pharyngeal and deep tendon reflexes, and with the onset of coma. No specific pharmacologic antagonist exists to reverse barbiturate-induced central nervous system depression, and the use of nonspecific stimulants is not encouraged. Depression of ventilation may be profound. As with opioid overdoses, maintenance of a patent upper airway, protection of the lungs from aspiration, and support of ventilation of the lungs using

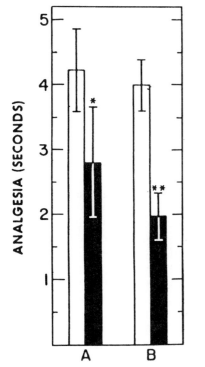

Figure 30–2 • Analgesic effects of nitrous oxide as determined by tail flick latency are decreased in rats (A, Long-Evans rats; B, Sprague-Dawley rats) tolerant to morphine (dark bars) compared to rats not treated with morphine (clear bars). Mean ± SE. *$p < 0.005$ compared with nontolerant rats. (From Berkowitz BA, Finck AD, Hynes MD, et al. Tolerance to N_2O anesthesia in rats and mice. Anesthesiology 1979;51:309–14, with permission.)

a cuffed tracheal tube may be necessary. Barbiturate overdoses may be associated with hypotension owing to central vasomotor depression, direct myocardial depression, and increased venous capacitance. This hypotension usually responds to infusion of fluids, although occasionally vasopressors or inotropic drugs are required. Hypothermia is frequent and may necessitate aggressive attempts to restore normothermia. Acute renal failure due to hypotension and rhabdomyolysis may occur. Forced diuresis and alkalinization of the urine promote elimination of phenobarbital but are of lesser value with many of the other barbiturates. Induced emesis or gastric lavage followed by administration of activated charcoal may be helpful in otherwise awake patients who ingested barbiturates less than 6 hours previously.

Withdrawal Syndrome

In contrast to opioid withdrawal, the abrupt cessation of excessive barbiturate ingestion is associated with potentially life-threatening responses. The time of onset, peak intensity, and duration of withdrawal symptoms for barbiturates are delayed compared to that seen with opioids (Table 30–13). Barbiturate withdrawal symptoms manifest initially as anxiety, skeletal muscle tremors, hyperreflexia, diaphoresis, tachycardia, and orthostatic hypotension. Cardiovascular collapse and hyperthermia may occur. The most serious problem associated with barbiturate withdrawal is the occurrence of grand mal seizures. Seizures are likely to be caused by abrupt decreases in circulating concentrations of drug. Many of the manifestations of barbiturate withdrawal, particularly seizures, are difficult to abort once they develop, in contrast to opioid withdrawal.

Pentobarbital may be administered if evidence of barbiturate withdrawal manifests. Typically, the initial oral dose is 200 to 400 mg, with subsequent doses titrated to effect, as tolerance may disappear rapidly in these patients. Phenobarbital and diazepam may also be useful for suppressing evidence of barbiturate withdrawal.

Management of Anesthesia

Although few data exist concerning management of anesthesia in chronic barbiturate abusers, it is predictable that cross-tolerance to depressant effects of anesthetic drugs occurs. For example, mice tolerant to thiopental awaken at higher barbiturate tissue concentrations than do control animals. Similarly, anecdotal reports describe the need for increased barbiturate doses for induction of anesthesia in chronic barbiturate abusers.[54] Although acute administration of barbiturates has been shown to decrease anesthetic requirements, there are no reports of increased anesthetic requirements (MAC) in chronic barbiturate abusers. Another concern is that chronic barbiturate abuse leads to induction of hepatic microsomal enzymes, introducing the potential for drug interactions with concomitantly administered medications (warfarin, digitalis, phenytoin, volatile anesthetics). Venous access is a likely problem in intravenous barbiturate abusers, as the alkalinity of the injected solutions is likely to sclerose veins.

Benzodiazepines

Benzodiazepine addiction probably requires ingestion of large doses (diazepam 80 to 120 mg for 40 to 50 days). As with barbiturates, tolerance and physical dependence occur with chronic benzodiazepine abuse. Benzodiazepines do not significantly induce microsomal enzymes. Symptoms of withdrawal generally occur later than with barbiturates and are less severe owing to the prolonged elimination half-times of most benzodiazepines and the fact that many of these drugs are metabolized to pharmacologically active metabolites that also have prolonged elimination half-times. Anesthetic considerations in chronic benzodiazepine abusers are similar to those described for chronic barbiturate abusers.

Acute benzodiazepine overdose is much less likely to produce depressed ventilation than barbiturate overdose. It should be recognized, however, that combinations of benzodiazepines and other

Table 30–13 • Time Course of Barbiturate Withdrawal Syndrome

Drug	Onset (hours)	Peak Intensity (days)	Duration (days)
Pentobarbital	12–24	2–3	7–10
Secobarbital	12–24	2–3	7–10
Phenobarbital	48–72	6–10	10+

central nervous system depressants, such as alcohol, have proved to be potentially fatal. Supportive treatment often suffices, whereas a specific benzodiazepine antagonist, flumazenil, is useful for managing profound overdoses. Seizure activity previously suppressed by benzodiazepines could be unmasked after administration of flumazenil.

Amphetamines

Amphetamines stimulate the release of catecholamines, resulting in increased cortical alertness with associated appetite suppression and decreased need for sleep. Approved uses of amphetamines are for treatment of narcolepsy, attention-deficit disorders, and hyperactivity associated with minimal brain dysfunction in children. Tolerance to the appetite suppressant effects develops within a few weeks, making these drugs poor substitutes for proper dieting techniques. Physiologic dependence on amphetamines is profound, and daily doses may be increased to several hundred times the therapeutic dose. Chronic abuse of amphetamines results in depletion of body stores of catecholamines. Such depletion may manifest as somnolence and anxiety or a psychotic-like state. Other physiologic abnormalities reported with long-term amphetamine abuse include systemic hypertension, cardiac dysrhythmias, and malnutrition. Amphetamines are most often abused orally or, in the case of methamphetamine, intravenously.

Overdose

Amphetamine overdose causes anxiety, a psychotic state, and progressive central nervous system irritability manifesting as hyperactivity, hyperreflexia, and occasionally seizures.[35] Other physiologic effects include increased systemic blood pressure and heart rate, cardiac dysrhythmias, decreased gastrointestinal motility, mydriasis, diaphoresis, and hyperthermia. Metabolic imbalances such as dehydration, lactic acidosis, and ketosis may occur.

Treatment of oral amphetamine overdoses is with induced emesis or gastric lavage followed by administration of activated charcoal and a cathartic. Phenothiazines may antagonize many of the acute central nervous system effects of amphetamines. Similarly, diazepam may be useful for controlling amphetamine-induced seizures. Acidification of the urine promotes elimination of amphetamines.

Withdrawal Syndrome

Abrupt cessation of excess amphetamine usage is accompanied by extreme lethargy, mental depression that may be suicidal, increased appetite, and weight gain. Benzodiazepines are useful in the management of withdrawal syndrome if sedation is needed, and β-adrenergic antagonists may be administered to control sympathetic nervous system hyperactivity. Postamphetamine mental depression may last for months and require treatment with antidepressant drugs. In this regard, tricyclic antidepressants such as desimpramine and imipramine are considerations, as they exert the most profound effects on neurotransmitter concentrations of norepinephrine.

Management of Anesthesia

Chronic pharmacologic doses of amphetamine administered for medically indicated uses (narcolepsy, attention-deficit disorder) need not be discontinued before elective surgery.[55] Patients requiring emergency surgery and who are acutely intoxicated from ingestion of amphetamines may exhibit systemic hypertension, tachycardia, increased body temperature, and increased requirements for volatile anesthetics. Even intraoperative intracranial hypertension and cardiac arrest has been attributed to amphetamine abuse.[55, 56] In animals, acute intravenous administration of dextroamphetamine produces dose-related increases in body temperature and anesthetic requirements.[57] For these reasons it seems prudent to monitor body temperature during the perioperative period. Chronic amphetamine abuse may be associated with markedly decreased anesthetic requirements, which are presumed to result from catecholamine depletion in the central nervous system. Refractory hypotension can reflect depletion of endogenous catecholamine stores. Direct-acting vasopressors, including phenylephrine and epinephrine, should be promptly available to treat hypotension, as responses to indirect-acting vasopressors such as ephedrine may be attenuated by amphetamine-induced catecholamine depletion. Intraoperative monitoring of systemic blood pressure using an intra-arterial catheter is a consideration. Postoperatively, there is the potential for orthostatic hypotension when these patients begin to ambulate.

Hallucinogens

Hallucinogens, as represented by lysergic acid diethylamine (LSD) and phencyclidine (PCP), are usually ingested orally. Although there is a high degree of psychological dependence, there is no evidence of physical dependence or withdrawal symptoms when LSD is acutely discontinued. Chronic use of hallucinogens is unlikely. The effects of these drugs develop within 1 to 2 hours and last 8 to 12 hours; they consist of visual, auditory, and tactile hallucinations and distortions of the surroundings and body images. The ability of the brain to suppress relatively unimportant stimuli is impaired by LSD. Evidence of sympathetic nervous system stimulation includes mydriasis, increased body temperature, systemic hypertension, and tachycardia. Tolerance to the behavioral effects of LSD occurs rapidly, whereas tolerance to the cardiovascular effects is less pronounced.

Overdose

Overdose of LSD has not been associated with death, although patients may suffer unrecognized injuries, reflecting intrinsic analgesic effects of the drug. On rare occasions LSD produces seizures and apnea. It can produce an acute panic reaction characterized by hyperactivity, mood lability, and in extreme cases overt psychosis. Patients are often placed in calm, quiet environments with minimal external stimuli. No specific antidote exists, although benzodiazepines may be useful for controlling agitation and anxiety reactions. Supportive care in the form of airway management, mechanical ventilation of the lungs, treating seizures, and controlling the manifestations of sympathetic nervous system hyperactivity is warranted. Forced diuresis and acidification of the patient's urine promotes elimination of phencyclidines but also introduces the risk of fluid overload and electrolyte abnormalities, especially hypokalemia.

Management of Anesthesia

Anesthesia and surgery have been reported to precipitate panic responses in these patients. In the event that such responses occur, diazepam is likely to be useful. Exaggerated responses to sympathomimetic drugs seem likely. Analgesic and pulmonary ventilatory depressant effects of opioids are prolonged by LSD. Inhibition of plasma cholinesterase activity by LSD is a theoretical possibility for which clinical evidence is lacking.

Marijuana

Marijuana is usually abused via smoking, which increases the bioavailability of the primary psychoactive component, tetrahydrocannabinol (THC), over that possible after oral ingestion. Inhalation of marijuana smoke produces euphoria, with signs of increased sympathetic nervous system activity and decreased parasympathetic nervous system activity. The most consistent cardiac change is an increased resting heart rate, although orthostatic hypotension may occur. Chronic marijuana abuse leads to increased tar deposits in the individual's lungs, impaired pulmonary defense mechanisms, and decreased pulmonary function. As such, an increased incidence of sinusitis and bronchitis is likely. In predisposed persons, marijuana may evoke seizures. Conjunctival reddening is evidence of the dilation of efferent blood vessels in the iris. Drowsiness is a common side effect. Tolerance to most of the psychoactive effects of THC has been observed. Although physical dependence on marijuana is not believed to occur, abrupt cessation after chronic use is characterized by mild withdrawal symptoms, such as irritability, insomnia, diaphoresis, nausea, vomiting, and diarrhea. A possible medical indication for marijuana is as an antiemetic in patients receiving cancer chemotherapy.

Pharmacologic effects of inhaled THC occur within minutes but rarely persist more than 2 to 3 hours, decreasing the likelihood that acutely intoxicated patients will be seen in the operating room. Management of anesthesia includes consideration of the known effects of THC on the heart, lungs, and central nervous system. Co-existing drug-induced drowsiness is consistent with animal studies demonstrating decreased dose requirements for volatile anesthetics following intravenous administration of THC.[58, 59] Barbiturate and ketamine sleep times are prolonged in THC-treated animals, and opioid-induced depression of ventilation may be potentiated.[60]

Tricyclic Antidepressant Overdose

Deliberate self-administration of overdoses of antidepressant drugs is a common cause of death due to drug ingestion. Because the usual indication for antidepressant drugs is mental depression, it is not surprising that deliberate overdose is a potential occurrence. Potentially lethal doses of these drugs may only be 5 to 10 times the daily therapeutic doses. Overdoses principally affect the central nervous system, parasympathetic nervous system, and cardiovascular system. Progression from being alert with mild symptoms to life-threatening changes (seizures, hypoventilation, hypotension, coma) may be rapid. Evidence of intense anticholinergic effects include tachycardia, mydriasis, flushed dry skin, urinary retention, and delayed gastric emptying. Cardiovascular toxicity with intractable myocardial depression or ventricular cardiac dysrhythmias, including ventricular fibrillation, are the most common causes of death. The likelihood of seizures and cardiac dysrhythmias is increased when the duration of QRS complexes on the ECG exceeds 100 ms.[61] Conversely, plasma concentrations of ingested tricyclic antidepressants do not predictably correlate with the likely occurrence of cardiac dysrhythmias or seizures. The comatose phase of tricyclic antidepressant overdoses lasts 24 to 72 hours. Even after this phase passes, the risk of life-threatening cardiac dysrhythmias persists for several days, often necessitating continued monitoring of the ECG in these patients.

Treatment of tricyclic antidepressant overdoses in the presence of preserved protective upper airway reflexes is initially with induced emesis and/or gastric lavage, even if as long as a 12-hour period has elapsed since drug ingestion, emphasizing the likely presence of drug-induced delays of gastric emptying. Depressed ventilation or coma may require tracheal intubation and mechanical support of ventilation. Pharmacologic treatment of overdose is directed toward the central nervous system and cardiovascular system (Table 30–14). Alkalinization of the plasma by intravenous administration of sodium bicarbonate or hyperventilation of the patient's lungs to a pH above 7.45 may attenuate drug-induced cardiac toxicity. Lidocaine is also useful for treating cardiac dysrhythmias. Patients who remain hypotensive after volume expansion and alkalinization may benefit from vasopressor or inotropic support, as guided by measurements of cardiac filling pressures and cardiac output. Diazepam may be useful for controlling seizures. Physostigmine is an unpredictable, nonspecific antagonist of tricyclic antidepressant effects on the central nervous system. It must be remembered that the duration of action of physostigmine is only 1 to 2 hours, so repeated doses of this drug may be necessary because of the long elimination half-times of tricyclic antidepressant drugs. Hemodialysis and forced diuresis are not effective, as high lipid solubility of tricyclic antidepressant drugs results in fixed, slow rates of excretion.

Salicylic Acid Overdose

Symptoms of salicylic acid overdose parallel salicylate blood levels, with plasma concentrations higher than 85 mg/dl indicating severe overdose. Hyperventilation is characteristic, reflecting increased carbon dioxide production and direct stimulation of the respiratory centers. Resulting respiratory alkalosis favors the water-soluble ionized fraction of salicylic acid, which may undergo renal elimination. Conversely, metabolic acidosis, which may also accompany salicylic acid overdose, favors the lipid-soluble nonionized fraction of the drug, which can leave the blood and enter tissues, including the brain, where toxic effects are produced. Hypoglycemia may occur after increased peripheral use of glucose or interference with gluconeogenesis. Hyperglycemia, when it occurs, may reflect the effect of epinephrine release secondary to stimulation of the central nervous system by salicylic acid. Noncardiogenic pulmonary edema often occurs during the first 24 hours after salicylic acid overdose. Other manifestations of salicylic acid overdose include tinnitus, vomiting, hyperthermia, seizures, and coma.

Treatment of salicylic acid overdose includes monitoring the arterial pH, as a decrease in pH to 7.2 doubles the fraction of lipid-soluble drug in the systemic circulation. Indeed, decreasing serum salicylate concentrations may reflect urinary excretion of salicylic acid or undesirable cellular penetration of this substance secondary to metabolic acidosis. Sodium bicarbonate administration may be necessary to maintain arterial pH above 7.4. Controlled ventilation of the patient's lungs through a tracheal tube is necessary if central nervous system depression and alveolar hyperventilation are prominent. Dehydration and electrolyte disturbances may require treatment. Hemodialysis may be indicated when potentially lethal serum concentrations of salicylic acid (higher than 100 mg/dl) are present.

Acetaminophen Overdose

Acetaminophen overdose manifests as vomiting, abdominal pain, and life-threatening centrilobular hepatic necrosis. Hepatic necrosis is most likely due to metabolism of acetaminophen to benzoquinonimine, which reacts with and destroys hepatocytes. Normally, this metabolite is inactivated by conjugation with endogenous glutathione, but the increased production owing to the acetaminophen overdose

Table 30–14 • Pharmacologic Treatment of Tricyclic Antidepressant Overdose

Side Effect	Treatment
Seizures	Diazepam
	Phenytoin
Cardiac dysrhythmias	Lidocaine
	Phenytoin
Heart block	Isoproterenol
Hypotension	Crystalloid or colloid solutions
	Sympathomimetics
	Inotropes

depletes glutathione stores. Depletion of glutathione stores allows this reactive intermediary metabolite to accumulate and destroy hepatocytes.

Treatment of acetaminophen overdose is with acetylcysteine, which provides sulfhydral groups that act as precursors for glutathione. Administration of acetylcysteine within 8 hours of acetaminophen overdose protects against the development of hepatotoxicity.[62]

Methyl Alcohol Ingestion

Methyl alcohol (methanol) is metabolized by alcohol dehydrogenase to formaldehyde and formic acid, resulting in metabolic acidosis. Toxic effects on the optic nerve produced by these metabolites are presumed to be responsible for blindness. Severe abdominal pain that mimics a surgical emergency or ureteral colic may occur.

Treatment of methyl alcohol poisoning includes attempts to decrease the metabolism of methyl alcohol by intravenous administration of alcohol, which competes with methyl alcohol for the enzyme alcohol dehydrogenase. Alternatively, the activity of alcohol dehydrogenase may be specifically inhibited by administration of methylpyrazole.[63] Metabolic acidosis is treated with intravenous administration of sodium bicarbonate, as guided by arterial pH measurements. Hemodialysis is also an effective treatment for removing methyl alcohol and preventing blindness and cerebral damage.

Ethylene Glycol Ingestion

Ethylene glycol (antifreeze is about 93% ethylene glycol) is metabolized by alcohol dehydrogenase to glycolic acid resulting in metabolic acidosis. Glycolate is then metabolized to oxalate, which may result in renal failure. Hypocalcemia due to oxalate chelation of calcium may also occur. Treatment of ethylene glycol ingestion is as described for methyl alcohol ingestion. In addition, treatment of hypocalcemia may be necessary.

Petroleum Product Ingestion

The morbidity associated with petroleum product ingestion (gasoline, kerosene, lighter fluid, furniture polish) is usually secondary to pulmonary aspiration during spontaneous vomiting or after induced emesis. Absorption from the gastrointestinal tract is not a likely cause of morbidity. Symptoms of hydrocarbon pneumonitis, which occur only if aspiration is present, range from coughing and dyspnea with tachypnea to life-threatening adult respiratory distress syndrome. Nearly all of the patients in whom hydrocarbon pneumonitis develops, exhibit radiographic changes within 12 hours of ingestion. Pneumonitis is presumably due to hydrocarbon-induced alterations in physical properties of pulmonary surfactant, leading to atelectasis and airway closure. Gastrointestinal symptoms of petroleum product ingestion include burning of the mouth and throat, nausea, vomiting, and diarrhea. Central nervous system symptoms are usually mild, with unconsciousness or seizures occurring only when aspiration leads to profound arterial hypoxemia. Renal function is not uniquely altered by petroleum product ingestion. Gasoline and glue sniffing have been implicated as causes of sudden, often fatal cardiac dysrhythmias. This may reflect sensitization of the myocardium to endogenous catecholamines.

Induced emesis is not recommended to treat petroleum product ingestion in view of the risk of pulmonary aspiration. Likewise, tracheal intubation performed only to permit gastric lavage is not recommended, as the seal provided by the tracheal tube cuff does not guarantee that aspiration of these low-density liquids will not occur. Activated charcoal and cathartics are not beneficial. The course and severity of hydrocarbon pneumonitis are not altered by administration of corticosteroids. Broad-spectrum antibiotics are indicated if bacterial infection is present.

Organophosphate Overdose

Organophosphate overdose is most likely to occur when insecticides that are potent inhibitors of the enzyme acetylcholinesterase (true cholinesterase) are ingested, inhaled, or absorbed through the skin.[64] Nerve agents, as developed for chemical warfare, are also inhibitors of this enzyme. Symptoms of organophosphate overdose reflect inhibition (irreversible phosphorylation) of acetylcholinesterase resulting in accumulation of acetylcholine at nicotinic (neuromuscular junctions) and cholinergic receptor sites (Table 30–15). The relative intensity of these manifestations is influenced by the route of absorption, with the most intense effects occurring after inhalation. Organophosphate overdose may be followed by delayed peripheral neuropathy involving the distal skeletal muscles of the extremities.[64] This neuropathy appears 2 to 5 weeks after the overdose. Skeletal muscle weakness developing 1 to 4 days after organophosphate overdose involves primarily proximal limb muscles, flexors of the necks, certain cranial nerves, and breathing muscles. Death from

Table 30–15 • Symptoms of Organophosphate (Insecticide) Overdose

Nicotinic effects (neuromuscular junction)
    Skeletal muscle fasciculations
    Skeletal muscle weakness
    Skeletal muscle paralysis (apnea)
Muscarinic effects
    Salivation
    Lacrimation
    Miosis
    Diaphoresis
    Bronchospasm
    Bradycardia
    Hyperperistalsis (diarrhea, urination)
Central nervous system effects
    Grand mal seizures
    Unconsciousness
    Apnea
    Hyperthermia

organophosphate overdose is usually the result of apnea.

Treatment of organophosphate overdose includes administration of anticholinergics, oximes, and benzodiazepines (Table 30–16). Atropine is the main antidote for overdose. The endpoint of atropine therapy is good control of airway secretions and the presence of an adequate tidal volume. Pralidoxime is an oxime that complexes with the organophosphate, resulting in its removal from the acetylcholinesterase enzyme. Such drug-induced removal of the organophosphate from acetylcholinesterase reactivates the enzyme, leading to restoration of normal enzymatic inactivation of acetylcholine and reestablishment of normal cholinergic neurotransmission. Diazepam is useful for controlling seizures induced by organophosphate overdoses. Weakness of the muscles of breathing may require mechanical support of ventilation.

Carbon Monoxide Poisoning

Carbon monoxide (product of incomplete combustion of hydrocarbons) poisoning is a common cause

Table 30–16 • Treatment of Organophosphate (Insecticide) Overdose

Drug	Dose
Atropine	2 mg IV until ventilation improves; usual dose for severe toxicity is 15–20 mg during first 3 hours
Pralidoxime	600 mg IV
Diazepam	5–10 mg IV; repeat until seizures are controlled

of morbidity due to poisoning in the United States.[65] Exposure may be accidental (fire-related smoke inhalation, poorly functioning heating systems, motor vehicle exhaust fumes, tobacco smoke) or intentional. Intraoperative increases in carboxyhemoglobin concentrations may reflect carbon monoxide formation as a result of degradation of volatile anesthetics that contain a CHF_2 moiety (desflurane, enflurane, and isoflurane but not halothane or sevoflurane) by the strong bases present in some (soda lime, Baralyme) but not all carbon dioxide absorbents.[66, 67] Motor vehicle exhaust fumes account for most accidental and intentional carbon monoxide poisoning that results in death (lethal concentrations of carboxyhemoglobin can be achieved within 10 minutes in the confines of a closed garage). Blood carboxyhemoglobin concentrations commonly reach levels of 10% in smokers compared with 1% to 3% in nonsmokers.

Pathophysiology

Carbon monoxide is a colorless, odorless, nonirritant gas that is easily absorbed through the lungs. Carbon monoxide toxicity appears to result from a combination of tissue hypoxia and direct carbon monoxide-mediated damage at the cellular level.[65] Carbon monoxide competes with oxygen for binding to hemoglobin. The affinity of hemoglobin for carbon monoxide is 200 to 250 times as great as its affinity for oxygen. The consequences of this competitive binding are a shift of the oxygen-hemoglobin dissociation curve to the left that changes it to a more hyperbolic shape (Fig. 30–3).[65] These changes result in impaired release of oxygen to tissues and cellular hypoxia. Nevertheless, the binding of carbon monoxide to hemoglobin does not account for all the pathophysiologic consequences related to carbon monoxide poisoning. For example, carbon monoxide-induced tissue hypoxia may be followed by reoxygenation injury to the central nervous system. Hyperoxygenation facilitates production of oxygen radicals, which in turn can oxidize proteins and nucleic acids, resulting in typical reperfusion injury. In addition, carbon monoxide exposure may cause degradation of unsaturated fatty acids with associated demyelination of central nervous system lipids. Carbon monoxide exposure has uniquely deleterious effects on parturients because of the greater sensitivity of the fetus to harmful effects of this gas.

Signs and Symptoms

The signs and symptoms of nonlethal carbon monoxide poisoning are nonspecific and may mimic

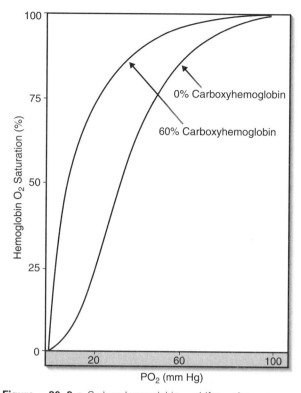

Figure 30–3 • Carboxyhemoglobin shifts the oxygen-hemoglobin dissociation curve to the left and changes it to a more hyperbolic shape. This results in decreased oxygen-carrying capacity and impaired release of oxygen at the tissue level. (From Ernst A, Zibrak JD. Carbon monoxide poisoning. N Engl J Med 1998;339:1603–8. Copyright 1998 Massachusetts Medical Society, with permission.)

nonspecific viral illnesses. Headache, nausea, vomiting, weakness, difficulty concentrating, and confusion are common symptoms. Tachycardia and tachypnea reflect cellular hypoxia. Syncope and seizures may result from cellular hypoxia and cerebral vasodilation, which can also lead to cerebral edema. Angina pectoris, cardiac dysrhythmias, and pulmonary edema may result from increased cardiac output caused by cellular hypoxia. Patients with underlying pulmonary or cardiac disease may experience exacerbations of their disease. The classic findings of cherry-red lips and cyanosis occur rarely. It is important to recognize that carboxyhemoglobin levels may not parallel the severity of symptoms. The duration of carbon monoxide exposure seems to be an important factor in mediating toxicity. If no dissolved carbon monoxide is present in the plasma, the symptoms can be minimal even with markedly increased carboxyhemoglobin concentrations.

Delayed neuropsychiatric syndrome, comprising cognitive dysfunction, personality changes, parkinsonism, dementia, and psychosis, occur in 10% to 30% of individuals following apparent recovery from carbon monoxide intoxication.[65] Delayed neuropsychiatric sequelae due to intraoperative exposure to carbon monoxide have been described as late as 21 days after anesthesia.[66, 67] No clinical or laboratory results predict which patients are at risk for this complication, but advanced age seems to be a risk factor. Cellular hypoxia is not sufficient to explain neuropsychiatric symptoms. Postischemic reperfusion injury and oxygen radical-mediated brain lipid peroxidation may have a role.

Diagnosis

The diagnosis of carbon monoxide poisoning requires a high index of suspicion, as there are no pathognomonic signs or symptoms. In most individuals, increased plasma concentrations of carboxyhemoglobin are diagnostic. Carbon monoxide poisoning is considered severe when blood concentrations of carboxyhemoglobin exceed 40%. Venous blood samples are adequate for measuring carboxyhemoglobin concentrations, which must be measured directly with a spectrophotometer. Pulse oximetry cannot distinguish carboxyhemoglobin from oxyhemoglobin such that SpO_2 values are likely to remain unchanged or falsely increased.[68] Nevertheless, there may be unexplained moderate decreases in SpO_2, which trigger measurement of arterial blood gases and further search (measurement of carboxyhemoglobin) for an explanation of the "desaturation" in the presence of normal PaO_2 values.[69] Calculation of SaO_2 from nomograms based on measured PaO_2 values results in erroneous conclusions. When unexplained SpO_2 decreases occur intraoperatively, it may be helpful to consider the possibility of carboxyhemoglobin accumulation, as general anesthesia otherwise masks the clinical signs and symptoms of carbon monoxide poisoning.

Treatment

Treatment consists of removing the individual from the source of the carbon monoxide production (often a fire that causes smoke inhalation) and immediate administration of 100% oxygen. Oxygen shortens the elimination half-time of carbon monoxide by competing at the binding sites for hemoglobin, and it improves tissue oxygenation. Oxygen administration is continued until the carboxyhemoglobin concentrations have become normal. The half-time of carboxyhemoglobin is 4 to 6 hours when victims are breathing air, 40 to 80 minutes when breathing 100% oxygen, and 15 to 30 minutes when breathing hyperbaric oxygen. Coma, carboxyhemoglobin concentrations higher than 40%, and pregnancy with carboxyhemoglobin concentrations higher than 15% are indications for hyperbaric oxygen therapy; use of hyperbaric oxygen in patients with mild to moderate cerebral dysfunction are disputed.[65] In patients with carbon monoxide poisoning who have been rescued from fires, special considerations should be given to the respiratory status and airway, as urgent or prophylactic tracheal intubation may be needed.

References

1. Alexander BH, Checkoway H, Nahahama SI, et al. Cause-specific mortality risks of anesthesiologists. Anesthesiology 2000;93:922–30
2. Potter WZ, Rudorfer MV, Manjii H. The pharmacologic treatment of depression. N Engl J Med 1991;325:633–42
3. Gram LF. Fluoxetine. N Engl J Med 1994;331:1354–61
4. Thompson TL, Moran MG, Nies AS. Psychotropic drug use in the elderly. N Engl J Med 1983;308:194–8
5. Veith RC, Raskind MA, Caldwell JH, et al. Cardiovascular effects of tricyclic antidepressants in depressed patients with chronic heart disease. N Engl J Med 1982;306:954–9
6. Roose SP, Glassman H, Giardina E-GV, et al. Nortriptyline in depressed patients with left ventricular impairment. JAMA 1986;256:521–6
7. Miller RD, Way WL, Eger EI. The effects of alpha-methyldopa, reserpine, guanethidine and iproniazid on minimum alveolar anesthetic requirement (MAC). Anesthesiology 1968;29:1153–8
8. Braverman B, McCarthy RJ, Ivankovich AD. Vasopressor challenges during chronic MAOI or TCA treatment in anesthetized dogs. Life Sci 1987;40:2587–95
9. Edwards RP, Miller RD, Roizen MF, et al. Cardiac responses to imipramine and pancuronium during anesthesia with halothane or enflurane. Anesthesiology 1979;50:421–5
10. Frommer DA, Kulig KW, Marx JA, et al. Tricyclic antidepressant overdose: a review. JAMA 1987;257:521–6
11. El-Ganzouri AR, Ivankovich AD, Braverman B, et al. Monoamine oxidase inhibitors: should they be discontinued preoperatively? Anesth Analg 1985;64:592–6
12. Wong KC. Preoperative discontinuation of monoamine oxidase inhibitor therapy: an old wives' tale. Semin Anesthesiol 1986;5:145–8
13. Stack CJ, Rogers P, Linter SPK. Monoamine oxidase inhibitors and anaesthesia. Br J Anaesth 1988;60:222–7
14. Wells DG, Bjorksten AR. Monoamine oxidase inhibitors revisited. Can J Anaesth 1989;36:64–74
15. Tordoff SG, Stubbing JF, Linter SPK. Delayed excitatory reaction following interaction of cocaine and monoamine oxidase inhibitor (phenelzine). Br J Anaesth 1991;66:516–8
16. Marks PJ. Electroconvulsive therapy: physiological and anesthetic considerations. Can Anaesth Soc J 1984;31:541–8
17. Selvin BL. Electroconvulsive therapy—1987. Anesthesiology 1987;67:367–85
18. Gaines GY, Rees EI. Electroconvulsive therapy and anesthetic considerations. Anesth Analg 1986;65:1345–56
19. Gerring JP, Shields HM. The identification and management of patients with a high risk for cardiac dysrhythmias during modified ECT. J Clin Psychiatry 1981;43:140–3
20. Khoury GF, Benedetti C. T-wave changes associated with electroconvulsive therapy. Anesth Analg 1989;69:677–9
21. Lee JT, Erbaugh PH, Stevens WC, et al. Modification of electroconvulsive therapy induced hypertension with nitroglycerin. Anesthesiology 1985;62:793–6
22. Weinger MB, Partridge BL, Hauger R, et al. Prevention of the cardiovascular and neuroendocrine response to electroconvulsive therapy. I. Effectiveness of pretreatment regimens on hemodynamics. Anesth Analg 1991;73:556–62
23. Lovac AL, Goto H, Pardo MP, et al. Comparison of two esmolol bolus doses on the hemodynamic response and seizure duration during electroconvulsive therapy. Can J Anaesth 1991;38:204–9
24. Rampton AJ, Griffin RM, Stuart CS, et al. Comparison of methohexital and propofol for electroconvulsive therapy: effects on hemodynamic responses and seizure duration. Anesthesiology 1989;70:412–7
25. Kellner CH, Monroe RR, Burns C, et al. Electroconvulsive therapy in a patient with a heart transplant. N Engl J Med 1991;325:663
26. Havdala HS, Borison RL, Diamond BI. Potential hazards and applications of lithium in anesthesiology. Anesthesiology 1979;50:534–7
27. Hill GE, Wong KC, Hodges MR. Lithium carbonate and neuromuscular blocking agents. Anesthesiology 1977;46:122–6
28. Kane JM. Schizophrenia. N Engl J Med 1996;334:34–41
29. Adnet P, Lestavel P, Krivosic-Horber R. Neuroleptic malignant syndrome. Br J Anaesth 2000;85:129–35
30. Tsujimoto S, Maeda K, Sugiyama T, et al. Efficacy of prolonged large-dose dantrolene for severe neuroleptic malignant syndrome. Anesth Analg 1998;86:1143–4
31. Geiduschek J, Cohen SA, Kahn A, et al. Repeated anesthesia for a patient with neuroleptic syndrome. Anesthesiology 1988;68:134–7
32. Caroff SN, Rosenberg H, Fletcher JE, et al. Malignant hyperthermia susceptibility in neuroleptic malignant syndrome. Anesthesiology 1987;67:20–5
33. Adams AP, Goroszeniuk T. Hysteria. a cause of failure to recover from anaesthesia. Anaesthesia 1991;46:932–4
34. Hyman SE. Drug abuse and addiction. Sci Am Med 1998;1–7
35. Jenkins LC. Anaesthetic problems due to drug abuse and dependence. Can Anaesth Soc J 1972;19:461–77
36. Morse RM, Flavin DK. The definition of alcoholism. JAMA 1992;268:1012–4
37. Fuller RK, Branchey L, Brightwell DR, et al. Disulfiram treatment of alcoholism: a Veterans Administration cooperative study. JAMA 1986;256:1449–53
38. Diaz JH, Hill GE. Hypotension with anesthesia in disulfiram-treated patients. Anesthesiology 1979;51:355–8
39. Cregler L, Mark H. Medical complications of cocaine abuse. N Engl J Med 1986;315:1495–1500
40. Lange RA, Cigarroa RG, Yancy CW, et al. Cocaine-induced coronary-artery vasoconstriction. N Engl J Med 1989;321:1557–62
41. Lange RA, Hillis D. Cardiovascular complications of cocaine use. N Engl J Med 2001;345:351–8
42. Levine SR, Brust JCM, Futrell N, et al. Cerebrovascular complications of the use of the "crack" form of alkaloidal cocaine. N Engl J Med 1990;323:699–704
43. Hollander J, Hoffman R, Gennis P, et al. Nitroglycerine in the treatment of cocaine associated chest pain clinical safety and efficacy. Clini Toxicol 1994;32:243–56
44. Lange R, Cigarroa R, Flores E, et al. Potentiation of cocaine-induced coronary vasoconstriction by beta-adrenergic blockade. Ann Intern Med 1990;112:897–903
45. Bernards CM, Teijeiro A. Illicit cocaine ingestion during anesthesia. Anesthesiology 1996;84:218–20
46. Stoelting RK, Creasser CW, Martz RC. Effects of cocaine administration on halothane MAC in dogs. Anesth Analg 1975;54:422–4
47. Gold MS, Pottash AC, Sweeney DR, et al. Opiate withdrawal using clonidine: a safe, effective, and rapid monopiate treatment. JAMA 1980;243:343–6

48. Gold CG, Cullen DJ, Gonzales S, et al. Rapid opioid detoxification during general anesthesia. a review of 20 patients. Anesthesiology 1999;91:1639–47

49. Whittington RA, Collins ED, Kleber HD. Rapid opioid detoxification during general anesthesia: is death not a significant outcome? Anesthesiology 2000;93:1363–4

50. Giuffrida JG, Bizzarri DV, Saure AC, et al. Anesthetic management of drug abusers. Anesth Analg 1970;49:273–82

51. Berkowitz BA, Finck AD, Hynes MD, et al. Tolerance to N_2O anesthesia in rats and mice. Anesthesiology 1979;51:309–14

52. Marck LC. Hypotension during anesthesia in narcotic addicts. NY State J Med 1966;66:2685–97

53. Johnson RE, Chutuape MA, Strain EC, et al. A comparison of levomethadyl acetate, buprenorphine and methadone for opioid dependence. N Engl J Med 2000;343:1290–7

54. Lee PKY, Cho MH, Dobkin AB. Effects of alcoholism, morphinism, and barbiturate resistance on induction and maintenance of general anesthesia. Can Anaesth Soc J 1974;11: 366–71

55. Fischer SP, Healzer JM, Brook MW, et al. General anesthesia in a patient on long-term amphetamine therapy: is there cause for concern? Anesth Analg 2000;91:758–9

56. Samuels SI, Maze A, Albright G. Cardiac arrest during cesarean section in a chronic amphetamine abuser. Anesth Analg 1979;58:528–30.

57. Johnston RR, Way WL, Miller RD. Alteration of anesthetic requirements by amphetamine. Anesthesiology 1972;36: 357–63

58. Stoelting RK, Martz RC, Gartner J, et al. Effects of delta-9-tetrahydrocannabinol on halothane MAC in dogs. Anesthesiology 1973;38:521–4

59. Vitez TS, Way WL, Miller RD, et al. Effects of delta-9-tetrahydrocannabinol on cyclopropane MAC in the rat. Anesthesiology 1973;38:525–7

60. Johnstone RC, Lief PL, Kulp RA, et al. Combination of delta-9-tetrahydrocannabinol with oxymorphine or pentobarbital. Anesthesiology 1975;42:674–9

61. Frommer DA, Kulig KW, Marx JA, Rumack B. Tricyclic antidepressant overdose: a review. JAMA 1987;257:521–6

62. Smilkstein MJ, Knapp GL, Kulig KW, et al. Efficacy of oral N-acetylcysteine in the treatment of acetaminophen overdose: analysis of the national multicenter study (1976–1985). N Engl J Med 1988;319:1557–62

63. Baud FJ, Galliot M, Astier A, et al. Treatment of ethylene glycol poisoning with intravenous 4-methylpyrazole. N Engl J Med 1988;319:97–100

64. Davies JE. Changing profile of pesticide poisoning. N Engl J Med 1987;316:807–8

65. Ernst A, Zibrak JD. Carbon monoxide poisoning. N Engl J Med 1998;339:1603–8

66. Fang ZX, Eger EI 2nd, Laster MJ, et al. Carbon monoxide production from degradation of desflurane, enflurane, isoflurane, halothane, and sevoflurane by soda lime and Baralyme. Anesth Analg 1995;80:1187–93

67. Baxter PJ, Kharasch ED. Rehydration of desiccated Baralyme prevents carbon monoxide formation from desflurane in an anesthesia machine. Anesthesiology 1997;86:1061–5

68. Baker SJ, Tremper KK. The effect of carbon monoxide inhalation on pulse oximetry and transcutaneous PO_2. Anesthesiology 1987;66:677–9

69. Gonzalez A, Gomez-Arnau J, Pensado A. Carboxyhemoglobin and pulse oximetry. Anesthesiology 1990;73:573

31

Diseases Associated with Pregnancy

Pregnancy and subsequent labor and delivery are accompanied by physiologic changes in multiple organ systems that may influence responses to anesthesia and the choice of anesthetic techniques. Furthermore, medical diseases unique to parturients may influence management of anesthesia, especially during labor and delivery.

PHYSIOLOGIC CHANGES ASSOCIATED WITH PREGNANCY

Cardiovascular System

Changes in the cardiovascular system during pregnancy provide for the needs of the developing fetus and prepare the mother for the events that accompany labor and delivery (Table 31–1). Decreased venous return due to obstruction of the inferior vena cava by the gravid uterus when the parturient assumes the supine position results in *supine hypotension syndrome* in about 10% of parturients as they approach term. The incidence of supine hypotensive syndrome can be minimized by nursing parturients in the lateral position or mechanically displacing the uterus to the left ("left uterine displacement") in supine parturients.

Respiratory Tract

Capillary engorgement of the mucosal lining of the upper respiratory tract emphasizes the need for gentleness during instrumentation of the upper airway. Vigorous oropharyngeal suctioning, placement of nasal, oral, or laryngeal mask airways, or trauma during direct laryngoscopy can result in bleeding and further edema. The combination of increased

Table 31–1 • Physiologic Changes Accompanying Pregnancy

Parameter	Average Change From Nonpregnant Value (%)
Intravascular fluid volume	+35
Plasma volume	+45
Erythrocyte volume	+20
Cardiac output	+40
Stroke volume	+30
Heart rate	+15
Peripheral circulation	
Systolic blood pressure	No change
Systemic vascular resistance	−15
Diastolic blood pressure	−15
Central venous pressure	No change
Femoral venous pressure	+15
Minute ventilation	+50
Tidal volume	+40
Breathing rate	+10
PaO$_2$	+10 mmHg
PaCO$_2$	−10 mmHg
pHa	No change
Total lung capacity	No change
Vital capacity	No change
Functional residual capacity	−20
Expiratory reserve volume	−20
Residual volume	−20
Airway resistance	−35
Oxygen consumption	+20
Renal blood flow and glomerular filtration rate	−50
Serum cholinesterase activity	−25

minute ventilation and decreased functional residual capacity in parturients speeds the rate at which changes in alveolar concentrations of inhaled anesthetics can be achieved. As a result, induction of anesthesia, emergence from anesthesia, and changes in the depth of anesthesia are notably faster in parturients. In addition, dose requirements for volatile anesthetic drugs (MAC) may be decreased during surgery. The combination of accelerated onset and decreased anesthetic requirements makes parturients susceptible to anesthetic overdoses. Induction of anesthesia in parturients may be associated with marked decreases in arterial oxygenation if apnea is prolonged, as during tracheal intubation, reflecting decreased oxygen reserves secondary to decreases in the functional residual capacity. These changes emphasize the potential value of preoxygenation before any anticipated period of apnea in parturients.

Gastrointestinal System

Gastrointestinal changes during pregnancy (enlarged uterus interferes with gastric emptying; pro-

gesterone prolongs gastric emptying time) make parturients vulnerable to aspiration of gastric contents. Parturients tend to develop hypoglycemia more readily than nonpregnant women, reflecting in part the prolonged fasting and increased metabolic demands that may be associated with labor and delivery. Mental status changes in parturients may reflect hypoglycemia, especially in the presence of epidural analgesia, which blunts the hyperglycemic response to pain and removes autonomic nervous system regulation of the adrenal medulla and hepatic glycogenolytic systems.[1]

Regional Anesthetic Techniques

The rational use of regional anesthetic techniques in parturients requires an understanding of the neural pathways responsible for the transmission of pain during labor and delivery (Fig. 31–1). The pain of

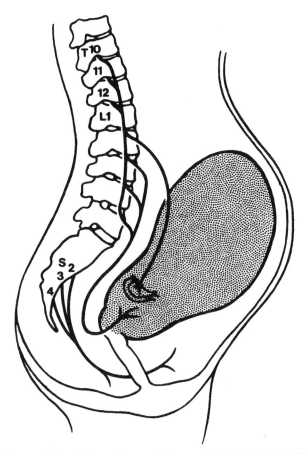

Figure 31–1 • Pain pathways during parturition. Afferent pain impulses from the cervix and uterus are carried by nerves that accompany sympathetic nervous system fibers and enter the spinal cord at T10-L1. Pain pathways from the perineum travel to S2-4 through the pudendal nerves.

labor arises primarily from receptors in uterine and perineal structures. Afferent pain impulses from the cervix and uterus travel in nerves that accompany sympathetic nervous system fibers and enter the spinal cord at T10-L1. Pain pathways from the perineum travel to S2-4 via the pudendal nerves. Pain during the first stage of labor (onset of regular contractions) results from dilation of the cervix, contraction of the uterus, and traction on the round ligament. The pain is visceral and is referred to dermatomes supplied by spinal cord segments T10-L1. During the second stage of labor (complete dilation of the cervix), pain is somatic and is produced by distension of the perineum and stretching of fascia, skin, and subcutaneous tissues.

Lumbar Epidural Anesthesia

When performing lumbar epidural techniques to provide analgesia during labor and delivery or anesthesia for cesarean section, it is important to confirm the absence of intravascular placement of the epidural catheter. In this regard it is common to administer a "test dose" of a solution containing the local anesthetic and epinephrine, 10 to 15 μg.[2, 3] An epinephrine-induced increase in the maternal heart rate alerts the anesthesiologist to the possible intravascular location of the epidural catheter. This test dose may be unreliable in parturients because of maternal heart rate variability. The incidence of false positive interpretations may be decreased by injecting the test dose immediately after a uterine contraction, which diminishes the likelihood of confusing epinephrine-induced tachycardia with pain-induced tachycardia.[3] Increasing progesterone concentrations during pregnancy have been implicated in enhancing the cardiotoxicity and dysrhythmogenic potential of bupivacaine but not of lidocaine and ropivacaine.[2] Hypotension caused by regional anesthesia administered to parturients during labor and delivery may require administration of small doses of ephedrine, 5 to 10 mg IV, or phenylephrine, 20 to 100 μg IV. Ephedrine is the preferred vasopressor for treating the hypotension that occurs in parturients with known uteroplacental insufficiency based on animal data suggesting that pure α-adrenergic agonists could further decrease uterine blood flow.[2] The effect of epidural analgesia on the progress of labor and the incidence of operative delivery is controversial but likely is influenced by the timing and extent of the block, the choice and concentration of the local anesthetic, and the addition of epinephrine or an opioid to the local anesthetic solution.[2]

Combined Spinal-Epidural Anesthesia

Combined spinal-epidural analgesia has been advocated as an alternative to epidural analgesia.[4] Advantages cited for the combined technique include more rapid onset of analgesia, increased reliability, effectiveness when instituted in a rapidly progressing labor, and production of minimal motor block, thus permitting parturients to ambulate during early labor. Subarachnoid placement of low doses of opioids such as fentanyl, 20 to 25 μg, or sufentanil, 5 to 10 μg, results in rapid (5 minutes), nearly complete pain relief during the first stage of labor. Low doses of local anesthetics such as bupivacaine, 2.5 mg, may also be added to the solution placed in the subarachnoid space. Disadvantages of the combined technique include increased technical complexity and the possible risk of postdural puncture headache. Inclusion of opioids may increase the incidence of pruritus and fetal bradycardia.

▮ PREGNANCY-INDUCED HYPERTENSION

Pregnancy-induced hypertension (PIH) encompasses a range of disorders collectively and formerly known as toxemia of pregnancy, which includes isolated systemic hypertension (nonproteinuric hypertension), preeclampsia (proteinuric hypertension), and eclampsia.[5] Occurring in 5% to 15% of all pregnancies, PIH is a major cause of obstetric and perinatal morbidity and mortality. The three principal mechanisms proposed for the etiology of PIH are vasospasm caused by abnormal sensitivity of vascular smooth muscles to catecholamines, antigen-antibody reactions between fetal and maternal tissues during the first trimester that initiates placental vasculitis, and an imbalance in the production of vasoactive prostaglandins (thromboxane A and prostacyclin), leading to vasoconstriction of small arteries and aggregation of platelets. The common pathologic features in the placenta, kidneys, and brain are vascular endothelial damage and dysfunction (Fig. 31–2).[5]

Gestational Hypertension

Gestational hypertension is characterized by the onset of systemic hypertension, without proteinuria or edema, during the last few weeks of gestation or during the immediate postpartum period.[6] Systemic hypertension is usually mild, and the outcome of pregnancy is not affected appreciably. Systemic blood pressure normalizes during the first few weeks postpartum, but systemic hypertension often recurs during subsequent pregnancies. It is believed that the risk of developing essential hypertension later in life is increased in these women. Chronic hypertension is considered to be present when sys-

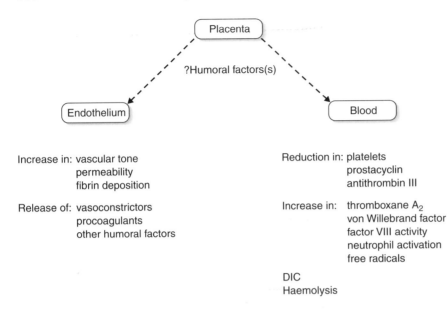

Figure 31–2 • Primary initiating change for the development of pregnancy-induced hypertension (pre-eclampsia) may be placental ischemia. DIC, disseminated intravascular coagulation. (From Mushambi MC, Halligan AW, Williamson K. Recent developments in the pathophysiology of pre-eclampsia. Br J Anaesth 1996; 76:133–48. © The Board of Management and Trustees of the British Journal of Anaesthesia. Reproduced by permission of Oxford University Press/British Journal of Anaesthesia.)

temic blood pressure is increased before 20 weeks of gestation and persists for more than 6 weeks postpartum.

Preeclampsia

Preeclampsia, a syndrome exhibited after 20 weeks of gestation, manifests as systemic hypertension, proteinuria, and generalized edema (Table 31–2). The generalized edema is not essential for the diag-

nosis, as edema is present in most normotensive parturients. Generalized edema associated with preeclampsia typically appears rather abruptly and is associated with accelerated weight gain. Signs and symptoms of preeclampsia usually abate within 48 hours following delivery. Systemic blood pressures higher than 140/90 mmHg with daily urine protein losses of more than 2 g are sufficient for the diagnosis of preeclampsia. Severe preeclampsia is present when systemic blood pressures exceed 160/110 mmHg with daily urine protein losses of more than 5 g. These patients are likely to complain of headaches, visual disturbances, and epigastric pain and consciousness may be altered.

HELLP Syndrome

*H*emolysis, *e*levated *l*iver transaminase enzymes, and *l*ow *p*latelet counts have been characterized as the HELLP syndrome, which represents a severe form of preeclampsia.[5, 7] It is estimated that the HELLP syndrome occurs in up to 20% of parturients who develop severe preeclampsia with many of the manifestations occurring in the postpartum period. Clinical signs and symptoms include epigastric pain, upper abdominal tenderness, systemic hypertension, proteinuria, nausea and vomiting, and jaundice. The disease may progress to pulmonary edema, pleural effusions, cerebral edema, hematuria, oliguria, acute tubular necrosis, and panhypopituitarism. Disseminated intravascular coagulation is a risk. Maternal and perinatal mortality are increased.

Treatment of the HELLP syndrome may include urgent delivery of the fetus by cesarean section. Vaginal delivery is acceptable, but the presence of fetal

Table 31–2 • Manifestations and Complications of Preeclampsia

Systemic hypertension
Congestive heart failure
Decreased colloid osmotic pressure
Pulmonary edema
Arterial hypoxemia
Laryngeal edema
Cerebral edema (headaches, visual disturbances, changes in levels of consciousness)
Grand mal seizures
Cerebral hemorrhage
Hypovolemia
HELLP syndrome (hemolysis, elevated liver enzymes, low platelets)
Disseminated intravascular coagulation
Proteinuria
Oliguria
Acute tubular necrosis
Epigastric pain
Decreased uterine blood flow
Intrauterine growth retardation
Premature labor and delivery
Abruptio placentae

thrombocytopenia could make it hazardous. Platelet transfusions may be necessary before delivery. Packed red blood cell transfusions may be considered if anemia due to hemolysis is severe. The bladder is catheterized to monitor urine output, and central venous pressure monitoring may be helpful.

Management of anesthesia and the choice of regional techniques or general anesthesia is influenced by the condition of the parturient and the fetus.[5] Regional techniques may be avoided because of coagulation defects. Selection of drugs is influenced by the presence of renal or hepatic dysfunction that could alter drug clearance, metabolism, and elimination. Blood glucose concentrations may be monitored, as severe hypoglycemia has been observed in parturients developing the HELLP syndrome.

Pathophysiology

Preeclampsia, a syndrome that affects virtually all maternal organ systems, is associated with placental ischemia. Subsequently, the abnormal placenta may release factors that produce generalized vascular

endothelial cell damage, leading to multiple organ system dysfunction (Figs. 31–2 and 31–3).[5,8]

Cardiovascular System

Systemic hypertension is an early sign of preeclampsia and may result partly from severe vasospasm and generalized arterial vasoconstriction. Increased afterload can lead to left ventricular failure and pulmonary edema. Responses to circulating catecholamines and angiotensin II are exaggerated, reflecting increased sensitivity to these hormones. Decreased intravascular fluid volume is common, especially in parturients with severe preeclampsia. Hypovolemia may result in an increased hematocrit and so obscure the presence of anemia.

Pulmonary System

Pulmonary edema is a common feature of severe preeclampsia that occurs most often in parturients manifesting multiple organ system dysfunction. Low colloid osmotic pressure due to urinary loss of albumin and increased capillary permeability lead

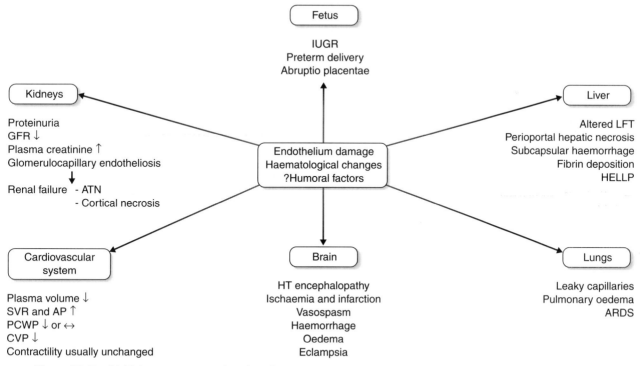

Figure 31–3 • Multiple organ system function changes accompany preeclampsia. AP, arterial pressure; ARDS, acute respiratory distress syndrome; ATN, acute tubular necrosis; CVP, central venous pressure; GFR, glomerular filtration rate; HELLP, hemolysis, elevated liver enzymes, low platelets; HT, hypertensive; IUGR, intrauterine growth retardation; LFT, liver function tests; PCWP, pulmonary capillary wedge pressure; SVR, systemic vascular resistance. (From Mushambi MC, Halligan AW, Williamson K. Recent developments in the pathophysiology and management of pre-eclampsia. Br J Anaesth 1996;76:133–48. © The Board of Management and Trustees of the British Journal of Anaesthesia. Reproduced by permission of Oxford University Press/British Journal of Anaesthesia.)

to interstitial accumulation of fluid in the lungs. Decreased PaO$_2$ is evidence of interstitial pulmonary edema. These parturients may be at increased risk of the development of pulmonary edema in response to intravenous fluid administration. Edema of the upper airway and larynx, which accompanies normal gestation, is exaggerated in these parturients. This change may influence the size of the tube selected for tracheal intubation.

Central Nervous System

Visual disturbances (photophobia, diplopia, blurred vision) may accompany preeclampsia. Ischemia caused by vasospasm of the posterior cerebral arteries or cerebral edema in the occipital regions may be the cause of visual disturbances. Headache and hyperreflexia are warning signs of increased cerebral irritation. Grand mal seizures may occur and most likely reflect the effects of cerebral ischemia due to vasospasm, cerebral edema, and microinfarcts.[5] The effectiveness of magnesium sulfate, a known cerebral vasodilator, for controlling seizures lends support to the occurrence of cerebral vasospasm. A relation between seizures and the degree of maternal systemic hypertension is questionable.[5] Coma in association with increased intracranial pressure may follow seizures. Cerebral hemorrhage may be a fatal event in these patients.

Kidney

Preeclampsia is likely to be associated with decreased renal blood flow and glomerular filtration rate, with corresponding increases in serum creatinine concentrations. Although oliguria is common, progression to acute renal failure is rare. Acute tubular necrosis is often the cause of reversible renal failure. Abruptio placentae, disseminated intravascular coagulation, and hypovolemia usually precede acute renal failure.

Liver

Impaired hepatic function in patients with severe preeclampsia may impair clearance of drugs metabolized by the liver. Spontaneous hepatic rupture is a rare but likely fatal event. Abnormal liver function tests accompany the HELLP syndrome.

Coagulation

Thrombocytopenia is a common finding in parturients experiencing preeclampsia and most likely reflects low grade disseminated intravascular coagulation. Increased circulating concentrations of fibrin degradation products are consistent with disseminated intravascular coagulation. Thrombocytopenia is also thought to involve autoimmune mechanisms as evidenced by increased immunoglobulin G levels. The effect of thrombocytopenia on bleeding is not clear, as prolonged bleeding times do not always parallel the platelet counts. Nevertheless, bleeding times and platelet counts may correlate when platelet counts are less than 100,000 cells/mm^3.

Maternal vascular prostacyclin concentrations are decreased with preeclampsia, and platelet thromboxane A$_2$ production is increased. The resulting imbalance between prostacyclin and thromboxane is likely to contribute to enhanced platelet activity and vascular damage. Aspirin inhibits cyclooxygenase, which is required for prostaglandin and thromboxane production, and thus decreases thromboxane generation and platelet activation. Aspirin also inhibits vascular prostacyclin production, and this action may not be desirable. However, in low doses aspirin may have selective action and block thromboxane production without affecting the systemic vascular prostacyclin. Platelets appear to play a significant role in the pathogenesis of preeclampsia. Indeed, the known effects of aspirin on platelets were the rationale for the notion that this drug might be effective in preventing preeclampsia. Nevertheless, an aspirin-induced protective effective against developing preeclampsia has not been shown to occur.[5]

Ureteroplacental Circulation

An impaired placental circulation caused by placental disease and vasospasm is the most likely explanation for the high incidence of intrauterine fetal death, intrauterine growth retardation, and perinatal mortality associated with preeclampsia. Placental abruption is also more common. Decreased uterine blood flow predisposes to a hyperactive uterus, and premature labor is common. Small and premature infants are vulnerable to depression from drugs administered to provide maternal analgesia. Meconium aspiration is a common problem in neonates born to these parturients.

Eclampsia

Eclampsia is present when seizures are superimposed on preeclampsia. Eclampsia is associated with a maternal mortality of about 10%. Causes of maternal mortality due to eclampsia include congestive heart failure and cerebral hemorrhage. Eclampsia without generalized edema is a recognized phenomenon and may be associated with a poor prognosis.

Although signs and symptoms of preeclampsia usually precede the onset of eclampsia, it is possible for eclampsia to develop without warning.

Treatment

Definitive treatment of PIH is delivery of the fetus and placenta. Until delivery is possible, treatment is based on managing the signs and symptoms of the secondary effects of preeclampsia. It is designed to decrease maternal and fetal complications.[5]

Systemic Hypertension

Cerebral hemorrhage is a major cause of maternal death due to preeclampsia and eclampsia. When the mean arterial pressure exceeds 140 mmHg (180/120 mmHg) there is a significant risk of maternal cerebral hemorrhage. For these reasons it is recommended that maternal systemic blood pressures higher than 170/110 mmHg be treated with the goal of maintaining systemic blood pressures below 170/110 mmHg and above 130/90 mmHg. This goal should decrease the risk of cerebral hemorrhage and preserve placental perfusion. Precipitous decreases in systemic blood pressure are not desirable. For this reason, it is common to provide intravascular fluid volume expansion before initiating drug therapy of hypertension.

Acute Treatment

Hydralazine is most commonly administered for the acute pharmacologic treatment of systemic hypertension due to preeclampsia (Table 31–3).[5] The onset

---

Table 31–3 • Treatment of Systemic Hypertension Associated with Preeclampsia

Maintain diastolic blood pressure < 110 mmHg
  Hydralazine 5–10 mg IV every 20–30 minutes
  Hydralazine 5–20 mg/hr IV as a continuous infusion
    following administration of 5 mg IV
  Labetalol 50 mg IV or 100 mg PO
  Labetalol 20–160 mg/hr IV as a continuous infusion
  Nitroglycerin 10 μg/min IV titrated to response
  Nitroprusside 0.25 μg/kg/min IV titrated to response
Prevent seizures
  Magnesium 4–6 g IV followed by 1–2 g/hr IV as a
    continuous infusion (goal is to maintain serum
    concentrations of 2.0–3.5 mEq/L)
  Toxicity
    4.0–6.5 mEq/L associated with nausea, vomiting,
      diplopia, somnolence, loss of patellar reflex
    6.5–7.5 mEq/L associated with skeletal muscle
      paralysis, apnea
    10 mEq/L or higher associated with cardiac arrest

---

of action of hydralazine is 20 to 30 minutes, which must be considered when timing repeat injections of the drug. Possible disadvantages of hydralazine are headaches, tremors, and vomiting, which mimic symptoms of impending eclampsia. Labetalol may be a satisfactory alternative to hydralazine and is relatively free of maternal side effects (Table 31–3).[5] Labetalol should be used with caution in patients with asthma. Administration of β-adrenergic antagonists in the presence of severe preeclampsia impairs the ability of the fetus to respond to intrauterine stress and may attenuate heart rate changes suggestive of fetal distress. Intravenous administration of nitroprusside or nitroglycerin effectively decrease maternal blood pressure, but there is a risk that excessive hypotension could adversely decrease the uteroplacental blood flow even further. High doses of nitroglycerin (more than 7 μg/kg/min IV) may result in methemoglobinemia. Fetal cyanide toxicity in response to nitroprusside administration has not been shown to occur, and short-term administration of this drug is acceptable. Intra-arterial monitoring of systemic blood pressure may be helpful whenever nitroprusside or nitroglycerin is administered.

Chronic Treatment ∅ ACEI

Many antihypertensive drugs (methyldopa, β-adrenergic antagonists, nifedipine) have been used for chronic treatment of systemic hypertension due to preeclampsia. Angiotensin-converting enzyme inhibitors are associated with teratogenic effects on the fetus (renal tubular agenesis, decreased skull ossification) and are not recommended.[9] Methyldopa is effective in most patients and has been documented to be safe for newborns.[5] Labetalol has theoretical advantages, particularly for the uteroplacental vasculature, because of its α-adrenergic blocking properties.

Hypovolemia noncardiogenic pulm edema

Correction of intravascular fluid volume may be recommended before administering antihypertensive drugs. Fluid replacement is complicated by the presence of low colloid osmotic pressure and increased capillary permeability such that noncardiogenic pulmonary edema may accompany attempts to restore the intravascular fluid volume. Colloid solutions may improve colloid osmotic pressure, but there is no evidence that this improves outcome. Crystalloid solutions are often administered at 1 to 2 ml/kg/hr IV with adjustments in the infusion rate based on the patient's clinical condition, urine output, and central venous pressure measurements, if available. In selected patients it may be useful to place a pulmonary artery catheter to monitor cardiac filling pressures in response to fluid infusion. Infusion of crystalloids alone further decreases the colloid osmotic pressure, whereas the use of colloids may increase the central venous pressure and result in pulmonary edema. If pulmonary edema occurs, it is treated conventionally with supplemental oxygen, diuretics, decreased afterload and preload, fluid restriction, and intermittent positive pressure ventilation.

Oliguria

Many parturients with urine output transiently decreased to less than 30 ml/hr resume normal urine output without therapy. When oliguria persists, an intravenous fluid challenge of 500 to 1000 ml of crystalloid solution is recommended. If there is no response to this fluid challenge, it is common to measure the central venous pressure and use the changes in this value as a guide to subsequent fluid infusion. Repetitive unmonitored fluid administration should be avoided, as it may lead to pulmonary edema. Dopamine may be considered for some oliguric parturients.

Seizures

Magnesium is the most commonly prescribed anticonvulsant drug in the United States for prophylaxis against seizures and for treating seizures associated with eclampsia.[5] The efficacy of magnesium sulfate is unclear, as this drug is not an anticonvulsant. Magnesium sulfate is thought to reverse cerebral vasoconstriction by blocking calcium influx via N-methyl-D-asparate subtypes of glutamate channels.[5] Magnesium sulfate also decreases the presynaptic release of acetylcholine and the sensitivity of postjunctional membranes to acetylcholine. In addition, magnesium sulfate has mild relaxant effects on vascular and uterine smooth muscles. Uterine relaxation is beneficial, as uterine blood flow is improved.

Magnesium sulfate is administered intravenously or intramuscularly, with the goal of achieving therapeutic concentrations of 2.0 to 3.5 mEq/L (Table 31–3).[5] Serum concentrations higher than 4 mEq/L may cause toxicity, which is treated with intravenous administration of calcium gluconate. Patients with poor renal function require slower magnesium sulfate infusion rates as magnesium is excreted by the kidneys. Monitoring parturients receiving magnesium sulfate includes measuring the serum magnesium concentrations and assessing tendon reflexes for the appearance of hyporeflexia. Marked depression of patellar reflexes is an indication of impending magnesium toxicity. Serum magnesium levels in toxic ranges can result in life-threatening side effects (Table 31–3).[5]

Potentiation of both depolarizing and nondepolarizing muscle relaxants by magnesium is clinically significant. This potentiation introduces the need for careful titration of the doses of muscle relaxants and for monitoring their effects at the neuromuscular junction. Parturients experiencing severe preeclampsia may manifest decreased serum cholinesterase activity greater than that normally associated with pregnancy, resulting in potentiation of the effects of succinylcholine independent of magnesium sulfate therapy.[10] Doses of sedatives and opioids may be decreased, as magnesium can potentiate their effects. Because magnesium readily crosses the placenta, it seems possible that neonatal skeletal muscle tone could be decreased at birth. Nevertheless, the deleterious effects of maternal magnesium sulfate therapy do not occur in nonasphyxiated fullterm neonates, suggesting that the depressed ventilation previously attributed to magnesium was due to asphyxia and/or prematurity. Conversely, hypomagnesemia may cause postpartum neurologic dysfunction, which may be erroneously attributed to regional anesthetic techniques used during labor and delivery.[11]

Management of Anesthesia

Vaginal delivery in the presence of PIH and in the absence of fetal distress is acceptable. Cesarean section is necessary in the presence of fetal distress reflecting progressive deterioration of the uteroplacental circulation. Regardless of the choice of anesthetic technique, it is important to continue fetal heart rate monitoring, especially if fetal distress is present.

Emergency Cesarean Section and Choice of Anesthesia

General anesthesia is indicated for preeclamptic parturients undergoing cesarean section who refuse regional anesthesia or who present with cardiovascular disorders in which an abrupt decrease in systemic vascular resistance might be poorly tolerated (aortic stenosis, pulmonary hypertension). Historically, parturients requiring emergency cesarean section for fetal distress have been managed most often with general anesthesia based on the notion that the time spent instituting regional anesthesia would be detrimental to the well-being of the fetus. Nevertheless, there is growing recognition that spinal anesthesia can be established in a timely manner, thereby avoiding the possible depressant effects of drugs on the fetus and the risk of failed or difficult tracheal intubation. Even epidural anesthesia is appropriate if a tested and functional epidural catheter is already in place at the time fetal distress occurs and the decision is made to perform an emergency cesarean section. General anesthesia is selected when hemorrhage or sepsis is the reason for an emergency cesarean section. In the presence of fetal distress, it is helpful to monitor the fetal heart rate continuously while placing the block or preparing for induction of anesthesia.

Epidural Analgesia

Management of anesthesia for labor and delivery in volume-repleted preeclamptic parturients is often with continuous lumbar epidural analgesia utilizing combinations of opioids and local anesthetics. Continuous epidural infusions of the drug-containing solutions may be associated with less hypotension than that produced by intermittent injections of the drugs. Thrombocytopenia is common and may influence the selection of regional anesthesia in these parturients. Nevertheless, there is controversy regarding the reliability of platelet counts for predicting the risk of epidural hemorrhage. There is evidence from thromboelastography that severely preeclamptic parturients with platelet counts of less than 100,000 cells/mm³ are hypocoagulable when compared to healthy parturients and other preeclamptic parturients.[12] There is no evidence that epidural anesthesia is associated with epidural hematomas when administered to parturients with platelet counts below 100,000 cells/mm³. Epidural analgesia negates the need for maternal opioids and thus their possible adverse effects on a preterm fetus. The absence of maternal pushing decreases the likelihood of associated systemic blood pressure increases. Furthermore, vasodilating effects produced by epidural analgesia and anesthesia may improve placental blood flow and could conceivably increase renal blood flow.

Before continuous lumbar epidural anesthesia is instituted, parturients should be hydrated with intravenous crystalloids (1 to 2 L of lactated Ringer's solution), as guided by central venous pressure monitoring. Furthermore, coagulation studies should be performed before placing a lumbar epidural catheter, particularly if the preeclampsia is severe. Epidural analgesia is accomplished with (1) incremental or continuous infusions of local anesthetic solutions containing ropivacaine, bupivacaine, or lidocaine while maintaining left uterine displacement and (2) fetal heart rate monitoring. Adding a small dose of opioid (fentanyl 50 to 100

μg) to the local anesthetic solution may be useful. Initially, a segmental band of anesthesia (T10-L1) provides analgesia for uterine contractions. As the second stage of labor is entered, lumbar epidural analgesia can be extended to provide perineal analgesia. Because of hypersensitivity of the maternal vasculature to catecholamines, it seems prudent not to add epinephrine to local anesthetic solutions used for epidural analgesia, although use of epinephrine-containing local anesthetic solutions has not produced predictable adverse circulatory responses in these parturients.[13]

Spinal Anesthesia

Spinal anesthesia may be discouraged in parturients with preeclampsia because of the risk of severe hypotension. Nevertheless, the magnitude of maternal blood pressure decreases are similar following spinal or epidural anesthesia for cesarean section in patients with severe preeclampsia (Fig. 31–4).[14] As with lumbar epidural techniques, institution of intravenous hydration before performing spinal anesthesia is desirable. Should systolic blood pressure decrease more than 30% from the preblock value, treatment is with left uterine displacement and an increased rate of fluid infusion. If hypotension persists, a small dose of ephedrine, 2.5 mg IV, is appropriate. Addition of small doses of opioid to the local anesthetic solutions provides several hours of postoperative analgesia. A T4 sensory level is needed for performance of cesarean section, keeping in mind that anesthetic requirements are decreased in parturients. In this regard, lidocaine (70 to 80 mg)

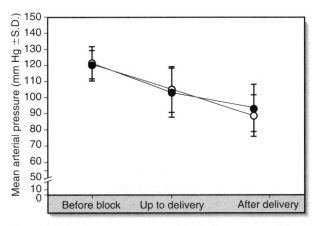

Figure 31–4 • Lowest mean arterial blood pressures did not differ between severely preeclamptic patients receiving spinal (open circles) or epidural (closed circles) anesthesia for cesarean section. (From Hood DD, Curry R. Spinal versus epidural anesthesia for cesarean section in severely preeclamptic patients. Anesthesiology 1999;90:1276–82. © 1999, Lippincott Williams & Wilkins, with permission.)

or bupivacaine (12 to 15 mg) is adequate to achieve the desired T4 sensory level and provides 60 minutes (lidocaine) to 120 minutes (bupivacaine) of anesthesia.

General Anesthesia

The risks of general anesthesia in parturients with preeclampsia include potentially difficult tracheal intubation owing to laryngeal edema, potential aspiration of gastric contents, increased sensitivity to nondepolarizing muscle relaxants, exaggerated pressor responses to direct laryngoscopy and tracheal intubation, and impaired placental blood flow. Mortality from general anesthesia in parturients is almost exclusively due to difficult airway management or failed tracheal intubation.

Induction of Anesthesia

Before induction of anesthesia, attempts are made to restore intravascular fluid volume. Continuous monitoring of intra-arterial blood pressure, cardiac filling pressures, urine output, and fetal heart rate is useful. Induction of anesthesia is often with thiopental, (3 to 5 mg/kg IV) plus succinylcholine, (1.0 to 1.5 mg/kg IV) to facilitate tracheal intubation. Use of defasciculating doses of nondepolarizing muscle relaxants before administration of succinylcholine may not be necessary, as magnesium therapy is likely to attenuate fasciculations produced by succinylcholine. Cricoid pressure may be provided by an assistant until the trachea is successfully intubated and the cuff inflated.

Airway Management

Exaggerated edema of the upper airway structures may interfere with visualization of the glottic opening (swollen tongue and epiglottis), and laryngeal swelling may result in the need to insert a smaller tracheal tube than anticipated. Laryngeal edema often occurs as part of the generalized edema and facial swelling that accompanies preeclampsia, but it may also occur with few warning signs.[5] It is important to avoid repeated direct laryngoscopy in attempts to place a tracheal tube, as this may worsen the existing edema. In preeclamptic parturients with impaired coagulation, any trauma associated with direct laryngoscopy could result in bleeding.

Systemic blood pressure responses to direct laryngoscopy and tracheal intubation are likely to be exaggerated in preeclamptic parturients, thereby increasing the risk of cerebral hemorrhage or pulmonary edema. Short duration laryngoscopy is the most predictable method for minimizing the magnitude and duration of blood pressure and heart rate responses evoked by tracheal intubation. Hydralazine, (5 to 10 mg IV administered 10 to 15 minutes before induction of anesthesia) or nitroglycerin (1 to 2 μg/kg IV just before initiating direct laryngoscopy) has also been administered to attenuate systemic blood pressure responses. Interventions with other drugs (opioids, esmolol, labetalol) intended to blunt pressor and heart rate responses to tracheal intubation must be balanced against potential lingering effects in the mother and the effects on a fetus who may be depressed at birth.

Maintenance of Anesthesia

Low doses of volatile anesthetics (0.5 to 1.0 MAC) with or without 50% nitrous oxide can be used for maintenance of anesthesia. Determinants of neonatal depression are a prolonged interval between the uterine incision and delivery, with the duration of anesthesia being important only with prolonged duration of administration (longer than 20 minutes) prior to delivery. After delivery the anesthesia is typically supplemented with opioids. Potentiation of muscle relaxants by magnesium must be considered and a peripheral nerve stimulator used to monitor activity at the neuromuscular junction. Administration of synthetic oxytocics to treat uterine atony after delivery is done cautiously in view of the parturient's hypersensitive peripheral vasculature. Laryngeal edema may also develop during the intraoperative period and interfere with successful tracheal extubation. Tracheal extubation is performed when protective upper airway reflexes have returned.

PREGNANCY AND CO-EXISTING MEDICAL DISEASES

Co-existing medical diseases may accompany pregnancy and thus assume importance out of proportion to the implications of the disease in the absence of pregnancy.

Heart Disease

Maternal heart disease is estimated to be present in about 1.6% of all parturients. The two most common causes are congenital malformations and acquired valvular heart disease due to rheumatic fever. Many of the signs and symptoms of normal pregnancy can mimic those of cardiac disease. For example, dyspnea associated with interstitial pulmonary edema due to left ventricular failure may be difficult to distinguish from the labored breathing typical of normal pregnancy. Leg edema from congestive heart failure can be mistaken for venous stasis due to aortocaval compression. The presence of congestive heart failure is suggested by hepatomegaly and jugular venous distension, as these changes do not accompany normal pregnancy. It may be difficult to differentiate heart murmurs due to organic lesions from those due to increased blood flow. Rotation of the maternal heart, which occurs because of elevation of the diaphragm as pregnancy progresses, can be mistaken for cardiac hypertrophy.

Circulatory Changes and Co-Existing Heart Disease

Pregnancy and labor may result in adverse effects on the already diseased cardiovascular system. For example, cardiac output is increased about 40% during gestation and can be increased an additional 30% to 45% above prelabor values during labor and delivery. After delivery, relief of aortocaval obstruction contributes to even further increases in cardiac output above prelabor values. These increases, well tolerated by parturients with normal hearts, may result in congestive heart failure in the presence of co-existing heart disease. Indeed, in nearly 50% of patients with symptoms of heart disease during minimal activity or at rest, congestive heart failure develops during pregnancy. Drugs used to treat heart disease (lidocaine, propranolol, digoxin) readily cross the placenta and may affect the fetus. For example, maternal blood lidocaine concentrations in excess of 5 μg/ml may be associated with neonatal depression. Propranolol may produce fetal bradycardia and hypoglycemia. Elimination half-times of digoxin are likely to be significantly longer in the fetus. Electrical cardioversion, as is used to treat paroxysmal atrial tachycardia, has no adverse effects on the fetus.

Detection and evaluation of heart disease is crucial when planning management of anesthesia during labor and delivery. For most heart diseases, no one anesthetic technique is specifically indicated or contraindicated. Nevertheless, analgesia produced by continuous lumbar epidural techniques can minimize the adverse effects of increased cardiac output due to pain or anxiety. Inhalation analgesia or anesthesia is usually selected when sudden decreases in systemic blood pressure would be detrimental.

Invasive monitoring during labor and delivery is probably not necessary in the absence of cardiac symptoms due to co-existing heart disease. Exceptions are parturients with pulmonary hypertension, right-to-left intracardiac shunts, or coarctation of the aorta. In these patients the ability to measure cardiac output and cardiac filling pressures, as well as to calculate systemic and pulmonary vascular resis-

tance, is helpful. Because the hemodynamic changes seen during labor and delivery can persist into the postpartum period, it is logical to continue invasive cardiac monitoring for several hours after delivery.

Mitral Stenosis

Mitral stenosis is the most common type of cardiac valvular defect present during pregnancy. Parturients with mitral stenosis have an increased incidence of pulmonary edema, atrial fibrillation, and paroxysmal atrial tachycardia. Continuous lumbar epidural techniques producing segmental analgesia are useful for labor and vaginal delivery, as this approach minimizes the undesirable effects of pain on the maternal heart rate and cardiac output. Perineal analgesia prevents the parturient's urge to push and eliminates the deleterious effects of the Valsalva maneuver on venous return. General or regional anesthesia can be provided for cesarean section. If general anesthesia is selected, drugs that produce tachycardia and events that increase pulmonary vascular resistance (arterial hypoxemia, hypoventilation) must be avoided.

Mitral Regurgitation

Mitral regurgitation is the second most common cardiac valvular defect present during pregnancy. In contrast to parturients with mitral stenosis, these patients usually tolerate pregnancy well. Indeed, clinical symptoms related to mitral regurgitation do not usually develop until after the age of childbearing.

Continuous lumbar epidural analgesia is recommended for labor and vaginal delivery, as this technique decreases the peripheral vasoconstriction associated with pain and thus helps to maintain forward left ventricular stroke volume. Regional techniques, however, also increase venous capacitance, such that intravenous fluids may be required to maintain the filling volume of the left ventricle. General anesthesia is acceptable when cesarean section is planned.

Aortic Regurgitation

Complications of aortic regurgitation, like those of mitral regurgitation, usually develop after the childbearing years. Therefore these patients usually have an uneventful pregnancy, although congestive heart failure may develop in a small percentage. Decreased systemic vascular resistance and increased heart rate during pregnancy may decrease the regurgitant flow and the intensity of cardiac murmurs associated with aortic regurgitation. Conversely, increased systemic vascular resistance associated with pain during labor and vaginal delivery can lead to decreased forward left ventricular stroke volume. As with mitral regurgitation, continuous lumbar epidural techniques are recommended for analgesia during labor and vaginal delivery. General anesthesia is acceptable when cesarean section is planned.

Aortic Stenosis

The rarity of aortic stenosis during pregnancy reflects the typical 35- to 40-year latent period between acute rheumatic fever and symptoms of aortic stenosis. Asymptomatic parturients are not at increased risk during labor and delivery. Because of the fixed orifice valve lesion, however, these parturients are vulnerable to decreased stroke volume and hypotension if systemic vascular resistance is abruptly decreased. Therefore if regional techniques are selected, a gradual onset of analgesia produced by continuous lumbar epidural anesthesia is useful in view of the hazards of hypotension. Techniques using systemic medication, pudendal block, and inhalation analgesia may be selected for labor and vaginal delivery. General anesthesia is acceptable when cesarean section is planned.

Tetralogy of Fallot

Pregnancy increases the morbidity and mortality associated with tetralogy of Fallot. For example, pain during labor and vaginal delivery may increase pulmonary vascular resistance, leading to an increase in the right-to-left intracardiac shunt, with decreased pulmonary blood flow and accentuation of arterial hypoxemia. In addition, normal decreases in systemic vascular resistance that accompany pregnancy can also increase right-to-left shunts and accentuate arterial hypoxemia. Indeed, most cardiac complications develop immediately postpartum, when systemic vascular resistance is lowest.

Analgesia for labor and vaginal delivery is often provided with a pudendal block. Regional anesthesia must be used with caution because of the hazards of decreased systemic blood pressure due to peripheral sympathetic nervous system blockade. Therefore general anesthesia is usually selected for cesarean section. Invasive monitoring, including continuous measurement of arterial and cardiac filling pressures, is helpful. Easy access to arterial blood facilitates determination of the PaO_2 and early detection of increased arterial hypoxemia, which can occur if the magnitude of right-to-left shunting is accentuated by decreased systemic blood pressure. Pulse oximetry also reflects changes in arterial oxygenation.

Eisenmenger Syndrome

Eisenmenger syndrome consists of obliterative pulmonary vascular disease with resultant pulmonary hypertension, right-to-left intracardiac shunts, and arterial hypoxemia. This combination of problems is not amenable to surgical correction, and pregnancy is not well tolerated. Indeed, maternal mortality can approach 30%, with the highest comparable mortality about 4% among parturients with coarctation of the aorta or tetralogy of Fallot.[15]

The major hazards facing parturients with Eisenmenger syndrome are decreased systemic vascular resistance, (can lead to an increase in the magnitude of the right-to-left intracardiac shunt) and thromboembolism (may interfere with an already decreased pulmonary blood flow). Indeed, the magnitude of the intracardiac shunt can be accentuated by even the normal decrease in systemic vascular resistance that accompanies pregnancy or the widespread pulmonary vasoconstriction that accompanies even small pulmonary emboli. The greatest risk to these patients is during delivery and immediately postpartum.

The principle of any analgesia or anesthesia technique chosen for patients with Eisenmenger syndrome is to avoid decreases in systemic vascular resistance or cardiac output. Likewise, events that could further increase pulmonary vascular resistance (hypercarbia, increased arterial hypoxemia) must be avoided. Meticulous attention is required to prevent infusion of air through tubing used to deliver intravenous fluids, as the possibility of paradoxical air embolism is great.

Vaginal delivery is an acceptable goal. Analgesia provided with continuous lumbar epidural techniques avoids the stress of exhausting, painful labor. If epidural analgesia is selected, however, it is crucial that decreases in systemic vascular resistance be minimized. Epinephrine probably should not be added to local anesthetic solutions, as decreased systemic vascular resistance can be accentuated by the peripheral β-adrenergic effects of epinephrine absorbed from the epidural space. Alternatively, management of parturients with Eisenmenger syndrome has also been described using intrathecal morphine to provide analgesia for the first stage of labor followed by pudendal nerve block to provide anesthesia for the second stage of labor.[16] Analgesia for vaginal delivery may also be provided with inhaled drugs.

Delivery by cesarean section is most often accomplished using general anesthesia. Extensive peripheral sympathetic nervous system blockade is the major disadvantage of epidural or spinal anesthesia. Nevertheless, epidural anesthesia has been used successfully for elective cesarean section in these patients.[15] Regardless of the anesthetic technique selected, antibiotics should be given during the perioperative period as protection against infective endocarditis. It should be recognized that arm-to-brain circulation times are rapid owing to right-to-left intracardiac shunts. Therefore drugs given intravenously have a rapid onset of action. Ketamine has a theoretical advantage over barbiturates in these patients because it does not decrease systemic vascular resistance, although an increase in pulmonary vascular resistance is theoretically possible. In contrast to parenteral drugs, the rate of rise of arterial concentrations of inhaled drugs is slow owing to decreased pulmonary blood flow. Despite the slow onset, myocardial depressant and vasodilating actions of volatile drugs emphasizes the potential hazards of using these anesthetics in patients with Eisenmenger syndrome. Even nitrous oxide can have adverse effects, as this drug has been shown to increase pulmonary vascular resistance. It must be appreciated that positive-pressure ventilation of the lungs can decrease pulmonary blood flow. Invasive monitoring of arterial and cardiac filling pressures is helpful. Because the right ventricle is at greater risk of dysfunction than the left ventricle, measuring the right atrial pressure is uniquely useful. The value of pulmonary artery catheter monitoring in these patients is unclear.[17]

Coarctation of the Aorta

Coarctation of the aorta, like aortic stenosis, represents a fixed obstruction to the forward ejection of left ventricular stroke volume. Increases in cardiac output can be achieved primarily by increasing the heart rate. During periods of high demand, as during labor or acute increases in intravascular fluid volume produced by uterine contractions, the heart rate may not be able to increase to the extent necessary to maintain adequate cardiac output. This sequence of events may result in acute left ventricular failure. Another hazard during labor and vaginal delivery is damage to the vascular wall of the aorta. Specifically, with the increased heart rate and myocardial contractility that accompany the pain of labor, the rate of ejection of blood from the left ventricle increases and may lead to dissection of the aorta.

Maintenance of heart rate, myocardial contractility, and systemic vascular resistance are important considerations in the management of anesthesia. As with aortic stenosis, analgesia for labor and vaginal delivery is often provided with systemic medica-

tions or inhalation analgesia and pudendal block. Likewise, general anesthesia is recommended for cesarean section. Invasive monitoring of arterial and cardiac filling pressures is helpful.

Primary Pulmonary Hypertension

Primary pulmonary hypertension is seen predominantly in young women. Pain during labor and vaginal delivery is especially detrimental because it may further increase pulmonary vascular resistance and decrease venous return. Continuous lumbar epidural anesthesia is useful for preventing pain-induced increases in pulmonary vascular resistance, although careful titration of the local anesthetic solution is important for minimizing decreases in systemic vascular resistance.[18] Addition of opioids to the local anesthetic solutions may be useful. General anesthesia is often recommended for cesarean section, although epidural anesthesia has also been utilized successfully.[19] Spinal anesthesia is not recommended for cesarean section because of the potential for sudden decreases in systemic vascular resistance associated with the high sensory levels required for this operation. Potential risks of general anesthesia in these patients include increased pulmonary artery pressures during laryngoscopy and tracheal intubation, the adverse effects of positive-pressure ventilation on venous return, and the negative inotropic effects of volatile anesthetics. Nitrous oxide may further increase pulmonary vascular resistance. Predelivery assessment of the effects of vasodilators, inotropes, oxytocin, and fluid administration may be of value during subsequent anesthetic management. In addition to oxygen, the administration of isoproterenol may be useful for decreasing pulmonary vascular resistance.[18] Hemodynamic monitoring, including systemic and pulmonary arterial pressures is indicated in these patients. Pulmonary artery rupture and thrombosis are risks with the use of pulmonary artery catheters in the presence of pulmonary hypertension, but the benefits in these critically ill patients appear to offset these potential hazards.[20] Maternal mortality is more than 50%, with most deaths due to congestive heart failure that occurs during labor and the early postpartum period.

Cardiomyopathy of Pregnancy

Left ventricular failure late in the course of pregnancy or during the first 6 weeks postpartum has been termed cardiomyopathy of pregnancy. If such failure persists despite diuretics and digitalis, it is recommended that analgesia for labor and vaginal delivery be provided with continuous lumbar epidural techniques. Acute increases in systemic vascular resistance should be avoided. In about one-half of these parturients, heart failure is transient and recurs only during subsequent pregnancies. In the remaining parturients, idiopathic congestive cardiomyopathy persists and death is likely, especially if another pregnancy is allowed to progress to term.

Dissecting Aneurysm of the Aorta

There is a recognized association between pregnancy and dissecting aneurysms of the aorta. Indeed, nearly 50% of such aneurysms in women younger than 40 years of age occur in association with pregnancy. A continuous lumbar epidural anesthetic is recommended to maintain a pain-free state and normal to slight decreased systemic blood pressure in parturients in whom this disorder is known to have developed.

Prosthetic Valve Replacement

Prosthetic valve replacement usually requires anticoagulation to decrease the likelihood of thromboembolism. Typically, a coumarin anticoagulant is replaced with heparin at 6 to 12 weeks of gestation, as it does not cross the placenta. The presence of anticoagulation limits the use of spinal or epidural anesthesia in these patients.

Diabetes Mellitus

The insulin requirements in parturients with diabetes mellitus change markedly during pregnancy. For example, less insulin is needed during the first trimester and more during the second trimester. Maternal insulin requirements decrease precipitously during the postpartum period. Insulin does not cross the placenta. Conversely, oral hypoglycemic drugs, especially sulfonylurea drugs and metformin, readily cross the placenta and can induce hypoglycemia in neonates. Glyburide, a sulfonylurea drug, does not cross the placenta in appreciable amounts and is an effective alternative to insulin for maintaining normoglycemia in parturients with gestational diabetes mellitus.[21]

Blood glucose concentrations during pregnancy in nondiabetic parturients are lower than nonpregnant levels. Therefore blood glucose concentrations are often maintained lower than the normal level in parturients with diabetes mellitus. Accomplishing this goal may require multiple injections of insulin and strict adherence to diet. Diabetic parturients are at increased risk for the development of ketoacidosis during the second and third trimesters. PIH is also more common in the presence of diabetes mellitus. Neonates born to diabetic mothers are often large for gestational age and are at increased risk for the development of respiratory distress syndrome. A common goal in the prenatal management of diabetic parturients is to ensure continuation of pregnancy to near term to permit maximal fetal lung maturation. Elective cesarean section is often performed in attempts to avoid the high incidence of fetal death seen during the third trimester.

The preferred technique of anesthesia for diabetic parturients undergoing elective cesarean section near term is not defined. Fetal acidosis following cesarean section has been observed with epidural or spinal anesthesia that was complicated by maternal hypotension.[22, 23] Nevertheless, regional anesthetic techniques in diabetic parturients provide the advantages of avoiding hyperglycemic responses to surgery, monitoring the parturient's central nervous system status, and providing anesthesia without added drug depression should operative delivery be difficult. Regardless of the technique selected for anesthesia, blood glucose concentrations should be monitored during the early neonatal period for infants born to diabetic parturients.

Myasthenia Gravis

The course of myasthenia gravis during gestation is highly variable and unpredictable.[24] Exacerbations are most likely to take place during the first trimester or within the first 10 days of the postpartum period. Anticholinesterase drugs should be continued during pregnancy and labor. Theoretically, these drugs increase uterine contractility but without increasing the incidence of spontaneous abortion or premature labor.

Myasthenia gravis does not affect the course of labor. The use of sedatives should be avoided in view of the limited margin of reserve in these patients. Continuous lumbar epidural anesthesia is acceptable for labor and vaginal delivery. Outlet forceps are frequently used to shorten the second stage of labor, thereby minimizing skeletal muscle fatigue associated with expulsive efforts. Regional anesthesia can be used safely for cesarean section, but it is important to recognize that co-existing skeletal muscle weakness may lead to hypoventilation during anesthesia.

Neonatal myasthenia gravis occurs transiently in 20% to 30% of babies born to mothers with this disorder. Manifestations usually occur within 24 hours of birth and are characterized by generalized skeletal muscle weakness and expressionless facies. When breathing efforts are inadequate, tracheal intubation and mechanical ventilation of the infant's lungs should be initiated. Anticholinesterase therapy in neonates is usually necessary for about 21 days after birth.

Cocaine Abuse

Cocaine abuse among parturients is associated with multiple organ involvement, including the cardiovascular, respiratory, neurologic, and hematologic systems (Fig. 31–5).[25] Cocaine is associated with maternal cardiovascular complications including systemic hypertension, myocardial ischemia and infarction, cardiac dysrhythmias, and sudden death.[25,26] Sudden increases in systemic blood pressure may be the primary etiology of cerebral hemorrhage. Alternatively, cerebrovascular spasm can produce local ischemia and infarction. Subarachnoid hemorrhage, intercerebral bleeding, aneurysmal rupture, and seizures have been associated with cocaine use during pregnancy. Thrombocytopenia may occur following cocaine use resulting in prolonged bleeding times. The incidence of acquired immunodeficiency syndrome (AIDS) and syphilis is increased among cocaine-abusing parturients. Maternal use of cocaine may lead to metabolic and endocrine changes in both fetus and mother, presumably reflecting cocaine-induced release of catecholamines. Pulmonary complications (asthma, chronic cough, dyspnea, pulmonary edema) occur most often in parturients who smoke free base cocaine.

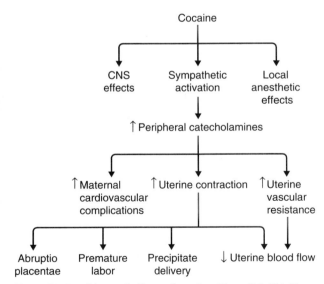

Figure 31–5 • Maternal effects of cocaine. (From Kain ZN, Rimar S, Barash PG. Cocaine abuse in the parturient and effects on the fetus and neonate. Anesth Analg 1993;77:835–45. © 1993, Lippincott Williams & Wilkins, with permission.)

Table 31–4 • Obstetric Complications Associated with Cocaine Abuse During Pregnancy

Spontaneous abortion
Preterm labor
Premature rupture of membranes
Abruptio placentae
Precipitous delivery
Stillbirth
Maternal hypertension
Meconium aspiration
Low Apgar scores at birth

Obstetrical Complications

An increased incidence of significant obstetric complications occur in parturients who abuse cocaine during pregnancy (Table 31–4).[25] The incidence of spontaneous abortion, stillborn birth, and preterm labor is increased. High spontaneous abortion rates may be related to cocaine-induced vasoconstriction, enhanced uterine contractions, and abrupt changes in systemic blood pressure. Cocaine use during the third trimester may result in immediate uterine contractions, increased fetal activity, abruptio placentae, and preterm labor. Uteroplacental insufficiency results in decreased birth weight, intrauterine growth retardation, microcephaly, and prematurity. Cocaine administered during organogenesis is associated with fetal anomalies. Maternal systemic hypertension and vasoconstriction may be the cause of the increased incidence of abruptio placentae in cocaine-abusing parturients. Cocaine effects on the fetus may manifest as an increased incidence of meconium staining and low Apgar scores at birth.

Management of Anesthesia

Identification of parturients abusing cocaine is difficult, as urine checks detect metabolites of cocaine for only 14 to 60 hours after use.[25] The single most important predictor of cocaine abuse is the absence of perinatal care. Evaluation of parturients suspected of cocaine abuse includes an electrocardiogram and possibly echocardiography for evidence of valvular heart disease. In parturients presenting with severe cocaine-induced cardiovascular toxicity, hemodynamic stabilization is established before induction of anesthesia. Cocaine-induced thrombocytopenia is considered if regional anesthesia is planned. Epidural anesthesia is instituted gradually, with attention to hydration and left uterine displacement to prevent hypotension. Hypotension due to rapid sequence induction of general anesthesia or institution of regional anesthesia usually responds to ephedrine, although chronic cocaine abuse could deplete catecholamines and theoretically blunt responses to indirect-acting vasopressors. Ester-based local anesthetics, which undergo metabolism by plasma cholinesterase, may compete with cocaine, resulting in decreased metabolism for both drugs. The relation between AIDS and cocaine abuse must be considered when caring for cocaine-abusing parturients. Body temperature increases and sympathomimetic effects associated with cocaine may mimic malignant hyperthermia. Cocaine-exposed newborns must be monitored postoperatively for apnea, and for this reason they may not be ideal candidates for outpatient surgery.

PREGNANCY AND CO-EXISTING SURGICAL DISEASES

It is estimated that 1% to 2% of parturients in the United States undergo surgical procedures unrelated to pregnancy.[27] Furthermore, women may undergo elective or emergency surgery at times when pregnancy is unrecognized. The most frequent nonobstetric operations are excision of ovarian cysts, appendectomy, breast biopsy, and surgery required because of trauma. Treatment of an incompetent cervix (cervical cerclage) requires anesthesia typically early in pregnancy (during the first trimester). The objectives for managing anesthesia in parturients undergoing nonobstetric operative procedures is preservation of maternal safety, avoidance of intrauterine fetal hypoxia and acidosis due to decreased uterine blood flow, avoidance of teratogenic drugs, and prevention of premature labor from the surgical procedure or drugs administered during anesthesia. In most circumstances, the fetus is a passive recipient of anesthesia administered to the mother, experiences no blood loss, and undergoes passive changes rather than direct stress or hemodynamic alterations caused by surgery (Fig. 31–6).[27]

Maternal Safety

During pregnancy, maternal anatomic and physiologic changes occur that result in implications for anesthetic management.[27] Minute ventilation and oxygen consumption increase, and residual volume and functional residual capacity decrease; therefore the oxygen reserve decreases, and parturients develop arterial hypoxemia and hypercarbia more rapidly with hypoventilation or apnea. Airway management by face mask, laryngeal mask airway, or tracheal intubation can be technically difficult in parturients because of breast enlargement, laryngeal

edema, and weight gain that affects the soft tissues of the neck. From mid-gestation, parturients are at risk for aortic and vena caval compression (supine hypotension syndrome) by the gravid uterus. Physiologic compensation for aortocaval compression can be compromised by anesthetic techniques (spinal, epidural, general) that interfere with sympathetic nervous system activity. Resulting hypotension and associated decreases in uterine blood flow must be minimized. Manual left lateral displacement of the uterus is important for minimizing interference with venous return. Pregnancy decreases the anesthetic requirements for inhaled anesthetics, and parturients may be more susceptible to axonal block by local anesthetics. Transient neurologic symptoms following spinal anesthesia with lidocaine in parturients are unlikely, suggesting a protective effect of pregnancy.[28] Mechanical and hormonal changes that accompany pregnancy (decreased esophageal sphincter tone) place parturients at increased risk for pulmonary aspiration with induction of anesthesia. Although gastric motility remains normal during pregnancy, the administration of opioids and onset of painful uterine contractions results in slowed gastric emptying.

Avoidance of Intrauterine Fetal Hypoxia and Acidosis

Intrauterine fetal hypoxia and acidosis are minimized by avoiding maternal hypotension, arterial hypoxemia, and excessive changes in the $PaCO_2$ thereby preserving uterine blood flow and fetal oxygen delivery. The asphyxiated fetus cannot increase oxygen extraction; rather, compensation is by redistribution of blood flow to vital organs.[27] Treatment of maternal hypotension with vasopressors or inotropes may increase maternal blood pressure while uterine blood flow remains decreased. When maternal hypotension occurs, the initial steps are left uterine displacement, intravenous fluid administration, and elevation of the parturient's legs. Pharmacologic management of maternal hypotension is initially with ephedrine. When ephedrine is not considered ideal (valvular cardiac lesions, co-existing tachycardia, no response to ephedrine), it is acceptable to administer small doses of phenylephrine.[27] Maternal administration of supplemental oxygen increases fetal oxygenation, but the fetus is not at risk for hyperoxia (retrolental fibroplasia, premature closure of the ductus arteriosus) because fetal oxygen partial pressures do not exceed 65 mmHg. This reflects the high oxygen consumption of the placenta and uneven distribution of maternal and fetal blood flow in the placenta. Maternal hyperventilation

Mother: Active changes

Fetus: Passive changes

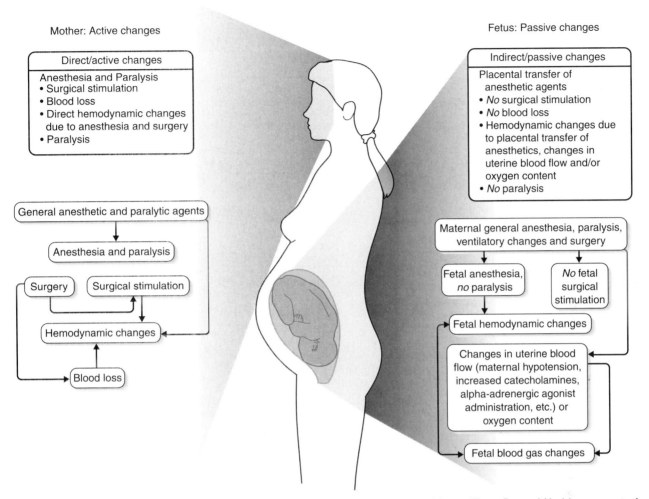

Figure 31–6 • Effects of anesthetic drugs and muscle relaxants on the paturient and fetus. (From Rosen MA. Management of anesthesia for the pregnant surgical patient. Anesthesiology 1999;91:1159–63. © 1999, Lippincott Williams & Wilkins, with permission.)

should be avoided intraoperatively, as positive airway pressure may decrease uterine blood flow and any resulting respiratory alkalosis increases the maternal hemoglobin affinity for oxygen, resulting in the release of less oxygen to the fetus at the placenta.

Avoidance of Teratogenic Drugs

Despite the greater risk to the fetus from maternal hypotension or arterial hypoxemia, considerable concern exists regarding the potential for drugs administered during anesthesia to have teratogenic effects or to result in abortion.[27] For a drug to be teratogenic, it must be given to a susceptible species in an appropriate dose and during a specific period of organ development. Each organ system undergoes a critical stage of development during which vulnerability to teratogens is greatest. In humans the critical period of organogenesis is between 15 and 56 days of gestation. Despite the frequency of expressed concerns, fewer than 30 drugs have been proven to be teratogenic in humans when used in clinically effective doses, and even fewer are currently in clinical use (Table 31–5).[9]

To date, no study has demonstrated that inhalation anesthesia given to parturients has had any teratogenic effect on the fetus. Available evidence suggests that administration of volatile anesthetics, nitrous oxide, opioids, regional anesthesia, or local anesthetics to parturients does not have deleterious effects on embryonic or fetal development.[27] Special

Table 31–5 • Examples of Drugs with Documented Teratogenic Effects when Administered in Clinical Doses to Humans

Drug	Teratogenic Effect
Angiotensin-converting enzyme inhibitors	Renal tubular dysgenesis
	Decreased skull ossification
Anticholinergic drugs	Neonatal meconium ileus
Antithyroid drugs (propylthiouracil, methimazole)	Fetal and neonatal goiter
Carbamazepine	Neural tube defects
Cyclophosphamide	Central nervous system malformation
Danazol	Masculinization of female fetuses
Diethylstilbestrol*	Vaginal cancer in female offspring
	Genitourinary defects
Hypoglycemic drugs	Neonatal hypoglycemia
Lithium	Ebstein's anomaly
Methotrexate	Central nervous system malformations
	Limb malformations
Misoprostol	Möbius syndrome
Nonsteroidal antiinflammatory drugs (except sulindac)	Constriction of the ductus arteriosus
	Necrotizing enterocolitis
Paramethadione*	Central nervous system defects
	Facial defects
Phenytoin	Central nervous system defects
	Growth retardation
Psychoactive drugs (opioids, benzodiazepines, barbiturates)	Neonatal withdrawal syndrome when drug is taken during late pregnancy
Systemic retinoids	Central nervous system defects
	Craniofacial defects
	Cardiovascular defects
Tetracycline	Skeletal and dental anomalies
Thalidomide	Limb-shortening defects
	Internal organ defects
Trimethadione*	Central nervous system defects
	Facial defects
Valproic acid	Neural tube defects
Warfarin	Central nervous system defects
	Skeletal defects

* Not in clinical use.
Adapted from: Koren G, Pastuszak A, Ito S. Drugs in pregnancy. N Engl J Med 1998;338:1128–37.

concerns regarding possible teratogenic effects of nitrous oxide were based on animal studies and the known ability of this drug to interfere with methionine synthetase activity. Extrapolating animal data on nitrous oxide to humans may not be justified, however, as there are differences between species with regard to susceptibility to specific teratogens. Current evidence suggests that parturients may be exposed to nitrous oxide during clinical anesthesia without risk.[2] No anesthetic, opioid, sedative-hypnotic, or anxiolytic drug appears to be teratogenic or safer than another drug. The previous concern regarding administration or benzodiazepines, especially during the first trimester, has been dispelled.[9] Likewise, the highly effective antiemetic drug bendectin has been shown not to be a teratogen.[9]

Neuromuscular blocking drugs do not cross the placenta in significant amounts. Parturients have decreased serum cholinesterase concentrations and increased volumes of distribution, suggesting that the onset, duration, and clearance of these drugs could be altered compared with that in nonpregnant patients. For these reasons, monitoring the responses to neuromuscular blocking drugs with a peripheral nerve stimulator seems prudent. Pharmacologic antagonism of nondepolarizing muscle relaxants with anticholinesterase drugs is acceptable, although there is the theoretical risk that these drugs could stimulate uterine contractions. Nitroprusside, nitroglycerin, and β-adrenergic blocking drugs have been used safely in parturients. High doses of esmolol have been associated with fetal bradycardia, but this drug is not considered to be contraindicated during pregnancy.

There is concern that subteratogenic doses of some psychoactive drugs, such as anesthetics, could produce behavioral and learning defects without causing gross morphologic changes. This concern is based on the fact that development of the central nervous system is not complete even at birth. Nevertheless, there is no evidence establishing the validity of the assertion that anesthesia administered to parturients adversely affects later mental and neurologic development of the offspring. There is no evidence that any anesthetic drug is carcinogenic to the fetus.

Premature Labor

There is no evidence that specific anesthetic drugs or techniques are associated with a higher or lower incidence of premature delivery.[27] It is the underlying disease and/or the site of surgery that determines the onset of premature labor. For example, premature labor occurs in 28% to 40% of parturients undergoing cervical cerclage, whereas orthopedic, neurosurgical, or plastic surgical procedures are not associated with premature labor. Laparoscopy is considered safe during the first half of gestation.[27] During laparoscopy it is recommended that pneumoperitoneum be produced with nitrous oxide rather than carbon dioxide to minimize the development of fetal respiratory acidosis and use of the lowest-pressure pneumoperitoneum possible to avoid exacerbation of vena caval compression. Whenever possible, the fetus should be shielded from radiographic exposure.

Premature labor can be treated with selective β_2-agonists such as terbutaline or ritodrine. These drugs relax uterine smooth muscle, resulting in inhibition of uterine contractions. Relaxation of the uterus also contributes to improved uteroplacental blood flow and fetal well-being. It is important to realize that significant maternal side effects, including pulmonary edema, cardiac dysrhythmias, and hypokalemia, can accompany administration of these drugs.[29] The drugs also cross the placenta and can cause fetal tachycardia and hypoglycemia. The mechanism for altered maternal serum potassium concentrations is not known. It is presumed that β_2-agonists stimulate both glycolysis and insulin release, resulting in shifts of potassium into the intracellular spaces. It is important to be aware that hypokalemia observed during administration of β_2-agonists may persist despite potassium chloride supplementation. Serum potassium concentrations return to preinfusion levels about 30 minutes after β_2-agonist infusions are discontinued. Therefore it may be prudent to discontinue these infusions about 30 minutes before initiation of anesthesia for obstetric delivery.[29] Unexpected hyperkalemia and cardiac arrest have been observed following succinylcholine administration to parturients being treated with magnesium and ritodrine.[30] Continuous monitoring of the electrocardiogram and avoidance of intraoperative hyperventilation of the parturient's lungs are useful principles for managing anesthesia. Intravenous alcohol has also been used to stop premature labor. Maternal and fetal central nervous system depression are undesirable side effects of this treatment.

Management of Anesthesia

Women of child-bearing age should be asked about their last menstrual period, informed of potential risks, and offered pregnancy testing if their menstrual history is uncertain or if they request it to avoid undergoing elective surgical procedures during early gestation.[27] Despite the lack of clinical evidence, delaying surgery until the second trimester, when possible, may decrease the risk of teratogenicity and spontaneous abortion.[27] Elective surgery other than postpartum tubal ligation is deferred until about 6 weeks after delivery, when the physiologic changes of pregnancy have passed (Fig. 31–7).[27] After about 16 weeks of gestation, fetal heart rate monitoring during surgery is useful, but in some circumstances access is difficult. When monitoring by external abdominal ultrasonography is not logistically feasible, it is possible to use a sterile sleeve on a transabdominal ultrasound transducer. Another alternative is a transvaginal ultrasound probe, particularly during early gestation. Although not considered a necessity for the intraoperative management of most parturients, preoperative and postoperative monitoring of the fetal heart rate and uterine activity is advocated.[27]

Emergency surgery during the first trimester is often performed with lumbar epidural or spinal anesthesia. Spinal anesthesia is useful, as it minimizes fetal drug exposure. Nevertheless, there is no evidence that inhaled anesthetics cause adverse responses when administered to parturients undergoing nonobstetric surgery.[27] When inhalation anesthesia is selected, it should be appreciated that low concentrations of volatile anesthetics are not associated with significant decreases in uterine blood flow because of concomitant decreases in uterine vascular resistance. Regardless of the anesthetic technique selected, supplemental oxygen administration is indicated.

Postpartum Tubal Ligation

Postpartum tubal ligation is the most common type of surgery performed during the early postpartum

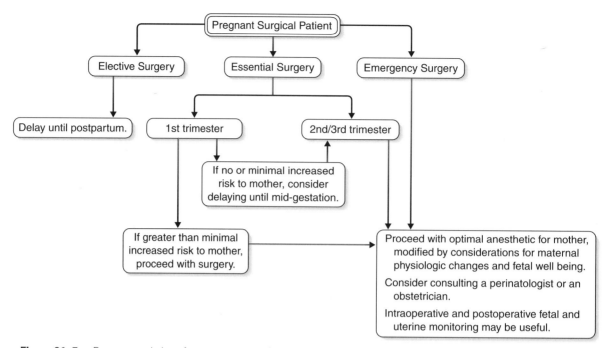

Figure 31–7 • Recommendations for management of parturients and surgical procedures. (From Rosen MA. Management of anesthesia for the pregnant surgical patient. Anesthesiology 1999;91:1159–63. © 1999, Lippincott Williams & Wilkins, with permission.)

period. The risk of aspiration and timing of surgery is resolved to a great extent if the surgery has been anticipated and continuous epidural anesthesia or spinal anesthesia is used for delivery. Residual anesthesia from the delivery is used to perform the intra-abdominal procedure, which necessitates a T5 sensory level to ensure patient comfort. When epidural or spinal anesthesia has not been used for delivery, it is common practice to wait 8 to 12 hours after delivery before inducing anesthesia for tubal ligation. This time interval is useful to allow parturients to reach cardiovascular stability, and it increases the likelihood of gastric emptying. Nevertheless, there is no demonstrable difference in gastric fluid volume and pH when parturients are studied 1 to 8 hours after vaginal delivery.[27]

If general anesthesia is selected for patients undergoing postpartum tubal ligation, many recommend administration of antacids or H_2-antagonists before induction of anesthesia and subsequent placement of a cuffed tube in the trachea. Spinal anesthesia provides rapid onset anesthesia compared with epidural anesthesia, and it is technically easier to accomplish. The incidence and severity of hypotension and occurrence of nausea and vomiting are less after postpartum tubal ligation than after cesarean section, reflecting the decreased size of the uterus. Avoiding spinal anesthesia in preference to epidural anesthesia, based on a concern that headache may follow the former, is questionable, considering the low incidence of this side effect when small-gauge needles are used to puncture the dura and the likely occurrence of a severe headache if the dura is accidentally punctured during performance of epidural anesthesia with a large bore needle.

In Vitro Fertilization

It is unclear if nitrous oxide or other anesthetics have undesirable effects on the outcome of in vitro fertilization and gamete intrafallopian transfer procedures.[2] Anesthetics have been detected in the follicular fluid during aspiration of oocytes and could affect the reproductive potential of such ova. The data for the effect of inhaled anesthetics on the success of in vitro fertilization procedures are conflicting.[31]

COMPLICATIONS ASSOCIATED WITH DELIVERY

Complications associated with delivery include abnormal presentations, multiple births, hemorrhagic complications, uterine rupture, and amniotic fluid embolism.

Abnormal Presentations and Multiple Births

The presentation of the fetus is determined by the presenting part and the anatomic portion of the fetus felt through the cervix by manual examination. The description of the fetal position is based on the relation of the fetal occiput, chin, or sacrum to the left or right side of the parturient. Approximately 90% of deliveries are cephalic presentations in either the occiput transverse or occiput anterior position. All other presentations and positions are considered abnormal.

Persistent Occiput Posterior Presentation

During active labor the occiput undergoes internal rotation to the occiput anterior position. If this rotation does not occur, the persistent occiput posterior position results, and labor becomes prolonged and painful. For example, severe back pain reflects pressure on the posterior sacral nerves by the fetal occiput. Spontaneous delivery requires more uterine and abdominal work. The incidence of cervical and perineal lacerations and postpartum bleeding is increased. Although spontaneous delivery may occur, the need for manual or forceps rotation and extraction is likely. A prolonged second stage of labor or difficult midforceps rotation is associated with increased birth trauma, intracranial hemorrhage, and birth asphyxia in neonates.

Regional anesthetic techniques that relax the maternal perineal muscles are best avoided until there is spontaneous internal rotation of the fetal head. Analgesia can be provided with a segmental (T10-L1) lumbar epidural technique. If back pain persists, analgesia may be extended to sacral areas by injecting dilute concentrations of local anesthetic solutions containing bupivacaine or ropivacaine, 0.125% to 0.25%, which should not paralyze the skeletal muscles necessary for internal rotation of the fetal head. Complete analgesia and perineal relaxation is appropriate when midforceps rotation is planned.

Breech Presentation

Breech rather than cephalic presentations characterizes about 3.5% of all pregnancies. Causes of breech presentations are unknown, but factors that seem to predispose to this presentation include prematurity, placenta previa, multiple gestations, and uterine anomalies. Fetal abnormalities, including hydrocephalus and polyhydramnios, are associated with breech presentations.

Breech deliveries result in increased maternal morbidity. Compared with cephalic presentations, there is a greater likelihood of cervical lacerations, perineal injury, retained placenta, and shock due to hemorrhage. Neonatal morbidity and mortality are increased. These infants are more likely to experience arterial hypoxemia and acidosis during delivery because of umbilical cord compression. Prolapse of the umbilical cord occurs with increased frequency in breech presentations and is presumed to reflect failure of the presenting part to fill the lower uterine segment.

Cesarean Delivery

Fetuses in breech presentations are often delivered by elective cesarean section. If cesarean section is planned, regional or general anesthesia may be selected. It should be appreciated that during regional anesthesia there may be difficulty extracting the infant through the uterine incision. If uterine hypertonus is the cause, it is necessary to induce general anesthesia rapidly, perform tracheal intubation, and produce uterine relaxation with volatile anesthetics. Alternatively, intravenous nitroglycerin may provide prompt uterine relaxation.

Vaginal Delivery

For vaginal delivery of breech presentations, parturients must be able to expel the fetus until the umbilicus is visible. The obstetrician then completes the delivery manually or with forceps. Analgesia during labor is often provided with intramuscular or intravenous medications followed by perineal infiltration of a local anesthetic solution or by performing a pudendal nerve block. Inhalation analgesia may also be administered. Rapid induction of general anesthesia, with tracheal intubation, may be necessary if perineal muscle relaxation is inadequate for delivery of the after-coming fetal head or if the lower uterine segment contracts and traps the head. Alternatives to local anesthetic infiltration or inhalation analgesia are lumbar epidural anesthesia techniques. Continuous lumbar epidural anesthesia, for example, provides analgesia and maximal perineal relaxation for delivery of the fetal head. The ability of parturients to push during delivery can be preserved by administering minimal concentrations of local anesthetics and providing constant maternal encouragement. Indeed, the incidence of breech extraction is not increased in the presence of epidural analgesia. If uterine relaxation is needed to facilitate breech extraction during vaginal delivery, it is necessary to induce general anesthesia and perform tracheal intubation.

Multiple Gestations

The incidence of twin gestations is approximately 1 in 90 births. PIH, anemia, premature labor, breech presentations, and hemorrhage are more common in multiple gestations. Approximately 60% of twins are premature. The large uterus associated with multiple gestations produces more aortocaval compression, predisposing parturients to a higher incidence of severe supine hypotension. This hypotension may be even further exaggerated if sympathetic nervous system blockade is produced by spinal or epidural anesthesia. Blood loss during twin delivery is twice that of a single gestation, and manual extraction of the placenta is required twice as often. It must be appreciated that the second twin is more likely to be depressed, presumably reflecting periods of fetal arterial hypoxemia and acidosis due to contraction of the uterus or to premature separation of the placenta after the first neonate is delivered.

The choice of anesthesia in the presence of multiple gestations is related to the frequent occurrence of prematurity and breech presentations. Preparations must be made for the possibility of providing anesthesia for version, extraction, breech delivery, cesarean section, or midforceps delivery. Pudendal nerve blocks with or without inhalation analgesia introduces minimal depression to the fetus, but maternal analgesia is often inadequate, and relaxation of the perineal muscles is absent. Continuous lumbar epidural anesthesia provides good analgesia and eliminates the need to administer opioids to parturients, which is particularly important for avoiding depression in premature neonates. Segmental lumbar epidural anesthesia with bupivacaine or ropivacaine, 0.25%, provides adequate analgesia and preserves sufficient abdominal muscle strength for the parturient to assist in delivery. In addition, forceps deliveries, which are likely with multiple gestations, are more easily accomplished in the presence of perineal muscle relaxation provided by epidural anesthesia. Intravenous infusions of fluids and left uterine displacement are important for minimizing aortocaval compression when peripheral sympathetic nervous system blockade is produced.

Hemorrhage in Obstetric Patients

Hemorrhage remains the leading cause of maternal mortality. Although bleeding can occur at any time during pregnancy, third-trimester hemorrhage is the most threatening to maternal and fetal well-being (Table 31–6). Placenta previa and abruptio placentae are the major causes of bleeding during the third trimester. Uterine rupture can be responsible for uncontrolled hemorrhage that manifests during active labor. Postpartum hemorrhage occurs after 3% to 5% of all vaginal deliveries and is typically due to retained placenta, uterine atony, or cervical or vaginal laceration.

Placenta Previa

Placenta previa (abnormally low implantation of the placenta in the uterus) occurs in up to 1% of full-term pregnancies (Table 31–6). The cause of placenta previa is not known, although there is an association with advancing age of the parturient and with high parity. Placenta previa is classified as "complete"

Table 31–6 • Differential Diagnosis of Third-Trimester Bleeding

Parameter	Placenta Previa	Abruptio Placentae	Uterine Rupture
Signs and symptoms	Painless vaginal bleeding	Abdominal pain Bleeding partially or wholly concealed Uterine irritability Shock Coagulopathy Acute renal failure Fetal distress	Severe abdominal pain Shock Disappearance of fetal heart tones
Predisposing conditions	Advanced age Multiple parity	Multiple parity Uterine anomalies Compression of the inferior vena cava Chronic systemic hypertension	Previous uterine incision Rapid spontaneous delivery Excessive uterine stimulation Cephalopelvic disproportion Multiple parity Polyhydramnios Spontaneous

when the entire cervical os is covered by placental tissue, "partial" when the internal cervical os is covered by placental tissue when closed but not when fully dilated, and "marginal" when placental tissue encroaches on or extends to the margin of the internal cervical os. Nearly 50% of parturients with placenta previa have marginal implantations.

The cardinal symptom of placenta previa is painless vaginal bleeding, which usually stops spontaneously. Bleeding typically manifests around week 32 of gestation, when the lower uterine segment begins to form. When this diagnosis is suspected, the position of the placenta is confirmed by ultrasonography or radioisotope scan.

Abruptio Placentae

Abruptio placentae is premature separation of a normally implanted placenta after 20 weeks of gestation (Table 31–6). The causes are unknown, but the incidence is increased with high parity, uterine anomalies, compression of the inferior vena cava, PIH, and cocaine abuse. Abruptio placentae accounts for about one-third of third trimester hemorrhages.

Signs and symptoms of abruptio placentae depend on the site and extent of the placental separation, but abdominal pain is always present. When the separation involves only placental margins, the escaping blood can appear as vaginal bleeding. Alternatively, large volumes of blood loss can remain concealed in the uterus. Severe blood loss from abruptio placentae presents as maternal hypotension, uterine irritability and hypertonia and fetal distress or even demise. Clotting abnormalities can occur that resemble disseminated intravascular coagulation. The classic hemorrhagic picture includes thrombocytopenia, depletion of fibrinogen, and prolonged plasma thromboplastin times. Acute renal failure may accompany disseminated intravascular coagulation, reflecting fibrin deposition in renal arterioles. Fetal distress reflects loss of functional placenta and decreased uteroplacental perfusion because of maternal hypotension.

Definitive treatment of abruptio placentae is delivery of the fetus. If maternal hypotension is absent, clotting studies are acceptable, and there is no evidence of fetal distress due to uteroplacental insufficiency, the use of continuous lumbar epidural techniques is useful for providing analgesia for labor and vaginal delivery. When the magnitude of placental separation and resulting hemorrhage is severe, emergency cesarean section is necessary; most often general anesthesia is used, as regional anesthesia in a hemodynamically unstable patient may be unwise. Ketamine, 1 mg/kg IV, is useful for induction of anesthesia, followed by the addition of nitrous oxide until the fetus is delivered. It is predictable that neonates born under these circumstances will be hypovolemic.

It is not uncommon for blood to dissect between layers of myometrium after premature separation of the placenta. As a result, the uterus is unable to contract adequately after delivery, and postpartum hemorrhage occurs. Uncontrolled hemorrhage may require an emergency hysterectomy. Bleeding may be exaggerated by a coagulopathy, in which case infusion of fresh frozen plasma and platelets may be helpful for replacing deficient clotting factors. Clotting parameters usually revert to normal within a few hours after delivery of the neonate.

Uterine Atony

Uterine atony after vaginal delivery is an important cause of postpartum bleeding and a potential cause of maternal mortality. A completely atonic uterus may result in 2000 ml blood loss in 5 minutes. Conditions associated with uterine atony include multiple parity, multiple births, polyhydramnios, a large fetus, and a retained placenta. Low concentrations of volatile anesthetics are unlikely to cause sustained uterine atony. Uterine atony may occur immediately after delivery or may manifest several hours later. Treatment is with intravenous oxytocin to cause contraction of the uterus. In rare instances it is necessary to perform an emergency hysterectomy.

Retained Placenta

Retained placenta occurs in about 1% of all vaginal deliveries and usually necessitates manual exploration of the uterus. If epidural or spinal anesthesia has not been used for vaginal delivery, manual removal of the retained placenta may be first attempted under continuous epidural analgesia. General anesthesia, including administration of volatile anesthetics to provide uterine relaxation, is required if the uterus remains firmly contracted around the placenta. Tracheal intubation is necessary when general anesthesia is used to relax the uterus. Ketamine in doses exceeding 1 mg/kg IV is not recommended in view of the dose related increases in uterine tone produced by this drug.

Asherman Syndrome

Asherman syndrome (traumatic intrauterine synechiae) most often follows postpartum or postabortion curettage. Although infertility is likely, conception can occur and pregnancy is associated with a high incidence of complications, the most serious of which is antepartum and postpartum hemorrhage due to accretion of the placenta. Placenta accreta describes any condition in which the placenta adheres to, invades, or penetrates the uterine myometrium. A diagnosis of placenta accreta usually mandates emergency hysterectomy, which, considering the highly vascular gravid uterus, may be associated with substantial blood loss. For this reason, selection of regional anesthetic techniques with their associated sympathetic nervous system blockade may be questionable in laboring parturients with Asherman syndrome and the likely presence of placenta accreta.[32]

Uterine Rupture

Uterine rupture occurs in up to 0.1% of full-term pregnancies and may be associated with separation of previous uterine surgical scars, rapid spontaneous delivery, excessive oxytocin stimulation, or multiple parity with cephalopelvic disproportion or unrecognized transverse presentations. Overall, however, more than 80% of uterine ruptures are spontaneous without obvious explanations. Furthermore, uterine rupture and dehiscence represent a spectrum ranging from incomplete rupture or gradual dehiscence of surgical scars to explosive rupture with intraperitoneal extrusion of uterine contents.

Signs and symptoms of uterine rupture include severe abdominal pain, often referred to the shoulder due to subdiaphragmatic irritation by intra-abdominal blood, maternal hypotension, and disappearance of fetal heart tones. Parturients with previous cesarean sections may be allowed to deliver vaginally. In these parturients, use of continuous lumbar epidural analgesia could mask abdominal pain due to uterine rupture. Nevertheless, this theoretical concern has not been confirmed by clinical experience; and with the proper precautions (continuous fetal monitoring, avoidance of oxytocic stimulation of the uterus), epidural analgesia produced by dilute concentrations of local anesthetics may be utilized safely in parturients who have delivered previously by cesarean section.[33]

Amniotic Fluid Embolism

Amniotic fluid embolism is a rare catastrophic and life-threatening complication of pregnancy that occurs in the setting of a disrupted barrier between the amniotic fluid and maternal circulation.[34–36] The three most common sites for entry of amniotic fluid into the maternal circulation are the endocervical veins, the placenta, and a uterine trauma site. Multiparous parturients experiencing tumultuous labors are at increased risk for amniotic fluid embolism.

Signs and Symptoms

The onset of signs and symptoms of amniotic fluid embolism are dramatic and abrupt, classically manifesting as dyspnea, arterial hypoxemia, cyanosis, seizures, loss of consciousness, and hypotension disproportionate to the blood loss. Fetal distress is present at the same time. More than 80% of these parturients experience cardiopulmonary arrest.[36] Coagulopathy resembling disseminated intravascular coagulation with associated bleeding is common and may be the only presenting symptom.[36]

Pathophysiology

The principal defect created by amniotic fluid embolism is mechanical blockage of part of the pulmonary circulation and vasoconstriction of the remaining vessels perhaps through the release of undefined chemicals such as prostaglandins, leukotrienes, serotonin, or histamine (Fig. 31–8).[34] As a result, pulmonary artery pressures increase, arterial hypoxemia occurs owing to ventilation-to-perfusion mismatching, and hypotension reflects decreased cardiac output and congestive heart failure due to

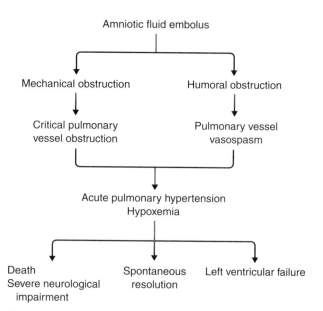

Figure 31–8 • Hemodynamic pathophysiology of amniotic fluid embolism. (From Davie S. Amniotic fluid embolus: a review of the literature. Can J Anesth 2001;48:88–98, with permission.)

right ventricular outflow obstruction and acute cor pulmonale.

Diagnosis

Diagnosis of amniotic fluid embolism is based on clinical signs and symptoms, increased pulmonary artery pressures and decreased cardiac output as determined by measurements from invasive monitors, and ultimately confirmation of amniotic fluid material in the parturient's blood aspirated from a central venous or pulmonary artery catheter.[37] Blood smears are examined in parturients suspected of experiencing an amniotic fluid embolism. The presence of fetal squamous cells, fat, and mucin in samples of the paturient's blood are indicative of amniotic fluid embolism. In this regard, it is not possible to differentiate between fetal and maternal squamous cells, and squamous cells have been identified in blood aspirated from pulmonary artery catheters in nonpregnant patients. The presence of mucin, however, seems to be a more sensitive indicator of amniotic fluid embolism.

Conditions that can mimic amniotic fluid embolism include inhalation of gastric contents, pulmonary embolism, venous air embolism, and local anesthetic toxicity. Pulmonary aspiration is more likely when bronchoconstriction accompanies the clinical signs and symptoms. Indeed, bronchospasm is rare in parturients who experience amniotic fluid embolism. Pulmonary embolism is usually accompanied by chest pain. High sensory levels produced by spinal or epidural anesthesia may be confused with amniotic fluid embolism (Table 31–7).[35]

Treatment

Treatment of amniotic fluid embolism includes tracheal intubation and mechanical ventilation of the parturient's lungs with 100% oxygen, inotropic support as guided by central venous or pulmonary artery catheter monitoring, and correction of coagulopathy.[36] Positive end-expiratory pressure is often helpful for improving oxygenation. Dopamine, dobutamine, and norepinephrine have been recommended as inotropes to treat acute left ventricular dysfunction and associated hypotension. Fluid therapy is guided by central venous pressure monitoring, keeping in mind that these patients are vulnerable to developing pulmonary edema. Treatment of disseminated intravascular coagulation may include administration of fresh frozen plasma, cryoprecipitate, and platelets. Even with immediate and

Table 31–7 • Differential Diagnosis of Amniotic Fluid Embolism

Signs and Symptoms	Amniotic Fluid Embolism	High Epidural Anesthesia	Total Spinal Anesthesia
Oxygenation	Arterial hypoxemia Not responsive to oxygen	Arterial hypoxemia Responsive to oxygen	Arterial hypoxemia Responsive to oxygen
Ventilation	Hypoventilation Respiratory distress Cough	Hypoventilation Respiratory distress Cannot cough	Hypoventilation Respiratory distress Cannot cough
Onset	Sudden onset Coincident with open uterine veins	Slow onset	Fast onset
Central nervous system	Loss of consciousness Agitation Seizures	Awake Some agitation No seizures	Loss of consciousness No movement No seizures
Cardiovascular system	Profound shock	Normal to decreased systemic blood pressure	Normal to decreased systemic blood pressure
	Difficult to resuscitate Cardiac arrest common	Easy to resuscitate Cardiac arrest uncommon	Easy to resuscitate Cardiac arrest uncommon
	Pulmonary hypertension	Normal pulmonary artery pressure	Normal pulmonary artery pressure
	Left and right heart failure Increased central venous pressure	Normal cardiac function Low central venous pressure	Normal cardiac function Low central venous pressure
Coagulation	Disseminated intravascular coagulation	Normal	Normal

Adapted from: Noble WH, St-Amand J. Amniotic fluid embolus. Can J Anaesth 1993;40:971–80.

aggressive treatment, mortality due to amniotic fluid embolism remains higher than 80%.[35]

■ FETAL DISTRESS

Causes

Fetal distress due to intrauterine hypoxia and acidosis is most likely to occur when uterine blood flow decreases with each uterine contraction. Indeed, a placenta with borderline function before the onset of labor may not be able to maintain fetal well-being when gas transfer across the placenta is further compromised by decreased uterine blood flow associated with vigorous contractions of the uterus.

Electronic Fetal Monitoring

Electronic fetal monitoring permits evaluation of fetal well-being by following changes in fetal heart rate, as recorded using an external monitor (Doppler) or fetal scalp electrode. The basic principle of electronic fetal monitoring is to correlate changes in fetal heart rate with fetal well-being and uterine contractions. For example, fetal well-being is evaluated by determining the beat-to-beat variability of the fetal heart rate, as computed from the RR intervals on the fetal electrocardiogram.[38] Another method is to evaluate the fetal heart rate decelerations associated with uterine contractions.[39] The three major fetal heart rate decelerations are classified as early, late, and variable. Fetal scalp sampling is indicated when an abnormal fetal heart rate pattern persists. It has been observed that the fetus is usually depressed when one or more fetal scalp pH values are near 7.0.

Beat-to-Beat Variability

The fetal heart rate varies 5 to 20 beats/min, with a normal heart rate ranging between 120 and 160 beats/min. This normal heart rate variability is thought to reflect the integrity of neural pathways from the fetal cerebral cortex through the medulla, vagus nerve, and cardiac conduction system. Fetal well-being is ensured when beat-to-beat variability is present. Conversely, fetal distress due to arterial hypoxemia, acidosis, or central nervous system damage is associated with minimal to absent beat-to-beat variability.

Drugs administered to parturients may blunt or eliminate fetal heart rate variability, even in the absence of fetal distress. Drugs most frequently associated with loss of beat-to-beat variability are benzodiazepines, opioids, barbiturates, anticholinergics, and local anesthetics, as used for continuous lumbar epidural analgesia. These drug-induced effects do not appear to be deleterious but may cause difficulty when interpretating the fetal heart rate monitoring results. In addition, the absence of heart rate variability may be normally present in the premature fetus and during fetal sleep cycles.

Early Decelerations

Early decelerations are characterized by the slowing of the fetal heart rate that begins with the onset of uterine contractions (Fig. 31–9). Slowing is maximum at the peak of the contraction, returning to near baseline at its termination. Decreases in heart rate are usually not more than 20 beats/min or below an absolute rate of 100 beats/min. This deceleration pattern is thought to be caused by vagal stimulation secondary to compression of the fetal head. Early decelerations are not prevented by increasing the fetal oxygenation but are blunted by the administration of atropine. Most important, this fetal heart rate pattern is not associated with fetal distress.

Late Decelerations

Late decelerations are characterized by the slowing of the fetal heart rate that begins 10 to 30 seconds after the onset of uterine contractions. Maximum slowing occurs after the peak intensity of the contractions (Fig. 31–10). A mild late deceleration is classified as a decrease in heart rate of less than 20 beats/min; profound slowing is present when the decrease is more than 40 beats/min. Late decelerations are associated with fetal distress, most likely reflecting myocardial hypoxia secondary to uteroplacental insufficiency. Primary factors contributing to the appearance of late decelerations include maternal hypotension, uterine hyperactivity, and chronic uteroplacental insufficiency, such as may be seen with diabetes mellitus or hypertension. When this pattern persists, there is a predictable correlation with the development of fetal acidosis.[39] Late decelerations can be corrected by improving fetal oxygenation. When beat-to-beat variability persists despite late decelerations, the fetus is still likely to be born vigorous.

Variable Decelerations

Variable decelerations are the most common pattern of fetal heart changes observed during the intrapartum period. As the term indicates, these decelerations are variable in magnitude, duration, and time

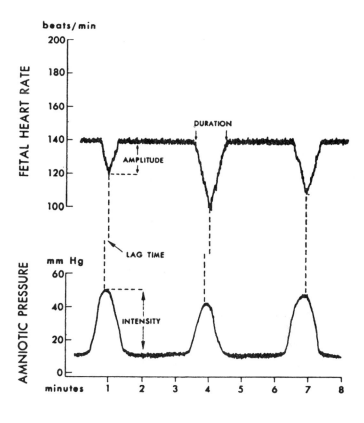

Figure 31-9 • Early decelerations of the fetal heart rate are characterized by a short lag time between the onset of uterine contractions and the beginning of fetal heart rate slowing. Maximum heart rate slowing is usually less than 20 beats/min and occurs at the peak intensity of the contraction. Heart rate returns to normal by the time the contraction has ceased. The most likely explanation for this early deceleration is a vagal reflex response to compression of the fetal head. (From Shnider SM. Diagnosis of fetal distress: fetal heart rate. In: Shnider SM, editor. Obstetrical Anesthesia: Current Concepts and Practice. Baltimore, Williams & Wilkins 1970;197–203, with permission.)

of onset relative to uterine contractions (Fig. 31–11). For example, this pattern may begin before, with, or after the onset of uterine contractions. Characteristically, deceleration patterns are abrupt in onset and cessation. The fetal heart rate almost invariably falls below 100 beats/min. Variable decelerations are thought to be caused by umbilical cord compression. Atropine diminishes the severity of variable decelerations, but administration of oxygen to the mother is without effect. If deceleration patterns are not severe and repetitive, there are usually only minimal alterations in the fetal acid-base status. Severe variable deceleration patterns that persist for 15 to 30 minutes are associated with fetal acidosis.

■ EVALUATION OF THE NEONATE

The importance of assessment immediately after birth is that depressed neonates who require active resuscitation are identified promptly. As a guide to identifying and treating depressed neonates, the Apgar score has not been surpassed.[40]

The Apgar score assigns a numerical value to five vital signs measured or observed in neonates 1 minute and 5 minutes after delivery (Table 31–8). Of the five criteria, the heart rate and the quality of the respiratory effort are the most important factors; color is the least informative for identifying distressed neonates. A heart rate of less than 100 beats/min generally signifies arterial hypoxemia. Disappearance of cyanosis is often rapid when ventilation and circulation are normal. Nevertheless, many healthy neonates still have cyanosis at 1 minute owing to peripheral vasoconstriction in response to cold ambient temperatures in the delivery room. Acidosis and pulmonary vasoconstriction are the most likely causes of persistent cyanosis.

Apgar scores correlate well with acid-base measurements performed immediately after birth. When scores are above 7, neonates are either normal or have mild respiratory acidosis. Infants with scores of 4 to 6 are moderately depressed; those with scores of 3 or below have combined metabolic and respiratory acidosis. Mildly to moderately depressed infants (Apgar scores 3 to 7) frequently improve in response to oxygen administered by face mask, with or without positive-pressure ventilation of the lungs. Tracheal intubation and perhaps external cardiac massage are indicated when Apgar scores are less than 3. Apgar scores are not sufficiently sensitive to detect drug-related changes reli-

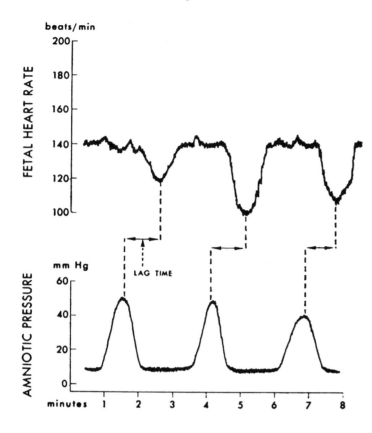

Figure 31–10 • Late decelerations of the fetal heart rate are characterized by a delay (lag time) between the onset of the uterine contraction and the beginning of fetal heart rate slowing. The fetal heart rate does not return to normal until after the contraction has ceased. A mild late deceleration pattern is present when slowing is less than 20 beats/min; profound slowing is present when the fetal heart rate slows more than 40 beats/min. Late fetal heart rate decelerations indicate fetal distress owing to uteroplacental insufficiency. (From Shnider SM. Diagnosis of fetal distress: fetal heart rate. In: Shnider SM, editor. Obstetrical Anesthesia: Current Concepts and Practice. Baltimore, Williams & Wilkins 1970;197–203, with permission.)

ably or to provide data necessary to evaluate the subtle effects of obstetric anesthetic techniques on neonates.

■ IMMEDIATE NEONATAL PERIOD

Major changes in the neonatal cardiovascular system and respiratory system must occur immediately after delivery. For example, with clamping of the umbilical cord at birth, systemic vascular resistance increases, left atrial pressure increases, and flow through the foramen ovale ceases. Expansion of the lungs decreases pulmonary vascular resistance, and the entire right ventricular output is diverted to the lungs. In normal newborns, increases in PaO_2 to above 60 mmHg causes vasoconstriction and functional closure of the ductus arteriosus. When adequate oxygenation and ventilation are not established after delivery, a fetal circulation pattern persists characterized by increased pulmonary vascular resistance and decreased pulmonary blood flow. Furthermore, the ductus arteriosus and foramen ovale remain open, resulting in large right-to-left intracardiac shunts with associated arterial hypoxemia and acidosis.

A high index of suspicion must be maintained for serious abnormalities, which can be present at birth or manifest shortly after delivery. They include meconium aspiration, choanal stenosis and atresia, diaphragmatic hernia, hypovolemia, hypoglycemia, tracheoesophageal fistula, laryngeal anomalies, and Pierre Robin syndrome (see Chapter 32).

Meconium Aspiration

Meconium is the breakdown product of swallowed amniotic fluid, gastrointestinal cells, and secretions. It is seldom present before 34 weeks of gestation. After about 34 weeks, intrauterine arterial hypoxemia can result in increased gut motility and defecation. Gasping associated with arterial hypoxemia causes the fetus to inhale amniotic fluid and debris into the lungs. If delivery is delayed, meconium is broken down and excreted from the lungs. If birth occurs within 24 hours after aspiration, the meconium is still present in the major airways and is distributed to the lung periphery with the onset of spontaneous breathing. Obstruction of small airways causes ventilation-to-perfusion mismatching. The breathing rate may be more than 100 breaths/min, and lung compliance decreases to levels seen in infants with respiratory distress syndrome. In severe cases, pulmonary hypertension and right-to-left shunting through the patent foramen ovale and

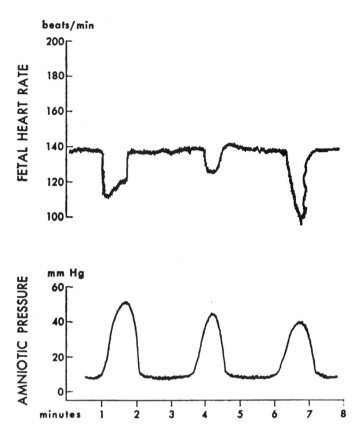

Figure 31-11 • Variable decelerations of the fetal heart rate are characterized by decreases in the heart rate of varying magnitude and duration that do not show a consistent relation to uterine contractions. This pattern of fetal heart rate slowing is associated with umbilical cord compression. (From Shnider SM. Diagnosis of fetal distress: fetal heart rate. In: Shnider SM, editor. Obstetrical Anesthesia: Current Concepts and Practice. Baltimore, Williams & Wilkins, 1970:197–203, with permission.)

ductus arteriosus (persistent fetal circulation) lead to severe arterial hypoxemia. Pneumothorax is also a common problem in the presence of meconium aspiration.

In the past, treatment of meconium aspiration consisted of placing a tracheal tube immediately after delivery and attempting to suction meconium from the newborn's airways. Currently, a more conservative approach is recommended because routine tracheal intubation of all infants with meconium staining (approximately 10% of all newborns) may cause unnecessary airway complications. Routine oropharyngeal suctioning is recommended at the time of delivery, but tracheal intubation and suctioning is performed selectively, depending on the infant's condition (those with Apgar scores above 7 are managed conservatively). Infants with low Apgar scores or who are clinically obstructed with meconium require active resuscitation, including tracheal intubation and attempts to remove meconium via suctioning.

Choanal Stenosis and Atresia

Nasal obstruction should be suspected in neonates who have good breathing efforts but in whom air entry is absent. Cyanosis develops if these infants are forced to breathe with their mouths closed. Unilateral or bilateral choanal stenosis is diagnosed

Table 31-8 • Evaluation of Neonates Using the Apgar Score

Parameter	0	1	2
Heart rate (beats/min)	Absent	< 100	> 100
Respiratory effort	Absent	Slow Irregular	Crying
Reflex irritability	No response	Grimace	Crying
Muscle tone	Limp	Flexion of extremities	Active
Color	Pale Cyanotic	Body pink Extremities cyanotic	Pink

based on the failure to pass a small catheter through each naris; such failure may reflect congenital (anatomic) obstruction or more commonly functional atresia due to blood, mucus, or meconium. The congenital form of choanal atresia must be treated surgically during the neonatal period. An oral airway may be necessary until surgical correction can be accomplished. Functional choanal atresia is treated by nasal suctioning. Opioids such as heroin often cause congestion of the nasal mucosa and obstruction. Such congestion can be treated with phenylephrine nosedrops.

Diaphragmatic Hernia

Severe respiratory distress at birth, associated with cyanosis and a scaphoid abdomen, suggests a diaphragmatic hernia (see Chapter 32). Chest radiographs demonstrate abdominal contents in the thorax. Initial treatment in the delivery room includes tracheal intubation and ventilation of the lungs with oxygen. A pneumothorax on the side opposite the hernia is likely if attempts are made to expand the ipsilateral lung.

Hypovolemia

Newborns with mean arterial pressures below 50 mmHg at birth are likely to be hypovolemic. Poor capillary refill, tachycardia, and tachypnea are present. Hypovolemia frequently follows intrauterine fetal distress, during which larger than normal portions of fetal blood are shunted to the placenta and remain there after delivery and clamping of the umbilical cord. Umbilical cord compression is also frequently associated with hypovolemia.

Hypoglycemia

Hypoglycemia can manifest as hypotension, tremors, and seizures. Infants with intrauterine growth retardation and those born to diabetic mothers or after severe intrauterine fetal distress are vulnerable to hypoglycemia.

Tracheoesophagal Fistula

Tracheoesophagal fistula should be suspected when polyhydramnios is present (see Chapter 32). An initial diagnosis in the delivery room is suggested when a catheter is inserted into the esophagus but cannot be passed into the stomach. Copious amounts of oropharyngeal secretions are usually present. Chest radiographs with the catheter in place confirm the diagnosis.

Laryngeal Anomalies

Stridor is present at birth as a manifestation of laryngeal anomalies and subglottic stenosis. Insertion of a tube into the trachea beyond the obstruction alleviates the symptoms. Vascular rings are anomalies of the aorta that may compress the trachea, producing both inspiratory and expiratory obstruction (see Chapter 3). It may be difficult to advance a tracheal tube beyond the obstruction produced by vascular rings.

Pierre Robin Syndrome

Pierre Robin syndrome is characterized by glossoptosis and micrognathia in all patients and the presence of cleft palate in more than one-half of patients. Respiratory obstruction occurs when the tongue is sucked against the posterior pharyngeal wall by negative intrapharyngeal pressures. Initial treatment in the delivery room consists of establishing a patent upper airway by inserting an oral airway or by pulling the tongue forward with a clamp. The prone position also helps displace the tongue away from the posterior pharyngeal wall. A small tube passed through the naris into the posterior pharynx may be required to vent negative intraoral pressures. Under no circumstances should these infants be given muscle relaxants in attempts to perform tracheal intubation, as skeletal muscle paralysis may make ventilation of the lungs impossible.

References

1. Jacobs JS, Vallejo R, DeSouza GJ, et al. Severe hypoglycemia after labor epidural analgesia. Anesth Analg 2000;90:892–3
2. Santos AC, Pededrsen H. Current controversies in obstetric anesthesia. Anesth Analg 1994;78:753–60
3. Birnbach DJ, Chestnut DH. The epidural test dose in obstetric patients: has it outlived its usefulness? Anesth Analg 1999;88:971–2
4. Eisenach JC. Combined spinal-epidural analgesia in obstetrics. Anesthesiology 1999;91:299–302
5. Mushambi MC, Halligan AW, Williamson K. Recent developments in the pathophysiology and management of preeclampsia. Br J Anaesth 1996;76:133–48
6. Cunningham FG, Lindheimer MD. Hypertension in pregnancy. N Engl J Med 1992;326:927–32
7. Patterson KW, O'Toole DP. HELLP syndrome: a case report with guidelines for diagnosis and management. Br J Anaesth 1991;66:513–5
8. Wright JP. Anesthetic considerations in preeclampsia-eclampsia. Anesth Analg 1983;63:590–6

9. Koren G, Pastuszak A, Ito S. Drugs in pregnancy. N Engl J Med 1998;338:1128–37

10. Kambam JRF, Mouton S, Entman S, et al. Effect of preeclampsia on plasma cholinesterase activity. Can J Anaesth 1987;34:509–11

11. Ravindran RS, Carelli A. Neurologic dysfunction of postpartum patients caused by hypomagnesemia. Anesthesiology 1987;66:391–2

12. Sharma SK, Philip J, Whitten CW, et al. Assessment of changes in coagulation in parturients with preeclampsia using thromboelastography. Anesthesiology 1999;90:385–90

13. Heller PJ, Goodman C. Use of local anesthetics with epinephrine for epidural anesthesia in preeclampsia. Anesthesiology 1986;65:224–6

14. Hood DD, Curry R. Spinal versus epidural anesthesia for cesarean section in severely preeclamptic patients. Anesthesiology 1999;90:1276–82

15. Spinnato JA, Kraynack BJ, Cooper MW. Eisenmenger's syndrome in pregnancy: epidural anesthesia for elective cesarean section. N Engl J Med 1981;304:1215–6

16. Pollack KL, Chestnut DH, Wenstrom KD. Anesthetic management of a parturient with Eisenmenger's syndrome. Anesth Analg 1990;70:212–5

17. Robinson S. Pulmonary artery catheters in Eisenmenger's syndrome: many risks, few benefits. Anesthesiology 1983;58:588–9

18. Slomka F, Salmeron S, Zetlaoui P, et al. Primary pulmonary hypertension and pregnancy: anesthetic management for delivery. Anesthesiology 1988;69:959–61

19. Breen TW, Tanzen JA. Pulmonary hypertension and cardiomyopathy: anaesthetic management for caesarean section. Can J Anaesth 1991;38:895–9

20. Weeks SK, Smith JB. Obstetric anaesthesia in patients with primary pulmonary hypertension. Can J Anaesth 1991;38:814–6

21. Langer O, Conway DL, Berkus MD, et al. A comparison of glyburide and insulin in women with gestational diabetes mellitus. N Engl J Med 2000;343:1134–8

22. Datta S, Brown WU, Ostheimer GW, et al. Epidural anesthesia for cesarean section in diabetic parturients: maternal and neonatal acid-base status and bupivacaine concentration. Anesth Analg 1981;60:574–8

23. Datta S, Brown WU. Acid-base status in diabetic mothers and their infants following general or spinal anesthesia for cesarean section. Anesthesiology 1977;47:272–6

24. Rolbin SH, Levinson G, Shnider SM, et al. Anesthetic considerations for myasthenia gravis and pregnancy. Anesth Analg 1978;57:441–7

25. Kain ZN, Rimar S, Barash PG. Cocaine abuse in the parturient and effects on the fetus and neonate. Anesth Analg 1993;77:835–45

26. Livingston JC, Mabie BC, Ramanthan J. Crack cocaine, myocardial infarction, and troponin I levels at the time of cesarean delivery. Anesth Analg 2000;91:913–5

27. Rosen MA. Management of anesthesia for the pregnant surgical patient. Anesthesiology 1999;91:1159–63

28. Aouad MT, Siddik SS, Jalbout MI, et al. Does pregnancy protect against intrathecal lidocaine-induced transient neurologic symptoms? Anesth Analg 2001;92:401–4

29. Ravindran R, Viegas OJ, Padilla LM, et al. Anesthetic considerations in pregnant patients receiving terbutaline therapy. Anesth Analg 1980;59:402–3

30. Sato K, Nishiwaki K, Kuno N, et al. Unexpected hyperkalemia following succinylcholine administration in prolonged immobilized parturients treated with magnesium and ritodrine. Anesthesiology 2000;93:1539–41

31. Rosen MA, Roizen MF, Eger EI, et al. The effect of nitrous oxide on in vitro fertilization success rate. Anesthesiology 1987;67:42–4

32. Smith CE, Weeks SK. Anesthesia for cesarean section in a patient with Asherman's syndrome. Anesthesiology 1988;68:615–8

33. Carlsson C, Nybell-Lincahl G, Ingemarsson I. Extradural block in patients who had previously undergone cesarean section. Br J Anaesth 1980;52:827–30

34. Davies S. Amniotic fluid embolus: a review of the literature. Can J Anesth 2001;48:88–98

35. Noble WH, St-Amand J. Amniotic fluid embolus. Can J Anaesth 1993;40:971–80

36. Bastien JL, Graves JR, Bailey S. Atypical presentation of amniotic fluid embolism. Anesth Analg 1998;87:124–6

37. Schaerf RHM, deCampo T, Civetta JA. Hemodynamic alterations and rapid diagnosis in a case of amniotic fluid embolus. Anesthesiology 1977;46:155–7

38. Finster M, Petrie RH. Monitoring of the fetus. Anesthesiology 1976;45:198–215

39. Paul RH, Suidan AK, Yeh SY, et al. Clinical fetal monitoring. VII. The evaluation and significance of intrapartum baseline FHR variability. Am J Obstet Gynecol 1975;123:206–10

40. Casey BM, McIntire DD, Leveno KJ. The continuing value of the Apgar score for the assessment of newborn infants. N Engl J Med 2001;344:467–71

32

Diseases Presenting in Pediatric Patients

Pediatric patients present unique anatomic, physiologic, and pharmacologic considerations for the management of anesthesia in the presence of diseases that occur exclusively or with increased frequency in this age group. Neonates (up to 28 days of age) and infants (1 to 6 months) comprise the age groups in which differences from adults are most marked. Neonates are more likely to experience adverse perioperative cardiopulmonary events.[1]

UNIQUE CONSIDERATIONS IN PEDIATRIC PATIENTS

Pediatric patients deserve special consideration with respect to anatomic, physiologic, and pharmacologic differences from adults.

Airway Anatomy

The large head and tongue, mobile epiglottis, and anterior position of the larynx characteristic of neonates makes tracheal intubation easier with the neonate's head in a neutral or slightly flexed position than with the head hyperextended. Because the infant's larynx is higher in the neck than in adults, the infant's tongue obstructs the airway more easily. The cricoid cartilage is the narrowest portion of the larynx in pediatric patients and necessitates the use of tracheal tubes that minimize risks of trauma to the airway and subsequent development of subglottic edema. As in adults, angulation of the right main stem bronchus favors right endobronchial intubation if the tracheal tube is inserted beyond the carina.

Physiology

Physiologic differences between children and adults are important determinants when planning management of anesthesia in pediatric patients. Monitoring vital signs and organ function during the perioperative period is especially important, as neonates and infants have decreased physiologic reserves.

Respiratory System

The single most important difference that physiologically distinguishes pediatric patients from adult patients is oxygen consumption. Oxygen consumption of neonates is more than 6 ml/kg, which is about twice that of adults on a weight basis (Table 32–1). To satisfy this high demand, alveolar ventilation is doubled compared with that in adults. Because the tidal volume on a weight basis is similar for infants and adults, the increased alveolar ventilation is accomplished by an increased breathing rate. PaO_2 increases rapidly after birth, but several days are needed to achieve the levels present in older children.

Cardiovascular System

Birth and the initiation of spontaneous ventilation initiate circulatory changes, permitting neonates to survive in an extrauterine environment.[2] Fetal circulation is characterized by high pulmonary vascular resistance, low systemic vascular resistance (placenta), and right-to-left shunting of blood through the foramen ovale and ductus arteriosus. The onset of spontaneous ventilation at birth is associated with decreased pulmonary vascular resistance and increased pulmonary blood flow. As the left atrial pressure increases, the foramen ovale functionally closes. Anatomic closure of the foramen ovale occurs between 3 months and 1 year of age, although 20%

to 30% of adults have probe-patent foramen ovales.[3] Functional closure of the ductus arteriosus normally occurs 10 to 15 hours after birth, with anatomic closure taking place in 4 to 6 weeks. Constriction of the ductus arteriosus occurs in response to increased arterial oxygenation that develops after birth. Nevertheless, the ductus arteriosus may reopen during periods of arterial hypoxemia. In addition, certain conditions, such as diaphragmatic hernia, meconium aspiration, pulmonary infections, and polycythemia, are associated with high pulmonary vascular resistance and persistence of fetal circulatory patterns. A diagnosis of persistent fetal circulation can be confirmed by measuring the PaO_2 in blood samples obtained simultaneously from preductal (right radial) and postductal (umbilical, posterior tibial, dorsalis pedis) arteries. The presence of PaO_2 differences of more than 20 mmHg in these simultaneously obtained blood samples confirms the diagnosis.

Neonates are highly dependent on heart rate to maintain cardiac output and systemic blood pressure. Vasoconstrictive responses to hemorrhage are less in neonates than in adults. For example, a 10% decrease in intravascular fluid volume is likely to cause a 15% to 30% decrease in mean arterial pressure in neonates. The hypotension that accompanies administration of volatile anesthetics to premature neonates is most likely due to decreased intravascular fluid volume and/or anesthetic overdose.

Distribution of Body Water

Total body water content and extracellular fluid (ECF) volume are increased proportionately in neonates. The ECF volume is equivalent to about 40% of body weight in neonates compared with about 20% in adults. By 18 to 24 months of age, the proportion of ECF volume relative to body weight is similar to that in adults. The increased metabolic rate characteristic of neonates results in accelerated turn-

Table 32–1 • Mean Pulmonary Function Values

Parameter	Neonates (3 kg)	Adults (70 kg)
Oxygen consumption (ml/kg/min)	6.4	3.5
Alveolar ventilation (ml/kg/min)	130	60
Carbon dioxide production (ml/kg/min)	6	3
Tidal volume (ml/kg)	6	6
Breathing frequency (min)	35	15
Vital capacity (ml/kg)	35	70
Functional residual capacity (ml/kg)	30	35
Tracheal length (cm)	5.5	12
PaO_2 (room air, mmHg)	65–85	85–95
$PaCO_2$ (room air, mmHg)	30–36	36–44
pH	7.34–7.40	7.36–7.44

Table 32–2 • Intraoperative Fluid Therapy for Pediatric Patients

Procedure	5% Glucose in Lactated Ringer's Solution (ml/kg/hr)		
	Maintenance	Replacement	Total
Minor surgery (herniorrhaphy)	4	2	6
Moderate surgery (pyloromyotomy)	4	4	8
Extensive surgery (bowel resection)	4	6	10

overs of ECF and dictates meticulous attention to intraoperative fluid replacement. Intraoperative fluid replacement often includes glucose, although the clinical impression that pediatric patients are more susceptible than adults to hypoglycemia during fasting periods has been challenged (Table 32–2).[4,5]

Renal Function

The glomerular filtration rate is greatly decreased in term neonates but increases nearly fourfold by 3 to 5 weeks. Preterm neonates may show delayed increases in the glomerular filtration rate. Neonates are obligate sodium losers and cannot concentrate urine as effectively as adults. Therefore, adequate exogenous sodium and water must be provided during the perioperative period. Conversely, neonates are likely to excrete volume loads more slowly than adults and are therefore more susceptible to fluid overload. Decreased renal function can also delay excretion of drugs dependent on renal clearance for elimination.

Hematology

Characteristics of fetal hemoglobin (HbF) influence oxygen transport. For example, HbF has a P_{50} of 19 mmHg compared with 26 mmHg for adults, which results in a leftward shift of the fetal oxyhemoglobin dissociation curve. Subsequent increased affinity of hemoglobin for oxygen manifests as decreased oxy-

gen release to peripheral tissues. This decreased release is offset by increased oxygen delivery provided by the increased hemoglobin concentrations characteristic of neonates (Table 32–3). By 2 to 3 months of age, however, physiologic anemia results. After 3 months there are progressive increases in erythrocyte mass and hematocrit. By 4 to 6 months, the oxyhemoglobin dissociation curve approximates that of adults. In view of the decreased cardiovascular reserve of neonates and the leftward shift of the oxyhemoglobin dissociation curve, it may be useful to maintain the neonate's hematocrit closer to 40% than 30%, as is often accepted for older children. Calculation of the estimated erythrocyte mass and the acceptable erythrocyte loss provides a useful guide for intraoperative blood replacement (Table 32–4).[6]

The need for routine preoperative hemoglobin determinations is controversial.[7] Routine preoperative hemoglobin determinations in children less than 1 year of age results in the detection of only a small number of patients with hemoglobin concentrations below 10 g/dl, and this rarely influences management of anesthesia or delays planned surgery. Because of the potential benefit of identifying anemia during infancy, preoperative hemoglobin testing may be justifiable only in this age group.

Thermoregulation

Neonates and infants are vulnerable to the development of hypothermia during the perioperative pe-

Table 32–3 • Normal Hemogram Values in Neonates, Infants, and Children

Age	Hemoglobin (g/dl)	Hematocrit (%)	Leukocytes (cells/mm³)
1 Day	19.0	61	18,000
2 Weeks	17.3	54	12,000
1 Month	14.2	43	
2 Months	10.7	31	
6 Months	12.3	36	10,000
1 Year	11.6	35	
6 Years	12.7	38	
10–12 Years	13.0	39	8,000

Table 32–4 • Estimation of Acceptable Blood Loss*

A 3.2 kg term neonate is scheduled for intra-abdominal surgery. The preoperative hematocrit is 50%. What is the acceptable intraoperative blood loss to maintain the hematocrit at 40%?

Parameter	Calculation
Estimated blood volume	85 ml/kg × 3.2 kg = 272 ml
Estimated erythrocyte mass	272 ml × 0.5 = 136 ml
Estimated erythrocyte mass to maintain hematocrit at 40%	272 ml × 0.4 = 109 ml
Acceptable intraoperative erythrocyte loss	136 ml − 109 ml = 27 ml
Acceptable intraoperative blood loss to maintain hematocrit at 40%	27 × 2[†] = 54 ml

* These calculations are only guidelines and do not consider the potential impact of intravenous infusion of crystalloid or colloid solutions on the hematocrit.
[†] Factor to correct the original hematocrit to 50%.

riod. Body heat is lost more rapidly in this age group than in older children or adults because of the large body surface area relative to body weight, the thin layer of insulating subcutaneous fat, and a decreased ability to produce heat. Shivering is of little significance during heat production in neonates, whose primary mechanism is nonshivering thermogenesis mediated by brown fat. Brown fat is a specialized adipose tissue located in the neonate's posterior neck, in the interscapular and vertebral areas, and surrounding the kidneys and adrenal glands. Metabolism of brown fat is stimulated by norepinephrine and results in triglyceride hydrolysis and thermogenesis. An important mechanism for loss of body heat in operating rooms is radiation. Steps designed to decrease loss of body heat include transporting neonates in heated modules, increasing the ambient temperature of operating rooms, and humidifying and warming inspired gases.

Pharmacology

Pharmacologic responses to drugs may differ in pediatric patients and adults. They manifest as differences in anesthetic requirements, responses to muscle relaxants, and pharmacokinetics.

Anesthetic Requirements

Full-term neonates require lower concentrations of volatile anesthetics than do infants 1 to 6 months of age. For example, the minimal alveolar concentration (MAC) is about 25% less in neonates than in infants.[8] Furthermore, MAC in preterm neonates less than 32 weeks' gestational age is less than MAC in preterm neonates 32 to 37 weeks' gestational age, and MAC for both of these age groups is less than that in full-term neonates (Fig. 32–1).[9] Decreased anesthetic requirements in neonates may be related to immaturity of the central nervous system and to increased circulating concentrations of progesterone and β-endorphins. MAC steadily increases until 2 to 3 months of age; but after 3 months the MAC steadily declines with aging, although there are slight increases at puberty.

Muscle Relaxants

Morphologic and functional maturation of the neuromuscular junctions are not complete until about 2 months of age, but the implications of this initial immaturity on the pharmacodynamics of muscle relaxants are not clear.[10] Infants may be more sensitive to the effects of nondepolarizing muscle relaxants, but the relatively large volume of distribution results in initial doses that are similar to those for adults.[11] Immaturity of hepatic or renal function could prolong the duration of action of muscle relaxants that are highly dependent on these mechanisms for their clearance. Antagonism of neuromuscular blockade seems to be reliable and in infants may

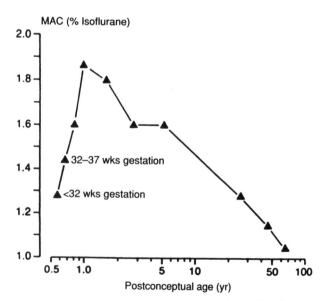

Figure 32–1 • Anesthetic requirements (minimum alveolar concentration, MAC) of isoflurane and postconceptual age. (From LeDez KM, Lerman J. The minimum alveolar concentration (MAC) of isoflurane in preterm neonates. Anesthesiology 1987;67: 301–7, with permission.)

be associated with decreased dose requirements for anticholinesterase drugs.[12]

Neonates and infants require more succinylcholine on a body weight basis than do older children to produce comparable degrees of neuromuscular blockade.[13] Presumably this response reflects increased ECF volumes characteristic of this age group, resulting in larger volumes of distribution of succinylcholine. The incidence of adverse side effects of succinylcholine (myoglobinuria, malignant hyperthermia) limits the administration of this drug to children.

Pharmacokinetics

Pharmacokinetics differ in neonates and infants compared with adults. For example, uptake of inhaled anesthetics is more rapid in infants than in older children or adults.[14] This accelerated uptake most likely reflects the infant's high alveolar ventilation relative to functional residual capacity. More rapid uptake may unmask negative inotropic effects of volatile anesthetics resulting in an increased incidence of hypotension in neonates and infants during administration of volatile anesthetics.[15, 16] Considering these factors, a decreased margin of safety when volatile anesthetics are administered to infants is predictable.

An immature blood–brain barrier and decreased ability to metabolize drugs could increase the sensitivity of neonates to the effects of barbiturates and opioids. As a result, neonates might require lower doses of barbiturates for induction of anesthesia. Nevertheless, children between the ages of 5 and 15 years require somewhat higher doses of thiopental and methohexital than do adults for induction of anesthesia.[17, 18] Decreased hepatic and renal clearance of drugs, which is characteristic of neonates, can produce prolonged drug effects. Clearance rates increase to adult levels by 5 to 6 months of age and during early childhood may even exceed adult rates. Protein binding of many drugs is decreased in infants, which could result in high circulating concentrations of unbound and pharmacologically active drugs.

Monitoring

Decreased cardiovascular reserve, altered anesthetic requirements, and exaggerated hypotensive responses during general anesthesia make monitoring the systemic blood pressure especially important in neonates and infants during the perioperative period. Oscillometric methods for noninvasive mea-surement of systemic blood pressure are reliable for pediatric patients. Selecting the proper cuff size is critical, as a cuff that is too large for the patient's arm results in falsely low readings. A catheter placed in a peripheral artery may be the method selected to monitor systemic blood pressure and to obtain blood samples for analysis of blood gases and pH. The peripheral artery selected in neonates is uniquely important, as blood sampled from an artery that arises distal to the ductus arteriosus (left radial artery, umbilical artery, posterior tibial artery) may not accurately reflect the PaO_2 being delivered to the retina or brain in the presence of a patent ductus arteriosus (Fig. 32–2). If retinopathy of the newborn is a consideration, a preductal artery, such as the right radial artery or temporal artery (risk of cerebral embolism with retrograde flushing) should be cannulated.

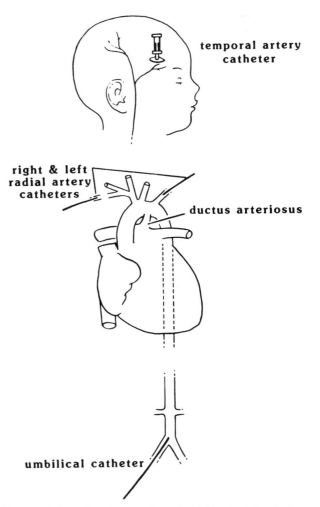

Figure 32–2 • Sites for sampling arterial blood relative to the ductus arteriosus.

Monitoring body temperature is useful during the perioperative period to detect the development of hypothermia as well as the rare patient manifesting malignant hyperthermia. Hypothermia, as is likely to occur in neonates or infants during anesthesia, results in increased total body oxygen consumption, depression of ventilation, bradycardia, metabolic acidosis, and hypoglycemia. Monitoring end-tidal carbon dioxide concentrations is reliable in children, although there are some limitations in neonates and infants. For example, because of small tidal volumes and high inspired gas flows, exhaled carbon dioxide concentrations may be diluted, producing falsely low values when measuring end-tidal carbon dioxide concentrations.

■ NEONATAL MEDICAL DISEASES

Technologic and medical advances have resulted in improved survival of low-birth-weight preterm neonates. Perioperative care of preterm and term neonates is based on knowledge of the disorders common or unique to this age group (Table 32–5).

Respiratory Distress Syndrome

Respiratory distress syndrome (RDS), or hyaline membrane disease, is responsible for 50% to 75% of deaths that occur in preterm neonates. This syndrome is caused by deficiencies in alveoli of surface-active phospholipids known as surfactant. The function of surfactant is to maintain alveolar stability. Without surfactant alveoli collapse, leading to right-to-left shunting, arterial hypoxemia, and metabolic acidosis. Surfactant is produced by type II pneumocytes. Before 26 weeks' gestation, however, there are not enough type II pneumocytes to produce an adequate amount of surfactant, although by 35 weeks there are large numbers of type II cells capable of sufficient surfactant synthesis. Until adequate surfactant can be produced, arterial oxygenation

---

Table 32–5 • Neonatal Medical Diseases

Respiratory distress syndrome
Bronchopulmonary dysplasia
Intracranial hemorrhage
Retinopathy of prematurity
Apnea spells
Sudden infant death syndrome
Kernicterus
Hypoglycemia
Hypocalcemia
Sepsis

---

must be maintained using supplemental oxygen, with or without mechanical ventilation of the lungs. Under certain circumstances, antenatal corticosteroids administered to the mother may accelerate maturation of the fetal lungs and prevent the development of RDS in preterm infants. Tracheal administration of human surfactant to preterm infants may be helpful.

During anesthesia in the presence of RDS, the PaO_2 is maintained near its preoperative levels. In this regard, volatile anesthetics can alter arterial oxygenation by decreasing cardiac output. Ideally, the PaO_2 is monitored from blood obtained from a catheter placed in a preductal artery (Fig. 32–2). For brief surgical procedures or when arterial cannulation is not feasible, monitoring oxygenation using pulse oximetry is satisfactory. The degree of pulmonary dysfunction in neonates with RDS is highly variable. The least afflicted neonates may require only supplemental oxygen for short periods of time. Severely afflicted neonates may require mechanical ventilation with high inspired oxygen concentrations and positive end-expiratory pressure. Pneumothorax is an ever-present danger and should be considered if oxygenation deteriorates abruptly in neonates being treated for RDS. An alternative to mechanical ventilation of the neonate's lungs is high-frequency ventilation. Hypotension is a frequently encountered problem during anesthesia. Administration of albumin, 1 g/kg IV, to preterm neonates with RDS is likely to increase the blood volume and glomerular filtration rate. The neonate's hematocrit is often maintained near 40% to optimize oxygen delivery to tissues. Fluid administration must be monitored because excess hydration may reopen the ductus arteriosus.

Bronchopulmonary Dysplasia

Bronchopulmonary dysplasia is a chronic pulmonary disorder that usually afflicts children with a history of RDS. Although the precise mechanism is unknown, certain risk factors have been identified. For example, increased inspired oxygen concentrations and positive-pressure ventilation of the lungs, as used for the treatment of RDS, may be etiologic factors. Indeed, a substantial percentage of neonates with RDS requiring supplemental oxygen for more than 24 hours show development of bronchopulmonary dysplasia.

Bronchopulmonary dysplasia is characterized by increased airway reactivity and resistance, decreased pulmonary compliance, ventilation-to-perfusion mismatch, decreased arterial oxygenation, and tachypnea.[19] Oxygen consumption is increased by as much as 25%. It should be assumed that children with a history of RDS requiring supplemental oxygen and mechanical ventilation of the lungs probably have some degree of residual pulmonary disease. The clinical consequences of this dysfunction are unknown; but the prognosis for children surviving the first year of life is good.

The choice of drugs for anesthesia in patients with bronchopulmonary dysplasia is not as important as management of the airway. For example, management of anesthesia in these children includes tracheal intubation, delivery of increased inspired concentrations of oxygen, and mechanical ventilation of the lungs. The possible presence of airway hyperreactivity suggests the need to establish a surgical level of anesthesia before instrumentation of the airway is initiated. Although these children may appear clinically well, pulmonary compliance is usually decreased. It should be appreciated, however, that pulmonary dysfunction in these patients is most marked during the first year of life.

Intracranial Hemorrhage

The four types of intracranial hemorrhage that occur during the neonatal period are subdural, primary subarachnoid, periventricular-intraventricular, and intercellular. The most frequent and important type is periventricular-intraventricular hemorrhage.

Periventricular-Intraventricular Hemorrhage

The incidence of periventricular-intraventricular hemorrhage is 40% to 45% in neonates less than 35 weeks' gestational age. Newborn prematurity is the single most important risk factor for intracranial hemorrhage. Severe respiratory complications and infections are associated with intracranial hemorrhage. Other factors that predispose preterm neonates to this type of hemorrhage are impaired autoregulation of cerebral blood flow, increased central venous pressure, and immaturity of neonatal cerebral capillary beds. The degree of autoregulation of cerebral blood flow in normal neonates is unknown, although impaired autoregulation of cerebral blood flow has been demonstrated in stressed neonates. When autoregulation is impaired, increased systemic blood pressure causes increased cerebral blood flow, which may result in periventricular-intraventricular hemorrhage. Arterial hypoxemia and hypercapnia during asphyxia associated with delivery can also result in this type of hemorrhage. The diagnosis of periventricular-intraventricular hemorrhage can be made by maintaining a high index of suspicion in susceptible neonates and by

clinical and radiologic features. Clinical features can range from subtle and not easily elicited neurologic aberrations to catastrophic deterioration with rapid onset of coma. Ultrasound scanning and computed tomography provide useful modalities for identifying periventricular-intraventricular hemorrhage.

Although the effects of anesthesia on cerebral blood flow in neonates are unknown, some recommendations can be made concerning the management of anesthesia. Certainly, factors known to precipitate periventricular-intraventricular hemorrhage, such as arterial hypoxemia and hypercapnia, should be avoided. In view of the altered autoregulation of cerebral blood flow, systolic blood pressures should be maintained within normal ranges to decrease the risk of cerebral overperfusion. To accomplish these goals, careful monitoring of oxygenation, ventilation, and systemic blood pressure is useful.

Retinopathy of Prematurity

Retinopathy of prematurity (retrolental fibroplasia) is probably due to multiple interacting events. The most significant risk factor is prematurity. The risk of retinopathy is inversely related to birth weight, with significant risk occurring in infants weighing less than 1500 g.[20] Retinal development and maturation is a complicated process. Our understanding of the process and factors that may alter development of the retinal vasculature is poor. Under normal circumstances, retinal vasculature develops from the optic disc toward the periphery of the retina. During arterial hyperoxia, retinal vasoconstriction occurs and normal retinal development is disturbed. When normal oxygen partial pressures return, vascularization of the retina resumes in an abnormal fashion, with resultant neovascularization and scarring. Although 80% to 90% of retinal changes regress spontaneously, 10% to 20% of children are left with some visual impairment. Cryotherapy, and possible laser surgery to ablate the avascular peripheral retina, arrests the progression of the disease in many cases and decreases visual impairment.

There are many unanswered questions concerning retinopathy. It is not known precisely what magnitude or duration of arterial hyperoxia produces adverse effects on the retinal vasculature. Exposure to a PaO_2 higher than 80 mmHg for prolonged periods (premature infants 500 to 1300 g) may be associated with an increased incidence and severity of retinopathy.[20] Although retinopathy may be a result of the interaction between vasoconstriction and an immature retina, it is also possible that direct effects of oxygen produce retinal damage. Retinopathy has even occurred in preterm infants who did not receive supplemental oxygen and in infants with cyanotic congenital heart disease. Free-radical scavengers such as vitamin E may attenuate oxygen damage but increase the risk of sepsis and necrotizing enterocolitis.[21] Genetics may play a role is some infants. There is no evidence that ambient light in the neonatal intensive care unit causes or contributes to retinopathy of prematurity.[21] Clearly, arterial hyperoxia is an important risk factor in the development of retinopathy, but prematurity must also be present. The risk of retinopathy is negligible 44 weeks after conception. Therefore preterm infants born after 36 weeks of gestation probably remain at risk of retinopathy until after 8 weeks of age. Retinopathy of prematurity appears not to be a preventable disease caused by the misuse of oxygen but, rather, a disease of prematurity in which several factors, including oxygen, can injure the retinal vessels.[20]

Management of anesthesia in patients with retinopathy of prematurity introduces the dilemma of trying to minimize oxygen administration to a group of patients who are also susceptible to arterial hypoxemia. To decrease the risk of retinopathy in susceptible neonates, it is recommended that the PaO_2 be maintained between 60 and 80 mmHg. During anesthesia it is useful to dilute the concentrations of oxygen delivered using nitrous oxide and/or air. The concentrations of oxygen delivered can be confirmed with an oxygen analyzer. Although it may be desirable to monitor arterial oxygenation in blood sampled from preductal arteries, the use of pulse oximetry is an acceptable alternative (Fig. 32–2). It is also important to recognize that arterial hypoxemia is a significant threat to these neonates. Certainly, attempts to prevent arterial hyperoxia must be tempered with the realization that arterial hypoxemia can result in irreversible brain damage.

Apnea Spells

Apnea spells are defined as cessation of breathing that lasts at least 30 seconds and produces cyanosis and bradycardia. An estimated 20% to 30% of preterm infants experience apnea spells during the first month of life.[22] The more premature the neonate, the greater is the likelihood of apnea spells. Preterm infants may also have RDS and bronchopulmonary dysplasia in addition to apnea spells. Inguinal hernia and incarceration of an inguinal hernia are common in preterm infants. Consequently, many preterm infants require inguinal hernia repair. Even though infant inguinal hernia repair is a minor sur-

gical procedure, up to 33% of such preterm infants have complications (apnea spells, atelectasis) during the perioperative period.[23] The incidence of postoperative apnea in preterm infants less than 60 weeks postconception age undergoing inguinal hernia repair may be increased when the preoperative hematocrit is less than 30%.[24] For these reasons, it is helpful to seek information about prematurity and RDS during the preoperative interview with the child's parents.

Inhaled and injected anesthetics affect the control of breathing and contribute to upper airway obstruction, thus increasing the likelihood of apnea spells during the postoperative period, especially in preterm infants less than 60 weeks postconception age.[23] Regional anesthesia may also be associated with apnea spells.[25] Consequently, preterm infants with a history of apnea spells are probably not suitable candidates for outpatient surgery. It is recommended that these patients be monitored in the hospital for at least 12 hours after surgery.[25, 26] The risk of postoperative apnea spells seems to be decreased beyond 60 weeks after conception, leading some to recommend postponement of nonessential surgery in preterm infants until after this age.

Sudden Infant Death Syndrome

Sudden infant death syndrome (SIDS) is the most frequent cause of death in infants 1 to 12 months of age. Those at increased risk of SIDS include premature infants, infants who had bronchopulmonary dysplasia, and those with infant apnea syndrome (not to be confused with apnea resulting from prematurity, which disappears as the infant matures). There may be a link between the long QT syndrome and SIDS (see Chapter 4). There is no evidence that general anesthesia triggers SIDS.

Kernicterus

Kernicterus is the term applied to a syndrome caused by the toxic effects of unconjugated bilirubin on the central nervous system. The gross clinical features of kernicterus include hypertonicity, opisthotonos, and spasticity. It is also evident that bilirubin encephalopathy can produce more subtle changes, such as dyslexia, hyperactivity, and decreased intellectual development.

Bilirubin is not lipophilic and does not readily cross the blood–brain barrier. Nevertheless, the blood–brain barrier of neonates, especially preterm neonates, is immature, which may explain the ability of bilirubin to enter the brain and produce cell damage. In addition, alterations in the blood–brain barrier by arterial hypoxemia, hypercapnia, or acidosis may facilitate passage of bilirubin into the central nervous system. Rapid changes in cerebral blood flow, such as may occur during exchange transfusions or rapid blood transfusions, may also disrupt the blood–brain barrier and permit entry of both bound and unbound bilirubin into the central nervous system. Neonates with other diseases, such as RDS and sepsis, may have decreased bilirubin-binding capacity and be at increased risk of kernicterus.

Treatment of hyperbilirubinemia includes phototherapy, exchange blood transfusions, and drugs. Phototherapy converts bilirubin to photobilirubin. Photobilirubin is water-soluble and does not bind to albumin. Although exchange blood transfusions are usually performed when serum bilirubin concentrations exceed 18 mg/dl, other risk factors, such as low birth weight, decreased serum albumin concentrations, acidosis, arterial hypoxemia, and hypothermia, must also be considered and may necessitate exchange blood transfusions at lower serum bilirubin concentrations. There are no data concerning effects of anesthesia on the serum concentrations of bilirubin in preterm infants.

Hypoglycemia

In contrast to adults, neonates have poorly developed systems for maintaining adequate serum glucose concentrations and therefore are susceptible to the development of hypoglycemia (see "Congenital Hyperinsulinism"). By definition, hypoglycemia is a serum glucose concentration less than 25 mg/dl for preterm neonates and less than 35 mg/dl for neonates younger than 3 days of age. Serum glucose concentrations at 3 days of age should be higher than 45 mg/dl for term neonates.

Signs of hypoglycemia in neonates include irritability, seizures, bradycardia, hypotension, and apnea. Many of these signs are nonspecific, and a high index of suspicion must be maintained. Manifestations of hypoglycemia may be attenuated by anesthetic drugs, suggesting the potential value for intraoperative monitoring of blood glucose concentrations in at-risk neonates. Maintenance of adequate serum glucose concentrations in neonates may require intravenous infusions of solutions containing glucose. The immediate treatment of hypoglycemia is administration of glucose, 0.5 to 2.0 g/kg IV, or continuous infusions of glucose, 8 mg/kg/min IV. Hyperglycemia must also be avoided, as serum glucose concentrations in excess of 125

mg/dl can produce osmotic diuresis, with resultant dehydration.

Hypocalcemia

Fetal calcium stores are largely achieved during the last trimester of gestation. Preterm neonates may therefore be susceptible to the development of hypocalcemia. Hypocalcemia in neonates is defined as serum calcium concentrations less than 3.5 mEq/L or serum ionized calcium concentrations less than 1.5 mEq/L. Signs of hypocalcemia are nonspecific and include irritability, hypotension, and seizures. Neonates with hypocalcemia exhibit increased skeletal muscle tone and twitching, in contrast to skeletal muscle hypotonia associated with hypoglycemia.

Hypocalcemia can occur with rapid intraoperative infusions of citrate, as may occur during exchange transfusions or infusions of citrated blood or fresh frozen plasma. Hypotensive effects of citrate-induced hypocalcemia can be minimized by administering calcium gluconate, 1 to 2 mg IV, for each milliliter of blood transfused.

Sepsis

Sepsis in neonates is associated with mortality approaching 50%. Presumably, this high mortality reflects the neonate's immature immune system. The clinical presentation of sepsis in neonates is nonspecific. Consequently, evaluation of sepsis has become an integral part of the evaluation of critically ill neonates. Suggestive signs of sepsis in neonates include lethargy, skeletal muscle hypotonia, hypoglycemia, and ventilatory distress. In contrast to adults, increased body temperature or leukocytosis may be absent in neonates. Positive blood cultures are important for confirming the diagnosis. Common sequelae of untreated neonatal sepsis incude meningitis and disseminated intravascular coagulation. Most neonates presenting for surgery are already receiving antibiotics, as the risk of sepsis is great. Nevertheless, the occurrence of pulmonary dysfunction during the postoperative period should arouse suspicion as to the possible presence of sepsis.

■ NEONATAL SURGICAL DISEASES

Neonatal surgical diseases during the first days of life may require life-saving surgery or be best managed by stabilizing the neonate followed by corrective sur-

	Table 32–6 • Neonatal Surgical Diseases
	Congenital diaphragmatic hernia
	Esophageal atresia
	Abdominal wall defects
	Omphalocele
	Gastroschisis
	Hirschsprung's disease
	Imperforate anus
	Pyloric stenosis
	Necrotizing enterocolitis
	Congenital hyperinsulinism
	Lobar emphysema

gery (Table 32–6).[27,28] In addition to physiologic aberrations produced by the disease process, incomplete adaptation to the extrauterine environment may further complicate perioperative management.

Congenital Diaphragmatic Hernia

Congenital diaphragmatic hernias are present in about 1 in every 2500 neonates.[28] This defect is usually characterized by pulmonary hypoplasia due to intrauterine compression of the developing lungs by the herniated viscera. In addition to the effects of lung compression, there may also be an underlying primary abnormality in airway branching that results in pulmonary hypoplasia. There is incomplete embryologic closure of the diaphragm. Although herniation of abdominal contents into the thorax can occur at several sites, the most common diaphragmatic defect occurs through the left posterolateral pleuroperitoneal canal (foramen of Bochdalek). The degree of pulmonary hypoplasia is related to the timing of the herniation of abdominal contents into the thorax. Early diaphragmatic herniation causes more pulmonary hypoplasia, resulting in a less favorable prognosis. Hypoplasia of the left ventricle may also occur, contributing to postnatal cardiac insufficiency. Despite significant progress in pediatric surgery and anesthesia, perioperative mortality is still substantial, with death most often due to pulmonary hypoplasia or persistent pulmonary hypertension.

Signs and Symptoms

Signs and symptoms of a congenital diaphragmatic hernia evident soon after birth include scaphoid abdomen, barrel-shaped chest, detection of bowel sounds during auscultation of the chest, and profound arterial hypoxemia. Chest radiographs show loops of intestine in the thorax and a shift of the mediastinum to the opposite side. Arterial hypoxemia reflects the presence of right-to-left shunting through the ductus arteriosus as manifestations of persistent fetal circulation. Increased pulmonary vascular resistance is further aggravated by arterial hypoxemia, hypercarbia, and acidosis, ensuring that the ductus arteriosus remains patent and fetal circulation patterns persist. There is a high incidence of congenital heart disease and intestinal malrotation in neonates with congenital diaphragmatic hernia.

Treatment

Immediate treatment of neonates with suspected congenital diaphragmatic hernias includes decompression of the stomach with an orogastric or nasogastric tube and administration of supplemental oxygen. Positive-pressure ventilation by mask should be avoided, as the passage of gas into the esophagus may increase stomach volume and further compromise pulmonary function. Indeed, awake tracheal intubation should be performed if the need for mechanical ventilation of the neonate's lungs is anticipated for any sustained period of time. After tracheal intubation, positive airway pressures during mechanical ventilation of the lungs should not exceed 25 to 30 cmH$_2$O, as excessive airway pressures can result in damage to the neonate's normal lung, manifesting as pneumothorax.

Congenital diaphragmatic hernias do not require immediate surgery, as the primary problem after birth is not herniation of abdominal viscera into the chest but, rather, severe pulmonary hypoplasia and associated pulmonary hypertension. Preoperative stabilization (skeletal muscle paralysis, mechanical ventilation of the lungs, extracorporeal membrane oxygenation) for a period of hours or days may decrease the mortality rate among unstable patients. Extracorporeal membrane oxygenation may improve survival in selected neonates. Permissive hypercapnia with gentle ventilation is used to minimize airway inflation pressures and decrease barotrauma associated with ventilatory treatment of severe pulmonary hypoplasia. Inhaled nitric oxide has not been effective in infants with congenital diaphragmatic hernias.[28]

Management of Anesthesia

Management of anesthesia for neonates with a congenital diaphragmatic hernia consists of awake tracheal intubation after preoxygenation. In addition to routine monitors, the right radial or temporal artery (preductal artery) is often cannulated for monitoring systemic blood pressure, blood gases, and pH. Anesthesia can be induced and maintained with low concentrations of volatile drugs. Nitrous oxide should be avoided, as its diffusion into loops of intestine present in the chest may result in distension of these loops and subsequent compression of functioning lung tissue. If the level of arterial oxygenation permits, the delivered concentrations of oxygen can be diluted by adding air to the oxygen until the desired concentrations of oxygen are attained, as reflected by an oxygen analyzer. Because prolonged postoperative ventilation of the lungs is required by almost all neonates with congenital diaphragmatic hernia, an alternative approach to inhaled drugs for anesthesia is the use of opioids such as fentanyl plus muscle relaxants. This regimen can also be continued during the postoperative period. Advantages of this technique include minimization of the postoperative hormonal responses to stress. Mechanical ventilation of the lungs is recommended, but airway pressures should be monitored and maintained below 25 to 30 cmH$_2$O to minimize the risk of pneumothorax. Reduction of the diaphragmatic hernia is accomplished through an abdominal surgical approach. After reduction an attempt to inflate the hypoplastic lung is not recommended, as it is unlikely to expand and the normal lung may be damaged by excessive positive airway pressures. In addition to a hypoplastic lung, these neonates are likely to have an underdeveloped abdominal cavity, such that a tight surgical abdominal closure causes increased intra-abdominal pressure, with cephalad displacement of the diaphragm, decreased functional residual capacity, and compression of the inferior vena cava. To prevent excessively tight abdominal surgical closures, it is often necessary to create ventral hernias, which can be surgically repaired later.

Postoperative Management

Postoperative management of neonates with congenital diaphragmatic hernias presents significant challenges. The prognosis of these neonates is ultimately determined by the degree of pulmonary hypoplasia. There is no effective treatment for pulmonary hypoplasia, other than keeping these neonates alive with the hope that lung maturation will occur. Extracorporeal membrane oxygenation has been used successfully in selected neonates for this purpose.

The postoperative course, after surgical reduction of congenital diaphragmatic hernias, is often characterized by rapid improvement, followed by sudden deterioration with profound arterial hypoxemia, hypercapnia, and acidosis, resulting in death. The mechanism for this deterioration is the reappearance of fetal circulation patterns, with right-to-left shunting through the foramen ovale and ductus arteriosus. If shunting occurs through the ductus arteriosus, there is a 20 mmHg or more difference in the PaO$_2$ measured in samples obtained simultaneously from preductal and postductal arteries. If the shunting is predominantly through the foramen ovale, no such gradient exists.

Esophageal Atresia

Esophageal atresia affects about 1 in 4000 neonates, with the most common form of the disorder manifesting as a blind upper esophageal pouch and a distal esophagus that forms a tracheoesophageal fistula (Fig. 32–3).[27, 28] Survival of neonates with esophageal atresia and no associated defects approaches 100%. Nevertheless, about 20% of neonates with esophageal atresia have major co-existing cardiovascular anomalies (ventricular septal defect, tetralogy of Fallot, coarctation of the aorta, atrial septal defect), and 30% to 40% are born before term. The highest risk of death is in those neonates weighing less than 1500 g at birth and those with associated

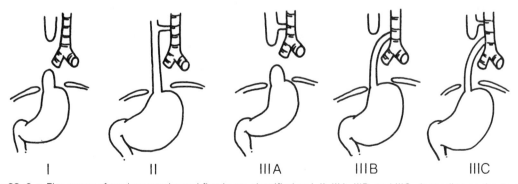

Figure 32–3 • Five types of tracheoesophageal fistula are classified as I, II, IIIA, IIIB, and IIIC, depending on the anatomic characteristics of the trachea and esophagus. A blind upper esophageal pouch and a fistula connecting the stomach to the trachea (IIIB) is the most common type of tracheoesophageal fistula. (From Dierdorf SF, Krishna G. Anesthetic management of neonatal surgical emergencies. Anesth Analg 1981;60:204–15, with permission.)

cardiac or chromosomal anomalies. Early deaths are the result of cardiac or chromosomal abnormalities, whereas later deaths are usually the result of respiratory complications. Survival among infants with other anomalies is decreased.

Signs and Symptoms

Esophageal atresia is usually diagnosed soon after birth when an oral catheter cannot be passed into the stomach or when the neonate exhibits cyanosis and coughing during oral feedings. Pulmonary aspiration is likely to occur. After a diagnosis of esophageal atresia is suspected, the blind upper pouch is decompressed and the neonate is placed in a head-up position. Gastric distension can be of sufficient magnitude to impair diaphragmatic excursion. Should life-threatening gastric distension occur, one-lung ventilation may be necessary until the stomach can be decompressed.[29]

Treatment

The preferred surgical approach to the treatment of newborns with esophageal atresia is ligation of the defect and primary anastomosis of the esophageal segments by an extrapleural approach. Neonates with this disorder who are premature may exhibit significant associated anomalies or have pneumonitis. In these neonates a staged surgical approach with an initial gastrostomy created under local anesthesia may be selected. Definitive repair of the tracheoesophageal fistula can then be delayed until the neonate's condition has improved.

Management of Anesthesia

Proper placement of the tracheal tube is critical; it should be above the carina but below the tracheoesophageal fistula. It is important that the tracheal tube be above the carina, as the right lung is compressed during thoracotomy. Accidental right main stem bronchus placement of the tracheal tube results in a precipitous decrease in arterial oxygenation, especially during surgical retraction of the lung. If the neonate does not have a gastrostomy, care must be exercised to avoid excessive airway pressures and further gastric distension. After tracheal intubation, the use of a pediatric fiberoptic bronchoscope is valuable for confirming the proper position of the tracheal tube.

Selection of anesthetic drugs for administration during surgical correction of esophageal atresia depends on the physiologic status of the neonates. Volatile anesthetics may be used if neonates are adequately hydrated. Nitrous oxide is used with caution in neonates without a gastrostomy, as diffusion of this gas into the distended stomach would be undesirable. If nitrous oxide is not administered, it may be necessary to dilute the concentrations of oxygen delivered to neonates with air to avoid arterial hyperoxia and the risk of retinopathy of prematurity. In addition to routine monitors, a catheter placed in a peripheral artery permits continuous monitoring of systemic blood pressure and measurement of arterial blood gases and pH. Pulse oximetry is useful for detecting acute changes in arterial oxygenation.

A consistent pathologic finding in neonates with esophageal atresia is decreased tracheal cartilage. This decreased support can result in tracheal collapse after tracheal extubation, requiring immediate reintubation of the trachea. By contrast, in some neonates symptomatic tracheal compression develops several months after repair of a tracheoesophageal fistula. Chronic gastroesophageal reflux and aspiration pneumonitis can follow corrective surgery, necessitating antireflux surgical procedures at a later time in life.

Abdominal Wall Defects

Omphalocele and gastroschisis are congenital defects of the anterior abdominal wall that permit external herniation of abdominal viscera.

Omphalocele

Omphalocele manifests as external herniation of abdominal viscera through the base of the umbilical cord.[27] The incidence is about 1 in every 5000 to 10,000 live births, with a male predominance. Omphalocele is associated with a 75% incidence of other congenital defects, including cardiac anomalies, Down syndrome, and Beckwith syndrome (omphalocele, organomegaly, macroglossia, hypoglycemia). About 33% of neonates with omphaloceles are preterm. Cardiac defects and prematurity are the major causes of the 30% mortality among newborns with an omphalocele.

Gastroschisis

Gastroschisis manifests as external herniation of abdominal viscera through a 2- to 5-cm defect in the anterior abdominal wall lateral to the normally inserted umbilical cord.[27] Unlike the omphalocele, a hernial sac does not cover the herniated abdominal viscera. Gastroschisis is rarely associated with other congenital anomalies. The incidence of preterm birth, however, is higher than in neonates with omphaloceles.

Preoperative Preparation

Factors that must be considered during preoperative preparation of the neonate with an omphalocele or gastroschisis are prevention of infections and minimization of fluid and heat loss from exposed abdominal viscera. Covering exposed viscera with moist dressings and a plastic bowel bag and maintaining neutral thermal environments are effective methods of decreasing fluid and heat loss. The stomach should be decompressed with an orogastric tube to decrease the risk of regurgitation and pulmonary aspiration. Adequate hydration during the preoperative period is essential. The initial fluid requirement in these neonates is increased and ranges from 6 to 12 ml/kg. These neonates experience considerable protein loss and third-space translocation. Hypovolemia is evidenced by hemoconcentration and metabolic acidosis. Plasma albumin concentrations and colloid oncotic pressures are decreased. To maintain normal oncotic pressures, protein-containing solutions should constitute about 25% of the replacement fluids. Sodium bicarbonate administration to correct metabolic acidosis should be guided by arterial pH measurements.

Management of Anesthesia

Important aspects of management of anesthesia for surgical treatment of omphalocele and gastroschisis include maintenance of body temperature and continuation of fluid replacement. After decompression of the stomach and preoxygenation, awake tracheal intubation is often recommended. Opioids such as fentanyl or sufentanil or volatile anesthetics may be used. Because of co-existing hypovolemia, anesthetics must be carefully titrated to avoid hypotension. The use of nitrous oxide may be questioned, as this gas could diffuse into the intestinal tract and interfere with the ease of returning exposed, distended loops of bowel to the neonate's abdomen. If nitrous oxide is not used, delivered concentrations of oxygen are adjusted by dilution with air, as these often preterm neonates are vulnerable to the development of retinopathy of prematurity. Muscle relaxants must be administered judiciously, as excessive skeletal muscle relaxation may make it difficult to determine whether primary surgical abdominal wall closure is feasible. It must be remembered that these neonates have an underdeveloped abdominal cavity; tight surgical abdominal closure can result in decreased diaphragmatic excursion and compression of the inferior vena cava. Monitoring airway

pressures is helpful for detecting changes in pulmonary compliance due to abdominal closure. High intra-abdominal pressure interferes with abdominal organ perfusion.[30] If primary surgical abdominal closure is not possible, the wound is temporarily covered with a Dacron-reinforced Silastic silo. The hernia is then gradually reduced over 1 to 2 weeks.

Intensive intraoperative and postoperative monitoring is recommended. Direct monitoring of arterial blood gases and pH is helpful for guiding fluid therapy, minimizing the risk of the development of retinopathy of prematurity, and recognizing previously undiagnosed cardiac anomalies. Mechanical ventilation of the neonate's lungs is often necessary for 24 to 48 hours following omphalocele or gastroschisis repair. Refinements of the techniques used for postoperative mechanical ventilation of the lungs and availability of total parenteral nutrition have increased the survival of neonates with omphalocele to about 75%.

Hirschsprung's Disease

Hirschsprung's disease is characterized by the absence of ganglion cells in the rectum.[28] This disorder may extend proximally for some distance but is usually limited to the rectum and distal colon. In rare cases it extends the entire length of the gastrointestinal tract, a condition that is often fatal. There may be deficiencies of nitric oxide synthase activity in the affected intestinal walls. The lack of nitric oxide-producing nerve fibers in the aganglionic bowel probably contributes to the inability of intestinal smooth muscle to relax appropriately, thereby impairing peristalsis.

Surgical treatment designed to bring ganglionated bowel down to the anus usually provides satisfactory long-term results. A single-stage repair through a transanal or combined abdominoperineal approach during the newborn period may be utilized, thereby eliminating the need for a preliminary colostomy. Alternatively, a laparoscopy assisted approach may be utilized.

Imperforate Anus

Imperforate anus is often associated with other congenital anomalies, especially genitourinary abnormalities and a tethered spinal cord.[28] Preliminary treatment is a diverting colostomy followed by a posterior sagittal surgical approach that facilitates placing the rectum within the pelvic muscles and allows division and closure of the rectourinary or rectovaginal fistula.

Pyloric Stenosis

Pyloric stenosis occurs in about 1 of every 500 live births. It generally manifests in male infants 2 to 5 weeks of age. Pyloric stenosis is as common in preterm neonates as it is in term neonates.

Signs and Symptoms

Pyloric stenosis is characterized by persistent vomiting, resulting in the loss of hydrogen ions from the stomach. As hydrogen ions are lost, the kidneys secrete potassium in exchange for hydrogen ions in an effort to maintain normal arterial pH. In addition, the kidneys begin exchanging potassium and hydrogen ions, as the infants become sodium-depleted from vomiting. The result is dehydrated infants with hypokalemic, hypochloremic metabolic alkalosis. Measurements of serum electrolyte concentrations, arterial blood gases, and pH may help quantitate the degree of the metabolic abnormality.

Treatment

Surgical treatment of pyloric stenosis is not an emergency.[31] Infants with this disorder should be treated initially with intravenous fluids containing sodium and potassium chloride. Surgery is performed electively after 24 to 48 hours of intravenous fluid therapy.

Management of Anesthesia

Pulmonary aspiration of gastric fluid is a definite risk in infants with pyloric stenosis. This risk is further increased in infants with pyloric stenosis who have undergone radiographic examination of the upper gastrointestinal tract using barium. Therefore the stomach should be emptied as completely as possible with large-bore catheters before induction of anesthesia. Awake tracheal intubation is indicated for less vigorous infants. Tracheal intubation after rapid-sequence induction of anesthesia with intravenous sedative drugs followed by succinylcholine or mivacurium can be used for more vigorous infants. Maintenance of anesthesia with volatile drugs, with or without nitrous oxide, is acceptable. Skeletal muscle relaxation, as provided by muscle relaxants, is usually not needed during maintenance of anesthesia. Mechanical ventilation of the lungs is recommended during the operation. If skeletal muscle relaxation is needed, administration of short-acting drugs such as succinylcholine or mivacurium are considerations.

Postoperative Management

Postoperative depression of ventilation often occurs in infants with pyloric stenosis. The cause is unknown but may be related to cerebrospinal fluid alkalosis and intraoperative hyperventilation of the infant's lungs. For this reason, infants should be fully awake and should display acceptable patterns of ventilation before tracheal extubation is considered. Hypoglycemia may occur 2 to 3 hours after surgical correction of pyloric stenosis.

Necrotizing Enterocolitis

Necrotizing enterocolitis is primarily a disease of small preterm neonates, resulting in substantial perinatal morbidity and mortality.[28] Neonates at greatest risk are those less than 32 weeks' gestation and weighing less than 1500 g. Survivors of necrotizing enterocolitis often have significant long-term nutritional and developmental problems.

The etiology of necrotizing enterocolitis is multifactorial. The combination of an immature gastrointestinal mucosal barrier with an immature immune system plays an important role in the etiology of necrotizing enterocolitis. Perinatal asphyxia, infections, umbilical artery catheterization, exchange blood transfusions, hyperosmolar feedings, and cyanotic congenital heart disease have all been implicated as causes. The common feature of this disease is hypoperfusion of the gastrointestinal tract, with subsequent mucosal and bowel wall ischemia. Initial mucosal ischemia may make the neonate's bowel more susceptible to bacterial damage and to the effects of hyperosmolar feedings.

Signs and Symptoms

The most common initial signs of necrotizing enterocolitis are abdominal distension and bloody feces. Apnea spells, lethargy, and thermal instability also occur. Hypovolemic shock and metabolic acidosis may occur secondary to generalized peritonitis due to multiple bowel perforations. A hemorrhagic diathesis secondary to thrombocytopenia is often present. Bowel gas frequently penetrates the damaged mucosa and enters the submucosal region; as a result, gas may gain access to the mesenteric veins and the portal venous system. Gas in the intestinal submucosa results in the classic *pneumatosis intestinalis* seen on radiographs of the abdomen. RDS requiring mechanical ventilation of the neonate's lungs frequently co-exists.

Treatment

Medical treatment, consisting of gastric decompression, intravenous fluids, and antibiotics, is often successful in the management of neonates with necrotizing enterocolitis. Surgery is reserved for neonates in whom medical treatment fails, as evidenced by sepsis (peritonitis), bowel perforation, and progressive metabolic acidosis. Bedside placement of peritoneal drains has been used initially in place of laparotomy for the management of gastrointestinal perforation in the smallest neonates (less than 1000 g).[28]

Management of Anesthesia

Neonates with necrotizing enterocolitis are frequently hypovolemic and require vigorous fluid resuscitation with crystalloid and colloid solutions before induction of anesthesia. Blood and platelet transfusions are often necessary. Adequate monitoring of fluid resuscitation is critical. A catheter placed in a peripheral artery provides the ability to measure systemic blood pressure continuously and to monitor arterial blood gases, pH, hematocrit, and electrolytes. It must be appreciated that rapid fluid administration to preterm neonates may cause intracranial hemorrhage or reopening of the ductus arteriosus.

Volatile anesthetics can produce significant hypotension in these neonates, particularly if hypovolemia is present. Therefore decreased doses of ketamine, fentanyl, or sufentanil plus nondepolarizing muscle relaxants may be selected for the maintenance of anesthesia. Nitrous oxide should be avoided, as it may increase the size of gas bubbles in the mesenteric veins and in the portal venous system. Gas embolism can also occur if portal venous gas bubbles traverse the ductus venosus and enter the inferior vena cava.[32] Postoperative mechanical ventilation of the neonate's lungs is usually required because of abdominal distension and coexisting RDS.

Congenital Hyperinsulinism

Congenital hyperinsulinism is characterized by excessive secretion of insulin and is the most common cause of recurrent hypoglycemia in neonates.[28] Irreversible brain damage may occur. Genetic abnormalities of the potassium channels may be responsible for impaired control of insulin secretion. Neonates with hyperinsulinism may have diffuse involvement of pancreatic beta cells or focal adenomatous islet cell hyperplasia. Diffuse disease often requires near-total pancreatectomy, which is associated with a long-term risk of diabetes mellitus. Conversely, focal disease may be cured with a partial pancreatectomy, with little risk of the subsequent development of diabetes mellitus.

Lobar Emphysema

Lobar emphysema is a rare cause of respiratory distress in neonates. Pathologic causes of congenital lobar emphysema include collapse of bronchi due to hypoplasia of supporting cartilage, bronchial stenosis, mucous plugs, obstructing cysts, and vascular compression of bronchi. Acquired lobar emphysema may be a result of bronchopulmonary dysplasia. The left upper and right middle lobes are most commonly affected by lobar emphysema.

Signs and Symptoms

Regardless of the cause of lobar emphysema, the end-result is an overdistended lobe that produces compression atelectasis of normal lung parenchyma, mediastinal shift, and impaired venous blood return, with subsequent arterial hypoxemia and hypotension. About one-half of affected children exhibit evidence of lobar emphysema during the first months of life. Signs and symptoms of lobar emphysema include tachypnea, tachycardia, cyanosis, wheezing, and asymmetrical breath sounds. Chest radiographs demonstrate hyperinflated lobes with mediastinal shifts. The presence of bronchovascular markings in the hyperinflated lobes helps differentiate lobar emphysema from pneumothorax.

Management of Anesthesia

Management of anesthesia for surgical lobectomy when treating lobar emphysema must consider cardiovascular and pulmonary changes that can occur with mechanical ventilation of the lungs.[33] In this regard, infants may be at greatest risk during induction of anesthesia, as positive-pressure ventilation of the lungs before the chest is open may cause rapid expansion of emphysematous lobes (gas enters but cannot leave), with sudden mediastinal shifts and cardiac arrest. For this reason, maintenance of spontaneous breathing with minimal positive airway pressures is recommended.[34] General anesthesia may be supplemented with local anesthesia until the chest is opened and the emphysematous lobes are delivered. Thereafter, these infants may be paralyzed and their lungs mechanically ventilated. Nitrous oxide should not be used, as its diffusion into the diseased lobes can cause further distension. Severely decompensated infants may require emergency needle aspiration or thoractomy for decompression of the affected lobe or lobes.

▌ INTRAUTERINE FETAL SURGERY

Congenital defects (omphalocele, gastroschisis, bowel obstruction, diaphragmatic hernia, obstructive uropathy, neural tube defects, neck masses, sacrococcygeal teratomas, adrenal neuroblastoma) can be detected by ultrasonography and ultrafast fetal magnetic resonance imaging.[35] Most correctable anomalies are managed with medical and surgical treatment after full-term delivery. If a congenital malformation is life-threatening, fetal surgery may be performed utilizing minimally invasive or fetoscopic procedures. Surgical repair of myelomeningocele before 25 weeks' gestation may preserve neurologic function.

■ MINIMALLY INVASIVE SURGERY

Many operations that previously required laparotomy or thoracotomy in children can be performed with minimally invasive surgical techniques.[28] High-resolution cameras and telescopes (2 to 10 mm in diameter) are introduced into the abdomen or thorax through small incisions. Instruments have been adapted for use through endoscopic ports to perform the needed surgical procedures. Potential advantages of endoscopic surgical approaches compared with thoracotomy or laparotomy include less likelihood of adhesion formation, decreased postoperative pain, more rapid recovery, and shorter hospitalization.

Gastroesophageal reflux in children (esophagitis, aspiration pneumonia, esophageal strictures, anemia, failure to thrive) can be treated with laparoscopic fundoplication. Laparoscopic splenectomy for treatment of hematologic disease may be superior to open splenectomy. As an alternative to open inguinal exploration, laparoscopy can be used to rule out the presence of an unrecognized contralateral inguinal hernia. Laparoscopic cholecystectomy is a common approach. Laparoscopy may be useful for evaluating children with chronic abdominal pain. Although not routinely utilized, the laparoscopic approach to the surgical treatment of appendicitis, pyloric stenosis, and inguinal hernia is possible. A minimally invasive approach to the correction of pectus excavatum involves insertion of a stainless steel strut across the anterior mediastinum under thoracoscopic guidance to elevate the sternum. Thoracoscopic decortication may be an alternative to long-term antibiotic treatment and hospitalization for pneumonia complicated by empyema formation. Thoracoscopy is suited for lung biopsy. Surgical closure of a patent ductus arteriosus may be accomplished by placing a metal clip across the patent ductus under thoracoscopic guidance.

■ TRAUMA

Trauma is the leading cause of death in children older than 1 year of age.[35, 36] Blunt head injury from motor vehicle accidents is responsible for most injuries and deaths. Child abuse must be considered in all children with injuries that do not appear to be consistent with the reported cause. Most preventable deaths are due to airway obstruction, pneumothorax, intra-abdominal bleeding, or an expanding intracranial hematoma. The most important indicator of intracranial bleeding and the need for prompt surgical intervention is a decrease in the level of consciousness as documented by a low Glasgow Coma Scale score (see Table 17–4). The Glasgow Coma Scale may have to be modified for children who are too young to talk. There is a trend toward nonoperative treatment of blunt abdominal injury (hepatic, splenic, pancreatic), including children with head injuries, based on a diagnosis using computed tomography.[35]

Much of the progress in the care of children with trauma has been in prevention, rather than management, of injury.[35] The use of safety helmets decreases the severity of head injuries from bicycle accidents. Airbag deployment, although effective in adults, may cause injuries in front seat restrained children when the release of the airbag drives the infant's head into the back of the automobile seat. Legislative efforts directed at gun safety seem useful for reducing violence involving firearms.

■ NERVOUS SYSTEM

Diseases of the nervous system that afflict pediatric patients include cerebral palsy, hydrocephalus, myelomeningocele, craniostenosis, seizure disorders (epilepsy), Down syndrome (trisomy 21), and neurofibromatosis. Management of these patients during the perioperative period is facilitated by understanding the pathophysiology of these diseases.

Cerebral Palsy

Cerebral palsy is a symptom complex rather than a specific disease. It comprises a group of nonprogressive, but often changing, motor impairment syndromes secondary to lesions or anomalies of the brain that arise during the early stages of development.[37] Cerebral palsy is classified according to the extremity involved (monoplegia, hemiplegia, diplegia, quadriplegia) and the characteristics of the neurologic dysfunction (spastic, hypotonic, dystonic, athetotic). The high frequency of epilepsy (approximately one-third of children with cerebral palsy) and cognitive disorders among individuals with this disease suggests that these disorders have common or related origins.

Incidence and Risk Factors

The prevalence of moderately severe or severe cerebral palsy is 1.5 to 2.5 per 1000 live births.[37] It has been assumed that problems during the birth process (midforceps delivery) and signs and symptoms that were present in newborn infants (low Apgar scores) are related to the subsequent development of cerebral palsy. This theory remains unproven, and it is likely that the characteristics associated with cerebral palsy may be consequences of the processes leading to the disease and not its cause. For example, recurrent neonatal seizures, which predict later cerebral palsy better than other perinatal characteristics, may be a consequence, rather than a cause, of the processes that lead to cerebral palsy. Risk factors for cerebral palsy may be classified according to whether they occur before pregnancy, during pregnancy, or during the perinatal period (Table 32–7).[37] The rate of later cerebral palsy is 25 to 31 times higher among infants who weigh less than 1500 g at birth than among full-size newborns.[37] Babies whose birth weight is less than 2500 g account for about one-third of all those who later develop signs and symptoms of cerebral palsy. Despite the perceived association between a multitude of factors and cerebral palsy, the cause of most cases of cerebral palsy is unknown.[38]

Signs and Symptoms

The most common manifestation of cerebral palsy is skeletal muscle spasticity. Extrapyramidal cerebral palsy is associated with choreoathetosis and dystonia, and cerebellar ataxia is characteristic of atonic cerebral palsy. Varying degrees of mental retardation and speech defects can accompany cerebral palsy. Seizure disorders co-exist in approximately one-third of individuals afflicted with cerebral palsy.

Children with cerebral palsy may have varying degrees of spasticity of different skeletal muscle groups, resulting in contractures and fixed deformities of several joints of both upper and lower extremities. They include fixed flexion and internal rotation deformities of the hip joint due to involved adductor and flexor muscles and plantar flexion of the ankles due to involvement of the Achilles tendon. These children often undergo elective orthopedic corrective procedures, such as Achilles tendon lengthening, hip adductor and iliopsoas release, and derotational osteotomy of the femur. Stereotactic surgery may be performed in attempts to decrease skeletal muscle rigidity, spasticity, and dyskinesia. Dental restorations requiring general anesthesia are frequently necessary in children with cerebral palsy. Gastroesophageal reflux is common in children with central nervous system disorders, and antireflux operations may be recommended.

Children with cerebral palsy frequently receive antiseizure medications and dantrolene for relief of skeletal muscle spasticity. Phenytoin may lead to gingival hyperplasia and megaloblastic anemia. Phenobarbital stimulates hepatic microsomal enzymatic activity and may lead to altered responses to drugs that undergo metabolism in the liver.

Management of Anesthesia

Management of anesthesia in children with cerebral palsy includes tracheal intubation because of the propensity for gastroesophageal reflux and poor function of laryngeal and pharyngeal reflexes. Although children with cerebral palsy have skeletal muscle spasticity, succinylcholine does not produce abnormal potassium release.[39] Body temperature should be monitored, as these children may be susceptible to the development of hypothermia during the intraoperative period. Emergence from anesthesia may be quite slow because of cerebral damage due to cerebral palsy and the presence of hypothermia. Tracheal extubation should be delayed until these children are fully awake and body temperature has returned toward normal. Postoperatively, these children have a high incidence of pulmonary complications.

Hydrocephalus

Hydrocephalus in pediatric patients is due to increased cerebrospinal fluid volume, resulting in enlarged cerebral ventricles and increased intracranial pressure. Hydrocephalus due to overproduction or abnormal absorption of cerebrospinal fluid is classi-

---

Table 32–7 • Factors Identified in Epidemiologic Studies as Associated with Cerebral Palsy

Before pregnancy
  History of fetal wastage
  Long menstrual cycles
During pregnancy
  Low social class
  Congenital malformations
  Fetal growth retardation
  Twin gestation
  Abnormal fetal presentation
During labor and delivery
  Premature separation of the placenta
During the early postnatal period
  Newborn encephalopathy

Adapted from: Kuban KCK, Leviton A. Cerebral palsy. N Engl J Med 1994;330:188–95.

fied as nonobstructive or communicating hydrocephalus, as there is no obstruction to the flow of cerebrospinal fluid. Obstructive hydrocephalus is present when there is obstruction to the flow of cerebrospinal fluid and its absorption from the subarachnoid space. This obstruction can be due to congenital, neoplastic, posttraumatic, or postinflammatory lesions. Congenital causes of obstructive hydrocephalus include Arnold-Chiari malformations, in which the basilar subarachnoid pathways are underdeveloped, aqueductal stenosis between the third and fourth ventricles, and Dandy-Walker syndrome, with occlusion at the outlet of the fourth ventricle by a congenital membrane. Ventricular dilation commonly follows periventricular-intraventricular hemorrhage, which most often occurs in preterm infants.

Signs and Symptoms

Signs and symptoms of hydrocephalus depend on the age of the child and the rapidity with which intracranial pressure increases. For example, the prominent feature of congenital hydrocephalus is abnormal enlargement of the head, which may present at birth or soon after birth. The enlargement is usually prominent in the frontal area of the skull. The cranial vault transilluminates in affected areas, and the cranial sutures are separated. Percussion of the skull produces a resonant note. The child's eyes are often deviated inferiorly. Scalp veins are dilated, and the skin is thin and shiny. Optic atrophy due to compression of the optic nerves can occur in chronic and untreated cases of hydrocephalus. Late-onset hydrocephalus may not produce an enlarged head but, instead, may cause significantly increased intracranial pressure. Hydrocephalus due to Arnold-Chiari malformation or aqueductal stenosis can lead to medullary and lower cranial nerve dysfunction, resulting in swallowing abnormalities, stridor, and atrophy of the tongue. Hydrocephalic children may have varying degrees of intellectual dysfunction; the dysfunction does not always correlate with the size of the ventricles or the thinness of the cortical mantle. Serial head circumference measurements skull radiographs, and computed tomography confirm the diagnosis.

Treatment

Treatment depends on the mechanisms responsible for hydrocephalus. Operative excision of lesions responsible for obstructing flow of cerebrospinal fluid is performed if feasible. A shunting procedure is necessary if the obstruction cannot be relieved surgically. The shunt system employs a one-way valve, that directs flow of cerebrospinal fluid away from the ventricles. Shunting procedures include ventriculocisternostostomy (Torkildsen's procedure) and ventriculoatrial and ventriculoperitoneal shunts. Less common are ventriculocholecystostomy, and ventriculospinal shunts.

Ventriculoatrial shunts are performed for nonobstructive or obstructive hydrocephalus. The distal end of the catheter is placed in the right atrium, as indicated by monitoring the changes in venous pressure wave patterns while advancing the catheter into the right atrium from the superior vena cava. Complications from atrial catheterization include thrombosis of the internal jugular vein or superior vena cava, septicemia, meningitis, pleural effusion, pulmonary embolism, and pulmonary hypertension. Furthermore, growth of these children displaces the cardiac end of the catheter into the superior vena cava, necessitating either revision of the shunt or its conversion to a ventriculoperitoneal shunt. Erosion of a ventriculoperitoneal catheter into a bronchus, with development of a ventriculobronchial fistula, has been described.[40]

Management of Anesthesia

Operative procedures in children with hydrocephalus are likely to be necessary for placement, revision, or removal of a cerebrospinal fluid shunt system. Some of these children have increased intracranial pressure, for which precautions should be taken during anesthesia. This is particularly important in children in whom a shunt is to be inserted before craniotomy to excise an intracranial tumor. For hydrocephalic infants and children with normal intracranial pressures, induction of anesthesia with short-acting induction drugs plus muscle relaxants to facilitate tracheal intubation, followed by maintenance of anesthesia with volatile anesthetics or opioids plus nitrous oxide, is acceptable. In the presence of co-existing intracranial hypertension, it is important to consider the potential for further increases in intracranial pressure in association with the use of succinylcholine. Nevertheless, succinylcholine-induced increases in intracranial pressure do not always occur, and avoidance of this drug is not necessary if the benefits of a rapid onset of skeletal muscle paralysis justify its administration. It should be appreciated that sudden hypotension sometimes occurs when tensely distended cerebral ventricles are decompressed. Furthermore, venous air embolism and increased blood loss can occur when large neck veins are opened to place an atrial catheter. Postoperatively, these patients are maintained in a slightly head-up position, to permit free drainage of cerebrospinal fluid.

During surgery in children with ventriculoperitoneal shunts, excessive pressure on the skin of the scalp overlying the shunt should be avoided by rotating the head to the side opposite the shunt. Pressure over the ventricular reservoir can produce skin necrosis and possibly cause shunt malfunction.

Myelomeningocele

The neural tube of the embryo is formed from the ectodermal neural crest. The neural crest deepens to form the neural groove, the margins of which fuse to form the neural tube. Failure of the caudal end of the neural tube to close can result in spina bifida (characterized by defects of the vertebral arches), meningocele (characterized by a sac that contains meninges), and myelomeningocele (characterized by a sac that contains neural elements).

Signs and Symptoms

Children with meningoceles are usually born without neurologic deficits; those with myelomeningoceles are likely to have varying degrees of motor and sensory deficits. For example, children with lumbosacral myelomeningoceles exhibit flaccid paraplegia, loss of sensation to pinprick, and loss of anal, urethral, and vesicle sphincter tone. Associated congenital anomalies include clubfoot, hydrocephalus, dislocation of the hips, extrophy of the bladder, prolapsed uterus, Klippel-Feil syndrome, and congenital cardiac defects. Severe dilation of the upper urinary tract may develop in these children, necessitating urinary diversion procedures such as vesicostomy, cutaneous ureterostomy, and ileal or colon conduit construction. They are likely to experience recurrent urinary tract infections, which may be complicated by gram-negative sepsis. The need for corrective orthopedic procedures on the lower extremities is predictable. As these patients mature, they have a tendency to develop varying degrees of scoliosis, often requiring posterior spinal fusion. Replacement or revision of a ventriculoperitoneal or ventriculoatrial shunt is frequently needed because of infections involving the shunt or malfunction due to malposition of the distal end of the catheter, reflecting normal patient growth.

Management of Anesthesia

The absence of skin covering a myelomeningocele introduces the risk of infection, necessitating surgical closure within a few hours of birth. Closure is performed during local or general anesthesia. If general anesthesia is selected, awake tracheal intubation may be performed with these children in the lateral decubitus position to avoid pressure on the meningocele sac. Anesthesia may also be induced with neonates in the supine position with the meningocele sac protected by elevating it on a doughnut-shaped support. Maintenance of anesthesia is with inhaled anesthetics delivered using mechanical ventilation of the lungs. The operative procedures are performed with these neonates in a prone position. Although succinylcholine may be used to facilitate tracheal intubation, long-acting nondepolarizing muscle relaxants are avoided, as the surgeon may need to use a nerve stimulator to identify functional neural elements. The surgical closure of a myelomeningocele sac must be tight enough to prevent leakage of cerebrospinal fluid, as confirmed by increasing the pressure in the sac with positive airway pressure. Postoperatively, neonates should be maintained in the prone position, with a high index of suspicion maintained for the development of increased intracranial pressure.

Older children with a myelomeningocele require numerous corrective procedures, primarily involving the urologic and musculoskeletal systems. Although myelomeningoceles produce both upper and lower motor neuron dysfunction, succinylcholine does not elicit a hyperkalemic response.[41] Inhaled anesthetics or opioids may be used for maintenance of anesthesia. Neonates with a myelomeningocele, however, may have an abnormal ventilatory response to hypoxia and hypercarbia. These neonates often have gastroesophageal reflux and abnormal vocal cord motility, emphasizing the need to take precautions against aspiration.

Latex Allergy

Children with a myelomeningocele have an increased incidence of sensitivity to latex (natural rubber), which manifests as intraoperative cardiovascular collapse and bronchospasm.[42] It is possible that chronic exposure to indwelling catheters results in sensitization to latex. A preoperative history of itching, rashes, or wheezing after wearing latex gloves or inflating toy balloons is suggestive of latex allergy (see Chapter 29).

Craniostenosis

Craniostenosis (craniosynostosis) is a congenital disorder resulting in a variety of deformities due to premature closure of one or more cranial sutures. Premature closure of the sagittal sutures is most common. The incidence of craniostenosis is 1 in every 1000 live births.

Signs and Symptoms

Craniostenosis results in deformity of the skull, which may lead to exophthalmos, optic atrophy, blindness, increased intracranial pressure, seizures, and mental retardation. Congenital cardiac defects and hydrocephalus may also be associated with craniostenosis. The shape of the deformed skull depends on the location of the suture that closes prematurely, as the cranial vault can compensate and grow only in areas with patent sutures. Skull radiographs and computed tomography confirm the diagnosis.

Treatment

Craniectomy is the surgical procedure effective for treatment of craniostenosis. This operation is usually performed as soon as the diagnosis is confirmed, as prompt correction is associated with fewer complications and better cosmetic results. When multiple cranial sutures are involved, craniectomy is performed as a staged procedure. Craniectomy involves removing linear strips of bone on either side of the involved sutures and extending them across the adjoining normal cranial sutures. The adjacent periosteum is stripped widely to retard new bone formation.

Management of Anesthesia

The possibility of increased intracranial pressure must be considered in children with craniostenosis. Nevertheless, most of these children have normal intracranial pressures, and induction of anesthesia is performed with intravenous administration of rapid-acting sedative drugs followed by succinylcholine or rapid-acting nondepolarizing muscle relaxants to facilitate tracheal intubation. When selecting drugs for maintenance of anesthesia, one must consider the likelihood that the surgeon will infiltrate the incision area with local anesthetic solutions containing epinephrine to minimize blood loss associated with the incision. Continuous monitoring of arterial blood pressure through a catheter in a peripheral artery is useful. Sudden and rapidly exsanguinating blood loss from the longitudinal sinus is possible during craniectomy. Most of the blood loss, however, occurs during bone stripping and is gradual. Because most of these children are in a prone position, care should be taken to prevent pressure damage to the face and eyes. Patients are often tilted into slight head-up positions to minimize blood loss from venous oozing. Depending on the degree of tilt and area of surgery, intraoperative venous air embolism is a distinct possibility; precautions

should be taken to prevent, recognize, and acutely treat such episodes.

Postoperatively, blood is likely to ooze into the wound, and these patients often require additional blood transfusions. They must be closely monitored for the onset of hypotension or localizing neurologic signs indicative of an epidural hematoma.

Epilepsy

Causes of epilepsy in children are often unknown, but recognized etiologies include metabolic disorders (phenylketonuria, hypoglycemia, kernicterus, tuberous sclerosis) and organic cerebral disorders (brain tumors, cerebral injuries) (see Chapter 17). The Lennox-Gastaut syndrome is a severe epileptic encephalopathy (multiple types of seizure) that affects children and constitutes about 5% of childhood epilepsies. It is difficult to control the seizures in these patients, even with multiple anticonvulsant drugs, and progressive mental retardation is likely.

Down Syndrome (Trisomy 21)

Down syndrome occurs in about 0.15% of live births. It is estimated that 80% of conceptions that would lead to Down syndrome end in spontaneous abortion. The abnormality in these children is due to the presence of an extra chromosome 21 (trisomy). The risk of having a child with Down syndrome increases with maternal age. For example, the 20-year-old mother has a risk of about 1 in 2000, but the risk increases to about 1 in 400 by age 35 and 1 in 40 after age 45.

Signs and Symptoms

Children with Down syndrome are readily recognized by their characteristic flat facies with oblique palpebral fissures (hence the term "mongolism"), single palmar crease (simian crease), and dysplastic middle phalanx of the fifth finger. Several features alter the upper airway in these children. For example, the nasopharynx is narrow and the tonsils and adenoids unusually large. The tongue is normal at birth but later becomes enlarged due to hypertrophy of the papillae. To compensate for their restricted airways, these children habitually hold their mouths open, with their tongues slightly protruding. Chronic upper airway obstruction, which may lead to arterial hypoxemia, is a result of airway changes characteristic of Down syndrome.

Congenital heart disease occurs in about 40% of patients with Down syndrome. Endocardial cushion defects account for about one-half of the total, and ventricular septal defects occur in about one-fourth of these children. Other abnormalities include tetralogy of Fallot, patent ductus arteriosus, and atrial septal defect of the secundum type. Surgical correction of congenital heart disease in children with Down syndrome is associated with increased morbidity (postoperative atelectasis and pneumonia) and mortality, presumably due to increased susceptibility to recurrent infections and an increased incidence of co-existing pulmonary hypertension. It has been suggested that impaired development of alveoli and the pulmonary vasculature, combined with arterial hypoxemia due to chronic upper airway obstruction, predisposes patients with Down syndrome to preoperative pulmonary hypertension and postoperative pulmonary complications.[43]

Congenital duodenal atresia occurs 300 times more frequently in patients with Down syndrome. Microcephaly and small brain mass may be present. Mental retardation in noninstitutionalized children tends to be mild to moderate, and measurement of social and vocational adjustment tends to be within the low-normal range. Behavioral traits are subject to great individual variability, but infants with Down syndrome are most often described as being good babies. Later, they are often characterized as content, good-natured, and affectionate. They may also be noted for their extreme stubbornness.

Oblique palpebral fissures and the presence of Brushfield spots (light-colored slightly elevated spots near the periphery of the iris) are characteristic of the eyes in children with Down syndrome. There is a high incidence of cataracts and strabismus, often necessitating surgical correction. Otitis media and hearing loss are common, necessitating frequent ear examinations and myringotomies. Dental hygiene may be deficient, and surgical repair of multiple caries may be needed.

Numerous musculoskeletal changes may be present in children with Down syndrome. For example, about 20% of these children have asymptomatic dislocation of the atlas on the axis. Although spinal cord compression is rare, this potential hazard must be remembered if the child's head and neck is forcefully manipulated during direct laryngoscopy for tracheal intubation.[44] Screening for atlantoaxial instability includes lateral radiographs of the neck in the flexed, extended, and neutral positions. If the distance between the anterior arch of the atlas and the adjacent odontoid process exceeds 5 mm, the diagnosis of atlantoaxial instability is likely.[44] Posterior cervical spine fusion is required for children who are symptomatic because of this subluxation.

Most hematologic parameters are within normal limits, although polycythemia has been observed.

Leukemia occurs in 1% of children with Down syndrome, but an increased incidence of other malignancies is not observed. Serum concentrations of norepinephrine are normal, and the sympathetic nervous system responds appropriately to stress. Pharmacologic responses to atropine are unusual in that mydriasis occurs more rapidly in these children, although the degree and duration of pupillary dilation is normal. Furthermore, cardiovascular responses to atropine are not altered. Thyroid function is normal in the presence of Down syndrome.

Management of Anesthesia

Preoperative medication of children with Down syndrome may include anticholinergic drugs, such as atropine or glycopyrrolate, to decrease upper airway secretions. As with other patients with mental retardation, responses to sedatives may be unpredictable. Oral midazolam is a common preoperative medication in the pediatric population. Occasionally, small doses of intramuscular ketamine facilitate preparation for induction of anesthesia in unusually obstinate children. Obesity and folds of skin at the wrist and ankles characteristic of Down syndrome may make venous cannulation technically difficult.

Patency of the upper airway may be difficult to maintain after the induction of anesthesia, reflecting the short neck, small mouth, narrow nasopharynx, and large tongue characteristic of these children. Nevertheless, tracheal intubation is usually not difficult, keeping in mind that asymptomatic dislocation of the atlas on the axis is present in about 20% of these patients. For this reason, extreme movement of the patient's head and neck during direct laryngoscopy for tracheal intubation is avoided if possible. Some recommend preoperative neurologic evaluation of children with Down syndrome as well as cervical spine films in the neutral, flexion, and extension positions.[45] In the absence of congenital heart disease, most commonly used inhaled or intravenous techniques of general anesthesia are acceptable. Otherwise, the selection of anesthetic drugs is influenced by the pathophysiology of the congenital cardiac lesion (see Chapter 3).

Neurofibromatosis

Neurofibromatosis is a congenital progressive disease of supportive tissues of the nervous system, with an incidence of 1 in every 3000 live births (see Chapter 17). It is estimated that neurofibromatosis develops in 40% of children with an affected parent.

CRANIOFACIAL ABNORMALITIES

Craniofacial abnormalities are of consequence to pediatric patients because of the cosmetic appearance. Indeed, these children often present for major reconstructive surgical procedures. The abnormalities are also important because they may be associated with airway obstruction. Craniofacial abnormalities likely to require surgical correction include cleft lip and palate, mandibular hypoplasia, and hypertelorism.

Cleft Lip and Palate

Cleft lip and palate, considered together, constitute the third most common congenital anomaly that requires surgical correction at an early age. About 50% of these children have cleft lip and palate, and associated congenital anomalies are common, especially congenital heart disease. Infants with cleft lip and palate have problems with deglutition and frequently experience pulmonary aspiration. Furthermore, the incidence of upper respiratory tract infections is increased, resulting in chronic otitis media. Anemia is often present, reflecting poor nutrition due to feeding problems.

Treatment

Surgical treatment of cleft lip (cheiloplasty) is based on variations of a Z-plasty. Palatoplasty is performed by midline closure of the cleft after adequate mobilization of the tissues of the hard and soft palate with bilateral relaxing incisions. Pushback palatoplasty is a procedure performed to add length to the soft palate with a local soft tissue flap. Posterior pharyngeal flap is another procedure, wherein a flap of mucosa and muscle is raised from the posterior pharyngeal wall and attached to the posterior aspect of the soft palate. Cheiloplasty is usually performed when infants are 2 to 3 months of age, but palatoplasty is delayed until infants are about 18 months of age.

Management of Anesthesia

Induction of anesthesia for children with cleft lip and/or palate is influenced by the degree of airway abnormality. For example, induction of anesthesia for children with no other airway anomalies can be safely accomplished by intravenous administration of rapid-acting sedative drugs followed by muscle relaxants to facilitate tracheal intubation. Conversely, administration of volatile anesthetics and tracheal intubation during spontaneous ventilation are recommended for children with associated anomalies such as Pierre Robin syndrome. Tracheal intubation may be difficult in infants with large cavernous defects of the palate if the blade of the laryngoscope slips into the cleft, presenting problems when manipulating the blade. Inserting a small piece of gauze or dental roll to fill the gap decreases the likelihood of this problem. The tracheal tube should be taped to the lower lip in the midline to minimize distortion of facial anatomy. The use of preformed tracheal tubes (RAE tubes) decreases the likelihood of tracheal tube occlusion by the palate retractor during palatoplasty.

Maintenance of Anesthesia

Maintenance of anesthesia is most often accomplished with volatile anesthetics plus nitrous oxide. The presence of associated congenital heart disease may influence the selection of anesthetic drugs and muscle relaxants and the management of ventilation. In addition, when selecting volatile anesthetics one must consider the likelihood that the surgical site will be infiltrated with local anesthetic solutions containing epinephrine. Nevertheless, in contrast to adults, children seem to tolerate large doses of exogenous epinephrine without developing cardiac dysrhythmias.[46] A high index of suspicion for accidental dislodgement of the tube from the trachea must be maintained during the operative procedure. Capnography is useful for confirming continued tracheal placement of the tube during intraoral surgery. Conjunctivitis and corneal abrasions are hazards; therefore the eyes are often lubricated with ophthalmic ointment and protected with eye covers. Blood loss requiring transfusions is uncommon during cheiloplasty or palatoplasty.

Postoperative Care

Postoperative airway problems are common following palatoplasty. For this reason, a suture may be placed through the middle of the tongue and taped to the child's cheek. In case of upper airway obstruction, the tongue can be pulled forward with the suture and the patency of the upper airway reestablished. Children with anomalies associated with small oral cavities may also have significant postoperative upper airway obstruction because of surgical edema, including macroglossia.[47] Tracheal intubation for 48 to 72 hours postoperatively is necessary in some children.

Mandibular Hypoplasia

Mandibular hypoplasia is a prominent feature of several syndromes that affect pediatric patients.

With these syndromes, the small mandible leaves little room for the tongue and makes the larynx appear to be anterior. Therefore upper airway obstruction and difficult tracheal intubation are likely.

Pierre Robin Syndrome

Pierre Robin syndrome consists of micrognathia usually accompanied by glossoptosis (posterior displacement of the tongue) and cleft palate. Mandibular hypoplasia may be responsible for displacement of the tongue into the pharynx, which subsequently prevents fusion of the palate. Acute upper airway obstruction can occur in neonates or infants with Pierre Robin syndrome. Feeding problems, failure to thrive, and cyanotic episodes are other early complications of this syndrome. Associated congenital heart disease is frequent. Fortunately, sufficient mandibular growth during early childhood markedly reduces the degree of airway problems in later years.

Treacher Collins Syndrome

Treacher Collins syndrome is the most common of the mandibulofacial dysostoses. Inheritance of this syndrome is as an autosomal dominant trait with variable expression. A lethal prenatal defect occurs frequently, as fetal wastage is common in affected families. Miller syndrome has facial features similar to those associated with Treacher Collins syndrome as well as severe deformities of the extremities.

Micrognathia results in early airway problems similar to those experienced by infants with Pierre Robin syndrome. About 30% of children with Treacher Collins syndrome have an associated cleft palate. Congenital heart disease, particularly a ventricular septal defect, frequently accompanies this syndrome. Other features include malar hypoplasia, colobomas (notching of the lower eyelids), and an antimongoloid slant of the palpebral fissures. Ear tags and gross deformities of the external ear canals and ossicular chain are common. Mental retardation is not a primary feature of Treacher Collins syndrome but may result from hearing loss. Tracheal intubation, as in infants with Pierre Robin syndrome, is difficult and sometimes impossible, especially once full dentition has been achieved. Patients with Treacher Collins syndrome may present for upper airway management, palatoplasty, treatment of chronic otitis media, and correction of congenital heart defects. In addition, some patients with Treacher Collins syndrome undergo extensive craniofacial osteotomies to correct cosmetic deformities (see "Hypertelorism").

Goldenhar Syndrome

Goldenhar syndrome is characterized by unilateral mandibular hypoplasia. Associated anomalies include eye, ear, and vertebral abnormalities on the affected side. Ease of tracheal intubation is highly variable. Some patients present little difficulty for tracheal intubation, whereas for others intubation is extremely difficult.

Nager Syndrome

Nager syndrome is a rare form of acrofacial dysostosis that includes characteristic craniofacial abnormalities (malar hypoplasia, severe micrognathia).[48] These children are likely to require multiple surgical interventions early in life to correct orthopedic and craniofacial abnormalities.

Preoperative Evaluation

Preoperative evaluation of children with severe mandibular hypoplasia begins with evaluation of the upper airway and formulation of plans for tracheal intubation. In addition, preoperative assessment should focus on the cardiovascular system and the hemoglobin concentrations. Some patients with chronic airway obstruction experience chronic arterial hypoxemia and develop pulmonary hypertension. Inclusion of anticholinergic drugs in the preoperative medication is recommended to decrease upper airway secretions. Opioids and other ventilatory depressants are often avoided in the preoperative medication. Oral administration of H_2-receptor antagonists may be a logical addition to the preoperative regimen in infants and children at risk of aspiration during induction of anesthesia and tracheal intubation.

Tracheal Intubation

Several approaches to tracheal intubation may be considered, but alternative methods must be immediately available, including facilities for emergency bronchoscopy, cricothyrotomy, or tracheostomy. Attempts at direct laryngoscopy may be preceded by intravenous administration of atropine to minimize the likelihood of vagal stimulation and resultant bradycardia. Preoxygenation before initiation of direct laryngoscopy is recommended. Administration of muscle relaxants to these patients is not recommended until mechanical ventilation of the lungs is established through a tracheal tube. Awake tracheal intubation with the aid of fiberoptic laryngoscopy can sometimes be accomplished by the oral or nasal route after adequate topical anesthesia has been established. Awake tracheal intubation may produce undue trauma to the child's upper airway and does not eliminate the risk of pulmonary aspiration. More often, fiberoptic tracheal intubation is accomplished after induction of anesthesia with volatile anesthetics, such as sevoflurane, provided a patent upper airway can be maintained until an adequate depth of anesthesia is attained. Spontaneous ventilation is desirable during induction of anesthesia to ensure continuous airway control and to avoid inflating the child's stomach with air. Fiberoptic laryngoscopy should not be attempted until a sufficient depth of anesthesia has been established. Transtracheal injection of lidocaine decreases the risk of laryngospasm during laryngoscopy. Forward traction of the tongue may facilitate maintenance of a patent upper airway until a sufficient depth of anesthesia can be obtained. Use of laryngeal mask airways may be an alternative to tracheal intubation in selected patients or when tracheal intubation proves impossible.[49] Tracheostomy during local anesthesia may be required when all other attempts to maintain the airway have failed. Tracheostomy in these children may be technically difficult, however, and associated with immediate and delayed complications. Risks of pneumothorax, bleeding, venous air embolism, and poor positioning of the tracheostomy site are increased in struggling children.

Tracheal extubation following surgery is delayed until these patients are fully awake and alert. Equipment for urgent tracheal reintubation must be immediately available.

Hypertelorism

Hypertelorism is an increased distance between the eyes and is associated with many craniofacial anomalies, such as Crouzon's disease and Apert syndrome. Crouzon's disease consists of hypertelorism, craniostenosis, shallow orbits with marked proptosis, and midface hypoplasia. Apert syndrome is characterized by essentially the same features, with the addition of syndactyly of all extremities. Other anomalies associated with hypertelorism are cleft palate, synostosis of the cervical spine, hearing loss, and mental retardation. Hypertelorism is representative of many craniofacial disorders amenable to facial reconstructive surgery.

Treatment

Correction of major craniofacial deformities may involve mandibular osteotomies, craniotomy with wide exposure of the frontal lobes, maxillary osteotomies with forward displacement of the maxilla, medial displacement of the orbits, and multiple rib grafts. Such complex operations may require several hours for completion and involve more than 100 separate surgical steps. Surgical correction is often performed during infancy, before ossification of the facial bones occurs.

Management of Anesthesia

Management of anesthesia for craniofacial surgery in children with hypertelorism is a complex undertaking that begins with meticulous preoperative assessment and preparation and extends into the postoperative period for several days. Craniofacial surgery should be attempted only by qualified teams of physicians under ideal circumstances recognizing the possibility of multiple potential anesthetic problems (Table 32–8).

Management of the patient's airway must not interfere with the exposure required to perform the corrective surgery. Predictably, tracheal intubation may be difficult. Intraoperatively, the tracheal tube may become dislodged or kinked during maxillary advancement, mandibular osteotomy, or repositioning of the head and neck. In addition, the tracheal tube may be displaced into a main stem bronchus when the child's neck is flexed, or the tube may be accidentally cut by the osteotome. Dry or inadequately humidified inspired gases are likely to lead to mucus plugs in the tracheal tube during these long operations, especially if small-diameter tubes are required.

Blood loss generally occurs in a steady ooze from multiple osteotomies and bone graft donor sites, averaging about 1.2 blood volumes. Quantitation of blood loss is difficult because of the diffuse oozing. Measurement of serial hematocrits, central venous pressure, and urine output are helpful for estimating blood loss and guiding intravenous fluid replacement. The availability of appropriate amounts of whole blood, platelets, and fresh frozen plasma should be confirmed before surgery. Intravenous catheters must be of sufficient number and diameter to permit rapid transfusions of blood.

Table 32–8 • Anesthetic Considerations in Management of Craniofacial Surgery

Difficult tracheal intubation versus elective
  tracheostomy
Excessive blood loss
Hypothermia
Intracranial hypertension
Corneal abrasions
Invasive monitoring
Postoperative mechanical ventilation of the lungs

Blood loss may be decreased by positioning the patient in a 15- to 20-degree head-up position. In addition, controlled hypotension, using nitroprusside during phases of surgery when major hemorrhage is anticipated, is useful. The mean arterial pressure, as measured at the level of the circle of Willis, should probably not be decreased below about 50 mmHg during controlled hypotension. Blood must be filtered, warmed, and, if given rapidly to small children, accompanied by calcium gluconate, 1 to 2 mg IV for every milliliter of blood infused, to decrease the possibility of citrate intoxication.

Complex craniofacial reconstruction surgeries are predictably prolonged. Hypothermia during these lengthy operations can be minimized by placing children on warming blankets, warming intravenous fluids and blood, and using warmed, humidified inspired gases. Pressure necrosis and nerve injuries can be minimized by careful positioning and padding, with an emphasis on avoiding traction on the patient's brachial plexus. Despite these precautions, peripheral nerve injury may still occur (especially ulnar neuropathy) in the absence of an obvious explanation (see Chapter 17). Venous stasis can be minimized by wrapping the child's legs with elastic bandages.

Hyperventilation of the lungs to maintain the $PaCO_2$ between 30 to 35 mmHg, maintenance of the head-up position, and administration of furosemide, mannitol, and corticosteroids are used to minimize brain swelling. Free water is limited by administering 5% dextrose in lactated Ringer's solution at a rate of 4 ml/kg/hr IV. An anesthetic technique that minimizes brain blood volume (nitrous oxide plus opioids) is useful. Intraoperative brain swelling can be minimized by continuous drainage of lumbar cerebrospinal fluid. Many reconstructive procedures are extracranial, and cerebral edema is not a consideration.

Corneal abrasions are likely in children when ocular proptosis is pronounced. Therefore eye ointment should be used and the eyelids sutured closed. In addition, ocular or orbital manipulations can evoke the oculocardiac reflex. Release of pressure on the orbits or administration of small doses of atropine, rapidly blocks the reflex.

In addition to routine monitors, a catheter placed in a peripheral artery for continuous measurement of systemic blood pressure is mandatory. Blood from the arterial catheter also permits determination of arterial blood gases, pH, hematocrit, electrolytes, and plasma osmolarity. A central venous catheter and a Foley catheter are helpful for evaluating the adequacy of intravenous fluid replacement. Capnography is useful for following the adequacy of

ventilation and prompt recognition of dislodgement of the tube from the trachea.

Postoperatively, the entire head may be wrapped in a pressure dressing, through which only the tracheal tube protrudes. The child's mouth may be wired shut. Pharyngeal bleeding, laryngeal edema, and increased intracranial pressure may be present. Therefore no attempt is made to reverse opioid or muscle relaxant effects at the end of the operation. Indeed, mechanical ventilation of the lungs should be maintained for several days postoperatively.

■ DISORDERS OF THE UPPER AIRWAY

Numerous pathologic processes may involve the upper airway and respiratory tract of pediatric patients (Table 32–9).

Acute Epiglottitis (Supraglottitis)

Acute epiglottitis is a short-lived disease that presents most often in boys 2 to 8 years of age with characteristic signs and symptoms (Table 32–10).[50] Adults may also develop acute epiglottitis.[51] The onset of acute epiglottitis may be abrupt, progressing to respiratory obstruction in a matter of hours. At times, however, classic signs and symptoms are not present, and it may be difficult to differentiate acute epiglottitis from laryngotracheobronchitis. Acute epiglottitis can be fatal if upper airway obstruction is not treated promptly. Edema of supraglottic tissues and the epiglottis is the reason some prefer to designate this disease acute supraglottitis rather than acute epiglottitis.

Signs and Symptoms

Classically, children with acute epiglottitis present with a history of acute difficulty swallowing, high fever, and inspiratory stridor. These signs and symptoms have usually developed over a period of less than 24 hours. In addition, there may be exces-

Table 32–9 • Disorders of the Pediatric Upper Airway

Acute epiglottitis (supraglottitis)
Laryngotracheobronchitis
Postintubation laryngeal edema
Foreign body aspiration
Laryngeal papillomatosis
Lung abscess

Table 32–10 • Clinical Features of Acute Epiglottitis (Supraglottitis) and Laryngotracheobronchitis

Parameter	Acute Epiglottitis	Laryngotracheobronchitis
Age group affected	2–8 years (most often in boys)	< 2 years
Incidence	Accounts for 5% of children with stridor	Accounts for about 80% of children with stridor
Etiologic agent	Bacterial (*Haemophilus influenzae*)	Viral
Onset	Rapid over 24 hours	Gradual over 24–72 hours
Signs and symptoms	Inspiratory stridor	Inspiratory stridor
	Pharyngitis	"Barking" cough
	Drooling	Rhinorrhea
	Fever (often > 39°C)	Fever (rarely > 39°C)
	Lethargic to restless	
	Insists on sitting up and leaning forward	
	Tachypnea	
	Cyanosis	
Laboratory	Neutrophilia	Lymphocytosis
Lateral radiographs of the neck	Swollen epiglottis	Narrowing of the subglottic area
Treatment	Oxygen	Oxygen
	Urgent tracheal intubation or tracheostomy during general anesthesia	Aerosolized racemic epinephrine
		Humidity
	Fluids	Fluids
	Antibiotics	Corticosteroids
	Corticosteroids (?)	Tracheal intubation for severe airway obstruction

sive drooling, a muffled voice, neutrophilia, and the characteristic posture of sitting upright and leaning forward. In fact, changes in posture may cause increased degrees of upper airway obstruction. Pulmonary edema, pericarditis, meningitis, or septic arthritis may accompany acute epiglottitis.

Diagnosis

Acute epiglottitis is a medical emergency. It is mandatory that children with suspected acute epiglottitis be admitted to the hospital. The diagnosis of acute epiglottitis is based principally on clinical signs. The history can be quickly obtained and the child examined for signs of upper airway obstruction. Attempts to visualize the epiglottis should not be undertaken as any instrumentation, even a tongue blade, may provoke laryngospasm. Unless acute respiratory distress is present, a lateral view chest radiograph is obtained. If the film does not demonstrate swelling of the epiglottis and aryepiglottic folds, indirect laryngoscopy can be undertaken. If epiglottitic edema is present, however, the diagnosis is confirmed, and instrumentation is unnecessary. The etiologic agent of acute epiglottitis is most often *Haemophilus influenzae*.

Treatment

When airway obstruction is impending it is common to bring the child to the operating room, where prep-

arations are completed for tracheal intubation and possible emergency tracheostomy. It should be remembered that total upper airway obstruction can occur at any time, especially with instrumentation of the upper airway, perhaps reflecting glottic obstruction by the edematous epiglottis, laryngospasm from aspirated saliva, and respiratory muscle fatigue. Physicians skilled in tracheal intubation and positive-pressure ventilation of the lungs with a face mask should accompany these children at all times.

Definitive treatment of acute epiglottitis includes administration of antibiotics effective against *Haemophilus influenzae* and establishment of a secure airway until inflammation of the epiglottis has subsided. Ampicillin is the antibiotic most often selected. Corticosteroids are of unproven efficacy for decreasing epiglottic edema. Translaryngeal tracheal intubation during general anesthesia is the recommended approach for securing the child's airway.[50] Although acute epiglottitis is primarily a disease of children, there are increasing numbers of reports of epiglottitis in adults.[51] A difference between adults and children with this disease is the appearance of the epiglottis, which in children is "cherry red" and in adults is only mildly erythematous or even has a pale, watery, edematous appearance. Management of acute epiglottitis in children is similar to that for adults, although the routine need for tracheal intubation in adults is unclear.[52–54] Rather than routine tracheal intubation, adults may be closely monitored, and provision is made for tracheal intubation or tracheostomy only if respiratory distress becomes evident.

Management of Anesthesia

Induction and maintenance of anesthesia for tracheal intubation is accomplished with volatile anesthetics, most often sevoflurane or halothane, in oxygen.[55] High inspired concentrations of oxygen permitted by the use of volatile anesthetics facilitate optimal oxygenation in these patients. Before induction of anesthesia, preparations are made for an emergency cricothyrotomy or tracheostomy, which may be required if airway obstruction suddenly occurs and translaryngeal tracheal intubation is not possible. An intravenous catheter is placed before induction of anesthesia, and administration of anticholinergic drugs to decrease secretions may be useful.

Inhalation induction of anesthesia is initiated with the child in the sitting position. After the onset of drowsiness, the child is placed supine, and ventilation of the lungs is assisted as necessary. When adequate depths of anesthesia have been established, direct laryngoscopy is performed, and the tube is placed in the child's trachea. After successful tracheal intubation, a thorough direct laryngoscopy is performed to confirm the diagnosis of acute epiglottitis. The next step is to replace the orotracheal tube with a nasotracheal tube under direct vision. A nasotracheal tube is more comfortable for awake children. After nasotracheal intubation is accomplished, the child is allowed to awaken from the anesthetic. Usually tracheal intubation is required for 48 to 96 hours, although periods as brief as 8 to 12 hours may be adequate.

Tracheal Extubation

Tracheal extubation may be considered when the child's fever and other signs of infection such as neutrophilia have waned. A clinical sign of resolution of the epiglottic swelling is the development of air leaks around the tracheal tube. Regardless of the clinical impression, it is often recommended that these children be examined by direct laryngoscopy in the operating room during general anesthesia to confirm that inflammation of the epiglottis and other supraglottic tissues has resolved before tracheal extubation is accomplished.

Laryngotracheobronchitis

Laryngotracheobronchitis ("croup") is a viral infection of the upper respiratory tract that typically af-

flicts children younger than 2 years of age (Table 32–10).[50] Parainfluenza, adenovirus, myxovirus, and influenza A virus have been implicated as causative agents. Laryngotracheobronchitis and acute epiglottitis share certain clinical features and at times are difficult to differentiate (Table 32–10).[50]

Signs and Symptoms

Laryngotracheobronchitis, in contrast to acute epiglottitis, has a gradual onset over 24 to 72 hours. There are signs of upper respiratory tract infection, such as rhinorrhea and lowgrade fever. Leukocyte counts are normal or only slightly increased, with lymphocytosis. The cough has a characteristic "barking" or "brassy" quality.

Treatment

Treatment of laryngotracheobronchitis includes administration of supplemental oxygen and racemic epinephrine as well as humidification of inspired gases. For example, hourly treatment with aerosolized racemic epinephrine has been shown to alleviate airway obstruction secondary to laryngotracheobronchitis effectively, thereby decreasing the need for tracheal intubation. Administration of corticosteroids, such as dexamethasone, 0.5 to 1.0 mg/kg IV or inhalation of budesonide is effective in relieving symptoms of croup.[56] Tracheal intubation is required if physical exhaustion occurs, as evidenced by increased $PaCO_2$. If tracheal intubation is required, a smaller than normal tracheal tube should be used to minimize the edema due to intubation. In the event that a smaller than normal tracheal tube fits too tightly in the subglottic area, a tracheostomy may be required. Although laryngotracheobronchitis is generally a short-lived illness, airway hyperreactivity may persist.

Postintubation Laryngeal Edema

Postintubation laryngeal edema is a potential complication of tracheal intubation in all children, although the incidence is highest in children between the ages of 1 and 4 years. Studies to delineate the etiology of postintubation laryngeal edema are lacking, but certain predisposing factors seem predictable. For example, mechanical trauma to the child's upper airway during tracheal intubation and placing a tube that produces a tight fit are possible causes. Postintubation laryngeal edema may be less likely if the size of the tube in the trachea is such that an audible air leak occurs around it during positive airway pressures equivalent to 15 to 25 cmH$_2$O. Another predisposing factor to the development of postintubation laryngeal edema may be co-existing upper respiratory tract infections, especially in neonates or infants in whom airway edema secondary to tracheal intubation results in greater decreases in the cross-sectional area of the trachea than those seen in older children. Indeed, the incidence of postintubation laryngeal edema seems to be increased in infants with upper respiratory tract infections and whose tracheas are intubated for elective operations.[57]

Treatment of postintubation laryngeal edema is with humidification of the inspired gases and hourly administration of aerosolized racemic epinephrine until symptoms subside. The aerosolized dose of racemic epinephrine is 0.05 ml/kg (maximum 0.5 ml) in 2.0 ml of saline. For most cases of postintubation laryngeal edema, one or two treatments with racemic epinephrine produce significant improvement. Reintubation of the trachea or a tracheostomy is rarely needed. Although administration of dexamethasone, 0.1 to 0.2 mg/kg IV, as a single dose has been used for prevention and treatment of airway edema, its efficacy for this purpose is undocumented. In adults, dexamethasone administered intravenously 1 hour before tracheal extubation does not influence the incidence of laryngeal edema.[58]

Foreign Body Aspiration

Foreign body aspiration into the airways, with its resultant airway obstruction, can produce a wide range of responses.[59] For example, complete obstruction at the level of the larynx or trachea can result in death from asphyxiation. At the opposite end of the spectrum, passage of a foreign body into distal airways may elicit only mild symptoms, which may go unnoticed. Because of their curiosity and newly found locomotion ability, children 1 to 3 years of age are most susceptible to foreign body aspiration.

Signs and Symptoms

Common clinical features of foreign body aspiration are cough, wheezing, and decreased air entry into the affected lung. The most frequent site of aspiration is the right bronchus. Foreign body aspiration often presents with the misdiagnosis of upper respiratory tract infections, asthma, or pneumonia. Chest radiography provides direct evidence if the aspirated object is radiopaque. If the aspirated foreign body is radiolucent, indirect evidence can be obtained by demonstrating hyperinflation of the affected lung on chest radiographs with atelectasis distal to the foreign body. Chest radiographs during exhalation may accentuate this hyperinflation. Measurement of the PaO$_2$ is helpful for evaluating the degree of right-to-left intrapulmonary shunting due to airway obstruction.

The type of foreign body aspirated can influence the clinical course. For example, nuts and certain vegetable materials are highly irritating to the bronchial tree. Nuts also tend to result in multiple-site aspiration. Inert substances, such as plastics, are relatively nonirritating and produce minimal inflammatory reactions.

Treatment

Treatment for aspirated foreign bodies requires endoscopic removal utilizing pediatric fiberoptic bronchoscopy. The goal is to remove the foreign body within 24 hours after aspiration. Risks of leaving the foreign body in the airways for longer than 24 hours include migration of the aspirated material, pneumonia, and residual pulmonary disease.

Management of Anesthesia

Few cases demand as much flexibility on the part of the anesthesiologist as do children with aspirated foreign bodies. Each child mandates individualization of the technique of anesthesia to fit the clinical situation. Techniques for induction of anesthesia depend on the severity of the airway obstruction. When airway obstruction is present, induction of anesthesia using only volatile anesthetics such as sevoflurane in oxygen is useful. Induction of anesthesia with intravenous induction drugs followed by inhalation of volatile anesthetics is acceptable if the airway is less tenuous. After an adequate depth of anesthesia has been attained, direct laryngoscopy is performed, and the larynx may be sprayed with a solution containing lidocaine. This topical anesthesia is effective in preventing laryngospasm when endoscopic manipulation is performed. Administration of atropine, 6 to 10 μg/kg IV, or glycopyrrolate, 3 to 5 μg/kg IV, is useful to decrease the likelihood of bradycardia from vagal stimulation during endoscopy. Muscle relaxants are often avoided during bronchoscopy, as spontaneous ventilation is desirable, providing greater flexibility and additional time for the endoscopist. Furthermore, positive airway pressures could contribute to distal migration of foreign bodies, complicating their extraction. In addition, if foreign bodies produce a ball-valve phenomenon, the use of positive-pressure ventilation of the lungs could contribute to hyperinflation and possibly pneumothorax. Despite the concerns that adverse effects of aspirated foreign bodies may be influenced by the method of ventilation selected during anesthesia (spontaneous versus controlled ventilation), there is no evidence that outcomes during and following bronchial or tracheal foreign body removal are influenced by the ventilatory management strategy employed.[59] During bronchoscopy, anesthesia is maintained with volatile anesthetics in oxygen. Skeletal muscle paralysis produced with succinylcholine or short-acting nondepolarizing muscle relaxants may be required to remove the bronchoscope and foreign body if the object is too large to pass through the moving vocal cords.

Complications that may occur during bronchoscopy include airway obstruction, fragmentation of the foreign body, arterial hypoxemia, and hypercapnia. Trauma to the tracheobronchial tree due to the foreign body and instrumentation can result in subglottic edema. After bronchoscopy, inhalation of aerosolized racemic epinephrine and intravenous administration of dexamethasone may decrease subglottic edema. Chest radiographs should be obtained after bronchoscopy to detect atelectasis or pneumothorax. Postural drainage and chest percussion enhance clearance of secretions and decrease the subsequent risk of infections.

Laryngeal Papillomatosis

Laryngeal papillomatosis is the most common benign laryngeal tumor of childhood. The likely cause is a tissue response to a virus. Malignant degeneration of juvenile papillomas is rare but can occur in older children. A change in the character of the child's voice is the most common symptom of papillomatosis. Most children with papillomatosis present with symptoms before the age of 7 years. Some degree of airway obstruction is present in more than 40% of patients. Papillomas usually regress spontaneously at puberty.

Treatment

Various forms of treatment for laryngeal papillomatosis have been used, including surgical excision, cryosurgery, topical 5-fluorouracil, exogenous interferon, and laser ablation. Because the disease is ultimately self-limiting, the complications of therapy must be avoided. For example, seeding of the distal airways can occur after tracheostomy. Surgical therapy with laser coagulation has been useful. Because papillomas recur, frequent laser coagulation is required until there is spontaneous remission.

Management of Anesthesia

Management of anesthesia for removal of laryngeal papillomas depends on the severity of the airway obstruction. Awake tracheal intubation is recommended for severe airway obstruction. Children with severe airway obstruction should not be given muscle relaxants in an attempt to facilitate tracheal intubation. Indeed, in some children the glottic opening can be identified only with the child breathing spontaneously. A rigid bronchoscope is readily available, and it may be the only means to secure an airway in some children. It should be appreciated that the degree of airway obstruction can vary greatly in the same patient for different surgical procedures.

Induction and maintenance of anesthesia is often achieved with volatile anesthetics, such as sevoflurane delivered in high inspired concentrations of oxygen. Surgical therapy for papillomatosis, by laser ablation or forceps excision, is usually done as a microlaryngoscopic procedure. During microlaryngoscopy the vocal cords must be quiescent. Skeletal muscle paralysis or deep anesthesia therefore is required to produce acceptable operating conditions. Short-acting nondepolarizing muscle relaxants are useful for this purpose. Cuffed tracheal tubes of smaller than predicted diameters should be utilized for tracheal intubation and should improve visualization of the glottis by the endoscopist. In some instances, apneic oxygenation techniques with temporary removal of the tracheal tube are useful. The usual safety precautions concerning laser use should be observed for laser ablation of papillomas. These precautions include utilization of appropriate tracheal tubes, consideration of inflation of the tracheal tube cuff with saline, protection of the child's face and eyes, and delivery of the lowest supplemental concentrations of oxygen compatible with adequate oxygenation, keeping in mind that nitrous oxide may support combustion. After resection of papillomas, the tracheal tube should be removed only when the child is fully awake and laryngeal bleeding has ceased. After tracheal extubation, inhalation of aerosolized racemic epinephrine and intravenous administration of dexamethasone may decrease subglottic edema.

Lung Abscess

Lung abscess in a child is most likely the result of inhalation of secretions containing disease-producing bacteria. In addition, bronchial obstruction by tumor may result in lung abscesses distal to sites of airway obstruction.

Surgical excision of the abscess cavity is indicated for the cases that do not respond to antibiotic therapy. Nevertheless, surgical intervention introduces the risk of rupture of the lung abscess and flooding of the tracheobronchial tree with large amounts of purulent material.

Placing a double-lumen endobronchial tube is often utilized to minimize the risk of contamination of the lungs and airways with purulent material from the lung abscess. High inspired concentrations of oxygen are necessary, as one-lung anesthesia may result in increased right-to-left intrapulmonary shunting, resulting in decreased PaO_2. The $PaCO_2$ is not influenced by one-lung anesthesia if minute ventilation is maintained.

Jeune Syndrome

Jeune syndrome is an inherited autosomal recessive disorder that occurs in a neonatal form (asphyxiating thoracic dystrophy) and a childhood form (diffuse interstitial fibrosis of the kidneys). In its neonatal form the deformity of the thoracic wall prevents normal intercostal movement, and ventilatory failure ensures. Lung volumes are predictably decreased. Pulmonary hypoplasia and persistent pulmonary hypertension may be present. Even if normoxic at rest, these infants are susceptible to profound arterial hypoxemia when stimulated because of asynchronous rib and abdominal movements. Cor pulmonale is a sequela of chronic arterial hypoxemia. Hepatic fibrosis and myocardial dysfunction have also been observed.

These children may require anesthesia for thoracoplasty, renal transplantation, bronchoscopy, and tracheostomy.[60] Older children undergoing renal transplantation also have the typical thoracic deformity, although it is less severe than in neonates. During the intraoperative period, peak airway pressures should be minimized to decrease the likelihood of barotrauma. The choice of drugs for anesthesia is influenced by known effects on pulmonary, cardiovascular, and renal function. Infants undergoing thoracoplasty require prolonged mechanical support of ventilation.

▪ MALIGNANT HYPERTHERMIA

Malignant hyperthermia is an example of a pharmocogenetic disease. Susceptible patients have a genetic predisposition for the development of this disorder, which does not manifest until they are exposed to triggering agents or stressful environmental factors.[61] Volatile inhalation anesthetics (halothane is the most potent, but all volatile drugs may trigger malignant hyperthermia) are the most commonly implicated pharmacologic triggers of malignant hyperthermia. Indeed, there are no verified cases of death due to malignant hyperthermia

where potent volatile anesthetics have not been used.[61]

The recognized modes of inheritance for malignant hyperthermia susceptibility are autosomal dominant, autosomal recessive, or multifactorial and unclassified. The gene for malignant hyperthermia is located on human chromosome 19, which is also the genetic coding site for the calcium release channels of skeletal muscle sarcoplasmic reticulum (ryanodine receptors). It is presumed that a defect in the calcium release channels results in malignant hyperthermia susceptibility. Indeed, in swine a single mutation in the ryanodine receptor gene can account for all cases of malignant hyperthermia. By contrast, a series of different mutations or even a lack of linkage between malignant hyperthermia and mutations of the ryanodine receptor gene in some patients indicates a heterogeneous genetic basis for the human syndrome.

Susceptible patients should be thoroughly educated with respect to the potential hazards and implications of malignant hyperthermia. Malignant hyperthermia has an estimated incidence of 1 in 12,000 pediatric anesthesias and 1 in 40,000 adult anesthesias. The incidence is higher when succinylcholine is used with other triggering agents.[62] The incidence has an apparent geographic variation, as it is more prevalent in certain areas of the United States. Malignant hyperthermia usually occurs in children and young adults but has been reported at the extremes of age, ranging from 2 months to 70 years. Two-thirds of patients susceptible to malignant hyperthermia manifest this syndrome during administration of their first general anesthetic and the remaining one-third during administration of subsequent anesthetics.

Signs and Symptoms

There are no clinical features that are specific for malignant hyperthermia, and the diagnosis depends on a knowledge of features that can occur during it (Table 32–11).[61] Malignant hyperthermia is characterized by signs and symptoms of hypermetabolism (up to 10 times normal). The clinical features of this disorder are nonspecific and include tachycardia, tachypnea, arterial hypoxemia, hypercarbia, metabolic and respiratory acidosis, hyperkalemia, cardiac dysrhythmias, hypotension, skeletal muscle rigidity (trismus or masseter spasm) after administration of succinylcholine, and increased body temperature.

The earliest signs of malignant hyperthermia are those related to enormous increases in the patient's metabolic rate reflecting the ability of triggering drugs to cause an imbalance in calcium homeostasis

Table 32–11 • Clinical Features of Malignant Hyperthermia

Timing	Clinical Signs	Changes in Monitored Variables	Biochemical Changes
Early	Masseter spasm		
	Tachypnea	Increased minute ventilation	
	Rapid exhaustion of soda lime	Increasing end-tidal carbon dioxide concentrations	Increased $PaCO_2$
	Warm soda lime canister		
	Tachycardia		Acidosis
	Irregular heart rate	Cardiac dysrhythmias	Hyperkalemia
		Peaked T waves on the ECG	
Intermediate	Patient warm to touch	Increasing core body temperature	
	Cyanosis	Decreasing hemoglobin oxygen saturation	
	Dark blood in surgical site		
	Irregular heart rate	Cardiac dysrhythmias	Hyperkalemia
		Peaked T waves on the ECG	
Late	Generalized skeletal muscle rigidity		Increased creatine kinase concentrations
	Prolonged bleeding		
	Dark urine		Myoglobinuria
	Oliguria		
	Irregular heart rate	Cardiac dysrhythmias	Hyperkalemia
		Peaked T waves on the ECG	

Adapted from: Hopkins PM. Malignant hyperthermia: advances in clinical management and diagnosis. Br J Anaesth 2000;85:118–28.

in skeletal muscle cells. In some patients metabolic stimulation is evident clinically within 10 minutes of administration of volatile anesthetics, whereas in others several hours may elapse. Increased intracellular calcium concentrations stimulate metabolism both directly, through activation of phosphorylase to increase glycolysis, and indirectly, because of increased demands for adenosine triphosphate production. Hypermetabolism leads to increased carbon dioxide production with associated tachypnea. In addition, lactic acidosis develops, and the presence of mixed respiratory and metabolic acidosis stimulates sympathetic nervous system activity with associated tachycardia. Increased carbon dioxide production occurs early, emphasizing the value of continuous capnography. Cardiac dysrhythmias, such as ventricular bigeminy, multifocal ventricular premature beats, and ventricular tachycardia, may also occur, especially when hyperkalemia resulting from rhabdomyolysis and sympathetic nervous system stimulation accompany this syndrome. Cutaneous changes may vary from flushing, caused by vasodilation, to blanching secondary to intense vasoconstriction.

In the absence of a family history of malignant hyperthermia, the first indication that an individual may be susceptible to malignant hyperthermia is the development of exaggerated initial responses to succinylcholine, manifesting as increased tension of the masseter muscles. If sufficiently sensitive measuring equipment is used, jaw stiffness after administration of succinylcholine can be detected in most patients but is often more pronounced in children. When skeletal muscle spasm is severe, it may be impossible to open the child's mouth to perform direct laryngoscopy for tracheal intubation. Conversely, in others, drug-induced masseter spasm is mild and transient or even absent. It is recommended that signs of hypermetabolism (metabolic and respiratory acidosis, increased body temperature) should be sought after masseter spasm is noted before a diagnosis of malignant hyperthermia is contemplated.[63] In the absence of other definitive signs of hypermetabolism, it does not seem justifiable to subject patients to skeletal muscle biopsies on the basis of masseter spasm alone.[64] It has been suggested, however, that children in whom masseter spasm develops have a 50% incidence of susceptibility to malignant hyperthermia.[65,66] Generalized skeletal muscle rigidity during administration of an anesthetic that includes halothane or succinylcholine may be a more specific predictor of malignant hyperthermia susceptibility than is masseter spasm after administration of succinylcholine.[67] Skeletal muscle biopsies are positive for malignant hyperthermia susceptibility in all patients in whom plasma creatine kinase (CK) concentrations exceed 20,000 IU/L after succinylcholine-induced masseter spasm.[65]

Body temperature increases are often late manifestations of malignant hyperthermia. Indeed the diagnosis of malignant hyperthermia should not depend on increased body temperature. Nevertheless, increased body temperature may be precipitous, increasing at a rate of 0.5°C every 15 minutes and reaching levels as high as 46°C.

Analysis of arterial and central venous blood reveals arterial hypoxemia, hypercarbia ($PaCO_2$ 100 to 200 mmHg), respiratory and metabolic acidosis (pH 7.15 to 6.80), and marked central venous oxygen desaturation. Hyperkalemia may occur early in the course of malignant hyperthermia; but after normothermia returns, the serum potassium concentrations decrease rapidly. Serum concentrations of transaminase enzymes and CK are markedly increased, although peak levels may not occur for 12 to 24 hours after acute episodes. Plasma and urine myoglobin concentrations (gives urine a color similar to that caused by hemoglobin) are also increased, reflecting massive rhabdomyolysis. Late complications of untreated malignant hyperthermia include disseminated intravascular coagulation, pulmonary edema, and acute renal failure. Central nervous system damage may manifest as blindness, seizures, coma, or paralysis. Perioperative and postoperative rhabdomyolysis has been described in patients who were subsequently determined to be susceptible to malignant hyperthermia, suggesting that unexpected development of rhabdomyolysis may be an unusual manifestation of malignant hyperthermia.[68, 69]

Treatment

Successful treatment of malignant hyperthermia depends on early recognition of the diagnosis and institution of a preplanned therapeutic regimen (Table 32–12).[70] Maintenance of appropriate equipment and drugs in central locations in the operating room can save valuable time. Treatment of malignant hyperthermia can be categorized as etiologic or symptomatic. Etiologic treatment is directed at correcting the underlying causative mechanisms. Symptomatic treatment is directed toward maintaining renal function and correcting hyperthermia, acidosis, and arterial hypoxemia.

Etiologic Treatment

Dantrolene, administered intravenously, is the only drug that is reliably effective for the treatment of malignant hyperthermia (Table 32–12).[70] Availability of intravenous dantrolene preparations has decreased mortality due to malignant hyperthermia from more than 70% to less than 5%. Treatment of acute episodes of malignant hyperthermia is with dantrolene, 2 to 3 mg/kg IV. This dose is repeated every 5 to 10 minutes to maximum doses of 10 mg/kg, depending on the patient's temperature and

Table 32–12 • Treatment of Malignant Hyperthermia

Etiologic treatment
    Dantrolene (2–3 mg/kg IV) as an initial bolus, followed with repeat doses every 5–10 minutes until symptoms are controlled (rarely need total dose >10 mg/kg)
    Prevent recrudescence (dantrolene 1 mg/kg IV every 6 hours for 72 hours)
Symptomatic treatment
    Immediately discontinue inhaled anesthetics and conclude surgery as soon as possible
    Hyperventilate the lungs with 100% oxygen
    Initiate active cooling (iced saline 15 ml/kg IV every 10 minutes, gastric and bladder lavage with iced saline, surface cooling)
    Correct metabolic acidosis (sodium bicarbonate 1–2 mEq/kg IV based on arterial pH)
    Maintain urine output (hydration, mannitol 0.25 g/kg IV, furosemide 1 mg/kg IV)
    Treat cardiac dysrhythmias (procainamide 15 mg/kg IV)
    Monitor in an intensive care unit (urine output, arterial blood gases, pH, electrolytes)

metabolic responses. Typically, dantrolene, 2 to 5 mg/kg IV, is required for treatment of acute episodes of malignant hyperthermia. Occasionally, doses higher than 10 mg/kg IV may be needed. In addition, dantrolene should be continued during the postoperative period to prevent possible recrudescence of malignant hyperthermia. One approach is to administer dantrolene, 1 mg/kg IV, every 6 hours for 72 hours after resolution of the acute episode.

Symptomatic Treatment

Symptomatic treatment for malignant hyperthermia includes immediate termination of the administration of the inhaled anesthetics and prompt conclusion of the surgical procedure (Table 32–12).[70] Under no circumstances should the administration of volatile anesthetics be continued with the false hope that anesthetic-induced vasodilation will aid in cooling or that high concentrations of these drugs will decrease the metabolic rate. The patient's lungs are hyperventilated with 100% oxygen, and active cooling is initiated. Active cooling may be done with surface cooling and intracavitary lavage of the stomach and bladder using cold saline solutions. Intravenous saline solutions infused through peripheral intravenous catheters should also be cooled. Cooling is discontinued when body temperature decreases to 38°C. Other symptomatic therapy includes intravenous administration of sodium bicarbonate to correct metabolic acidosis and hyperkalemia, hydration with saline, and maintenance of urine output at 2 ml/kg/hr with administration of osmotic or tubular diuretics. Intravenous administration of glucose with regular insulin helps drive potassium intracellularly and provides an exogenous energy source with which to replace depleted cerebral metabolic substrates. Failure to maintain diuresis may result in acute renal failure due to deposition of myoglobin in the renal tubules. Procainamide, 15 mg/kg IV, can be administered to treat the ventricular dysrhythmias that may occur during malignant hyperthermia.

After recovery from acute episodes of malignant hyperthermia, patients should be closely monitored in an intensive care unit for up to 72 hours. Urine output, arterial blood gases, pH, and serum electrolyte concentrations should be determined frequently. It must be appreciated that malignant hyperthermia may recur in the intensive care unit in the absence of obvious triggering events.[71]

Identification of Susceptible Patients

The advantages of detecting patients susceptible to malignant hyperthermia before anesthesia are obvious. Detailed medical and family histories, with particular reference to previous anesthetic experiences, should be obtained. Prior uneventful anesthetic experiences do not necessarily indicate that patients are not susceptible to malignant hyperthermia. Environmental stress, a consistent trigger of malignant hyperthermia in animals, is also a trigger in humans. Therefore a history of the patient's response to physical exertion may be helpful. The physical examination should focus on the musculoskeletal and cardiac systems. Two distinct myopathic syndromes result in an increased risk of malignant hyperthermia. The first type of myopathy features wasting of the distal ends of the vastus muscles and hypertrophy of the proximal femoris muscles of the thigh. The second myopathy features cryptorchidism, pectus carinatum, kyphosis, lordosis, ptosis, and hypoplastic mandible. The incidence of malignant hyperthermia is increased in patients with Duchenne muscular dystrophy (see Chapter 26). Malignant hyperthermia has also been observed in patients with Burkitt's lymphoma, osteogenesis imperfecta, myotonia congenita, neuroleptic malignant syndrome, and myelomeningocele. There is evidence of cardiac muscle involvement in patients susceptible to malignant hyperthermia. Cardiac findings include ventricular dysrhythmias and abnormal myocardial imaging with radionuclides.

The CK level should be measured in patients being evaluated for susceptibility to malignant hyper-

thermia. About 70% of susceptible patients have increased resting plasma concentrations of CK. By contrast, persons in some families with susceptibility to malignant hyperthermia have normal CK levels. Other conditions, such as muscular dystrophy and skeletal muscle trauma, also produce increased CK concentrations. For these reasons, measurement of CK levels is not a definitive screening test for malignant hyperthermia. Electromyographic changes are present in 50% of patients susceptible to malignant hyperthermia. These findings include an increased incidence of polyphasic action potentials and fibrillation potentials. Patients with exercise-induced rhabdomyolysis may be considered for skeletal muscle biopsies and in vitro contracture tests to determine malignant hyperthermia susceptibility.[72] The complexity of the molecular genetics of malignant hyperthermia precludes DNA-based diagnosis of malignant hyperthermia susceptibility.

Skeletal muscle biopsies with in vitro contracture testing provides definitive confirmation of susceptibility to malignant hyperthermia. Biopsy specimens are typically obtained from the vastus muscles of the thighs using local or regional anesthesia. Histologic changes in skeletal muscles from malignant hyperthermia susceptible patients are not diagnostic. The two most widely used protocols for the diagnosis of malignant hyperthermia susceptibility using in vitro skeletal muscle contracture tests both utilize separate exposures to halothane and caffeine.[73] The combined caffeine-halothane test is associated with a high incidence of false-positive results. The ryanodine contracture test using skeletal muscle biopsies may be the most specific diagnostic test for malignant hyperthermia susceptibility.

Management of Anesthesia

No anesthetic regimen has been shown to be reliably safe for malignant hyperthermia susceptible patients. Nevertheless, certain guidelines should be followed for management of these patients.

Dantrolene Prophylaxis

Prophylaxis for malignant hyperthermia-susceptible patients may be provided with dantrolene, 5 mg/kg PO, in three or four divided doses every 6 hours with the last dose 4 hours preoperatively. This regimen results in therapeutic plasma concentrations of dantrolene at induction of anesthesia and for at least 6 hours (Fig. 32–4).[74] Alternatively, dantrolene 2.4 mg/kg IV, may be administered over 10 to 30 minutes as prophylaxis just prior to induction

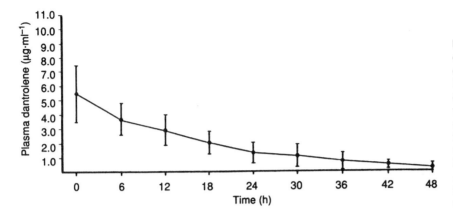

Figure 32-4 • Serum dantrolene concentrations (mean ± SD) at the induction of anesthesia (0) and for the next 48 hours in patients receiving a total dantrolene dose of 5 mg/kg PO in three or four divided doses every 6 hours, with the last dose administered 4 hours preoperatively. (From Allen BC, Cattran CB, Peterson RG, et al. Plasma levels of dantrolene following oral administration in malignant hyperthermia-susceptible patients. Anesthesiology 1988;69:900–4, with permission.)

of anesthesia; and for continued protection, one-half the dose is repeated in 6 hours (Fig. 32–5).[75] Diuresis may accompany intravenous administration of dantrolene, reflecting the addition of mannitol to the dantrolene powder in an effort to make the solution isotonic. For this reason, it is recommended that patients receiving intravenous dantrolene also have a urinary catheter in place. Large doses of dantrolene administered acutely for prophylaxis against malignant hyperthermia may cause nausea, diarrhea, blurred vision, and skeletal muscle weakness, the latter of which skeletal may be sufficient to interfere with adequate ventilation or protection of the lungs from aspiration of gastric fluid.[76] In the absence of signs of malignant hyperthermia intraoper-

atively, it is probably not necessary to continue administration of dantrolene into the postoperative period. Despite prophylaxis with dantrolene, malignant hyperthermia may still develop in the occasional susceptible patient.[77] In view of the potential adverse effects associated with dantrolene therapy, some have concluded that prophylactic use of dantrolene therapy is not necessary in patients suspected to be susceptible to malignant hyperthermia provided all known triggering drugs are avoided.[78, 79]

Drug Selections

Patients susceptible to malignant hyperthermia should be well sedated before induction of anesthesia. Preoperative medication should not include anticholinergic drugs to avoid confusion regarding heart rate changes or possible interference with normal body heat loss. All preparations for the treatment of malignant hyperthermia must be made before induction of anesthesia (see "Treatment"). Drugs that can trigger malignant hyperthermia include volatile anesthetics and succinylcholine. Administration of calcium entry blocking drugs in the presence of dantrolene has been associated with the development of hyperkalemia and myocardial depression.[80] Drugs considered safe for administration to malignant hyperthermia susceptible patients include barbiturates, propofol, opioids, benzodiazepines, ketamine, droperidol, and nondepolarizing muscle relaxants (Table 32–13). Prolonged neuromuscular blockade in response to nondepolarizing muscle relaxants may occur in patients susceptible to malignant hyperthermia who have been pretreated with dantrolene.[81] Nitrous oxide is probably a safe drug to administer to these patients, although its use has been implicated in the onset of malignant hyperthermia.[77] Conceivably, nitrous oxide could influence the course of malignant hyperthermia

DANTROLENE

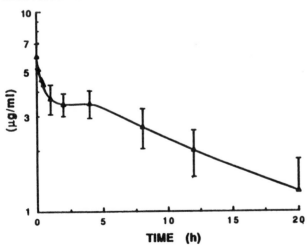

Figure 32-5 • Serum concentrations of dantrolene during the 20 hours following administration of dantrolene 2.4 mg/kg IV to 10 children. (From Lerman J, McLeond ME, Strong HA. Pharmacokinetics of intravenous dantrolene in children. Anesthesiology 1989;70:625–9, with permission.)

Table 32–13 • Nontriggering Drugs for Malignant Hyperthermia

Barbiturates
Propofol
Etomidate
Benzodiazepines
Opioids
Droperidol
Nitrous oxide (?)
Nondepolarizing muscle relaxants
Anticholinesterases
Anticholinergics
Sympathomimetics
Local anesthetics (esters and amides)

indirectly through its capacity to stimulate the sympathetic nervous system. Antagonism of nondepolarizing muscle relaxants has not been shown to trigger malignant hyperthermia in susceptible patients. Vasopressors, digitalis, and methylxanthines are acceptable when specific indications for their use are present.

Anesthesia Machine

No studies have confirmed that malignant hyperthermia can be triggered by residual concentrations of volatile anesthetics delivered from previously used anesthesia machines. Nevertheless, some have advocated use of a "dedicated" anesthesia machine that has never been used to deliver volatile anesthetics for administration of anesthesia to patients susceptible to malignant hyperthermia. A more practical, acceptable alternative is to use a conventional anesthesia machine with a disposable anesthesia breathing circuit and fresh gas outlet hoses, fresh carbon dioxide absorbent, no vaporizers (removed), and a continuous flow of oxygen at 10 L/min for 5 to 20 minutes before using the machine to deliver anesthesia to patients susceptible to malignant hyperthermia.[79, 82]

Regional Anesthesia

Regional anesthesia is an acceptable choice for anesthesia in malignant hyperthermia susceptible patients. In the past, avoidance of amide-based local anesthetics was recommended, as it was believed that these drugs could trigger malignant hyperthermia in susceptible patients. This opinion, however, is probably not valid, and ester- and amide-based local anesthetics are considered acceptable for regional or local anesthesia, as may be needed to perform skeletal muscle biopsies.[79, 83] It must be appreciated that regional anesthesia may not protect against

triggering of malignant hyperthermia due to stress in susceptible patients. Therefore anxiety should be alleviated by sedating these children during regional anesthesia.

Postoperative Discharge Home

Children otherwise suitable for same-day discharge after elective surgical procedures may be admitted to the hospital for overnight observation solely because they are known to be malignant hyperthermia susceptible. There is no evidence to support this practice. Discharge home after minor surgery is not associated with increased risk in these patients.[84]

▌ FAMILIAL DYSAUTONOMIA

Familial dysautonomia (Riley-Day syndrome) is a rare inherited disorder of the central nervous system found almost exclusively in children of Eastern European Jewish ancestry. Inheritance of this syndrome is as an autosomal recessive trait, with symptoms appearing during infancy or early childhood. Approximately 50% of these children die by 4 years of age, usually as the result of respiratory complications. Nevertheless, as a result of improved treatment of this disease, many afflicted children survive to adulthood.

Signs and Symptoms

Dysfunction of the autonomic nervous system is the most apparent manifestation of familial dysautonomia. Vasomotor instability is characterized by sudden alterations in systemic blood pressure, ranging from hypertension to hypotension. Orthostatic hypotension with syncope may occur and reflect defective baroreceptor reflex activity and/or deficient release of norepinephrine. Characteristic findings in these children include failure of the heart rate to increase in response to decreases in systemic blood pressure and an absence of increases in circulating serum concentrations of norepinephrine in response to exercise or on assuming the standing position. Ventilatory responses to arterial hypoxemia and hypercarbia are also depressed. Episodes of systemic hypertension and hyperthermia, often in response to emotional stress, are thought to reflect exaggerated responses to catecholamines (denervation hypersensitivity) and an inability to enlist compensatory parasympathetic nervous system responses. The presence of systemic hypertension distinguishes this disease from Shy-Drager syndrome.

Pain perception is decreased to absent in affected children. There may be a history of repeated episodes of unrecognized trauma. Split-thickness skin grafts have been harvested from these children without anesthesia. Corneal anesthesia and the absence of tears predisposes to corneal ulceration. Taste and thermal discrimination are invariably defective, as evidenced by an inability of these children to distinguish tap water from ice water. The tongue is smooth owing to the absence of fungiform papillae.

The gag reflex and esophageal motility are markedly impaired, predisposing these patients to recurrent pulmonary aspiration. A vomiting crisis characterized by convulsive retching that occurs as often as every 15 to 20 minutes over periods of 1 to 5 days, in association with systemic hypertension and diaphoresis, is a common reason for hospitalizing children with familial dysautonomia. Dehydration and pulmonary aspiration of vomitus may occur during these crises. Hematemesis complicates about 25% of these crises, for which surgical intervention may be necessary. Chlorpromazine, 0.5 to 1.0 mg/kg IM, may be useful for decreasing anxiety and the systemic blood pressure while also acting as an antiemetic.

Temperature control in children with autonomic dysautonomia is erratic. Early morning body temperatures may be 35°C or lower. Conversely, mild infections may trigger marked increases in body temperature and the appearance of febrile seizures. By contrast, major infections may not be accompanied by febrile responses.

Kyphoscoliosis occurs in nearly 90% of these children, reflecting neuromuscular imbalance. Severe kyphoscoliosis may result in restrictive lung disease, culminating in arterial hypoxemia and pulmonary hypertension. About 40% of these patients have a history of epilepsy, most often attributed to fever. Emotional lability and immature, dependent, behavior are characteristic of these patients. Mild mental retardation may be secondary to chronic illness, motor incoordination, and sensory deprivation, rather than being a primary feature of the disease.

Management of Anesthesia

Preoperative assessment of children with familial dysautonomia often includes evaluation of pulmonary function (arterial blood gases, pulmonary function tests), especially if surgery to correct kyphoscoliosis is being planned. Recurrent aspiration may be accompanied by preoperative evidence of pneumonia. Fluid and electrolyte status are of special interest in children with a recent history of protracted vomiting. Atropine, as administered for preoperative medication, does not prevent bradycardia or hypotension during induction of anesthesia in these patients. Use of opioids in the preoperative medication is not recommended, as these children are relatively insensitive to pain. Furthermore, opioids may serve to depress further already blunted ventilatory responses to arterial hypoxemia and hypercarbia.

Induction of anesthesia with conventional intravenous drugs is acceptable. Nitrous oxide plus muscle relaxants are often sufficient for maintenance of anesthesia in children who are relatively insensitive to pain. Nevertheless, fentanyl anesthesia has also been recommended in these children.[85] Stimulation, as associated with tracheal intubation, may result in exaggerated systemic hypertension. In this regard, intermittent administration of volatile anesthetics may be useful, keeping in mind that these drugs can produce precipitous hypotension.[85, 86] Use of nondepolarizing muscle relaxants with minimal circulatory effects seems prudent. Succinylcholine has been administered to these children, although the risk of increased potassium release in patients with progressive neurologic diseases is a consideration. Systemic blood pressure is critically dependent on blood volume in these patients, emphasizing the need for monitoring and prompt replacement of fluid losses. Hypotension is treated with intravenous infusions of crystalloid solutions or administration of small doses of direct-acting vasopressors such as phenylephrine, recognizing that exaggerated increases in systemic blood pressure could accompany the administration of sympathomimetics. Continuous monitoring of systemic blood pressure, cardiac rhythm, and body temperature is important in these patients. Particular care should be taken to avoid corneal abrasions in view of the likely decrease in sensation and tear production in these children. A central venous or pulmonary artery catheter is helpful during major surgery, particularly when cardiopulmonary function is already marginal. Regional anesthesia does not seem to be an attractive choice in view of the cardiovascular instability characteristic of this disease.

Postoperative Management

Complications during the postoperative period include persistent vomiting, pulmonary aspiration, hyperthermia, labile systemic blood pressure, arterial hypoxemia, hypoventilation, and seizures. Increased inspired concentrations of oxygen should be routinely administered to these patients. Continuous monitoring of arterial oxygenation with pulse oximetry and measurement of arterial blood gases and pH is indicated if there is any question regarding the adequacy of oxygenation and/or ventilation. A need for opioids to produce postoperative analgesia is unlikely, as these children have decreased sensory perception. Chlorpromazine has been useful for controlling nausea, hyperthermia, and systemic hypertension during the postoperative period.

■ SOLID TUMORS

Cancer is second only to accidental trauma as a cause of death in children age 1 to 14 years.[35] Although treatment of acute lymphoblastic leukemia was the first recognized success of pediatric oncology, similar success is now being achieved with treatment of malignant solid tumors. Dramatic improvements in survival have been achieved with multimodal therapy (coordination of surgery, chemotherapy, and radiation therapy). In addition to anesthesia for primary tumor excision, there is a continually increasing need for anesthesia for patients undergoing diagnostic and supportive procedures.

Solid tumors that develop in infants and children may be intra-abdominal or retroperitoneal in origin. Nearly 60% of intra-abdominal tumors in children reflect leukemia involving the liver and spleen. Conversely, most intra-abdominal tumors in infants are benign and of renal origin. Retroperitoneal solid tumors are also likely to be of renal origin. Two-thirds of these renal masses are cystic lesions, such as hydronephrosis, and the remainder are nephroblastomas (Wilms' tumors). Neuroblastoma is another example of a solid tumor that tends to occur in the retroperitoneal space.

Neuroblastoma

Neuroblastoma is the most common extracranial solid tumor in infants and children, resulting from malignant proliferation of sympathetic ganglion cell precursors. These tumors may arise anywhere along the sympathetic ganglion chain, but 60% to 75% occur in the adrenal medulla and the retroperitoneal area.

Signs and Symptoms

Children with neuroblastomas typically present with protuberant abdomens, often discovered by the parents. On clinical examination, neuroblastomas are large, firm, nodular, sometimes painful flank masses that are usually fixed to surrounding structures. Ptosis and periorbital ecchymosis secondary to periorbital metastases may be present.

Some children present with pulmonary metastases. Paraspinal neuroblastomas may extend through the neural foramina into the epidural space, producing paralysis. Enlarged peripheral lymph nodes, Horner syndrome, complete to partial absence of the iris, and metastatic enlargement of the liver may also be present. Neuroblastomas may secrete a vasoactive intestinal peptide, which is responsible for persistent watery diarrhea with loss of fluid and electrolytes. These tumors also synthesize catecholamines, but the incidence of hypertension is low.

Diagnosis

Ultrasonography, computed tomography, and magnetic resonance imaging are the primary diagnostic procedures for evaluating abdominal masses in children. Arteriography is helpful for delineating the extent of involvement of the great vessels by the tumors and their resectability. In some children the great vessels are entrapped by tumors such that attempts at complete resection would risk major blood loss. A sonogram may be necessary to demonstrate the extent of involvement of these vessels by tumor. Urinary excretion of vanillylmandelic acid is increased in most children with neuroblastomas, reflecting the metabolism of catecholamines produced by these tumors. Unfortunately, tumors with distant metastases are present in 50% of children at the time of diagnosis. The survival rate for children with neuroblastoma is about 30%.

Treatment

Treatment of neuroblastoma consists of surgical removal, including local metastases and involved lymph nodes. If the tumor cannot be resected completely, a biopsy is performed. Complete resection is delayed until after completion of chemotherapy and/or radiation therapy. Children presenting with signs of spinal cord compression and varying degrees of paralysis may require laminectomy to remove tumors that have extended into the epidural space. Radiation therapy can be given as a palliative or a therapeutic measure. Drugs used for chemotherapy, in varied combinations, include cyclophosphamide, vincristine, and doxorubicin. Possible adverse effects of chemotherapy must be considered during the preoperative evaluation of these patients (see Chapter 28).

Management of Anesthesia

Management of anesthesia for resection of neuroblastomas is as described for children with nephroblastomas.

Nephroblastoma

Nephroblastoma (Wilms' tumor) is the most common malignant renal tumor in children, accounting for 10% of all solid tumors.[35] One-third of these tumors occur in children younger than 1 year of age, and three-fourths are diagnosed by 4 years. The incidence is about 1 in every 13,500 births.

Signs and Symptoms

Nephroblastomas typically present as asymptomatic flank masses in otherwise healthy children. The mass is usually accidentally discovered by the parents or by a physician during a routine physical examination. Nephroblastomas vary in size and are usually firm, nontender, and free from surrounding structures. Pain, fever, and hematuria are usually late manifestations. These children may exhibit malaise, weight loss, anemia, disturbed micturition, and symptoms such as vomiting or constipation due to compression of adjacent portions of the gastrointestinal tract by tumor. Systemic hypertension may be a manifestation of nephroblastoma, particularly if the tumor involves both kidneys. Increases in systemic blood pressure are usually mild; but on rare occasions hypertension is so severe encephalopathy and congestive heart failure develop. Systemic hypertension may reflect renin production by the tumor or indirect stimulation of renin release due to compression of the renal vasculature. Secondary hyperaldosteronism and hypokalemia may be present. Hypertension usually disappears after nephrectomy but may recur if metastases develop.

Diagnosis

Radiography of the abdomen demonstrates a renal mass and occasional calcification. Intravenous pyelography shows distortion of the renal collecting system and occasionally absence of excretion by the involved kidney. This diagnostic test also assesses the function of the contralateral kidney. An inferior vena cavagram may indicate tumor invasion of this blood vessel. An arteriogram shows the extent of the tumor and involvement of the contralateral kidney. Chest radiographs or liver scans may demonstrate metastatic disease.

Treatment

Treatment of nephroblastomas consists of nephrectomy, with or without subsequent radiation and chemotherapy, depending on the stage of involvement. Combined treatment of nephroblastomas is associated with a survival rate approaching 90%.

Extensive tumor may necessitate radical en bloc resection, including portions of the inferior vena cava, pancreas, spleen, and diaphragm. The presence of metastases may require multiple surgical procedures. If the tumor is inoperable at the initial exploration or if the child is in poor clinical condition, radiation therapy is given initially to shrink the tumor, and the child is then surgically reexplored. Prior radiation therapy may produce radiation nephritis of the normal kidney, especially when given in association with chemotherapy. In other patients, renal sparing procedures (partial nephrectomy, enucleation of tumor nodules) before or after chemotherapy are acceptable.[35]

Bilateral nephroblastomas occur in 3% to 10% of children. Two-thirds of these tumors occur at the same time; in the remainder, involvement of the contralateral kidney occurs at a later date. Depending on the magnitude of the tumor involvement, surgical treatment can consist of bilateral partial nephrectomy or bilateral total nephrectomy followed by dialysis and eventually renal transplantation.

Management of Anesthesia

Infants or children scheduled for exploration and resection of neuroblastomas or nephroblastomas are in varying degrees of general health. For example, if the tumor is diagnosed at a late stage, it is likely that the anemia is severe. In addition, adverse effects related to chemotherapy must be considered (see Chapter 28). Anemia is corrected to a hemoglobin concentration of about 10 g/dl. Children scheduled for surgery after radiation and chemotherapy may have a low platelet count, requiring transfusion of platelets before induction of anesthesia. Adequate amounts of blood should be cross-matched preoperatively, as resection of neuroblastomas or nephroblastomas may be associated with excessive surgical blood loss. These children must be well hydrated preoperatively, and their electrolyte and acid-base imbalances must be corrected, especially in the presence of excessive fluid and electrolyte losses due to diarrhea.

In addition to routine monitoring, placing a catheter in a peripheral artery may be recommended to permit constant monitoring of systemic blood pressure and frequent determination of arterial blood gases and pH. Intraoperative hypotension is not uncommon owing to sudden surgical blood loss, which is most likely to occur during dissection of the tumor from around major blood vessels. Catheters for infusion of intravenous fluids should be placed in the upper extremities or the external jugular veins. Lower extremity veins should be avoided, as it may be necessary to ligate or partially resect the inferior vena cava. Measurement of central venous pressure is helpful for evaluating intravascular fluid volume and the adequacy of fluid replacement. Likewise, a Foley catheter to facilitate monitoring urine output aids maintaining an optimal intravascular fluid volume.

Precautions should be taken during induction of anesthesia to prevent pulmonary aspiration, particularly if tumors are causing compression of the gastrointestinal tract. In children in poor general condition, sudden hypotension may develop during the induction of anesthesia, particularly if intravascular fluid volume has not been restored by preoperative infusion of crystalloid or colloid solutions. Systemic hypertension, as is present in some of these children, must be considered and measures taken to prevent excessive increases in systemic blood pressure during tracheal intubation. Although this is usually not a troublesome feature in these patients compared with patients with a pheochromocytoma, it is conceivable that catecholamine-secreting neuroblastomas could cause systemic hypertension similar to that produced by pheochromocytomas. In addition, systemic hypertension may reflect manipulation of the adrenal medulla during resection of the tumor. Manipulation of the inferior vena cava containing metastatic tumor can result in a tumor embolism to the heart or pulmonary artery.[87] This may result in varying degrees of obstruction of blood flow at the level of the right atrium, producing signs characteristic of pulmonary embolism including precipitous hypotension, cardiac dysrhythmias, and cardiac arrest.

Maintenance of anesthesia is acceptably provided with nitrous oxide plus volatile anesthetics or opioids. Muscle relaxants are necessary to optimize surgical exposure. The stomach may be decompressed through a nasogastric tube.

■ ONCOLOGIC EMERGENCIES

Life-threatening oncologic emergencies may develop in children with cancer.

Superior Mediastinal Syndrome

Mediastinal lymph nodes that surround the superior vena cava and trachea may cause compression of these structures if the nodes become invaded by tumor. Although it is desirable to obtain tissue specimens before initiation of therapy, the severity of the airway obstruction may preclude this goal. Most lymphomas are highly sensitive to radiation therapy and radiation can dramatically reduce the size of the tumor. Unfortunately, it may also evoke tissue changes that interfere with a precise histologic diagnosis.

The risk of anesthesia for pediatric patients with untreated mediastinal masses is that ventilation of the lungs may become impossible after loss of consciousness, even with properly placed tracheal tubes.[88] The inability to ventilate the child's lungs through a tracheal tube may require emergent insertion of a rigid bronchoscope beyond the site of obstruction.

Spinal Cord Compression

Spinal cord compression by tumor occurs in about 4% of children with cancer. Tumors most likely to produce this effect are sarcomas, neuroblastomas, lymphomas, and leukemias. Definitive treatment requires radiation therapy or surgery.

Tumor Lysis Syndrome

Tumor lysis syndrome may appear 1 to 5 days after initiation of chemotherapy for highly responsive tumors (lymphomas, leukemias), manifesting as hyperuricemia, hyperkalemia, and hyperphosphatemia. The syndrome is produced by the sudden systemic overload of uric acid and potassium. Uric acid and phosphate deposition in renal tubules may lead to acute renal failure. Hydration and the administration of allopurinol are frequently instituted in attempts to prevent the adverse manifestations of this syndrome. Anesthesia may be necessary for insertion of dialysis access catheters.

■ BURN (THERMAL) INJURIES

Burn (thermal) injuries cause many complications and deaths, with the victims often younger than 15 years of age.[89-91] Survival after burn injuries depends on the patient's age and the percentage of body area burned, with young patients most likely to survive. Burns are classified according to the total body surface area involved, the depth of the burn, and the presence or absence of inhalation injury. The total body surface area burned is calculated using the rule of nines, which accurately predicts the body surface area involved in adults, even modified versions of the rule of nines, however, appear to underestimate the extent of burn injury in children (Figs.

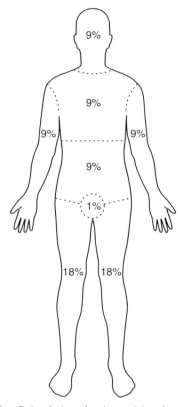

Figure 32–6 • Rule of nines for determining the percentage of body surface area burned in adults. (From MacLennan N, Heimbach DM, Cullen BF. Anesthesia for major thermal injury. Anesthesiology 1998;89:749–70. © 1998, Lippincott Williams & Wilkins, with permission.)

32–6, 32–7).[90] Classification of burn injuries and outcomes are based on the depth of the burn (Table 32–14).[90] Definitions of major burn injuries are based on the percentage of body surface area burned and the area of the body burned (Table 32–15).[91]

Pathophysiology

Burn injuries produce predictable pathophysiologic responses (Table 32–16).[90] Mediators released from the burn wound contribute to local inflammation and burn wound edema.[90] With minor burns, the inflammatory process is limited to the burned area. With major burns, local injury triggers the release of circulating mediators, resulting in systemic responses characterized by hypermetabolism, immunosuppression, and the systemic inflammatory response syndrome (Fig. 32–8).[90] Cytokines appear to be the primary mediators of systemic inflammation after burn injuries. These responses must be considered when formulating plans for management of anesthesia for burned patients.

Cardiac Output

Cardiac output decreases dramatically during the immediate postburn period. The initial decrease precedes any measurable loss of intravascular fluid volume and may reflect the presence of circulating low-molecular-weight myocardial depressant factors.[92] Subsequently, cardiac output is even more profoundly depressed by acute hypovolemia, which occurs as third-space fluid shifts lead to decreased intravascular fluid volume. Although prompt fluid resuscitation results in the return of urine flow within 3 hours, cardiac output remains decreased until the beginning of the second postburn day. Intense vasoconstriction, increased metabolic demands, and hemolysis of erythrocytes further strain the myocardium. Sudden circulatory decompensation may occur if the depressant effects of volatile anesthetics are superimposed.

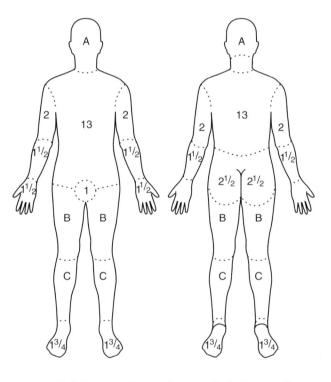

Relative percentages of areas affected by growth (age in years)

Area	0	1	5	10	15	Adult
A: Half of head	$9^{1}/_{2}$	$8^{1}/_{2}$	$6^{1}/_{2}$	$5^{1}/_{2}$	$4^{1}/_{2}$	$3^{1}/_{2}$
B: Half of thigh	$2^{3}/_{4}$	$3^{1}/_{4}$	4	$4^{1}/_{4}$	$4^{1}/_{2}$	$4^{3}/_{4}$
C: Half of leg	$2^{1}/_{2}$	$2^{1}/_{2}$	$2^{3}/_{4}$	3	$3^{1}/_{4}$	$3^{1}/_{2}$

Figure 32–7 • Methods to determine the percentage of body surface area burned in children. (From MacLennan N, Heimbach DM, Cullen BF. Anesthesia and major thermal injury. Anesthesiology 1998;89:749–70. © 1998, Lippincott Williams & Wilkins, with permission.)

Table 32-14 • Classification of Burn Injuries

Classification	Depth of Burn Injury	Outcome and Treatment
First degree (superficial)	Epidermis	Heals spontaneously
Second degree (partial thickness)		
Superficial dermal burn	Epidermis and upper dermis	Heals spontaneously
Deep dermal burn	Epidermis and deep dermis	Requires excision and grafting for rapid return of function
Third-degree (full thickness)	Destruction of epidermis and dermis	Wound excision and grafting required Some limitation of function and scar formation
Fourth degree	Skeletal muscles Fascia Bone	Complete excision Limited function

Adapted from: MacLennan N, Heimbach DM, Cullen BF. Anesthesia for major thermal injury. Anesthesiology 1998;89:749–70.

After the initial 24 hours of fluid resuscitation the circulatory system enters a hyperdynamic state that persists well into the postburn period. The systemic blood pressure and heart rate are increased, and cardiac output stabilizes at about twice normal. Pulmonary artery occlusion pressures are within low-normal ranges unless high-output congestive heart failure supervenes. Pulmonary edema is rare during the initial few days of fluid resuscitation but is encountered later during the first postburn week, when edema fluid is being resorbed and intravascular fluid volume is maximally increased.

Systemic Hypertension

Approximately 30% of children with extensive thermal injury become hypertensive during the postburn period. The onset of systemic hypertension is usually within the first 2 weeks. Males younger than 10 years of age are at greatest risk for the development of systemic hypertension. Systemic hypertension is usually transient but on occasion persists

several weeks. Indeed, left untreated, hypertensive encephalopathy manifesting as irritability and headache, with or without seizures, develops in about 10% of these children. The etiology of systemic hypertension is unknown but may be related to increased serum concentrations of catecholamines and/or activation of the renin-angiotensin system. Treatment with antihypertensive drugs, such as hydralazine or nitroprusside, is needed in some children.

Intravascular Fluid Volume

Intravascular fluid volume deficits after thermal injury are roughly proportional to the extent and depth of the burn injury. After burn injuries fluid accumulates rapidly in the injured area and to a lesser extent in unburned tissues. If burn injuries involve at least 10% to 15% of the total body surface area, hypovolemic shock develops unless there is effective, rapid intervention.[91]

On the first postburn day, the vascular compartment becomes permeable to plasma proteins, including fibrinogen. This increased permeability exists throughout the vascular system but is most pronounced in the area of the burn injury. Extravasated plasma proteins exert an osmotic pressure that can hold large volumes of fluid in an extravascular third space. Severe hypoproteinemia is the primary cause of tissue edema. Pulmonary capillary permeability does not increase unless smoke inhalation occurs. Consequently, colloids do not need to be withheld during the early phases of resuscitation. The loss of fluid from the vascular compartment on the first postburn day is about 4 mg/kg for each percent of body surface burned. For example, in a 40 kg child with a 50% burn, fluid needed for the first 24 hours would be 8000 ml. The most effective restoration of intravascular fluid volume occurs

Table 32-15 • Definition of Major Burns

Third-degree (full-thickness) burn injuries involving more than 10% of the total body surface area

Second-degree (partial-thickness) burn injuries involving more than 25% of the total body surface area in adults (at extremes of age 20% of total body surface area)

Burn injuries involving the face, hands, feet, or perineum

Inhalation burn injuries

Chemical burn injuries

Electrical burn injuries

Burn injuries in patients with serious co-existing medical diseases

Adapted from: MacLennan N, Heimbach DM, Cullen BF. Anesthesia for major thermal injury. Anesthesiology 1998;89:749–70.

Table 32–16 • Pathophysiologic Responses Evoked by Burn Injuries

Cardiovascular responses
  Early
    Hypovolemia (burn shock)
    Impaired myocardial contractility
  Late
    Systemic hypertension
    Tachycardia
    Increased cardiac output
Pulmonary responses
  Early direct effects
    Upper airway obstruction (burns)
    Effects of smoke inhalation (chemical pneumonitis, carbon monoxide)
    Asphyxia
  Early indirect effects
    Effects of inflammatory mediators
    Pulmonary edema (complication of resuscitation)
  Late direct effects
    Chest wall restriction (thoracic burn injuries)
  Late indirect effects (complications of ventilation and airway management)
    Oxygen toxicity
    Barotrauma
    Infections
    Laryngeal damage
    Tracheal stenosis
Metabolism and thermoregulation
  Increased metabolic rate
  Increased carbon dioxide production
  Increased oxygen utilization
  Impaired thermoregulation
Renal and electrolyte responses
  Early
    Decreased renal blood flow
    Myoglobinuria
    Hyperkalemia (tissue necrosis)
  Late
    Increased renal blood flow
    Variable drug clearance
    Hypokalemia (diuresis)
Endocrine responses
  Increased serum norepinephrine concentrations
  Hyperglycemia (susceptible to development of nonketotic hyperosmolar coma)
Gastrointestinal responses
  Stress ulcers
  Impaired gastrointestinal barrier to bacteria
  Endotoxemia
Coagulation and rheology
  Early
    Activation of thrombotic and fibrinolytic systems
    Hemoconcentration
    Hemolysis
  Late
    Anemia
Immune responses
  Impaired immune function (sepsis, pneumonia)
  Endotoxemia
  Multiple organ system failure

Adapted from: MacLennan N, Heimbach DM, Cullen BF. Anesthesia for major thermal injury. Anesthesiology 1998;89:749–70.

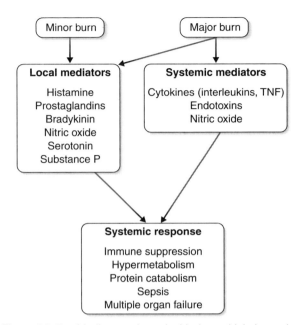

Figure 32–8 • Mediators released with thermal injuries and responses to their release. (From MacLennan N, Heimbach DM, Cullen BF. Anesthesia for major thermal injury. Anesthesiology 1998;89:749–70. © 1998, Lippincott Williams & Wilkins, with permission.)

when two-thirds of this fluid is given within the first 8 hours after the burn.

On the second postburn day, capillary integrity is largely restored, and fluid and plasma protein losses are markedly decreased. Decreasing amounts of fluid are required to maintain the intravascular fluid volume. Further rapid administration of electrolyte solutions at this time may result in edema in excess of any gain in circulatory dynamics. Therefore infusion of crystalloid solutions are decreased after the first postburn day, and colloid solutions are administered.

Airway

Direct burn injuries to the airway, with the exception of steam inhalation, does not occur below the level of the vocal cords, reflecting the low thermal capacity of air and the efficient cooling ability of the upper air passages. Burn or chemical injuries of the upper airway, however, can cause severe edema. Laryngeal edema manifesting as hoarseness, stridor, and tachypnea demand prompt airway evaluation, as swelling of supraglottic tissues can result in sudden, complete upper airway obstruction within hours after the original thermal injury. Fiberoptic laryngoscopy is indicated if the diagnosis of upper airway edema is in doubt. The airway should be secured before respiratory decompensation occurs, as translaryngeal tracheal intubation after progression of edema of the airway is likely to be difficult. Tracheal intubation may be required for several days until edema subsides. The small caliber of the child's airway accentuates the impact of airway edema on resistance to breathing. If tracheal intubation is required for a child, a nasotracheal tube may be preferred, as this placement is more comfortable and easily secured than an oral tube.

Tracheostomy is reserved for patients who show late pulmonary complications that require prolonged ventilatory support. Performance of a tracheotomy in burned children with swelling of the face and neck is a formidable surgical challenge. Early complications of tracheostomy in burn patients include hemorrhage, pneumothorax, and malposition of the tracheostomy tube; late complications are related to mechanical factors (displacement of the cannula) and to cannula erosion into blood vessels with massive hemorrhage.

Smoke Inhalation

Inhalation of suspended particles (smoke) and toxic products of incomplete combustion results in chemical pneumonitis similar to that resulting from aspiration of acidic gastric fluid. Most individuals with smoke inhalation have associated face and neck burns or a history of being trapped in a closed space. Smoke inhalation victims often experience asymptomatic periods lasting as long as 48 hours before respiratory distress becomes overt. Initial chest radiographs may be clear, but the PaO_2 is consistently decreased while these individuals are breathing room air. Production of carbonaceous sputum and detection of wheezes and rales during auscultation of the chest herald impending ventilatory failure.

Treatment of respiratory distress related to smoke inhalation is symptomatic. Administration of warm humidified oxygen and bronchodilators is indicated. Early institution of positive-pressure ventilation of the lungs with positive end-expiratory pressure should be considered if the PaO_2 is less than 60 mmHg while breathing room air. Prophylactic antibiotic administration is not beneficial, and the value of corticosteroids is controversial. Extracorporeal membrane oxygenation has been attempted, but the results have not been encouraging. A catheter placed in a peripheral artery is useful for monitoring patients with symptomatic smoke inhalation injury. The presence of cardiac dysfunction in association with ventilatory distress is often an indication to place a pulmonary artery catheter.

Carbon Monoxide

Carbon monoxide poisoning often complicates burns that occur in closed spaces and is the most common immediate cause of death from fires (see Chapter 30). Measurement of carboxyhemoglobin concentrations can serve as a useful diagnostic marker of smoke inhalation.[91] The best treatment for carbon monoxide poisoning is ventilation of the victim's lungs with 100% oxygen, which decreases the half-life of carboxyhemoglobin from 4 to 6 hours to 40 to 80 minutes.

Restrictive Burn Injuries

Mechanical factors resulting from burn injuries may interfere with pulmonary function. For example, circumferential burns of the chest and upper abdomen can lead to restricted chest wall motion, as the eschar contracts and hardens. This restriction is further aggravated by ileus and abdominal distension. Escharotomies may be necessary to relieve the restriction.

Metabolism and Thermoregulation

The metabolic rate increases in proportion to the extent of burn injury. The metabolic rate can be more than doubled in individuals with burn injury involving 50% of the body surface area. Total parenteral nutrition may be required to meet these increased metabolic requirements. Accompanying these hypermetabolic responses, the metabolic thermostat is reset upward so burn patients tend to increase skin and core temperatures somewhat above normal, regardless of the environmental temperatures. Early enteral alimentation of burn patients has several benefits, including attenuation of the hypermetabolic responses to burn injury.[93] Early enteral feedings also maintains intestinal integrity and retards the absorption of bacteria and endotoxins.

Thermoregulatory functions of the skin, including vasoactivity, sweating, piloerection, and insulation, are abolished or diminished by thermal injury. In addition, skin no longer functions as an effective water vapor barrier, resulting in the loss of ion-free water. It is estimated that daily evaporative water loss is equivalent to 4000 ml/m² of burn surface in children, compared with 2500 ml/m² in adults.[93] Assuming that 0.58 calories is lost for each milliliter of evaporative water loss, a 4000 ml water loss would represent daily energy losses of about 2400 calories. Failure of occlusive dressings or increased ambient temperatures to lower the metabolic rate substantially confirms that the hypermetabolism of burn patients does not relate exclusively to loss of water and heat through the areas of burn injury. In children, intense vasoconstriction in the nonburned areas of skin can result in an increased body temperature sufficient to cause febrile seizures. Conversely, when metabolism and peripheral vasoconstriction are depressed, as during general anesthesia, children with burn injuries may experience a rapid decrease in body temperature.

Gastrointestinal Tract

Adynamic ileus is virtually universal after burn injuries of more than 20% of the body surface area. Therefore, early decompression of the stomach through a nasogastric tube is indicated. Acute ulceration of the stomach or duodenum, known as Curling's ulcer, is the most frequent life-threatening gastrointestinal complication. The precise etiology of Curling's ulcer is unknown, but it occurs most frequently in patients with sepsis or extensive burn injuries. Duodenal ulcers occur twice as frequently in children with burn injuries as in adults (14% versus 7%). Most patients with Curling's ulcer can be managed conservatively with antacids or H_2-antagonist drugs, but occasional patients require vagotomy with or without partial gastrectomy.

Acalculous cholecystitis may occur during the second or third postburn week. Prompt cholecystectomy is indicated to treat this complication. A superior mesenteric artery syndrome may occur at the time of maximum weight loss in burn patients. If conservative therapy fails, duodenojejunostomy or other intra-abdominal surgery may be required.

Renal Function

Immediately after burn injury, cardiac output and intravascular fluid volume decrease and plasma catecholamine concentrations increase, resulting in decreased renal blood flow and glomerular filtration rates. Diminished renal blood flow activates the renin-angiotensin-aldosterone system and stimulates the release of antidiuretic hormone. The net effect on renal function is retention of sodium and water and exaggerated losses of potassium, calcium, and magnesium. Later, after adequate fluid resuscitation, renal blood flow and glomerular filtration may increase dramatically.

Hourly urine output remains the most readily available guide to the adequacy of fluid resuscitation. For example, urine output should be about 1.0 ml/kg/hr in adequately hydrated children. Renal failure is rare in children who have received adequate fluid resuscitation unless there are extensive electrical burns or massive burn injuries of skeletal muscles. In the latter circumstance, hemochromogens may be released into the circulation and precipitate in renal tubules, leading to acute tubular necrosis.

Electrolytes

Increased serum potassium concentrations due to tissue necrosis and hemolysis are common during the first two postburn days. This is followed over the next several days by marked hypokalemia due to accentuated renal loss of potassium. Diarrhea and gastric suction further exaggerate the potassium loss. Cardiac dysrhythmias may occur in hypokalemic patients who receive drugs that promote intracellular movement of potassium (insulin, glucose, sodium bicarbonate) or drugs that oppose the myocardial conduction effects of potassium (calcium). Digitalis administration is particularly hazardous in these patients and should not be used prophylactically.

Serum concentrations of ionized calcium may be decreased during postburn periods. Because children are more sensitive than adults to the effects of citrate and potassium in stored blood, children with extensive burn injuries who are receiving large volumes of rapidly infused whole blood should receive 1 to 2 mg of calcium gluconate, for every milliliter of infused blood.

Endocrine Responses

Endocrine responses to burn injuries are characterized by massive outpourings of corticotropin, antidiuretic hormone, renin, angiotensin, aldosterone, glucagon, and catecholamines. Serum concentrations of insulin may be increased or decreased. Nevertheless, serum glucose concentrations are increased owing to increased concentrations of glucagon and catecholamine-induced glycogenolysis in the liver and skeletal muscles. Indeed, glycosuria occurs frequently in nondiabetic burn patients. Burn patients may be particularly susceptible to the development of nonketotic hyperosmolar coma, especially if total parenteral nutrition is being used.

Maximum increases in serum norepinephrine levels occur 3 to 4 days after the burn and may remain increased for several days. Peak serum concentrations of norepinephrine may be 26 times normal. These markedly increased serum catecholamine concentrations produce intense vasoconstriction of the skin and splanchnic vessels. Increased serum norepinephrine levels have been implicated as a causative factor for many of the adverse manifestations of burn injuries in children, including ischemia of the gastrointestinal tract, liver dysfunction, Curling's ulcer, oliguria, disseminated intravascular coagulation, cardiac dysfunction, hypertensive crises, and increased body temperature. Occasionally, peripheral vasodilators, such as hydralazine, are infused during the early postburn period to offset vasoconstriction and improve tissue perfusion.

Rheology

Blood viscosity increases acutely after thermal injury and remains increased for several days after the burn, even after the hematocrit has returned to normal. After transient decreases, increased serum concentrations of fibrinogen and factors V and VIII persist for several weeks. This hypercoagulable state may give rise to disseminated intravascular coagulation, the diagnosis of which is difficult, as serum concentrations of fibrin split products are almost invariably increased following thermal injury.

Hemolysis of erythrocytes in response to burn injuries is not extensive. Therefore early transfusions of whole blood or packed erythrocytes, in the absence of other indications, is rarely necessary. Nevertheless, generalized suppression of erythrocyte production and decreased erythrocyte survival time follow burn injuries and may persist well into the postburn period. Therefore transfusions of erythrocytes is often needed by about the fifth postburn day to maintain the hemoglobin concentration above 10 g/dl.

Immunology

Leukocyte function is depressed, and levels of immunoglobulins G and M are low after burn injuries. Gram-negative bacteremia is associated with increased mortality. Pneumonia, suppurative thrombophlebitis, and bacterial invasion of the burn eschar are likely explanations for sepsis. Aseptic technique must be strictly observed by all those participating in the care of burned children.

Liver Function

Liver function tests are frequently abnormal in burn patients, even when the areas of burn injury are small. Overt liver failure is uncommon, however, unless the postburn course is complicated by hypotension, sepsis, or multiple blood transfusions.

Management of Anesthesia

Successful anesthesia for excision and grafting of burn injuries requires preoperative assessment and preparation (Table 32–17).[90] Historic information regarding the time and type of burn injury is pertinent for the management of anesthesia in acutely burned children.[94] For example, the time of burn injury is important, as initial fluid requirements are based

Table 32–17 • Anesthetic Considerations for Excision and Grafting of Major Burn Injuries

Preoperative medication
    Provide adequate analgesia
    Limit period of fluid fasting
Vascular access
    Establish appropriate intravenous access
    Consider invasive monitoring
Airway management
    Consider alternatives to direct laryngoscopy
    Consider awake fiberoptic intubation (neck or facial contractures)
Ventilation
    Minute ventilation requirements increased (increased metabolic rate, parenteral hyperalimentation)
    Mechanical ventilation (smoke inhalation, acute respiratory failure)
Fluids and blood
    Anticipate possibility of rapid and large blood loss
    Evaluate coagulation status
Temperature regulation
    Increase ambient temperatures of the operating rooms
    Warm intravenous fluids
Anesthetic drugs
    Include opioids
    Consider effects of increased circulating catecholamine concentrations
Muscle relaxants
    Avoid succinylcholine
    Anticipate resistance to neuromuscular blocking effects of nondepolarizing muscle relaxants
Postoperative period
    Anticipate increased analgesic (opioids) requirements

Adapted from: MacLennan N, Heimbach DM, Cullen BF. Anesthesia for major thermal injury. Anesthesiology 1998;89:749–70.

on the time elapsed since the burn occurred. Children who were trapped in closed spaces are likely to have experienced smoke inhalation injury. Electrical burns may produce far more tissue destruction than the surface burns indicate (see ''Electrical Burns'').

The physical examination should focus on the status of the patient's airway. Head and neck burns, burned nasal hairs, and hoarseness are signs that supraglottic edema may develop or is already present. Carbonaceous sputum, wheezing, or diminished breath sounds suggest the presence of smoke inhalation injury. Abdominal distension may indicate ileus, warranting special precautions during the induction of anesthesia to decrease the risk of pulmonary aspiration. A careful search should be made during the preoperative evaluation for sites suitable for placing intravenous catheters and monitoring devices.

Measurement of arterial blood gases and pH and evaluation of chest radiographs are indicated in patients suspected of having experienced smoke inhalation. Serum carboxyhemoglobin concentrations are helpful only for the first few hours after burn injuries. In the presence of carboxyhemoglobin, the pulse oximeter may overestimate saturation of hemoglobin with oxygen, emphasizing the need for caution in relying solely on this monitor in patients who have recently experienced carbon monoxide exposure.[95] Serum glucose concentrations and osmolarity are determined, particularly if burn patients are receiving total parenteral nutrition. Measures of renal function are indicated after extensive electrical burns. The adequacy of fluid replacement can be judged by urine output, which should be about 1 ml/kg/hr. Coagulation profiles should be obtained in patients in whom extensive intraoperative blood loss is anticipated.

Establishing intravenous infusion lines may be difficult in severely burned individuals. In some instances, it is necessary to use veins in areas that have escaped burn injury, such as the axilla, scalp, or web spaces between the digits. Reliable intravenous catheters of sufficient caliber are essential for patients undergoing excision of burn eschars, as large amounts of blood can be lost in brief periods of time. Even split-thickness skin grafts are associated with about 80 ml of blood loss for each 100 cm² of skin that is harvested for grafting.[92]

Children with extensive burn injuries may require intensive monitoring, yet not have an unburned limb available for placing a blood pressure cuff. Catheters placed in peripheral arteries occasionally must be inserted through burn eschars. Septic complications are likely, such that catheters placed through eschars should be removed as soon as possible. Venous cannulation sites are likewise vulnerable to septic complications. Decreases in body temperature are exaggerated during the intraoperative period, reflecting the loss of the insulating properties of the skin, evaporative loss of water from eschars, and depression of the metabolic rate by general anesthesia. Routine measures for decreasing heat loss include the use of warming blankets and radiant overhead warmers. Inspired gases may be warmed and humidified, and intravenous fluids are administered through a warmer. Ambient temperatures of the operating room should be maintained near 25°C. Plastic or paper drapes decrease evaporative and convective heat losses.

A number of pathophysiologic alterations produced by burn injuries affect drug responses.[90] Immediately after burn injury, organ and tissue blood flow is decreased as a result of hypovolemia, depressed myocardial function, and release of vasoactive substances. Absorption of drugs administered by any route other than intravenously is predictably delayed. Intravenous and inhaled drugs may have increased effects on the brain and heart because of relative increases in blood flow to these organs. After adequate fluid resuscitation, the hypermetabolic phase begins about 48 hours after burn injury. During this time oxygen and glucose consumption are markedly increased. Serum albumin concentrations are decreased after burn injuries; thus albumin-bound drugs (benzodiazepines, anticonvulsants) have increased circulating free and pharmacologically active fractions. Conversely, serum concentrations of α_1-acid glycoprotein are increased, so drugs bound to this protein (muscle relaxants, tricyclic antidepressant drugs) have decreased free fractions. Pharmacologic alterations may persist after recovery from burn injuries. It has been shown that thiopental requirements are increased in children for more than 1 year after burn injuries (Fig. 32–9).[96] Opioid requirements may also be decreased in burn patients.

Of all the classes of drugs, the effects of burn injury on muscle relaxants have been studied most extensively. Hyperkalemic responses to succinylcholine are well known. The risk of hyperkalemia is probably related to the severity of the burn injury and the time elapsed from the burn injury to succinylcholine administration. The greatest risk appears to be 10 to 50 days after the burn injury. Nevertheless, these zones are poorly defined, and the safest recommendation may be to avoid succinylcholine. Several studies have shown that burn patients develop marked resistance (up to threefold increases in dose requirements) to nondepolarizing muscle relaxants (Fig. 32–10).[94, 97, 98] Approximately 30% or more of the body must be burned to produce resistance to nondepolarizing muscle relaxants, manifesting about 10 days after burn injury, peaking at 40 days, and declining after about 60 days.[97] Despite this typical time sequence, one report described prolonged resistance to the effects of nondepolarizing muscle relaxants that was still present after 463 days.[98] Pharmacodynamic explanations as the principal mechanisms for resistance to effects of nondepolarizing muscle relaxants are documented by the need to achieve higher serum drug concentrations to produce given degrees of twitch suppression in burn-injured patients compared with non-burn-injured patients.[99] It is speculated that proliferation of extrajunctional cholinergic receptors is responsible for this resistance to the effects produced by nondepolarizing muscle relaxants. This increased number of extrajunctional cholinergic receptors would also increase the available sites for potassium exchange to occur after administration of succinylcholine to burn-injured patients, leading to the possibility of hyperkalemia. Despite these theories, there is evidence that burn injuries are not associated with an increased number of extrajunctional cholinergic re-

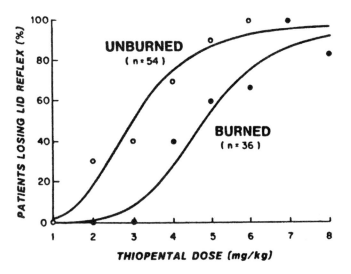

Figure 32–9 • Doses of thiopental administered intravenously to produce loss of the lid reflex were increased in burned children (more than 15% body surface area burn and more than 1 year after injury) compared with those in unburned children. (From Cote CJ, Petkau AJ. Thiopental requirements were increased in children reanesthetized at least 1 year after recovery from extensive thermal injury. Anesth Analg 1985;64:1156–60, with permission.)

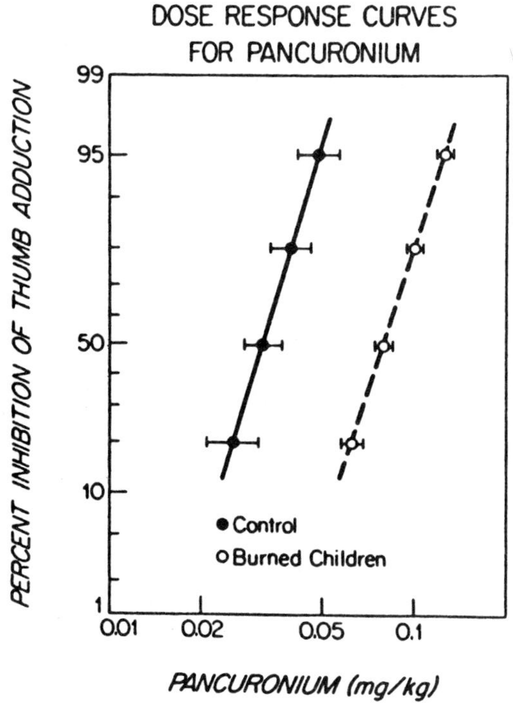

DOSE RESPONSE CURVES FOR PANCURONIUM

PERCENT INHIBITION OF THUMB ADDUCTION

PANCURONIUM (mg/kg)

● Control
○ Burned Children

Figure 32–10 • Doses of pancuronium administered intravenously to produce inhibition of thumb adduction were greater in burned children [body surface area burn 4%–85% and studied 34 ± 7.9 (mean ± SE) days after injury] than in control children. (From Martyn JAJ, Liu LMP, Szyfelbein SK, et al. The neuromuscular effects of pancuronium in burned children. Anesthesiology 1983;59:561–4, with permission.)

ceptors.[100] Instead, altered affinity of cholinergic receptors for acetylcholine or nondepolarizing muscle relaxants may be the basis for burn injury-induced resistance to these drugs. Responses to mivacurium in patients with burn injuries are normal.[101]

Ketamine has been utilized for years for anesthesia in burn injury patients, especially for dressing changes and escharotomy. The drug can be administered intravenously or intramuscularly with good effect. Administration of ketamine is often preceded by anticholinergic drugs, as excessive salivation is likely. Ketamine, 1 to 2 mg/kg IV, provides excellent somatic analgesia for skin grafting procedures. Recovery of consciousness from single intravenous doses of ketamine is usually rapid, allowing early return to oral nutritional support. Nitrous oxide can be administered to decrease random motion of the patient's limbs, which often accompanies ketamine anesthesia. The incidence of postoperative delirium after administration of ketamine to pediatric patients appears to be minimal; but if central nervous system effects occur, they can be at least partially reversed by administration of physostigmine, 30 μg/kg IV. Excessive movement during emergence from anesthesia may dislodge skin grafts or promote hemorrhage, resulting in early graft loss. Sevoflurane is the most likely inhaled drug to be used for anesthesia in children with burn injuries. This volatile anesthetic permits maintenance of spontaneous ventilation and administration of high inspired concentrations of oxygen, if necessary. The depth of anesthesia can be adjusted for the surgical stimulus, such that increased delivered concentrations of sevoflurane can be administered during high-intensity stimulation associated with harvesting skin grafts. Application of skin grafts is essentially painless, and concentrations of sevoflurane can be decreased during this time.

■ ELECTRICAL BURNS

High-voltage electrical currents cause tissue damage by conversion to thermal energy. The amount of thermal energy transferred to tissues depends on the voltage of the electrical source, the skin resistance of the victim, and the duration of the contact with the source of the electrical current. Tissue damage is greatest where the electrical current is most concentrated, as occurs at points of entry and exit, and where the involved extremities are narrowest. Visceral injuries due to electrical current are unlikely.

Signs and Symptoms

Deep tissue destruction produced by electrical burns is often extensive, as these tissues cannot dissipate thermal energy as rapidly as more superficial tissues. This makes the extent of damage produced by electrical currents difficult to judge from the extent of visible superficial injuries. Fasciotomies, multiple débridements of wounds, and arteriograms to define the level of viability of affected limbs may be necessary.

Cardiopulmonary arrest requiring cardiopulmonary resuscitation may have occurred at the time of the electrical injury. Cardiac dysrhythmias occur in one of every six patients who experience electrical burns. These patients should be monitored by continuous displays of the electrocardiogram for at least the first 48 hours after the burn.

Renal failure may accompany electrical burns, reflecting precipitation of myoglobin from injured skeletal muscles in renal tubules. Furthermore, the extent of superficial tissue damage may result in underestimating the initial fluid requirements. Nevertheless, with recognition of deep tissue injuries accompanying electrical burns and concurrent administration of fluids and diuretics to maintain urine output close to 1 mg/kg/hr, renal failure should be uncommon.

Neurologic complications following electrical burns are common. Peripheral nerve deficits or spinal cord deficits can occur early, reflecting direct injury of nerves, or later as a result of perineural scarring or neural ischemia. Neuropathies may involve nerves far removed from the points of electical contact and may progress for several years after the

injury. Cataract formation is another late sequela of electrical burn injury.

A common type of electrical burn in children occurs when the child bites through an electrical cord. The resulting burn usually involves the oral commissures. Subsequent scar formation can narrow the oral opening, leading to difficulty maintaining the upper airway or accomplishing tracheal intubation during corrective surgery.

Lightning

Injuries due to lightning represent a special form of electrical burn. Lightning tends to flow around the exterior of its victim, resulting in superficial flash burns rather than deep tissue burn injuries, as are characteristic of electrical burns. Transient neurologic deficits and cardiac dysrhythmias are common after injuries due to lightning. Most deaths associated with lightning are due to cardiopulmonary arrest at the time of the injury.

■ SEPARATION OF CONJOINED TWINS

Surgical separation of conjoined twins requires thorough preoperative preparation and discussion among surgeons, pediatricians, and anesthesiologists.[102–104] Detailed rehearsals of the entire procedure, beginning with transportation to the operating room, serve to emphasize the needs and responsibilities of all involved. Preoperative evaluation demonstrates whether there are shared organ systems. Management of anesthesia requires two teams and separate anesthsia machines, delivery systems, ventilators, and monitoring systems. Ultimately, a second operating room table is required.

Awake tracheal intubation before administration of muscle relaxants is often recommended but not mandatory.[102] Monitoring must be extensive and invasive (central venous pressure, intra-arterial blood pressure) to facilitate prompt, appropriate replacement of fluid and blood losses and to provide indications of the adequacy of oxygenation and ventilation. Maintenance of body temperature is important. Monitoring the serum concentrations of ionized calcium and appropriate replacement are useful for maintaining myocardial contractility and optimizing coagulation.[103] Color coding of all vascular lines, monitors, apparatus, records, and personnel is useful. The presence of cross-circulation means that drugs administered to one infant are likely to produce detectable effects in the other infant. The magnitude of cross-circulation may vary from minute to minute, making prediction of drug effects difficult.

Aggressive efforts are required to maintain normothermia. Metabolic acidosis may be prominent and require treatment with sodium bicarbonate. The need for continued support of ventilation of the separated twin's lungs is likely during the postoperative period.

References

1. Morray JP, Geiduschek JM, Ramamoorthy C, et al. Anesthesia-related cardiac arrest in children. Anesthesiology 2000;93:6–14
2. Pang LM, Mellins RB. Neonatal cardiorespiratory physiology. Anesthesiology 1975;43:171–96
3. Hagen PT, Scholz DG, Edwards WD. Incidence and size of patent foramen ovale during the first 10 decades of life on autopsy study of 965 normal hearts. Mayo Clin Proc 1984;59:17–20
4. Leelanukrom R, Cunliffe AM. Intraoperative fluid and glucose management in children. Paediatr Anaesth 2000;10:353–9
5. Sieber FE, Smith DS, Traystman FJ, et al. Glucose: a reevaluation for its intraoperative use. Anesthesiology 1987;67:72–81
6. Furman EB, Roman DG, Lemmer LAS, et al. Specific therapy in water, electrolyte, and blood volume replacement during pediatric surgery. Anesthesiology 1975;42:187–93
7. Roy WL, Lerman J, McIntyre BG. Is preoperative haemoglobin testing justified in children undergoing minor elective surgery? Can J Anaesth 1991;38:700–3
8. Lerman J, Robinson S, Willis MM, et al. Anesthetic requirement for halothane in young children 0–1 month and 1–6 months of age. Anesthesiology 1983;59:421–4
9. LeDez KM, Lerman J. The minimum alveolar concentration (MAC) of isoflurane in preterm neonates. Anesthesiology 1987;67:301–7
10. Goudsouzian NG. Maturation of neuromuscular transmission in the infant. Br J Anaesth 1980;50:203–8
11. Fisher DM, Campbell PC, Spellman MJ, et al. Pharmacokinetics and pharmacodynamics of atracurium in infants and children. Anesthesiology 1990;73:33–7
12. Fisher DM, Cronnelly R, Miller RD, et al. The neuromuscular pharmacology of neostigmine in infants and children. Anesthesiology 1983;59:220–5
13. Liu LMP, DeCook TH, Goudsouzian NG, et al. Dose response to succinylcholine in children. Anesthesiology 1981;55:599–602
14. Cook DR. Newborn anaesthesia: pharmacological considerations. Can Anaesth Soc J 1986;33:38–42
15. Friesen RH, Lichtor JL. Cardiovascular effects of inhalation induction with isoflurane in the infant. Anesth Analg 1983;62:411–4
16. Murray DJ, Forbes RB, Mahoney LT. Comparative hemodynamic depression of halothane versus isoflurane in neonates and infants: an echocardiographic study. Anesth Analg 1992;74:329–37
17. Cote CJ, Goudsouzian NG, Liu LMP, et al. The dose response of intravenous thiopental for induction of general anesthesia in unpremedicated children. Anesthesiology 1981;55:703–5
18. Westrin P, Jonmarker C, Werner O. Thiopental requirements for induction of anesthesia in neonates and infants one to six months of age. Anesthesiology 1989;71:344–6
19. Northway WH, Moss RB, Carlisle KB, et al. Late pulmonary sequelae of bronchopulmonary dysplasia. N Engl J Med 1990;323:1793–9
20. Phelps DL. Retinopathy of prematurity. N Engl J Med 1992;326:1078–80
21. Reynolds JD, Hardy RJ, Kennedy KA, et al. Lack of efficacy of light reduction in preventing retinopathy of prematurity. N Engl J Med 1998;338:1572–6
22. Gregory GA, Steward DJ. Life-threatening perioperative apnea in the ex-''premie.'' Anesthesiology 1983;59:495–8
23. Kurth CD, LeBard SE. Association of postoperative apnea, airway obstruction, and hypoxemia in former premature infants. Anesthesiology 1991;75:22–6
24. Welborn LG, Hannallah RS, Luban NLC, et al. Anemia and postoperative apnea in former preterm infants. Anesthesiology 1991;74:1003–6
25. Welborn LG, Rice LJ, Hannallah RS, et al. Postoperative apnea in former preterm infants: prospective comparison of spinal and general anesthesia. Anesthesiology 1990;72:838–42
26. Liu LMP, Cote CJ, Goudsouzian NG, et al. Life-threatening apnea in infants recovering from anesthesia. Anesthesiology 1983;59:506–10
27. Dierdorf SF, Krishna G. Anesthetic management of neonatal surgical emergencies. Anesth Analg 1981;60:204–15
28. Adzick NS, Nance ML. Pediatric surgery. N Engl J Med 2000;342:1651–7
29. Baraka A, Akel S, Haroun S, Yazigi A. One lung ventilation of the newborn with tracheoesophageal fistula. Anesth Analg 1988;67:189–91
30. Yaster M, Buck JR, Dudgeon DL, et al. Hemodynamic effects of primary closure of omphalocele/gastroschisis in human newborns. Anesthesiology 1988;69:84–8
31. Bissonnette B, Sullivan PJ. Pyloric stenosis. Can J Anaesth 1991;38:668–76
32. Haselby KA, Dierdorf SF, Krishna G, et al. Anesthetic implications of neonatal necrotizing enterocolitis. Can Anaesth Soc J 1982;29:255–9
33. Al-Salem AH, Adu-Gyamfi Y, Grant CS. Congenital lobar emphysema. Can J Anaesth 1990;37:377–9
34. Cote CJ. The anesthetic management of congenital lobar emphysema. Anesthesiology 1978;49:296–8
35. Adzick NS, Nance ML. Pediatric surgery. N Engl J Med 2000;343:1726–32
36. Jaffe D, Wesson D. Emergency management of blunt trauma in children. N Engl J Med 1991;324:1477–82
37. Kuban KCK, Leviton A. Cerebral palsy. N Engl J Med 1994;330:188–95
38. Nelson KB, Ellenberg JH. Antecedents of cerebral palsy. N Engl J Med 1986;315:81–6
39. Dierdorf SF, McNiece WL, Rao CC, et al. Effect of succinylcholine on plasma potassium in children with cerebral palsy. Anesthesiology 1985;62:88–90
40. Rao CC, Krishna G, Haselby K, et al. Ventriculobronchial fistula complicating a ventriculoperitoneal shunt. Anesthesiology 1977;47:388–90
41. Dierdorf SF, McNiece WL, Rao CC, et al. Failure of succinylcholine to alter plasma potassium in children with myelomeningocele. Anesthesiology 1986;64:272–3
42. Vautrin-Moneret DA, Laxenaire MC, Bavoux F. Allergic shock to latex and ethylene oxide during surgery for spina bifida. Anesthesiology 1990;73:556–8
43. Morray JP, MacGillivrary R, Duker G. Increased perioperative risk following repair of congenital heart disease in Down's syndrome. Anesthesiology 1986;65:221–4
44. Williams JP, Somerville GM, Miner ME, et al. Atlanto-axial subluxation and trisomy-21: another perioperative complication. Anesthesiology 1987;67:253–4
45. Popitz MD. Anesthetic implications of chronic disease of the cervical spine. Anesth Analg 1997;84:672–83

46. Karl HW, Swedlow DB, Lee KW, et al. Epinephrine-halothane interactions in children. Anesthesiology 1983;58:142–5

47. Bell C, Oh TH, Loeffler JR. Massive macroglossia and airway obstruction after cleft palate repair. Anesth Analg 1988;67:71–4

48. Przybylo HJ, Stevenson BW, Vicari FA, et al. Retrograde fiberoptic intubation in a child with Nager's syndrome. Can J Anaesth 1996;43:697–9

49. Chadd GD, Crane DL, Phillips RM, et al. Extubation and reintubation guided by the laryngeal mask airway in a child with the Pierre-Robin syndrome. Anesthesiology 1992;76:640–1

50. Diaz JH. Croup and epiglottitis in children. Anesth Analg 1985;64:621–33

51. Ames WA, Ward VMM, Tranter RMD, et al. Adult epiglottitis: an under-recognized, life-threatening condition. Br J Anaesth 2000;85:795–7

52. Mayo-Smith MF, Hirsch PJ, Wodzinski SF, et al. Acute epiglottitis in adults. N Engl J Med 1986;314:1133–9

53. Muller BJ, Fliegel JE. Acute epiglottitis in a 79-year-old man. Can Anaesth Soc J 1985;32:415–7

54. Crosby E, Reid D. Acute epiglottitis in the adult: is intubation mandatory? Can J Anaesth 1991;38:914–8

55. Spalding MB, Ala-Kokko TI. The use of inhaled sevoflurane for endotracheal intubation in epiglottitis. Anesthesiology 1998;89:1025–6

56. Koka BV, Jeon IS, Andre JM, et al. Postintubation croup in children. Anesth Analg 1977;56:501–5

57. Cohen MM, Cameron CB. Should you cancel the operation when a child has an upper respiratory tract infection? Anesth Analg 1991;72:282–4

58. Damron J-Y, Rauss A, Dreyfuss D, et al. Evaluation of risk factors for laryngeal edema after tracheal extubation in adults and its prevention by dexamethasone. Anesthesiology 1992;77:245–51

59. Litman RS, Ponnuri J, Trogan I. Anesthesia for tracheal or bronchial foreign body removal in children: an analysis of ninety-four cases. Anesth Analg 2000;91:1389–91

60. Borland LM. Anesthesia for children with Jeune's syndrome (asphyxiating thoracic dystrophy). Anesthesiology 1987;66:86–8

61. Hopkins PM. Malignant hyperthermia: advances in clinical management and diagnosis. Br J Anaesth 2000;85:118–28

62. Ording H. Incidence of malignant hyperthermia in Denmark. Anesth Analg 1985;64:700–4

63. Van der Spek AF, Reynolds PIO, Fang WB, et al. Changes in resistance to mouth opening induced by depolarizing and nondepolarizing neuromuscular blockers. Br J Anaesth 1990;64:21–7

64. Saddler JM. Jaw stiffness: an ill understood condition. Br J Anaesth 1991;67:515–6

65. Rosenberg H, Fletcher JE. Masseter muscle rigidity and malignant hyperthermia susceptibility. Anesth Analg 1986;65:161–4

66. Allen GC, Rosenberg H. Malignant hyperthermia susceptibility in adult patients with masseter muscle rigidity. Can J Anaesth 1990;37:31–5

67. Larach MG, Rosenberg H, Larach DR, et al. Prediction of malignant hyperthermia susceptibility by clinical signs. Anesthesiology 1987;66:547–50

68. Harwood TN, Nelson TE. Massive postoperative rhabdomyolysis after uneventful surgery: a case report of subclinical malignant hyperthermia. Anesthesiology 1998;88:265–8

69. Fierobe L, Nivoche Y, Mantz J, et al. Perioperative severe rhabdomyolysis revealing susceptibility to malignant hyperthermia. Anesthesiology 1998;88:263–5

70. Britt BAA. Dantrolene. Can Anaesth Soc J 1984;31:61–75

71. Mathieu A, Bogosian AJ, Ryan JF, et al. Recrudescence after survival of an initial episode of malignant hyperthermia. Anesthesiology 1979;51:454–5

72. Wappler F, Fiege M, Steinfath M, et al. Evidence for susceptibility to malignant hyperthermia in patients with exercise-induced rhabdomyolysis. Anesthesiology 2001;94:95–100

73. Lynch C, Gronert GA. Complex pharmacology of malignant hyperthermia. Anesthesiology 1996;84:1275–9

74. Allen GC, Cattraikn CB, Peterson RG, et al. Plasma levels of dantrolene following oral administration in malignant hyperthermia-susceptible patients. Anesthesiology 1988;67:900–4

75. Lerman J, McLoen ME, Strong HA. Pharmacokinetics of intravenous dantrolene in children. Anesthesiology 1989;70:625–9

76. Watson CB, Reierson N, Norfleet EA. Clinically significant muscle weakness induced by oral dantrolene sodium prophylaxis for malignant hyperthermia. Anesthesiology 1986;65:312–4

77. Ruhland B, Hinkle AJ. Malignant hyperthermia after oral and intravenous pretreatment with dantrolene in a patient susceptible to malignant hyperthermia. Anesthesiology 1984;60:159–60

78. Hackl W, Maurtiz W, Winkler M, et al. Anaesthesia in malignant hyperthermia susceptible patients without dantrolene prophylaxis: a report of 30 cases. Acta Anaesthesiol Scand 1990;34:534–7

79. Lucy SJ. Anaesthesia for caesarean delivery of a malignant hyperthermia susceptible patient. Can J Anaesth 1994;41:1220–6

80. Rubin AS, Zablocki AD. Hyperkalemia, verapamil, and dantrolene. Anesthesiology 1987;66:246–9

81. Dreissen JJ, Wuis EW, Gielen PM. Prolonged vecuronium neuromuscular blockade in a patient receiving orally administered dantrolene. Anesthesiology 1965;62:523–4

82. Beebe JJ, Sessler DI. Preparation of anesthesia machines for patients susceptible to malignant hyperthermia. Anesthesiology 1988;69:395–400

83. Berkowitz A, Rosenberg H. Femoral block with mepivacaine for muscle biopsy in malignant hyperthermia patients. Anesthesiology 1985;62:651–2

84. Yentis SM, Levine MF, Hartley EJ. Should all children with suspected or confirmed malignant hyperthermia susceptibility be admitted after surgery? A 10-year review. Anesth Analg 1992;75:345–50

85. Beilin B, Maayan CH, Vatashsky E, et al. Fentanyl anesthesia in familial dysautonomia. Anesth Analg 1985;64:72–6

86. Stirt JA, Frantz RA, Gunz EF, et al. Anesthesia, catecholamines, and hemodynamics in autonomic dysfunction. Anesth Analg 1982;61:701–4

87. Milne B, Cervenko FW, Morales A, et al. Massive intraoperative pulmonary tumor embolus from renal cell carcinoma. Anesthesiology 1981;54:253–5

88. Ferrari LR, Bedrod RF. General anesthesia prior to treatment of anterior mediastinal masses in pediatric cancer patients. Anesthesiology 1990;72:991–5

89. Smith EI. Acute management of thermal burns in children. Surg Clin North Am 1970;50:807–14

90. MacLennan N, Heimbach DM, Cullen BF. Anesthesia for major thermal injury. Anesthesiology 1998;89:749–70

91. Monafo WW. Initial management of burns. N Engl J Med 1996;335:1581–6

92. Demling RH. Burns. N Engl J Med 1985;313:1389–98

93. Deitch EA. The management of burns. N Engl J Med 1990;323:1249–53

94. Martyn J. Clinical pharmacology and drug therapy in the burned patient. Anesthesiology 1986;65:67–75

95. Barker SJ, Tremper KK. The effect of carbon monoxide inhalation on pulse oximetry and transcutaneous PO₂. Anesthesiology 1987;66:677–9

96. Cote CJ, Petkau AJ. Thiopental requirements may be increased in children reanesthetized at less than one year after recovery from extensive thermal injury. Anesth Analg 1985;64:1156–60

97. Martyn JAJ, Liu MLP, Szyfelbein SK, et al. The neuromuscular effects of pancuronium in burned children. Anesthesiology 1983;59:561–4

98. Martyn JAJ, Matteo RS, Szyfelbein SK, et al. Unprecedented resistance to neuromuscular blocking effects of metocurine with persistence after complete recovery in a burned patient. Anesth Analg 1982;61:614–7

99. Marathe PH, Dwersteg JF, Pavlin EG, et al. Effect of thermal injury on the pharmacokinetics and pharmacodynamics of atracurium in humans. Anesthesiology 1989;70:752–5

100. Marathe PH, Haschke RH, Slattery JT, et al. Acetylcholine receptor density and acetylcholinesterase activity in skeletal muscle of rats following thermal injury. Anesthesiology 1989;70:654–9

101. Martyn JAJ, Goudsouzian NG, Chang YC, et al. Neuromuscular effects of mivacurium in 2 to 12-year-old children with burn injury. Anesthesiology 2000;92:31–7

102. Hoshima H, Tanaka O, Obara H, et al. Thoracopagus conjoined twins: management of anesthetic induction and postoperative chest wall defect. Anesthesiology 1987;66:424–6

103. Georges LS, Smith KW, Wong KC. Anesthetic challenges in separation of craniopagus twins. Anesth Analg 1987;66:783–7

104. Diaz JH, Furman ER. Perioperative management of conjoined twins. Anesthesiology 1987;67:965–73

33

Diseases Associated with Aging

Aging is accompanied by unavoidable alterations in organ system function (physiologic decline) that predisposes elderly patients to homeostatic failure, chronic diseases, and loss of independence in the performance of daily activities (functional decline).[1] Decreased organ system function can often be demonstrated only by stress testing. For example, cardiac function sufficient for sedentary life may become inadequate during the perioperative period if anemia or infection occurs. It is important to recognize that there is not necessarily a correlation between biologic and chronologic age.

PHYSIOLOGIC CHANGES ASSOCIATED WITH AGING

Aging is accompanied by unavoidable declines in organ system function and responses to drugs.[3] As part of the normal aging process, most organ systems lose approximately 1% of their function per year beginning at around 30 years of age. Nevertheless, there is considerable variability in decline. The hallmark of aging is not so much a decline in the resting levels of performance but, rather, lack of functional reserve and inability of organ systems to respond to external stress.[2] Exercise tolerance best reflects the biologic age and is one of the most important predictors of perioperative outcome in elderly surgical patients.

Organ System Function

Changes in organ system function are manifested as decreased margins of reserve. In fact, old age can be characterized as a continuation of life with a decreasing capacity for adaptation.[3]

Nervous System

Aging is associated with progressive declines in central nervous system activity and loss of neurons, particularly in the cerebral cortex. The conduction velocity in peripheral nerves gradually slows with advancing age, and there may be decreased numbers of fibers in the spinal cord tracts. These changes are consistent with the decreased dose requirements for injected and inhaled anesthetics that accompany aging. Disturbances in the sleep patterns characterized by a decrease in slow-wave sleep are common in elderly patients. Increased nighttime wakefulness in elderly patients is mirrored by increased daytime fatigue and the likelihood of falling asleep during the day.

Cardiovascular System

The most clinically relevant alterations in cardiovascular physiology that accompany aging are increased myocardial and vascular stiffness; blunted β-adrenergic receptor-mediated modulation of inotropy, chronotropy, and vasomotor tone; and autonomic nervous system reflex dysfunction.[3] Despite evidence of impaired diastolic and systolic function in elderly men, overall cardiac performance is adequately maintained at rest during advancing age. Age-related alterations in cardiovascular responses to changes in posture or exercise are caused more by autonomic nervous system dysfunction and blunted β-adrenergic receptor responsiveness with advancing age than by impaired myocardial function.

Elderly individuals who maintain physical fitness may sustain relatively unchanged cardiac output despite progressive aging.[4] The aged heart shows less chronotropic response to catecholamines, presumably reflecting decreased β-adrenergic receptor responsiveness. The heart rate decreases with age, suggesting a predominance of parasympathetic nervous system activity, degenerative changes that involve the sinus node and/or cardiac conduction system. The systemic blood pressure increases with aging, reflecting the development of thickened elastic fibers in the walls of the large arteries. As a result, blood vessels become poorly compliant, and systolic and diastolic blood pressures increase.

Congestive heart failure is a common problem among elderly individuals. Determining whether there is predominantly a systolic or a diastolic component to congestive heart failure is important in elderly individuals because many of them have pre-served diastolic function. Congestive heart failure is often associated with essential hypertension or ischemic heart disease. Atrial fibrillation is the most common supraventricular dysrhythmia in individuals older than 65 years of age. This dysrhythmia often impairs cardiac performance because aging individuals become progressively dependent on atrial contractions for diastolic filling.

Autonomic Nervous System

Aging is accompanied by alterations in autonomic nervous system function manifesting as increased sympathetic nervous system activity and decreased parasympathetic nervous system activity.[3] Increased basal sympathetic nervous system outflow and serum norepinephrine concentrations suggest up-regulation of sympathetic nervous system outflow. This increased activity is presumed to result in desensitization (down-regulation) of β-adrenergic receptors, which is consistent with the blunted postsynaptic responsiveness of β-adrenergic receptors that accompanies aging. The autonomic nervous system control of cardiovascular function changes with aging, manifesting as decreased parasympathetic nervous system influences on sinus node function. Age-related decreases in baroreceptor reflex function (heart rate responses to changes in systemic blood pressure) may compromise compensatory responses to abrupt changes in intravascular fluid volume, institution of positive-pressure ventilation, and changes in body position. Blunted baroreceptor reflex responses may contribute to sinus node depression and syncope in elderly patients.

Respiratory System

Elderly individuals are prone to develop acute postoperative respiratory failure. Older patients are more likely to develop apnea, periodic breathing, and respiratory depression after administration of opioids and benzodiazepines. Mechanical ventilatory function and the efficiency of gas exchange deteriorate with aging. Mechanical ventilatory function is impaired because of decreased elasticity of the lungs and decreased maximal movements of the thorax. Progressive decreases in PaO_2 accompany aging, likely reflecting airway closure and decreased cardiac output leading to ventilation-to-perfusion mismatching. At rest, elderly individuals may not exhibit symptoms of pulmonary dysfunction, but pulmonary changes produced by surgery superimposed on the already present changes of aging can result in symptoms because of a decreased margin of reserve. Nocturnal respiratory dysfunction (sleep apnea syndrome) is common in elderly individuals.

Renal Function

Advancing age is associated with progressive declines in renal blood flow and the glomerular filtration rate, paralleling decreased cardiac output. As a result, elderly patients are vulnerable to fluid overload and the cumulative effects of drugs that depend on renal clearance mechanisms (digoxin, antibiotics, certain nondepolarizing muscle relaxants). Despite this deteriorated renal function, plasma creatinine concentrations often do not increase, presumably reflecting decreased production of creatinine that parallels the decreased skeletal muscle mass that accompanies aging. Decreased urine-concentrating ability that accompanies aging means that elderly patients are less able to concentrate urine after fluid deprivation, and the ability to secrete acid loads is decreased. Elderly individuals' ability to conserve sodium is impaired, making this age group vulnerable to hyponatremia, particularly when acute illness leads to decreased oral intake of sodium.

Hepatic, Gastrointestinal, and Endocrine Function

The decreased hepatic blood flow that accompanies aging and parallels cardiac output possibly influences clearance of drugs that depend on hepatic metabolism. Decreased rates of gastric emptying may accompany aging, and the incidence of diabetes mellitus increases with aging, perhaps reflecting decreased insulin release or insensitivity of insulin receptors. Subclinical hypothyroidism manifesting solely as increased plasma thyrotropin concentrations is present in more than 13% of healthy elderly individuals, especially women.[5]

Management of Anesthesia

Preoperative Evaluation

Preoperative evaluation of elderly patients includes consideration of the likely presence of co-existing diseases independent of the reasons for surgery (Table 33–1). In fact, many of the findings considered

to be typical of aging actually represent disease processes that have a higher incidence among the elderly. Alcoholism may be an unexpected finding in elderly patients. Recent changes in mental function should not be attributed to aging until cardiac or pulmonary disease has been eliminated as an etiology. Hazards of co-existing diseases are emphasized by the increased postoperative mortality among elderly patients, especially when emergency surgery is necessary. The likelihood of adverse drug interactions is increased by alterations in the pharmacokinetics and pharmacodynamics that accompany aging. Furthermore, elderly patients are likely to be taking several drugs, which can result in adverse effects or drug interactions (Table 33–2).

Functional Reserve

Preoperative evaluation of the elderly patient's functional reserves and airway should consider the presence of changes characteristic of aging.[3] The age-related changes in cardiovascular performance most relevant to perioperative management are the stiffened myocardium and vasculature, blunted β-adrenergic receptor responsiveness, and impaired autonomic nervous system reflex control of the heart rate. These changes may be of little clinical significance when elderly patients are at rest but have considerable consequences during superimposed cardiovascular stress. Preoperative assessment of organ system functional reserves is uniquely important in elderly patients. Poor functional reserve or high risk surgical procedures may justify preoperative cardiac assessment with noninvasive testing (dipyridamole-thallium myocardial perfusion imaging, dobutamine stress echocardiography). Perioperative myocardial infarction is associated with an increased risk of mortality in elderly patients. Anemia and orthostatic hypotension are common preoperative findings in elderly patients.

Airway

The potential presence of vertebrobasilar arterial insufficiency can be evaluated by determining the effects of extension and rotation of the patient's head on mental status. Poor dentition or the presence of dentures may influence the approach to induction of anesthesia. For example, if maintenance of anesthesia by mask is anticipated, it may be useful to ask edentulous patients to wear dentures to the operating room. Cervical osteoarthritis or rheumatoid arthritis may interfere with visualizing the glottic opening during direct laryngoscopy.

Table 33–1 • Co-Existing Diseases That Often Accompany Aging

Essential hypertension
Ischemic heart disease
Cardiac conduction disturbances
Congestive heart failure
Chronic pulmonary disease
Diabetes mellitus
Subclinical hypothyroidism
Rheumatoid arthritis
Osteoarthritis

Table 33-2 • Drugs Commonly Prescribed for Elderly Patients

Drug	Adverse Effects or Drug Interactions
Diuretics	Hypokalemia
	Hyperkalemia
Digitalis	Cardiac dysrhythmias
	Cardiac conduction disturbances
β-Adrenergic antagonists	Bradycardia
	Congestive heart failure
	Bronchospasm
	Attenuation of autonomic nervous system activity
Centrally acting antihypertensives	Attenuation of autonomic nervous system activity
	Decreased MAC
Tricyclic antidepressants	Anticholinergic effects
	Cardiac dysrhythmias
	Cardiac conduction disturbances
	Increased MAC
Lithium	Cardiac dysrhythmias
	Prolongation of muscle relaxants
Cardiac antidysrhythmics	Prolongation of muscle relaxants
Antibiotics	Prolongation of muscle relaxants
Oral hypoglycemics	Hypoglycemia
Alcohol	Increased MAC
	Delirium tremens

MAC, minimum alveolar concentration.

Blood Volume

Elderly patients are often volume-depleted during the preoperative period, reflecting decreased thirst, age-related decreased renal capacity to conserve water and sodium, and frequent use of diuretics. Because of decreased left ventricular compliance and limited β-adrenergic receptor responsiveness, elderly patients are predictably more sensitive to fluid overload. Assessment of intravascular fluid volume status is important prior to the induction of anesthesia in elderly patients.

Skin

Senile atrophy with collagen loss and decreased elasticity makes the skin more sensitive to injury from adhesive tape and monitoring electrodes, as used for recording the electrocardiogram or eliciting responses to a peripheral nerve stimulator.

Preoperative Medication

Preoperative medication in elderly patients may be best achieved during a preoperative visit when events that are going to occur during the perioperative period are described. If additional anxiety relief is desired, benzodiazepines are often selected. Anticholinergic drugs such as atropine may contribute to postoperative confusion in elderly patients. In this regard, glycopyrrolate, which does not easily cross the blood-brain barrier, is probably less likely to cause undesirable central nervous system effects if anticholinergic drugs are included in the preoperative medication of elderly patients.

General Anesthesia

Selection of drugs and techniques for induction of anesthesia in elderly patients must consider changes in organ system function that are likely to accompany aging, as well as altered responses to drugs because of age-related changes in pharmacokinetics or pharmacodynamics. Decreased cardiac output and delayed clearance of drugs may contribute to a slow onset of drug effects followed by prolonged drug effects. The combination of decreased anesthetic requirements and decreased cardiac output could increase the risk of anesthetic overdose, especially with volatile anesthetics. Induction of anesthesia decreases sympathetic nervous system activity on which aged patients with impaired cardiac performance may depend to maintain perfusion pressures. This response in the presence of anesthetic drug-induced negative inotropic effects may manifest as hypotension during the induction of anesthesia in elderly patients.

There is no evidence that specific inhaled or injected anesthetic drugs are preferable for induction and maintenance of anesthesia in elderly patients. Progressive decreases in the reactivity of protective upper airway reflexes with aging plus the high incidence of hiatal hernia in elderly patients may increase the importance of protecting the lungs from aspiration by placing a cuffed tube in the patient's trachea. An increased heart rate associated with administration of isoflurane is less likely to occur in the elderly than in young adults. Cardiac performance in elderly patients is progressively dependent on preload, and acute decreases in intravascular fluid volume and venous return can result in evidence of left ventricular failure, including decreased arterial oxygenation and development of pulmonary edema. Transesophageal echocardiography and pulmonary artery catheter monitoring may be useful. This is especially true for elderly patients with limited exercise tolerance who are undergoing major surgical procedures associated with cardiovascular stress and extensive intravascular fluid volume changes.

Regional Anesthesia

Regional anesthesia is an acceptable alternative to general anesthesia in selected elderly patients, especially those undergoing transurethral resection of the prostate, gynecologic procedures, inguinal herniorrhaphy, or treatment of hip fractures. A T8 sensory level is desirable for these operations. A prerequisite when selecting regional anesthesia techniques is an alert, cooperative patient. Maintenance of consciousness during surgery permits prompt recognition of acute changes in cerebral function or the onset of angina pectoris. Apprehension despite adequate anesthesia may require intravenous administration of sedative drugs (propofol, midazolam), keeping in mind that elderly patients may require low doses to achieve the desired effects. On occasion, regional and general anesthesia techniques may be combined, as in elderly patients undergoing hip surgery.

Prolongation of spinal anesthesia in elderly patients may reflect decreased vascular absorption of local anesthetics owing to decreased blood flow in atherosclerotic blood vessels surrounding the subarachnoid space. Doses of local anesthetics required to achieve given sensory levels during epidural anesthesia are often perceived to be less with aging, although not all reports describe a linear relation between doses and age.[6] There are also data demonstrating that cephalad spread is more extensive and the duration of epidural sensory and motor blockade is shorter in the elderly than in younger patients.[7] Decreased dose requirements in elderly patients are thought to be due in part to anatomic changes in the epidural space characterized by progressive occlusion of intervertebral foramina with connective tissue. As a result, less local anesthetic solution escapes through the intervertebral foram-

ina, and there is increased spread in the epidural space. This change would also result in an increased surface area for absorption of local anesthetic solutions from the epidural space, consistent with the higher peak serum concentrations of lidocaine observed after epidural placement in elderly patients compared with young adults.[6] There is clinical evidence that regional anesthesia in elderly patients decreases the magnitude of perioperative blood loss and decreases the incidence of postoperative deep vein thrombosis and pulmonary embolism (see "Gait Disturbances").

Postoperative Period

During the postoperative period, attention to the development of arterial hypoxemia or myocardial ischemia is important. Early ambulation is recommended in efforts to decrease the likelihood of pneumonia or deep vein thrombosis. Postoperative confusion and impaired memory may contribute to morbidity in elderly patients (see "Postoperative Delirium").

▌ GERIATRIC SYNDROMES

Geriatric syndromes reflect the presence of common chronic disorders in the elderly population (Table 33–3).[3] These syndromes increase in frequency and clinical importance with advanced age, growing more prevalent in patients older than 75 years of age.[4] Cognitive dysfunction due to delirium, dementia, and mental depression is a prominent feature of many geriatric syndromes.

Table 33–3 • Examples of Geriatric Syndromes

Cognitive dysfunction
  Delirium
  Postoperative delirium
  Dementia
Gait disturbances
Urinary and/or bowel incontinence
Immobility
Pressure ulcers
Malnutrition
Dehydration
Sensory impairment
  Hearing
  Vision (cataracts, glaucoma, macular degeneration)
Iatrogenic illness
  Polypharmacy
  Nosocomial infections
Progeria

Delirium

Delirium is a transient, potentially reversible disorder of cognition and attention characterized by an acute onset with a fluctuating course and the presence of an underlying organic derangement (Table 33–4).[1,8] Delirium is common in hospitalized elderly patients and may be misdiagnosed as other psychiatric illnesses. Postoperative delirium occurs in 10% to 15% of elderly general surgical patients and in 30% to 50% of elderly patients admitted with hip fractures or who are undergoing knee arthroplasty. The use of psychoactive drugs and the presence of azotemia, hip fractures, or electrolyte disturbances (most often sodium) are independent risk factors for the development of delirium in elderly hospitalized patients. Co-existing dementia or cognitive impairment is the single most important risk factor for delirium, perhaps reflecting impaired brain homeostasis in these highly susceptible patients. Precipitating factors for delirium in hospitalized elderly patients include the use of physical restraints, administration of more than three medications added to the patient's routine drug regimen, bladder catheterization, and any iatrogenic event such as an accidental injury.[1] Delirium is a significant cause of morbidity (prolonged hospitalizations, falls, persistent functional declines) and mortality in elderly patients. Delirium frequently is an irreversible, terminal event that complicates care at the end of life.[8]

Causes

Virtually any acute physical stress can precipitate delirium in elderly patients, particularly those with known risk factors. In elderly hospitalized patients, delirium is most commonly associated with acute infection (pneumonia, bladder infection), arterial hypoxemia, hypotension, and administration of psychoactive drugs (benzodiazepines, opioids, drugs with anticholinergic effects). Drugs with anticholinergic effects include many cardiac antidysrhythmics, tricyclic antidepressants, gastrointestinal medications, and antihistamines. Antibiotics, nonsteroidal antiinflammatory drugs, and H_2-receptor antagonists have been associated with delirium. Other causes of delirium include alcohol withdrawal and neurologic events such as stroke.

The pathophysiology of delirium is complex and poorly understood. The most frequently proposed explanation for delirium is disturbed neurotransmitter function, especially as related to cholinergic function. Decreased cholinergic activity is caused by decreased acetylcholine synthesis or enhanced anticholinergic activity. Neurotransmitters other than acetylcholine that may play roles in the development of delirium include γ-aminobutyric acid, serotonin, dopamine, and norepinephrine.

Diagnosis

Delirium should be considered in elderly patients who experience changes in cognitive function (Table 33–4).[1] Patients with delirium often present with acute changes in mental status with features of disturbed consciousness, impaired cognition, and a fluctuating course. Patients have decreased ability to focus, associated with incoherent or erratic thought processes. Perceptual disturbances, such as misperceptions and hallucinations, may be accompanied by increased psychomotor activity. Alternatively,

Table 33–4 • Differential Diagnosis of Delirium and Dementia

Feature	Delirium	Dementia
Onset	Abrupt	Insidious
Duration	Hours to days	Persistent
Attention span	Decreased	Normal
Awareness	Impaired	Normal
Alertness	Fluctuates	Normal
Consciousness	Depressed	Normal
Memory	Impaired (especially short term)	Impaired (especially remote)
Language	Normal or incorrect naming	Aphasia Anomia Paraphasia
Perception	Illusions Hallucinations Misperceptions	Delusions
Psychomotor activity	Increased to decreased	Normal
Sleep–wake cycle	Disrupted (reversed)	Normal or fragmented

Adapted from: Palmer RM. Management of common clinical disorders in geriatric patients. Sci Am Med 1998;1–16.

elderly patients with delirium may be best characterized as exhibiting "quiet confusion." Delirium is often misdiagnosed as dementia, mental depression, or functional psychosis. In this regard, the clinical features of delirium and dementia and altered levels of consciousness and the duration of the symptoms usually lead to a correct diagnosis (Table 33–4).[1] Psychosis caused by schizophrenia or major mental depression is not characterized by impaired attention, altered levels of consciousness, or fluctuating mental status. Although many depressed patients perform poorly on formal tests of cognition, they remain alert and attentive and do not display the characteristics of delirium.

Treatment

Treatment of the obvious potential causes of delirium (pneumonia, arterial hypoxemia, electrolyte derangements, polypharmacy) is the first step in the evaluation and management of elderly patients. Continuity of nursing care to provide familiarity decreases anxiety and agitation; and correcting sensory impairments by providing personal interactions with family members is often helpful. Promotion of normal sleep cycles through noise control, dim lighting at night, and avoidance of unnecessary interruptions during the normal sleep time are recommended. Use of restraints may paradoxically increase agitation. Pharmacologic interventions are indicated for patients with specific indications such as hallucinations or aggressive behavior. Haloperidol, 0.5 to 1.0 mg PO or IM, is most often utilized. For treatment of anxiety and sleep disturbances, lorazepam, 0.5 to 1.0 mg PO, is a consideration. Haloperidol or lorazepam may be useful for preparing patients for neuroimaging procedures or when an invasive procedure, such as central line placement, is required. Patients experiencing delirium secondary to alcohol withdrawal are most often treated with benzodiazepines. The adverse effects of haloperidol include extrapyramidal effects, dystonic reactions, and cardiac dysrhythmias, whereas paradoxical confusion, amnesia, and gait disturbances may result from benzodiazepines.

Postoperative Delirium

Postoperative delirium (postoperative cognitive dysfunction, postoperative confusion) is a transient global disorder that develops in 10% to 60% of patients 65 years of age or older admitted to hospitals with hip fractures or undergoing knee arthroplasty.[1, 9, 10] Postoperative cognitive dysfunction, which may be persistent, is common following cardiac surgery that requires cardiopulmonary bypass; proposed explanations include decreased cerebral perfusion due to hypotension or loss of pulsatile perfusion during cardiopulmonary bypass, altered autoregulation, and microemboli (air, particulate matter).[11] Transpulmonary passage of microemboli may occur, accounting for cerebral infarctions in the absence of a documented patent foramen ovale. Elderly patients undergoing cataract surgery are especially vulnerable to development of postoperative delirium because of loss of vision and the common use of anticholinergic drugs, often as topical eyedrops.

Signs and Symptoms

The distinguishing features of postoperative delirium are impaired cognition, fluctuating levels of consciousness, altered psychomotor activity, and a disturbed sleep-wake cycle. Delirium usually manifests on the first or second postoperative day, and symptoms are often exacerbated at night. The condition may be silent and go unnoticed, or it may be misdiagnosed as mental depression. Postoperative delirium can result in increased morbidity, delayed functional recovery, and a prolonged hospital stay.

Causes

Possible risk factors for the development of postoperative delirium include polypharmacy, preoperative administration of anticholinergic drugs, intraoperative hypotension, perioperative arterial hypoxemia, postoperative use of opioids or benzodiazepines, and the development of postoperative surgical complications. Another potentially important cause of postoperative delirium in elderly patients is the sleep disturbance that invariably accompanies the postoperative period.[12] In older adults undergoing elective total knee replacement, the incidence of delirium or other cognitive impairments are not related to the type of anesthesia (general or epidural).[13]

Postoperative cognitive deficits following major abdominal, noncardiac thoracic, or orthopedic surgery performed in patients older than 60 years of age were documented to be present in nearly 26% of patients at 7 days postoperatively, and these deficits persisted in nearly 10% after 3 months.[14] In that report, only patient age was identified as a predictor of postoperative cognitive dysfunction, whereas arterial hypoxia and/or hypotension were not independent predictors for the occurrence of this deficit.[14] Nevertheless, there may be subgroups of elderly patients who have little reserve for maintenance of normal cognitive function, and these individuals may be vulnerable to perioperative effects of arterial hypoxemia and hypotension.

It is presumed that alterations in the central cholinergic system are important to the development of postoperative cognitive dysfunction. It is speculated that memory deficits seen after operations in patients of all ages could result from the anticholinergic effects of atropine, as used for preoperative medication or pharmacologic antagonism of nondepolarizing muscle relaxants.[10] This notion is consistent with the observation that patients with parkinsonism may experience deterioration should they receive anticholinergic drugs.

Dementia

Dementia is the clinical syndrome characterized by acquired persistent impairment of cognitive (intellectual) and emotional abilities severe enough to interfere with daily functioning and quality of life.[15, 16] It is important to differentiate dementia from delirium (acute, usually reversible, metabolically induced state), recognizing that delirium is a common complication of chronic dementia (Table 33–4).[1]

Signs and Symptoms

Intellectual impairment in patients with dementia may manifest in the spheres of language, memory, abstract thinking, and judgment. A specific cause or pathologic process is not implied by the designation dementia, as multiple diseases may be causative. Dementia occurs primarily late in life, the prevalence being about 1% at age 60, doubling every 5 years, reaching 30% to 50% by 85 years of age.[15] Cortical dementias are represented by Alzheimer's disease, Pick's disease, and frontal lobe degeneration. Subcortical dementias are associated with Parkinson's disease, Huntington's disease, and Creutzfeldt-Jakob disease. Potentially treatable dementias due to hypothyroidism, acquired immunodeficiency syndrome (AIDS), neurosyphilis, and vitamin B_{12} deficiency must be differentiated from irreversible, degenerative dementias. It may be difficult to differentiate dementia from mental depression, and in some patients it is appropriate to administer antidepressant drugs as a therapeutic trial.

Alzheimer's Disease

Alzheimer's disease is the most common of the progressive cortical dementias, accounting for about 70% of the dementias in individuals older than 55 years of age. The characteristic cognitive features of Alzheimer's disease are progressive memory impairment, predominantly loss of short-term memory. Progressive disorientation with respect to time and place is always present. Language impairment is an important symptom of Alzheimer's disease, manifesting as difficulty finding words for spontaneous speech. Performance of daily tasks such as meal preparation and personal hygiene becomes impaired. Symptoms of mental depression and anxiety may be prominent. About one-half of nursing home beds are occupied by patients with Alzheimer's disease.

Diagnosis

A diagnosis of Alzheimer's disease is probable when the dementing illness is characterized by insidious onset, progressive worsening of memory, and a normal level of consciousness. Computed tomography typically shows ventricular dilation and marked cortical atrophy. Positron emission tomography may demonstrate areas of decreased cerebral blood flow. Cholinergic neurons in the brain may be selectively destroyed early in the course of the disease; the activity of choline acetyltransferase, which catalyzes the synthesis of acetylcholine, is decreased as much as 90%. The definitive diagnosis of Alzheimer's disease can be made only after examining brain tissue and demonstrating proteins or protein fragments precipitated as amyloid and fibrillar aggregates.

Treatment

There are no proven preventive therapies for Alzheimer's disease, and drugs are not consistently effective for preventing progression of the disease. Symptomatic therapy is helpful during the early stages, especially if mental depression is prominent. Drugs with anticholinergic effects are avoided when treating mental depression. Anticholinesterase drugs such as tacrine or donepezil (once a day dosing) appear to have beneficial effects for some patients early in the disease. The typical course is one of progressive decline; and the median survival after the onset of dementia is 3.3 years.

Management of Anesthesia

Management of anesthesia is influenced by the pathophysiology of Alzheimer's disease. Challenges during the perioperative period often are related to dealing with patients who are unable to comprehend their environment or to cooperate with those responsible for providing their medical care. Sedative drugs, as might be used for preoperative medication, should rarely be administered to these patients, as further mental confusion could result.

Centrally acting anticholinergic drugs are not recommended for inclusion in the preoperative medication, whereas pharmacologic antagonism of nondepolarizing neuromuscular blocking drugs might logically include glycopyrrolate, rather than atropine. Maintenance of anesthesia can be acceptably achieved with inhaled or injected drugs. Possible advantages of inhaled drugs would be more predictable returns to co-existing levels of consciousness during the early postoperative period. Possible drug interactions based on co-existing treatments with centrally acting anticholinesterase drugs are considerations.

Vascular Dementia

Permanent cognitive impairment resulting from cerebrovascular disease is the second most common form of dementia.[15] Vascular dementia typically has a fluctuating course. The rate of deterioration is determined by the underlying cerebrovascular disease (multiple infarcts, infectious vasculitis, autoimmune vasculitis), and there is no effective treatment.

Pick's Disease

Pick's disease is cortical dementia characterized by impaired ability to plan and initiate goals and the development of disinhibited behavior ("dementia of the frontal lobe type").[15] Most patients have little awareness of these changes and emphatically deny that there are any cognitive changes present. Apathy is common and difficult to distinguish from mental depression. Abundant unfocused speech (logorrhea), echo-like spontaneous repetition of words or phrases (echolalia), and compulsive repetition of phrases (palilalia) are seen in conjunction with behavioral disturbances that characterize this form of frontal lobe dementia. Pick's disease is less common than Alzheimer's disease.[16]

Subcortical Dementias

The dementia that accompanies Parkinson's disease is characterized by rapid progression in association with psychomotor slowing, delusions, and hallucinations. Creutzfeldt-Jakob disease is a rare, rapidly progressive infectious dementia (see Chapter 27). Normal-pressure hydrocephalus is associated with dementia manifesting as gait disturbances, urinary incontinence, and cognitive declines. Each of these three symptoms is relatively common in elderly patients, making the diagnosis difficult. The likelihood of cognitive improvement following shunting is best when the dementia is of short duration.

Gait Disturbances

Disorders of balance and gait increase with advancing age and predispose elderly individuals to falls and injuries, including hip fractures, subdural hematomas, cervical fractures, and soft tissue damage (bruises, lacerations, hematomas).[1] The incidence of falls and serious injuries increases to at least 50% among persons 80 years of age and older. Gait or balance disorders associated with syncope, vertigo, and postural hypotension are risk factors for falls and injuries.

Hip fractures are a major cause of disability, functional impairment, and death in elderly individuals. Hip fractures are often associated with poor bone mineral density (osteoporosis), gait disturbances (drugs, confusion, visual impairment), physical inactivity, and poor general health. In most cases of hip fracture, the immediate cause of the fracture is a sideways fall with direct impact on the greater trochanter of the proximal femur. In elderly individuals considered to be at high risk for falls and resulting hip fractures, the use of hip protectors designed to protect the hips (so at the time of a fall the force and energy of the impact are attenuated and shunted away from the trochanter) may decrease the likelihood of fracture.[17]

The choice of anesthesia (general or regional) in elderly patients for repair of hip fractures has not been shown to influence postoperative morbidity (congestive heart failure, myocardial infarction, pneumonia, confusion) or mortality.[18] In one report there was a decreased incidence of deep vein thrombosis and mortality 1 month postoperatively and a tendency toward a lower incidence of myocardial infarction, confusion, and postoperative arterial hypoxemia in elderly patients undergoing hip fracture surgery under regional anesthesia, whereas patients receiving general anesthesia experienced less hypotension and fewer cerebral vascular events.[19] These authors concluded that there were marginal advantages for regional anesthesia compared to general anesthesia for hip fracture patients in terms of early mortality and risk of deep vein thrombosis.

Urinary and Bowel Incontinence

Urinary incontinence results from neurologic defects (stroke) or anatomic defects (prostatic hyperplasia) that interfere with normal bladder function. It is estimated that 25% of men and women older than 85 years of age experience urinary incontinence.[1] Bladder suspension surgery may be considered in elderly women who develop stress incontinence. Stress incontinence in men is most often related to prior prostatectomy and may respond to placing an artificial urethral sphincter. Long-term indwelling urinary catheterization is usually reserved for patients who cannot be catheterized intermittently because of discomfort or terminal illness. Bowel incontinence is present in nearly 50% of hospitalized elderly patients. Chronic constipation and fecal impaction are often associated with inadequate dietary fiber intake and inactivity.

Immobility

Prolonged bed rest produces many physiologic changes, including decreased circulating plasma volume and cardiac output, orthostatic hypotension, arterial hypoxemia, skeletal muscle atrophy, and generalized skeletal muscle weakness.[1] These physiologic effects are reversed by physical activity, aerobic exercises, and low-impact resistive exercises.

Pressure Ulcers

Pressure ulcers occur when persistent external pressure on the skin damages underlying tissues, especially over bony prominences. About 80% of pressure ulcers that develop in nursing home patients occur over the sacrum, coccyx, hips, and heels. Impaired mobility, incontinence, malnutrition, and impaired consciousness are significant risk factors for the development of pressure ulcers. Aging skin is more susceptible to sheer forces, has decreased vascularity, and in malnourished patients has decreased subcutaneous fat. Pressure ulcers often present as skin blisters that evolve to ulceration with exudate or plaque eschar. Ischemic injury associated with pressure ulcers extends to subcutaneous tissues, and sinus tracts may develop. Pressure ulcers may become infected, resulting in cellulitis or bacteremia, especially in immunocompromised patients.

Prevention of pressure ulcers begins with decreasing pressure at risk sites. Pressure-reducing devices, such as air-fluidized beds, and low-air-loss beds, are useful. Necrotic tissue is a barrier to epithelialization and serves as a nidus for infection, emphasizing the value of surgical débridement.

Malnutrition

Protein-calorie malnutrition is present in 20% to 40% of elderly patients admitted to hospitals for a medical illness.[1] Malnutrition is an independent predictor of subsequent mortality. Indicators of malnutrition include weight loss, low weight for height, decreases in mid-arm circumference, the presence of nutrition-related disorders (osteoporosis, vitamin B_{12} deficiency, folate deficiency), unexplained normocytic anemia, and serum albumin concentrations less than 3.5 g/dl. The most common medical conditions predisposing to malnutrition are congestive heart failure, chronic obstructive pulmonary disease, and cancer. Nutritional enteral supplements improve the outcomes of hospitalization for patients admitted with hip fractures and pulmonary infections. Elderly patients who are acutely ill, delirious, or demented are at risk for aspiration pneumonia.

Specific nutrient deficiencies result from dietary imbalance, chronic disease, or medications.[1] The most commonly recognized examples are vitamin B_{12}, iron, and calcium deficiencies. Dietary calcium deficiency is common among elderly women. Iron deficiency anemia is more common among the elderly because of long-term internal or external blood loss.

Dehydration

Dehydration is the most common fluid and electrolyte disorder in the long-term care setting and is often associated with infections.[20] Risk factors for the development of dehydration in elderly individuals are decreased fluid intake and increased fluid losses. Physiologic reasons for the development of dehydration include decreased ability of the kidneys to concentrate urine, altered thirst sensations, and relative resistance to vasopressin. Changes in functional status, delirium, dementia, mental depression, medications, and mobility disorders further place elderly individuals at risk for developing dehydration. Aging can decrease cardiovascular responses to volume depletion. Mortality may exceed 50% if dehydration is not treated.

Classification

Several forms of dehydration may occur and must be distinguished, as the type of dehydration influences the treatment. Isotonic dehydration results from the balanced losses of water and sodium that occur during a complete fast. Vomiting and diarrhea, because of large amounts of water and electrolytes in gastric contents, result in isotonic dehydration. Hypertonic dehydration (serum sodium concentrations higher than 145 mEq/L, serum osmolarity higher than 300 mOsm/L) results if water losses exceed sodium losses. Fever results in water losses through the lungs and skin and, when combined with a limited ability to increase fluid intake, hypertonic dehydration. Hypotonic dehydration (serum sodium concentrations lower than 135 mEq/L, serum osmolarity lower than 285 mOsm/L) occurs when sodium losses exceed water losses. This type of dehydration occurs primarily with administration of diuretics that stimulate sodium excretion. Hyponatremic and hypernatremic dehydration may develop during the postoperative period.

Diagnosis

Dehydration is suggested by rapid weight loss that is more than 3% of the individual's body weight.[20] Signs and symptoms of dehydration and volume depletion may be vague, imprecise, or absent in elderly individuals. General clinical evaluation and cardiovascular assessment of systemic blood pressure and heart rate are the principal objective parameters for diagnosing dehydration. Skin turgor and urine specific gravity are not reliable assessments of dehydration. Orthostatic hypotension (systolic blood pressure decreases of 20 mmHg after 1 minute) or orthostatic heart rate increases (10 to 20 beats/min) may be a sign of dehydration especially in the presence of intake and output records that document inadequate fluid intake or increased fluid losses. Blood urea nitrogen to serum creatinine concentration ratios of 25 or higher suggests dehydration, although other conditions often present in elderly individuals (renal vascular disease, obstructive uropathy) can produce similar changes in the absence of dehydration.

Treatment

Supplemental oral fluids may be sufficient treatment of dehydration, keeping in mind that daily water requirements in individuals weighing between 50 and 80 kg are 1500 to 2000 ml. Estimated daily fluid requirements in adults older than 65 years of age are about 30 ml/kg. Sports replacement drinks or equivalent commercial products (carbonated beverages, fruit juices) are readily absorbed by the stomach and rapidly correct hypertonic dehydration. When replacing fluid orally, patients are monitored for signs of developing fluid overload (dyspnea, confusion), which is generally reversible with administration of diuretics. Intravenous administration of fluids may be required but has the disadvantage of not being easily performed in nursing home environments. For patients with significant volume depletion due to isotonic fluid losses (vomiting, diarrhea), replacement is with isotonic saline.

Sensory Impairment

Hearing and visual losses are the most important and common sensory impairments in elderly individuals. Sensory impairment adversely affects the elderly individual's physical, cognitive, and social functioning.

Hearing Impairment

Hearing loss is categorized as sensorineural or conductive.[1] Sensorineural hearing loss, caused by cochlear or retrocochlear disease, is characterized by decreased thresholds for both air and bone conduction. Presbycusis is the most common cause of sensorineural hearing loss in the elderly, especially men. Hearing aids are the usual treatment for sensorineural hearing loss. The most common causes of conduction hearing loss are cerumen impaction and otosclerosis.

Vision Impairment

Age-related changes in vision, especially presbyopia or farsightedness, are common causes of increasing vision impairment. Other important aging changes that affect vision include decreased pupillary dilation (contributes to poor night vision) and changes in the vitreous fluid (produces dots in the individual's visual field). Major causes of visual impairment associated with poor correctability or blindness in elderly individuals include cataracts, glaucoma, macular degeneration, and diabetic retinopathy. Diabetic retinopathy is the leading cause of blindness in patients 25 to 74 years of age.[21]

Cataracts

Cataracts are opacities of the crystalline lens that may affect visual acuity, contrast sensitivity, and light perception. The prevalence of opacification of the lens increases with aging to nearly 100% in those older than 90 years of age, although functional impairment typically occurs in about only half of these individuals.[1]

Treatment. Surgical removal is the only effective therapy for visual impairment caused by cataracts. Cataract surgery is the most commonly performed operation in elderly patients. Microsurgical techniques to remove cataracts include extracapsular cataract extraction and phacoemulsification. Cataract extraction is usually followed by placing an intraocular lens.

Preoperative Evaluation. Cataract surgery is performed almost exclusively as an outpatient procedure. The rates of perioperative morbidity and mortality associated with cataract surgery are low. Nevertheless, because patients with cataracts are usually elderly and have co-existing medical diseases (systemic hypertension, atherosclerosis, diabetes mellitus), there is controversy as to the need for a detailed medical history and physical examination with laboratory testing (electrocardiogram, hemoglobin, electrolytes, creatinine, glucose) before patients can be considered eligible for cataract surgery. A large prospective study was unable to document a measurable increase in safety when routine medical testing preceded cataract surgery.[22] The most frequent medical events during cataract surgery in this large study were treatment for systemic hypertension and cardiac dysrhythmias, principally bradycardia. Based on this study, it was concluded that routine ordering of medical tests before elective cataract surgery is not necessary. Tests should be ordered only if the history or medical findings on physical examination indicates a need for the test.

Management of Anesthesia. Cataract extraction may be performed under local anesthesia utilizing a retrobulbar block with or without intravenous sedation (propofol, midazolam, remifentanil) or under general anesthesia (etomidate, fentanyl, isoflurane). There is evidence that only minor psychomotor deficits are present 2 hours after general anesthesia for cataract surgery in elderly patients and that psychomotor function recovers completely 24 hours after surgery.[23] Placement of the retrobulbar block may be preceded by intravenous doses of propofol and/or opioids (remifentanil) to ensure patient comfort. Risks of retrobulbar block include bleeding and passage of local anesthetic along the optic nerve sheath into the subarachnoid space, leading to apnea. Preoperative use of aspirin or nonsteroidal anti-inflammatory drugs has not been shown to increase the incidence of hemorrhage following performance of retrobulbar blocks.[24] Increased resistance encountered during injection of local anesthetic solutions during performance of a retrobulbar block may reflect an incorrect position of the needle in the optic nerve sheath, rather than proper placement in the retrobulbar adipose tissues. Continued injection of local anesthetic solutions should the needle be in the neural sheath may result in high spinal anesthesia.[25] Continuous intravenous sedation may be provided with remifentanil, 0.5 to 1.0 μg/kg IV, followed by continuous intravenous infusions of remifentanil, 0.05 to 0.10 μg/kg/min IV, with or without 1 to 2 mg of midazolam IV.[26]

Patients who require general anesthesia for cataract extraction are likely to be elderly with one or more co-existing medical diseases. General anesthesia must ensure patient immobility, as sudden movements or attempts to cough when the lens is exposed could result in extrusion of vitreous and permanent ocular damage. Adequate depths of anesthesia, with or without skeletal muscle paralysis, are recommended. Although succinylcholine increases the intraocular pressure, this increase is transient. Nevertheless, the use of rapid-onset, short-acting nondepolarizing muscle relaxants such as mivacurium may be a useful alternative. Modest hyperventilation of the patient's lungs to produce hypocarbia and a 10- to 15-degree head-up tilt to promote venous drainage likely can decrease intraocular pressure during intraocular surgery. It is important to minimize the possibility of stimulation due to the endotracheal tube at the conclusion of surgery. In this regard, tracheal extubation may be considered before airway depression from anesthetic drugs has waned. If the tracheal tube is left in place as the patient awakens, it may be helpful to administer lidocaine, 0.5 to 1.5 mg/kg IV, in attempts to attenuate tracheal reflex responses to the presence of the tube.

It is helpful to minimize the likelihood of vomiting during the postoperative period. In this regard, use of opioids during the perioperative period may be avoided. Routine aspiration of the stomach with an orally inserted tube at the conclusion of general anesthesia serves not only to remove gastric fluid but also to decrease gastric distension, which could contribute to postoperative nausea and vomiting. Use of propofol for induction of anesthesia may exert an antiemetic effect during the postoperative period. In addition, prophylactic administration of antiemetic drugs is frequently utilized.

Incidence of Perioperative Myocardial Ischemia. Cataract surgery in elderly patients with risk factors for coronary artery disease is associated with perioperative evidence of myocardial ischemia in about one-third of patients.[27] Intraoperative myocardial ischemia is most likely to be associated with tachycardia (more than 20% increase above the preoperative baseline), whereas postoperative myocardial ischemia changes are likely to be independent of the patient's heart rate. The incidence of perioperative myocardial ischemia events is similar in patients receiving general or local anesthesia for the cataract extraction, although the number of ischemic episodes, including those that occur intraoperatively, is higher during general anesthesia than with local anesthesia.[27]

Glaucoma

Glaucoma is the leading cause of irreversible blindness in the world. Glaucoma is an optic neuropathy with peripheral vision loss occurring before loss of central vision. Diagnosis before vision loss is by ophthalmoscopic examination of the optic nerve to detect cupping. Patients at increased risk for developing glaucoma are the elderly and those with increased intraocular pressures (higher than 21 mmHg). Glaucoma may be classified anatomically as open-angle glaucoma (chronic and more common) and narrow-angle (acute) glaucoma based on the mechanism for poor aqueous outflow. Acute angle-closure glaucoma can be precipitated by the use of dilating eyedrops and is a medical emergency. In contrast, primary open-angle glaucoma is an insidious disease most often discovered during routine eye examination (intraocular pressures higher than 21 mmHg).

Treatment. Treatment of glaucoma is lowering of intraocular pressure by decreasing the amount of aqueous humor produced by the ciliary bodies or by increasing its outflow through the trabecular meshwork, the uveoscleral pathway, or a surgically created pathway. Medical treatment of glaucoma includes topical eyedrops to manage the open-angle glaucoma. The β-adrenergic blocking drug timolol is administered as topical eyedrops resulting in decreased aqueous production by the ciliary bodies. Although topical β-blockers may be absorbed systemically resulting in bronchospasm, cardiovascular side effects from these drugs are uncommon. Cardioselective β-adrenergic blockers such as betaxolol may be less likely to cause systemic side effects. Miotic topical eyedrops, such as the parasympathomimetic pilocarpine, constrict the pupils to enhance aqueous outflow. The production of miotic pupils interferes with night vision. Acetazolamide is a carbonic anhydrase inhibitor that decreases the production of aqueous from the ciliary bodies, but its use is limited by systemic side effects. Latanoprost is a synthetic prostaglandin that decreases intraocular pressure and does not exacerbate asthma or cardiovascular symptoms.

Surgical treatment of glaucoma includes iridectomy to enhance outflow of aqueous when used to treat angle-closure glaucoma; and for open-angle glaucoma, argon laser therapy is used to improve outflow through the trabecular meshwork. Surgery for glaucoma is usually reserved for patients in whom acceptable intraocular pressures cannot be obtained with medical therapy.

Management of Anesthesia. Management of anesthesia for patients with glaucoma includes maintenance of miosis by continuing topical miotic therapy throughout the perioperative period. This practice decreases the likelihood of attacks of acute narrow-angle glaucoma. Inclusion of anticholinergic drugs in the preoperative medication is acceptable, as the amount of drug reaching the eye via the circulation is too little to dilate the pupils. Furthermore, the use of anticholinergic drugs in combination with anticholinesterases to pharmacologically antagonize nondepolarizing muscle relaxants is acceptable. For example, it is estimated that administration of atropine, 2 mg IV, results in the delivery of only 4 μg to the patient's eyes. Despite these assurances, it seems reasonable to limit administration of anticholinergic drugs in patients with glaucoma. Indeed, scopolamine, 0.4 mg IM, produces significant increases in the diameter of the pupils in healthy subjects and therefore may not be the best drug to administer to patients with glaucoma. By contrast, the same dose of atropine does not alter the size of the pupils. Although not evaluated, glycopyrrolate, administered systemically, predictably should have minimal effects on the diameter of the pupils. Administration of anticholinergic drugs in combination with drugs that produce miosis (opioids, anticholinesterases) may prevent dilating effects on the pupils normally produced by anticholinergic drugs.

Prevention of increased intraocular pressure is an important goal during management of patients with glaucoma. Succinylcholine-induced increases in intraocular pressure are maximal 2 to 4 minutes after administering the drug, returning to baseline values in about 6 minutes. These increases in intraocular pressure are not reliably obscured by any method, including prevention of drug-induced fasciculations by prior administration of nonparalyzing doses of nondepolarizing muscle relaxants. Implications of this drug-induced increase in intraocular pressure in patients with glaucoma are unknown. Presumably, patients with adequate medical control of glaucoma would not be jeopardized by the transient increases in intraocular pressure produced by succinylcholine. Intraocular pressure is lowered by hypocarbia and decreased central venous pressure, as produced by drug-induced osmotic diuresis, opioids, and volatile anesthetic drugs. Fluctuations in systemic blood pressure and skeletal muscle paralysis produced by nondepolarizing muscle relaxants exert only a minor influence on intraocular pressure.

Interactions of drugs administered during anesthesia with those used to treat glaucoma are considered in the management of anesthesia. Bradycardia and exaggerated hypotension have been attributed to β-blockade produced by chronic topical administration of timolol.[28] Postoperatively, patients with glaucoma are observed for dilated pupils that are irregular and asymmetrical, as these changes suggest an acute episode of narrow-angle glaucoma. Patients experiencing such attacks are likely to complain of pain in and around the eye as well as loss of vision. By contrast, patients with corneal abrasions complain of pain only in the eye.

Macular Degeneration

Age-related macular degeneration is deterioration of the central portion of the retina.[29] Typically there is slow, insidious loss of central vision, with initial symptoms of decreased visual perception and visual sensitivity to light and gradual progression to legal blindness despite preservation of peripheral vision. Cigarette smoking is associated with an increased incidence of macular degeneration. Some patients with macular degeneration benefit from laser photocoagulation therapy.

Retinal Detachment

Retinal detachment is separation between the photoreceptors and retinal pigment epithelium in the retina resulting in accumulation of fluid or blood in the potential space.[21] Rhegmatogenous retinal detachment (hole in the retina allows fluid from the vitreous cavity to enter the subretinal space) is most often spontaneous, especially in predisposed individuals such as those with a high degree of myopia. Traction on the peripheral retina induced by cataract extraction may produce retinal defects with eventual detachment months after the surgery. Occurrence of a hole in the retina is typically perceived as a sudden burst of flashing lights or sparks followed by numerous small spots in the field of vision. The subsequent detachment of the retina is perceived by the patient as a "dark curtain" progressing across the visual field.

Surgical reattachment usually results in visual improvement. Laser therapy to coagulate holes in the retina is effective. To maintain retinal attachment during the postoperative period while laser-induced chorioretinal adhesions develop, perfluoropropane gas, sulfur hexafluoride gas, or silicone oil is placed in the eye at the conclusion of surgery to maintain a long-term tamponade effect. Nitrous oxide is avoided for general anesthesia administered to patients undergoing retinal detachment surgery, as this gas could diffuse into any remaining air bubbles in the globe.

Iatrogenic Illnesses

The most commonly recognized causes of iatrogenic illness in elderly individuals include complications of drug therapy and diagnostic or therapeutic procedures, nosocomial infections, fluid and electrolyte disorders, and trauma.[1] Iatrogenic illness in elderly patients is often associated with falls secondary to gait disturbances and delirium due to medications.

Polypharmacy

The most frequently documented causes of iatrogenic illnesses are adverse drug reactions, usually associated with polypharmacy. The incidence of adverse drug reactions increases with advancing age and the number of chronic illnesses requiring drug therapy. The concomitant use of several drugs increases the risk of drug interactions, unwanted side effects, and adverse reactions.[1]

There are age-related changes in pharmacokinetics and pharmacodynamics. Many medications should be used with special caution in elderly individuals because of changes in drug pharmacokinetics and pharmacodynamics.[1]

Drug distribution is altered by aging principally because of body composition changes characterized by decreased total body water and lean body mass and relative increases in body fat. Consequently, water-soluble drugs achieve higher serum concentrations, whereas lipid-soluble drugs have prolonged elimination half-times. These changes are especially important for lipid-soluble drugs such as diazepam that penetrate the blood-brain barrier. Differences in the pharmacokinetics of propofol in elderly patients may be gender-specific.[30] Although concentrations of serum proteins are not significantly altered by aging, many elderly individuals experience malnutrition-induced decreases in serum albumin concentrations. As a result, displacement of a drug from albumin by one that also binds to albumin increases the risk of adverse reactions (warfarin toxicity may occur when phenytoin is administered).

Drug metabolism and clearance may be altered by changes that accompany aging. For example, aging-induced decreases in hepatic blood flow decrease the rate of metabolism of drugs that undergo high degrees of first-pass hepatic extraction (propranolol). Aging may slow hepatic microsomal mixed function oxidase system metabolism (phase I hepatic metabolism). As a result, active metabolites of drugs that undergo phase I metabolism may prolong the effects of the parent drug (diazepam) and explain the increased risk of cognitive impairment and falls that accompany administration of this drug to elderly individuals. Age-associated decreases in renal function, which results in decreased creatinine clearance, necessitates lower maintenance doses of renally excreted drugs in elderly patients.

The effects of aging on target organ (receptor) responsiveness are not well established.[1] Decreased β-adrenergic receptor responsiveness and increased opioid receptor responsiveness does accompany aging. Many elderly patients seem more sensitive to the adverse effects of anticholinergic drugs.

Nosocomial Infections

Nosocomial pathogens are primarily transmitted through contact with hospital or nursing home personnel. Urinary tract, pulmonary, and wound infections are the most common examples of nosocomial infections. Patients at greatest risk for development of nosocomial infections are those with physical debility, prolonged hospitalizations, and exposures to broad-spectrum antibiotics.

Progeria

Progeria (Hutchinson-Gilford syndrome) is characterized by premature aging. This disease is inherited as an autosomal recessive disorder, with clinical manifestations becoming apparent after about 6 months of age. These patients acquire all the diseases of old age during the first or second decades of life. For example, ischemic heart disease, essential hypertension, cerebrovascular disease, osteoarthritis, and diabetes mellitus are common. The mean survival age is 13 years, with death usually occurring by 25 years of age from congestive heart failure or myocardial infarction.

Management of anesthesia for patients with progeria is based on changes in organ system function that predictably accompany aging.[31] In addition, the presence of mandibular hypoplasia and micrognathia may lead to difficulty with airway management and tracheal intubation. The presence of a narrow glottic opening and the need for a small tracheal tube are suggested by the typical high-pitched voice characteristic of these patients. Even minimal laryngeal edema can compromise the patency of the airway. Careful movement and positioning of patients with progeria are necessary to minimize the likelihood of injury to thin, fragile extremities.

SKELETAL CHANGES LIKELY TO ACCOMPANY AGING

Osteoarthritis and osteoporosis are skeletal changes that are likely to accompany aging. Chronic disease of the cervical spine has important implications for the management of anesthesia.

Osteoarthritis

Osteoarthritis (degenerative joint disease) is a common form of arthritis characterized by degeneration of articular cartilage and reactive changes in surrounding bones and periarticular tissues.[32] Pathologic findings suggest that articular cartilage is the site of the primary abnormality in osteoarthritis. These changes result in pain and dysfunction of affected joints and are a major cause of disability. Radiographic changes of osteoarthritis are present in the hands of nearly all patients older than 65 years of age. Symptomatic osteoarthritis is present in 17% of men and 30% of women older than 60 years of age.

Classification

Patients without specific inflammatory or metabolic conditions known to be associated with arthritis and without a history of injury or trauma are considered to have primary osteoarthritis. In most patients involvement is limited to one or a small number of joints or joint areas. Secondary osteoarthritis is associated with conditions that cause damage to articular cartilage through a variety of mechanisms, including trauma and inflammatory and metabolic processes. Acute trauma, particularly intra-articular fractures and meniscal tears, can result in articular instability and the development of osteoarthritis years after injury.

Risk Factors

Age is the factor most strongly associated with osteoarthritis. Obesity is associated with osteoarthritis of the knees. An association between increased bone density and osteoarthritis is reflected by the observation that women with osteoporosis and hip fractures have a decreased risk of osteoarthritis. The chronic repetitive impact on joints may cause degenerative changes in articular cartilage. Many individuals with osteoarthritis have positive family histories, and multiple genetic factors may be responsible for various forms of osteoarthritis.

Diagnosis

Characteristic radiographic features that are corroborated by compatible clinical symptoms confirm the diagnosis of osteoarthritis. Laboratory studies such as the erythrocyte sedimentation rate, rheumatoid factor, and routine hematologic and biochemical parameters are normal in patients with osteoarthritis. Synovial fluid from involved joints is noninflammatory. Gout usually affects foot and ankle joints and is not often confused with osteoarthritis. Rheumatoid arthritis can usually be distinguished from osteoarthritis on the basis of different patterns of joint disease, more prominent morning stiffness, and soft tissue swelling and warmth on physical examination.

Signs and Symptoms

Typical signs and symptoms of osteoarthritis include pain, stiffness, swelling, deformity, and loss of function.[32] The pain is usually chronic and localized to the involved joint or joints. Pain is made worse with activity and improves with rest. Morning stiffness is not as prolonged as in patients with inflammatory diseases, usually lasting less than an hour. Swelling tends to be mild or moderate and is often related to bony enlargement rather than soft tissue edema. Deformity and loss of function are later manifestations that occur after many years of disease. The physical findings of osteoarthritis are pain on motion, bony enlargement, and periarticular tenderness. Synovial effusions may be present, especially in the knee.

Osteoarthritis is a slowly progressive condition with a variable prognosis. Radiographically, most joints remain stable or gradually worsen over a 5- to 15-year period.[30] In most patients symptoms evolve over many years and may spontaneously remit for long periods without explanation. Progression of osteoarthritis of the hand is particularly difficult to measure because pain levels frequently improve after the involved joints become fused. Disease may progress more rapidly in the hips and knees of older women with osteopenic bones.

Specific Joint Involvement and Spinal Canal Stenosis

Osteoarthritis has a characteristic pattern of involvement in most joints. The most commonly affected joints in the hands are the distal and proximal interphalangeal joints, resulting in bony enlargement of these joints, referred to as Heberden's and Bouchard's nodes, respectively. The progressive enlargement of these joints occurs slowly over many years, is frequently familial, and occurs most often in middle-aged or elderly women. Osteoarthritis frequently involves the knees and/or hips and is a common cause of significant disability. Spondylosis is the term used to describe osteoarthritis of the cervical and lumbar spine. Intervertebral disk spaces or the posterior spinal facet joints may be affected and cause chronic neck or back pain that is worse with activity and better with rest. Disc degeneration may be complicated by protrusion of

the nucleus pulposus, causing nerve root compression with radicular pain or skeletal muscle weakness. Stenosis of the spinal canal can occur in patients with extensive degenerative changes, resulting in compression of the cervical spine or of the cauda equina in the lumbar region. Lumbar spinal canal stenosis, causing chronic radicular leg pain that is worse with activity and better with rest ("neurogenic claudication") is a common complication in elderly patients.

Radiographic Changes

Typical radiographic findings of osteoarthritis include joint space narrowing, subchondral bone sclerosis, subchondral cysts, and osteophytes (bone spurs).[30] Joint space narrowing, resulting from loss of cartilage, is often asymmetrical and may be the only finding early in the disease process. Central erosion may be seen within the joint spaces of the small interphalangeal joints of the fingers; they should be easily distinguishable from the periarticular erosions of rheumatoid arthritis.

Treatment

Treatment of osteoarthritis is based on relieving symptoms and improving function. Exercise is an important part of treatment. For example, quadriceps muscle weakness contributes significantly to disability in patients with osteoarthritis of the knees, and exercises designed to strengthen the quadriceps muscles are useful. Weight loss may decrease the risk of developing symptoms in patients predisposed to osteoarthritis.

The primary goal of pharmacologic therapy in osteoarthritis is to relieve pain. In some patients simple analgesics, such as acetaminophen, may be as effective as nonsteroidal antiinflammatory drugs. Patients taking large doses of acetaminophen should be advised to limit alcohol ingestion and be warned about the increased risk of acetaminophen hepatotoxicity. Opioids are rarely utilized in the management of osteoarthritis. Intra-articular corticosteroid injections may be useful for treating selected joints, particularly during exacerbations characterized by increased pain and effusion.

Total joint replacement is an effective option in patients with badly damaged knees and hips. Patients experience significant pain relief, and some have improved ranges of motion. Some patients with osteoarthritis of the knees may be helped by arthroscopic débridement, particularly when mechanical symptoms suggesting internal derangement are present.

Cervical Spine Disease

Cervical spine disease may interfere with airway management and render direct laryngoscopy for tracheal intubation difficult.[33] Spinal cord compression can be secondary to hyperextension or hyperflexion of the patient's neck in the presence of spinal canal stenosis. Maintenance of a neutral cervical spine position is the goal. Adverse respiratory events in patients with chronic cervical spine disease can occur throughout the perioperative period. With aging, loss of flexibility and extensibility of the cervical spine increases the distance from the posterior portion of the cricoid ring to the anterior portion of the vertebral body. Because of this change and the decreased mobility of the laryngeal cartilage, it may be difficult to apply effective cricoid pressure. It may also be more difficult to displace the laryngeal aperture posteriorly with external pressure applied over the patient's anterior neck. With increasing age, the intervertebral foramina become narrowed, osteophytes are formed, and the ligamentum flavum bulges. Extension and flexion of the neck are diminished, and there is decreased elasticity of the atlanto-occipital ligaments. For every decade of life after age 30, there is approximately 10 degrees loss in the range of flexion and extension of the cervical spine. The incidence of spinal canal stenosis approaches 100% in elderly individuals.[33]

Treatment

The goals of cervical spine surgery include stabilizing the spine and decompressing the spinal cord or nerve roots.[33] Patients with cervical spinal canal stenosis associated with myelopathy (cord damage) and/or radiculopathy (nerve root damage) are candidates for surgery. Surgical management of radiculopathy with nerve root compression secondary to cervical spinal canal stenosis includes posterior cervical laminectomy, laminotomy-foraminotomy, anterior cervical fusion, or anterior discectomy. For myelopathy due to cervical cord compression, the surgical procedure is anterior cervical fusion or laminectomy.

Anterior Discectomy with Fusion

Complications of anterior discectomy with fusion include damage to the recurrent laryngeal nerves with vocal cord paresis or paralysis and damage to the thoracic duct. Less common complications of anterior fusion are carotid or vertebral artery injury; esophageal, pharyngeal, or tracheal perforation; and airway obstruction secondary to hematoma or severe edema formation. An advantage of the anterior surgical approach is use of the supine position, thereby eliminating the need for placing patients in the prone position. Depending on the presence of spinal cord impingement preoperatively, fiberoptic tracheal intubation may be indicated. Hyperextension of the patient's neck may exacerbate or lead to acute cord compression. If patients remain awake during tracheal intubation, neurologic impairment may be detected or excluded prior to induction of anesthesia. If cervical cord compression is evident preoperatively, an awake fiberoptic tracheal intubation is a consideration. Facilitation of graft placement may be provided by applying axial cranial traction. Reactions to the tracheal tube must be prevented, as this response could expel the bone graft.

Posterior Fusion

Posterior fusion is the most common surgical treatment for cervical spine instability in patients with rheumatoid arthritis. Cervical fusion, or arthrodesis, usually is performed for C1-2 instability. These patients are usually in neutral cervical positions as maintained by halo traction devices. Awake fiberoptic tracheal intubation is a likely approach. This surgical procedure requires placing patients in the prone position.

Laminotomy-Foraminotomy

Laminotomy-foraminotomy is performed to enlarge the bony openings through which the nerve roots exit from the spinal cord. This surgery is most commonly performed with patients in the prone position.

Management of Anesthesia

Awake fiberoptic tracheal intubation is often indicated in patients with cervical spinal canal stenosis, keeping in mind the importance of avoiding extremes of neck range of motion. Monitoring the somatosensory evoked potentials is useful for early recognition of spinal cord compression and resulting brain stem ischemia during the surgical procedure. Neutral head, neck, and shoulder positioning is indicated. Abrupt or persistent atypical changes in head positions may be associated with brain ischemia. The extracranial vertebral artery is vulnerable to injury from manipulation, sudden neck motion, and hyperextension with rotation of the cervical spine, perhaps because of decreased vertebral artery blood flow and the resulting hypoperfusion and ischemia.

Osteoporosis

Osteoporosis, a systemic skeletal disease, is characterized by low bone mass and microarchitectural deterioration, with consequent increased bone fragility and susceptibility to fracture.[34] Risk factors for the development of osteoporosis and subsequent fractures include family history, low body weight, inactivity, and cigarette smoking. Bone mineral density (lumbar spine) is measured in women with strong risk factors for the development of osteoporosis. Women with osteoporosis often present with acute pain due to vertebral fractures. The tendency for elderly individuals to fall enhances the risk of fracture in the presence of osteoporosis.

Treatment of osteoporosis is intended to decrease the likelihood of fractures (vertebral fractures and nonvertebral). Most of the drugs used to treat osteoporosis act by decreasing bone resorption and are referred to as antiresorptive drugs (estrogens, bisphosphonates, calcitonin). Some drugs used to treat osteoporosis act by increasing bone formation (fluoride). Antiresorptive drugs result in a 5% to 10% increase in bone mineral density of the lumbar spine within 24 months in women with postmenopausal osteoporosis. In addition to preventing bone loss and fractures, estrogen therapy in postmenopausal women is helpful for preventing ischemic heart disease and dementia. The risks associated with this therapy are uterine bleeding, breast tenderness, breast cancer, migrane headaches, deep vein thrombosis, and pulmonary embolism. Raloxifene is a mixed estrogen agonist-antagonist that decreases bone resorption and increases bone mineral density in the lumbar spine, hip, and total body. This drug does not stimulate endometrial growth.

References

1. Palmer RM. Management of common clinical disorders in geriatric patients. Sci Am Med 1998;1–16
2. Peibe H-J. The aged cardiovascular risk patient. Br J Anaesth 2000;85:763–78
3. Prinz PN, Vitello MV, Raskind MA, et al. Geriatrics: sleep disorders and aging. N Engl J Med 1990;323:520–6
4. Craig DB, McLeskey CH, Mitenko PA, et al. Geriatric anaesthesia. Can J Anaesth 1987;34:156–67
5. Cooper DS. Subclinical hypothyroidism. JAMA 1987;258:246–7
6. Finucane BT, Hammonds WD, Welch MB. Influence of age on vascular absorption of lidocaine from the epidural space. Anesth Analg 1987;66:843–6
7. Nydahl P-A, Philipson L, Axelsson K, et al. Epidural anesthesia with 0.5% bupivacaine: influence of age on sensory and motor blockade. Anesth Analg 1991;73:780–6
8. Lawlor PG, Fainsinger RL, Bruera ED. Delirium at the end of life: critical issues in clinical practice and research. JAMA 2000;284:2427–9
9. Parikh SS, Chung F. Postoperative delirium in the elderly. Anesth Analg 1995;80:1223–32
10. Dodds C, Allison J. Postoperative cognitive deficit in the elderly surgical patient. Br J Anaesth 1998;81:449–62
11. Newman MF, Kirchner JL, Phillips-Bute B, et al. Longitudinal assessment of neurocognitive function after coronary-artery bypass surgery. N Engl J Med 2001;344:395–402
12. Rosenberg-Adamsen S, Kehlet H, Dodds C, et al. Postoperative sleep disturbances: mechanisms and clinical implications. Br J Anaesth 1996;76:552–9
13. Williams-Russo P, Sharrock NE, Mattis S, et al. Cognitive effects after epidural vs. general anesthesia in older adults: a randomized trial. JAMA 1995;274:44–8
14. Moller JT, Cluitmans P, Rasmussen LS, et al. Prolonged postoperative cognitive dysfunction in the elderly. Lancet 1998; 351:857–61
15. Geldmacher DS, Whitehouse PJ. Evaluation of dementia. N Engl J Med 1996;335:330–6
16. Roses AD, Saunders AM. Alzheimer disease and the dementias. Sci Am Med 2000;1–10
17. Kannus P, Parkkari J, Niemi S, et al. Prevention of hip fracture in elderly people with the use of a hip protector. N Engl J Med 2000;343:1506–13
18. O'Hara DA, Duff A, Berlin JA, et al. The effect of anesthetic technique on postoperative outcomes in hip fracture repair. Anesthesiology 2000;92:947–57
19. Urwin SC, Parker MJ, Griffiths R. General versus regional anaesthesia for hip fracture surgery: a meta-analysis of randomized trials. Br J Anaesth 2000;84:450–5
20. Weinberg AD, Minaker KL, Council on Scientific Affairs, American Medical Association. Dehydration: evaluation and management in older adults. JAMA 1995;274:1552–6
21. D'Amico DJ. Diseases of the retina. N Engl J Med 1994; 331:95–106
22. Schein OD, Katz J, Bass EB, et al. The value of rotuine preoperative medical testing before cataract surgery. N Engl J Med 2000;342:168–75
23. Kubitz J, Epple J, Bach A, et al. Psychomotor recovery in very old patients after total intravenous or balanced anesthesia for cataract surgery. Br J Anaesth 2001;86:203–8
24. Kallio H, Paloheimo M, Maunuksela E-L. Haemorrhage and risk factors associated with retrobulbar/peribulbar block: a prospective study in 1383 patients. Br J Anaesth 2000; 85:708–11
25. Wang BC, Bogart B, Hillman DE, et al. Subarachnoid injection: a potential complication of retrobulbar block. Anesthesiology 1989;71:845–7
26. Gold MI, Watkins WD, Sung Y-F, et al. Remifentanil versus remifentanil/midazolam for ambulatory surgery during monitored anesthesia care. Anesthesiology 1997;87:51–7
27. Glantz L, Drenger B, Gozal Y. Perioperative myocardial ischemia in cataract surgery patients: general versus local anesthesia. Anesth Analg 2000;91:1415–9
28. Mishra P, Calvey TN, Williams NE, et al. Intraoperative bradycardia and hypotension associated with timolol and pilocarpine eye drops. Br J Anaesth 1983;55:897–9
29. Fine SL, Berger JW, Maguire MG, et al. Age-related macular degeneration. N Engl J Med 2000;342:483–92
30. Vuyk J, Oostwouder J, Vletter AA, et al. Gender differences in the pharmacokinetics of propofol in elderly patients during and after continuous infusion. Br J Anaesth 2001;86:183–8
31. Chapin JW, Kahre J. Progeria and anesthesia. Anesth Analg 1979;58:424–5
32. Wise C. Osteoarthritis. Sci Am Med 1999;1–7
33. Popitz MD. Anesthetic implications of chronic disease of the cervical spine. Anesth Analg 1997;84:672–83
34. Eastell R. Treatment of postmenopausal osteoporosis. N Engl J Med 1998;338:736–46

Index

Note: Page numbers followed by the letter *f* refer to figures and those followed by *t* refer to tables.

ISBN 0-443-06604-3